Nutrition for Health and Health Care

Fourth Edition

Ellie Whitney

Linda Kelly DeBruyne

Kathryn Pinna

Sharon Rady Rolfes

WADSWORTH
CENGAGE Learning

Australia • Brazil • Japan • Korea • Mexico • Singapore • Spain • United Kingdom • United States

WADSWORTH
CENGAGE Learning™

**Nutrition for Health and Health Care,
Fourth Edition**
Ellie Whitney, Linda Kelly DeBruyne,
Kathryn Pinna, Sharon Rady Rolfes

Publisher: Yolanda Cossio

Acquisitions Editor: Peggy Williams

Developmental Editor: Elesha Feldman

Assistant Editor: Elesha Feldman

Editorial Assistant: Alexis Glubka

Media Editor: Miriam Myers

Marketing Manager: Laura McGinn

Marketing Assistant: Elizabeth Wong

Marketing Communications Manager: Linda Yip

Senior Content Project Manager: Carol Samet

Creative Director: Rob Hugel

Art Director: John Walker

Print Buyer: Rebecca Cross

Rights Acquisitions Account Manager, Text:
    Roberta Broyer

Rights Acquisitions Account Manager, Image:
    Dean Dauphinais

Production Service: Elm Street Publishing Services

Text Designer: Riezebos Holzbaur Design Group

Photo Researcher: Scott Rosen, Bill Smith Group

Copy Editor: Elm Street Publishing Services

Cover Designer: Yvo Riezebos Design Group

Cover Image: Michael Balderas/Istockphoto.com

Compositor: Integra Software Services Pvt. Ltd.

For product information and technology assistance, contact us at
Cengage Learning Customer & Sales Support, 1-800-354-9706

For permission to use material from this text or product,
submit all requests online at **www.cengage.com/permissions**
Further permissions questions can be e-mailed to
permissionrequest@cengage.com

Library of Congress Control Number: 2010928384

ISBN-13: 978-0-538-73357-1

ISBN-10: 0-538-73357-8

Wadsworth
20 Davis Drive
Belmont, CA 94002-3098
USA

Cengage Learning is a leading provider of customized learning
solutions with office locations around the globe, including
Singapore, the United Kingdom, Australia, Mexico, Brazil, and Japan.
Locate your local office at **www.cengage.com/global**

Cengage Learning products are represented in Canada by
Nelson Education, Ltd.

To learn more about Wadsworth, visit
www.cengage.com/Wadsworth

Purchase any of our products at your local college store or at our
preferred online store **www.cengagebrain.com**

Printed in the United States of America
1 2 3 4 5 6 7 14 13 12 11 10

To the memory of my parents, Edith Tyler Noss and Henry H. B. Noss, who supported me with love, discipline, and pride.
ELLIE WHITNEY

To my husband Tom, thanks for the music, the magic, and the memories.
LINDA KELLY DEBRUYNE

To my Nutrition 12 students at San Francisco City College, who have challenged and inspired me over my many years of teaching: I write these pages with your interests, questions, and concerns in mind.
KATHRYN PINNA

To my son Lyle, whose smile makes my heart smile.
SHARON RADY ROLFES

ELLIE WHITNEY, PH.D., grew up in New York City and received her B.A. and Ph.D. degrees in English and Biology at Radcliffe/Harvard University and Washington Universities, respectively. She has taught at both Florida State University and Florida A&M University, has written newspaper columns on environmental matters for the *Tallahassee Democrat*, and has authored almost a dozen college textbooks on nutrition, health, and related topics, many of which have been revised multiple times over the years. In addition to teaching and writing, she has spent the past three-plus decades exploring outdoor Florida and studying its ecology. Her latest book is *Priceless Florida: The Natural Ecosystems* (Pineapple Press, 2004).

LINDA KELLY DEBRUYNE, M.S., R.D., received her B.S. in 1980 and her M.S. in 1982 in nutrition and food science at the Florida State University. She is a founding member of Nutrition and Health Associates, an information resource center in Tallahassee, Florida, where her specialty areas are life cycle nutrition and fitness. Her other publications include the textbooks *Nutrition and Diet Therapy* and *Health: Making Life Choices* and a multimedia CD-ROM called *Nutrition Interactive*. As a consultant for a group of Tallahassee pediatricians, she teaches infant nutrition classes to parents. She is a registered dietitian and maintains a professional membership in the American Dietetic Association.

KATHRYN PINNA received her M.S. and Ph.D. degrees in nutrition from the University of California at Berkeley. She has taught nutrition, food science, and human biology courses in the San Francisco Bay area for over 20 years and currently teaches nutrition classes at City College of San Francisco. She has also worked as an outpatient dietitian, Internet consultant, and freelance writer. Her other publications include the textbooks *Understanding Normal and Clinical Nutrition* and *Nutrition and Diet Therapy*. She is a registered dietitian and a member of the American Society for Nutrition and the American Dietetic Association.

SHARON RADY ROLFES, M.S., R.D., received her M.S. in nutrition and food science from Florida State University. She is a founding member of Nutrition and Health Associates, an information resource center that maintains a research database on over 1000 nutrition-related topics. Her other publications include the college textbooks *Understanding Normal and Clinical Nutrition* and *Nutrition for Health and Health Care* and a multimedia CD-ROM called *Nutrition Interactive*. In addition to writing, she occasionally teaches at Florida State University and serves as a consultant for various educational projects. Her volunteer work includes serving on the board of Working Well, a community initiative dedicated to creating a healthy workforce. She maintains her registration as a dietitian and membership in the American Dietetic Association.

CONTENTS

CHAPTER 6

Energy Balance and Body Composition 141

CHAPTER 7

Weight Management: Overweight and Underweight 167

CHAPTER 8

The Vitamins 200

CHAPTER 9

Water and the Minerals 237

PREFACE

Whether for the prevention of disease or appropriate treatment of illness, health professionals and patients rank nutrition among their most serious concerns. Moreover, medical personnel are often called upon to answer questions about foods and diets or provide nutrition care. This fourth edition of *Nutrition for Health and Health Care* provides a solid foundation in nutrition science and the role of nutrition in clinical care. Although much of the material has been written for nursing students and is relevant to nursing care, this textbook can be useful for students of other health-related professions, including nursing assistants, physician assistants, dietitians, dietary technicians, and health educators.

Each chapter of this textbook includes essential nutrition concepts along with practical information for addressing nutrition concerns and solving nutrition problems. The introductory chapters (Chapters 1–2) provide an overview of the nutrients and nutrition recommendations and describe the process of digestion and absorption. Chapters 3 through 5 introduce the attributes and functions of carbohydrates, lipids, and protein and explain how appropriate intakes of these nutrients support health. Chapters 6 and 7 introduce the concepts of energy balance and weight management and describe the health effects of overweight, underweight, and eating disorders. Chapters 8 and 9 introduce the vitamins and minerals, describing their roles in the body, appropriate intakes, and food sources. Chapters 10 through 12 explain how nutrient needs change throughout the life cycle. Chapters 13 and 14 explore how nurses can use information from nursing assessments to identify and address a patient's nutrient needs. The remaining chapters (Chapters 15–23) examine nutrition therapy and its role in the prevention and treatment of medical conditions.

Special Features

Students of nutrition often begin a nutrition course with some practical knowledge of nutrition; after all, they may purchase food, read food labels, and be familiar with common nutrition problems such as obesity or lactose intolerance. After just a few weeks of class, however, the nutrition student realizes that nutrition is a biological and chemical science with a fair amount of new terminology and new concepts to learn. This book contains abundant pedagogy to help students master the subject matter. Within each chapter, definitions and notes in the margins clarify nutrition information, remind readers of previously defined terms, and provide cross-references. How To skill boxes help readers work through calculations or give practical suggestions for

applying nutrition advice. The Nursing Diagnosis feature enables nursing students to correlate nutrition care with nursing care. Review Notes summarize the information following each major heading; these summaries can be used to preview or review key chapter concepts. The Self Check at the end of each chapter provides questions to help review chapter information. Each chapter concludes with a Nutrition on the Net feature, which lists websites relevant to the topics covered in the chapter.

In the clinical chapters, Case Studies guide readers in applying nutrition therapy to patient care. Diet-Drug Interaction boxes identify important nutrient-drug and food-drug interactions. Clinical Applications encourage readers to practice mathematical calculations, synthesize information from previous chapters, or understand how dietary adjustments affect patients. Nutrition Assessment Checklists remind readers of assessment parameters relevant to specific stages of the life cycle or medical problems.

The Nutrition in Practice sections that follow chapters explore issues of current interest, advanced topics, or specialty areas such as dental health or dialysis. Examples of topics covered include foodborne illness, the glycemic index, vegetarian diets, alcohol in health and disease, nutritional genomics, the metabolic syndrome, and childhood obesity and chronic disease.

Appendixes

The appendixes support the book with a wealth of information on the nutrient contents of thousands of foods, Canadian nutrient recommendations and food choices, U.S. nutrient intake recommendations and the exchange system, physical activity and energy requirements, nutrition assessments, eternal formulas, aids to calculations, and answers to Self Check questions.

New to This Edition

Due to the rapid pace of nutrition research, staying current is a primary concern. Each chapter of this book has been substantially updated to reflect advances in research and clinical practice since the third edition. In addition, we have made the following changes:

CHAPTER 1

- Introduced the Physical Activity Guidelines for Americans, 2008
- Expanded the nutrient density discussion
- Revised the discussion of Healthy People in anticipation of Healthy People 2020
- Added a new table of metric/household measures

CHAPTER 2

- Revised glossaries of gastrointestinal terms and digestive glands
- Revised a figure on the gastrointestinal tract
- Created a new Nutrition in Practice about food safety

CHAPTER 3

- Revised and updated a figure on added sugars
- Added a new figure on sugar alternatives on food labels
- Changed a table about fiber to a figure, adding photos and additional explanation
- Added information about the herbal sweetener stevia
- Changed and updated a table on U.S. approved sweeteners
- Moved a Nutrition in Practice about oral health to chapter 17
- Created a Nutrition in Practice about the glycemic index

CHAPTER 4

- Added information pertaining to *trans* fat
- Expanded the tables on functions of fats in the body and in food
- Added a new table ranking omega-3 fatty acids in different types of fish
- Revised the section on fish oil supplements

CHAPTER 5

- Reorganized the section on roles of body proteins
- Added a new section about structural functions of proteins
- Revised and reorganized the sections about protein turnover and nitrogen balance
- Enhanced the discussion on protein excess
- Added a new table about vegetarian sources of key nutrients

CHAPTER 6

- Expanded the section about the health risks of obesity and added information about the health hazards of central (abdominal) obesity
- Included a new figure on abdominal obesity
- Defined several new terms, including insulin resistance, adipokines, subcutaneous fat, and inflammation
- Streamlined and simplified the Nutrition in Practice

CHAPTER 7

- Added a brief discussion of adiponectin
- Added a brief discussion about cognitive skills and weight management
- Added a new table of physical activity strategies for weight management from a 2009 position paper by the American College of Sports Medicine
- Added strategies for successful weight maintenance

CHAPTER 8

- Added a new table of strategies to minimize nutrient losses during food preparation and storage
- Enhanced the discussion of vitamin A's role in vision
- Added a second photo to the vitamin D deficiency figure
- Added a list of factors that may limit vitamin D synthesis in the skin

CHAPTER 9

- Added a new table that lists the percentage of water in selected foods
- Included a brief discussion of iron deficiency and obesity
- Enhanced the discussion of zinc

CHAPTER 10

- Enhanced the discussion about weight gain during pregnancy, addressing the current concern about obesity during pregnancy
- Added a discussion about weight loss after pregnancy
- Included the new pregnancy weight gain guidelines for obese women
- Added a discussion about the frequency and duration of breastfeeding
- Redesigned the figure pertaining to spina bifida

CHAPTER 11

- Enhanced the discussion about nutrient needs during childhood
- Moved (into the chapter) and expanded the section on childhood obesity from the Nutrition in Practice; the Practice now focuses on later diseases related to childhood obesity, including coronary heart disease, hypertension, and diabetes
- Created a figure that includes MyPyramid for Preschoolers and MyPyramid for Kids
- Created a figure showing trends in childhood obesity
- Added a new figure showing a physical activity pyramid for children
- Included new information about food skills for preschoolers
- Created a table of foods and beverages that meet recommended standards for nutrition in schools

CHAPTER 12

- Created a new table on signs of dementia
- Expanded the section on Alzheimer's disease, and included a list of signs of normal memory loss compared with memory loss related to Alzheimer's
- Added a new box showing how to turn convenience foods into nutritious meals

CHAPTER 13

- Reorganized the section on identifying malnutrition risk
- Added a new table on the medical problems associated with malnutrition
- Revised the discussion about determination of healthy body weight
- Added a table showing the rates of involuntary weight loss associated with nutritional risk
- Added information about epigenetics to the Nutrition in Practice

CHAPTER 14

- Added a new table showing examples of nutrition interventions

- Revised the table on incorporating nutrition care into the nursing care plan
- Added a section about determining energy requirements, including a new table with sample equations and a box showing how to determine the energy needs of hospital patients
- Moved the information about foodservice from the former Nutrition in Practice to the chapter
- Revised the tables listing grapefruit juice–drug interactions and foods high in tyramine
- Moved the Nutrition in Practice about complementary and alternative medicine from Chapter 23 to here, and added a new table on herb–drug interactions and some information about detoxification treatments

CHAPTER 15
- Revised and reorganized the section on enteral formulas
- Added photos to show the difference between transnasal and gastrostomy tube feedings and to compare open feeding systems and closed feeding systems
- Revised and reorganized the table on the causes and management of tube feeding complications
- Expanded the section about transitioning from tube feedings to table foods
- Added a box explaining how to express the osmolar concentration of solutions
- Added a figure showing a parenteral nutrition order form
- Expanded descriptions of the metabolic complications associated with parenteral nutrition
- Revised the box showing how to calculate the nutrient content of parenteral solutions

CHAPTER 16
- Added a new table showing how to estimate energy needs in critical care patients
- Revised the sections on nutrient needs and approaches to nutrition care for patients undergoing acute stress
- Clarified the descriptions of chronic bronchitis and emphysema
- Modified the discussions about the causes and nutrition care for respiratory failure

CHAPTER 17
- Revised the table on dysphagia diets, including new listings of foods to avoid in each type of diet
- Eliminated descriptions of the rarely performed vagotomy and pyloroplasty procedures
- Expanded the section on bariatric surgery, including a new figure that shows both the gastric banding and gastric bypass surgeries
- Moved the Nutrition in Practice about nutrition and oral (dental) health from Chapter 3 to here, and added discussions about periodontal disease and the relationships between dental diseases and other illnesses

CHAPTER 18
- Modified the section on diarrhea and revised the table listing foods that affect diarrhea
- Reorganized the section on malabsorption, revised the table listing foods to include and restrict in a fat-controlled diet, and added a new figure showing a sample menu for a fat-controlled diet
- Reorganized and revised the sections on pancreatitis and cystic fibrosis
- Revised the table describing a gluten-free diet and added a new figure showing a sample menu
- Added a photo of a case of diverticulosis as seen in a colonoscopy
- Created a new Nutrition in Practice about probiotics and intestinal health

CHAPTER 19
- Expanded descriptions of the different types of hepatitis viruses
- Revised the sections on the medical treatment and nutrition therapy for cirrhosis

CHAPTER 20
- Added the glycated hemoglobin measure to the section on diagnosis of diabetes
- Revised the discussion about type 2 diabetes in children and adolescents
- Added a section about prevention of type 2 diabetes
- Expanded the discussion about microvascular complications of diabetes
- Added information about the fructosamine test to the discussion of long-term glycemic control
- Extended the list of antidiabetic drugs to include recently approved medications for diabetes

CHAPTER 21
- In the section on causes of atherosclerosis, included small, dense low-density lipoproteins (LDLs) and advanced glycation end products in the discussions about LDLs and diabetes, respectively
- Added a paragraph about symptoms in the section on coronary heart disease
- In the section on therapeutic lifestyle changes, added a paragraph about polyunsaturated and monounsaturated fat, eliminated the discussion about soy protein due to ambiguous research results, and expanded the discussions about alcohol and weight reduction
- Distinguished between right-sided and left-sided heart failure in the section on consequences of heart failure
- Expanded the discussion about the medical management of heart failure

CHAPTER 22
- Revised the table on foods to include and restrict in a sodium-controlled diet

- Replaced the terms *acute renal failure* and *chronic renal failure* with the more current terms *acute kidney injury* and *chronic kidney disease*
- Added a new table showing the approximate potassium content of common fruits and vegetables
- Expanded the section on formation of kidney stones

CHAPTER 23

- Expanded the section on consequences of HIV infection to include neurological and other types of complications
- Expanded the table listing antiretroviral drugs to include recently approved medications for HIV infection
- Reorganized and revised the section on nutrition therapy for HIV infection, including new paragraphs on weight management and overweight/obesity

Instructor Tools

A number of helpful ancillary materials are available for instructors, including a Power Lecture DVD-ROM that includes figures and photos from the text as well as PowerPoint lecture presentations, a test bank, and an instructor's manual. A printed version of the instructor's manual and test bank is also available.

Student Ancillaries

A printed study guide for students provides chapter outlines, nutrition applications exercises, multiple choice and discussion questions, math exercises, and case study problems to help students master chapter concepts. The book's website **www.cengage.com/nutrition/whitney/nhhc4e** provides additional study tools.

We hope that as you discover the many fascinating aspects of nutrition science and nutrition therapy, you will enthusiastically apply the concepts in both your personal and professional life.

Ellie Whitney
Linda Kelly DeBruyne
Kathryn Pinna
Sharon Rady Rolfes

ACKNOWLEDGMENTS

Among the most difficult words to write are those that express the depth of our gratitude to the many dedicated people whose efforts have made this book possible. We extend special thanks to Fran Webb for her expertise and valuable contributions throughout this text. Thanks also to Eric Arima at Elm Street for his careful attention to the numerous details involved in production, John Walker and Yvo Riezebos for designing these pages, Dean Dauphinais and Sue Howard for their help in securing permissions, Scott Rosen at the Bill Smith Group for selecting photographs, and the folks at Axxya for compiling the food composition appendix. We are indebted to our editorial team, Peggy Williams and Elesha Feldman, and to our production manager, Carol Samet, for seeing this project through from start to finish. We would also like to thank those who helped to prepare the many supplements available with the text: Lynn Earle of Old Dominion University, Beth Fontenot of McNeese State University, Phyllis Magaletto of Cochran School of Nursing, Jillann Neely of Onondaga Community College, Karen Schmitz of Madonna University, Lynn Thomas of the University of South Carolina School of Medicine, and Elesha Feldman and Miriam Myers, who managed the preparation of the print and media supplements. We would also like to acknowledge Laura McGinn for her marketing efforts. To the many others involved in designing, indexing, typesetting, dummying, and marketing, we offer our thanks. We are especially grateful to our associates, family, and friends for their continued encouragement and support, and to the following reviewers who offered excellent suggestions for improving the text.

Reviewers

Alena M. Clark, *University of Northern Colorado*

Crystal Day-Black, *Coppin State University School of Nursing*

L. L. Earle, *Old Dominion University*

Phyllis Magaletto, *Cochran School of Nursing & Pace University*

Donna H. Mueller, *Drexel University*

Karen J. Schmitz, *Madonna University*

Lynn K. Thomas, *University of South Carolina School of Medicine*

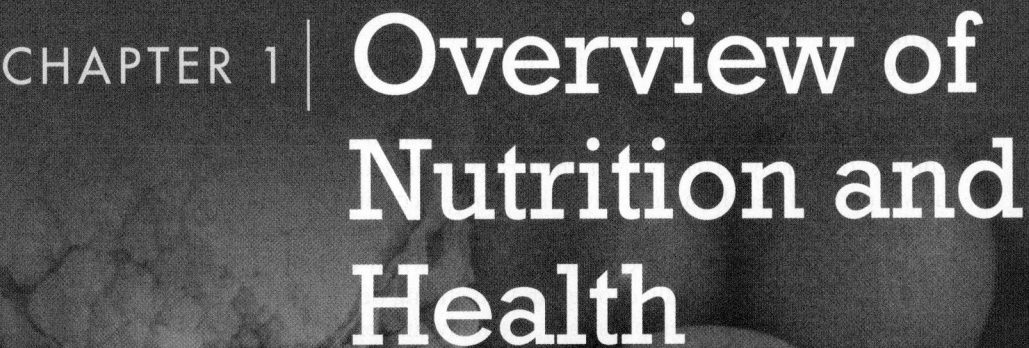

CHAPTER 1 | Overview of Nutrition and Health

© Rosenfeld/Corbis

CONTENTS

EVERY DAY, SEVERAL TIMES A DAY, YOU MAKE CHOICES THAT WILL EITHER improve your **health** or harm it. Each choice may influence your health only a little, but when these choices are repeated over years and decades, their effects become significant.

The choices people make each day affect not only their physical health but also their **wellness**—all the characteristics that make a person strong, confident, and able to function well with family, friends, and others. People who consistently make poor lifestyle choices, on a daily basis, increase their risks of developing diseases. Figure 1-1 shows how a person's health can fall anywhere along a continuum, from maximum wellness on the one end to total failure to function (death) on the other.

As nurses or other health care professionals, when you take responsibility for your own health by making daily choices and practicing behaviors that enhance your well-being, you prepare yourself physically, mentally, and emotionally to meet the demands of your profession. As health care professionals, however, you have a responsibility to your clients (✚) as well as to yourselves. You have unique opportunities to make your clients aware of the benefits of positive health choices and behaviors, to show them how to change their behaviors and make daily choices to enhance their own health, and to serve as role models for those behaviors.

This text focuses on how nutrition choices affect health and disease. The early chapters introduce the basics of nutrition to support good health. The later chapters emphasize diet therapy and its role in supporting health and treating diseases and symptoms.

FIGURE 1-1 | The Health Line

Wellness—optimal physical, mental, emotional, spiritual, and social health

Person takes responsibility for all health areas and meets all needs.

Superior level of health

Good level of health

Person covers most needs well, but some areas lack attention.

Most people function near here—they meet needs at a minimum to prevent symptoms.

Moderate level of health

Person is physically, mentally, emotionally, spiritually, or socially nonfunctional.

Person relies on medicine to treat symptoms; needs are not met.

Marginal level of health

Death from disease

Poor level of health

Person meets needs only to reverse symptoms as they appear.

No matter how well you maintain your health today, you may still be able to improve tomorrow. Likewise, a person who is well today can slip by failing to maintain health-promoting habits.

✚ Nurses generally use either *client* or *patient* when referring to an individual under their care. The first 12 chapters of this text emphasize the nutrition concerns of people in good health; therefore, the term *client* is used in these chapters.

health: a range of states with physical, mental, emotional, spiritual, and social components. At a minimum, health means freedom from physical disease, mental disturbances, emotional distress, spiritual discontent, social maladjustment, and other negative states. At a maximum, health means *wellness*.

wellness: maximum well-being; the top range of health states; the goal of the person who strives toward realizing his or her full potential physically, mentally, emotionally, spiritually, and socially.

Food Choices

Sound **nutrition** throughout life does not ensure good health and long life, but it can certainly help to tip the balance in their favor. Nevertheless, most people choose foods for reasons other than their nourishing value. Even people who claim to choose foods primarily for the sake of health or nutrition will admit that other factors also influence their food choices. Because food choices become an integral part of people's lifestyles, they sometimes find it difficult to change their eating habits. Health care professionals who help clients make diet changes must understand the dynamics of food choices because people will alter their eating habits only if their preferences are honored.

Nutrition is only one of the many factors that influence people's food choices.

Preference Why do people like certain foods? One reason, of course, is their preference for certain tastes. Some tastes are widely liked, such as the sweetness of sugar and the zest of salt. Research suggests that genetics influence people's taste preferences, a finding that may eventually have implications for clinical nutrition.[1] For example, sensitivity to bitter taste is an inheritable trait. People born with great sensitivity to bitter tastes tend to avoid foods with bitter flavors such as broccoli, cabbage, brussels sprouts, spinach, and grapefruit juice. These foods, as well as many other fruits and vegetables, contain **bioactive food components**: **phytochemicals** and nutrients, which may reduce the risk of cancer. (✚) Thus, the role that genetics may play in food selection is gaining importance in cancer research.

Habit Sometimes habit dictates people's food choices. People eat a sandwich for lunch or drink orange juice at breakfast simply because they have always done so.

Associations People also like foods with happy associations—foods eaten in the midst of warm family gatherings on traditional holidays or given to them as children by someone who loved them. By the same token, people can attach intense and unalterable dislikes to foods that they ate when they were sick or that were forced on them when they weren't hungry.

Ethnic Heritage and Tradition Every country, and every region of a country, has its own typical foods and ways of combining them into meals. The **foodways** of North America reflect the many different cultural and ethnic backgrounds of its inhabitants. Many foods with foreign origins are familiar items on North American menus: tacos, egg rolls, lasagna, and gyros, to name a few. Still others, such as spaghetti and croissants, are almost staples in the "American diet." North American regional cuisines like Cajun and TexMex blend the traditions of several cultures. Table 1-1 (p. 4) presents selected **ethnic diets** and food choices.

Values People's values, environmental ethics, religious beliefs, and political views also influence their food choices. By choosing to eat some foods or to avoid others, people make statements that reflect their values. For example, people may select only foods that come in containers that can be reused or recycled. A concerned consumer may boycott fruit or vegetables picked by migrant workers who have been exploited. People may buy vegetables from local farmers to save the fuel and environmental costs of foods shipped from far away. Labels on some foods carry statements or symbols—known as ecolabels—that imply that the foods have been produced in ways that are considered environmentally favorable. One of the most successful ecolabels is "Certified Organic," meaning the food was grown and processed according to regulations defining the use of synthetic fertilizers, herbicides, pesticides, and other chemical ingredients.

Religion also influences many people's food choices. Jewish law sets forth an extensive set of dietary rules. Many Christians forgo meat on Fridays during Lent, the period prior to Easter. In Islamic dietary laws, permitted or lawful foods are called *halal*. Other faiths prohibit some dietary practices and promote others. Diet planners can foster sound nutrition practices only if they respect and honor each person's values.

✚ Nutrition in Practice 8 addresses phytochemicals and their role in disease prevention.

nutrition: the science of foods and the nutrients and other substances they contain, and of their ingestion, digestion, absorption, transport, metabolism, interaction, storage, and excretion. A broader definition includes the study of the environment and of human behavior as it relates to these processes.

bioactive food components: components in foods, either nutrients or phytochemicals, that alter physiological processes in the body.

phytochemical (FIGH-toe-CHEM-ih-cals): compounds in plants that confer color, taste, and other characteristics. Some phytochemicals are bioactive food components in functional foods. Nutrition in Practice 8 provides details.

foodways: the eating habits and culinary practices of a people, region, or historical period.

ethnic diets: foodways and cuisines typical of national origins, races, cultural heritages, or geographic locations.

TABLE 1-1	Selected Ethnic Cuisines and Food Choices				
	Grains	Vegetables	Fruits	Meats, Poultry, Fish, Legumes, Eggs, and Nuts	Milk
Asian	Barley, buckwheat, millet, rice, wheat, rice or wheat noodles	Amaranth, baby corn, bamboo shoots, bok choy, cabbages, mung bean sprouts, scallions, seaweed, snow peas, straw mushrooms, water chestnuts, wild yam	Kumquats, loquats, lychee, mandarin oranges, melons, pears, persimmon, plums	Beef, pork, poultry, fish and other seafood, squid, soybeans, tofu, duck eggs, cashews, peanuts	Soymilk
Mediterranean	Bulgur, couscous, focaccia, Italian bread, pastas, pita pocket bread, polenta, rice	Cucumbers, eggplant, grape leaves, onions, peppers, tomatoes	Dates, figs, grapes, lemons, melons, olives, raisins	Beef, gyros, lamb, pork, sausage, chicken, fish and other seafood, fava beans, lentils, almonds, walnuts	Feta, goat, mozzarella, parmesan, provolone, and ricotta cheeses; yogurt
Mexican	Taco shells, tortillas (corn or flour), rice	Cactus, cassava, chayote, chilies, corn, jicama, onions, tomatoes, tomato salsa, yams	Avocado, bananas, guava, lemons, limes, mango, oranges, papaya, plantain	Beef, chorizo, chicken, fish, refried beans, eggs	Cheese, flan (caramel custard)

© Becky Luigart-Stayner/Corbis

© PhotoDisc, Inc.

© PhotoDisc, Inc.

Ethnic meals and family gatherings nourish the spirit as well as the body.

Social Interaction Social interaction is another powerful influence on people's food choices. Meals are social events, and the sharing of food is part of hospitality. It is often considered rude to refuse food or drink being shared by a group or offered by a host. Food brings people together for many different reasons: to celebrate a holiday or special event, to renew an old friendship, to make new friends, to conduct business, and many more. Sometimes food defines status. Lobster and caviar are often associated with wealth; peanut butter and jelly, with children. Sometimes food is used to influence or impress someone. For example, a business executive invites a prospective new client out to dinner in hopes of edging out the competition. In each case, for whatever the purpose, food plays an integral part of the social interaction.

Emotional State People may eat in response to emotional stimuli—for example, to relieve boredom or depression or to calm anxiety. A lonely person may choose to eat rather than to call a friend and risk rejection. A person who has returned home from an exciting evening out may unwind with a late-night snack. Eating in response to emotions can easily lead to overeating and obesity but may be appropriate at times. For example, sharing food at times of bereavement serves both the giver's need to provide comfort and the receiver's need to be cared for and to interact with others.

In contrast, some people do not eat at all, or eat very little, in response to emotions. A depressed person may simply have no appetite for food. A person overcome with grief can easily lose all interest in food. As long as a person's appetite or interest in food returns quickly, little harm is done.

Availability, Convenience, and Economy The influence of these factors on people's food selections is clear. You cannot eat foods if they are not available, if you cannot get to the grocery store, if you do not have the time or skill to prepare them,

Overview of Nutrition and Health

or if you cannot afford them. Consumers today value convenience so highly that they are willing to spend half of their food budget on meals that require little or no preparation. They frequently eat out, bring home ready-to-eat meals, cook meals ahead at storefront meal preparation sites, or have food delivered.[2] Along with convenience, however, consumers want great taste and quality—foods that are fast, delicious, and nutritious. The demand for fully prepared ready-to-eat foods or foods that can be easily prepared in a microwave oven demonstrates this influence. Consumer demand for microwavable foods that taste and smell as though they were prepared in a conventional oven has prompted manufacturers to expand the variety of microwavable foods available and to change the formulation and packaging of the foods.[3] Food processors are developing many more microwavable meals and snacks for use at home and the office—rising-crust pizzas, chicken and fish dishes, precooked entrées, and side dishes such as french fries and rice. Many of the new products are packaged in single-serve containers.

Age
Age influences people's food choices. Infants, for example, depend on others to choose foods for them. Older children also rely on others but become more active in selecting foods that taste sweet and are familiar to them and rejecting those whose taste or texture they dislike. In contrast, the links between taste preferences and food choices in adults are less direct than in children. Adults often choose foods based on health concerns such as body weight. Indeed, adults may avoid sweet or familiar foods because of such concerns.

Occupation
Some people have jobs that keep them away from home for days at a time, require them to conduct business in restaurants or at conventions, or involve hectic schedules that allow little or no time for meals at home. For these people, the kinds of restaurants available to them and the cost of eating out so often may limit food choices.

Body Weight and Image
Sometimes people select certain foods and supplements that they believe will improve their physical appearance and avoid those they believe might be detrimental. Such decisions can be beneficial when based on sound nutrition and fitness knowledge but may undermine good health when based on fads or carried to extremes. (✚)

Medical Conditions
Sometimes medical conditions and their treatments (including medications) limit the foods a person can select. For example, a person with heart disease might need to adopt a diet low in certain types of fats. The chemotherapy needed to treat cancer can interfere with a person's appetite or limit food choices by causing vomiting. Allergy to certain foods can also limit choices. The second half of this text discusses how diet can be modified to accommodate different medical conditions.

Health and Nutrition
Consumers today cite nutrition as a primary concern in making food choices, yet the foods they choose do not always reflect this concern. Food manufacturers and restaurant chefs have responded to scientific findings linking health with nutrition by offering an abundant selection of health-promoting foods and beverages. Foods that provide health benefits beyond their nutrient contributions are called **functional foods**.[4] Whole foods—as natural and familiar as oatmeal or tomatoes—are the simplest functional foods. In other cases, foods have been modified through fortifications, enrichment, or enhancement. Examples of these functional foods include orange juice fortified with calcium to build strong bones, bread enriched with folate to promote normal fetal development, and margarine enhanced with a plant sterol to lower blood cholesterol. (✚)

Consumers typically welcome new foods into their diets, provided that these foods are reasonably priced, clearly labeled, easy to find in the grocery store, and convenient to prepare. These foods must also taste good—as good as the traditional choices. Of course, a person need not eat any "special" foods to enjoy a healthy diet; many "regular" foods provide numerous health benefits as well. In fact, foods such as whole grains; vegetables and legumes; fruits; meats, fish, and poultry; and milk products are among the healthiest choices a person can make.

✚ Eating disorders are the topic of Nutrition in Practice 7.

✚ Nutrition in Practice 8 offers more discussion of functional foods.

functional foods: whole or modified foods that contain bioactive food components believed to provide health benefits, such as reduced disease risks, beyond the benefits that their nutrients contribute. All whole foods are functional in some ways because they provide at least some needed substances, but certain foods stand out as rich sources of bioactive food components.

The Nutrients

You are a collection of molecules that move. All these moving parts are arranged in patterns of extraordinary complexity and order—cells, tissues, and organs. Although the arrangement remains constant, the parts are continually changing, using **nutrients** and energy derived from nutrients.

Almost any food you eat is composed of dozens or even hundreds of different kinds of materials. Spinach, for example, is composed mostly of water (95 percent), and most of its solid materials are the compounds carbohydrates, fats (properly called lipids), and proteins. If you could remove these materials, you would find a tiny residue of minerals, vitamins, and other compounds.

SIX CLASSES OF NUTRIENTS

➕ The six classes of nutrients are water, carbohydrates, fats, proteins, vitamins, and minerals.

➕ *Metabolism* is the set of processes by which nutrients are rearranged into body structures or broken down to yield energy.

➕ Food energy can also be measured in kilojoules (kJ). The kilojoule is the international unit of energy. One kcalorie equals 4.2 kJ.

nutrients: substances obtained from food and used in the body to provide energy and structural materials and to serve as regulating agents to promote growth, maintenance, and repair. Nutrients may also reduce the risks of some diseases.

essential nutrients: nutrients a person must obtain from food because the body cannot make them for itself in sufficient quantities to meet physiological needs.

organic: carbon containing. The four organic nutrients are carbohydrate, fat, protein, and vitamins.

energy-yielding nutrients: the nutrients that break down to yield energy the body can use. The three energy-yielding nutrients are carbohydrate, protein, and fat.

inorganic: not containing carbon or pertaining to living things.

calories: units by which energy is measured. Food energy is measured in **kilocalories** (1000 calories equal 1 kilocalorie), abbreviated **kcalories** or kcal. One kcalorie is the amount of heat necessary to raise the temperature of 1 kilogram (kg) of water 1°C. The scientific use of the term *kcalorie* is the same as the popular use of the term *calorie.*

Water, carbohydrates, fats, proteins, vitamins, and minerals are the six classes of nutrients commonly found in spinach and other foods. (➕) Some of the other materials in foods, such as the pigments and other phytochemicals, are not nutrients but may still be important to health. The body can make some nutrients for itself, at least in limited quantities, but it cannot make them all, and it makes some in insufficient quantities to meet its needs. Therefore, the body must obtain many nutrients from foods. The nutrients that foods must supply are called **essential nutrients.**

Carbohydrates, Fats, and Proteins Four of the six classes of nutrients (carbohydrates, fats, proteins, and vitamins) contain carbon, which is found in all living things. They are therefore **organic** (meaning, literally, "alive"). During metabolism, three of these four (carbohydrates, fats, and proteins) provide energy the body can use. (➕) These **energy-yielding nutrients** continually replenish the energy you spend daily. Carbohydrates and fats meet most of the body's energy needs; proteins make a significant contribution only when other fuels are unavailable.

Vitamins, Minerals, and Water Vitamins are organic but do not provide energy to the body. They facilitate the release of energy from the three energy-yielding nutrients. In contrast, minerals and water are **inorganic** nutrients. Minerals yield no energy in the human body, but, like vitamins, they help to regulate the release of energy, among their many other roles. As for water, it is the medium in which all of the body's processes take place.

kCALORIES: A MEASURE OF ENERGY

The amount of energy that carbohydrates, fats, and proteins release can be measured in **calories**—tiny units of energy so small that a single apple provides tens of thousands of them. To ease calculations, energy is expressed in 1,000-calorie metric units known as **kilocalories** (shortened to **kcalories**, but commonly called "calories"). When you read in popular books or magazines that an apple provides "100 calories," understand that it means 100 kcalories. This book uses the term *kcalorie* and its abbreviation *kcal* throughout, as do other scientific books and journals. (➕) kCalories are not constituents of foods; they are a measure of the energy foods provide. The energy a food provides depends on how much carbohydrate, fat, and protein the food contains.

Overview of Nutrition and Health

To calculate the energy available from a food, multiply the number of grams of carbohydrate, protein, and fat by 4, 4, and 9, respectively. Then add the results together. For example, one slice of bread with 1 tablespoon of peanut butter on it contains 16 grams of carbohydrate, 7 grams of protein, and 9 grams of fat:

$$16 \text{ g carbohydrate} \times 4 \text{ kcal/g} = 64 \text{ kcal}$$
$$7 \text{ g protein} \times 4 \text{ kcal/g} = 28 \text{ kcal}$$
$$9 \text{ g fat} \times 9 \text{ kcal/g} = 81 \text{ kcal}$$
$$\text{Total} = 173 \text{ kcal}$$

From this information, you can calculate the percentage of kcalories each of the energy nutrients contributes to the total. To determine the percentage of kcalories from fat, for example, divide the 81 fat kcalories by the total 173 kcalories:

$$81 \text{ fat kcal} \div 173 \text{ total kcal} = 0.468 \text{ (rounded to 0.47)}$$

Then multiply by 100 to get the percentage:

$$0.47 \times 100 = 47\%$$

Dietary recommendations that urge people to limit fat intake to 20 to 35 percent of kcalories refer to the day's total energy intake, not to individual foods. Still, if the proportion of fat in each food choice throughout a day exceeds 35 percent of kcalories, then the day's total surely will, too. Knowing that this snack provides 47 percent of its kcalories from fat alerts a person to the need to make lower-fat selections at other times that day.

Carbohydrate yields 4 kcalories of energy from each gram, and so does protein. Fat yields 9 kcalories per gram. Thus, fat has a greater **energy density** than either carbohydrate or protein. (✚) If you know how many grams of each nutrient a food contains, you can derive the number of kcalories potentially available from the food. Simply multiply the carbohydrate grams times 4, the protein grams times 4, and the fat grams times 9, and add the results together (the accompanying "How to" describes how to calculate the energy a food provides).

Energy Nutrients in Foods Practically all foods contain mixtures of the energy-yielding nutrients, although foods are sometimes classified by their predominant nutrient. To speak of meat as "a protein" or of bread as "a carbohydrate," however, is inaccurate. Each is rich in a particular nutrient, but a protein-rich food such as beef contains a lot of fat along with the protein, and a carbohydrate-rich food such as cornbread also contains fat (corn oil) and protein. Only a few foods are exceptions to this rule, the common ones being sugar (which is pure carbohydrate) and oil (which is pure fat).

Energy Storage in the Body The body first uses the energy-yielding nutrients to build new compounds and fuel metabolic and physical activities. Excesses are then rearranged into storage compounds, primarily body fat, and put away for later use. Thus, if you take in more energy than you expend, whether from carbohydrate, fat, or protein, the result is an increase in energy stores and weight gain. Similarly, if you take in less energy than you expend, the result is a decrease in energy stores and weight loss.

Alcohol, Not a Nutrient One other substance contributes energy: alcohol. The body derives energy from alcohol at the rate of 7 kcalories per gram. Alcohol is not a nutrient, however, because it cannot support the body's growth, maintenance, or repair. Nutrition in Practice 19 discusses alcohol's effects on nutrition.

Review Notes

- Foods provide nutrients—substances that support the growth, maintenance, and repair of the body's tissues.
- The six classes of nutrients are water, carbohydrates, fats, proteins, vitamins, and minerals.
- Vitamins, minerals, and water facilitate a variety of activities in the body.
- Foods rich in the energy-yielding nutrients (carbohydrates, fats, and proteins) provide the major materials for building the body's tissues and yield energy the body can use or store.
- Energy is measured in kcalories.

✚ Chapter 7 comes back to energy density with regard to weight management.

energy density: a measure of the energy a food provides relative to the amount of food (kcalories per gram).

Appendix B presents nutrient recommendations developed by the World Health Organization.

Dietary Reference Intakes (DRI): a set of values for the dietary nutrient intakes of healthy people in the United States and Canada. These values are used for planning and assessing diets.

Recommended Dietary Allowances (RDA): a set of values reflecting the average daily amounts of nutrients considered adequate to meet the known nutrient needs of practically all healthy people in a particular life stage and gender group; a goal for dietary intake by individuals.

Adequate Intakes (AI): a set of values that are used as guides for nutrient intakes when scientific evidence is insufficient to determine an RDA.

requirement: the lowest continuing intake of a nutrient that will maintain a specified criterion of adequacy.

deficient: in regard to nutrient intake, describes the amount below which almost all healthy people can be expected, over time, to experience deficiency symptoms.

Nutrient Recommendations

Nutrient recommendations are used as standards to evaluate healthy people's energy and nutrient intakes. (✚) Nutrition experts use the recommendations to assess nutrient intakes and to guide people on amounts to consume. Individuals can use them to decide how much of a nutrient they need to consume.

DIETARY REFERENCE INTAKES

Defining the amounts of energy, nutrients, and other dietary components that best support health is a huge task. Nutrition experts have produced a set of standards that define the amounts of energy, nutrients, other dietary components, and physical activity that best support health. These recommendations are called **Dietary Reference Intakes (DRI)** and reflect the collaborative efforts of scientists in both the United States and Canada.*[5] The DRI values are presented on the inside front covers.

Setting Nutrient Recommendations: RDA and AI
One advantage of the DRI is that they apply to the diets of individuals. The DRI committee offers two sets of values to be used as nutrient intake goals by individuals: a set called the **Recommended Dietary Allowances (RDA)** and a set called **Adequate Intakes (AI)**.

Based on solid experimental evidence and other reliable observations, the RDA are the foundation of the DRI. The AI values are based on less extensive scientific findings and rely more heavily on scientific judgment. The committee establishes an AI value whenever scientific evidence is insufficient to generate an RDA.[6] To see which nutrients have an AI and which have an RDA, turn to the inside front cover.

In the last several decades, abundant new research has linked nutrients in the diet with the promotion of health and the prevention of chronic diseases. An advantage of the DRI is that, where appropriate, they take into account disease prevention as well as an adequate nutrient intake. For example, the AI for calcium is based on intakes thought to reduce the likelihood of osteoporosis-related fractures later in life.

To ensure that the vitamin and mineral recommendations meet the needs of as many people as possible, the recommendations are set near the top end of the range of the population's estimated average requirements (see Figure 1-2). Small amounts above the daily **requirement** do no harm, whereas amounts below the requirement may lead to health problems. When people's intakes are consistently **deficient**, their nutrient stores decline, and over time this decline leads to deficiency symptoms and poor health.

Facilitating Nutrition Research and Policy: EAR
In addition to the RDA and AI, the DRI committee has established another set of values: **Estimated Average Requirements (EAR)**. These values establish average requirements for given life stage and gender groups that researchers and nutrition policymakers use in their work. Nutrition scientists may use the EAR as standards in research. Public health officials may use them to assess nutrient intakes of populations and make recommendations. The EAR values form the scientific basis on which the RDA are set.

Establishing Safety Guidelines: UL
The DRI committee also establishes upper limits of intake for nutrients posing a hazard when consumed in excess. These values, the **Tolerable Upper Intake Levels (UL)**, are indispensable to consumers who take supplements. Consumers need to know how much of a nutrient is too much. The UL are also of value to public health officials who set allowances for nutrients that are added to foods and water. The UL values are listed on the inside front cover.

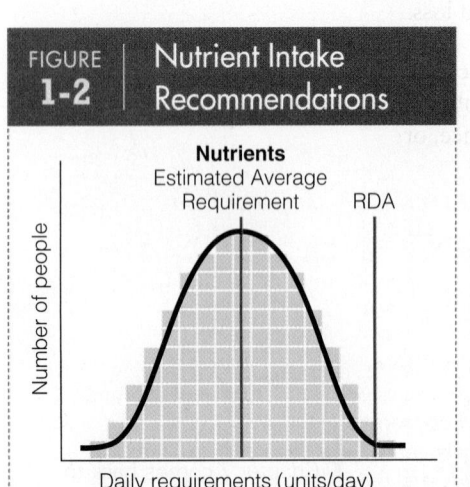

FIGURE 1-2 Nutrient Intake Recommendations

The nutrient intake recommendations are set high enough to cover nearly everyone's requirements (the boxes represent people).

---

*The DRI reports are produced by the Food and Nutrition Board, Institute of Medicine of the National Academies, with active involvement of scientists from Canada.

Overview of Nutrition and Health

Using Nutrient Recommendations Each of the four DRI categories serves a unique purpose. For example, the EAR are most appropriately used to develop and evaluate nutrition programs for *groups* such as schoolchildren or military personnel. The RDA (or AI, if an RDA is not available) can be used to set goals for *individuals*. The UL help to keep nutrient intakes below the amounts that increase the risk of toxicity. With these understandings, professionals can use the DRI for a variety of purposes.

In addition to understanding the unique purposes of the DRI, it is important to keep their uses in perspective. Consider the following:

- The values are recommendations for safe intakes, not minimum requirements; except for energy, they include a generous margin of safety. Figure 1-3 presents an accurate view of how a person's nutrient needs fall within a range, with marginal and danger zones both below and above the range.
- The values reflect daily intakes to be achieved on average, over time. They assume that intakes will vary from day to day, and they are set high enough to ensure that body nutrient stores will meet nutrient needs during periods of inadequate intakes lasting a day or two for some nutrients and up to a month or two for others.
- The values are chosen in reference to specific indicators of nutrient adequacy, such as blood nutrient concentrations, normal growth, and reduction of certain chronic diseases or other disorders when appropriate, rather than prevention of deficiency symptoms alone.
- The recommendations are designed to meet the needs of most healthy people. Medical problems alter nutrient needs, as later chapters describe.
- The recommendations are specific for people of both genders as well as various ages and stages of life: infants, children, adolescents, men, women, pregnant women, and lactating women.

Setting Energy Recommendations In contrast to the vitamin and mineral recommendations, the recommendation for energy, called the **Estimated Energy Requirement (EER)**, is not generous because excess energy cannot be excreted and is eventually stored as body fat. Rather, the key to the energy recommendation is balance. For a person who has a body weight, body composition, and physical activity level consistent with good health, energy intake from food should match energy expenditure, so the person achieves energy balance. Enough energy is needed to sustain a healthy, active life, but too much energy leads to obesity. The EER is therefore set at a level of energy intake predicted to maintain energy balance in a healthy adult of a defined age, gender, weight, height, and physical activity level.* Another difference between the requirements for other nutrients and those for energy is that each person has an obvious indicator of whether energy intake is inadequate, adequate, or excessive: body weight. Because *any* amount of energy in excess of need leads to weight gain, the DRI committee did not set a Tolerable Upper Intake Level.

ACCEPTABLE MACRONUTRIENT DISTRIBUTION RANGES (AMDR)

As noted earlier, the DRI committee considers prevention of chronic disease as well as nutrient adequacy when establishing recommendations. To that end, the committee established healthy ranges of intakes for the energy-yielding nutrients—carbohydrate, fat, and protein—known as **Acceptable Macronutrient Distribution Ranges (AMDR)**. Each of these three energy-yielding nutrients contributes to a person's total energy

---

Estimated Average Requirements (EAR): the average daily nutrient intake levels estimated to meet the requirements of half of the healthy individuals in a given age and gender group; used in nutrition research and policymaking and as the basis on which RDA values are set.

Tolerable Upper Intake Levels (UL): a set of values reflecting the highest average daily nutrient intake levels that are likely to pose no risk of toxicity to almost all healthy individuals in a particular life stage and gender group. As intake increases above the UL, the potential risk of adverse health effects increases.

Estimated Energy Requirement (EER): the dietary energy intake level that is predicted to maintain energy balance in a healthy adult of a defined age, gender, weight, and physical activity level consistent with good health.

Acceptable Macronutrient Distribution Ranges (AMDR): ranges of intakes for the energy-yielding nutrients that provide adequate energy and nutrients and reduce the risk of chronic disease.

FIGURE 1-3 | Naive versus Accurate View of Nutrient Intakes

The RDA or AI for a given nutrient represents a point that lies within a range of appropriate and reasonable intakes between toxicity and deficiency. Both of these recommendations are high enough to provide reserves in times of short-term dietary inadequacies but not so high as to approach toxicity. Nutrient intakes above or below this range may be equally harmful.

---

*The EER for children, pregnant women, and lactating women includes energy needs associated with the deposition of tissue or the secretion of milk at rates consistent with good health.

(kcalorie) intake, and those contributions vary in relation to each other. The DRI committee has determined that a diet that provides the energy-yielding nutrients in the following proportions provides adequate energy and nutrients and reduces the risk of chronic disease:

- 45 to 65 percent from carbohydrate
- 20 to 35 percent from fat
- 10 to 35 percent from protein

National Nutrition Surveys

How do nutrition experts know whether people are meeting nutrient recommendations? The Dietary Reference Intakes and other major reports that examine the relationships between diet and health depend on information collected from nutrition surveys. Researchers use nutrition surveys to learn which foods people are eating and which supplements they are taking, to assess people's nutritional health, and to determine people's knowledge, attitudes, and behaviors about nutrition and how these relate to health. The resulting wealth of information can be used for a variety of purposes. For example, Congress uses this information to establish public policy on nutrition education, assess food assistance programs, and regulate the food supply. The food industry uses the information to guide decisions in public relations and product development. Scientists use the information to establish research priorities. One of the first nutrition surveys, taken before World War II, suggested that up to a third of the U.S. population might be eating poorly. Programs to correct **malnutrition** have been evolving ever since.

COORDINATING NUTRITION SURVEY DATA

The National Nutrition Monitoring program coordinates the many nutrition-related activities of various federal agencies. All major reports that examine the contribution of diet and nutrition status to the health of the people of the United States depend on information collected and coordinated by this national program. The integration of two major national surveys provides comprehensive data efficiently. One portion of the survey collects data on the kinds and amounts of foods people eat.* Researchers then calculate the energy and nutrients in the foods and compare the amounts consumed with standards such as the DRI. The other portion of the survey examines the people themselves, using nutrition assessment methods.† The data provide valuable information on several nutrition-related conditions such as growth retardation, heart disease, and nutrient deficiencies. These data also provide the basis for developing and monitoring national health goals.

NATIONAL HEALTH GOALS

Healthy People is a program that identifies the nation's health priorities and guides policies that promote health and prevent disease. At the start of each decade, the program sets goals for improving the nation's health during the following 10 years. Nutrition is one of many focus areas, each with numerous objectives. Table 1-2 lists the nutrition and overweight objectives.

malnutrition: any condition caused by deficient or excess energy or nutrient intake or by an imbalance of nutrients.

Healthy People: a national public health initiative under the jurisdiction of the U.S. Department of Health and Human Services (DHHS) that identifies the most significant preventable threats to health and focuses efforts toward eliminating them.

---

*This survey was formerly called the Continuing Survey of Food Intakes by Individuals (CSFII), conducted by the U.S. Department of Agriculture (USDA).
†This survey is known as the National Health and Nutrition Examination Survey (NHANES).

TABLE 1-2	Healthy People Nutrition and Overweight Objectives

- Increase the proportion of adults who are at a *healthy weight*.

- Reduce the proportion of adults who are *obese*.

- Reduce the proportion of children and adolescents who are *overweight* or *obese*.

- Reduce *growth retardation* among low-income children under age 5 years.

- Increase the proportion of persons aged 2 years and older who consume at least two daily servings of *fruit*.

- Increase the proportion of persons aged 2 years and older who consume at least three daily servings of *vegetables*, with at least one-third being dark green or orange vegetables.

- Increase the proportion of persons aged 2 years and older who consume at least six daily servings of *grain products*, with at least three being whole grains.

- Increase the proportion of persons aged 2 years and older who consume less than 10 percent of kcalories from *saturated fat*.

- Increase the proportion of persons aged 2 years and older who consume no more than 30 percent of kcalories from *total fat*.

- Increase the proportion of persons aged 2 years and older who consume 2400 milligrams or less of *sodium*.

- Increase the proportion of persons aged 2 years and older who meet dietary recommendations for *calcium*.

- Reduce *iron deficiency* among young children, females of childbearing age, and pregnant females.

- Reduce *anemia* among low-income pregnant females in their third trimester.

- Increase the proportion of children and adolescents aged 6 to 19 years whose intake of *meals and snacks at school* contributes to good overall dietary quality.

- Increase the proportion of schools that teach all essential *nutrition education* topics in one course.

- Increase the proportion of worksites that offer *nutrition or weight management classes or counseling*.

- Increase the proportion of primary care providers who provide nutrition *assessment* when appropriate and who formulate a diet plan for those who need *intervention*.

- Increase the proportion of physician office visits made by patients with a diagnosis of cardiovascular disease, diabetes, or hyperlipidemia that include *counseling or education related to diet and nutrition*.

- Increase *food security* among U.S. households and in so doing reduce hunger.

Note: "Nutrition and Overweight" is one of 28 focus areas, each with numerous objectives. Several of the other focus areas have nutrition-related objectives.

Source: Healthy People 2010, www.healthypeople.gov

overnutrition: overconsumption of food energy or nutrients sufficient to cause disease or increased susceptibility to disease; a form of malnutrition.

undernutrition: underconsumption of food energy or nutrients severe enough to cause disease or increased susceptibility to disease; a form of malnutrition.

chronic diseases: diseases characterized by slow progression, long duration, and degeneration of body organs due in part to such personal lifestyle elements as poor food choices, smoking, alcohol use, and lack of physical activity.

adequacy: the characteristic of a diet that provides all the essential nutrients, fiber, and energy necessary to maintain health and body weight.

balance: the dietary characteristic of providing foods of a number of types in proportion to each other, such that foods rich in some nutrients do not crowd out foods that are rich in other nutrients.

kcalorie (energy) control: management of food energy intake.

Review Notes

- The Dietary Reference Intakes (DRI) are a set of nutrient intake values that can be used to plan and evaluate dietary intakes for healthy people.
- The Estimated Energy Requirement (EER) defines the energy intake level needed to maintain energy balance in a healthy adult of a defined age, gender, weight, height, and physical activity level.
- The Acceptable Macronutrient Distribution Ranges (AMDR) define the proportions contributed by carbohydrate, fat, and protein to a healthy diet.
- Nutrition surveys measure people's food consumption and evaluate the nutrition status of populations.
- Information gathered from nutrition surveys serves as the basis for many major diet and nutrition reports, including Healthy People.

Dietary Guidelines and Food Guides

Today, government authorities are as much concerned about **overnutrition** as they once were about **undernutrition**. Research confirms that dietary excesses, especially of energy, certain fats, and alcohol, contribute to many **chronic diseases**, including heart disease, cancer, stroke, diabetes, and liver disease.[7] Only two common lifestyle habits have more influence on health than a person's choice of diet: smoking and other tobacco use, and excessive drinking of alcohol. Table 1-3 lists the leading causes of death in the United States; notice that the top three are nutrition related (and related to tobacco use). Note, however, that although diet is a powerful influence on these diseases, they cannot be prevented by a healthy diet alone; genetics, physical activity, and lifestyle also play a role. Within the range set by genetic inheritance, however, disease development is strongly influenced by the foods a person chooses to eat.

So how can health care professionals help people select foods to create a diet that supplies all the needed nutrients in amounts consistent with good health? The principle is simple enough: encourage clients to eat a variety of foods that supply all the nutrients the body needs. In practice, how do people do this? It helps to keep in mind that a nutritious diet achieves six basic ideals.

DIETARY IDEALS

A nutritious diet has six characteristics. (✚) The first, **adequacy**, was already addressed in the earlier discussion on the DRI. An adequate diet has enough energy and enough of every nutrient (as well as fiber) to meet the needs of healthy people. Second is **balance**: the food choices do not overemphasize one nutrient or food type at the expense of another. (✚)

The essential minerals calcium and iron illustrate the importance of dietary balance. Meats, fish, and poultry are rich in iron but poor in calcium. Conversely, milk and milk products are rich in calcium but poor in iron. Use some meat or meat alternatives for iron; use some milk and milk products for calcium; and save some space for other foods, too, because a diet consisting of milk and meat alone would not be adequate. For other nutrients, people need to consume whole grains, vegetables, and fruit.

The third characteristic is **kcalorie control**: the foods provide the amount of energy needed to maintain a healthy body weight—not more, not less. The key to kcalorie control is to select foods that deliver the most nutrients for the least food energy. This fourth characteristic is known as **nutrient density**. Consider foods containing calcium, for example. You can get about 300 milligrams of calcium from either 1½ ounces of

TABLE 1-3	Leading Causes of Death in the United States

The diseases in bold italics are nutrition related.

1. *Heart disease*
2. *Cancers*
3. *Strokes*
4. Chronic lung diseases
5. Accidents
6. Alzheimer's disease
7. *Diabetes mellitus*
8. Pneumonia and influenza
9. Kidney disease
10. Infections of the blood

Source: National Center for Health Statistics, 2009.

cheddar cheese or 1 cup of fat-free milk, but the cheese delivers about twice as much food energy (kcalories) as the milk. The fat-free milk, then, is twice as calcium dense as the cheddar cheese; it offers the same amount of calcium for half the kcalories. Both foods are excellent choices for adequacy's sake alone, but to achieve adequacy while controlling kcalories, (✚) the fat-free milk is the better choice. (Alternatively, a person could select a low-fat cheddar cheese providing kcalories comparable to fat-free milk.)

Just as a financially responsible person pays for rent, food, clothes, and tuition on a limited budget, healthy people obtain iron, calcium, and all the other essential nutrients on a limited energy (kcalorie) allowance. Success depends on getting many nutrients for each kcalorie "dollar." For example, a can of cola and handful of grapes may both provide about the same number of kcalories, but grapes deliver many more nutrients. A person who makes nutrient-dense choices, such as fruit instead of cola, can meet daily nutrient needs on a lower energy budget. Such choices support good health.

Foods that are notably low in nutrient density—such as potato chips, candy, and colas—are sometimes called **empty-kcalorie foods**. The kcalories these foods provide are called "empty" because they deliver energy (from sugar, fat, or both) with little or no protein, vitamins, or minerals.

The fifth characteristic of a nutritious diet is **moderation**. (✚) Foods rich in fat and sugar provide enjoyment and energy but relatively few nutrients. In addition, they promote weight gain when eaten in excess. A person who practices moderation eats such foods only on occasion and regularly selects foods low in solid fats and added sugars, a practice that automatically improves nutrient density. Returning to the example of cheddar cheese and fat-free milk, the milk not only offers more calcium for less energy, but it contains far less fat than the cheese.

Finally, the sixth characteristic of a nutritious diet is **variety**: the foods chosen differ from one day to the next. A diet may have all the virtues just described and still lack variety if a person eats the same foods day after day. People should select foods from each of the food groups daily and vary their choices within each food group from day to day for a couple of reasons. First, different foods within the same group contain different arrays of nutrients. Among the fruits, for example, strawberries are especially rich in vitamin C while apricots are rich in vitamin A. Variety improves nutrient adequacy.[8] Second, no food is guaranteed entirely free of substances that, in excess, could be harmful. The strawberries might contain trace amounts of one contaminant, the apricots another. By alternating fruit choices, a person will ingest very little of either contaminant.

DIETARY GUIDELINES FOR AMERICANS

The *Dietary Guidelines for Americans* originated from convincing scientific evidence that nutritious food, kcalorie control, and physical activity promote health and reduce the risk of chronic disease.[9] In general, the *Guidelines* answer the question, "What should an individual eat to stay healthy?" Table 1-4 (p. 14) presents the nine *Guideline* topics with their key recommendations. The first three topics focus on choosing nutrient-rich foods within energy needs, maintaining a healthy body weight, and engaging in regular physical activity. The fourth topic, "Food Groups to Encourage," focuses on the selection of a variety of fruits and vegetables, whole grains, and milk. The next four topics advise people to choose sensibly in their use of fats, carbohydrates, salt, and alcoholic beverages for those who partake. Finally, consumers are reminded to keep food safe. Together, the *Dietary Guidelines* point the way toward better health.

✚ A nutritious diet has the following characteristics:
- Adequacy
- Balance
- kCalorie control
- Nutrient density
- Moderation
- Variety

✚ Balance in the diet helps to ensure adequacy.

✚ Nutrient density promotes adequacy and kcalorie control.

✚ Moderation contributes to adequacy, balance, and kcalorie control.

nutrient density: a measure of the nutrients a food provides relative to the energy it provides. The more nutrients and the fewer kcalories, the higher the nutrient density.

empty-kcalorie foods: a popular term used to denote foods that contribute energy but lack protein, vitamins, and minerals.

moderation: providing enough, but not too much, of a substance.

variety (dietary): eating a wide selection of foods within and among the major food groups (the opposite of monotony).

Review Notes

- A well-planned diet delivers adequate nutrients, a balanced array of nutrients, and an appropriate amount of energy.
- A well-planned diet is based on nutrient-dense foods, moderate in substances that can be detrimental to health, and varied in its selections.
- The Dietary Guidelines apply these principles, offering practical advice on how to eat for good health.

Adequate Nutrients within Energy Needs

Consume a variety of nutrient-dense foods and beverages within and among the basic food groups; limit intakes of saturated and *trans* fats, cholesterol, added sugars, salt, and alcohol.

Meet recommended intakes within energy needs by adopting a balanced eating pattern, such as the USDA Food Guide (Figure 1-4, pp. 18–19).

Weight Management

To maintain body weight in a healthy range, balance kcalories from foods and beverages with kcalories expended (see Chapters 6 and 7).

To prevent gradual weight gain over time, make small decreases in food and beverage kcalories and increase physical activity.

Physical Activity

Engage in regular physical activity and reduce sedentary activities to promote health, psychological well-being, and a healthy body weight.

To reduce the risk of chronic disease in adulthood, engage in at least 30 minutes of moderate-intensity physical activity, above usual activity, at home or work on most days of the week.

For most people, greater health benefits can be obtained by engaging in physical activity of more vigorous intensity or longer duration.

Achieve physical fitness by including cardiovascular conditioning, stretching exercises for flexibility, and resistance exercises or calisthenics for muscle strength and endurance.

Food Groups to Encourage

Consume a sufficient amount of fruits, vegetables, milk and milk products, and whole grains while staying within energy needs.

Select a variety of fruits and vegetables each day, including selections from all five vegetable subgroups (dark green, orange, legumes, starchy vegetables, and other vegetables) several times a week. Make at least half of the grain selections whole grains. Select fat-free or low-fat milk products.

Fats

Consume less than 10 percent of kcalories from saturated fats and less than 300 milligrams of cholesterol per day, and keep *trans* fat consumption as low as possible (see Chapter 4).

Keep total fat intake between 20 and 35 percent of kcalories; choose from mostly polyunsaturated and monounsaturated fat sources such as fish, nuts, and vegetable oils.

Select and prepare foods that are lean, low fat, or fat free and low in saturated and/or *trans* fat.

Carbohydrates

Choose fiber-rich fruits, vegetables, and whole grains often.

Choose and prepare foods and beverages with little added sugars (see Chapter 3).

Reduce the incidence of dental caries by practicing good oral hygiene and consuming sugar- and starch-containing foods and beverages less frequently.

Sodium and Potassium

Choose and prepare foods with little salt (less than 2300 milligrams sodium or approximately 1 teaspoon salt). At the same time, consume potassium-rich foods, such as fruits and vegetables (see Chapter 9).

Alcoholic Beverages

Those who choose to drink alcoholic beverages should do so sensibly and in moderation.

Some individuals should not consume alcoholic beverages (see Nutrition in Practice 19).

Food Safety

To avoid microbial foodborne illness, keep foods safe: clean hands, food contact surfaces, and fruits and vegetables; separate raw, cooked, and ready-to-eat foods; cook foods to a safe internal temperature; chill perishable food promptly; and defrost food properly.

Avoid unpasteurized milk and products made from it; raw or undercooked eggs, meat, poultry, fish, and shellfish; unpasteurized juices; and raw sprouts.

Note: These guidelines are intended for adults and healthy children ages 2 and older.
Source: The *Dietary Guidelines for Americans 2005,* available at www.healthierus.gov/dietaryguidelines.

FITNESS GUIDELINES

The *Dietary Guidelines for Americans* (see Table 1-4) encourage people not only to make wiser food choices but also to balance kcalories from food with kcalories expended and, in general, to be more physically active to promote health and reduce the risk of chronic disease. What does a person have to do to reap the health rewards of physical activity? The *Physical Activity Guidelines for Americans, 2008* (see Table 1-5) specify the minimum amount of **aerobic physical activity** people need to gain substantial *health* benefits.[10] The guidelines recommend longer or shorter times for activity depending on whether the activity is **moderate-intensity physical activity** or **vigorous-intensity physical activity**. For clarity and effectiveness, a minimum length of 10 minutes for short bouts of aerobic physical activity is recommended.[11] The *Physical Activity Guidelines 2008*, the American College of Sports Medicine (ACSM), and the DRI Committee, however, all advise that greater aerobic physical activity brings more extensive health benefits such as maintaining a healthy body weight (BMI of 18.5 to 24.9) and further reducing the risk of chronic diseases.

For many people, the health benefits of regular, moderate physical activity are reward enough. Others, however, seek the kinds and amount of physical activity that will improve their physical fitness or their performance in sports, as well as benefit health. To develop and maintain *fitness*, the ACSM recommends the types and amounts of physical activities presented in Table 1-6 (p. 16). The kinds and amounts of physical activity that improve physical fitness also provide still greater health benefits (substantially lower risk of premature death compared with those who are inactive and improved body composition, for example).[12]

Extensive evidence confirms that regular physical activity promotes health and reduces the risk of developing a number of diseases.[13] Despite an increasing awareness of the health benefits that physical activity confers, however, about half of adults in the United States are not regularly active, and about 20 percent are completely inactive.[14] A sedentary lifestyle is linked to the major degenerative diseases—heart disease, cancer, stroke, diabetes, and hypertension—the primary killers of adults in developed countries.[15] Therefore, one of the most important challenges health care professionals face is to motivate more people to become physically active. To motivate others, health care professionals must first become more physically active themselves, thereby enhancing their own health. Second, they can include regular physical activity as a component of therapy for their clients. As a person becomes physically fit, the health of the entire body improves. In general, physically fit people enjoy:

- *Restful sleep.* Rest and sleep occur naturally after periods of physical activity. During rest, the body repairs injuries, disposes of wastes generated during activity, and builds new physical structures.
- *Nutritional health.* Physical activity expends energy and thus allows people to eat more food. If they choose wisely, active people will consume more nutrients and be less likely to develop nutrient deficiencies.

aerobic physical activity: activity in which the body's large muscles move in a rhythmic manner for a sustained period of time. Aerobic activity, also called *endurance activity*, improves cardiorespiratory fitness. Brisk walking, running, swimming, and bicycling are examples.

moderate-intensity physical activity: physical activity that requires some increase in breathing and/or heart rate and expends 3.5 to 7 kcalories per minute. Walking at a speed of 3 to 4.5 miles per hour (about 15 to 20 minutes to walk one mile) is an example.

vigorous-intensity physical activity: physical activity that requires a large increase in breathing and/or heart rate and expends more than 7 kcalories per minute. Walking at a very brisk pace (>4.5 miles per hour) or running at a pace of at least 5 miles per hour are examples.

TABLE 1-5	Physical Activity Guidelines for Americans, 2008

- For substantial health benefits, adults should do at least 150 minutes (2 hours and 30 minutes) a week of moderate-intensity aerobic physical activity, or 75 minutes (1 hour and 15 minutes) a week of vigorous-intensity aerobic activity, or an equivalent combination of moderate- and vigorous-intensity aerobic activity. Aerobic activity should be performed in episodes of at least 10 minutes, and, preferably, it should be spread throughout the week.

- For additional and more extensive health benefits, adults should increase their aerobic physical activity to 300 minutes (5 hours) a week of moderate-intensity, or 150 minutes a week of vigorous-intensity aerobic physical activity, or an equivalent combination of moderate- and vigorous-intensity activity. Additional health benefits are gained by engaging in physical activity beyond this amount.

- Adults should also do muscle-strengthening activities that are moderate or high intensity and involve all major muscle groups on 2 or more days a week, as these activities provide additional health benefits.

Source: Key Guidelines for Adults" from http://www.health.gov/paguidelines/guidelines/summary.aspx

TABLE
1-6
Guidelines for Physical Fitness

	Cardiorespiratory	Strength	Flexibility
Type of activity	Aerobic activity that uses large-muscle groups and can be maintained continuously	Resistance activity that is performed at a controlled speed and through a full range of motion	Stretching activity that uses the major muscle groups
Frequency	3 to 5 days per week	2 or more nonconsecutive days per week	2 to 7 days per week
Intensity	Moderate (equivalent to walking at a pace of 3 to 4 miles per hour)ᵃ	Enough to enhance muscle strength and improve body composition	Enough to develop and maintain a full range of motion
Duration	At least 30 minutes	8 to 12 repetitions of 8 to 10 different exercises (minimum)	2 to 4 repetitions of 15 to 30 seconds per muscle group
Examples	Running, cycling, swimming, inline skating, rowing, power walking, cross-country skiing, kickboxing, jumping rope; sports activities such as basketball, soccer, racquetball, tennis, volleyball	Pull-ups, push-ups, weight lifting, pilates	Yoga

ᵃFor those who prefer vigorous-intensity aerobic activity such as walking at a very brisk pace (>4.5 mph) or running (≥5 mph), a minimum of 20 minutes per day, 3 days per week is recommended.

Source: Adapted from W. L. Haskell and coauthors, Physical activity and public health: Updated recommendation for adults from the American College of Sports Medicine and the American Heart Association, *Medicine & Science in Sports & Exercise* 39 (2007): 1423–1434.

- *Optimal body composition.* A balanced program of physical activity limits body fat and increases or maintains lean tissue. Thus, physically active people have relatively less body fat than sedentary people at the same body weight.[16]
- *Optimal bone density.* Weight-bearing physical activity builds bone strength and protects against osteoporosis.[17]
- *Resistance to colds and other infectious diseases.* Fitness enhances immunity.*[18]
- *Low risks of some types of cancers.* Lifelong physical activity may help to protect against colon cancer, breast cancer, and some other cancers.[19]
- *Strong circulation and lung function.* Physical activity that challenges the heart and lungs strengthens the circulatory system.
- *Low risk of cardiovascular disease.* Physical activity lowers blood pressure, slows resting pulse rate, and lowers blood cholesterol, thus reducing the risks of heart attacks and strokes.[20] Some research suggests that physical activity may reduce the risk of cardiovascular disease in another way as well—by reducing intra-abdominal fat stores.[21]

*Moderate physical activity can stimulate immune function. Intense, vigorous, prolonged activity such as marathon running, however, may compromise immune function.

- *Low risk of type 2 diabetes.* Physical activity normalizes glucose tolerance.[22] Regular physical activity reduces the risk of developing type 2 diabetes and benefits those who already have the condition.
- *Reduced risk of gallbladder disease.* Regular physical activity reduces the risk of gallbladder disease—perhaps by facilitating weight control and lowering blood lipid levels.[23]
- *Low incidence and severity of anxiety and depression.* Physical activity may improve one's mood and enhance the quality of life by reducing depression and anxiety.[24]
- *Strong self-image.* The sense of achievement that comes from meeting physical challenges promotes self-confidence.
- *Long life and high quality of life in the later years.* Active people live longer, healthier lives than sedentary people do.[25] Even a two-mile walk daily can add years to a person's life. In addition to extending longevity, physical activity supports independence and mobility in later life by reducing the risk of falls and minimizing the risk of injury should a fall occur.[26]

© Warren Morgan/Corbis

Physical activity helps you look good, feel good, and have fun, and it brings many long-term health benefits as well.

Review Notes

- Regular physical activity promotes health and reduces risk of chronic disease.
- The *Physical Activity Guidelines 2008,* the ACSM, and the DRI committee recommend at least 30 minutes of physical activity each day for health benefits and 60 minutes or more for maintaining body weight and still greater health benefits.
- The ACSM has issued recommendations for physical activity to develop and maintain physical fitness.

THE USDA FOOD GUIDE

To help people achieve the goals set forth by the *Dietary Guidelines for Americans* (see Table 1-4), the USDA provides a **food group plan**—the **USDA Food Guide**—that builds a diet from categories of foods that are similar in vitamin and mineral content. (✚) Thus, each group provides a set of nutrients that differs somewhat from the nutrients supplied by the other groups. Selecting foods from each of the groups eases the task of creating an adequate and balanced diet.

Figure 1-4 (on pp. 18–19) presents the USDA Food Guide. The USDA Food Guide assigns foods to five major food groups and recommends daily amounts of foods from each group to meet nutrient needs. (✚) The judicious use of oils, solid fats, and added sugars is also described in the USDA Food Guide. In addition to presenting the food groups, the figure indicates the most notable nutrients of each group and lists some foods within each group sorted by nutrient density. (✚)

Recommended amounts for fruits, vegetables, and milk are given in cups and those for grains and meats, in ounces. Figure 1-4 provides equivalent measures for foods that are not readily measured in cups and ounces. For example, 1 ounce of grains is considered equivalent to 1 slice of bread or ½ cup of cooked rice.

Recommended Daily Food Amounts All food groups offer valuable nutrients, and people should make selections from each group daily. Table 1-7 (p. 20) specifies the amounts of food needed from each group daily to create a healthful diet for several energy (kcalorie) levels. (✚) Estimated daily kcalorie needs for sedentary and active men and women are shown in Table 1-8 (p. 21). For example, a person needing 2000 kcalories a day would select 2 cups of fruit; 2½ cups of vegetables (dispersed among the vegetable subgroups); 6 ounces of grain foods (with at least half coming from whole grains); 5½ ounces of meat, poultry, or fish, or the equivalents of **legumes**, eggs, seeds, or nuts; and 3 cups of milk or yogurt, or the equivalent of cheese or fortified soy products. Additionally, a small amount of unsaturated oil, such as vegetable oil or the oils of nuts, olives, or fatty fish, is required to supply needed nutrients.

✚ The DASH Eating Plan, presented in Chapter 21, is another dietary pattern that meets the goals of the *Dietary Guidelines for Americans.*

✚ Five food groups:
- Fruits
- Vegetables
- Grains
- Meat, poultry, fish, legumes, eggs, and nuts
- Milk, yogurt, and cheese

✚ Chapter 11 provides a food guide for children, and Appendix B presents Canada's food group plan, *Eating Well with Canada's Food Guide.*

✚ Chapter 6 explains how to determine energy needs.

food group plan: a diet-planning tool that sorts foods into groups based on nutrient content and then specifies that people should eat certain amounts of food from each group.

USDA Food Guide: the USDA's food group plan for ensuring dietary adequacy that assigns foods to five major food groups.

legumes (lay-GYOOMS, LEG-yooms): plants of the bean and pea family with seeds that are rich in protein compared with other plant-derived foods.

FIGURE
1-4

USDA Food Guide

Key:

● Foods generally high in nutrient density (choose most often)

△ Foods lower in nutrient density (limit selections)

GRAINS

© Polara Studios, Inc.

Make at least half of the grain selections whole grains.

These foods contribute folate, niacin, riboflavin, thiamin, iron, magnesium, selenium, and fiber.

> 1 oz grains is equivalent to 1 slice bread; ½ c cooked rice, pasta, or cereal; 1 oz dry pasta or rice; 1 c ready-to-eat cereal; 3 c popped popcorn.

● Whole grains (amaranth, barley, brown rice, buckwheat, bulgur, millet, oats, quinoa, rye, wheat) and whole-grain, low-fat breads, cereals, crackers, and pastas; popcorn.

● Enriched bagels, breads, cereals, pastas (couscous, macaroni, spaghetti), pretzels, rice, rolls, tortillas.

△ Biscuits, cakes, cookies, cornbread, crackers, croissants, doughnuts, french toast, fried rice, granola, muffins, pancakes, pastries, pies, presweetened cereals, taco shells, waffles.

VEGETABLES

Choose a variety of vegetables each day, and choose from all five subgroups several times a week.

These foods contribute folate, vitamin A, vitamin C, vitamin K, vitamin E, magnesium, potassium, and fiber.

> 1 c vegetables is equivalent to 1 c cut-up raw or cooked vegetables; 1 c cooked legumes; 1 c vegetable juice; 2 c raw, leafy greens.

Vegetable subgroups

● 1. Dark green vegetables: Broccoli and leafy greens such as arugula, beet greens, bok choy, collard greens, kale, mustard greens, romaine lettuce, spinach, and turnip greens.

● 2. Orange and deep yellow vegetables: Carrots, carrot juice, pumpkin, sweet potatoes, and winter squash (acorn, butternut).

● 3. Legumes: Black beans, black-eyed peas, garbanzo beans (chickpeas), kidney beans, lentils, navy beans, pinto beans, soybeans and soy products such as tofu, and split peas.

● 4. Starchy vegetables: Cassava, corn, green peas, hominy, lima beans, and potatoes.

● 5. Other vegetables: Artichokes, asparagus, bamboo shoots, bean sprouts, beets, brussels sprouts, cabbages, cactus, cauliflower, celery, cucumbers, eggplant, green beans, iceberg lettuce, mushrooms, okra, onions, peppers, seaweed, snow peas, tomatoes, vegetable juices, zucchini.

△ Baked beans, candied sweet potatoes, coleslaw, french fries, potato salad, refried beans, scalloped potatoes, tempura vegetables.

FRUITS

© Polara Studios, Inc.

Consume a variety of fruits and no more than one-half of the recommended intake as fruit juice.

These foods contribute folate, vitamin A, vitamin C, potassium, and fiber.

> 1 c fruit is equivalent to 1 c fresh, frozen, or canned fruit; ½ c dried fruit; 1 c fruit juice.

● Apples, apricots, avocados, bananas, blueberries, cantaloupe, cherries, grapefruit, grapes, guava, kiwi, mango, nectarines, oranges, papaya, peaches, pears, pineapples, plums, raspberries, strawberries, tangerines, watermelon; dried fruit (dates, figs, raisins); unsweetened juices.

△ Canned or frozen fruit in syrup; juices, punches, ades, and fruit drinks with added sugars; fried plantains.

(Continued)

FIGURE 1-4 | USDA Food Guide *(Continued)*

MILK, YOGURT, AND CHEESE

© Polara Studios, Inc.

Make fat-free or low-fat choices. Choose lactose-free products or other calcium-rich foods if you don't consume milk.

These foods contribute protein, riboflavin, vitamin B$_{12}$, calcium, magnesium, potassium, and, when fortified, vitamin A and vitamin D.

> 1 c milk is equivalent to 1 c fat-free milk or yogurt; 1½ oz fat-free natural cheese; 2 oz fat-free processed cheese.

- Fat-free milk and fat-free milk products such as buttermilk, cheeses, cottage cheese, yogurt; fat-free fortified soy milk.

△ 1% low-fat milk, 2% reduced-fat milk, and whole milk; low-fat, reduced-fat, and whole-milk products such as cheeses, cottage cheese, and yogurt; milk products with added sugars such as chocolate milk, custard, ice cream, ice milk, milk shakes, pudding, sherbet; fortified soy milk.

MEAT, POULTRY, FISH, LEGUMES, EGGS, AND NUTS

© Polara Studios, Inc.

Make lean or low-fat choices. Prepare them with little, or no, added fat.

Meat, poultry, fish, and eggs contribute protein, niacin, thiamin, vitamin B$_6$, vitamin B$_{12}$, iron, magnesium, potassium, and zinc; legumes and nuts are notable for their protein, folate, thiamin, vitamin E, iron, magnesium, potassium, zinc, and fiber.

> 1 oz meat is equivalent to 1 oz cooked lean meat, poultry, or fish; 1 egg; ¼ c cooked legumes or tofu; 1 tbs peanut butter; ½ oz nuts or seeds.

- Poultry (no skin), fish, shellfish, legumes, eggs, lean meat (fat-trimmed beef, game, ham, lamb, pork); low-fat tofu, tempeh, peanut butter, nuts (almonds, filberts, peanuts, pistachios, walnuts) or seeds (flaxseeds, pumpkin seeds, sunflower seeds).

△ Bacon; baked beans; fried meat, fish, poultry, eggs, or tofu; refried beans; ground beef; hot dogs; luncheon meats; marbled steaks; poultry with skin; sausages; spare ribs.

OILS

Matthew Farruggio

Select the recommended amounts of oils from among these sources.

These foods contribute vitamin E and essential fatty acids (see Chapter 4), along with abundant kcalories.

> 1 tsp oil is equivalent to 1 tbs low-fat mayonnaise; 2 tbs light salad dressing; 1 tsp vegetable oil; 1 tsp soft margarine.

- Liquid vegetable oils such as canola, corn, flaxseed, nut, olive, peanut, safflower, sesame, soybean, and sunflower oils; mayonnaise, oil-based salad dressing, soft *trans*-free margarine.

- Unsaturated oils that occur naturally in foods such as avocados, fatty fish, nuts, olives, seeds (flaxseeds, sesame seeds), and shellfish.

SOLID FATS AND ADDED SUGARS

Matthew Farruggio

Limit intakes of food and beverages with solid fats and added sugars.

Solid fats deliver saturated fat and *trans* fat, and intake should be kept low. Solid fats and added sugars contribute abundant kcalories but few nutrients, and intakes should not exceed the discretionary kcalorie allowance—kcalories to meet energy needs after all nutrient needs have been met with nutrient-dense foods. Alcohol also contributes abundant kcalories but few nutrients, and its kcalories are counted among discretionary kcalories. See Table 1-7 for some discretionary kcalorie allowances.

△ Solid fats that occur in foods naturally such as milk fat and meat fat (see △ in previous lists).

△ Solid fats that are often added to foods such as butter, cream cheese, hard margarine, lard, sour cream, and shortening.

△ Added sugars such as brown sugar, candy, honey, jelly, molasses, soft drinks, sugar, and syrup.

△ Alcoholic beverages include beer, wine, and liquor.

TABLE 1-7	Recommended Daily Amounts from Each Food Group							
FOOD GROUP	1600 kcal	1800 kcal	2000 kcal	2200 kcal	2400 kcal	2600 kcal	2800 kcal	3000 kcal
Fruits	1½ c	1½ c	2 c	2 c	2 c	2 c	2½ c	2½ c
Vegetables	2 c	2½ c	2½ c	3 c	3 c	3½ c	3½ c	4 c
Grains	5 oz	6 oz	6 oz	7 oz	8 oz	9 oz	10 oz	10 oz
Meat and legumes	5 oz	5 oz	5½ oz	6 oz	6½ oz	6½ oz	7 oz	7 oz
Milk	3 c	3 c	3 c	3 c	3 c	3 c	3 c	3 c
Oils	5 tsp	5 tsp	6 tsp	6 tsp	7 tsp	8 tsp	8 tsp	10 tsp
Discretionary kcalorie allowance	132 kcal	195 kcal	267 kcal	290 kcal	362 kcal	410 kcal	426 kcal	512

© Matthew Farruggio

A portion of grains is 1 ounce, yet most bagels today weigh 4 ounces or more—meaning that a single bagel can easily supply four or more portions of grains, not one, as many people assume.

+ The USDA nutrients of concern are vitamins A, C, and E; the minerals calcium, magnesium, and potassium; and fiber.

All vegetables provide an array of vitamins, fiber, and the mineral potassium, but some vegetables are especially good sources of certain nutrients and beneficial phytochemicals. For this reason, the USDA Food Guide sorts the vegetable group into subgroups. The dark green vegetables deliver the B vitamin folate; the orange vegetables provide abundant vitamin A; legumes supply iron and protein; the starchy vegetables contribute abundant carbohydrate energy; and the other vegetables fill in the gaps and add more of these same nutrients.

In a 2000-kcalorie diet, then, the recommended 2½ cups of daily vegetables should be spread among the subgroups over a week's time, as shown in Table 1-9. In other words, eating 2½ cups of potatoes or even spinach every day for seven days would *not* meet the recommended vegetable intakes. Potatoes and spinach make excellent choices when consumed in balance with other vegetables from other subgroups. Intakes of vegetables are appropriately averaged over a week's time—it isn't necessary to include every subgroup every day.

Notable Nutrients As Figure 1-4 notes, each food group contributes key nutrients. This feature provides flexibility in diet planning: a person can select any food from a food group and receive similar nutrients. For example, a person can choose milk, cheese, or yogurt and receive the same key nutrients the milk group offers. Legumes are included in the meat, fish, and poultry group because these foods are notable for their contributions of protein, iron, and zinc. Legumes are unique, however, because they are also grouped with the vegetables by virtue of their fiber and vitamins. Thus, legumes can count in either the meat and legumes group or the vegetable group. Importantly, foods provide not only the nutrients for which each group is noted but small amounts of other nutrients and phytochemicals as well.

The USDA Food Guide encourages greater consumption from certain food groups to provide the nutrients most often lacking in the diets of Americans. (+) In general, most people need to eat:

- *More* dark green vegetables, orange vegetables, legumes, fruits, whole grains, and low-fat milk and milk products.
- *Fewer* refined grains, total fats (especially saturated fat, *trans* fat, and cholesterol), added sugars, and total kcalories.

Overview of Nutrition and Health

Nutrient Density

The USDA Food Guide provides a foundation for a healthy diet by emphasizing nutrient-dense options within each food group. By consistently selecting nutrient-dense foods, a person can both obtain all the nutrients needed and keep kcalories under control. In contrast, eating foods that are low in nutrient density makes it difficult to get enough nutrients without exceeding energy needs and gaining weight. For this reason, consumers should select low-fat foods from each group and foods without added fats or sugars—for example, fat-free milk instead of whole milk, baked chicken without the skin instead of hot dogs, green beans instead of french fries, orange juice instead of fruit punch, and whole-wheat bread instead of biscuits. Notice that Figure 1-4 provides a key indicating which foods *within each group* are high or low in nutrient density. Oil is a notable exception: even though oil is pure fat and therefore rich in kcalories, a small amount of oil from sources such as nuts, fish, or vegetable oils is necessary every day to provide nutrients lacking from other foods. Consequently, these high-fat foods are listed among the nutrient-dense foods (see Nutrition in Practice 4 to learn why).

Discretionary kCalorie Allowance

At each kcalorie level, people who consistently choose nutrient-dense foods may be able to meet their nutrient needs without consuming their full allotment of kcalories. This difference between the kcalories needed to supply nutrients and those needed for energy—known as the **discretionary kcalorie allowance**—is illustrated in Figure 1-5 (p. 22).

Table 1-7 (p. 20) includes the discretionary kcalorie allowance for several kcalorie levels. A person with discretionary kcalories available might choose to:

- Eat additional nutrient-dense foods, such as an extra serving of skinless chicken or a second ear of corn.
- Select a few foods with fats or added sugars, such as reduced-fat milk or sweetened cereal.
- Add a little fat or sugar to foods, such as butter or jelly on toast.
- Consume some alcohol. (Nutrition in Practice 19 explains why this may not be a good choice for some individuals.)

Alternatively, a person wanting to lose weight might choose to:
- Omit the kcalories available from the discretionary kcalorie allowance.

TABLE 1-8	Estimated Daily kCalorie Needs for Adults		
		Sedentary[a]	Active[b]
Women			
19–30 yr		2000	2400
31–50 yr		1800	2200
51+ yr		1600	2100
Men			
19–30 yr		2400	3000
31–50 yr		2200	2900
51+ yr		2000	2600

Note: In addition to gender, age, and activity level, energy needs vary with height and weight (see Chapter 6).

[a]*Sedentary* describes a lifestyle that includes only the activities typical of day-to-day life.

[b]*Active* describes a lifestyle that includes physical activity equivalent to walking more than 3 miles per day at a rate of 3 to 4 miles per hour, in addition to the activities typical of day-to-day life. kCalorie values for active people reflect the midpoint of the range appropriate for age and gender, but within each group older adults may need fewer kcalories and younger adults may need more.

discretionary kcalorie allowance: the kcalories remaining in a person's energy allowance after consuming enough nutrient-dense foods to meet all nutrient needs for a day.

TABLE 1-9 Recommended Weekly Amounts from the Vegetable Subgroups								
Vegetable Subgroups	1600 kcal	1800 kcal	2000 kcal	2200 kcal	2400 kcal	2600 kcal	2800 kcal	3000 kcal
Dark green	2 c	3 c	3 c	3 c	3 c	3 c	3 c	3 c
Orange and deep yellow	1½ c	2 c	2 c	2 c	2 c	2½ c	2½ c	2½ c
Legumes	2½ c	3 c	3 c	3 c	3 c	3½ c	3½ c	3½ c
Starchy	2½ c	3 c	3 c	6 c	6 c	7 c	7 c	9 c
Other	5½ c	6½ c	6½ c	7 c	7 c	8½ c	8½ c	10 c

Table 1-7 specifies the recommended amounts of total vegetables per *day*. This table shows those amounts dispersed among five vegetable subgroups per week.

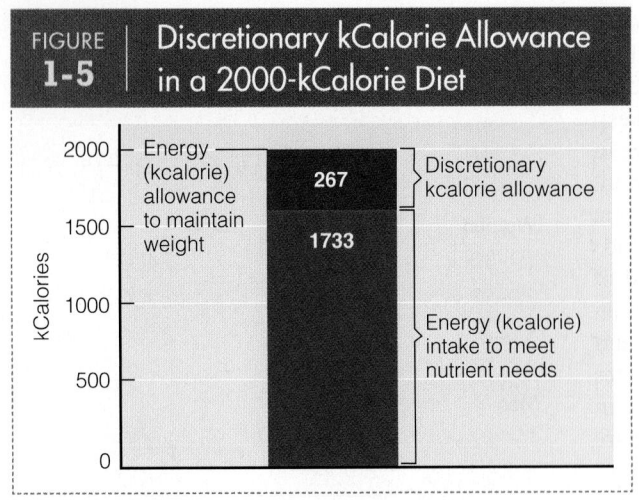

FIGURE 1-5 Discretionary kCalorie Allowance in a 2000-kCalorie Diet

267 — Discretionary kcalorie allowance

Energy (kcalorie) allowance to maintain weight

1733 — Energy (kcalorie) intake to meet nutrient needs

Compared with physically active adults, sedentary adults have lower kcalorie needs, so they have a lower discretionary kcalorie allowance. Physically active adults expend more energy and therefore have a higher energy need and a greater discretionary allowance.

Added fats and sugars are always counted as discretionary kcalories. The kcalories from the fat in higher-fat milks and meats are also counted among discretionary kcalories. It helps to think of fat-free milk as "milk," and whole milk or reduced-fat milk as "milk with added fat." Similarly, "meats" should be the leanest; other cuts are "meats with added fat." Puddings and other desserts made from whole milk provide discretionary kcalories from both the sugar added to sweeten them and the naturally occurring fat in the whole milk they contain. Even fruits, vegetables, and grains can carry discretionary kcalories into the diet in the form of peaches canned in syrup, french fries, or high-fat crackers.

Discretionary kcalories must be counted separately from the kcalories of the nutrient-dense foods of which they may be a part. A fried chicken leg, for example, provides discretionary kcalories from two sources: the naturally occurring fat of the chicken skin and the added fat absorbed during frying. The kcalories of the skinless chicken underneath are not discretionary kcalories—they are necessary to provide the nutrients of chicken.

Portion Control To control kcalories, the diet planner must also learn to control food portions (USDA serving equivalents were listed in Figure 1-4). The trend in the United States has been toward consuming larger food portions, especially of foods rich in fat and sugar. At the same time, body weights have been steadily creeping upward, suggesting an increasing need to control portion sizes. In contrast to the random-size (and often large) helpings offered in restaurants, fast-food franchises, and elsewhere, the quantities recommended in the USDA Food Guide are specific, precise, and reliable for delivering certain amounts of key nutrients in food. The margin offers some tips for estimating portion sizes. (✚)

Mixtures of Foods Some foods—such as casseroles, soups, and sandwiches—fall into two or more food groups. With a little practice, users can learn to divide these foods into food groups. From the USDA Food Guide point of view, a taco represents four different food groups: the taco shell from the grains group; the onions, lettuce, and tomatoes from the "other vegetable" group; the ground beef from the meat group; and the cheese from the milk group.

Vegetarian Food Guide Vegetarian diets rely mainly on plant foods: grains, vegetables, legumes, fruits, seeds, and nuts. Some vegetarian diets include eggs, milk products, or both. People who do not eat meats or milk products can still use the USDA Food Guide to create an adequate diet.[27] The food groups are similar, and the recommended amounts of foods remain the same. Vegetarians select *meat alternates* from the meat group—foods such as legumes, seeds, nuts, tofu, and, for those who eat them, eggs. Legumes and at least one cup of dark green leafy vegetables help to supply the iron that meats usually provide. Vegetarians who do not drink cow's milk can use soy "milk"—a product made from soybeans that provides similar nutrients if it has been fortified with calcium, vitamin D, and vitamin B_{12}. Nutrition in Practice 5 presents a Food Guide for Vegetarians, defines vegetarian terms, and provides more information on vegetarian diet planning.

Ethnic Food Choices People can use the USDA Food Guide and still enjoy a diverse array of culinary styles by sorting ethnic foods into their appropriate food groups. For example, a person eating Mexican foods would find tortillas in the grains group, jicama in the vegetable group, and guava in the fruit group. Table 1-1 (p. 4) features ethnic food choices.

✚ For quick and easy estimates, visualize each portion as being about the size of a common object:
- ¼ c dried fruit = a golf ball
- 3 oz meat = a deck of cards
- 1½ oz cheese = a nine-volt battery
- ½ c ice cream = a racquetball
- four small cookies = four poker chips

FIGURE
1-6 | MyPyramid

The multiple colors of the pyramid illustrate variety: each color represents one of the five food groups, plus one for oils. Different widths of colors suggest the proportional contribution of each food group to a healthy diet.

The name, slogan, and website present a personalized approach.

MyPyramid
STEPS TO A HEALTHIER YOU
MyPyramid.gov

A person climbing steps reminds consumers to be physically active each day.

The narrow slivers of color at the top imply moderation in foods rich in solid fats and added sugars.

The wide bottom represents nutrient-dense foods that should make up the bulk of the diet.

Greater intakes of grains, vegetables, fruits, and milk are encouraged by the width of orange, green, red, and blue, respectively.

GRAINS   VEGETABLES   FRUITS   OILS   MILK   MEAT & BEANS

MYPYRAMID

The USDA created an educational tool called MyPyramid to illustrate the concepts presented in the *Dietary Guidelines* and the USDA Food Guide. Figure 1-6 presents a graphic image of MyPyramid, which was designed to encourage consumers to make healthy food and physical activity choices every day.

An abundance of material supporting MyPyramid is available to consumers who want to find the kinds and amounts of foods to eat each day (www.MyPyramid.gov). In addition to creating a personal plan, consumers can find tips to help them improve their diet and lifestyle by taking small steps each day.

Review Notes

- Food group plans such as the USDA Food Guide serve as the basis for planning adequate, balanced, and varied diets.
- Each food group contributes key nutrients, a feature that provides flexibility in diet planning.
- The USDA Food Guide emphasizes nutrient-dense foods within each group.
- The discretionary kcalorie allowance is the difference between the kcalories needed to meet nutrient needs and those needed for energy.
- MyPyramid is an educational tool used to illustrate the concepts presented in the *Dietary Guidelines* and the USDA Food Guide.

Food Labels

Today, consumers know more about the links between diet and disease than they did in the past, and they are demanding still more information on disease prevention. Many people rely on food labels to help them select foods with less saturated fat, *trans* fat, cholesterol, and sodium and more vitamins, minerals, and dietary fiber. Food labels appear on virtually all processed foods, and posters or brochures provide similar nutrition information for fresh meats, fruits, and vegetables. Figure 1-7 illustrates the requirements for label information. A few foods need not carry nutrition labels: those contributing few nutrients, such as plain coffee, tea, and spices; foods produced by small businesses; and foods prepared and sold in the same establishment as long as the foods do not make nutrient or health claims.§

THE INGREDIENT LIST

All packaged foods must list *all* ingredients on the label in descending order of predominance by weight. Knowing that the first ingredient predominates by weight, consumers can glean much information. Compare these products, for example:

---

§For example, restaurants need not provide complete nutrition information unless they are making "heart-healthy" claims for menu items.

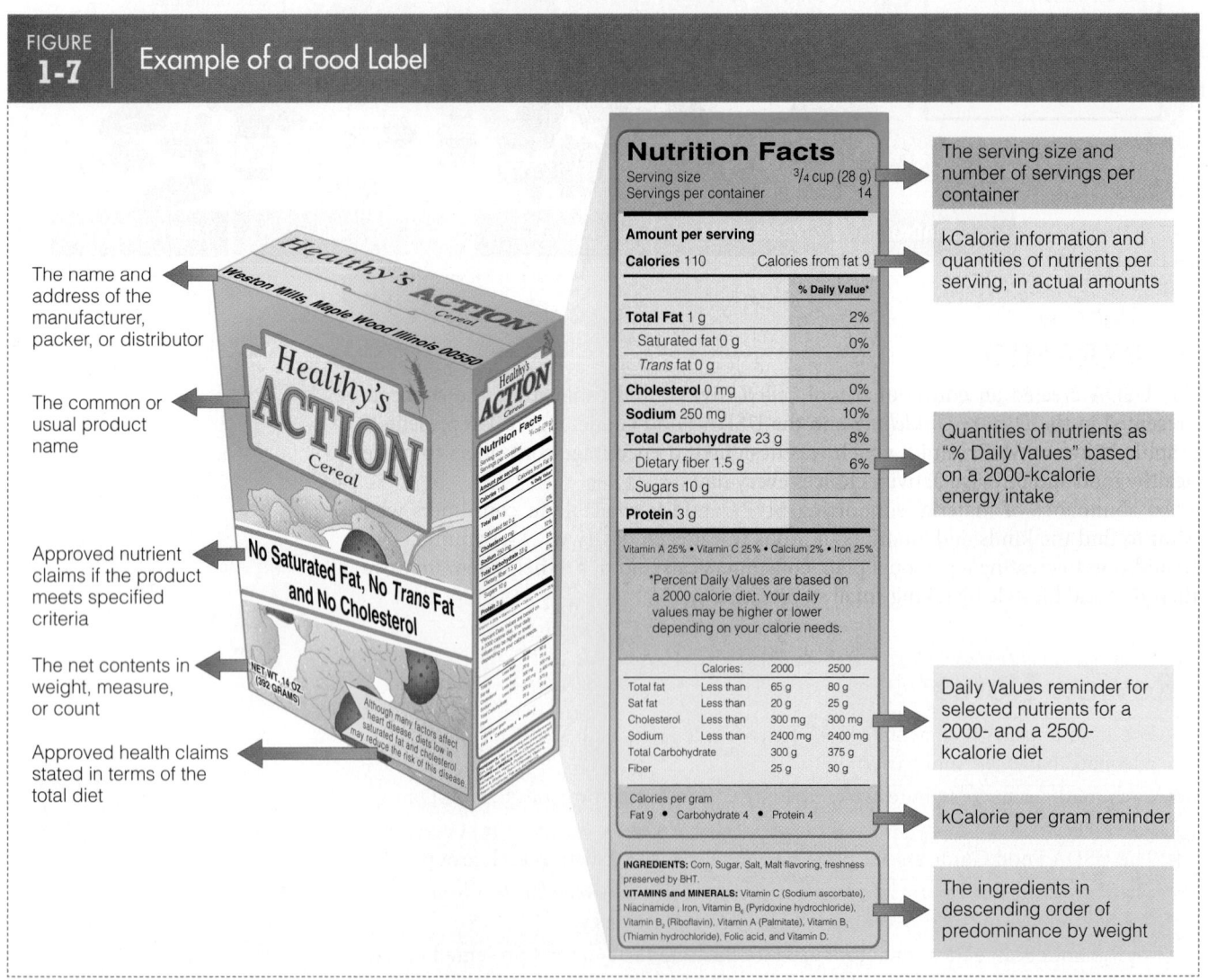

FIGURE 1-7 Example of a Food Label

The serving size and number of servings per container

kCalorie information and quantities of nutrients per serving, in actual amounts

Quantities of nutrients as "% Daily Values" based on a 2000-kcalorie energy intake

Daily Values reminder for selected nutrients for a 2000- and a 2500-kcalorie diet

kCalorie per gram reminder

The ingredients in descending order of predominance by weight

The name and address of the manufacturer, packer, or distributor

The common or usual product name

Approved nutrient claims if the product meets specified criteria

The net contents in weight, measure, or count

Approved health claims stated in terms of the total diet

- A beverage powder that contains "sugar, citric acid, natural flavors …" versus a juice that contains "water, tomato concentrate, concentrated juices of carrots, celery. …"
- A cereal that contains "puffed milled corn, sugar, corn syrup, molasses, salt …" versus one that contains "100 percent rolled oats. …"

In each comparison, consumers can tell that the second product is the more nutrient dense.

NUTRITION FACTS PANEL

The FDA requires food labels to include key nutrition facts. The "Nutrition Facts" panel provides such information as serving sizes, Daily Values, and nutrient quantities.

Serving Sizes Because labels present nutrient information per serving, they must identify the size of a serving. The Food and Drug Administration (FDA) has established specific serving sizes for various foods and requires that all labels for a given product use the same serving size. For example, the serving size for all ice creams is ½ cup and for all beverages, 8 fluid ounces. This facilitates comparison shopping. Consumers can see at a glance which brand has more or fewer kcalories or grams of fat, for example. Standard serving sizes are expressed in both common household measures, such as cups, and metric measures, such as milliliters, to accommodate users of both types of measures (see Table 1-10).

When examining the nutrition information on a food label, consumers need to consider how the serving size compares with the actual quantity eaten. If it is not the same, they will need to adjust the quantities accordingly. For example, if the serving size is four cookies and you only eat two, then you need to cut the nutrient and kcalorie values in half; similarly, if you eat eight cookies, then you need to double the values. Notice, too, that small bags or individually wrapped items, such as chips or candy bars, may contain more than a single serving. The number of servings per container is listed just below the serving size.

The Daily Values To help consumers evaluate the information found on labels, the FDA created a set of nutrient standards called the **Daily Values** specifically for use on food labels. The Daily Values do two things: they set adequacy standards for nutrients that are desirable in the diet such as protein, vitamins, minerals, and fiber, and they also set moderation standards for other nutrients that must be limited, such as fat, saturated fat, cholesterol, and sodium.

The "% Daily Value" column on a label provides a ballpark estimate of how individual foods contribute to the total diet. It compares key nutrients in a serving of food with the daily goals of a person consuming 2000 kcalories. Most labels list, at the bottom, Daily Values for both a 2000-kcalorie and a 2500-kcalorie diet, but the "% Daily Value" column on all labels applies only to a 2000-kcalorie diet. Although the Daily Values are based on a 2000-kcalorie diet, people's actual energy intakes vary widely; some people need fewer kcalories, and some people need many more. This makes the Daily Values most useful for comparing one food with another and less useful as nutrient intake targets for individuals. By examining a food's general nutrient profile, however, a person can determine whether the food contributes "a little" or "a lot" of a nutrient, whether it contributes "more" or "less" than another food, and how well it fits into the consumer's overall diet.

Nutrient Quantities In addition to the serving size and the servings per container, the FDA requires that the "Nutrition Facts" panel on a label present nutrient information in two ways—in quantities (such as grams) and as percentages of the Daily

TABLE 1-10	Household and Metric Measures

- 1 teaspoon (tsp) = 5 milliliters (mL)
- 1 tablespoon (tbs) = 15 mL
- 1 cup (c) = 240 mL
- 1 fluid ounce fl (fl oz) = 30 mL
- 1 ounce (oz) = 28 grams (g)

Note: The Aids to Calculation section at the back of the book provides additional weights and measures.

Daily Values: reference values developed by the FDA specifically for use on food labels.

Values. The Nutrition Facts panel must provide the nutrient amount, percent Daily Value, or both for the following:

- Total food energy (kcalories)
- Food energy from fat (kcalories)
- Total fat (grams and percent Daily Value)
- Saturated fat (grams and percent Daily Value)
- *Trans* fat (grams)
- Cholesterol (milligrams and percent Daily Value)
- Sodium (milligrams and percent Daily Value)
- Total carbohydrate, including starch, sugar, and fiber (grams and percent Daily Value)
- Dietary fiber (grams and percent Daily Value)
- Sugars (grams), including both those naturally present in and those added to the food
- Protein (grams)

The labels must also present nutrient content information as a percentage of the Daily Values for the following vitamins and minerals:

- Vitamin A
- Vitamin C
- Iron
- Calcium

TABLE 1-11 | Daily Values for Food Labels

Food labels must present the "% Daily Value" for these nutrients.

Food Component	Daily Value	Calculation Factors
Fat	65 g	30% of kcalories
Saturated fat	20 g	10% of kcalories
Cholesterol	300 mg	—
Carbohydrate (total)	300 g	60% of kcalories
Fiber	25 g	11.5 g per 1000 kcalories
Protein	50 g	10% of kcalories
Sodium	2400 mg	—
Potassium	3500 mg	—
Vitamin C	60 mg	—
Vitamin A	1500 µg	—
Calcium	1000 mg	—
Iron	18 mg	—

Note: Daily Values were established for adults and children over 4 years old. The values for energy-yielding nutrients are based on 2000 kcalories a day. For fiber, the Daily Value was rounded up from 23.

The FDA developed the Daily Values for use on food labels because comparing nutrient amounts against a standard helps make them meaningful to consumers. A person might wonder, for example, whether 1 milligram of iron or calcium is a little or a lot. As Table 1-11 shows, the Daily Value for iron is 18 milligrams, so 1 milligram of iron is enough to take notice of: it is more than 5 percent. But the Daily Value for calcium on food labels is 1000 milligrams, so 1 milligram of calcium is a negligible amount.

CLAIMS ON LABELS

In addition to the Nutrition Facts panel, consumers may find various claims on labels. These claims include nutrient claims, health claims, and structure-function claims.

Nutrient Claims The FDA defines the **nutrient claims** a label may use to describe the contents of a product (see Table 1-12). Definitions include the conditions under which each term can be used. For example, in addition to having less than 2 milligrams of cholesterol, a "cholesterol-free" product may not contain more than 2 grams of saturated fat and *trans* fat combined per serving.

Some descriptions imply that a food contains, or does not contain, a nutrient. Implied claims are prohibited unless they meet specified criteria. For example, a claim that a product "contains no oil" implies that the food contains no fat. If the product is truly fat free, then it may make the no-oil claim, but if it contains another source of fat, such as butter, it may not.

Health Claims Until recently, the FDA held manufacturers to the highest standards of scientific evidence before allowing them to place **health claims** on food labels.[28] When a label stated, "diets low in

TABLE 1-12 | Terms Used on Food Labels

GENERAL TERMS

free: "nutritionally trivial" and unlikely to have a physiological consequence; synonyms include *without, no,* and *zero.* A food that does not contain a nutrient naturally may make such a claim but only as it applies to all similar foods (for example, "applesauce, a fat-free food").

good source of: the product provides between 10 and 19 percent of the Daily Value for a given nutrient per serving.

healthy: a food that is low in fat, saturated fat, cholesterol, and sodium and that contains at least 10 percent of the Daily Values for vitamin A, vitamin C, iron, calcium, protein, or fiber.

high: 20 percent or more of the Daily Value for a given nutrient per serving; synonyms include *rich in* or *excellent source.*

less: at least 25 percent less of a given nutrient or kcalories than the comparison food (see individual nutrients); synonyms include *fewer* and *reduced.*

light or **lite:** one-third fewer kcalories than the comparison food; 50 percent or less of the fat or sodium than the comparison food; any use of the term other than as defined must specify what it is referring to (for example, "light in color" or "light in texture").

low: an amount that would allow frequent consumption of a food without exceeding the Daily Value for the nutrient. A food that is naturally low in a nutrient may make such a claim but only as it applies to all similar foods (for example, "fresh cauliflower, a low-sodium food"); synonyms include *little, few,* and *low source of.*

more: at least 10 percent more of the Daily Value for a given nutrient than the comparison food; synonyms include *added* and *extra.*

organic: on food labels, that at least 95 percent of the product's ingredients have been grown and processed according to USDA regulations defining the use of fertilizers, herbicides, insecticides, fungicides, preservatives, and other chemical ingredients.

ENERGY

kcalorie-free: fewer than 5 kcalories per serving.

low kcalorie: 40 kcalories or less per serving.

reduced kcalorie: at least 25 percent fewer kcalories per serving than the comparison food.

FAT AND CHOLESTEROL[a]

percent fat free: may be used only if the product meets the definition of *low fat* or *fat free* and must reflect the amount of fat in 100 grams (for example, a food that contains 2.5 grams of fat per 50 grams can claim to be "95 percent fat free").

fat free: less than 0.5 gram of fat per serving (and no added fat or oil); synonyms include *zero-fat, no-fat,* and *nonfat.*

low fat: 3 grams or less fat per serving.

less fat: 25 percent or less fat than the comparison food.

saturated fat free: less than 0.5 gram of saturated fat and 0.5 gram of *trans* fat per serving.

low saturated fat: 1 gram or less saturated fat and less than 0.5 gram of *trans* fat per serving.

less saturated fat: 25 percent or less saturated fat and *trans* fat combined than the comparison food.

***trans* fat free:** less than 0.5 gram of *trans* fat and less than 0.5 gram of saturated fat per serving.

cholesterol-free: less than 2 milligrams cholesterol per serving and 2 grams or less saturated fat and *trans* fat combined per serving.

low cholesterol: 20 milligrams or less cholesterol per serving and 2 grams or less saturated fat and *trans* fat combined per serving.

less cholesterol: 25 percent or less cholesterol than the comparison food (reflecting a reduction of at least 20 milligrams per serving), and 2 grams or less saturated fat and *trans* fat combined per serving.

extra lean: less than 5 grams of fat, 2 grams of saturated fat and *trans* fat combined, and 95 milligrams of cholesterol per serving and per 100 grams of meat, poultry, and seafood.

lean: less than 10 grams of fat, 4.5 grams of saturated fat and *trans* fat combined, and 95 milligrams of cholesterol per serving and per 100 grams of meat, poultry, and seafood. For mixed dishes such as burritos and sandwiches, less than 8 grams of fat, 3.5 grams of saturated fat, and 80 milligrams of cholesterol per reference amount customarily consumed.

(Continued)

Overview of Nutrition and Health   27

TABLE 1-12	Terms Used on Food Labels *(Continued)*

CARBOHYDRATES: FIBER AND SUGAR

high fiber: 5 grams or more fiber per serving. A high-fiber claim made on a food that contains more than 3 grams fat per serving and per 100 grams of food must also declare total fat.

sugar-free: less than 0.5 gram of sugar per serving.

SODIUM

sodium-free and **salt-free:** less than 5 milligrams of sodium per serving.

low sodium: 140 milligrams or less per serving.

very low sodium: 35 milligrams or less per serving.

ªFoods containing more than 13 grams total fat per serving or per 50 grams of food must indicate those contents immediately after a cholesterol claim. As you can see, all cholesterol claims are prohibited when the food contains more than 2 grams saturated fat and *trans* fat combined per serving.

sodium may reduce the risk of high blood pressure," for example, consumers could be sure that the FDA had examined much scientific evidence and found substantial support for the claim. Such reliable health claims make up the FDA's "A" list (see Table 1-13).

TABLE 1-13	Food Label Health Claims—The "A" List

- Calcium and reduced risk of osteoporosis

- Sodium and reduced risk of hypertension

- Dietary saturated fat and cholesterol and reduced risk of coronary heart disease

- Dietary fat and reduced risk of cancer

- Fiber-containing grain products, fruits, and vegetables and reduced risk of cancer

- Fruits, vegetables, and grain products that contain fiber, particularly soluble fiber, and reduced risk of coronary heart disease

- Fruits and vegetables and reduced risk of cancer

- Folate and reduced risk of neural tube defects

- Sugar alcohols and reduced risk of tooth decay

- Soluble fiber from whole oats and from psyllium seed husk and reduced risk of heart disease

- Soy protein and reduced risk of heart disease

- Whole grains and reduced risk of heart disease and certain cancers

- Plant sterol and plant stanol esters and reduced risk of heart disease

- Potassium and reduced risk of hypertension and stroke

TABLE 1-14	The FDA's Health Claims Report Card	
Grade	Level of Confidence in Health Claim	Required Label Disclaimers
A	High: significant scientific agreement	These health claims do not require disclaimers; see Table 1-13 for examples.
B	Moderate: evidence is supportive but not conclusive	"[Health claim.] Although there is scientific evidence supporting this claim, the evidence is not conclusive."
C	Low: evidence is limited and not conclusive	"Some scientific evidence suggests [health claim]. However, FDA has determined that this evidence is limited and not conclusive."
D	Very low: little scientific evidence supporting this claim	"Very limited and preliminary scientific research suggests [health claim]. FDA concludes that there is little scientific evidence supporting this claim."

These reliable health claims still appear on some food labels, but finding them may be difficult now that the FDA has created three additional categories of allowable health claims that are supported by evidence that is less conclusive. Each claim receives a letter grade reflecting the degree to which the claim is backed by science (see Table 1-14). The FDA can no longer demand that only health claims with the highest degree of scientific support appear on food labels.

The reliable health claims shown in Table 1-13 receive an "A" grade. Claims with a "B," "C," or "D" grade are called "qualified" health claims because they must bear a statement explaining the degree of scientific evidence backing them up. The FDA is relying on consumers to notice these printed disclaimers.

Structure-Function Claims Consumers need to be aware that a different kind of claim, known as a "structure-function" claim, may also appear on food or dietary supplement labels. **Structure-function claims** are statements about a food substance's effect on a structure or function of the body—for example, "antioxidants support heart health." Structure-function claims are not required to have FDA approval, but the claims may not refer to the reduction of disease risk. The claims must be carefully worded to avoid any mention of a specific disease. Typical claims are "slows aging," "improves memory," and "builds strong bones." To make a more specific claim such as "prevents osteoporosis," the manufacturer would have to submit to the rigorous requirements for health claims or meet the even stricter safety and efficacy standards applied to drugs. These rules ensure that consumers can have confidence that when a claim names a specific disease, there is substantial scientific agreement that the food, in the context of a healthy diet, may help protect against that disease.

Review Notes

- Food labels provide consumers with information they need to select foods that will help them meet their nutrition and health goals.
- Daily Values are a set of nutrient standards created by the FDA for use on food labels.
- Health claims that are graded "A" are backed by the highest standards of scientific evidence. Health claims with a "B," "C," or "D" grade are supported by less conclusive scientific evidence than those graded with an "A."

structure-function claims: statements that describe how a product may affect a structure or function of the body; for example, "calcium builds strong bones." Structure-function claims do not require FDA authorization.

Self Check

1. When people eat the foods typical of their families or geographic region, their choices are influenced by:
   a. occupation.
   b. nutrition.
   c. emotional state.
   d. ethnic heritage or tradition.

2. The energy-yielding nutrients are:
   a. fats, minerals, and water.
   b. minerals, proteins, and vitamins.
   c. carbohydrates, fats, and vitamins.
   d. carbohydrates, fats, and proteins.

3. The inorganic nutrients are:
   a. proteins and fats.
   b. vitamins and minerals.
   c. minerals and water.
   d. vitamins and proteins.

4. Alcohol is not a nutrient because:
   a. the body derives no energy from it.
   b. it is organic.
   c. it is converted to body fat.
   d. it does not contribute to the body's growth or repair.

5. DRI stands for:
   a. Daily Recommended Intakes.
   b. Dietary Requirements for Individuals.
   c. Dietary Reference Intakes.
   d. Daily Recommendations for Individuals.

6. Which of the following is consistent with the *Dietary Guidelines for Americans*?
   a. Limit intakes of fruits, vegetables, and whole grains.
   b. Engage in regular physical activity and reduce sedentary activities to promote health, psychological well-being, and a healthy body weight.
   c. Choose a diet with plenty of whole-milk products.
   d. Eat an abundance of foods to ensure nutrient adequacy.

7. In a food group plan such as the USDA Food Guide, foods within a given food group are similar in their contents of:
   a. energy.
   b. proteins and fibers.
   c. vitamins and minerals.
   d. carbohydrates and fats.

8. A slice of apple pie supplies 350 kcalories with 3 grams of fiber; an apple provides 80 kcalories and the same 3 grams of fiber. This is an example of:
   a. kcalorie control.
   b. nutrient density.
   c. variety.
   d. essential nutrients.

9. Which of the following statements does *not* apply to a person's discretionary kcalorie allowance?
   a. Compared with physically active adults, sedentary adults have a lower discretionary kcalorie allowance.
   b. It is the difference between the kcalories needed to supply nutrients and those needed for energy.
   c. Compared to physically active adults, sedentary adults have a higher discretionary kcalorie allowance.
   d. A person with discretionary kcalories available can, if he or she chooses to, select a few foods with added fat or sugar.

10. Food labels list ingredients in:
    a. alphabetical order.
    b. ascending order of predominance by weight.
    c. descending order of predominance by weight.
    d. manufacturer's order of preference.

Answers to these questions appear in Appendix H.

Clinical Applications

1. Make a list of the foods and beverages you've consumed in the past two days. Look at each item on your list and consider why you chose the particular food or beverage you did. Did you eat cereal for breakfast because that's what you always eat (habit), or because it was the easiest, quickest food to prepare (convenience)? Did you put fat-free milk on the cereal because you want to control your energy intake (nutrition)? In going down your list, you may be surprised to discover exactly why you chose certain foods.

2. As a nurse, you can uncover clues about a client's food choices by paying close attention. You may be surprised to discover why a client chooses certain foods, but you can then use this knowledge to serve the best interests of the client. For example, an elderly, undernourished widower may eat the same sandwich for lunch every day. In talking

with the client, you discover that this is what he and his wife fixed together each day. Consider ways you might be able to help the client learn to eat other foods and vary his choices.

3 • Using the list of foods and beverages from exercise #1, compare your day's intake with the USDA Food Guide. Did you vary your choices within each food group? Did your intake match the daily recommended amounts from each group? If not, list some changes you could have made to meet the recommendations.

Nutrition on the Net

For further study of the topics in this chapter, access these websites.

- Find updates and quick links to these and other nutrition-related sites at our website: www.cengage.com/nutrition/whitney/nhhc4e
- Search for "nutrition" at the U.S. government health information site: www.healthfinder.gov
- Review the Dietary Reference Intakes: www.nap.edu
- Review nutrient recommendations from the Food and Agriculture Organization and the World Health Organization: www.fao.org and www.who.int
- Learn more about the *Dietary Guidelines for Americans*: www.healthierus.gov/dietaryguidelines

- View Canadian information on nutrition guidelines and food labels: www.hc-sc.gc.ca
- Visit MyPyramid: www.mypyramid.gov
- See food pyramids for various ethnic groups at Oldways Preservation and Exchange Trust: www.oldwayspt.org
- View the Healthy People objectives for the nation: www.healthypeople.gov
- Learn more about food labeling from the Food and Drug Administration: www.fda.gov/food

Notes

1. J. R. Krebs, The gourmet ape: Evolution and human food preferences, *American Journal of Clinical Nutrition* 90 (2009): 707S–711S; Q. Y. Chen and coauthors, Perceptual variation in umami taste and polymorphisms in *TAS1R* taste receptor genes, *American Journal of Clinical Nutrition* 90 (2009): 770S–779S; B. J. Tepper, Nutritional implications of genetic taste variation: The role of PROP sensitivity and other taste phenotypes, *Annual Review of Nutrition* 28 (2008): 367–388; A. A. Bachmanov and G. K. Beauchamp, Taste receptor genes, *Annual Review of Nutrition* 27 (2007): 389–414; A. El-Sohemy and coauthors, Nutrigenomics of taste—Impact on food preferences and food production, *Forum of Nutrition* 60 (2007): 176–182; K. Keskitalo and coauthors, Same genetic components underlie different measures of sweet taste preference, *American Journal of Clinical Nutrition* 86 (2007): 1663–1669; M. R. Yeomans and coauthors, Human hedonic responses to sweetness: Role of taste genetics and anatomy, *Physiology and Behavior* 91 (2007): 264–273; A. Knaapila and coauthors, Food neophobia shows heritable variation in humans, *Physiology and Behavior* 91 (2007): 573–578.
2. J. E. Tillotson, Fast food—through the ages: Part 1, *Nutrition Today* 43 (2008): 70–74; J. Mathieu, Hey everyone, dinner's ready … two weeks ago, *Journal of the American Dietetic Association* 107 (2007): 26–27.
3. K. Bertrand, Microwavable foods satisfy need for speed and palatability, *Food Technology* 59 (2005): 30–34.
4. Position of the American Dietetic Association: Functional foods, *Journal of the American Dietetic Association* 109 (2009): 735–746.
5. Standing Committee on the Scientific Evaluation of Dietary Reference Intakes, *Food and Nutrition Board, Institute of Medicine, Dietary Reference Intakes for Water, Potassium, Sodium, Chloride, and Sulfate* (Washington, D.C.: National Academies Press, 2004); Standing Committee on the Scientific Evaluation of Dietary Reference Intakes, *Food and Nutrition Board, Institute of Medicine, Dietary Reference Intakes for Energy, Carbohydrate, Fiber, Fat, Fatty Acids, Cholesterol, Protein, and Amino Acids* (Washington, D.C.: National Academies Press, 2005); Standing Committee on the Scientific Evaluation of Dietary Reference Intakes, Food and Nutrition Board, Institute of Medicine, *Dietary Reference Intakes for Vitamin A, Vitamin K, Arsenic, Boron, Chromium, Copper, Iodine, Iron, Manganese, Molybdenum, Nickel, Silicon, Vanadium, and Zinc* (Washington, D.C.: National Academy Press, 2001); Standing Committee on the Scientific Evaluation of Dietary Reference Intakes, Food and

Nutrition Board, Institute of Medicine, *Dietary Reference Intakes for Vitamin C, Vitamin E, Selenium, and Carotenoids* (Washington, D.C.: National Academy Press, 2000); Standing Committee on the Scientific Evaluation of Dietary Reference Intakes, Food and Nutrition Board, Institute of Medicine, *Dietary Reference Intakes for Thiamin, Riboflavin, Niacin, Vitamin B₆, Folate, Vitamin B₁₂, Pantothenic Acid, Biotin, and Choline* (Washington, D.C.: National Academy Press, 1998); Standing Committee on the Scientific Evaluation of Dietary Reference Intakes, Food and Nutrition Board, Institute of Medicine, *Dietary Reference Intakes for Calcium, Phosphorus, Magnesium, Vitamin D, and Fluoride* (Washington, D.C.: National Academy Press, 1997).
6. Institute of Medicine, *Dietary Reference Intakes: The Essential Guide to Nutrient Requirements*, eds., J. J. Otten, J. P. Hellwig, and L. D. Meyers (Washington, D.C.: The National Academies Press, 2006), pp. 5–18.
7. F. Magkos and coauthors, Management of the metabolic syndrome and type 2 diabetes through lifestyle modification, *Annual Review of Nutrition* 29 (2009): 223–256; S. S. Gidding and coauthors, Implementing American Heart Association pediatric and adult nutrition guidelines: A scientific statement from the American Heart Association Nutrition Committee of the Council on Nutrition, Physical Activity and Metabolism, Council on Cardiovascular Disease in the Young, Council on Arteriosclerosis, Thrombosis and Vascular Biology, Council on Cardiovascular Nursing, Council on Epidemiology and Prevention, and Council for High Blood Pressure Research, *Circulation* 119 (2009): 1161–1175; A. Galimanis and coauthors, Lifestyle and stroke risk: A review, *Current Opinion in Neurology* 22 (2009): 60–68; World Cancer Research Fund/American Institute for Cancer Research, *Food, Nutrition, Physical Activity, and the Prevention of Cancer: A Global Perspective* (Washington, D.C.: World Cancer Research Fund/American Institute for Cancer Research, 2007), pp. 66–196.
8. S. P. Murphy and coauthors, Simple measures of dietary variety are associated with improved dietary quality, *Journal of the American Dietetic Association* 106 (2006): 425–429.
9. U.S. Department of Agriculture and U.S. Department of Health and Human Services, *Dietary Guidelines for Americans 2005*, available at www.healthierus.gov/dietaryguidelines.
10. Centers for Disease Control and Prevention, www.cdc.gov/physicalactivity/everyone, site updated October 7, 2008, and visited September 10, 2009.

11. W. L. Haskell and coauthors, Physical activity and public health: Updated recommendation for adults from the American College of Sports Medicine and the American Heart Association, *Medicine and Science in Sports and Exercise* 39 (2007): 1423–1434.

12. Centers for Disease Control and Prevention, www.health.gov/paguidelines/guidelines/chapter2.aspx; site updated October 7, 2008, and accessed September 10, 2009; Haskell and coauthors, 2007.

13. Centers for Disease Control and Prevention, www.cdc.gov/physicalactivity/everyone, site updated October 7, 2008, and accessed October 20, 2008; X. Yang and coauthors, The longitudinal effects of physical activity history on metabolic syndrome, *Medicine and Science in Sports and Exercise* 40 (2008): 1424–1431; L. B. Yates and coauthors, Exceptional longevity in men, *Archives of Internal Medicine* 168 (2008): 284–290; X. Sui and coauthors, Cardiorespiratory fitness and adiposity as mortality predictors in older adults, *Journal of the American Medical Association* 298 (2007): 2507–2516; D. E. Warburton, C. W. Nicol, and S. S. Bredin, Health benefits of physical activity: The evidence, *Canadian Medical Association Journal* 174 (2006): 801–809; T. S. Altena and coauthors, Lipoprotein subfraction changes after continuous or intermittent exercise training, *Medicine and Science in Sports and Exercise* 38 (2006): 367–372.

14. Centers for Disease Control and Prevention, Surveillance of certain health behaviors and conditions among states and selected local areas—Behavioral Risk Factor Surveillance System (BRFSS), United States, 2006, *Morbidity and Mortality Weekly Report* 57 (2008): 1–188; Centers for Disease Control and Prevention, Prevalence of regular physical activity among adults—United States, 2001 and 2005, *Morbidity and Mortality Weekly Report* 56 (2007): 1209–1212.

15. P. T. Katzmarzyk and coauthors, Sitting time and mortality from all causes, cardiovascular disease, and cancer, *Medicine and Science in Sports and Exercise* 41 (2009): 998–1005; A. R. Weinstein and coauthors, The joint effects of physical activity and body mass index on coronary heart disease risk in women, *Archives of Internal Medicine* 168 (2008): 884–890; N. Orsini and coauthors, Combined effects of obesity and physical activity in predicting mortality among men, *Journal of Internal Medicine* 264 (2008):442–451; P. Anand and coauthors, Cancer is a preventable disease that requires major lifestyle changes, *Pharmaceutical Research* 25 (2008): 2097–2116; X. Yang, The longitudinal effects of physical activity history on metabolic syndrome, *Medicine and Science in Sports and Exercise* 40 (2008): 1424–1431; R. D. Telford, Low physical activity and obesity: Causes of chronic disease or simply predictors? *Medicine and Science in Sports and Exercise* 39 (2007): 1233–1240.

16. S. J. Elder and S. B. Roberts, The effects of exercise on food intake and body fatness: A summary of published studies, *Nutrition Reviews* 65 (2007): 1–19; P. T. Williams, Maintaining vigorous activity attenuates 7-yr weight gain in 8340 runners, *Medicine and Science in Sports and Exercise* 39 (2007): 801–809; P. T. Williams and R. R. Pate, Cross-sectional relationships of exercise and age to adiposity in 60,617 male runners, *Medicine and Science in Sports and Exercise* 37 (2005): 1329–1337.

17. N. A. Lynch and coauthors, Older elite football players have reduced cardiac and osteoporosis risk factors, *Medicine and Science in Sports and Exercise* 39 (2007): 1124–1130; K. M. Shedd and coauthors, Quantifying leisure physical activity and its relation to bone density and strength, *Medicine and Science in Sports and Exercise* 39 (2007): 2189–2198; American College of Sports Medicine, Position stand: Physical activity and bone health, *Medicine and Science in Sports and Exercise* 36 (2004): 1985–1996.

18. M. Gleeson, Immune function in sport and exercise, *Journal of Applied Physiology* 103 (2007): 693–699; M. H. Arai, A. J. Duarte, and V. M. Natale, The effects of long-term training on the immune and endocrine systems of elderly men: The role of cytokines and anabolic hormones, *Immunity & Ageing* 3 (2006): 9.

19. World Cancer Research Fund/ American Institute for Cancer Research, *Food, Nutrition, Physical Activity, and the Prevention of Cancer: A Global Perspective* (Washington, D.C.: AICR, 2007), pp. 244–321; B. Tehard and coauthors, Effect of physical activity on women at increased risk of breast cancer: Results from the E3N cohort study, *Cancer Epidemiology, Biomarkers, and Prevention* 15 (2006): 57–64.

20. P. T. Williams, Reduced diabetic, hypertensive, and cholesterol medication use with walking, *Medicine and Science in Sports and Exercise* 40

(2008): 433–443; S. Kodama and coauthors, Effect of aerobic exercise training on serum levels of high-density lipoprotein cholesterol, *Archives of Internal Medicine* 167 (2007): 999–1008; M. M. Lockard and coauthors, Exercise training-induced changes in coagulation factors in older adults, *Medicine and Science in Sports and Exercise* 39 (2007): 587–592; L. K. Stewart and coauthors, the influence of exercise training on inflammatory cytokines and C-reactive protein, *Medicine and Science in Sports and Exercise* 39 (2007): 1714–1719; J. W. Starnes and R. P. Taylor, Exercise-induced cardioprotection: Endogenous mechanisms, *Medicine and Science in Sports and Exercise* 39 (2007): 1537–1543; T. Rankinen and coauthors, Cardiorespiratory fitness, BMI, and risk of hypertension: The HYPGENE Study, *Medicine and Science in Sports and Exercise* 39 (2007): 1687–1692; M. B. Conroy and coauthors, Past physical activity, current physical activity, and risk of coronary heart disease, *Medicine and Science in Sports and Exercise* 37 (2005): 1251–1256.

21. B. A. Irving and coauthors, Effect of exercise training intensity on abdominal visceral fat and body composition, *Medicine and Science in Sports and Exercise* 40 (2008): 1863–1872; M. Fogelholm, How physical activity can work? *International Journal of Pediatric Obesity* 3 (2008): 10–14; K. Wijndaele and coauthors, Muscular strength, aerobic fitness, and metabolic syndrome risk in Flemish adults, *Medicine and Science in Sports and Exercise* 39 (2007): 233–240.

22. C. Y. Jeon and coauthors, Physical activity of moderate intensity and risk of type 2 diabetes: A systematic review, *Diabetes Care* 30 (2007): 744–752; R. J. Sigal and coauthors, Effects of aerobic training, resistance training, or both on glycemic control in type 2 diabetes, *Annals of Internal Medicine* 147 (2007): 357–369; S. A. Kavouras and coauthors, Physical activity, obesity status, and glycemic control: The ATTICA Study, *Medicine and Science in Sports and Exercise* 39 (2007): 606–611.

23. A. M. Kriska and coauthors, Physical activity and gallbladder disease determined by ultrasonography, *Medicine and Science in Sports and Exercise* 39 (2007): 1927–1932; K. L. Storti and coauthors, Physical activity and decreased risk of clinical gallstone disease among postmenopausal women, *Preventive Medicine* 41 (2005): 772–777.

24. D. B. Nelson and coauthors, Effect of physical activity on menopausal symptoms among urban women, *Medicine and Science in Sports and Exercise* 40 (2008): 50–58; J. A. Blumenthal and coauthors, Exercise and pharmacotherapy in the treatment of major depressive disorder, *Psychosomatic Medicine* 69 (2007): 587–596; D. I. Galper and coauthors, Inverse association between physical inactivity and mental health in men and women, *Medicine and Science in Sports and Exercise* 38 (2006): 173–178; J. B. Bartholomew, D. Morrison, and J. T. Ciccolo, Effects of acute exercise on mood and well-being in patients with major depressive disorder, *Medicine and Science in Sports and Exercise* 37 (2005): 2032–2037.

25. L. B. Yates and coauthors, Exceptional longevity in men, *Archives of Internal Medicine* 168 (2008): 284–290; P. Kokkinos and coauthors, Exercise capacity and mortality in black and white men, *Circulation* 117 (2008): 614–622; X. Sui and coauthors, Cardiorespiratory fitness and adiposity as mortality predictors in older adults, *Journal of the American Medical Association* 298 (2007): 2507–2516; T. M. Manini and coauthors, Daily activity energy expenditure and mortality among older adults, *Journal of the American Medical Association* 296 (2006): 171–179.

26. M. E. Nelson and coauthors, Physical activity and public health in older adults: Recommendation from the American College of Sports Medicine and the American Heart Association, *Medicine and Science in Sports and Exercise* 39 (2007): 1435–1445; N. Takeshima and coauthors, Functional fitness gain varies in older adults depending on exercise mode, *Medicine and Science in Sports and Exercise* 39 (2007): 2036–2043; P. Aagaard and coauthors, Mechanical muscle function, morphology, and fiber type in lifelong trained elderly, *Medicine and Science in Sports and Exercise* 39 (2007): 1989–1996.

27. Position of the American Dietetic Association: Vegetarian diets, *Journal of the American Dietetic Association* 109 (2009): 1266–1282.

28. C. L. Taylor and V. L. Wilkening, How the nutrition food label was developed, part 2: The purpose and promise of nutrition claims, *Journal of the American Dietetic Association* 108 (2008): 618–623.

Finding the Truth about Nutrition

Nutrition and health receive so much attention on television, in the popular press, and on the Internet that it is easy to be overwhelmed with conflicting, confusing information. Determining whether nutrition information is accurate can be a challenging task. It is also an important task because nutrition affects a person both professionally and personally.

A person watches a nutrition report on television and then reads a conflicting report in the newspaper. Why do nutrition news reports and claims for nutrition products seem to contradict each other so often?

The problem of conflicting messages arises for several reasons:

- Popular media, often faced with tight deadlines and limited time or space to report new information, rush to present the latest "breakthrough" in a headline or a 60-second spot. They can hardly help omitting important facts about the study or studies that the "breakthrough" is based on.
- Despite tremendous advances in the past few decades, scientists still have much to learn about the human body and nutrition. Scientists themselves often disagree on their first tentative interpretations of new research findings, yet these are the very findings that the public hears most about.
- The popular media often broadcast preliminary findings in hopes of grabbing attention and boosting readership or television ratings.
- Commercial promoters turn preliminary findings into advertisements for products or supplements long before the findings have been validated—or disproved. The scientific process requires many experiments or trials to confirm a new finding. Seldom do promoters wait as long as they should to make their claims.
- Promoters are aware that consumers like to try new products or treatments even though they probably will not withstand the tests of time and scientific scrutiny.

So how can a person tell what claims to believe?

Valid nutrition information derives from scientific research, which has the following characteristics:

- Scientists test their ideas by conducting properly designed scientific experiments. They report their methods and procedures in detail so that other scientists can verify the findings through replication.
- Scientists recognize the inadequacy of personal testimonials.
- Scientists who use animals in their research do not apply their findings directly to human beings.
- Scientists may use specific segments of the population in their research. When they do, they are careful not to generalize the findings to all people.
- Scientists report their findings in respected scientific journals. Their work must survive a screening review by their peers before it is accepted for publication.

With each report from scientists, the field of nutrition changes a little—each finding contributes another piece to the whole body of knowledge. Table NP1-1 features ten red flags of junk science to help consumers distinguish valid from misleading nutrition information.[1]

TABLE NP1-1	Red Flags of Junk Science

1. Promises of a quick and easy fix.
2. Dire warnings of danger from a single product or regimen.
3. Too good to be true. The claim says what most people want to hear.
4. Enticingly simple conclusions drawn from a complex study.
5. Recommendations based on a single study.
6. Dramatic statements that are refuted by reputable scientific organizations.
7. Lists of "good" and "bad" foods.
8. Claims are made to help sell a product.
9. Claims or recommendations based on studies published without peer review.
10. Recommendations from studies that ignore differences among individuals or groups.

Source: Adapted from Position of the American Dietetic Association: Food and nutrition misinformation, *Journal of the American Dietetic Association* 106 (2006): 601–607. Used by permission of Elsevier, Inc.

Because nutrition misinformation harms the health and economic status of consumers, the American Dietetic Association (ADA) works with health care professionals and educators to present sound nutrition information to the public and to actively confront nutrition misinformation.[2] Table NP1-2 offers a list of credible sources of nutrition information.

What about nutrition and health information found on the Internet? How does a person know whether the websites are reliable?

With hundreds of millions of websites on the Internet, searching for nutrition and health information can be daunting. The Internet offers no guarantee of the accuracy of the information found there, and much of it is pure fiction. Websites must be evaluated for their accuracy, just like every other source. Table NP1-3 (p. 36) provides clues to identifying reliable nutrition information sites and lists some credible sites.

One of the most trustworthy sites used by scientists and others is the National Library of Medicine's PubMed (www.ncbi.nlm.nih.gov), which provides free access to more than 10 million abstracts (short descriptions) of research papers published in scientific journals around the world. Many abstracts provide links to websites where full articles are available.

Promoters of fraudulent "health" products use the Internet as a primary means to sell their wares. Agencies such as the Food and Drug Administration (FDA) take

---

TABLE NP1-2 | Credible Sources of Nutrition Information

Government agencies, volunteer associations, consumer groups, and professional organizations provide consumers with reliable health and nutrition information. Credible sources of nutrition information include:

- Nutrition and food science departments at a university or community college

- Local agencies such as the health department or County Cooperative Extension Service

- Government health agencies such as:
  - Department of Agriculture (USDA) — www.usda.gov
  - Department of Health and Human Services (DHHS) — www.os.dhhs.gov
  - Food and Drug Administration (FDA) — www.fda.gov
  - Health Canada — www.hc-sc.gc.ca/fn-an

- Volunteer health agencies such as:
  - American Cancer Society — www.cancer.org
  - American Diabetes Society — www.diabetes.org
  - American Heart Association — www.americanheart.org

- Reputable consumer groups such as:
  - American Council on Science and Health — www.acsh.org
  - Federal Citizen Information Center — www.pueblo.gsa.gov
  - International Food Information Council — www.ific.org

- Professional health organizations such as:
  - American Dietetic Association — www.eatright.org
  - American Medical Association — www.ama-assn.org
  - Dietitians of Canada — www.dietitians.ca

- Journals such as:
  - *American Journal of Clinical Nutrition* — www.ajcn.org
  - *Journal of the American Dietetic Association* — www.adajournal.org
  - *New England Journal of Medicine* — www.nejm.org
  - *Nutrition Reviews* — www.blackwellpublishing.com/nure

---

action against fraudulent marketing of supplements and health products on the Internet.[3] The latest actions target unscrupulous companies that use the Internet to promote products to the most vulnerable consumers—those with diseases such as cancer or AIDS. Of greatest concern are those products that not only make false promises but also are potentially dangerous. For example, herbal products touted as safe treatments for serious illnesses such as cancer may interact with and impair the effectiveness of medications. FDA advises consumers to be suspicious of:

- Claims that a product is "natural" or "nontoxic." "Natural" or "nontoxic" does not always mean safe.
- Claims that a product is a "scientific breakthrough," "miraculous cure," "secret ingredient," or "ancient remedy."
- Claims that a product cures a wide range of illnesses.
- Claims that use impressive-sounding medical terms.
- Claims of a "money-back" guarantee.

Consumers with questions or suspicions about fraud can contact the FDA on the Internet at www.FDA.gov or by telephone at (888) INFO-FDA.

Everyone seems to be giving advice on nutrition. How can a person tell whom to listen to?

Registered dietitians (RDs) and nutrition professionals with advanced degrees (M.S., Ph.D.) are experts (see the glossary). These professionals are probably in the best position to answer a person's nutrition questions. On the other hand, a "**nutritionist**" may be an expert or a quack, depending on which state the person practices in. Some states require people who use this title to meet strict standards. In other states, a "nutritionist" may be any individual who claims a career connection with the nutrition field. There is no accepted national definition for the term *nutritionist*.

Other purveyors of nutrition information may also lack credentials. A health food store owner may be in the nutrition business simply because it is a lucrative market. The owner may have a background in business or sales and no education in nutrition at all. Such a person is not qualified to provide nutrition information to customers. For accurate nutrition information, seek out a trained professional with a college education in nutrition—an expert in the field of **dietetics**.

What about nurses and other health care professionals?

All members of the health care team share responsibility for helping each client to achieve optimal health, but the registered dietitian is usually the primary nutrition expert. Each of the other team members has a related specialty. Some physicians are specialists in clinical nutrition and are also experts in the field. Other physicians, nurses, and **dietetic technicians** often assist dietitians in providing nutrition information and may help to administer direct nutrition care. Nurses play central roles in client care management and client relationships. Visiting nurses and home health care nurses may become intimately involved in clients' nutrition care at home, teaching them both theory and cooking techniques. Physical therapists can provide individualized exercise programs related to nutrition—for example, to help control obesity. Social workers may provide practical and emotional support.

What roles might these other health care professionals play in nutrition care?

Some of the responsibilities of the health care professional might be:

- Helping people understand why nutrition is important to them.
- Answering questions about food and diet.
- Explaining to clients how modified diets work.
- Collecting information about clients that may influence their nutritional health.

Glossary of Terms Associated with Nutrition Experts

dietetic technicians: persons who have completed a minimum of an associate's degree from an accredited college or university and an approved dietetic technician program. A **dietetic technician, registered (DTR)** has also passed a national examination and maintains registration through continuing professional education.

dietetics: the application of nutrition principles to achieve and maintain optimal human health.

nutritionists: all registered dietitians are nutritionists, but not all nutritionists are registered dietitians. Some state licensing boards set specific qualifications for holding the title. For states that regulate this title, the definition varies from state to state. There are

"nutritionist" credentials that require little more than payment to obtain.

registered dietitians (RDs): dietitians who have graduated from a university or college after completing a program of dietetics that has been accredited by the American Dietetic Association (or Dietitians of Canada). The dietitians must serve in an approved internship or coordinated program to practice the necessary skills, pass the association registration examination, and maintain competency through continuing education. Many states require licensing for practicing dietitians. Licensed dietitians (LDs) have met all *state* requirements to offer nutrition advice.

To judge whether an Internet site offers reliable nutrition information, answer the following questions.

Who is responsible for the site? Clues can be found in the three-letter "tag" that follows the dot in the site's name. For example, "gov" and "edu" indicate government and university sites, respectively, which are usually reliable sources of information.

Do the names and credentials of information providers appear? Is an editorial board identified? Many legitimate sources provide e-mail addresses or other ways to obtain more information about the site and the information providers behind it.

Are links with other reliable information sites provided? Reputable organizations almost always provide links with other similar sites because they want you to know of other experts in their area of knowledge. Caution is needed when you evaluate a site by its links, however. Anyone, even a quack, can link a web page to a reputable site without the organization's permission. Doing so may give the quack's site the appearance of legitimacy, just the effect for which the quack is hoping.

Is the site updated regularly? Nutrition information changes rapidly, and sites should be updated often.

Is the site selling a product or service? Commercial sites may provide accurate information, but they also may not. Their profit motive increases the risk of bias.

Does the site charge a fee to gain access to it? Many academic and government sites offer the best information, usually for free. Some legitimate sites do charge fees, but before paying up, check the free sites. Chances are good you will find what you are looking for without paying.

Some credible websites include:

National Council Against Health Fraud

www.ncahf.org

Stephen Barrett's Quackwatch

www.quackwatch.com

- Identifying clients at risk for poor nutrition status (see Chapter 13) and recommending or taking appropriate action.
- Recognizing when clients need extra help with nutrition problems (in such cases, the problems should be referred to a dietitian or physician).

Health care professionals may routinely perform these nutrition-related tasks:

- Obtaining diet histories.
- Taking weight and height measurements.
- Feeding clients who cannot feed themselves.
- Recording what clients eat or drink.
- Observing clients' responses and reactions to foods.

- Helping clients mark menus.
- Monitoring weight changes.
- Monitoring food and drug interactions.
- Encouraging clients to eat.
- Assisting clients at home in planning their diets and managing their kitchen chores.
- Alerting the physician or dietitian when nutrition problems are identified.
- Charting actions taken and communicating on these matters with other professionals as needed.

Thus, although the dietitian assumes the primary role as the nutrition expert on a health care team, other health care professionals play important roles in administering nutrition care.

Notes

1. Position of the American Dietetic Association: Food and nutrition misinformation, *Journal of the American Dietetic Association* 106 (2006): 601–607.
2. Position of the American Dietetic Association, 2006.

3. Food and Drug Administration, *FDA 101: Health Fraud Awareness*, FDA Consumer Health Information, May 2009, available at www.fda.gov.

CHAPTER 2 | Digestion and Absorption

© Envision/Corbis

CONTENTS

THE BODY'S ABILITY TO TRANSFORM THE FOODS A PERSON EATS INTO the nutrients that fuel the body's work is quite remarkable. Yet most people probably give little, if any, thought to all the body does with food once it is eaten. This chapter offers the reader the opportunity to learn how the body digests, absorbs, and transports the nutrients and how it excretes the unwanted substances in foods.

One of the beauties of the digestive tract is that it is selective. Materials that are nutritive for the body are broken down into particles that can be absorbed into the bloodstream. Most of the nonnutritive materials are left undigested and pass out the other end of the digestive tract.

Anatomy of the Digestive Tract

The **gastrointestinal (GI) tract** is a flexible muscular tube extending from the mouth to the anus. Figure 2-1 on pp. 40–41 traces the path followed by food from one end of the GI tract to the other. The accompanying glossary defines GI anatomical terms. In a sense, the human body surrounds the GI tract. Only when a nutrient or other substance passes through the cells of the digestive tract wall does it actually enter the body.

THE DIGESTIVE ORGANS

The process of **digestion** begins in the **mouth**. As you chew, your teeth crush and soften the food, while saliva mixes with the food mass and moistens it for comfortable swallowing. Saliva also helps dissolve the food so that you can taste it; only particles in solution can react with taste buds.

Glossary

These terms are listed in order from start to end of the digestive system.

mouth: the oral cavity containing the tongue and teeth.

pharynx (FAIR-inks): the passageway leading from the nose and mouth to the larynx and esophagus, respectively.

epiglottis (epp-ih-GLOTT-iss): cartilage in the throat that guards the entrance to the trachea and prevents fluid or food from entering it when a person swallows.

- *epi* = upon (over)
- *glottis* = back of tongue

esophagus (ee-SOFF-ah-gus): the food pipe; the conduit from the mouth to the stomach.

sphincter (SFINK-ter): a circular muscle surrounding, and able to close, a body opening. Sphincters are found at specific points along the GI tract and regulate the flow of food particles.

- *sphincter* = band (binder)

esophageal (ee-SOF-a-GEE-al) **sphincter:** a sphincter muscle at the upper or lower end of the esophagus. The *lower esophageal sphincter* is also called the *cardiac sphincter*.

stomach: a muscular, elastic, saclike portion of the digestive tract that grinds and churns swallowed food, mixing it with acid and enzymes to form chyme.

pyloric (pie-LORE-ic) **sphincter:** the circular muscle that separates the stomach from the small intestine and regulates the flow of partially digested food into the small intestine; also called *pylorus* or *pyloric valve*.

- *pylorus* = gatekeeper

small intestine: a 10-foot length of small-diameter intestine that is the major site of digestion of food and absorption of nutrients. Its segments are the duodenum, jejunum, and ileum.

duodenum (doo-oh-DEEN-um, doo-ODD-num): the top portion of the small intestine (about "12 fingers' breadth long" in ancient terminology).

- *duodecim* = twelve

jejunum (je-JOON-um): the first two-fifths of the small intestine beyond the duodenum.

ileum (ILL-ee-um): the last segment of the small intestine.

gallbladder: the organ that stores and concentrates bile. When it receives the signal that fat is present in the duodenum, the gallbladder contracts and squirts bile through the bile duct into the duodenum.

pancreas: a gland that secretes digestive enzymes and juices into the duodenum. (The pancreas also secretes hormones into the blood that help to maintain glucose homeostasis.)

ileocecal (ill-ee-oh-SEEK-ul) **valve:** the sphincter separating the small and large intestines.

large intestine or colon (COAL-un): the lower portion of intestine that completes the digestive process. Its segments are the ascending colon, the transverse colon, the descending colon, and the sigmoid colon.

- *sigmoid* = shaped like the letter S (sigma in Greek)

appendix: a narrow blind sac extending from the beginning of the colon that stores lymph cells.

rectum: the muscular terminal part of the intestine, extending from the sigmoid colon to the anus.

anus (AY-nus): the terminal outlet of the GI tract.

The tongue allows you not only to taste food but also to move food around the mouth, facilitating chewing and swallowing. When you swallow a mouthful of food, it passes through the **pharynx**, a short tube that is shared by both the **digestive system** and the respiratory system.

Mouth to the Esophagus

Once a mouthful of food has been chewed and swallowed, it is called a **bolus**. Each bolus first slides across your **epiglottis**, bypassing the entrance to your lungs. During each swallow, the epiglottis closes off your trachea, the air passageway to the lungs, so that you do not choke.

Esophagus to the Stomach

The **esophagus** has a **sphincter** muscle at each end. During a swallow, the upper **esophageal sphincter** opens. The bolus then slides down the esophagus, which conducts it through the diaphragm to the **stomach**. The lower esophageal sphincter closes behind the bolus so that it cannot slip back. The stomach retains the bolus for a while, adds juices to it (gastric juices are discussed on p. 44), and transforms it into a semiliquid mass called **chyme**. Then, bit by bit, the stomach releases the chyme through another sphincter, the **pyloric sphincter**, which opens into the **small intestine** and then closes after the chyme passes through.

The Small Intestine

At the beginning of the small intestine, the chyme passes by an opening from the common bile duct, which secretes digestive fluids into the small intestine from two organs outside the GI tract—the **gallbladder** and the **pancreas**. The chyme travels on down the small intestine through its three segments—the **duodenum**, the **jejunum**, and the **ileum**. Together, the segments amount to a total of about 10 feet of tubing coiled within the abdomen.* Digestion is completed within the small intestine.

The Large Intestine (Colon)

Having traveled the length of the small intestine, what remains of the intestinal contents passes through another sphincter, the **ileocecal valve**, into the beginning of the **large intestine (colon)** in the lower right-hand side of the abdomen. Upon entering the colon, the contents pass another opening. Should any intestinal contents slip into this opening, they would end up in the **appendix**, a blind sac about the size of your little finger. Normally, the contents bypass this opening, however, and travel up the right-hand side of the abdomen, across the front to the left-hand side, down to the lower left-hand side, and finally below the other folds of the intestines to the back side of the body above the **rectum**.

The Rectum

As the intestinal contents pass to the rectum, the colon withdraws water, leaving semisolid waste. The strong muscles of the rectum hold back this waste until it is time to defecate. Then the rectal muscles relax, and the last sphincter in the system, the **anus**, opens to allow the wastes to pass. Thus, food follows the path shown in the margin. (✚)

THE INVOLUNTARY MUSCLES AND THE GLANDS

You are usually unaware of all the activity that goes on between the time you swallow and the time you defecate. As is the case with so much else that happens in the body, the muscles and **glands** of the digestive tract meet internal needs without your having to exert any conscious effort to get the work done.

People consciously chew and swallow, but even in the mouth there are some processes over which you have no control. The salivary glands secrete just enough saliva to moisten each mouthful of food so that it can pass easily down your esophagus.

Gastrointestinal Motility

Once you have swallowed, materials are moved through the rest of the GI tract by involuntary muscular contractions. This motion, known as **gastrointestinal motility**, consists of two types of movement,

---

*The small intestine is almost two and a half times shorter in living adults than it is at death, when muscles are relaxed and elongated.

✚ The path of food through the digestive tract:
- Mouth
- Esophagus
- Lower esophageal sphincter (or cardiac sphincter)
- Stomach
- Pyloric sphincter
- Duodenum (common bile duct enters here), jejunum, ileum
- Ileocecal valve
- Large intestine (colon)
- Rectum
- Anus

digestive system: all the organs and glands associated with the ingestion and digestion of food.

bolus (BOH-lus): the portion of food swallowed at one time.

chyme (KIME): the semiliquid mass of partly digested food expelled by the stomach into the duodenum (the top portion of the small intestine).

gastrointestinal motility: spontaneous motion in the digestive tract accomplished by involuntary muscular contractions.

peristalsis (peri-STALL-sis): successive waves of involuntary muscular contractions passing along the walls of the GI tract that push the contents along.

peri = around
stellein = wrap

FIGURE
2-1
The Gastrointestinal Tract

FIBER	CARBOHYDRATE

Mouth and salivary glands

The mechanical action of the mouth and teeth crushes and tears fiber in food and mixes it with saliva to moisten it for swallowing.

The salivary glands secrete saliva into the mouth to moisten the food. The salivary enzyme amylase begins digestion:

$$\text{Starch} \xrightarrow{\text{amylase}} \text{small polysaccharides, maltose.}$$

Stomach

Fiber is unchanged.

Stomach acid inactivates salivary enzymes, halting starch digestion. To a small extent, stomach acid hydrolyzes maltose and sucrose.

Small intestine

Fiber is unchanged.

The pancreas produces enzymes and releases them through the pancreatic duct into the small intestine:

$$\text{Polysaccharides} \xrightarrow{\text{pancreatic amylase}} \text{disaccharides.}$$

Then enzymes on the surfaces of the small intestinal cells break disaccharides into monosaccharides, and the cells absorb them:

$$\text{Maltose} \xrightarrow{\text{maltase}} \text{glucose} + \text{glucose.}$$

$$\text{Sucrose} \xrightarrow{\text{sucrase}} \text{fructose} + \text{glucose.}$$

$$\text{Lactose} \xrightarrow{\text{lactase}} \text{galactose} + \text{glucose.}$$

Large intestine (colon)

Most fiber passes intact through the digestive tract to the large intestine. Here, bacterial enzymes digest some fiber:

$$\text{Some fiber} \xrightarrow{\text{bacterial enzymes}} \text{fatty acids, gas.}$$

Fiber holds water; regulates bowel activity; and binds cholesterol and some minerals, carrying them out of the body as it is excreted with feces.

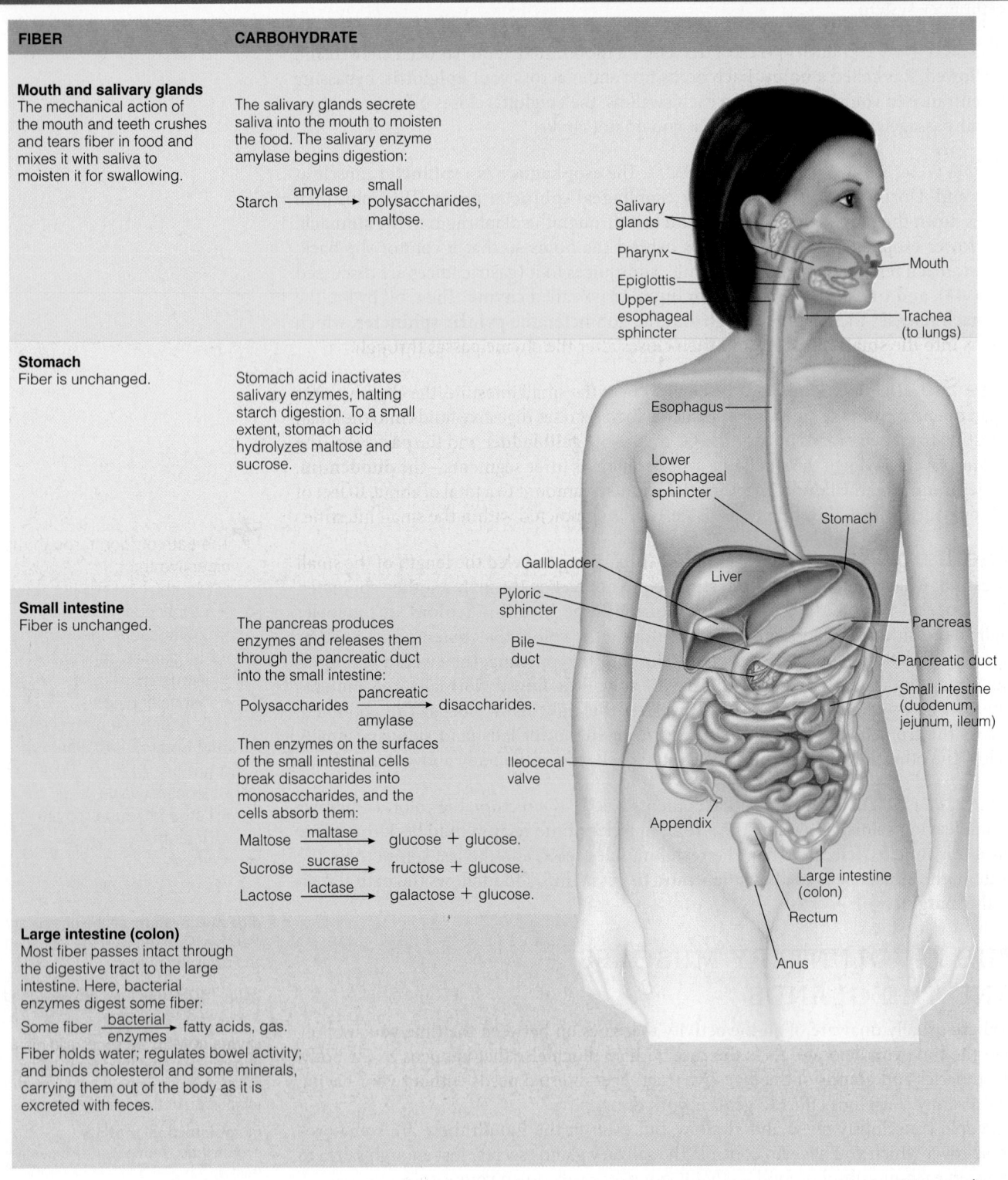

Salivary glands
Pharynx
Epiglottis
Upper esophageal sphincter
Mouth
Trachea (to lungs)
Esophagus
Lower esophageal sphincter
Stomach
Gallbladder
Liver
Pyloric sphincter
Bile duct
Pancreas
Pancreatic duct
Small intestine (duodenum, jejunum, ileum)
Ileocecal valve
Appendix
Large intestine (colon)
Rectum
Anus

(Continued)

peristalsis and segmentation (see Figure 2-2 on p. 42). Peristalsis propels, or pushes; segmentation mixes, with more gradual pushing.

Peristalsis **Peristalsis** begins when the bolus enters the esophagus. The entire GI tract is ringed with circular muscles, which are surrounded by longitudinal muscles.

FIGURE
2-1 | The Gastrointestinal Tract (Continued)

	FAT	PROTEIN	VITAMINS	MINERALS AND WATER
Mouth and salivary glands	The sublingual salivary gland in the base of the tongue secretes a fat-digesting enzyme known as lingual lipase. Some hard fats begin to melt as they reach body temperature.	Chewing and crushing moisten protein-rich foods and mix them with saliva to be swallowed.	No action.	The salivary glands add water to disperse and carry food.
Stomach	The acid-stable lingual lipase splits one bond of triglycerides to produce diglycerides and fatty acids. The degree of hydrolysis is slight for most fats but may be appreciable for milk fats. The stomach's churning action mixes fat with water and acid. A gastric lipase accesses and hydrolyzes a very small amount of fat.	Hydrochloric acid (HCL) uncoils protein strands and activates stomach enzymes: Protein $\xrightarrow[\text{HCl}]{\text{pepsin}}$ smaller polypeptides.	Intrinsic factor (see Chapter 8) attaches to vitamin B_{12}.	Stomach acid (HCl) acts on iron to reduce it, making it more absorbable. The stomach secretes enough watery fluid to turn a moist, chewed mass of solid food into liquid chyme.
Small intestine	Bile flows in from the liver and gallbladder (via the common bile duct): Fat $\xrightarrow{\text{bile}}$ emulsified fat. Pancreatic lipase flows in from the pancreas (via the pancreatic duct): Emulsified fat $\xrightarrow[\text{lipase}]{\text{pancreatic}}$ monoglycerides, glycerol, fatty acids (absorbed).	Polypeptides $\xrightarrow[\text{and intestinal proteases}]{\text{pancreatic}}$ tripeptides, dipeptides, amino acids. Then enzymes on the surface of the small intestinal cells hydrolyze these peptides and the cells absorb them. Peptides $\xrightarrow[\text{dipeptidases and tripeptidases}]{\text{intestinal}}$ amino acids (absorbed)	Bile emulsifies fat-soluble vitamins and aids in their absorption with other fats. Water-soluble vitamins are absorbed.	The small intestine, pancreas, and liver add enough fluid so that approximately 2 gallons are secreted into the intestine in a day. Many minerals are absorbed. Vitamin D aids in the absorption of calcium.
Large intestine	Some fat and cholesterol, trapped in fiber, exit in feces.		Bacteria produce vitamin K, which is absorbed.	More minerals and most of the water are absorbed.

When the rings tighten and the long muscles relax, the tube is constricted. When the rings relax and the long muscles tighten, the tube bulges. These actions alternate continually and push the intestinal contents along. If you have ever watched a bolus of food pass along the body of a snake, you have a good picture of how these muscles work. The waves of contraction ripple through the GI tract at varying rates and intensities

FIGURE 2-2 | Peristalsis and Segmentation

The small intestine has two muscle layers that work together in peristalsis and segmentation.

Circular muscles are inside.

Longitudinal muscles are outside.

Peristalsis

Chyme

The inner circular muscles contract, tightening the tube and pushing the food forward in the intestine.

When the circular muscles relax, the outer longitudinal muscles contract, and the intestinal tube is loose.

As the circular and longitudinal muscles tighten and relax, the chyme moves ahead of the constriction.

Segmentation

Chyme

Circular muscles contract, creating segments within the intestine.

As each set of circular muscles relaxes and contracts, the chyme is broken up and mixed with digestive juices.

These alternating contractions, occurring 12 to 16 times per minute, continue to mix the chyme and bring the nutrients into contact with the intestinal lining for absorption.

depending on the part of the GI tract and on whether food is present. Peristalsis, aided by the sphincter muscles located at key places, keeps things moving along. However, factors such as stress, medicines, and medical conditions may interfere with normal GI tract contractions.[1]

Segmentation The intestines not only push but also periodically squeeze their contents as if a string tied around the intestines were being pulled tight. This motion, called **segmentation**, forces the contents back a few inches, mixing them and promoting

segmentation: a periodic squeezing or partitioning of the intestine by its circular muscles that both mixes and slowly pushes the contents along.

close contact with the digestive juices and the absorbing cells of the intestinal walls before letting the contents slowly move along again.

Liquefying Process Besides forcing the intestinal contents along, the muscles of the GI tract help to liquefy them to chyme so that the digestive juices will have access to all their nutrients. The mouth initiates this liquefying process by chewing, adding saliva, and stirring with the tongue to reduce the food to a coarse mash suitable for swallowing. The stomach then further mixes and kneads the food.

Stomach Action The stomach has the thickest walls and strongest muscles of all the GI tract organs. In addition to circular and longitudinal muscles, the stomach has a third layer of diagonal muscles that also alternately contract and relax (see Figure 2-3). These three sets of muscles work to force the chyme downward, but the pyloric sphincter usually remains tightly closed so that the stomach's contents are thoroughly mixed and squeezed before being released. Meanwhile, the gastric glands are adding juices. When the chyme is thoroughly liquefied, the pyloric sphincter opens briefly, about three times a minute, to allow small portions through. At this point, the intestinal contents no longer resemble food in the least.

Review Notes

- As Figure 2-1 shows, food enters the mouth and travels down the esophagus and through the lower esophageal sphincter to the stomach, then through the pyloric sphincter to the small intestine, on through the ileocecal valve to the large intestine, past the appendix to the rectum, and ending at the anus.
- The wavelike contractions of peristalsis and the periodic squeezing of segmentation keep things moving at a reasonable pace.

FIGURE 2-3 | Stomach Muscles

Crisscrossed muscle layers create churning and mixing motions:

inner (diagonal)

middle (circular)

outer (longitudinal)

The pyloric sphincter controls the flow of chyme into the small intestine.

Small intestine (duodenum)

Esophagus

Folds inside stomach allow it to stretch and contract.

The stomach has three layers of muscles.

The Process of Digestion

One person eats nothing but vegetables, fruits, and nuts; another, nothing but meat, milk, and potatoes. How is it that both people wind up with essentially the same body composition? It all comes down to the body rendering food—whatever it is to start with—into the basic units that make up carbohydrate, fat, and protein. The body absorbs these units and builds its tissues from them.

To digest food, five different body organs secrete digestive juices: the salivary glands, the stomach, the small intestine, the liver (via the gallbladder), and the pancreas. These secretions enter the GI tract at various points along the way, bringing an abundance of water and a variety of enzymes. (✚) Each of the juices has a turn to mix with the food and promote its breakdown to small units that can be absorbed into the body. The accompanying glossary defines some of the digestive glands and their juices.

✚ Enzymes are formally introduced in Chapter 5, but for now a simple definition will suffice. An *enzyme* is a protein that facilitates a chemical reaction—making a compound, breaking down a compound, changing the arrangement of a compound, or exchanging parts. Enzymes themselves are not changed by the reactions they facilitate.

DIGESTION IN THE MOUTH

Digestion of carbohydrate begins in the mouth, where the **salivary glands** secrete **saliva**, which contains water, salts, and enzymes (including salivary **amylase**) that break the bonds in the chains of starch. Saliva also protects the tooth surfaces and linings of the mouth, esophagus, and stomach from attack by molecules that might harm them. The enzymes in the mouth do not, for the most part, affect the fats, proteins, vitamins, minerals, and fiber that are present in the foods people eat (review Figure 2-1).

DIGESTION IN THE STOMACH

Gastric juice, secreted by the **gastric glands**, is composed of water, enzymes, and **hydrochloric acid**. The acid is so strong that it burns the throat if it happens to reflux into the upper esophagus and mouth. The strong acidity of the stomach prevents bacterial

Glossary

These terms are listed in order from the beginning of the digestive tract to the end.

glands: cells or groups of cells that secrete materials for special uses in the body. Glands may be *exocrine* (EKS-oh-crin) *glands,* secreting their materials "out" (into the digestive tract or onto the surface of the skin), or *endocrine* (EN-doe-crin) *glands,* secreting their materials "in" (into the blood).

- *exo* = outside
- *endo* = inside
- *krine* = to separate

salivary glands: exocrine glands that secrete saliva into the mouth.

saliva: the secretion of the salivary glands. The principal enzyme is salivary amylase.

amylase (AM-uh-lace): an enzyme that splits amylose (a form of starch). Amylase is a carbohydrase. The ending *–ase* indicates an enzyme; the root tells what it digests. Other examples: protease, lipase.

gastric glands: exocrine glands in the stomach wall that secrete gastric juice into the stomach.

- *gastro* = stomach

gastric juice: the digestive secretion of the gastric glands containing a mixture of water, hydrochloric acid, and enzymes. The principal enzymes are pepsin (acts on proteins) and lipase (acts on emulsified fats).

hydrochloric acid (HCl): an acid composed of hydrogen and chloride atoms; normally produced by the gastric glands.

mucus (MYOO-cuss): a mucopolysaccharide (a relative of carbohydrate) secreted by cells of the stomach wall that protects the cells from exposure to digestive juices (and other destructive agents). The cellular lining of the stomach wall with its coat of mucus is known as the *mucous membrane.* (The noun is *mucus;* the adjective is *mucous.*)

pepsin: a protein-digesting enzyme (gastric protease) in the stomach. It circulates as a precursor, pepsinogen, and is converted to pepsin by the action of stomach acid.

intestinal juice: the secretion of the intestinal glands; contains enzymes for the digestion of carbohydrate and protein and a minor enzyme for fat digestion.

liver: the organ that manufactures bile. (The liver's other functions are described in Chapter 19.)

bile: an emulsifier that prepares fats and oils for digestion; made by the liver, stored in the gallbladder, and released into the small intestine when needed.

pancreatic (pank-ree-AT-ic) **juice:** the exocrine secretion of the pancreas, containing enzymes for the digestion of carbohydrate, fat, and protein. Juice flows from the pancreas into the small intestine through the pancreatic duct. The pancreas also has an endocrine function, the secretion of insulin and other hormones.

bicarbonate: an alkaline secretion of the pancreas; part of the pancreatic juice. (Bicarbonate also occurs widely in all cell fluids.)

Digestion and Absorption

growth and kills most bacteria that enter the body with food. You might expect that the stomach's acid would attack the stomach itself, but the cells of the stomach wall secrete **mucus**, a thick, slimy, white polysaccharide that coats and protects the stomach's lining.

The major digestive event in the stomach is the initial breakdown of proteins. Other than being crushed and mixed with saliva in the mouth, nothing happens to protein until it comes in contact with the gastric juices in the stomach. There, the acid helps to uncoil (denature) the protein's tangled strands so that the stomach enzymes can attack the bonds. Both the enzyme **pepsin** and the stomach acid itself act as catalysts in the process. Minor events are the digestion of some fat by a gastric lipase, the digestion of sucrose (to a very small extent) by the stomach acid, and the attachment of a protein carrier to vitamin B_{12}.

The stomach enzymes work most efficiently in the stomach's strong acid, but salivary amylase, which is swallowed with food, does not work in acid this strong. Consequently, the digestion of starch gradually ceases as the acid penetrates the bolus. In fact, salivary amylase becomes just another protein to be digested. The amino acids in amylase end up being absorbed and recycled into other body proteins.

DIGESTION IN THE SMALL AND LARGE INTESTINES

By the time food leaves the stomach, digestion of all three energy-yielding nutrients has begun, but the process gains momentum in the small intestine. There, the pancreas and the liver contribute additional digestive juices through the duct leading into the duodenum, and the small intestine adds **intestinal juice**. These juices contain digestive enzymes, bicarbonate, and bile.

Digestive Enzymes **Pancreatic juice** contributes enzymes that digest fats, proteins, and carbohydrates. Glands in the intestinal wall also secrete digestive enzymes. (Review the glossary of digestive glands and their secretions on p. 44 for details.)

Bicarbonate The pancreatic juice also contains sodium **bicarbonate**, which neutralizes the acidic chyme as it enters the small intestine. From this point on, the contents of the digestive tract are neutral or slightly alkaline. The enzymes of both the intestine and the pancreas work best in this environment.

Bile **Bile** is secreted continuously by the **liver** and is concentrated and stored in the gallbladder. The gallbladder squirts bile into the duodenum whenever fat arrives there. Bile is not an enzyme but an **emulsifier** that brings fats into suspension in water (see Figure 2-4 on p. 46). (✚) After the fats are emulsified, enzymes can work on them, and they can be absorbed. Thanks to all these secretions, all three energy-yielding nutrients are digested in the small intestine.

The Rate of Digestion The rate of digestion of the energy nutrients depends on the contents of the meal. If the meal is high in simple sugars, digestion proceeds fairly rapidly. On the other hand, if the meal is rich in fat, digestion is slower.

Protective Factors The intestines contain bacteria that produce a variety of vitamins, including biotin and vitamin K (although bacteria alone cannot meet the need for these vitamins). The GI bacteria also protect people from infections. Provided that the normal **intestinal flora** are thriving, infectious bacteria have a hard time getting established and launching an attack on the system. In addition, the small intestine and the entire GI tract manufacture and maintain a strong arsenal of defenses against foreign invaders. Several different types of defending cells are present there and confer specific immunity against intestinal diseases. (✚)

The Final Stage The story of how food is broken down into nutrients that can be absorbed is now nearly complete. The three energy-yielding nutrients—carbohydrate, fat, and protein—are disassembled to basic building blocks before they are absorbed. Most of the other nutrients—vitamins, minerals, and water—are absorbed as they are. Undigested residues, such as some fibers, are not absorbed but

✚ Mayonnaise, made from vinegar and oil, would separate as other vinegar-and-oil salad dressings do if food chemists did not blend in a third ingredient—an emulsifier. The emulsifier mixes well with the fatty oil and the watery vinegar. In the case of mayonnaise, the emulsifier is lecithin from egg yolks.

✚ Probiotics and intestinal health is the topic of Nutrition in Practice 18.

emulsifier: a substance that mixes with both fat and water and that disperses the fat in the water, forming an emulsion.

intestinal flora: the bacterial inhabitants of the GI tract. *flora* = plant growth

FIGURE
2-4 | Emulsification of Fat by Bile

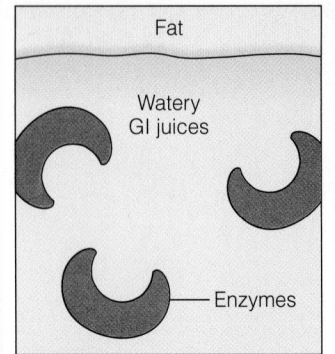

In the stomach, the fat and watery GI juices tend to separate. The enzymes are in the water and can't get at the fat.

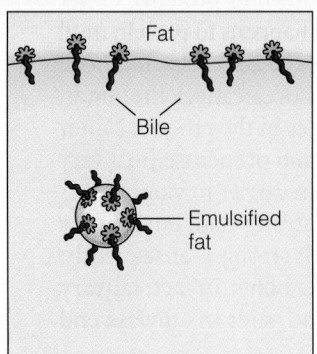

When fat enters the small intestine, the gallbladder secretes bile. Bile has an affinity for both fat and water, so it can bring the fat into the water.

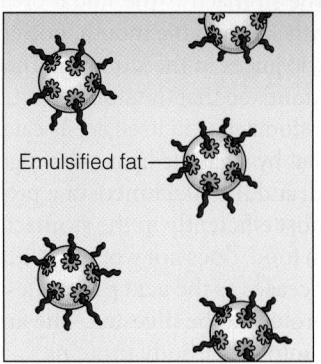

Bile's emulsifying action converts large fat globules into small droplets that repel each other.

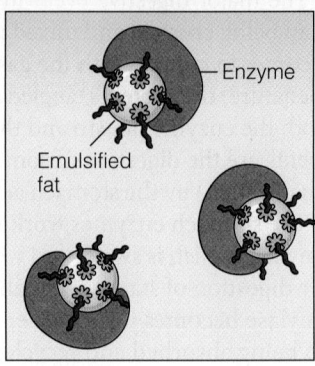

After emulsification, the enzymes have easy access to the fat droplets.

Like bile, detergents are emulsifiers and work the same way, which is why they are effective at removing grease spots from clothes. Molecule by molecule, the grease is dissolved out of the spot and suspended in water, where it can be rinsed away.

continue through the digestive tract as a semisolid mass that stimulates the tract's muscles, helping them remain strong and able to perform peristalsis efficiently. Fiber also retains water, keeping the stools soft, and carries some bile acids, sterols, and fat out of the body. Drinking plenty of water in conjunction with eating foods high in fiber supplies fluid for the fiber to take up. This is the basis for the recommendation to drink water and eat fiber-rich foods to relieve constipation.

The process of absorbing the nutrients into the body is discussed in the next section. For the moment, let us assume that the digested nutrients simply disappear from the GI tract as they are ready. Virtually all nutrients are gone by the time the contents of the GI tract reach the end of the small intestine. Little remains but water, a few salts and body secretions, and undigested materials such as fiber. These enter the large intestine (colon).

In the colon, intestinal bacteria degrade some of the fiber to simpler compounds. The colon itself retrieves from its contents the materials that the body is designed to recycle—water and dissolved salts. The waste that is finally excreted has little or nothing of value left in it. The body has extracted all that it can use from the food.

The Absorptive System

Within three or four hours after you have eaten a meal, your body must find a way to absorb millions of molecules one by one. The absorptive system is ingeniously designed to accomplish this task.

THE SMALL INTESTINE

Most absorption takes place in the small intestine. The small intestine is a tube about 10 feet long and about an inch across, yet it provides a surface comparable in area to a tennis court. When nutrient molecules make contact with this surface, they are absorbed and carried off to the liver and other parts of the body.

Villi and Microvilli How does the intestine manage to provide such a large absorptive surface area? Its inner surface looks smooth, but viewed through a microscope, it turns out to be wrinkled into hundreds of folds. Each fold is covered with thousands of fingerlike projections called **villi**. The villi are as numerous as the hairs on velvet fabric. A single villus, magnified still more, turns out to be composed of several hundred cells, each covered with microscopic hairs called **microvilli** (see Figure 2-5).

Review Notes

- To digest food, the salivary glands, stomach, pancreas, liver (via the gallbladder), and small intestine deliver fluids and digestive enzymes.

villi (VILL-ee or VILL-eye): fingerlike projections from the folds of the small intestine. The singular form is **villus**.
villus = shaggy hair

microvilli (MY-cro-VILL-ee or MY-cro-VILL-eye): tiny, hairlike projections on each cell of every villus that can trap nutrient particles and transport them into the cells. The singular form is **microvillus**.

FIGURE
2-5
The Small Intestinal Villi

Stomach

Small intestine

Folds with villi on them

A villus

Capillaries

Lymphatic vessel

The wall of the small intestine is wrinkled into thousands of folds and is carpeted with villi.

Muscle layers beneath folds

Between the villi are tubular glands that secrete enzyme-containing intestinal juice.

Artery

Vein

Lymphatic vessel

© D.W. Fawcet, The Cell, 2e

Microvilli

This is a photograph of part of an actual human intestinal cell with microvilli.

Three cells of a villus. Each cell is covered with microvilli.

Review Notes

- The many folds and villi of the small intestine dramatically increase its surface area, facilitating nutrient absorption.

- Nutrients pass through the cells of the villi and enter either the blood (if they are water soluble or small fat fragments) or the lymph (if they are fat soluble).

The villi are in constant motion. A thin sheet of muscle lines each villus so that it can wave, squirm, and wiggle like the tentacles of a sea anemone. Any nutrient molecule small enough to be absorbed is trapped among the microvilli and drawn into a cell beneath them. Some partially digested nutrients are caught in the microvilli, digested further by enzymes there, and then absorbed into the cells.

Specialization in the Intestinal Tract As you can see, the intestinal tract is beautifully designed to perform its functions. A further refinement of the system is that the cells of successive portions of the tract are specialized to absorb different nutrients. The nutrients that are ready for absorption early are absorbed near the top of the tract; those that take longer to be digested are absorbed farther down. The rate at which the nutrients travel through the GI tract is finely adjusted to maximize their availability to the appropriate absorptive segment of the tract when they are ready. The lowly "gut" turns out to be one of the most elegantly designed organ systems in the body.

The Myth of "Food Combining" Some popular fad diets advocate the idea that people should not eat certain food combinations (for example, fruit and meat) at the same meal, because the digestive system cannot handle more than one task at a time. This is a myth. The art of "food combining" (which actually emphasizes "food separating") is based on this idea, and it represents faulty logic and a gross underestimation of the body's capabilities. In fact, the opposite is often true: foods eaten together can enhance each other's use by the body. For example, vitamin C in a pineapple or citrus fruit can enhance the absorption of iron from a meal of chicken and rice or other iron-containing foods. Many other instances of mutually beneficial interactions are presented in later chapters.

ABSORPTION OF NUTRIENTS

Once a molecule has entered a cell in a villus, the next step is to transmit it to a destination elsewhere in the body by way of the body's two transport systems—the bloodstream and the **lymphatic system**. As Figure 2-5 shows, both systems supply vessels to each villus. Through these vessels, the nutrients leave the cell and enter either the **lymph** or the blood. In either case, the nutrients end up in the blood, at least for a while. The water-soluble nutrients (and the smaller products of fat digestion) are released directly into the bloodstream by way of the capillaries, but the larger fats and the fat-soluble vitamins find direct access into the capillaries impossible because these nutrients are insoluble in water (and blood is mostly water). They require some packaging before they are released.

The intestinal cells assemble the products of fat digestion into larger molecules called **triglycerides**. These triglycerides, fat-soluble vitamins (when present), and other large lipids (cholesterol and the phospholipids) are then packaged for transport. They cluster together with special proteins to form **chylomicrons**, one kind of **lipoproteins** (lipoproteins are described beginning on p. 50). Finally, the cells release the chylomicrons into the lymphatic system. They can then glide through the lymph spaces until they arrive at a point of entry into the bloodstream near the heart.

Transport of Nutrients

Once a nutrient has entered the bloodstream or the lymphatic system, it may be transported to any part of the body, from the tips of the toes to the roots of the hair, where it becomes available to any of the cells. The circulatory systems are arranged to deliver nutrients wherever they are needed.

THE VASCULAR SYSTEM

The vascular or blood circulatory system is a closed system of vessels through which blood flows continuously in a figure eight, with the heart serving as a pump at the crossover point. On each loop of the figure eight, blood travels a simple route: heart to arteries to capillaries to veins to heart.

The routing of the blood through the digestive system is different, however. The blood is carried to the digestive system (as it is to all organs) by way of an **artery**, which (as in all organs) branches into **capillaries** to reach every cell. Blood leaving the digestive system, however, goes by way of a **vein**. The **hepatic portal vein** directs blood not back to the heart but to another organ—the liver. This vein *again* branches into *capillaries* so that every cell of the liver has access to the newly absorbed nutrients that the blood is carrying. Blood leaving the liver then *again* collects into a vein, called the **hepatic vein**, which returns the blood to the heart. The route is thus heart to arteries to capillaries (in intestines) to hepatic portal vein to capillaries (in liver) to hepatic vein to heart. (✚)

An anatomist studying this system knows there must be a reason for this special arrangement. The liver is located in the circulation system at the point where it will have the first chance at the materials absorbed from the GI tract. In fact, the liver is the body's major metabolic organ (see Figure 2-6) and must prepare the absorbed nutrients for use by the rest of the body. Furthermore, the liver stands as a gatekeeper to waylay intruders that might otherwise harm the heart or brain. Chapter 19 offers more information about this noble organ.

THE LYMPHATIC SYSTEM

The lymphatic system is a one-way route for fluids to travel from tissue spaces into the blood. The lymphatic system has no pump; instead, lymph is squeezed from one portion of the body to another like water in a sponge, as muscles contract and create

✚ The artery that delivers oxygen-rich blood from the heart and lungs to the liver is the *hepatic artery*.

capillaries: small vessels that branch from an artery. Capillaries connect arteries to veins. Oxygen, nutrients, and waste materials are exchanged across capillary walls.

vein: a vessel that carries blood back to the heart.

hepatic portal vein: the vein that collects blood from the GI tract and conducts it to capillaries in the liver.
• *portal* = gateway

hepatic vein: the vein that collects blood from the liver capillaries and returns it to the heart.
• *hepatic* = liver

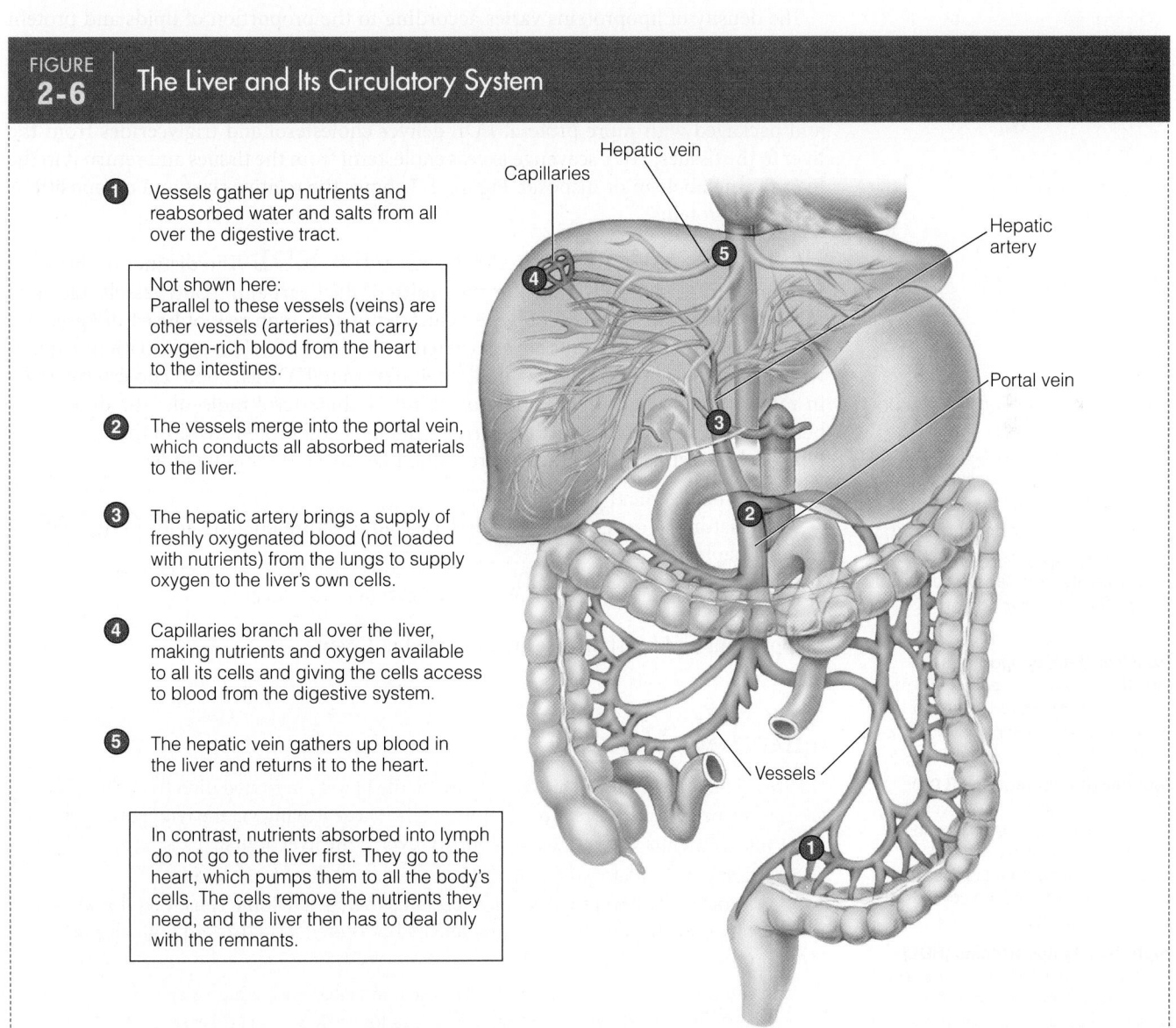

| FIGURE 2-6 | The Liver and Its Circulatory System |

❶ Vessels gather up nutrients and reabsorbed water and salts from all over the digestive tract.

Not shown here:
Parallel to these vessels (veins) are other vessels (arteries) that carry oxygen-rich blood from the heart to the intestines.

❷ The vessels merge into the portal vein, which conducts all absorbed materials to the liver.

❸ The hepatic artery brings a supply of freshly oxygenated blood (not loaded with nutrients) from the lungs to supply oxygen to the liver's own cells.

❹ Capillaries branch all over the liver, making nutrients and oxygen available to all its cells and giving the cells access to blood from the digestive system.

❺ The hepatic vein gathers up blood in the liver and returns it to the heart.

In contrast, nutrients absorbed into lymph do not go to the liver first. They go to the heart, which pumps them to all the body's cells. The cells remove the nutrients they need, and the liver then has to deal only with the remnants.

Hepatic vein

Capillaries

Hepatic artery

Portal vein

Vessels

pressure here and there. Ultimately, the lymph collects in a large duct behind the heart. This duct terminates in a vein that conducts the lymph into the heart. (✚) Thus, some materials from the GI tract enter the lymphatic system before entering the bloodstream.

TRANSPORT OF LIPIDS: LIPOPROTEINS

Within the circulatory system, lipids always travel from place to place bundled with protein, that is, as lipoproteins. When physicians measure a person's blood lipid profile, they are interested in both the types of fat present (such as triglycerides and cholesterol) and the types of lipoproteins that carry them.

VLDL, LDL, and HDL As mentioned earlier, chylomicrons transport newly absorbed (*diet-derived*) lipids from the intestinal cells to the rest of the body. As chylomicrons circulate through the body, cells remove their lipid contents, so the chylomicrons get smaller and smaller. The liver picks up these chylomicron remnants. When necessary, the liver can assemble different lipoproteins, which are known as **very-low-density lipoproteins (VLDL)**. As the body's cells remove triglycerides from the VLDL, the proportions of their lipid and protein contents shift. As this occurs, VLDL become cholesterol-rich **low-density lipoproteins (LDL)**. Cholesterol returning to the liver for metabolism or excretion from other parts of the body is packaged in lipoproteins known as **high-density lipoproteins (HDL)**. HDL are synthesized primarily in the liver.

The density of lipoproteins varies according to the proportion of lipids and protein they contain. The more lipids in the lipoprotein molecule, the lower the density; the more protein, the higher the density. Both LDL and HDL carry lipids around in the blood, but LDL are larger, lighter, and filled with more lipid; HDL are smaller, denser, and packaged with more protein. LDL deliver cholesterol and triglycerides from the liver to the tissues; HDL scavenge excess cholesterol from the tissues and return it to the liver for metabolism or disposal. Figure 2-7 shows the relative sizes and compositions of the lipoproteins.

Health Implications of LDL and HDL The distinction between LDL and HDL has implications for the health of the heart and blood vessels. Elevated LDL concentrations in the blood are associated with a high risk of heart disease, and elevated HDL concentrations are associated with a low risk.[2] These associations explain why some people refer to LDL as "bad" cholesterol and HDL as "good" cholesterol. Keep in mind, though, that there is only *one* kind of cholesterol molecule; the differences between LDL and HDL reflect *proportions* of lipids and proteins within them—not the type of cholesterol. Factors that improve the LDL-to-HDL ratio include:

- Weight management (see Chapter 7).
- Polyunsaturated or monounsaturated, instead of saturated, fatty acids in the diet (see Chapter 4).
- Soluble fibers (see Chapter 3).
- Physical activity.

Lipoproteins and heart disease are discussed in Chapter 21.

✚ The duct that conveys lymph toward the heart is the *thoracic* (thor-ASS-ic) *duct*. The *subclavian vein* connects this duct with the right upper chamber of the heart, providing a passageway by which lymph can be returned to the vascular system.

very-low-density lipoproteins (VLDL): the type of lipoproteins made primarily by liver cells to transport lipids to various tissues in the body; composed primarily of triglycerides.

low-density lipoproteins (LDL): the type of lipoproteins derived from VLDL as cells remove triglycerides from them. LDL carry cholesterol and triglycerides from the liver to the cells of the body and are composed primarily of cholesterol.

high-density lipoproteins (HDL): the type of lipoproteins that transport cholesterol back to the liver from peripheral cells; composed primarily of protein.

Review Notes

- Nutrients leaving the digestive system via the blood are routed directly to the liver before being transported to the body's cells. Those leaving via the lymphatic system eventually enter the vascular system but bypass the liver at first.
- Within the circulatory system, lipids travel bundled with proteins as lipoproteins. Different types of lipoproteins include chylomicrons, very-low-density lipoproteins (VLDL), low-density lipoproteins (LDL), and high-density lipoproteins (HDL).
- Elevated blood concentrations of LDL are associated with a high risk of heart disease. Elevated HDL are associated with a low risk of heart disease.

FIGURE
2-7 | The Lipoproteins

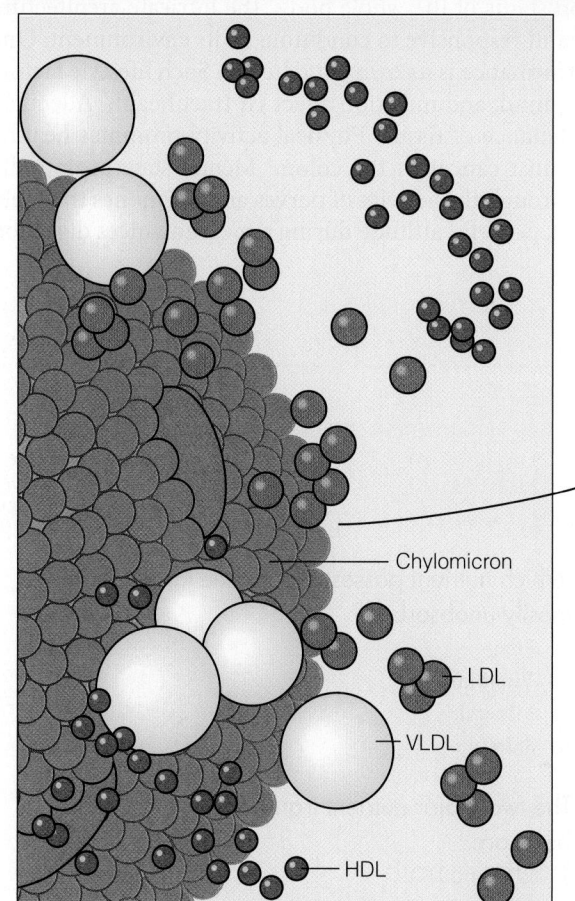

Phospholipid

Cholesterol

Triglyceride

Protein

A typical lipoprotein contains an interior of triglycerides and cholesterol surrounded by phospholipids. The phospholipids' fatty acid "tails" point toward the interior, where the lipids are. Proteins near the outer ends of the phospholipids cover the structure. This arrangement of hydrophobic molecules on the inside and hydrophilic molecules on the outside allows lipids to travel through the watery fluids of the blood.

Chylomicron

LDL

VLDL

HDL

This solar system of lipoproteins shows their relative sizes. Notice how large the fat-filled chylomicron is compared with the others and how the others get progressively smaller as their proportion of fat declines and protein increases.

Chylomicrons contain so little protein and so much triglyceride that they are the lowest in density.

Very-low-density lipoproteins (VLDL) are half triglycerides, accounting for their low density.

Low-density lipoproteins (LDL) are half cholesterol, accounting for their implication in heart disease.

High-density lipoproteins (HDL) are half protein, accounting for their high density.

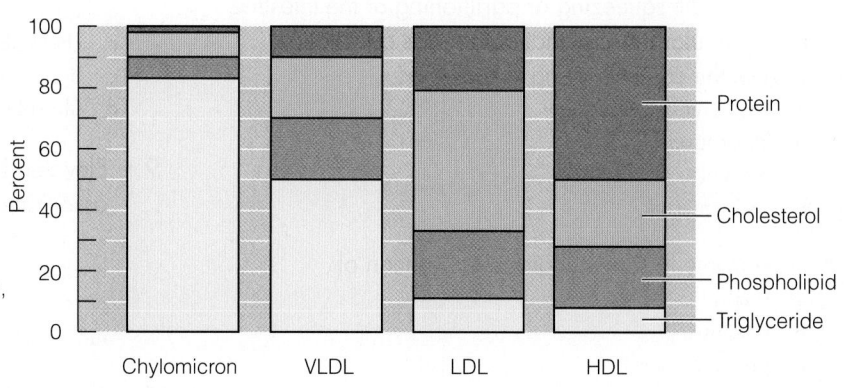

The System at Its Best

The GI tract is the first organ in the body to deal with the nutrients that will ultimately maintain the health and nutrition status of the whole body. The intricate architecture of the GI tract makes it sensitive and responsive to conditions in its environment. One condition indispensable to its performance is its own good health. Such lifestyle factors as sleep, physical activity, state of mind, and nutrition affect GI tract health. Adequate sleep allows for repair and maintenance of tissue. Physical activity promotes healthy muscle tone and may protect against cancer of the colon.[3] Mental state profoundly affects digestion and absorption through the activity of nerves and hormones that help regulate these processes. A relaxed, peaceful attitude during a meal enhances digestion and absorption.

Self Check

1 • Once food is swallowed, it travels through the digestive tract in this order:
   a. esophagus, stomach, large intestine, liver.
   b. esophagus, stomach, small intestine, large intestine.
   c. small intestine, stomach, esophagus, large intestine.
   d. small intestine, large intestine, stomach, esophagus.

2 • Once chyme travels the length of the small intestine, it passes through the ileocecal valve at the beginning of the:
   a. large intestine.
   b. stomach.
   c. esophagus.
   d. jejunum.

3 • The periodic squeezing or partitioning of the intestine by its circular muscles that both mixes and slowly pushes the contents along is known as:
   a. secretion.
   b. absorption.
   c. peristalsis.
   d. segmentation.

4 • An enzyme in saliva begins the digestion of:
   a. starch.
   b. vitamins.
   c. protein.
   d. minerals.

5 • Bile is:
   a. an enzyme that splits starch.
   b. an alkaline secretion of the pancreas.
   c. an emulsifier made by the liver that prepares fats and oils for digestion.
   d. a stomach secretion containing water, hydrochloric acid, and the enzymes pepsin and lipase.

6 • Which nutrient passes through the large intestine mostly unabsorbed?
   a. Fiber
   b. Vitamins
   c. Minerals
   d. Starch

7 • The two major nutrient transport systems in the body are:
   a. LDL and HDL.
   b. digestion and absorption.
   c. lipoproteins and chylomicrons.
   d. the vascular and lymphatic systems.

8 • Within the circulatory system, lipids always travel from place to place bundled with proteins as:
   a. microvilli.
   b. chylomicrons.
   c. lipoproteins.
   d. phospholipids.

9 • Elevated LDL concentrations in the blood are associated with:
   a. a high-protein diet.
   b. a low risk of diabetes.
   c. too much physical activity.
   d. a high risk of heart disease.

10 • Three factors that improve the LDL-to-HDL ratio include:
   a. polyunsaturated fat, rest, and dietary HDL.
   b. antioxidants, insoluble fibers, and dietary HDL.
   c. saturated fat, antioxidants, and insoluble fibers.
   d. weight control, soluble fibers, and physical activity.

Answers to these questions can be found in Appendix H.

Digestion and Absorption

Clinical Applications

1 ● People who experience malabsorption frequently have the most difficulty digesting fat. Considering the differences in fat, carbohydrate, and protein digestion and absorption, can you offer an explanation?

2 ● How might you explain the importance of dietary fiber to a client who frequently experiences constipation?

Nutrition on the Net

For further study of the topics in this chapter, access these websites.

- Find updates and quick links to these and other nutrition-related sites at our website: www.cengage.com/nutrition/whitney/nhhc4e
- Visit the Center for Digestive Health and Nutrition: www.gihealth.com

- Visit the Patient Information section of the American College of Gastroenterology: www.acg.gi.org

Notes

1. A. Stengel and Y. Taché, Neuroendocrine control of the gut during stress: Corticotropin-releasing factor signaling pathways in the spotlight, *Annual Review of Physiology* 71 (2009): 219–239; P. Holzer, Opioid receptors in the gastrointestinal tract, *Regulatory Peptides* 155 (2009): 11–17; J. López-Herce, Gastrointestinal complications in critically ill patients: What differs between adults and children? *Current Opinion in Clinical Nutrition and Metabolic Care* 12 (2009): 180–185; National Digestive Diseases Information Clearinghouse, *Irritable bowel syndrome*, NIH publication no. 07-693 (Bethesda, MD: National Institute of Diabetes and Digestive and Kidney Diseases, 2007).
2. A. K. Chhatriwalla and coauthors, Low levels of low-density lipoprotein cholesterol and blood pressure and progression of coronary atherosclerosis, *Journal of the American College of Cardiology* 53 (2009): 1110–1115;

A. H. Lichtenstein and coauthors, Diet and lifestyle recommendations revision 2006: A scientific statement from the American Heart Association Nutrition Committee, *Circulation* 114 (2006): 82–96; Expert Panel on Detection, Evaluation, and Treatment of High Blood Cholesterol in Adults (Adult Treatment Panel III), *Third Report of the National Cholesterol Education Program (NCEP)*, NIH publication no. 02-5215 (Bethesda, MD: National Heart, Lung, and Blood Institute, 2002) pp. II-1–II-61.
3. World Cancer Research Fund/American Institute for Cancer Research, *Food, Nutrition, Physical Activity, and the Prevention of Cancer: A Global Perspective* (Washington, D.C.: American Institute for Cancer Research, 2007), pp. 244–321.

NUTRITION IN PRACTICE

Food Safety

The Food and Drug Administration (FDA) lists **foodborne illness** as the leading food safety concern in the United States because episodes of food poisoning far outnumber episodes of any other kind of food contamination. The **CDC** estimates that 76 million people experience foodborne illness each year in the United States.[1] For some 5,000 people each year, the symptoms (Table NP2-1) can be so severe as to cause death. Most vulnerable are pregnant women; very young, very old, sick, or malnourished people; and those with a weakened immune system (as in AIDS). By taking the proper precautions, people can minimize their chances of contracting foodborne illnesses. The accompanying glossary defines related terms.

What is foodborne illness?

Foodborne illness can be caused by either an infection or an intoxication. Table NP2-2 summarizes the most common or severe foodborne illnesses, their food sources, general symptoms, and prevention methods.

What is the difference between foodborne infections and food intoxications?

Foodborne infections are caused by eating foods contaminated by infectious microbes. Two of the most common foodborne **pathogens** are *Campylobacter jejuni* and *Salmonella*, which enter the GI tract in contaminated foods such as undercooked poultry and unpasteurized milk.

TABLE NP2-1	Symptoms of Foodborne Illness

Get medical help when these symptoms occur:

- Bloody diarrhea
- Diarrhea lasting more than three days
- Prolonged vomiting that prevents keeping liquids down and can lead to dehydration
- Difficulty breathing
- Difficulty swallowing
- Double vision
- Fever lasting more than 24 hours
- Headache accompanied by muscle stiffness and fever
- Numbness, muscle weakness, and tingling sensations in the skin
- Rapid heart rate, fainting, and dizziness

Glossary

CDC (Centers for Disease control): a branch of the Department of Health and Human Services that is responsible for, among other things, monitoring foodborne diseases. *www.cdc.gov*

cross-contamination: the contamination of food by bacteria that occurs when the food comes into contact with surfaces previously touched by raw meat, poultry, or seafood.

foodborne illness: illness transmitted to human beings through food and water, caused by either an infectious agent (foodborne infection) or a poisonous substance (food intoxication); commonly known as **food poisoning**.

Hazard Analysis Critical Control Points (HACCP): a systematic plan to identify and correct potential microbial hazards in the manufacturing, distribution, and commercial use of food products; commonly referred to as "HASS-ip."

pasteurization: heat processing of food that inactivates some, but not all, microorganisms in the food; not a sterilization process. Bacteria that cause spoilage are still present.

pathogens (PATH-oh-jens): microorganisms capable of producing disease.

sushi: vinegar-flavored rice and seafood, typically wrapped in seaweed and stuffed with colorful vegetables. Some sushi is stuffed with raw fish; other varieties contain cooked seafood.

traveler's diarrhea: nausea, vomiting, and diarrhea caused by consuming food or water contaminated by any of several organisms, most commonly, *E. coli*, *Shigella*, *Campylobacter jejuni*, and *Salmonella*.

Disease and Organism that Causes It	Most Frequent Food Sources	Onset and General Symptoms	Prevention Methods [a]
Foodborne Infections			
Campylobacteriosis (KAM-pee-loh-BAK-ter-ee-OH-sis) *Campylobacter* bacterium	Raw and undercooked poultry, unpasteurized milk, contaminated water	Onset: 2 to 5 days. Diarrhea, vomiting, abdominal cramps, fever; sometimes bloody stools; lasts 2 to 10 days.	Cook foods thoroughly; use pasteurized milk; use sanitary food-handling methods.
Cryptosporidiosis (KRIP-toe-spo-rid-ee-OH-sis) *Crytosporidium parvum* parasite	Contaminated swimming or drinking water, even from treated sources; highly chlorine-resistant; contaminated raw produce and unpasteurized juices and ciders	Onset: 2 to 10 days. Diarrhea, stomach cramps, upset stomach, slight fever; symptoms may come and go for weeks or months.	Wash all raw vegetables and fruits before peeling; use pasteurized milk and juice; do not swallow drops of water while using pools, hot tubs, ponds, lakes, rivers, or streams for recreation.
Cyclosporiasis (sigh-clo-spore-EYE-uh-sis) *Cyclospora cayetanensis* parasite	Contaminated water, contaminated fresh produce	Onset: 1 to 14 days. Diarrhea, loss of appetite, weight loss, stomach cramps, nausea, vomiting, fatigue; symptoms may come and go for weeks or months.	Use treated, boiled, or bottled water; cook foods thoroughly; peel fruits.
***E. coli* infection** *Escherichia coli* [b] bacterium	Undercooked ground beef, unpasteurized milk and juices, raw fruits and vegetables, contaminated water, and person-to-person contact	Onset: 1 to 8 days. Severe bloody diarrhea, abdominal cramps, vomiting; lasts 5 to 10 days.	Cook ground beef thoroughly; use pasteurized milk; use sanitary food-handling methods; use treated, boiled, or bottled water.
Gastroenteritis[c] Norovirus	Person-to-person contact; raw foods, salads, sandwiches	Onset: 1 to 2 days. Vomiting; lasts 1 to 2 days.	Use sanitary food-handling methods.
Giardiasis (JYE-are-DYE-ah-sis) *Giardia intestinalis* parasite	Contaminated water; uncooked foods	Onset: 7 to 14 days. Diarrhea (but occasionally constipation), abdominal pain, gas.	Use sanitary food-handling methods; avoid raw fruits and vegetables where parasites are endemic; dispose of sewage properly.
Hepatitis (HEP-ah-TIE-tis) Hepatitis A virus	Undercooked or raw shellfish	Onset: 15 to 50 days (28 days average). Diarrhea, dark urine, fever, headache, nausea, abdominal pain, jaundice (yellowed skin and eyes from buildup of wastes); lasts 2 to 12 weeks.	Cook foods thoroughly.
Listeriosis (lis-TER-ee-OH-sis) *Listeria monocytogenes* bacterium	Unpasteurized milk; fresh soft cheeses; luncheon meats, hot dogs	Onset: 1 to 21 days. Fever, muscle aches; nausea, vomiting, blood poisoning, complications in pregnancy, and meningitis (stiff neck, severe headache, and fever).	Use sanitary food-handling methods; cook foods thoroughly; use pasteurized milk.

Perfringens (per-FRINGE-enz) food poisoning *Clostridium perfringens* bacterium	Meats and meat products stored at between 120°F and 130°F	Onset: 8 to 16 hours. Abdominal pain, diarrhea, nausea; lasts 1 to 2 days.	Use sanitary food-handling methods; use pasteurized milk; cook foods thoroughly; refrigerate foods promptly and properly.
Salmonellosis (sal-moh-neh-LOH-sis) *Salmonella* bacteria (>2300 types)	Raw or undercooked eggs, meats, poultry, raw milk and other dairy products, shrimp, frog legs, yeast, coconut, pasta, and chocolate	Onset: 1 to 3 days. Fever, vomiting, abdominal cramps, diarrhea; lasts 4 to 7 days; can be fatal.	Use sanitary food-handling methods; use pasteurized milk; cook foods thoroughly; refrigerate foods promptly and properly.
Shigellosis (shi-gel-LOH-sis) *Shigella* bacteria (>30 types)	Person-to-person contact, raw foods, salads, sandwiches, and contaminated water	Onset: 1 to 2 days. Bloody diarrhea, cramps, fever; lasts 4 to 7 days.	Use sanitary food-handling methods; cook foods thoroughly; use proper refrigeration.
Vibrio (VIB-ree-oh) infection *Vibrio vulnificus* [d] bacterium	Raw or undercooked seafood, contaminated water	Onset: 1 to 7 days. Diarrhea, abdominal cramps, nausea, vomiting; lasts 2 to 5 days; can be fatal.	Use sanitary food-handling methods; cook foods thoroughly.
Yersiniosis (yer-SIN-ee-OH-sis) *Yersinia enterocolitica* bacterium	Raw and undercooked pork, unpasteurized milk	Onset: 1 to 2 days. Diarrhea, vomiting, fever, abdominal pain; lasts 1 to 3 weeks.	Cook foods thoroughly; use pasteurized milk; use treated, boiled, or bottled water.

Food Intoxications

Botulism (BOT-chew-lizm) Botulinum toxin produced by *Clostridium botulinum* bacterium, which grows without oxygen, in low-acid foods, and at temperatures between 40°F and 120°F; the **botulinum** (BOT-chew-line-um) **toxin** responsible for botulism is called **botulin** (BOT-chew-lin).	Anaerobic environment of low acidity (canned corn, peppers, green beans, soups, beets, asparagus, mushrooms, ripe olives, spinach, tuna, chicken, chicken liver, liver pâté, luncheon meats, ham, sausage, stuffed eggplant, lobster, and smoked and salted fish)	Onset: 4 to 36 hours. Nervous system symptoms, including double vision, inability to swallow, speech difficulty, and progressive paralysis of the respiratory system; often fatal; leaves prolonged symptoms in survivors.	Use proper canning methods for low-acid foods; refrigerate homemade garlic and herb oils; avoid commercially prepared foods with leaky seals or with bent, bulging, or broken cans. Do not give infants honey because it may contain spores of *Clostridium botulinum*, which is a common source of infection for infants.
Staphylococcal (STAF-il-oh- KOK-al) **food poisoning** Staphylococcal toxin (produced by *Staphylococcus aureus* bacterium)	Toxin produced in improperly refrigerated meats; egg, tuna, potato, and macaroni salads; cream-filled pastries	Onset: 1 to 6 hours. Diarrhea, nausea, vomiting, abdominal cramps, fever; lasts 1 to 2 days.	Use sanitary food-handling methods; cook food thoroughly; refrigerate foods promptly and properly; use proper home-canning methods.

Note: Travelers' diarrhea is most commonly caused by *E. coli, Campylobacter jejuni, Shigella,* and *Salmonella.*

[a]Table NP2-3 on pp. 59-60 provides more details on the proper handling, cooking, and refrigeration of foods.

[b]The most serious strain is *E. coli* STEC O157.

[c]Gastroenteritis refers to an inflammation of the stomach and intestines but is the most common name used for illnesses caused by noroviruses.

[d]Most cases of *Vibrio vulnificus* infection occur in persons with underlying illness, particularly those with liver disorders, diabetes, cancer, and AIDS, and those who require long-term steroid use. The fatality rate is 50 percent for this population.

Symptoms generally include abdominal cramps, fever, vomiting, and diarrhea.

Norovirus, another leading cause of foodborne illness, illustrates the importance of personal hygiene.[2] Norovirus is passed in the stool and vomit of infected people. Thus, infected people who do not wash their hands adequately can pass the virus directly to other people, or they can pass it indirectly by way of contaminated food or water. Outbreaks in the United States are often linked to food touched by infected food handlers or to person-to-person contact in day care centers, nursing homes, and cruise ships.[3] People can also be infected with norovirus by eating raw shellfish such as oysters and clams that are grown in sewage-contaminated waters.

Food intoxications are caused by eating foods containing natural toxins or, more likely, microbes that produce toxins. The most common food toxin is produced by *Staphylococcus aureus;* it affects more than 1 million people each year. Less common, but more infamous, is *Clostridium botulinum,* an organism that produces a deadly toxin in anaerobic conditions such as improperly canned (especially home-canned) foods and homemade garlic or herb-flavored oils stored at room temperature. Botulism paralyzes muscles; consequently, seeing, speaking, swallowing, and breathing become difficult. Because death can occur within 24 hours of onset, botulism demands immediate medical attention. Even then, survivors may suffer the effects for months or years.

How do people get foodborne illness?

Transmission of foodborne illness has changed as our food supply and lifestyles have changed.[4] In the past, foodborne illness was caused by one person's error in a small setting, such as improperly refrigerated egg salad at a family picnic, and affected only a few victims. Today, we are eating more foods prepared and packaged by others. Consequently, when a food manufacturer or restaurant chef makes an error, foodborne illness can become epidemic. An estimated 80 percent of reported foodborne illnesses are caused by errors in a commercial setting, such as the improper **pasteurization** of milk at a large dairy.

In the early 2000s, a national food company had to recall more than 4 million pounds of poultry products after *Listeria* poisoning killed 7 people and made more than 50 others sick. In the 2006 *E. coli* outbreak from fresh spinach, nearly 200 people became sick, and two elderly women and a two-year-old boy died before consumers got the FDA message not to eat fresh spinach. In 2009, *Salmonella* was found in peanut butter that had been used in more than 2100 products made by more than 200 companies. These incidents and others focus the national spotlight on two important safety issues: disease-causing organisms are commonly found in foods, and safe food-handling practices can minimize harm from most of these foodborne pathogens.

What kinds of programs are in place to help keep foods safe?

To make our food supply safe for consumers, the U.S. Department of Agriculture (USDA), the FDA, and the food-processing industries have developed and implemented programs to control foodborne illness.* The **Hazard Analysis Critical Control Points (HACCP)** system requires food manufacturers to identify points of contamination and implement controls to prevent foodborne disease. For example, after tracing two large outbreaks of salmonellosis to imported cantaloupe, producers began using chlorinated water to wash the melons and to make ice for packing and shipping. Safety procedures such as this prevent hundreds of thousands of foodborne illnesses each year and are responsible for the decline in infections over the past decade.[5]

This example raises another issue regarding the safety of imported foods. Because FDA inspectors cannot keep pace with the increasing numbers of imported foods, the FDA is working with other countries to help them adopt the safe food-handling practices used in the United States.

Are foods bought in grocery stores and foods eaten in restaurants safe?

Canned and packaged foods sold in grocery stores are easily controlled, but rare accidents do happen. Batch numbering makes it possible to recall contaminated foods through public announcements via newspapers, television, and radio. In the grocery store, consumers can buy items before the "sell by" date and inspect the safety seals and wrappers of packages. A broken seal, bulging can lid, or mangled package fails to protect the consumer against microbes, insects, spoilage, or even vandalism.

State and local health regulations provide guidelines on the cleanliness of facilities and the safe preparation of foods for restaurants, cafeterias, and fast-food establishments. Even so, consumers can also take these actions to help prevent foodborne illnesses when dining out:

- Wash hands with hot, soapy water before meals.
- Expect clean tabletops, dinnerware, utensils, and food preparation areas.
- Expect cooked foods to be served piping hot and salads to be fresh and cold.
- Refrigerate take-home items within two hours.

Improper handling of foods can occur anywhere along the line from commercial manufacturers to large supermarkets to small restaurants to private homes. Maintaining a safe food supply requires everyone's efforts.

---

*In addition to HACCP, other programs initiated under the Food Safety Initiative include FoodNet, PulseNet, the Environmental Health specialists Network (EHS-Net), and Fight BAC!

What can people do to protect themselves from foodborne illness?

Whether microbes multiply and cause illness depends, in part, on a few key food-handling behaviors in the kitchen—whether the kitchen is in your home, a school cafeteria, a gourmet restaurant, or a canned goods manufacturer. Figure NP2-1 summarizes the four simple things that can help most to prevent foodborne illness:

- *Keep a clean, safe kitchen.* Wash countertops, cutting boards, hands, sponges, and utensils in hot, soapy water before and after each step of food preparation.

- *Avoid cross-contamination.* Keep raw eggs, meat, poultry, and seafood separate from other foods. Wash all utensils and surfaces (such as cutting boards or platters) that have been in contact with these foods with hot, soapy water before using them again. Bacteria inevitably left on the surfaces from the raw meat can recontaminate the cooked meat or other foods—a problem known as **cross-contamination.** Washing raw eggs, meat, and poultry is not recommended as the extra handling increases the risk of cross-contamination.

- *Keep hot foods hot.* Cook foods long enough to reach internal temperatures that will kill microbes, and maintain adequate temperatures to prevent bacterial growth until the foods are served.

- *Keep cold foods cold.* Go directly home upon leaving the grocery store and immediately unpack foods into the refrigerator or freezer upon arrival. After a meal, refrigerate any leftovers immediately.

Unfortunately, consumers commonly fail to follow these simple food-handling recommendations. See Table NP2-3 for additional food safety tips.

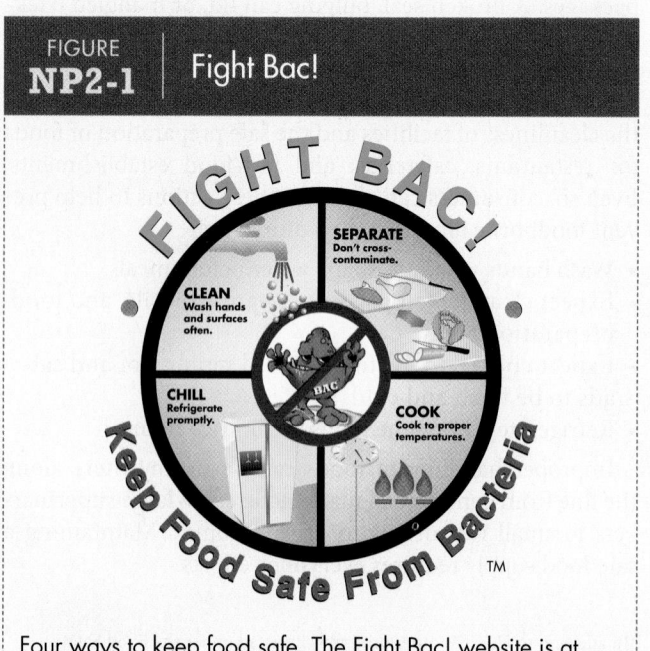

FIGURE NP2-1 | Fight Bac!

Four ways to keep food safe. The Fight Bac! website is at www.fightbac.org.

Wash your hands with warm water and soap before preparing or eating food to reduce the chance of microbial contamination.

What precautions need to be taken when preparing meat and poultry?

Figure NP2-2 (p. 61) presents label instructions for the safe handling of meat and poultry and two types of USDA seals. Meats and poultry contain bacteria and provide a moist, nutrient-rich environment that favors microbial growth. Ground meat is especially susceptible because it receives more handling than other kinds of meat and has more surface exposed to bacterial contamination. Consumers cannot detect the harmful bacteria in or on meat. For safety's sake, cook meat thoroughly, using a thermometer to test the internal temperature (see Figure NP2-3 on p. 61).

How can a person enjoy seafood safely?

Most seafood available in the United States and Canada is safe, but eating it undercooked or raw can cause severe illnesses—hepatitis, worms, parasites, viral intestinal disorders, and other diseases.[†] Rumor has it that freezing fish will make it safe to eat raw, but this is only partly true. Commercial freezing will kill mature parasitic worms, but only cooking can kill all worm eggs and other microorganisms that can cause illness. For safety's sake, all seafood should be cooked until it is opaque. Even **sushi** can be safe to eat when chefs combine cooked seafood and other ingredients into delicacies.

[†]Diseases caused by toxins from the sea include ciguatera poisoning, scombroid poisoning, and paralytic and neurotoxic shellfish poisoning.

Most foodborne illnesses can be prevented by following four simple rules: keep a clean kitchen, avoid cross-contamination, keep hot foods hot, and keep cold foods cold.

Keep a Clean Kitchen

- Wash fruits and vegetables in a clean sink with a scrub brush and warm water; store washed and unwashed produce separately.
- Use hot, soapy water to wash hands, utensils, dishes, nonporous cutting boards, and countertops before handling food and between tasks when working with different foods. Use a bleach solution on cutting boards (one capful per gallon of water).
- Cover cuts with clean bandages before food preparation; dirty bandages carry harmful microorganisms.
- Mix foods with utensils, not hands; keep hands and utensils away from mouth, nose, and hair.
- Anyone may be a carrier of bacteria and should avoid coughing or sneezing over food. A person with a skin infection or infectious disease should not prepare food.
- Wash or replace sponges and towels regularly.
- Clean up food spills and crumb-filled crevices.

Avoid Cross-Contamination

- Wash all surfaces that have been in contact with raw meats, poultry, eggs, fish, and shellfish before reusing.
- Serve cooked foods on a clean plate with a clean utensil. Separate raw foods from those that have been cooked.
- Don't use marinade that was in contact with raw meat for basting or sauces.

Keep Hot Foods Hot

- When cooking meats or poultry, use a thermometer to test the internal temperature. Insert the thermometer between the thigh and the body of a turkey or into the thickest part of other meats, making sure the tip of the thermometer is not in contact with bone or the pan. Cook to the temperature indicated for that particular meat (see Figure NP2-3 on p. 61); cook hamburgers to at least medium well done. If you have safety questions, call the USDA Meat and Poultry Hotline: (800) 535-4555.
- Cook stuffing separately, or stuff poultry just prior to cooking.
- Do not cook large cuts of meat or turkey in a microwave oven; it leaves some parts undercooked while overcooking others.
- Cook eggs before eating them (soft-boiled for at least 3 1/2 minutes; scrambled until set, not runny; fried for at least 3 minutes on one side and 1 minute on the other).
- Cook seafood thoroughly. If you have safety questions about seafood, call the FDA hotline: (800) FDA-4010.
- When serving foods, maintain temperatures at 140°F or higher.
- Heat leftovers thoroughly to at least 165°F.

Keep Cold Foods Cold

- When running errands, stop at the grocery store last. When you get home, refrigerate the perishable groceries (such as meats and dairy products) immediately. Do not leave perishables in the car any longer than it takes for ice cream to melt.
- Put packages of raw meat, fish, or poultry on a plate before refrigerating to prevent juices from dripping on food stored below.
- Buy only foods that are solidly frozen in store freezers.
- Keep cold foods at 40°F or less; keep frozen foods at 0°F or less (keep a thermometer in the refrigerator).
- Marinate meats in the refrigerator, not on the counter.
- Look for "Keep Refrigerated" or "Refrigerate after Opening" on food labels.
- Refrigerate leftovers promptly; use shallow containers to cool foods faster; use leftovers within three to four days.
- Thaw meats or poultry in the refrigerator, not at room temperature. If you must hasten thawing, use cool water (changed every 30 minutes) or a microwave oven.
- Freeze meat, fish, or poultry immediately if not planning to use within a few days.

In General

- Do not reuse disposable containers; use nondisposable containers or recycle instead.

- Do not taste food that is suspect. "If in doubt, throw it out."

- Throw out foods with danger-signaling odors. Be aware, though, that most food-poisoning bacteria are odorless, colorless, and tasteless.

- Do not buy or use items that have broken seals or mangled packaging; such containers cannot protect against microbes, insects, spoilage, or even vandalism. Check safety seals, buttons, and expiration dates.

- Follow label instructions for storing and preparing packaged and frozen foods; throw out foods that have been thawed or refrozen.

- Discard foods that are discolored, moldy, or decayed or that have been contaminated by insects or rodents.

For Specific Food Items

- *Canned goods.* Carefully discard food from cans that leak or bulge so that other people and animals will not accidentally ingest it; before canning, seek professional advice from the USDA Extension Service (check your phone book under U.S. government listings, or go online: www.crees.usda.gov.)

- *Milk and cheeses.* Use only pasteurized milk and milk products. Aged cheeses, such as cheddar and Swiss, do well for an hour or two without refrigeration, but they should be refrigerated or stored in an ice chest for longer periods.

- *Eggs.* Use clean eggs with intact shells. Do not eat eggs, even pasteurized eggs, raw; raw eggs are commonly found in Caesar salad dressing, eggnog, cookie dough, hollandaise sauce, and key lime pie. Cook eggs until whites are firmly set and yolks begin to thicken.

- *Honey.* Honey may contain dormant bacterial spores, which can awaken in the human body to produce botulism. In adults, this poses little hazard, but infants younger than 1 year should never be fed honey. Honey can accumulate enough toxin to kill an infant; it has been implicated in several cases of sudden infant death. (Honey can also be contaminated with environmental pollutants picked up by the bees.)

- *Mayonnaise.* Commercial mayonnaise may actually help a food to resist spoilage because of the acid content. Still, keep it refrigerated after opening.

- *Mixed salads.* Mixed salads of chopped ingredients spoil easily because they have extensive surface area for bacteria to invade, and they have been in contact with cutting boards, hands, and kitchen utensils that easily transmit bacteria to food (regardless of their mayonnaise content). Chill them well before, during, and after serving.

- *Picnic foods.* Choose foods that last without refrigeration, such as fresh fruits and vegetables, breads and crackers, and canned spreads and cheeses that can be opened and used immediately. Pack foods cold, layer ice between foods, and keep foods out of water.

- *Seafood.* Buy only fresh seafood that has been properly refrigerated or iced. Cooked seafood should be stored separately from raw seafood to avoid cross-contamination.

Cook hamburgers to 160°F; color alone cannot determine doneness. Some burgers will turn brown before reaching 160°F, while others may retain some pink color, even when cooked to 175°F.

Eating raw oysters can be dangerous for anyone, but people with liver disease and weakened immune systems are most vulnerable. At least 10 species of bacteria found in raw oysters can cause serious illness and even death.[‡] Raw oysters may also carry the hepatitis A virus, which can cause liver disease. Some hot sauces can kill many of these bacteria but not the virus; alcohol may also protect some people against some oyster-borne illnesses but not enough to guarantee protection (or to recommend drinking alcohol). Pasteurization of raw oysters—holding them at a specified temperature for a specified time—holds promise for killing bacteria without cooking the oyster or altering its texture or flavor.

As population density increases along the shores of seafood-harvesting waters, pollution inevitably invades the sea life there. Preventing seafood-borne illness is in large part a task of controlling water pollution. To help ensure a safe seafood market, the FDA requires processors to adopt

[‡]Raw oysters can carry the bacterium *Vibrio vulnificus*; see Table NP2-2 for details.

The voluntary "Graded by USDA" seal indicates that the product has been graded for tenderness, juiciness, and flavor. Beef is graded Prime (abundant marbling of the meat muscle), Choice (less marbling), and Select (lean). Similarly, poultry is graded A, B, and C.

The mandatory "Inspected and Passed by the USDA" seal ensures that meat and poultry products are safe, wholesome, and correctly labeled. Inspection does not guarantee that the meat is free of potentially harmful bacteria.

Safe Handling Instructions

THIS PRODUCT WAS PREPARED FROM INSPECTED AND PASSED MEAT AND/OR POULTRY. SOME FOOD PRODUCTS MAY CONTAIN BACTERIA THAT CAN CAUSE ILLNESS IF THE PRODUCT IS MISHANDLED OR COOKED IMPROPERLY. FOR YOUR PROTECTION, FOLLOW THESE SAFE HANDLING INSTRUCTIONS.

KEEP REFRIGERATED OR FROZEN.
THAW IN REFRIGERATOR OR MICROWAVE.

KEEP RAW MEAT AND POULTRY SEPARATE FROM OTHER FOODS. WASH WORKING SURFACES (INCLUDING CUTTING BOARDS), UTENSILS, AND HANDS AFTER TOUCHING RAW MEAT OR POULTRY.

COOK THOROUGHLY.

KEEP HOT FOODS HOT. REFRIGERATE LEFTOVERS IMMEDIATELY OR DISCARD.

The USDA requires that safe handling instructions appear on all packages of meat and poultry.

Inspection is mandatory; grading is voluntary. Neither guarantees that the product will not cause foodborne illnesses, but consumers can help to prevent foodborne illnesses by following the safe handling instructions.

170° — Well-done meats
165° — Stuffing, poultry; reheat leftovers
160° — Medium-done meats, raw eggs, egg dishes, pork, ground meats
145° — Medium-rare beef steaks, roasts, veal, lamb
140° — Hold hot foods
DANGER ZONE: Do not keep foods between 40°F and 140°F for more than 2 hours or for more than 1 hour when the air temperature is greater than 90°F.
40° — Refrigerator temperatures
0° — Freezer temperatures

Bacteria multiply rapidly at temperatures between 40°F and 140°F. Cook foods to the temperatures shown on this thermometer and hold them at 140°F or higher.

food safety practices based on the HACCP system mentioned earlier.

Chemical pollution and microbial contamination lurk not only in the water but also in the boats and warehouses where seafood is cleaned, prepared, and refrigerated. Seafood is one of the most perishable foods: time and temperature are critical to its freshness and flavor. To keep seafood as fresh as possible, people in the industry "keep it cold, keep it clean, and keep it moving." Wise consumers eat it cooked.

Do foods that are unsafe to eat smell bad?

Fresh food generally smells fresh. Not all types of food poisoning are detectable by odor, but some bacterial wastes produce "off" odors. If an abnormal odor exists, the food is spoiled. Throw it out or, if it was recently purchased, return it to the grocery store. Do not taste it. Table NP2-4 (p. 62) lists safe refrigerator storage times for selected foods.

Local health departments and the USDA Extension Service can provide additional information about food safety. Should precautions fail and mild foodborne illness develop, drink clear liquids to replace fluids lost through vomiting and diarrhea. If serious foodborne

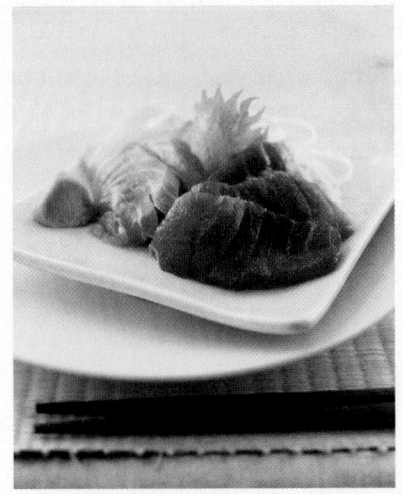

Eating raw seafood is a risky proposition.

TABLE NP2-4	Safe Refrigerator Storage Times (≤40°F)

One to Two Days

Raw ground meats, breakfast or other raw sausages, raw fish or poultry; gravies

Three to Five Days

Raw steaks, roasts, or chops; cooked meats, poultry, vegetables, and mixed dishes; lunchmeats (packages opened); mayonnaise salads (chicken, egg, pasta, tuna)

One Week

Hard-cooked eggs, bacon or hot dogs (opened packages); smoked sausages or seafood

Two to Four Weeks

Raw eggs (in shells); lunchmeats, bacon, or hot dogs (packages unopened); dry sausages (pepperoni, hard salami); most aged and processed cheeses (Swiss, brick)

Two Months

Mayonnaise (opened jar); most dry cheeses (Parmesan, Romano)

illness is suspected, first call a physician. Then wrap the remainder of the suspected food and label the container so that the food cannot be mistakenly eaten, place it in the refrigerator, and hold it for possible inspection by health authorities.

How can a person defend against foodborne illness when traveling to foreign countries?

People who travel to other countries have an estimated 40 percent chance of contracting a foodborne illness, commonly described as **travelers' diarrhea**.[6] Like many other foodborne illnesses, travelers' diarrhea is a sometimes serious, always annoying bacterial infection of the digestive tract. The risk is high because some countries' cleanliness standards for food and water may be lower than those in the United States and Canada. Also, every region's microbes are different, and while people are immune to those in their own neighborhoods, they have had no chance to develop immunity to the pathogens in places they are visiting for the first time. In addition to the food safety tips outlined on pp. 59–60, precautions while traveling include:

- Wash hands frequently with soap and hot water, especially before handling food or eating. Use antiseptic gel or hand wipes regularly.
- Eat only well-cooked and hot or canned foods. Eat raw fruits or vegetables only if washed in purified water and peeled with clean hands.
- Use purified, bottled water for drinking, making ice cubes, and brushing teeth. Alternatively, use disinfecting tablets or boil water.
- Refuse dairy products that have not been pasteurized and refrigerated properly.
- Travel with antidiarrheal medication in case efforts to avoid illness fail.

To sum up these recommendations, "Boil it, cook it, peel it, or forget it."

Notes

1. Position of the American Dietetic Association: Food and water safety, *Journal of the American Dietetic Association* 109 (2009): 1449–1460; Centers for Disease Control and Prevention, *FoodNet Surveillance Report for 2004*, June 2006.
2. Centers for Disease Control and Prevention, Surveillance for foodborne disease outbreaks—United States, 2006, *Morbidity and Mortality Weekly Report* 58 (2009): 609–614.
3. L. Verhoef and coauthors, Emergence of new norovirus variants on spring cruise ships and prediction of winter epidemics, *Emerging Infectious Diseases* 14 (2008): 238–243.
4. Position of the American Dietetic Association, 2009.
5. Centers for Disease Control and Prevention, *FoodNet Surveillance Report for 2004*, June 2006.
6. H. L. Koo and H. L. DuPont, Current and future developments in travelers' diarrhea therapy, *Expert Review of Anti-Infective Therapy* 4 (2006): 417–427.

CHAPTER 3 | # Carbohydrates

© photocuisine/Corbis

CONTENTS

Grains, vegetables, legumes, fruits, and milk offer ample carbohydrate.

© Polara Studios, Inc.

➕ Chapter 4 describes the roles of fats in health and disease.

➕ Diabetes, a disorder characterized by elevated blood glucose, is the topic of Chapter 20.

carbohydrates: energy nutrients composed of monosaccharides.
carbo = carbon
hydrate = water

monosaccharides (mon-oh-SACK-uh-rides): single sugar units.
mono = one
saccharide = sugar

disaccharides (dye-SACK-uh-rides): a pair of sugar units bonded together.
di = two

polysaccharides: long chains of monosaccharide units arranged as starch, glycogen, or fiber.
poly = many

glucose: a monosaccharide, the sugar common to all disaccharides and polysaccharides; also called *blood sugar* or *dextrose.*

fructose: a monosaccharide; sometimes known as *fruit sugar*. It is abundant in fruits, honey, and saps.
fruct = fruit

galactose: a monosaccharide; part of the disaccharide lactose.

homeostasis (HOME-ee-oh-STAY-sis): the maintenance of constant internal conditions (such as chemistry, temperature, and blood pressure) by the body's control system.
homeo = the same
stasis = staying

insulin: a hormone secreted by the pancreas in response to high blood glucose. It promotes cellular glucose uptake for use or storage.

MOST PEOPLE WOULD LIKE TO FEEL GOOD ALL THE TIME. PART OF THE secret of feeling good is replenishing the body's energy supply with food. That means choosing foods that contain the energy nutrients—carbohydrate and fat, primarily. But which to choose?

Carbohydrate is the preferred energy source for many of the body's functions. As long as carbohydrate is available, the human brain depends exclusively on it as an energy source. Athletes eat a "high-carb" diet to store as much muscle fuel as possible, and dietary recommendations urge people to eat carbohydrate-rich foods for better health. Many people, however, mistakenly think of carbohydrate-rich foods as "fattening" and avoid them. In truth, people who wish to lose fat and to maintain lean tissue and the health of the body can best do so by being physically active, paying close attention to portion sizes, and designing a diet based on foods that supply carbohydrate in balance with other energy nutrients.[1] Most unrefined plant foods—grains, vegetables, legumes, and fruits—provide ample carbohydrate and fiber with little or no fat. Milk is the only animal-derived food that contains significant amounts of carbohydrate.

Carbohydrate shares its fuel-providing responsibility with fat. Fat, however, normally is not used as fuel by the brain and central nervous system, and diets high in certain types of fat are associated with chronic diseases. (➕) The other energy sources available to the body—protein and alcohol—offer no advantage as fuels. Protein is best left to serve its own diverse functions, as discussed in Chapter 5. Alcohol, of course, has well-known undesirable side effects when used in excess. Alcohol and its relationships with health and disease are the subject of Nutrition in Practice 19.

The Chemist's View of Carbohydrates

The dietary **carbohydrates** include the sugars and starch and fiber.[2] Chemists describe the sugars as:

- **Monosaccharides** (single sugars).
- **Disaccharides** (double sugars).

Starch and fiber are:*

- **Polysaccharides**—compounds composed of chains of monosaccharide units.

All of these carbohydrates are composed of the single sugar **glucose** and other compounds that are much like glucose in composition and structure. Figure 3-1 shows the chemical structure of glucose.

MONOSACCHARIDES

Three monosaccharides are important in nutrition: glucose, **fructose,** and **galactose.** All three monosaccharides have the same number and kinds of atoms but in different arrangements.

Glucose Most cells depend on glucose for their fuel to some extent, and the cells of the brain and the rest of the nervous system depend almost exclusively on glucose for their energy. The body can obtain this glucose from carbohydrates. To function optimally, the body must maintain blood glucose within limits that allow the cells to nourish themselves. If blood glucose falls below normal, the person may become dizzy and weak; if it rises substantially above normal, the person may become fatigued. (➕) Left untreated, fluctuations to the extremes—either high or low—can be fatal. Blood glucose **homeostasis** is regulated primarily by two hormones: **insulin,** which moves glucose from the blood into the cells, and **glucagon,** which brings glucose out of storage when blood glucose falls (as occurs between meals).

---

*Monosaccharides and disaccharides (sugars) are sometimes called *simple carbohydrates,* and the polysaccharides (starch and fiber) are sometimes called *complex carbohydrates.*

Fructose Fructose is the sweetest of the sugars. Fructose occurs naturally in fruits, honey, and saps. Other sources include soft drinks, ready-to-eat cereals, and other products sweetened with high-fructose corn syrup. Glucose and fructose are the most common monosaccharides in nature.

Galactose The third single sugar, galactose, occurs mostly as part of lactose, a disaccharide also known as milk sugar. During digestion, galactose is freed as a single sugar.

DISACCHARIDES

In disaccharides, pairs of single sugars are linked together. Three disaccharides are important in nutrition: maltose, sucrose, and lactose. All three have glucose as one of their single sugars. As Table 3-1 shows, the other monosaccharide is either another glucose (in maltose), fructose (in sucrose), or galactose (in lactose). The shapes of the sugars in Table 3-1 reflect their chemical structures as drawn on paper.

Sucrose **Sucrose** (table, or white, sugar) is the most familiar of the three disaccharides and is what people mean when they speak of "sugar." This sugar is usually obtained by refining the juice from sugar beets or sugarcane to provide the brown, white, and powdered sugars available in the supermarket, but it occurs naturally in many fruits and vegetables.

When a person eats a food containing sucrose, enzymes in the digestive tract split the sucrose into its glucose and fructose components. Because the body can convert fructose to glucose, one molecule of sucrose can ultimately yield two molecules of glucose.

Lactose **Lactose** is the principal carbohydrate of milk. Most human infants are born with the digestive enzymes necessary to split lactose into its two monosaccharide parts, glucose and galactose, so as to absorb it. Breast milk thus provides a simple, easily digested carbohydrate that meets an infant's energy needs; many formulas do, too, because they are made from milk.(✚)

Maltose The third disaccharide, **maltose**, is a plant sugar that consists of two glucose units. Maltose is produced whenever starch breaks down—as happens in plants when they break down their stored starch for energy and start to sprout and in human beings during carbohydrate digestion.

POLYSACCHARIDES

Unlike the sugars, which contain the three monosaccharides—glucose, fructose, and galactose—in different combinations, the polysaccharides are composed almost entirely of glucose (and, in some cases, other monosaccharides). Three types of polysaccharides are important in nutrition: glycogen, starch, and fibers.

Glycogen is a storage form of energy for human beings and animals; starch plays that role in plants; and fibers provide structure in stems, trunks, roots, leaves, and skins of plants. Both glycogen and starch are built of entirely glucose units; fibers are composed of a variety of monosaccharides and other carbohydrate derivatives.

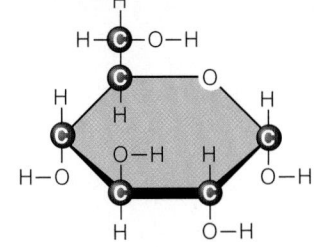

FIGURE 3-1 | Chemical Structure of Glucose

On paper, the structure of glucose has to be drawn flat, but in nature the five carbons and oxygen are roughly in a plane, with the H, OH, and CH2OH extending out above and below it.

✚ Many people lose the ability to digest lactose after infancy. This condition, known as lactose intolerance, is discussed in Chapter 18.

glucagon (GLOO-ka-gon): a hormone that is secreted by special cells in the pancreas in response to low blood glucose concentration and elicits release of glucose from storage.

sucrose: a disaccharide composed of glucose and fructose; commonly known as *table sugar*, *beet sugar*, or *cane sugar*.
sucro = sugar

lactose: a disaccharide composed of glucose and galactose; commonly known as *milk sugar*.
lact = milk

maltose: a disaccharide composed of two glucose units; sometimes known as *malt sugar*.

TABLE 3-1	The Major Sugars		
Monosaccharides		**Disaccharides**	
Glucose	⬡	Sucrose (glucose + fructose)	⬡⬡
Fructose	⬠	Lactose (glucose + galactose)	⬡⬡
Galactose	⬡ (found only as part of lactose)	Maltose (glucose + glucose)	⬡⬡

Glycogen

Glycogen molecules, which are also made of chains of glucose, are more highly branched than starch molecules. Glycogen is found in meats only to a limited extent and not at all in plants. *For this reason, glycogen is not a significant food source of carbohydrate, but it does play an important role in the body. The human body stores much of its glucose as glycogen in the liver and muscles.

After a meal, as blood glucose rises, the pancreas is the first organ to respond. It releases the hormone insulin, which signals the body's tissues to take up surplus glucose. Muscle and liver cells use some of this excess glucose to build glycogen. The muscles hoard two-thirds of the body's total glycogen and use it just for themselves during physical activity. The brain stores a tiny fraction of the total, thought to provide an emergency glucose reserve sufficient to fuel the brain for an hour or two in severe glucose deprivation.[3] The liver stores the remainder and is generous with its glycogen, making it available as blood glucose for the brain or other tissues when the supply runs low.

Starch

Starch is a long, straight, or branched chain of hundreds or thousands of glucose units linked together. These giant molecules are packed side by side in grains such as rice or wheat, in root crops and tubers such as yams and potatoes, and in legumes such as peas and beans. When a person eats the plant, the body splits the starch into glucose units (✚) and uses the glucose for energy.

All starchy foods come from plants. Grains are the richest food source of starch. In most human societies, people depend on a staple grain for much of their food energy: rice in Asia; wheat in Canada, the United States, and Europe; corn in much of Central and South America; and millet, rye, barley, and oats elsewhere. A second important source of starch is the legume (bean and pea) family. Legumes include peanuts and "dry" beans such as butter beans, kidney beans, "baked" beans, black-eyed peas (cowpeas), chickpeas (garbanzo beans), and soybeans. Root vegetables (tubers) such as potatoes and yams are a third major source of starch, and in many non-Western societies, they are the primary starch sources. Grains, legumes, and tubers not only are rich in starch but may also contain abundant dietary fiber, protein, and other nutrients.

Fibers

Dietary fibers are the structural parts of plants and thus are found in all plant-derived foods—vegetables, fruits, whole grains, and legumes. Most dietary fibers are polysaccharides—chains of sugars—just as starch is, but in fibers the sugar units are held together by bonds that human digestive enzymes cannot break. Consequently, most dietary fibers pass through the body providing little or no energy for its use. Figure 3-2 shows the difference between starch and the plant fiber cellulose. In addition to cellulose, fibers include the polysaccharides hemicellulose, pectins, gums, and mucilages, as well as the nonpolysaccharide lignins.

Cellulose is the main constituent of plant cell walls, so it is found in all vegetables, fruits, and legumes. Hemicellulose is the main constituent of cereal fibers. Pectins are abundant in vegetables and fruits, especially citrus fruits and apples. The food industry uses pectins to thicken jelly and keep salad dressing from separating. Gums and mucilages have similar structures and are used as additives or stabilizers by the food industry. Lignins are the tough, woody parts of plants; few foods people eat contain much lignin.

✚ The short chains of glucose units that result from the breakdown of starch are known as *dextrins*. The word sometimes appears on food labels because dextrins can be used as thickening agents in foods.

glycogen (GLY-co-gen): a polysaccharide composed of glucose, made and stored by liver and muscle tissues of human beings and animals as a storage form of glucose. Glycogen is not a significant food source of carbohydrate and is not counted as one of the polysaccharides in foods.

starch: a plant polysaccharide composed of glucose and digestible by human beings.

dietary fibers: a general term denoting in plant foods the polysaccharides cellulose, hemicellulose, pectins, gums and mucilages, as well as the nonpolysaccharide lignins, which are not digested by human digestive enzymes, although some are digested by GI tract bacteria.

FIGURE 3-2	Starch and Cellulose Molecules Compared (Small Segments)

Starch   Cellulose

The bonds that link the glucose units together in cellulose are different from the bonds in starch (and glycogen). Human enzymes cannot digest cellulose.

*Glycogen in animal muscles rapidly breaks down after slaughter.

Carbohydrates

A few starches are classified as fibers. Known as **resistant starches,** these starches escape digestion and absorption in the small intestine. Starch may resist digestion for several reasons, including the individual's efficiency in digesting starches and the food's physical properties. Resistant starch is common in whole or partially milled grains, legumes, raw potatoes, and unripe bananas.[4] Cooked potatoes, pasta, and rice that have been chilled also contain resistant starch. Similar to some fibers, resistant starch may support a healthy colon.[5]

Although cellulose and other dietary fibers are not broken down by human enzymes, some fibers can be digested by bacteria in the human digestive tract. Bacterial digestion of fibers can generate some absorbable products that can yield energy when metabolized. Food fibers, therefore, can contribute some energy (1.5 to 2.5 kcalories per gram), depending on the extent to which they break down in the body.

Fibers are divided into two general groups by their chemical and physical properties. *In the first group are fibers that dissolve in water (**soluble fibers**). These form gels (are **viscous**) and are easily digested by bacteria in the human large intestine (are easily fermented). Commonly found in barley, legumes, fruits, oats, and vegetables, these fibers are often associated with lower risks of chronic diseases (as discussed in a later section). In foods, soluble fibers add a pleasing consistency; for example, pectin puts the gel in jelly, and gums are added to salad dressings and other foods to thicken them.

Other fibers do not dissolve in water (**insoluble fibers**), do not form gels (are not viscous), and are less readily fermented. Insoluble fibers, such as cellulose and many hemicelluloses, are found in the outer layers of whole grains (bran), the strings of celery, the hulls of seeds, and the skins of corn kernels. These fibers retain their structure and rough texture even after hours of cooking. In the body, they aid the digestive system by easing elimination.[6]

© Brian Leatart/FoodPix/Jupiter Images

Starch- and fiber-rich foods are the foods to emphasize.

Review Notes

- Carbohydrate is the body's preferred energy source. Six sugars are important in nutrition: the three monosaccharides (glucose, fructose, and galactose) and the three disaccharides (sucrose, lactose, and maltose).
- The three disaccharides are pairs of monosaccharides; each contains glucose paired with one of the three monosaccharides. The polysaccharides (chains of monosaccharides) are glycogen, starches, and fibers.
- Both glycogen and starch are storage forms of glucose—glycogen in the body and starch in plants—and both yield energy for human use.
- The dietary fibers also contain glucose (and other monosaccharides), but their bonds cannot be broken by human digestive enzymes, so they yield little, if any, energy.

Health Effects of Sugars and Alternative Sweeteners

Fiber-rich carbohydrate foods such as vegetables, whole grains, legumes, and fruits should predominate in people's diets; concentrated sweets such as candy, cola beverages and other soft drinks, cookies, pies, cakes, and other foods with **added sugars** add kcalories, but few, if any, other nutrients. These foods therefore contribute discretionary kcalories to the diet. (✚) Estimated intakes of added sugars in the United States far exceed the allowance for discretionary kcalories, regardless of energy intake.[7]

The **naturally occurring sugars** in vegetables, fruits, grains, and milk are acceptable because they are accompanied by many nutrients. People who want to limit their use of sugar may choose from two sets of alternative sweeteners: sugar alcohols and artificial sweeteners.

✚ The *USDA Food Guide* distinguishes between naturally occurring and added sugars, designating the kcalories from added sugars as discretionary kcalories.

resistant starches: starches that escape digestion and absorption in the small intestine of healthy people.

soluble fibers: indigestible food components that readily dissolve in water and often impart gummy or gel-like characteristics to foods. An example is pectin from fruit, which is used to thicken jellies.

viscous: a gel-like consistency.

insoluble fibers: the tough, fibrous structures of fruits, vegetables, and grains; indigestible food components that do not dissolve in water.

added sugars: sugars and syrups added to a food for any purpose, such as to add sweetness or bulk or to aid in browning (baked foods). Also called *carbohydrate sweeteners*, they include glucose, fructose, corn syrup, concentrated fruit juice, and other sweet carbohydrates.

naturally occurring sugars: sugars that are not added to a food but are present as its original constituents, such as the sugars of fruit or milk.

---

*The DRI committee has proposed these fiber definitions: the term *dietary fibers* refers to naturally occurring fibers in intact foods, and *functional fibers* refers to added fibers that have health benefits; *total fiber* refers to the sum of fibers from both sources.

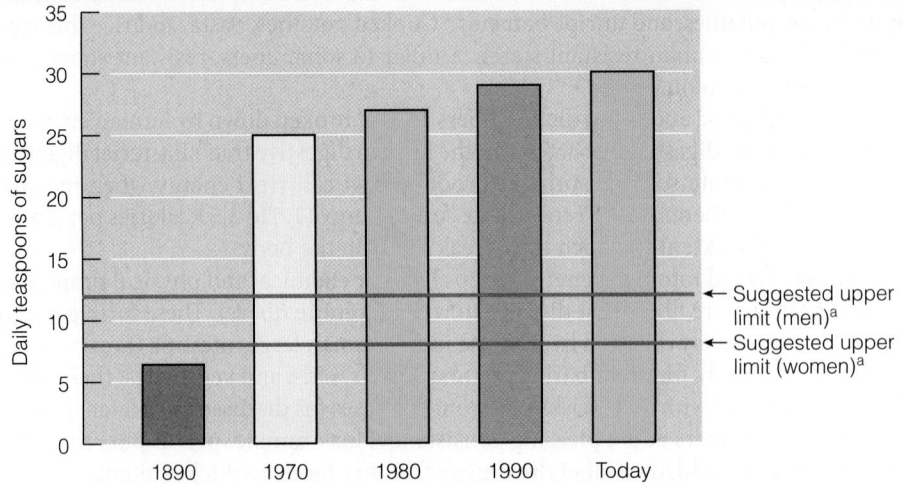

FIGURE 3-3 | Added Sugars: Average U.S. Supply per Person Compared with Suggested Upper Intake Limits

[a] These USDA suggested upper limits for added sugars reflect one-half of the average discretionary kcalorie allowance for sedentary men aged 19-30 consuming 2400 kcal/day and sedentary women aged 19-30 consuming 2000 kcal/day. The American Heart Association sets a prudent upper limit of 6 teaspoons of sugar for most women, and 9 for most men.

Sources: USDA Food Guide; R. K. Johnson and coauthors, Dietary sugars intake and cardiovascular health: A Scientific Statement from the American Heart Association, *Circulation* 120 (2009): 1011–1020.

SUGARS

Estimates are that each man, woman, and child in the United States consumes more than 100 pounds of sugar per year, or a little less than 2 pounds per week. Figure 3-3 depicts the dramatic upward trend in available added sugars in the U.S. diet and offers the American Heart Association prudent upper intake limits for added sugars for comparison. The steady upward trend in consumption of added sugars shown in Figure 3-3 is largely the result of a dramatic increase in consumption of commercially prepared foods and beverages that contain added sugars. Food manufacturers are adding the sugars to foods during processing. Soft drinks and other sugar-sweetened beverages are the main source of added sugars in the diets of U.S. consumers.[8] In contrast, people are adding less sugar in the kitchen. Note that the columns in the figure represent sugars in the food supply and do not account for waste, such as the syrup drained from sweet pickles or jam that molds and is thrown away. The usual amount of added sugars consumed in a day averages more than 22 teaspoons.[9] The committee that drafted the *Dietary Guidelines for Americans* offers clear advice on added sugars: treat them as discretionary kcalories.[10] In other words, fill the day's nutrient needs with foods contributing little or no added sugar. Most people can afford only a little added sugar in their diets if they are to meet nutrient needs within kcalorie limits.

The U.S. population is not alone in increasing sugar consumption. The trend is a worldwide phenomenon. In response, the World Health Organization has also taken a stand on sugar intake: consume no more than 10 percent of total kcalories from added sugars.*

The increase in sugar consumption has raised many questions about sugar's effects on health. Many accusations have been made against sugar, but the Food and Drug Administration (FDA) and the National Academy of Sciences have concluded that, in moderate amounts, sugars pose no major health risk. In excess, however, they can

Sugary soft drinks are the leading source of added sugars in the United States; cakes, cookies, pies, and other baked goods come next; and sweetened fruit drinks and punches follow closely behind.

*The World Health Organization uses the term *free sugars* to mean all monosaccharides and disaccharides added to foods by the manufacturer, cook, or consumer plus the naturally occurring sugars in honey, syrups, and fruit juices.

be detrimental in two ways. One, sugars can contribute to nutrient deficiencies by supplying energy (kcalories) without providing nutrients. Two, sugars contribute to tooth decay, or **dental caries**.

High intakes of added sugars, along with dramatically increasing rates of obesity, have raised concerns about the relationship between obesity and excessive sugar intake.[11] A later section in this discussion addresses this concern.

Sugar and Nutrient Deficiencies Empty-kcalorie foods that contain lots of added sugars such as cakes, candies, and sodas provide the body with glucose and energy, but few, if any, other nutrients.[12] By comparison, foods such as whole grains, vegetables, legumes, and fruits that contain some natural sugars and lots of starches and fibers also provide protein, vitamins, and minerals.

A person spending 200 kcalories of a day's energy allowance on a 16-ounce soda gets little of value for those kcalories. In contrast, a person using 200 kcalories on three slices of whole-wheat bread gets 9 grams of protein, 6 grams of fiber, plus several of the B vitamins with those kcalories. For the person who wants something sweet, a reasonable compromise might be two slices of bread with a teaspoon of jam on each. The amount of sugar a person can afford to eat depends on how many discretionary kcalories are available beyond those needed to deliver indispensable vitamins and minerals.

By following MyPyramid and making careful food selections, a typical adult can obtain all the needed nutrients within an allowance of about 1500 kcalories. Some people have more generous energy allowances. For example, an active teenage boy may need as many as 3000 kcalories a day. If he eats mostly nutritious foods, then he may have discretionary kcalories available for cola beverages and other "extras." In contrast, an inactive older woman who is limited to fewer than 1500 kcalories a day can afford to eat only the most nutrient-dense foods—with few, or no, discretionary kcalories available. As mentioned earlier, intakes of added sugars far exceed discretionary kcalorie allowances, regardless of energy needs.[13]

Sugar and Dental Caries Does sugar contribute to dental caries? The evidence says yes. Any carbohydrate-containing food, including bread, bananas, or milk, as well as sugar, can support bacterial growth in the mouth. These bacteria produce the acid that eats away tooth enamel. Of major importance is the length of time the food stays in the mouth. This, in turn, depends on the composition of the food, how sticky the food is, how often a person eats the food, and especially whether the teeth are brushed afterward.[14] (✚) Total sugar intake still plays a major role in caries incidence; populations whose diets provide no more than 10 percent of kcalories from sugar have a low prevalence of dental caries. Nutrition in Practice 17 discusses nutrition and oral health.

Sugar and Obesity Over the past several decades, as obesity rates increased sharply, consumption of added sugars reached an all-time high—much of it because high-fructose corn syrup use, especially in beverages, surged.[15] High-fructose corn syrup is composed of fructose and glucose in a ratio of about 50:50. Compared with sucrose, high-fructose corn syrup is less expensive, easier to use, and more stable. In addition to being used in beverages, high-fructose corn syrup sweetens candies, baked goods, and hundreds of other foods. The use of high-fructose corn syrup sweetener parallels unprecedented increases in the incidence of obesity, but does this mean that the increasing sugar intakes are responsible for the increase in body fat and its associated health problems?[16] Excess sugar in the diet may be associated with more fat on the body.[17] When eaten in excess of need, energy from added sugars contributes to body fat stores, just as excess energy from other sources does.[18] Added sugars provide excess energy, raising the risk of weight gain.[19] When total energy intake is controlled, however, *moderate* amounts of sugar do not *cause* obesity. A recent meta-analysis of sugar-sweetened beverage consumption and body mass index in children and adolescents showed no significant relationship.[20] The authors point out that sugar-sweetened beverages are a source of energy, and excess energy consumption promotes weight gain. Thus, to the extent that sugar contributes to an excessive energy intake, it can play a role in the development of obesity.

✚ *Dietary Guidelines for Americans*: Reduce the incidence of dental caries by practicing good oral hygiene and consuming sugar- and starch-containing foods and beverages less frequently.

dental caries: the gradual decay and disintegration of a tooth.

The USDA Food Guide suggests:*
- 3 tsp for 1,600 kcal
- 5 tsp for 1,800 kcal
- 8 tsp for 2,000 kcal
- 9 tsp for 2,200 kcal
- 12 tsp for 2,400 kcal

For perspective, each of these sources of concentrated sugars provides about 500 kcal:
- 40 oz cola
- 1/2 cup honey
- 125 jelly beans
- 23 marshmallows
- 30 tsp sugar

Recommended Sugar Intakes Moderate sugar intakes—enough for pleasure but not enough to displace more nutritious foods—are not harmful. Sugar is a delicious, concentrated source of food energy, but it contains no protein, vitamins, or minerals. Eaten in the place of nutrient- and fiber-rich foods, it makes malnutrition likely.

The *Dietary Guidelines for Americans* urge people to "choose and prepare foods and beverages with little added sugars." The USDA Food Guide suggests that, within kcalorie limits, small amounts of added sugars can be enjoyed as part of the discretionary kcalorie allowance in a nutrient-dense diet. (+) The USDA Food Guide recommendations represent about 5 to 10 percent of the day's total energy intake. The American Heart Association suggests a prudent upper limit of not more than half the discretionary kcalorie allowance (no more than 100 kcalories of added sugars for most women or 150 kcalories for most men). As noted earlier, the World Health Organization agrees that people should restrict their consumption of added sugars to 10 percent or less of total energy.

The DRI committee did not set a Tolerable Upper Intake Level for added sugars, but, as mentioned, excessive intakes can interfere with sound nutrition and dental health. Few people can eat lots of sugary treats and still meet all of their nutrient needs without exceeding their kcalorie allowance. Instead, the DRI committee suggests, as a rather high maximum, that added sugars should account for no more than 25 percent of the day's total energy intake.[21] For a person consuming 2000 kcalories a day, 25 percent represents 500 kcalories from added sugars—quite a lot of sugar. (+) Perhaps an athlete in training whose energy needs are high can afford the added sugars from sports drinks without compromising nutrient intake, but most people would do better following recommendations to limit added sugar consumption to less than 10 percent of the day's total energy intake.

Recognizing Sugars People often fail to recognize sugar in all its forms and so do not realize how much they consume. To help your clients estimate how much

Glossary

brown sugar: white sugar with molasses added; 95 percent pure sucrose.

concentrated fruit juice sweetener: a concentrated sugar syrup made from dehydrated, deflavored fruit juice, commonly grape juice; used to sweeten products that can then claim to be "all fruit."

confectioner's sugar: finely powdered sucrose; 99.9 percent pure.

corn sweeteners: corn syrup and sugar solutions derived from corn.

corn syrup: a syrup, mostly glucose, partly maltose, produced by the action of enzymes on cornstarch.

dextrose: an older name for glucose.

evaporated cane juice: raw sugar from which impurities have been removed.

fructose, galactose, glucose: the monosaccharides.

granulated sugar: common table sugar, crystalline sucrose, 99.9 percent pure.

high-fructose corn syrup (HFCS): a mixture of primarily fructose and glucose; the predominant sweetener used in processed foods today.

honey: a concentrated solution primarily composed of glucose and fructose; produced by enzymatic digestion of the sucrose in nectar by bees.

invert sugar: a mixture of glucose and fructose formed by the splitting of sucrose in an industrial process. Sold only in liquid form and sweeter than sucrose, invert sugar forms during certain cooking procedures and works to prevent crystallization of sucrose in soft candies and sweets.

lactose, maltose, sucrose: the disaccharides.

levulose: an older name for fructose.

maple sugar: a concentrated solution of sucrose derived from the sap of the sugar maple tree, mostly sucrose. This sugar was once common but is now usually replaced by sucrose and artificial maple flavoring.

molasses: a syrup left over from the refining of sucrose from sugarcane; a thick, brown syrup. The major nutrient in molasses is iron, a contaminant from the machinery used in processing it.

raw sugar: the first crop of crystals harvested during sugar processing. Raw sugar cannot be sold in the United States because it contains too much filth (dirt, insect fragments, and the like). Sugar sold as "raw sugar" is actually evaporated cane juice.

turbinado (ter-bih-NOD-oh) sugar: raw sugar from which the filth has been washed; legal to sell in the United States.

white sugar: pure sucrose, produced by dissolving, concentrating, and recrystallizing raw sugar.

---

*The amounts of added sugars suggested here are *not* specific recommendations for amounts of added sugars to consume but rather represent the amounts that can be included in the diet at each kcalorie level.

sugar they consume, tell them to treat all of the following concentrated sweets as equivalent to 1 teaspoon of white sugar (4 grams of carbohydrate):

- 1 teaspoon brown sugar, candy, jam, jelly, any corn sweetener, syrup, honey, molasses, or maple sugar
- 1 tablespoon catsup
- 11/2 ounces carbonated soft drink

These portions of sugar all provide about the same number of kcalories. Some are closer to 10 kcalories (for example, 14 kcalories for molasses), while some are more than 20 (22 kcalories for honey), so an average figure of 16 kcalories is an acceptable approximation. The accompanying glossary presents the multitude of names that denote sugar on food labels.

People often ask: What is the difference between honey and white sugar? Is honey, by virtue of being natural, more nutritious? Honey, like white sugar, contains glucose and fructose. The difference is that, in white sugar, the glucose and fructose are bonded together in pairs, whereas in honey some of them are paired and some are free single sugars. When you eat either white sugar or honey, though, your body breaks all of the sugars apart into single sugars. It ultimately makes no difference, then, whether you eat single sugars linked together, as in white sugar, or the same sugars unlinked, as in honey; they will end up as single sugars in your body.

Honey does contain a few vitamins and minerals but not many. Honey is denser than crystalline sugar, too, so it provides more energy per spoonful. Table 3-2 shows that

Mathew Farruggio

You receive about the same amount and kinds of sugars from an orange as from a tablespoon of honey, but the packaging makes a big nutrition difference.

TABLE 3-2	Sample Nutrients in Sugars and Other Foods

The indicated portion of any of these foods provides approximately 100 kcalories. Notice that—for a similar number of kcalories and grams of carbohydrate—milk, legumes, fruits, grains, and vegetables offer more of the other nutrients than do the sugars.

	Size of 100 kCal Portion	Carbohydrate (g)	Protein (g)	Calcium (mg)	Iron (mg)	Vitamin A (μg)	Vitamin C (mg)
Foods							
Milk, 1% low-fat	1 c	12	8	300	0.1	144	2
Kidney beans	½ c	20	7	30	1.6	0	2
Apricots	6	24	2	30	1.1	554	22
Bread, whole wheat	1½ slices	20	4	30	1.9	0	0
Broccoli, cooked	2 c	20	12	188	2.2	696	148
Sugars							
Sugar, white	2 tbs	24	0	trace	trace	0	0
Molasses, blackstrap	2½ tbs	28	0	343	12.6	0	0.1
Cola beverage	1 c	26	0	6	trace	0	0
Honey	1½ tbs	26	trace	2	0.2	0	trace

honey and white sugar are similar nutritionally—and both fall short of milk, legumes, fruits, grains, and vegetables. Honey may offer some health benefits, however: It seems to relieve nighttime coughing in children and reduce the severity of mouth ulcers in cancer patients undergoing chemotherapy or radiation.[22]

Some sugar sources are more nutritious than others, though. Consider a fruit such as an orange. The orange provides the same sugars and about the same energy as a tablespoon of sugar or honey, but the packaging makes a big difference in nutrient density. The sugars of the orange are diluted in a large volume of fluid that contains valuable vitamins and minerals, and the flesh and skin of the orange are supported by fibers that also offer health benefits. A tablespoon of honey offers no such bonuses. Of course, a cola beverage, containing many teaspoons of sugar, offers no advantages either. (✚)

Review Notes

- Sugars pose no major health threat except for an increased risk of dental caries.
- Excessive sugar intakes may displace needed nutrients and fiber and may contribute to obesity. A person deciding to limit daily sugar intake should recognize that not all sugars need to be restricted, just concentrated sweets with added sugars, which are high in kcalories and relatively lacking in other nutrients. Sugars that occur naturally in fruits, vegetables, and milk are acceptable.

ALTERNATIVE SWEETENERS: SUGAR ALCOHOLS

The **sugar alcohols** are carbohydrates, but they yield slightly less energy (2 to 3 kcalories per gram) than sucrose (4 kcalories per gram) because they are not absorbed completely.[23] The sugar alcohols are sometimes called **nutritive sweeteners** because they do yield some energy.

The sugar alcohols occur naturally in fruits and vegetables; they are also used by manufacturers to provide sweetness and bulk to cookies, sugarless gum, hard candies, and jams and jellies. Their sweetness relative to sugar is shown in Table 3-3. Unlike sucrose, sugar alcohols are fermented in the large intestine by intestinal bacteria. Consequently, side effects such as gas, abdominal discomfort, and diarrhea make the sugar alcohols less attractive than the artificial sweeteners.

The advantage of using sugar alcohols is that they do not contribute to dental caries. Bacteria in the mouth metabolize sugar alcohols much more slowly than sucrose, thereby inhibiting the production of acids that promote caries' formation. They are therefore valuable in chewing gums, breath mints, and other products that people keep in their mouths awhile. The FDA allows food labels to carry a health claim (see p. 28 in Chapter 1) about the relationship between sugar alcohols and the nonpromotion of dental caries as long as the FDA criteria for sugar-free status and other criteria are met. Figure 3-4 presents labeling information for products using sugar alternatives.

ALTERNATIVE SWEETENERS: ARTIFICIAL SWEETENERS

The **artificial sweeteners** are not carbohydrates. They yield virtually no energy in the amounts typically used and are sometimes called nonnutritive sweeteners. Like the sugar alcohols, artificial sweeteners make foods taste sweet without promoting tooth

✚ A 12 oz can of cola contains the equivalent of 8 tsp of sugar.

sugar alcohols: sugarlike compounds. Like sugars, they are sweet to taste but yield 2 to 3 kcal per gram, slightly less than sucrose. Examples are maltitol, mannitol, sorbitol, isomalt, lactitol, and xylitol.

nutritive sweeteners: sweeteners that yield energy, including both the sugars and the sugar alcohols.

artificial sweeteners: noncarbohydrate, nonkcaloric synthetic sweetening agents; sometimes called *nonnutritive sweeteners*.

Carbohydrates

TABLE
3-3 | Sugar Alcohols

Sugar Alcohols	Relative Sweetness*	Energy (kcal/g)	Approved Uses
Erythritol	0.7	0.2	Bulk sweetener in low-kcalorie foods
Isomalt	0.5	2.0	Candies, chewing gum, ice cream, jams and jellies, frostings, beverages, baked goods
Lactitol	0.4	2.0	Candies, chewing gum, frozen dairy desserts, jams and jellies, frostings, baked goods
Maltitol	0.9	2.1	Particularly good for candy coating
Mannitol	0.7	1.6	Bulking agent, chewing gum
Sorbitol	0.5	2.6	Special dietary foods, candies, gums, frozen desserts, baked goods
Xylitol	1.0	2.4	Chewing gum, candies, pharmaceutical and oral health products

*The relative sweetness depends on the temperature, acidity, and other flavors of the foods in which the substance occurs. The sweetness of pure sucrose is the standard with which the approximate sweetness of sugar substitutes is compared.

decay. Table 3-4 (p. 74) and the glossary (p. 75) offer details on artificial sweeteners of interest.

Saccharin   **Saccharin** has been used for more than 100 years in the United States and is currently used by millions of people, mainly in soft drinks and as the tabletop sweetener Sweet'n Low or SugarTwin. Questions about the safety of

FIGURE
3-4 | Sugar Alternatives on Food Labels

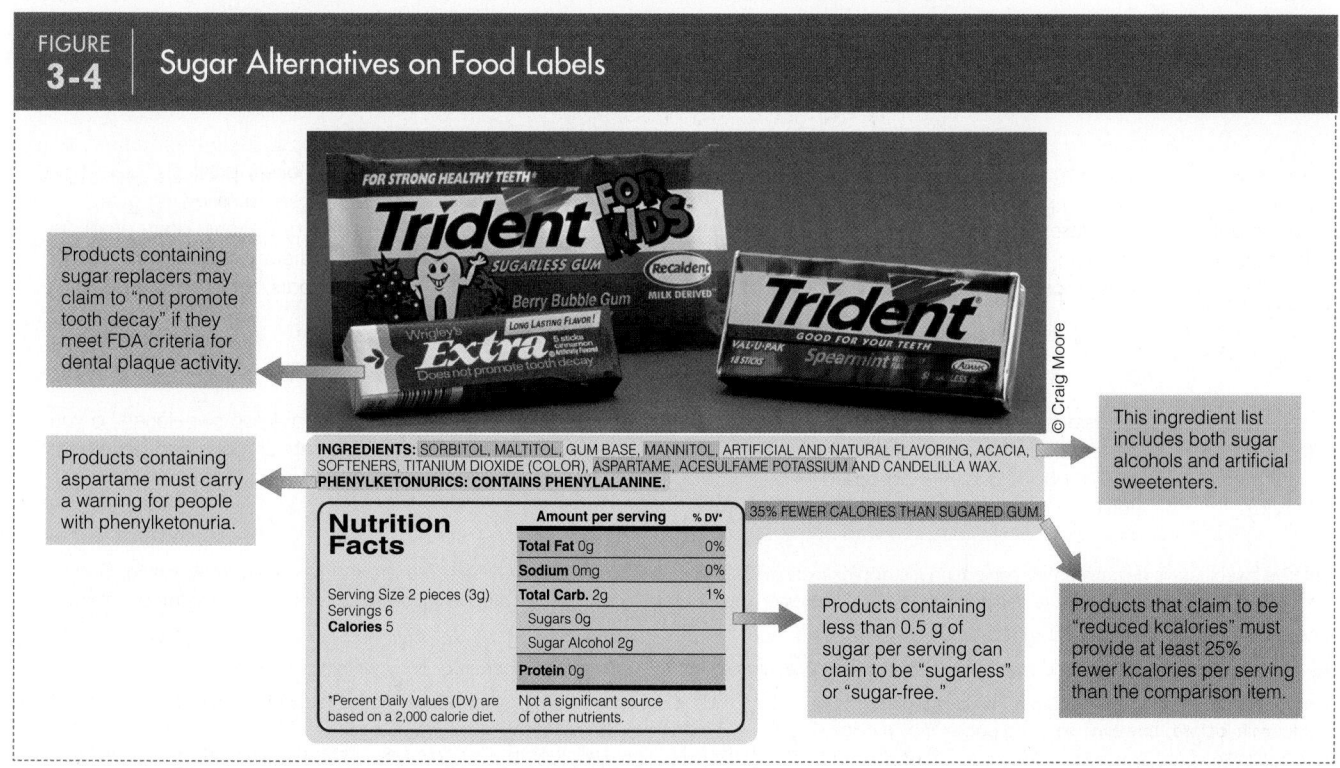

Products containing sugar replacers may claim to "not promote tooth decay" if they meet FDA criteria for dental plaque activity.

Products containing aspartame must carry a warning for people with phenylketonuria.

INGREDIENTS: SORBITOL, MALTITOL, GUM BASE, MANNITOL, ARTIFICIAL AND NATURAL FLAVORING, ACACIA, SOFTENERS, TITANIUM DIOXIDE (COLOR), ASPARTAME, ACESULFAME POTASSIUM AND CANDELILLA WAX. PHENYLKETONURICS: CONTAINS PHENYLALANINE.

This ingredient list includes both sugar alcohols and artificial sweetenters.

35% FEWER CALORIES THAN SUGARED GUM.

Nutrition Facts

Serving Size 2 pieces (3g)
Servings 6
Calories 5

Amount per serving	% DV*
Total Fat 0g	0%
Sodium 0mg	0%
Total Carb. 2g	1%
Sugars 0g	
Sugar Alcohol 2g	
Protein 0g	

*Percent Daily Values (DV) are based on a 2,000 calorie diet. Not a significant source of other nutrients.

Products containing less than 0.5 g of sugar per serving can claim to be "sugarless" or "sugar-free."

Products that claim to be "reduced kcalories" must provide at least 25% fewer kcalories per serving than the comparison item.

© Craig Moore

TABLE
3-4 | U.S.-Approved Sweeteners

Sweetener	Chemical Composition	Body's Response	Sweetness Relative to Sucrose[a]	Energy (kcal/g)	Acceptable Daily Intake (ADI) and (Estimated Equivalent[b])	Approved Uses
Artificial Sweeteners						
Acesulfame potassium or Acesulfame K (Sunette, Sweet One)	Potassium salt	Not digested or absorbed	200	0	15 mg/kg body[c] weight (30 cans diet soda)	Alcoholic beverages, baked goods, candies, chewing gum, desserts, gelatins, puddings, tabletop sweeteners
Aspartame (NutraSweet, Equal, others)	Amino acids (phenylalanine and aspartic acid) and a methyl group	Digested and absorbed	180	4[d]	50 mg/kg body[e] weight (18 cans diet soda)	General-purpose sweetener in all foods and beverages; warning to population with PKU
Neotame	Aspartame with an additional side group attached	Not digested or absorbed	7000	0	18 mg/day	Baked goods, beverages (nonalcoholic), candies, chewing gum, frosting, frozen desserts, gelatins, puddings, jams and jellies, syrups
Saccharin (SugarTwin, Sweet'N Low, others)	Benzoic sulfimide	Rapidly absorbed and excreted	300	0	5 mg/kg body weight (10 packets of sweetener)	Tabletop sweeteners, wide range of foods, beverages, cosmetics, and pharmaceutical products
Sucralose (Splenda)	Sucrose with Cl atoms instead of OH groups	Not digested or absorbed	600	0	5 mg/kg body weight (6 cans diet soda)	Baked goods, carbonated beverages, chewing gum, coffee and tea, dairy products, frozen desserts, fruit spreads, salad dressing, syrups, tabletop sweeteners
Tagatose (Nutralose, Nutrilatose, Tagatesse)	Monosaccharide similar in structure to fructose; naturally occurring or derived from lactose	Not well absorbed	0.9	1.5	7.5 g/day	Bakery products, beverages, cereals, chewing gum, confections, dairy products, dietary supplements, health bars, tabletop sweetener
Herbal Sweeteners						
Stevia (Sweetleaf, Truvia, PurVia)	Glyosides found in the leaves of the *Stevia rebaudiana* herb	Digested and absorbed	200–300	0	4 mg/kg body weight	Tabletop sweeteners, a variety of foods and beverages

[a]Relative sweetness is determined by comparing the approximate sweetness of a sugar substitute with the sweetness of pure sucrose, which has been defined as 1.0. Chemical structure, temperature, acidity, and other flavors of the foods in which the substance occurs all influence relative sweetness.

[b]Based on a person weighing 70 kg (154 lbs).

[c]Recommendations from the World Health Organization limit acesulfame-K intake to 9 mg per kilogram of body weight per day.

[d]Aspartame provides 4 kcal per gram, as does protein, but because so little is used, its energy contribution is negligible. In powdered form, it is sometimes mixed with lactose, however, so a 1-g packet may provide 4 kcal.

[e]Recommendations from the World Health Organization and in Europe and Canada limit aspartame intake to 40 mg per kilogram of body weight per day.

saccharin arose in 1977 when experiments suggested that large doses (equivalent to hundreds of cans of diet soda daily for a lifetime) increased the risk of bladder cancer in rats. The FDA proposed banning saccharin as a result. Public outcry in favor of saccharin was so loud that Congress imposed a moratorium on the ban, while additional safety studies were conducted. Products containing saccharin were required to carry a warning label until 2001, when studies concluded that saccharin did not cause cancer in humans. Common sense dictates that consuming large amounts of saccharin is probably not safe, but, at moderate intake levels, saccharin is currently assumed to be safe for most people. The FDA has set **Acceptable Daily Intake (ADI)** levels for the artificial sweeteners used in the United States.

Aspartame **Aspartame** is the active ingredient in NutraSweet, which is used in many commercially prepared foods, and in Equal, a tabletop sweetener. Aspartame is 200 times sweeter than sucrose and was approved by the FDA in 1981. Aspartame is one of the most studied of all food additives: extensive animal and human studies document its safety. Long-term consumption of aspartame is safe and is not associated with any adverse health effects.[24] Aspartame is approved for use in more than 100 countries.

The FDA's approval of aspartame is based on the assumption that no one will consume more than the ADI of 50 milligrams per kilogram of body weight in a day. This daily intake is indeed a lot: for a 150-pound adult, it adds up to 97 packets of Equal or 20 cans of soft drinks sweetened only with aspartame every day for a lifetime. Most users of aspartame consume between 2 and 10 milligrams per kilogram of body weight per day. Infants or toddlers under two years old should not be fed artificially sweetened foods and drinks.

Aspartame and PKU Although aspartame is considered safe for most people, individuals with the metabolic disorder phenylketonuria (PKU) are an exception. The labels of products that contain aspartame must include information for individuals with PKU. Aspartame contains the amino acid phenylalanine, and people with PKU cannot dispose of it efficiently (see Nutrition in Practice 15).

Acesulfame Potassium The FDA approved **acesulfame potassium (acesulfame-K)** in 1988 after reviewing more than 90 safety studies, conducted over 15 years. Marketed under the trade names Sunette and Sweet One, acesulfame-K is about as sweet as aspartame. It is used in chewing gum, beverages, instant coffee and tea, gelatins, and puddings, as well as for table use. Unlike aspartame, acesulfame-K holds up well during cooking.

Acceptable Daily Intake (ADI): the amount of an artificial sweetener that individuals can safely consume each day over the course of a lifetime without adverse effect. It includes a 100-fold safety factor.

Sucralose Sucralose received FDA approval in 1998 for use as a sweetener in the United States. Sucralose is the only artificial sweetener made from sucrose. Many years of testing have deemed sucralose safe to use and, specifically, not a cause of cancer. Sucralose is not recognized by the body as sugar and therefore passes through unchanged. Sucralose is heat stable and so is useful for cooking and baking; it is used in commercially prepared products and as the tabletop sweetener Splenda. Its sugarlike taste and versatility are earning sucralose some popularity among consumers.

Neotame In 2002, the FDA approved **neotame** on the strength of findings from more than 110 safety studies conducted on both animals and human beings. Neotame is so intensely sweet—about 7,000 times sweeter than sugar—that very little is needed to sweeten foods and beverages. Currently, neotame is available to food manufacturers for sweetening processed foods but not to consumers for home use.

A chemical cousin of aspartame, neotame also contains the amino acids phenylalanine and aspartic acid. Unlike aspartame, however, neotame is indigestible. Whereas digestive enzymes can separate the amino acids in aspartame, neotame's chemistry is sufficiently different to block the enzymes' action. This slight chemical difference makes neotame a better choice for people with phenylketonuria because it provides no phenylalanine to the body.

Tagatose The FDA has granted **tagatose**, a relative of fructose, the status of "generally recognized as safe," making it available as a lower-kcalorie sweetener for foods, beverages, confections, dietary supplements, and other uses. Tagatose is derived from lactose, but unlike fructose or lactose, 80 percent of tagatose remains unabsorbed until it reaches the large intestine. There the normal bacterial colonies of the intestine ferment tagatose, releasing gases and small products that are absorbed. At high doses, tagatose causes flatulence, rumbling, and loose stools. Otherwise, no adverse side effects have been noted by the maker.

Stevia—An Herbal Product Stevia sweeteners are extracted from the sweetest part of the stevia plant, whose leaves have long been used by the people of South America to sweeten their beverages. Until recently, stevia was sold in the United States only as a dietary supplement. Having recently been granted the status of "generally recognized as safe (GRAS)," stevia can now be used as an additive in a variety of foods and beverages and as a tabletop sweetener.

Cyclamate FDA approval for **cyclamate** is still pending. Cyclamate has been battling safety issues for 50 years. Approved by the FDA in 1949, cyclamate was banned in 1970 because of evidence indicating that it caused bladder cancer in rats. In 1985, the National Academy of Sciences concluded that evidence to date indicated that cyclamate did not cause cancer in human beings but that further studies were warranted. In Canada, cyclamate is restricted to use as a tabletop sweetener on the advice of a physician. In the United States, the FDA is currently reviewing a petition to reapprove the use of cyclamate.

Artificial Sweeteners and Weight Control Many people eat and drink products sweetened with artificial sweeteners to help them control weight. Does this work? Ironically, a few studies have reported that, after consuming such products, people experience heightened feelings of hunger. Despite these reports, most studies find that artificial sweeteners do not heighten feelings of hunger, enhance food intake, or cause weight gain in people.[25] When people reduce their energy intakes by replacing sugar in their diets with artificial sweeteners and then compensate for the reduced energy at later meals, energy intake may stay the same or increase. Using artificial sweeteners will not automatically lower energy intake; to successfully control energy intake, a person needs to make informed diet and activity decisions throughout the day.

Health Effects of Starch and Dietary Fibers

Despite dietary recommendations that people should eat generous servings of starch and fiber-rich carbohydrate foods for their health, many people still believe that carbohydrate is the "fattening" component of foods. Gram for gram, carbohydrates contribute fewer kcalories to the body than do dietary fats, so a moderate diet based on starch- and fiber-rich carbohydrate foods is likely to be lower in kcalories than a diet based on high-fat foods.

For health's sake, most people should increase their intakes of carbohydrate-rich foods such as whole grains, vegetables, legumes, and fruits—foods noted for their starch, fiber, and naturally occurring sugars. In addition, most people should also limit their intakes of foods with added sugars and the types of fats associated with heart disease (see Chapter 4). A diet that emphasizes whole grains, vegetables, legumes, and fruits is almost invariably moderate in food energy, low in fats that can harm health, and high in dietary fiber, vitamins, and minerals. All these factors working together can help reduce the risks of obesity, cancer, cardiovascular disease, diabetes, dental caries, gastrointestinal disorders, and malnutrition.

It is difficult to sort out which carbohydrates contribute to which health benefits. Starch and fibers almost always occur together in foods (except refined foods), so it is hard to distinguish their effects. Some health effects appear to be especially closely associated with fibers, however.

CARBOHYDRATES: DISEASE PREVENTION AND RECOMMENDATIONS

Fiber-rich carbohydrate foods benefit health in many ways. Foods such as whole grains, legumes, vegetables, and fruits supply valuable vitamins, minerals, and phytochemicals, along with abundant dietary fiber and little or no fat. The following paragraphs describe some of the health benefits of diets that emphasize a variety of these foods each day.

Heart Disease Diets rich in whole grains, legumes, and vegetables, especially those rich in whole grains, may protect against heart disease and stroke by lowering blood pressure, improving blood lipids, and reducing inflammation.[26] Such diets are low in animal fat and cholesterol and high in dietary fibers, vegetable proteins, and phytochemicals—all factors associated with a lower risk of heart disease. (✚) Foods rich in soluble fibers (such as oat bran, barley, and legumes) lower blood cholesterol by binding cholesterol compounds and carrying them out of the body with the feces.[27] High-fiber foods may also lower blood cholesterol indirectly by displacing fatty, cholesterol-raising foods from the diet. Even when dietary fat intake is low, research shows that high intakes of soluble fiber exert separate and significant blood cholesterol–lowering effects.

Diabetes High-fiber foods—and especially whole grains—play a key role in reducing the risk of **type 2 diabetes** (see Chapter 20).[28] The soluble fibers of foods such as oats and legumes can help regulate the blood glucose following a carbohydrate-rich meal. Soluble fibers trap nutrients and delay their transit through the digestive

✚ The role of animal fat and cholesterol in heart disease is discussed in Chapter 4. The role of vegetable proteins in heart disease is presented in Chapter 5. The benefits of phytochemicals in disease prevention are presented in Nutrition in Practice 8.

type 2 diabetes: the type of diabetes that accounts for 90 to 95 percent of diabetes cases and usually results from insulin resistance coupled with insufficient insulin secretion.

tract, slowing glucose absorption and preventing the glucose surge and rebound often associated with diabetes onset.

The term **glycemic response** refers to how quickly glucose is absorbed after a person eats, how high blood glucose rises, and how quickly it returns to normal. Slow absorption, a modest rise in blood glucose, and a smooth return to normal are desirable (a low glycemic response). Fast absorption, a surge in blood glucose, and an overreaction that plunges glucose below normal are less desirable (a high glycemic response). Different foods have different effects on blood glucose. The **glycemic index** is a method of classifying foods according to their potential to raise blood glucose and is the topic of Nutrition in Practice 3.

GI Health Dietary fibers may enhance the health of the large intestine. The healthier the intestinal walls, the better they can block absorption of unwanted constituents. Fibers that both enlarge and soften stools such as cellulose (in cereal brans, fruits, and vegetables) ease elimination for the rectal muscles and thereby alleviate or prevent constipation and hemorrhoids. Other fibers help to solidify watery stools.

Some fibers (again, such as cereal bran) help keep the contents of the intestinal tract moving easily. This action helps prevent compaction of the intestinal contents, which could obstruct the appendix and permit bacteria to invade and infect it. In addition, fibers stimulate the muscles of the gastrointestinal (GI) tract so that they retain their strength and resist bulging out in places, as occurs in diverticulosis.[29] Insoluble fiber seems to be most beneficial in lowering the risk of diverticulosis, which is described in Chapter 18.

Cancer Many studies show that, as people increase their dietary fiber intakes, their risk for colon cancer declines.[30] When the largest study of diet and cancer to date examined the diets of more than a half million people in 10 countries, the researchers found an inverse association between dietary fiber and colon cancer.[31] People who ate the most dietary fiber (35 grams per day) reduced their risk of colon cancer by 40 percent compared with those who ate the least fiber (15 grams per day). Importantly, the study focused on dietary fiber, not fiber supplements or additives. Fiber supplements and additives lack valuable nutrients and phytochemicals that also help protect against cancer.

When researchers examine other lifestyle factors, obesity, red and processed meat intake, cigarette smoking, and other factors emerge as associated with colon and rectal cancers, too.[32] More investigation into this important area of research is needed.

How fiber may help prevent colon cancer is under investigation. One focus of research is fiber's ability to dilute and speed removal of potential cancer-causing agents from the large intestine (colon). In addition, the colon's bacteria ferment soluble fibers, forming small fatlike molecules that lower the pH. (✚) These small fatlike molecules activate cancer-killing enzymes and inhibit inflammation in the colon.[33]

Other processes may also be at work. As research progresses, cancer experts recommend that fiber in the diet come from five to nine half-cup servings of vegetables and fruit, along with generous portions of whole grains and legumes.

Weight Management Fiber-rich foods tend to be low in fats and added sugars and, therefore, promote weight loss by delivering less energy per bite.[34] In addition, as fibers absorb water from the digestive juices, they swell, creating feelings of fullness, lowering food intake, and delaying hunger.[35] Recent research suggests that dietary fiber intake may not only protect against excess body fat but may offer specific protection against abdominal obesity, a risk factor for type 2 diabetes. In a study of overweight adolescents, a modest *decrease* (3 grams per 1,000 kcalories per day) in dietary fiber intake over one year was associated with a 21 percent increase in abdominal obesity compared with those who increased dietary fiber intake by the same modest amount.[36] The researchers concluded that public health messages and strategies focusing on increasing dietary fiber intake are especially urgent for young people at risk of obesity and other metabolic disorders.

Many weight-loss products on the market today contain bulk-inducing fibers such as methylcellulose, but buying pure fiber compounds like this is not advised. Besides adding bulk to the diet, high-fiber foods supply other nutrients as well. Most experts agree that the

✚ pH is the unit of measure expressing a substance's acidity or alkalinity. (Chapter 5 provides a more detailed definition.)

glycemic response: the extent to which a food raises the blood glucose concentration and elicits an insulin response.

glycemic index: a method of classifying foods according to their potential for raising blood glucose.

health benefits attributed to fiber may come from other constituents of fiber-containing foods and not from the fiber alone.[37] Therefore, to use fiber in a weight-loss plan, select fresh fruits, vegetables, legumes, and whole-grain foods. As a bonus, fiber-rich foods are often economical as well as nutritious. Figure 3-5 summarizes fibers and their health benefits.

Harmful Effects of Excessive Fiber Intake

Despite fiber's benefits to health, when too much fiber is consumed, some minerals may bind to it and be excreted with it without becoming available for the body to use. When mineral intake is adequate, however, a reasonable intake of high-fiber foods does not seem to compromise mineral balance.

People with marginal intakes who eat mostly high-fiber foods may not be able to take in enough food to meet energy or nutrient needs. The malnourished, the elderly, and young children adhering to all-plant (vegan) diets are especially vulnerable to this problem. Fibers also carry water out of the body and can cause dehydration. Advise clients to add an extra glass or two of water to go along with the fiber added to their diets. Athletes may want to avoid bulky, fiber-rich foods just prior to competition.

Adding purified fibers, such as oat bran or wheat bran, to foods can be taken to extremes. Too much fiber and too little fluid can obstruct the GI tract. Also, purified fiber may not affect the body the same way as the fiber in its original food product.

Recommended Intakes of Starches and Fibers

The DRI committee advises that carbohydrates should contribute about half (45 to 65 percent) of the energy requirement. A person consuming 2000 kcalories a day should therefore have 900 to 1300 kcalories of carbohydrate, or between 225 and 325 grams. (✚) This amount is more than adequate to meet the RDA for carbohydrate, which is set at 130 grams per day based on the average minimum amount of glucose used by the brain.[38] (✚)

When it established the Daily Values that appear on food labels, the FDA used a guideline of 60 percent of kcalories in setting the Daily Value for carbohydrate at 300 grams per day. (✚) For most people, this means increasing total carbohydrate intake.

✚ 45% of 2000 kcal:
2000 × 0.45 = 900 kcal.
900 kcal ÷ 4 kcal/g = 225 g

65% of 2,000 kcal:
2000 × 0.65 = 1300 kcal.
1300 kcal ÷ 4 kcal/g = 325 g

✚ RDA for carbohydrate:
130 g/day
45 to 65% of energy intake

✚ Daily Value:
300 g carbohydrate (based on 60% of 2,000 kcal diet)

FIGURE 3-5 | Characteristics, Sources, and Health Effects of Fibers

People who eat these foods...	obtain these types of fibers...	with these actions in the body...	and these probable health benefits...
	Viscous, soluble, more fermentable		
• Barley, oats, oat bran, rye, fruits (apples, citrus), legumes (especially young green peas and black-eyed peas), seaweeds, seeds and husks, many vegetables, fibers used as food additives	• Gums • Pectins • Psyllium[a] • Some hemicellulose	• Lower blood cholesterol by binding bile • Slow glucose absorption • Slow transit of food through upper GI tract • Hold moisture in stools, softening them • Yield small fat molecules after fermentation that the colon can use for energy • Increase satiety	• Lower risk of heart disease • Lower risk of diabetes • Lower risk of colon and rectal cancer • Increased satiety, and may help with weight management
	Nonviscous, insoluble, less fermentable		
• Brown rice, fruits, legumes, seeds, vegetables (cabbage, carrots, Brussels sprouts), wheat bran, whole grains, extracted fibers used as food additives	• Cellulose • Lignins • Resistant starch • Hemicellulose	• Increase fecal weight and speed fecal passage through colon • Provide bulk and feelings of fullness	• Alleviate constipation • Lower risk of diverticulosis, hemorrhoids, and appendicitis • Lower risk of colon and rectal cancer

[a] Psyllium, a soluble fiber derived from seeds, is used as a laxative and food additive.

To this end, the *Dietary Guidelines for Americans* encourage people to choose fiber-rich whole grains, vegetables, fruits, and legumes daily.

Recommendations for fiber encourage the same foods just mentioned: whole grains, vegetables, fruits, and legumes, which also provide vitamins, minerals, and phytochemicals. The FDA set the Daily Value for fiber at 25 grams, rounding up from the recommended 11.5 grams per 1000 kcalories for a 2000-kcalorie intake. (✚) The DRI recommendation is slightly higher, at 14 grams per 1000-kcalorie intake—roughly 25 to 35 grams of dietary fiber daily. (✚) These recommendations are about two times higher than the usual intake in the United States.[39]

As health care professionals, you can advise your clients that an effective way to add dietary fiber while lowering fat is to substitute plant sources of proteins (legumes) for some of the animal sources of protein (meats and cheeses) in the diet. Another way to add fiber is to encourage clients to consume the recommended amounts of fruits and vegetables each day. People choosing high-fiber foods are wise to seek out a variety of fiber sources and to drink extra fluids to help the fiber do its job. Many foods provide fiber in varying amounts, as Figure 3-6 shows.

As mentioned earlier, too much fiber is no better than too little. The World Health Organization recommends an upper limit of 40 grams of dietary fiber a day.

Review Notes

- A diet rich in starches and dietary fibers helps prevent heart disease, diabetes, GI disorders, and possibly some types of cancer. It also supports efforts to manage body weight.
- For these reasons, recommendations urge people to eat plenty of whole grains, vegetables, legumes, and fruits—enough to provide 45 to 65 percent of the daily energy from carbohydrate.

CARBOHYDRATES: FOOD SOURCES

A day's meals based on the USDA Food Guide not only meet carbohydrate recommendations but provide abundant fiber, too. Grains, vegetables, fruits, and legumes deliver fiber to the diet and are noted for their valuable energy-yielding starches and dilute sugars. Each class of foods makes its own typical carbohydrate contribution. The USDA Food Guide in Chapter 1 can help you and your clients obtain carbohydrate-rich foods.

Grains Most foods in this group—a slice of whole-wheat bread, half an English muffin or bagel, a 6-inch tortilla, or ½ cup of rice, pasta, or cooked cereal—provide about 15 grams of carbohydrate, mostly as starch.* Most grain choices should be low in fat and sugar. When extra kcalories are needed to meet energy needs, some selections higher in fat, preferably unsaturated fat (see Chapter 4), and sugar can supply discretionary kcalories. These choices include biscuits, muffins, and snack crackers.

Vegetables Some vegetables are major contributors of starch in the diet. Just a small white or sweet potato or 1/2 cup of cooked dry beans, corn, peas, plantain, or winter squash provides 15 grams of carbohydrate, as much as in a slice of bread, though as a mixture of sugars and starch. A 1/2-cup portion of carrots, okra, onions, tomatoes, cooked greens, and most other nonstarchy vegetables or a cup of salad greens provides about 5 grams as a mixture of starch and sugars. Each of these foods also contributes a little protein, some fiber, and no fat.

Fruits The size of a typical serving of fruit varies depending on the form of the fruit: ½ cup of juice; a small banana, apple, or orange; ½ cup of most canned or fresh fruit; or ¼ cup of dried fruit. A typical fruit serving contains an average of about

*Gram values in this section are adapted from the U.S. Food Exchange System.

FIGURE
3-6 Fiber in Selected Foods

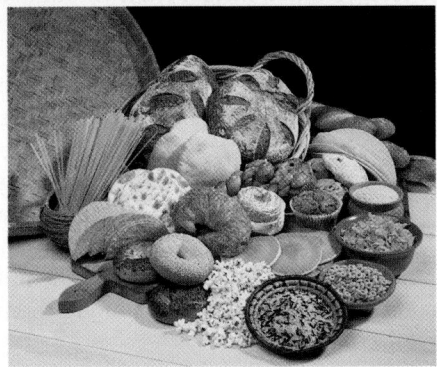

Grains

Whole-grain products provide 1 to 2 g of fiber or more per serving:

- 1 slice whole-wheat or rye bread (1 g).
- 1 slice pumpernickel bread (2 g).
- ½ c ready-to-eat 100% bran cereal (10 g).
- ½ c cooked barley, bulgur, grits, oatmeal (2 to 3 g).

Vegetables

Most vegetables contain 2 to 3 g of fiber per serving:

- 1 c raw bean sprouts.
- ½ c cooked broccoli, brussels sprouts, cabbage, carrots, cauliflower, collards, corn, eggplant, green beans, green peas, kale, mushrooms, okra, parsnips, potatoes, pumpkin, spinach, sweet potatoes, swiss chard, winter squash.
- ½ c chopped raw carrots, peppers.

Fruits

- Fresh, frozen, and dried fruits have about 2 g of fiber per serving:
- 1 medium apple, banana, kiwi, nectarine, orange, pear.
- ½ c applesauce, blackberries, blueberries, raspberries, strawberries.
- Fruit juices contain very little fiber.

Legumes and Nuts

Many legumes provide about 8 g of fiber per serving:

- ½ c cooked baked beans, black beans, black-eyed peas, kidney beans, navy beans, pinto beans.

Some legumes provide about 5 g of fiber per serving:

- ½ c cooked garbanzo beans, great northern beans, lentils, lima beans, split peas.

Most nuts and seeds provide 1 to 3 g of fiber per serving:

- 1 oz almonds, cashews, hazelnuts, peanuts, pecans, pumpkin seeds, sunflower seeds.

© Polara Studios, Inc. (all)

15 grams of carbohydrate, mostly as sugars, including the fruit sugar fructose. Fruits vary greatly in their water and fiber contents; therefore, their sugar concentrations vary also. No more than one-half of the day's fruit should come from juice. With the exception of avocado, which is high in fat, the fruits contain insignificant amounts of fat and protein.

Milk, Cheese, and Yogurt One cup of milk or yogurt or the equivalent (1 cup of buttermilk, ⅓ cup of dry milk powder, or ½ cup of evaporated milk) provides a generous 12 grams of carbohydrate. Among cheeses, cottage cheese provides about 6 grams of carbohydrate per cup, while most other types contain little, if any, carbohydrate. These foods also contribute high-quality protein as well as several important vitamins and minerals. Calcium-fortified soy beverages are options for providing calcium and about the same amount of carbohydrate as milk. All milk products vary in fat content, an important consideration in choosing among them; Chapter 4 provides the details.

Cream and butter, although dairy products, are not equivalent to milk because they contain little or no carbohydrate and insignificant amounts of the other nutrients important in milk. They are appropriately placed with the solid fats and added sugars.

Meat, Poultry, Fish, Legumes, Eggs, and Nuts With two exceptions, foods of this group provide almost no carbohydrate to the diet. The exceptions are nuts, which provide a little starch and fiber along with their abundant fat, and dry beans, which are excellent sources of both starch and fiber. Just a ½-cup serving of beans provides 15 grams of carbohydrate, an amount equal to the richest carbohydrate sources. Among sources of fiber, beans and other legumes are outstanding, providing as much as 8 grams in ½ cup. The carbohydrate content of a diet can be determined by using a nutrient composition table such as that found in Appendix A, the exchange list system described in Chapter 20, or a computer diet analysis program.

CARBOHYDRATES: FOOD LABELS AND HEALTH CLAIMS

Food labels list the amount, in grams, of total carbohydrate—including starch, fibers, and sugars—per serving. Fiber grams are also listed separately, as are the grams of sugars. (With this information, consumers can calculate starch grams by subtracting the grams of fibers and sugars from the total carbohydrate.) Sugars on the Nutrition Facts panel of a food label reflect both added sugars and those that occur naturally in foods. Total carbohydrate and dietary fiber are also expressed in the "% Daily Values" column for a person consuming 2000 kcalories; there is no Daily Value for sugars.

The FDA authorizes four health claims on food labels concerning fiber-rich carbohydrate foods. One is for "fiber-containing grain products, fruits, and vegetables and reduced risk of cancer." Another is for "fruits, vegetables, and grain products that contain fiber, and reduced risk of coronary heart disease." A third is for "soluble fiber from whole oats and from psyllium seed husk and reduced risk of coronary heart disease," and a fourth is for "whole grains and reduced risk of heart disease and certain cancers." Chapter 1 describes the criteria foods must meet to bear these health claims.

Review Notes

- Grains, vegetables, fruits, and legumes contribute dietary fiber and energy-yielding starches and dilute sugars to people's diets. One cup of milk or yogurt or the equivalent contributes a generous 12 grams of carbohydrate as well as protein and other important nutrients.
- Food labels list grams of total carbohydrate and also provide separate listings of grams of fiber and sugar.

Self Check

1. Carbohydrates are found in virtually all foods **except**:
   a. milks.
   b. meats.
   c. breads.
   d. vegetables.

2. Polysaccharides include:
   a. galactose, starch, and glycogen.
   b. starch, glycogen, and fiber.
   c. lactose, maltose, and glycogen.
   d. sucrose, fructose, and glucose.

3. The chief energy source of the body is:
   a. sucrose.
   b. starch.
   c. glucose.
   d. fructose.

4. The primary form of stored glucose in animals is:
   a. glycogen.
   b. cellulose.
   c. starch.
   d. lactose.

5. The polysaccharide that helps form the cell walls of plants is:
   a. cellulose.
   b. starch.
   c. glycogen.
   d. lactose.

6. Which of the following items may denote sugar on food labels?
   a. Corn syrup
   b. Aspartame
   c. Xylitol
   d. Cellulose

7. The two types of alternative sweeteners are:
   a. saccharin and cyclamate.
   b. sugar alcohols and artificial sweeteners.
   c. sorbitol and xylitol.
   d. sucrose and fructose.

8. A diet high in carbohydrate-rich foods such as whole grains, vegetables, fruits, and legumes is:
   a. most likely low in fat.
   b. most likely low in fiber.
   c. most likely poor in vitamins and minerals.
   d. most likely disease promoting.

9. A fiber-rich diet may help to prevent or control:
   a. diabetes.
   b. heart disease.
   c. constipation.
   d. all of the above.

10. The DRI fiber recommendation is:
    a. 10 grams per 1000 kcalories.
    b. 15 to 25 grams per day.
    c. 14 grams per 1000 kcalories.
    d. 40 to 55 grams per day.

Answers to these questions can be found in Appendix H.

Clinical Applications

1. Considering the health benefits of carbohydrate-rich foods, especially those that provide starch and fiber, what suggestions would you offer to a client who reports the following:
   - Eats only three servings of refined, sugary breads or cereals each day.
   - Eats one serving of vegetables (usually french fries) each day.
   - Drinks fruit juice once a day but never eats fruit.
   - Eats cheese at least twice a day but does not drink milk.
   - Eats large servings of meat at least twice a day.
   - Eats hard candy two or three times a day.

Nutrition on the Net

For further study of the topics in this chapter, access these websites.

- Find updates and quick links to these and other nutrition-related sites at our website: www.cengage.com/nutrition/whitney/nhhc4e
- Search for "artificial sweeteners" at the U.S. government health information site: www.healthfinder.gov
- Search for "sugars" and "fiber" at the International Food Information Council site: www.ific.org
- Learn more about dental caries from the American Dental Association and the National Institute of Dental and

Craniofacial Research: www.ada.org and www.nidcr.nih.gov
- Learn more about diabetes from the American Diabetes Association, the Canadian Diabetes Association, and the National Diabetes Information Clearinghouse: www.diabetes.org, www.diabetes.ca, and www.niddk.nih.gov

Notes

1. A. T. Merchant and coauthors, Carbohydrate intake and overweight and obesity among healthy adults, *Journal of the American Dietetic Association* 109 (2009): 1165–1172; Standing Committee on the Scientific Evaluation of Dietary Reference Intakes, Food and Nutrition Board, Institute of Medicine, *Dietary Reference Intakes for Energy, Carbohydrate, Fiber, Fat, Fatty Acids, Cholesterol, Protein, and Amino Acids* (Washington, D.C.: National Academies Press, 2005), pp. 265–338.

2. J. H. Cummings and A. M. Stephen, Carbohydrate terminology and classification, *European Journal of Clinical Nutrition* 61 (2007): S5–S18.

3. A. M. Brown and B. R. Ransom, Astrocyte glycogen and brain energy metabolism, *Glia* 55 (2007): 1263–1271; M. K. Dalsqaard and coauthors, High glycogen levels in the hippocampus of patients with epilepsy, *Journal of Cerebral Blood Flow and Metabolism* 27 (2007): 1137–1141.

4. M. M. Murphy, J. S. Douglass, and A. Birkett, Resistant starch intakes in the United States, *Journal of the American Dietetic Association* 108 (2008): 67–78.

5. S. S. Dronamraju and coauthors, Cell kinetics and gene expression changes in colorectal cancer patients give resistant starch: A randomised controlled trial, *Gut* 58 (2009): 413–420; M. Nofrarias and coauthors, Long-term intake of resistant starch improves colonic mucosal integrity and reduces gut apoptosis and blood immune cells, *Nutrition* 23 (2007): 861–870.

6. Position of the American Dietetic Association: Health implications of dietary fiber, *Journal of the American Dietetic Association* 108 (2008): 1716–1731.

7. R. K. Johnson and coauthors, Dietary sugars intake and cardiovascular health: A scientific statement from the American Heart Association, *Circulation* 120 (2009): 1011–1020.

8. Johnson and coauthors, 2009.

9. National Cancer Institute, Usual intake of added sugars, available at http://riskfactor.cancer.gov/diet/usualintakes/pop/t35.html.

10. U.S. Department of Agriculture and U.S. Department of Health and Human Services, *2005 Dietary Guidelines Committee Report*, 2005, available online at www.healthierus.gov/dietaryguidelines.

11. Johnson and coauthors, 2009.

12. A. Bhargava and A. Amialchuk, Added sugars displaced the use of vital nutrients in the National Food Stamp Program Survey, *Journal of Nutrition* 137 (2007): 453–460.

13. Johnson and coauthors, 2009; U.S. Department of Agriculture, MyPyramid.gov, available at www.mypramid.gov, accessed October 15, 2009.

14. Position of the American Dietetic Association: Oral health and nutrition, *Journal of the American Dietetic Association* 107 (2007): 1418–1428.

15. V. S. Malik, M. B. Schulze, and F. B. Hu, Intake of sugar-sweetened beverages and weight gain: A systematic review, *American Journal of Clinical Nutrition* 84 (2006): 274–288.

16. G. A. Bray, How bad is fructose? *American Journal of Clinical Nutrition* 86 (2007): 895–896; R. Dhingra and coauthors, Soft drink consumption and risk of developing cardiometabolic risk factors and the metabolic syndrome in middle-aged adults in the community, *Circulation* 116 (2007): 480–488; R. J. Johnson and coauthors, Potential role of sugar (fructose) in the epidemic of hypertension, obesity and the metabolic syndrome, diabetes, kidney disease, and cardiovascular disease, *American Journal of Clinical Nutrition* 86 (2007): 899–906; S. C. Larsson, L. Bergkvist, and A. Wolk, Consumption of sugar and sugar-sweetened foods and the risk of pancreatic cancer in a prospective study, *American Journal of Clinical Nutrition* 84 (2006): 1171–1176.

17. J. N. Davis and coauthors, Associations of dietary sugar and glycemic index with adiposity and insulin dynamics in overweight Latino youth, *American Journal of Clinical Nutrition* 86 (2007): 1331–1338.

18. R. A. Forshee and coauthors, A critical examination of the evidence relating high fructose corn syrup and weight gain, *Critical Reviews in Food Science and Nutrition* 47 (2007): 561–582.

19. L. R. Vartanian, M. B. Schwartz, and K. D. Brownell, Effects of soft drink consumption on nutrition and health: A systematic review and meta-analysis, *American Journal of Public Health* 97 (2007): 667–675.

20. R. A. Forshee, P. A. Anderson, and M. L. Storey, Sugar-sweetened beverages and body mass index in children and adolescents: A meta-analysis, *American Journal of Clinical Nutrition* 87 (2008): 1662–1671.

21. Standing Committee on the Scientific Evaluation of Dietary Reference Intakes, 2005, p. 770.

22. I. M. Paul and coauthors, Effect of honey, dextromethorphan, and no treatment on nocturnal cough and sleep quality for coughing children and their parents, *Archives of Pediatric and Adolescent Medicine* 161 (2007): 1140–1146; H. V. Worthington, J. E. Clarkson, and O. B. Eden, Interventions for preventing oral mucositis for patients with cancer receiving treatment, *Cochrane Database of Systematic Reviews* 4 (2007): CD000978.

23. Position of the American Dietetic Association: Use of nutritive and non-nutritive sweeteners, *Journal of the American Dietetic Association* 104 (2004): 255–275.

24. Position of the American Dietetic Association, 2004.

25. R. D. Mattes and B. M. Popkin, Nonnutritive sweetener consumption in humans: Effects on appetite and food intake and their putative mechanisms, *American Journal of Clinical Nutrition* 89 (2009): 1–14.

26. Position of the American Dietetic Association, 2008; M. T. Streppel and coauthors, Dietary fiber intake in relation to coronary heart disease and all-cause mortality over 40 y: The Zutphen Study, *American Journal of Clinical Nutrition* 88 (2008): 1119–1125; M. F. Chong, B. A. Fielding, and K. N. Frayn, Metabolic interaction of dietary sugars and plasma lipids with a focus on mechanisms and de novo lipogenesis, *Proceedings of the Nutrition Society* 66 (2007): 52–59; P. B. Mellen, T. F. Walsh, and D. M. Herrington, Whole grain intake and cardiovascular disease: A meta-analysis, *Nutrition, Metabolism and Cardiovascular Diseases* 18 (2008): 283–290; R. Solà and coauthors, Effects of soluble fiber (*Plantago ovata* husk) on plasma lipids, lipoproteins, and apolipoproteins in men with ischemic heart disease, *American Journal of Clinical Nutrition* 85 (2007): 1157–1163; P. B. Mellen and coauthors, Whole-grain intake and carotid artery atherosclerosis in a multiethnic cohort: The Insulin Resistance Atherosclerosis Study, *American Journal of Clinical Nutrition* 85 (2007): 1495–1502.

27. J. A. Nettleton and coauthors, Dietary patterns and incident cardiovascular disease in the MultiEthnic Study of Atherosclerosis, *American Journal of Clinical Nutrition* 90 (2009): 647–654; A. Mente and coauthors, A systematic review of the evidence supporting a causal link between dietary factors and coronary heart disease, *Archives of Internal Medicine* 169 (2009): 659–669; Streppel and coauthors, 2008; Position of the American Dietetic Association, 2008.

28. V. Vuksan and coauthors, Fiber facts: Benefits and recommendations for individuals with type 2 diabetes, *Current Diabetes Reports* 9 (2009): 405–411; H. Kim and coauthors, Glucose and insulin responses to whole grain breakfasts varying in soluble fiber, beta-glucan: A dose response study in

obese women with increased risk for insulin resistance, *European Journal of Nutrition* 48 (2009): 170–175; P. L. Lutsey and coauthors, Whole grain intake and its cross-sectional association with obesity, insulin resistance, inflammation, diabetes, and subclinical CVD: The MESA Study, *British Journal of Nutrition* 98 (2007): 397–405; M. B. Schulze and coauthors, Fiber and magnesium intake and incidence of type 2 diabetes, *Archives of Internal Medicine* 167 (2007): 956–965; J. S. de Munter and coauthors, Whole grain, bran, and germ intake and risk of type 2 diabetes: A prospective cohort study and systematic review, *PLoS Medicine* 4 (2007): e261.

29. J. R. Korzenik, Diverticulitits: New frontiers for an old country: Risk factors and pathogenesis, *Journal of Gastroenterology* 42 (2008): 1128–1129; Position of the American Dietetic Association, 2008; D. O. Jacobs, Diverticulitis, *New England Journal of Medicine* 357 (2007): 2057–2066.

30. L. B. Sansbury and coauthors, The effect of strict adherence to a high-fiber, high-fruit and -vegetable, and low-fat eating pattern on adenoma recurrence, *American Journal of Epidemiology* 170 (2009): 576–584; World Cancer Research Fund/American Institute for Cancer Research, *Food, Nutrition, Physical Activity, and the Prevention of Cancer: A Global Perspective* (Washington, D.C.: AICR, 2007), pp. 280–288.

31. S. Bingham, The fibre-folate debate in colo-rectal cancer, *Proceedings of the Nutrition Society* 65 (2006): 19–23; S. A. Bingham and coauthors, Dietary fibre in food and protection against colorectal cancer in the European Prospective Investigation into Cancer and Nutrition (EPIC): An observational study, *Lancet* 361 (2003): 1496–1501.

32. K. Wallace and coauthors, The association of lifestyle and dietary factors with the risk for serrated polyps of the colorectum, *Cancer Epidemiology, Biomarkers, and Prevention* 18 (2009): 2310–2317.

33. D. J. Rose and coauthors, Influence of dietary fiber on inflammatory bowel disease and colon cancer: Importance of fermentation pattern, *Nutrition Reviews* 65 (2007): 51–62.

34. L. A. Tucker and K. S. Thomas, Increasing total fiber intake reduces of weight and fat gains in women, *Journal of Nutrition* 139 (2009): 567–581.

35. M. Lyly and coauthors, Fiber in beverages can enhance perceived satiety, *European Journal of Nutrition* 48 (2009): 251–258; K. R. Juvonen and coauthors, Viscosity of oat bran-enriched beverages influences gastrointestinal hormonal responses in healthy humans, *Journal of Nutrition* 139 (2009): 461–466; R. A. Samra and G. H. Anderson, Insoluble cereal fiber reduces appetite and short-term food intake and glycemic response to food consumed 75 min later by healthy men, *American Journal of Clinical Nutrition* 86 (2007): 972–979.

36. J. N. Davis and coauthors, Inverse relation between dietary fiber intake and visceral adiposity in overweight Latino youth, *American Journal of Clinical Nutrition* 90 (2009): 1160–1166.

37. Davis and coauthors, 2009; Standing Committee on the Scientific Evaluation of Dietary Reference Intakes, 2005, pp. 391–399.

38. Standing Committee on the Scientific Evolution of Dietary Reference Intakes, 2005, p. 265.

39. Position of the American Dietetic Association, 2008.

The Glycemic Index in Nutrition Practice

Carbohydrate-rich foods vary in the degree to which they elevate both blood glucose and insulin concentrations. Chapter 3 introduced the *glycemic index (GI)*, a ranking of carbohydrate foods based on their glycemic effect after ingestion. The glycemic index may be of interest to people with diabetes who must regulate their blood glucose to protect their health. In diabetes treatment, however, the total amount of carbohydrate is more important than the type of carbohydrate consumed.[1] Thus, dietetics experts have debated the usefulness of the glycemic index for diabetes treatment. Despite some controversy, however, the American Diabetes Association encourages low-glycemic foods that are rich in fiber and other nutrients.[2] Furthermore, because recent research shows that a low-glycemic index diet can improve blood glucose control in type 2 diabetes, the use of low-glycemic diets for this purpose may be gaining credibility.[3]

Researchers are also trying to determine whether low-GI diets may be helpful for improving risk factors for a number of other chronic diseases.[4] This Nutrition in Practice will describe the factors that contribute to a food's glycemic effect and the results of research studies that have examined the potential benefits of selecting mainly low-GI foods.

How is the glycemic index measured?

The glycemic index is essentially a measure of how quickly the carbohydrate in a food is digested and absorbed. Although testing methods vary to some degree, the most common protocol is to feed the test food—which contains a measured quantity of digestible carbohydrate—to research subjects and then measure blood glucose levels for two or three hours after the feeding. The increase in blood glucose over the two- or three-hour period is then compared to the blood glucose rise after an identical amount of digestible carbohydrate is ingested from a reference food such as pure glucose or white bread. Figure NP3-1 illustrates the difference in the blood glucose response to a low-GI food and a high-GI food. The blood glucose curve displays the surge in blood glucose above normal fasting levels after the food is consumed and the subsequent fall over several hours. Table NP3-1 lists the GIs of various carbohydrate-containing foods, arranged from highest to lowest within each food group listed.

The *amount* of carbohydrate consumed also influences the glycemic response. A food's total glycemic effect—expressed as the *glycemic load (GL)*—is the product of its GI and the amount of available carbohydrate from the portion consumed, divided by 100.[5]

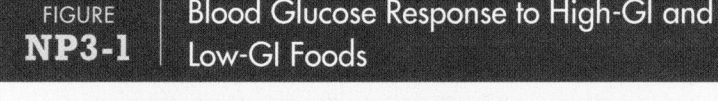

| FIGURE **NP3-1** | Blood Glucose Response to High-GI and Low-GI Foods |

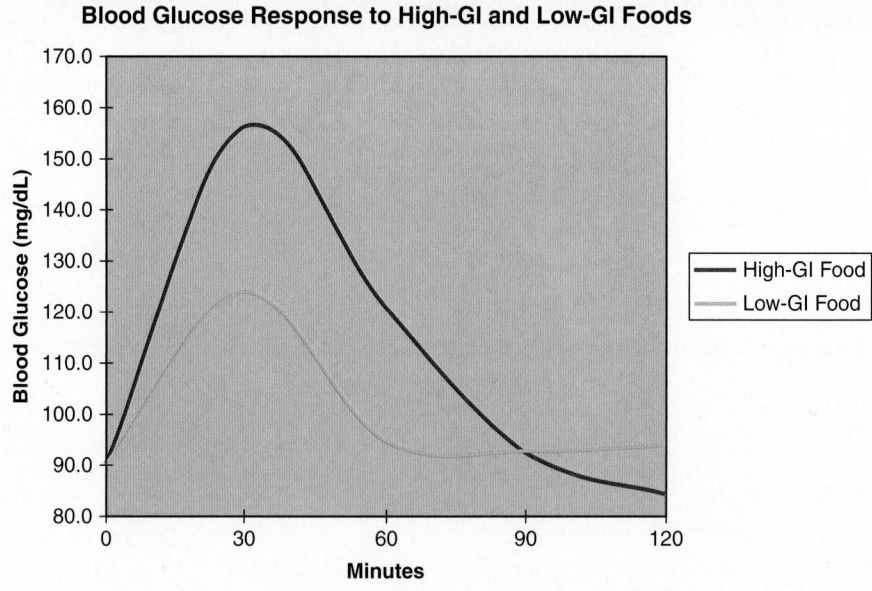

Foods that are digested slowly have a low glycemic index. These foods cause a gradual and more moderate response in blood glucose than do foods with a high glycemic index.

TABLE NP3-1 | Glycemic Index (GI) of Selected Foods[a]

Value	GI
High	≥70
Medium	56–69
Low	≤55

Food Item	Glycemic Index
Grains	
Cornflakes	81
Instant oatmeal, cooked	79
White bread, enriched	75
Whole wheat bread	74
White rice	73
Bagel, white	69
Brown rice	68
Couscous	65
Popcorn	65
Bran Flakes	63
Oatmeal, cooked	55
Spaghetti, white, boiled	49
Spaghetti, whole meal, boiled	48
Corn tortilla	46
Oat bran bread; 50% oat bran	44
Barley	28
Milk products	
Ice cream	51
Yogurt, fruit	41
Whole milk	39
Nonfat milk	37
Soy milk	34
Legumes	
Lentils	32
Garbanzo beans	28
Kidney beans	24
Soy beans	16

Food Item	Glycemic Index
Vegetables	
Russet potato, baked	111
Potato, instant mash	87
Potato, boiled	78
Pumpkin, boiled	64
Potato, french fries	63
Sweet potato, boiled	63
Taro	53
Sweet corn	52
Green peas, boiled	51
Carrots, boiled	39
Fruits	
Watermelon	76
Pineapple	59
Bananas	51
Mangoes	51
Orange juice	50
Oranges	43
Apple juice	41
Apples	36
Snack Foods/Beverages	
Fruit punch	67
Soft drink/soda	59
Chocolate	56
Potato chips	40
Sugars	
Sucrose	65
Honey	61
Fructose	15

[a] Reference food: glucose = 100

Source: F. S. Atkinson, K. Foster-Powell, and J. C. Brand-Miller, International tables of glycemic index and glycemic load values: 2008, *Diabetes Care* (2008): 2281–2283.

What factors influence a food's glycemic effect?

Table NP3-1 shows that starchy foods such as bread and potatoes tend to have high GI values, whereas many fruits and legumes have low GI values. The main factors that influence the GI value of a food include the following:

- *Starch structure.* Starch is present in foods as either a straight chain or branched chain of glucose molecules. Whereas digestion of the branched form tends to release glucose quickly, the straight chain is resistant to digestion. Thus, foods that contain mainly the branched form of starch tend to raise blood glucose levels more quickly and have a high GI value. Due to the subtle differences in starch among foods, different species of the same foods can have substantially different GI values; for example, current GI values for rice range from low (38 for parboiled white rice) to high (85 for Japanese sushi-style white rice).[6]
- *Fiber content.* Certain types of dietary fibers (primarily soluble fibers) increase the viscosity of chyme, slowing the passage of food in the stomach and upper intestine and making it more difficult for enzymes to digest the food. Therefore, foods such as beans, fruits, and vegetables, which contain soluble fibers, tend to have lower GI values.
- *Presence of fat and protein.* The fat in foods tends to slow stomach emptying, thus reducing the rate of digestion and absorption; hence, the presence of fat usually reduces a food's GI value. The protein in foods can also influence the GI because protein promotes insulin secretion, increasing the rate at which glucose is taken up from the blood.[7]
- *Food processing.* The manner in which a food is processed and cooked influences the interactions among starch, protein, and fiber and thus affects the final GI value. For example, both pasta and bread are prepared from wheat flour, but pasta (cooked *al dente*) has a lower GI because the starch granules in pasta are surrounded by a sturdy protein barrier that hampers starch digestion. Cooking the pasta for longer periods can break down its structure and raise the GI value. As another example, the GI values for oatmeal vary according to the size and thickness of the oats used to prepare it: oatmeal prepared from steel-cut oats has a lower GI value than oatmeal prepared from quick oats. This is because the steel-cut oats are solid particles of grain, whereas "quick oats" are small, thin flakes.
- *Mixture of foods in a meal.* Because foods are rarely consumed in isolation, the GI value of an individual food may be less important than the combination of foods consumed at a meal. For example, in a cheese sandwich, the high GI of the bread is lowered by the addition of fat and protein in the cheese.

© Brad Martin/The Image Bank

Pasta cooked *al dente* has a lower glycemic index than many other starchy foods.

- *Individual glucose tolerance.* Cellular responses to insulin vary; thus, individual variability affects the glycemic response to foods. Persons with diabetes or prediabetes exhibit higher blood glucose levels after ingesting carbohydrate foods than do healthy individuals.[8]

What evidence suggests that a low-GI diet may influence chronic disease risk?

Some research shows that low-GI diets may reduce the risks of developing diabetes, heart disease, and obesity and help individuals lose weight.[9] Other studies, however, do not support such findings.[10] Because of mixed findings so far, health practitioners do not routinely recommend that patients consume low-GI diets to prevent or treat disease. An abundance of ongoing research to reveal specific relationships between low-GI diets and chronic disease risk, however, may change such thinking. Examples of research include the following:

- *Diabetes prevention.* Some researchers have proposed that a high glycemic load can increase the body's demand for insulin and eventually reduce pancreatic function, resulting in inadequate insulin secretion. Indeed, results of several studies suggest that low-GI diets might prevent or delay the onset of type 2 diabetes in those at risk.[11] In fact, a summary of an international workshop on the glycemic index stated that "lower GI-diets are beneficial for those with impaired glucose metabolism, but that it is as yet unclear what such diets mean for healthy people."[12]

- *Heart disease risk.* Although some research suggests that low-GI diets may improve blood lipid levels, the majority of research shows no consistent effects of low-GI diets on heart disease risk.[13] One author concludes that there is a minimal role for the implementation of low-GI diets in the prevention or treatment of heart disease.[14]
- *Appetite and weight loss.* Research shows that low-GI foods can slow the after-meal rise in blood glucose, supporting the hypothesis that such foods may promote satiety and suppress hunger.[15] Research results are inconsistent, however, on whether low-GI diets assist in weight loss.[16]

Given the mixed results of research studies on chronic disease prevention, are there any benefits associated with consuming low-GI foods?

Yes, if the low-GI foods are nutrient-dense, high-fiber foods. Not all low-GI foods meet these criteria: note that cakes, cookies, and candy bars may have a low GI due to their high fat content. Thus, a food's GI should be considered along with other nutrient criteria when assessing the health benefits.

The GI can be a helpful tool for choosing the most healthful food from a food group. For example, low-GI breakfast cereals tend to be high in fiber and low in added sugars, whereas high-GI cereals tend to be those that contain refined flours and significant amounts of added sugars. In other words, low-GI foods are often wholesome foods that have been minimally processed.

In general, should people avoid consuming high-GI foods?

Some people assume that starchy foods such as breads and potatoes should be avoided due to their high GI values. As mentioned earlier, these foods are rarely consumed in isolation, and their GI values are reduced in a mixed meal. For example, breads often have a GI greater than 70, but adding cheese or peanut butter reduces the GI to 55 or 59, respectively. Also worth considering is that GI values often vary considerably. For example, published values for white potatoes range from 24 to 101, and many samples have values in the mid-50s.[17] For these reasons and others, some researchers believe more studies are needed to confirm whether the GI is practical or beneficial for healthy people.[18]

Given the complexity of the GI, what are the current recommendations?

The potential benefits associated with consuming low-GI diets are still under investigation. As discussed earlier, people with type 2 diabetes may benefit from limiting high-GI foods—those that produce too great a rise, or too sudden a fall, in blood glucose.[19] Additional research is needed to justify the use of diets based on the GI for preventing or treating diseases such as heart disease, obesity, or other medical problems.

At present, many nutrition scientists advocate consuming a plant-based diet that contains minimally processed grains, legumes, vegetables, and fruits. Such a diet would include abundant fiber and limited amounts of solid fats and added sugars. Undoubtedly, meals consisting of these foods would tend to have low or medium GI values.

Notes

1. American Diabetes Association, Position statement: Nutrition recommendations and interventions for diabetes, *Diabetes Care* 31 (2008): S61–78.
2. American Diabetes Association, 2008.
3. D. Thomas and E. J. Elliott, Low glycaemic index, or low glycaemic load, diets for diabetes mellitus, *Cochrane Database of Systematic Reviews* January 21, 2009, CD006296; Low glycaemic index diet and disposition index in type 2 diabetes (the Canadian trial of carbohydrates in diabetes): A randomized controlled trial, *Diabetologia* 51 (2009): 1607–1615; D. J. A. Jenkins and coauthors, Effect of a low-glycemic index or a high-cereal fiber diet on type 2 diabetes, *Journal of the American Medical Association* 300 (2008): 2742–2753; G. Riccardi, A. A. Rivellese, and R. Giacco, Role of glycemic index and glycemic load in the healthy state, in prediabetes, and in diabetes, *American Journal of Clinical Nutrition* 87 (2008): 269S–274S.
4. G. Radulian and coauthors, Metabolic effects of low glycaemic index diets, *Nutrition Journal* 8 (2009): 5; A. W. Barclay and coauthors, Glycemic index, glycemic load, and chronic disease risk—A meta-analysis of observational studies, *American Journal of Clinical Nutrition* 87 (2008): 627–637;

J. Brand-Miller and coauthors, Carbohydrates—the good, the bad and the whole grain, *Asia Pacific Journal of Clinical Nutrition* 17 (2008): 16–19.
5. H. Hare-Bruun and coauthors, Should glycemic index and glycemic load be considered in dietary recommendations? *Nutrition Reviews* 66 (2008): 569–590.
6. F. S. Atkinson, K. Foster-Powell, and J. C. Brand-Miller, International tables of glycemic index and glycemic load values: 2008, *Diabetes Care* 31 (2008): 228–2283.
7. A. Flint and coauthors, The use of glycaemic index tables to predict glycaemic index of composite breakfast meals, *British Journal of Nutrition* 91 (2004): 979–989.
8. Riccardi, Rivellese, and Giacco, 2008.
9. Radulian and coauthors, 2009; Brand-Miller and coauthors, 2008; Barclay and coauthors, 2008; Jenkins and coauthors, 2008; K. C. Maki and coauthors, Effects of a reduced-glycemic-load diet on body weight, body composition, and cardiovascular disease risk markers in overweight and obese adults, *American Journal of Clinical Nutrition* 85 (2007): 724–734; M. A. Pereira,

Weighing in on glycemic index and body weight, *American Journal of Clinical Nutrition* 84 (2006): 677–679.

10. N. R. Sahyoun and coauthors, Dietary glycemic index and glycemic load and the risk of type 2 diabetes in older adults, *American Journal of Clinical Nutrition* 87 (2008): 126–131; A. Mosdol and coauthors, Dietary glycemic index and glycemic load are associated with high-density-lipoprotein cholesterol at baseline but not with increased risk of diabetes in the Whitehall II Study, *American Journal of Clinical Nutrition* 86 (2007): 988–994; E. B. Levitan and coauthors, Dietary glycemic index, dietary glycemic load, and cardiovascular disease in middle-aged and older Swedish men, *American Journal of Clinical Nutrition* 85 (2007): 1521–1526; R. Sichieri and coauthors, An 18-mo randomized trial of a low-glycemic-index diet and weight change in Brazilian women, *American Journal of Clinical Nutrition* 86 (2007): 707–713.

11. Radulian and coauthors, 2009; Brand-Miller and coauthors, 2008.

12. J. Howlett and M. Ashwell, Glycemic response and health: Summary of a workshop, *American Journal of Clinical Nutrition* 87 (2008): 212S–216S.

13. J. M. Shikany and coauthors, Effects of low- and high-glycemic index/glycemic load diets on coronary heart disease risk factors in overweight/obese men, *Metabolism* 58 (2009): 1793–1801; E. B. Levitan and coauthors, Dietary glycemic index, dietary glycemic load, blood lipids, and C-reactive protein, *Metabolism* 58 (2009): 1793–1801: M. J. Franz, Is there a role for the glycemic index in coronary heart disease prevention or treatment? *Current Atherosclerosis Reports* 10 (2008): 497–502; J. E. Milton and coauthors, Relationship of glycaemic index with cardiovascular risk factors: Analysis of the National Diet and Nutrition Survey for people aged 65 and older, *Public Health Nutrition* 10 (2007): 1321–1335.

14. Franz, 2008.

15. R. C. Reynolds and coauthors, Effect of the glycemic index of carbohydrates on day-long (10 h) profiles of plasma glucose, insulin, cholecystokinin and ghrelin, *European Journal of Clinical Nutrition* 63 (2009): 872–878; S. Pal, S. Lim, and G. Egger, The effect of a low glycaemic index breakfast on blood glucose, insulin, lipid profiles, blood pressure, body weight, body composition and satiety in obese and overweight individuals: A pilot study, *Journal of the American College of Nutrition* 27 (2008): 387–393.

16. M. A. Mendez and coauthors, Glycemic load, glycemic index, and body mass index in Spanish adults, *American Journal of Clinical Nutrition* 89 (2009): 316–322; D. E. Thomas, E. J. Elliott, and L. Baur, Low glycaemic index or low glycaemic load diets for overweight and obesity, *Cochrane Database of Systematic Reviews*, July 18, 2007: CD005105; C. B. Ebbeling and coauthors, Effects of a low-glycemic load vs. low-fat diet in obese young adults, *Journal of the American Medical Association* 297 (2007): 2092–2102; R. Sichieri and coauthors, An 18-mo randomized trial of a low-glycemic-index diet and weight change in Brazilian women, *American Journal of Clinical Nutrition* 86 (2007): 707–713; S. K. Das and coauthors, Long-term effects of 2 energy-restricted diets differing in glycemic load on dietary adherence, body composition, and metabolism in CALERIE: A 10y randomized controlled trial, *American Journal of Clinical Nutrition* 85 (2007): 1023–1030.

17. Atkinson, Foster-Powell, and Brand-Miller, 2008.

18. H. Hare-Bruun and coauthors, Should glycemic index and glycemic load be considered in dietary recommendations? *Nutrition Reviews* 66 (2008): 569–590.

19. Riccardi, Rivellese, and Giacco, 2008.

© age fotostock/SuperStock

CHAPTER 4 | Lipids

CONTENTS

MOST PEOPLE KNOW THAT TOO MUCH FAT, ESPECIALLY CERTAIN KINDS OF fat, in the diet imposes health risks, but they may be surprised to learn that too little does, too. People in the United States, however, are more likely to eat too much fat than too little.

Fat is a member of the class of compounds called **lipids**. The lipids in foods and in the human body include triglycerides (**fats** and **oils**), phospholipids, and sterols.

Roles of Body Fat

Lipids perform many tasks in the body, but most importantly, they provide energy. A constant flow of energy is so vital to life that, in a pinch, any other function is sacrificed to maintain it. Chapter 3 described one safeguard against such an emergency—the stores of glycogen in the liver that provide glucose to the blood whenever the supply runs short. The body's stores of glycogen are limited, however. In contrast, the body's capacity to store fat for energy is virtually unlimited due to the fat-storing cells of the **adipose tissue**. The fat cells of the adipose tissue readily take up and store fat, growing in size as they do so. When extra energy storage is needed, new fat cells are readily produced. Fat cells are more than just storage depots, however; fat cells secrete hormones that help to regulate the appetite and influence other body functions.[1] Figure 4-1 shows a fat cell.

The fat stored in fat cells supplies 60 percent of the body's ongoing energy needs during rest. During some types of physical activity or prolonged periods of food deprivation, (✚) fat stores may make an even greater energy contribution. The brain and nerves, however, need their energy as glucose, and the body cannot convert fat to glucose. After a long period of glucose deprivation (during fasting or starvation), brain and nerve cells develop the ability to derive about half of their energy from a special form of fat known as **ketones**, but they still require glucose as well. This means that

✚ Chapter 6 discusses fat use during fasting.

lipids: a family of compounds that includes triglycerides (fats and oils), phospholipids, and sterols. Lipids are characterized by their insolubility in water.

fats: lipids that are solid at room temperature (70°F or 21°C).

oils: lipids that are liquid at room temperature (70°F or 21°C).

adipose tissue: the body's fat, which consists of masses of fat-storing cells called adipose cells.

ketones (KEY-tones): acidic, fat-related compounds formed from the incomplete breakdown of fat when carbohydrate is not available; technically known as *ketone* bodies.

| FIGURE 4-1 | A Fat Cell |

Muscle tissue

Fat tissue

Blood capillaries

FAT CELL

Lipids enter from blood

Lipids exit to blood

Nucleus

Cell membrane

Within the fat, or adipose, cell, lipid is stored in a droplet. This droplet can greatly enlarge, and the fat cell membrane will expand to accommodate its swollen contents.

TABLE
4-1 | The Functions of Fats in the Body

Fats in the body:

- *Energy stores.* Fats are the body's chief form of stored energy.

- *Muscle fuel.* Fats provide most of the energy to fuel muscular work.

- *Emergency reserve.* Fats serve as an emergency fuel supply in times of illness and diminished food intake.

- *Padding.* Fats protect the internal organs from shock through fat pads inside the body cavity.

- *Insulation.* Fats insulate against temperature extremes through a fat layer under the skin.

- *Cell membranes.* Fats form the major material of cell membranes.

- *Raw materials.* Fats are converted to other compounds, such as hormones, bile, and vitamin D, as needed.

people wanting to lose weight need to eat a certain minimum amount of carbohydrate to meet their energy needs, even when they are limiting their food intakes.

In addition to supplying energy, fat serves other roles in the body. Natural oils in the skin provide a radiant complexion; in the scalp, they help nourish the hair and make it glossy. The layer of fat beneath the skin insulates the body from extremes of temperature. A pad of hard fat beneath each kidney protects it from being jarred and damaged, even during a motorcycle ride on a bumpy road. The soft fat in a woman's breasts protects her mammary glands from heat and cold and cushions them against shock. The fat embedded in muscle tissue shares with muscle glycogen the task of providing energy when the muscles are active. The phospholipids and the sterol cholesterol are cell membrane constituents that help maintain the structure and health of all cells. Table 4-1 summarizes the major functions of fats in the body.

Echo/Jupiter Images

Body fat supplies much of the fuel that muscles need to do their work.

Review Notes

- Lipids in the body not only serve as energy reserves but also protect the body from temperature extremes, cushion the vital organs, and provide the major material of cell membranes.

The Chemist's View of Lipids

The diverse and vital functions that lipids play in the body reveal why eating too little fat can be harmful. As mentioned earlier, though, too much fat in the diet seems to be the greater problem for most people. To understand both the beneficial and harmful effects that fats exert on the body, a closer look at the structure and function of members of the lipid family is in order.

TRIGLYCERIDES

When people talk about fat—for example, "I'm too fat" or "That meat is fatty"—they are usually referring to triglycerides. Among lipids, **triglycerides** predominate—both in the diet and in the body. The name triglyceride almost explains itself: three (tri) **fatty acids** attached to a **glycerol** "backbone." Figure 4-2 (p. 94) shows how three fatty acids combine with glycerol to make a triglyceride.

triglycerides (try-GLISS-er-rides): one of the main classes of lipids; the chief form of fat in foods and the major storage form of fat in the body; composed of glycerol with three fatty acids attached.
tri = three
glyceride = a compound of glycerol

fatty acids: organic compounds composed of a chain of carbon atoms with hydrogen atoms attached and an acid group at one end.

glycerol (GLISS-er-ol): an organic compound, three carbons long, that can form the backbone of triglycerides and phospholipids.

FATTY ACIDS

When energy from any energy-yielding nutrient is to be stored as fat, the nutrient is first broken into small fragments. Then the fragments are linked together into chains known as fatty acids. The fatty acids are then packaged, three at a time, with glycerol to make triglycerides.

Chain Length and Saturation Fatty acids may differ from one another in two ways—in chain length and in degree of saturation. The chain length refers to the number of carbons in a fatty acid. Saturation also refers to its chemical structure—specifically, to the number of hydrogen atoms the carbons in the fatty acid are holding. If every available carbon is filled to capacity with hydrogen atoms, the chain is called a **saturated fatty acid**. A saturated fatty acid is fully loaded with hydrogen atoms and has only single bonds between the carbons. The first zigzag structure in Figure 4-3 represents a saturated fatty acid.

Unsaturated Fatty Acids In some fatty acids, including most of those in plants and fish, hydrogen atoms are missing in the fatty acid chains. The places where the hydrogen atoms are missing are called points of unsaturation, and a chain containing such points is called an **unsaturated fatty acid**. An unsaturated fatty acid has at least one double bond between its carbons. If there is one point of

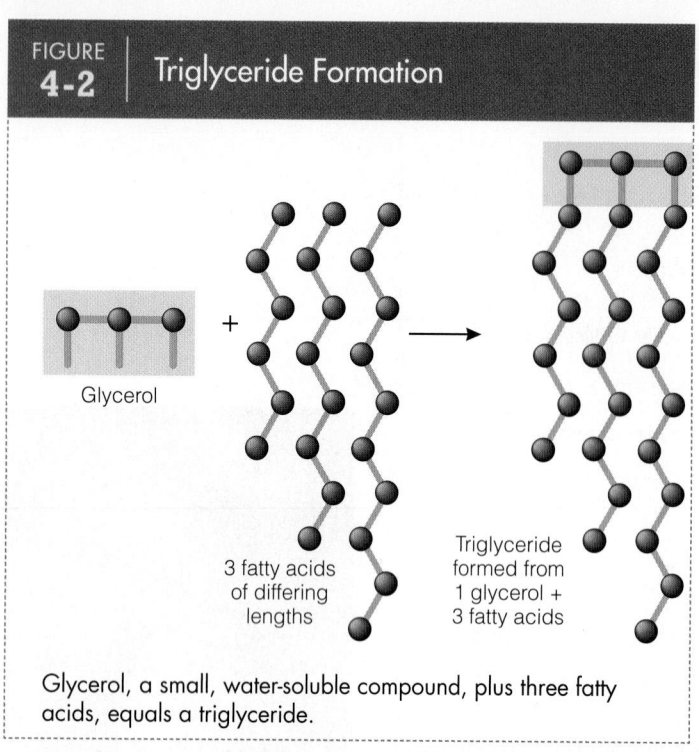

FIGURE 4-2 | Triglyceride Formation

Glycerol

+

3 fatty acids of differing lengths

Triglyceride formed from 1 glycerol + 3 fatty acids

Glycerol, a small, water-soluble compound, plus three fatty acids, equals a triglyceride.

saturated fatty acid: a fatty acid carrying the maximum possible number of hydrogen atoms (having no points of unsaturation).

unsaturated fatty acid: a fatty acid with one or more points of unsaturation where hydrogen atoms are missing (includes monounsaturated and polyunsaturated fatty acids).

monounsaturated fatty acid (MUFA): a fatty acid that has one point of unsaturation; for example, the oleic acid found in olive oil.

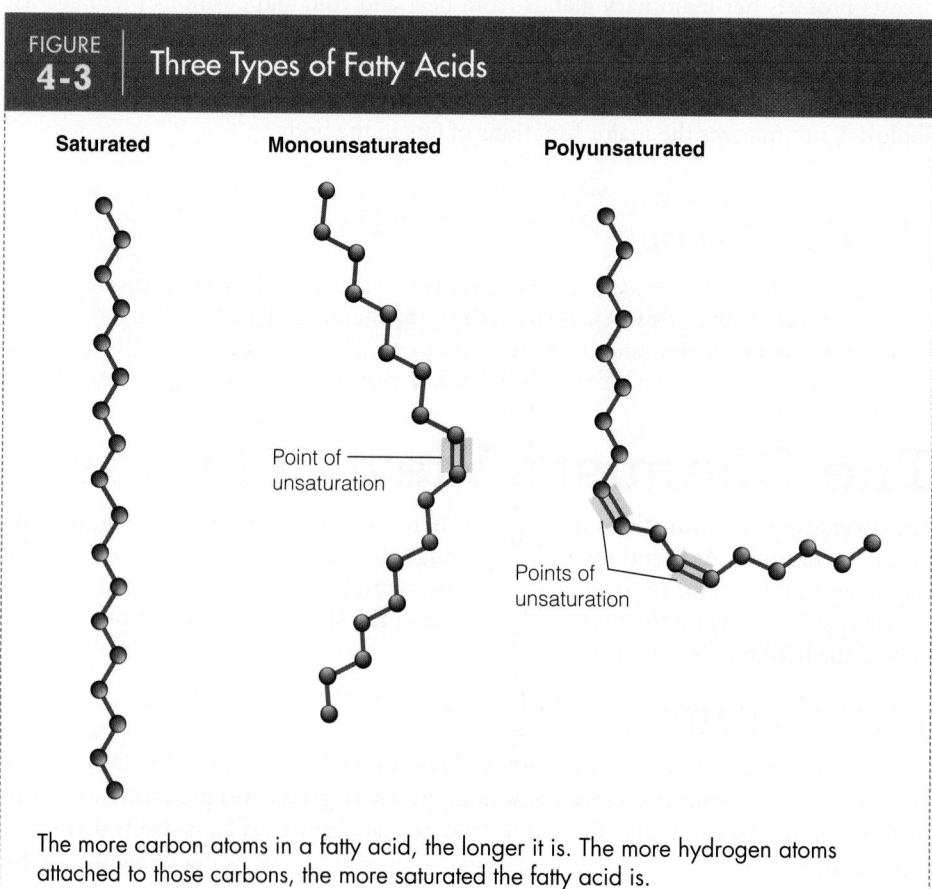

FIGURE 4-3 | Three Types of Fatty Acids

Saturated

Monounsaturated

Polyunsaturated

Point of unsaturation

Points of unsaturation

The more carbon atoms in a fatty acid, the longer it is. The more hydrogen atoms attached to those carbons, the more saturated the fatty acid is.

unsaturation, the chain is a **monounsaturated fatty acid**. The second structure in Figure 4-3 is an example. If there are two or more points of unsaturation, then the fatty acid is a **polyunsaturated fatty acid** (see the third structure in Figure 4-3).

Hard and Soft Fat A triglyceride can contain any combination of fatty acids—long chain or short chain and saturated, monounsaturated, or polyunsaturated. The degree of saturation of the fatty acids in a fat influences the health of the body (discussed in a later section) and the characteristics of foods. Fats that contain the shorter-chain or the more unsaturated fatty acids are softer at room temperature and melt more readily. A comparison of three fats—lard (which comes from pork), chicken fat, and safflower oil—illustrates these differences: lard is the most saturated and the hardest; chicken fat is less saturated and somewhat soft; and safflower oil, which is the most unsaturated, is a liquid at room temperature.

Stability Saturation also influences stability. Fats can become **rancid** when exposed to oxygen. Polyunsaturated fatty acids spoil most readily because their double bonds are unstable. The **oxidation** of unsaturated fats produces a variety of compounds that smell and taste rancid; saturated fats are more resistant to oxidation and thus less likely to become rancid. Other types of spoilage can occur due to microbial growth, however.

Manufacturers can protect fat-containing products against rancidity in three ways—none of them perfect. First, products may be sealed airtight and refrigerated—an expensive and inconvenient storage system. Second, manufacturers may add **antioxidants** to compete for the oxygen and thus protect the oil (examples are the additives **BHA** and **BHT** and vitamins C and E).* Third, manufacturers may saturate some or all of the points of unsaturation by adding hydrogen atoms—a process known as hydrogenation.

Hydrogenation **Hydrogenation** offers two advantages: it protects against oxidation (thereby prolonging shelf life) and also alters the texture of foods by increasing the solidity of fats. When partially hydrogenated, vegetable oils become spreadable margarine. Hydrogenated fats make piecrusts flaky and puddings creamy. A disadvantage is that hydrogenation makes polyunsaturated fats more saturated. Consequently, any health advantages of using polyunsaturated fats instead of saturated fats are lost in hydrogenation.

Trans-Fatty Acids Another disadvantage of hydrogenation is that some of the molecules that remain unsaturated after processing change shape from *cis* to *trans*. In nature, most unsaturated fatty acids are *cis*-fatty acids—meaning that the hydrogen atoms next to the double bonds are on the same side of the carbon chain. Only a few fatty acids in nature (notably a small percentage of those found in milk and meat products) are *trans*-**fatty acids**—meaning that the hydrogen atoms next to the double bonds are on opposite sides of the carbon chain (see Figure 4-4 on p. 96). These arrangements result in different configurations for the fatty acids, and this difference affects function: in the body, *trans*-fatty acids behave more like saturated fats than like unsaturated fats. The relationship between *trans*-fatty acids and heart disease is the subject of much ongoing research, as a later section describes.

Essential Fatty Acids The human body can synthesize all the fatty acids it needs from carbohydrate, fat, or protein except for two—**linoleic acid** and **linolenic acid**. Both linoleic acid and linolenic acid are polyunsaturated fatty acids. Because they cannot be made from other substances in the body, they must be obtained from food and are therefore called **essential fatty acids**. Linoleic acid and linolenic acid are found in small amounts in plant oils, and the body readily stores them, making deficiencies unlikely. From both of these essential fatty acids, the body makes important substances that help regulate a wide range of body functions: blood pressure, clot formation, blood lipid concentration, the immune response, the inflammatory response to injury, and many others.[2] These two essential nutrients also serve as structural components of cell membranes.

---

* BHA is butylated hydroxyanisole; BHT is butylated hydroxytolvene.

polyunsaturated fatty acids (PUFA): fatty acids with two or more points of unsaturation. For example, linoleic acid has two such points, and linolenic acid has three. Thus, polyunsaturated *fat* is composed of triglycerides containing a high percentage of PUFA.

rancid: the term used to describe fats when they have deteriorated, usually by oxidation. Rancid fats often have an "off" odor.

oxidation (OKS-ee-day-shun): the process of a substance combining with oxygen.

antioxidants: as a food additive, preservatives that delay or prevent rancidity of foods and other damage to food caused by oxygen.

BHA, BHT: preservatives commonly used to slow the development of "off" flavors, odors, and color changes caused by oxidation.

hydrogenation (high-dro-gen-AY-shun): a chemical process by which hydrogen atoms are added to monounsaturated or polyunsaturated fats to reduce the number of double bonds, making the fats more saturated (solid) and more resistant to oxidation (protecting against rancidity). Hydrogenation produces *trans*-fatty acids.

***trans*-fatty acids:** fatty acids in which the hydrogen atoms next to the double bond are on opposite sides of the carbon chain.

linoleic acid, linolenic acid: polyunsaturated fatty acids that are essential for human beings.

essential fatty acids: fatty acids that the body requires but cannot make in amounts sufficient to meet its physiological needs.

FIGURE
4-4 | *Cis-* and *Trans-*Fatty Acids Compared

*Cis-*fatty acid

*Trans-*fatty acid

+ Chemists use the term *omega*, the last letter of the Greek alphabet, to refer to the position of the last double bond in a fatty acid.

+ Reminder: Emulsifiers are substances that mix with both fat and water and are able to dispense the fat in the water, forming an emulsion.

omega-6 fatty acid: a polyunsaturated fatty acid with its endmost double bond six carbons back from the end of its carbon chain; long recognized as important in nutrition. Linoleic acid is an example.

omega-3 fatty acids: polyunsaturated fatty acids in which the endmost double bond is three carbons back from the end of the carbon chain; relatively newly recognized as important in nutrition. Linolenic acid is an example.

EPA, DHA: omega-3 fatty acids made from linolenic acid. The full name for EPA is *eicosapentaenoic* (EYE-cosa-PENTA-ee-NO-ick) *acid*. The full name for DHA is *docosahexaenoic* (DOE-cosa-HEXA-ee-NO-ick) *acid*.

phospholipids: one of the three main classes of lipids; compounds that are similar to triglycerides but have *choline* (or another compound) and a phosphorus-containing acid in place of one of the fatty acids.

lecithins: one type of phospholipid.

choline: a nonessential nutrient that can be made in the body from an amino acid.

TABLE 4-2	The Lipid Family

Triglycerides (fats and oils)
- Glycerol (1 per triglyceride)
- Fatty acids (3 per triglyceride)
  Saturated
  Monounsaturated
  Polyunsaturated
     Omega-6
     Omega-3

Phospholipids (such as the lecithins)

Sterols (such as cholesterol)

Linoleic Acid: An Omega-6 Fatty Acid

Linoleic acid is an **omega-6 fatty acid,** (+) found in the seeds of plants and in the oils produced from the seeds. Any diet that contains vegetable oils, seeds, nuts, and whole-grain foods provides enough linoleic acid to meet the body's needs. Researchers have long known and appreciated the importance of the omega-6 fatty acid family.

Linolenic Acid and Other Omega-3 Fatty Acids

Linolenic acid belongs to a family of polyunsaturated fatty acids known as **omega-3 fatty acids**, a family that also includes **EPA** and **DHA**. EPA and DHA are found primarily in fish oils. As mentioned, the human body cannot make linolenic acid, but given dietary linolenic acid, it can make EPA and DHA, although the process is slow.

The importance of omega-3 fatty acids was first recognized during the 1980s when research began to unveil impressive roles for EPA and DHA in metabolism and disease prevention. The brain has a high content of DHA, and both EPA and DHA are needed for normal brain development.[3] DHA is also especially active in the rods and cones of the retina of the eye.[4] Today, researchers know that these omega-3 fatty acids are essential for normal growth and development and that they may play an important role in the prevention and treatment of heart disease, diabetes, hypertension, arthritis, and cancer.[5]

PHOSPHOLIPIDS

Up to now, this discussion has focused on one class of lipids, the triglycerides (fats and oils), and their component parts, the fatty acids (see Table 4-2). Two other classes of lipids, the **phospholipids** and sterols, make up only 5 percent of the lipids in the diet, but they are nevertheless worthy of attention. Among the phospholipids, the lecithins are of particular interest.

Structure of Phospholipids

Like the triglycerides, the **lecithins** and other phospholipids have a backbone of glycerol; they differ from the triglycerides in having only two fatty acids attached to the glycerol. In place of the third fatty acid, they have a phosphate group (a phosphorus-containing acid) and a molecule of **choline** or a similar compound. The fatty acids make the phospholipids soluble in fat; the phosphate group enables them to dissolve in water. Such versatility benefits the food industry, which uses phospholipids as emulsifiers to mix fats with water in such products as mayonnaise and candy bars. (+)

Phospholipids in Foods

In addition to the phospholipids used by the food industry as emulsifiers, phospholipids are also found naturally in foods. The richest food sources of lecithin are eggs, liver, soybeans, wheat germ, and peanuts.

Roles of Phospholipids Lecithins and other phospholipids are important constituents of cell membranes. They also act as emulsifiers in the body, helping to keep other fats in solution in the watery blood and body fluids.

Phospholipids: Not Essential Lecithins periodically receive attention in the popular press. People may hear that lecithins are a major constituent of cell membranes (true), that the functioning of all cells depends on the integrity of the cell membranes (true), and that consumers must therefore take lecithin supplements (false). The body digests lecithins before it absorbs them, so the lecithins people eat do not reach the body tissues intact. Instead, the lecithins used for building cell membranes are made from scratch by the liver. In other words, the lecithins are not essential nutrients.

STEROLS

Sterols are large, complex molecules consisting of interconnected rings of carbon. Cholesterol is the most familiar sterol, but others, such as vitamin D and the sex hormones (for example, testosterone), are important, too.

Sterols in Foods Foods derived from both plants and animals contain sterols, but only those from animals—meats, eggs, fish, poultry, and dairy products—contain significant amounts of cholesterol. Organ meats, such as liver and kidneys, and eggs are richest in cholesterol; cheeses and meats have less. Shellfish contain many sterols but much less cholesterol than was previously thought.

Sterols other than cholesterol are naturally found in plants. Being structurally similar to cholesterol, plant sterols interfere with cholesterol absorption. By inhibiting cholesterol absorption, a diet rich in plant sterols lowers blood cholesterol levels.[6] Food manufacturers have fortified foods such as margarine with plant sterols, creating a functional food that helps to reduce blood cholesterol.

Cholesterol Synthesis Like the lecithins, cholesterol can be made by the body, so it is not an essential nutrient. Your liver is manufacturing it now, as you read. The raw materials that the liver uses to make cholesterol can all be taken from glucose or fatty acids. In other words, cholesterol can be made from either carbohydrate or fat. Most of the body's cholesterol ends up in the membranes of cells, where it performs vital structural and metabolic functions.

Cholesterol's Two Routes in the Body After being made, cholesterol leaves the liver by two routes:

1. It may be made into bile, stored in the gallbladder, and delivered to the intestine. (✚)
2. It may travel, via the bloodstream, to all the body's cells.

The bile that is made from cholesterol in the liver is released into the intestine to aid in the digestion and absorption of fat. After bile does its job, most of it is reabsorbed into the body and recycled; the rest is excreted in the feces.

Cholesterol Excreted While bile is in the intestine, some of it may be trapped by soluble fibers or by some medications, which carry it out of the body in feces. The excretion of bile reduces the total amount of cholesterol remaining in the body.

Cholesterol Transport Recall from Chapter 2 that some cholesterol, packaged with other lipids and protein, leaves the liver via the arteries and is transported to the body tissues by the blood. (✚) These packages of lipids and proteins are called lipoproteins. As the lipoproteins travel through the body, tissues can extract lipids from them. Cholesterol's harmful effects in the body occur when it forms deposits in the artery walls. These deposits contribute to **atherosclerosis**, a disease that can cause heart attacks and strokes.

✚ Reminder: Bile is a compound made by the liver from cholesterol and stored in the gallbladder. Bile prepares fat for digestion.

✚ Both the intestine and the liver make lipoproteins. Chapter 2 tells the story of lipid transport.

sterols: one of the main classes of lipids; includes cholesterol, vitamin D, and the sex hormones (such as testosterone).

atherosclerosis (ath-er-oh-scler-OH-sis): a type of artery disease characterized by accumulations of lipid-containing material on the inner walls of the arteries (see Chapter 21).

Review Notes

- Table 4-2 summarizes the members of the lipid family.
- The predominant lipids both in foods and in the body are triglycerides, which have glycerol backbones with three fatty acids attached.
- Fatty acids vary in the length of their carbon chains and their degree of saturation. Those that are fully loaded with hydrogen atoms are saturated; those that are missing hydrogen atoms and therefore have double bonds are unsaturated (monounsaturated or polyunsaturated).
- Most triglycerides contain more than one type of fatty acid.
- Fatty acid saturation affects the physical characteristics and storage properties of fats.
- Hydrogenation, which makes polyunsaturated fats more saturated, gives rise to trans-fatty acids, altered fatty acids that may have health effects similar to those of saturated fatty acids.
- Linoleic acid and linolenic acid are essential nutrients. In addition to serving as structural parts of cell membranes, they make powerful substances that help regulate blood pressure, blood clot formation, and the immune response.
- Phospholipids, including the lecithins, have a unique chemical structure that allows them to be soluble in both water and fat.
- In the body, phospholipids are major constituents of cell membranes; the food industry uses phospholipids as emulsifiers.
- Sterols include cholesterol, bile, vitamin D, and the sex hormones.
- Only animal-derived foods contain significant amounts of cholesterol.

Health Effects and Recommended Intakes of Fats

Of all the dietary factors related to chronic diseases prevalent in developed countries, high intakes of certain fats are by far the most significant. The person who chooses a diet too high in saturated fats or *trans* fats invites the risk of **cardiovascular disease (CVD)**, and heart disease is the number one killer of adults in the United States and Canada. As for cancer, evidence is less compelling than for heart disease, but it does suggest that a diet high in certain kinds of fat is associated with a greater-than-average risk of developing some types of cancer.[7] Conversely, some research suggests that omega-3 fatty acids from fish may protect against some cancers.[8] Nutrition and cancer is a topic of Chapter 23. Obesity carries serious risks to health, and the high energy density of fatty foods makes it easy for people to exceed their energy needs and so gain unneeded weight. The health risks of obesity are described in Chapter 6, and Chapter 7 focuses on weight management. The links between diet and disease are the focus of much research. Some points about fats and heart health are presented here because they underlie dietary recommendations concerning fats. Nutrition and heart disease is the topic of Chapter 21.

FATS AND HEART HEALTH

As noted earlier and described in Chapter 2, cholesterol travels in the blood within lipoproteins. Two of the lipoproteins, LDL and HDL, play major roles with regard to heart health and are the focus of most recommendations made for reducing the risk of heart disease. A high blood LDL cholesterol concentration is a predictor of the likelihood of suffering a fatal heart attack or stroke, and the higher the LDL, the earlier the episode is expected to occur. Conversely, high HDL cholesterol signifies a *lower* disease risk.

cardiovascular disease (CVD): a general term for all diseases of the heart and blood vessels (see Chapter 21).

Most people realize that elevated blood cholesterol is an important risk factor for heart disease. Most people may not realize, though, that cholesterol in *food* is not the main influential factor in raising *blood* cholesterol.

Saturated Fats and Blood Cholesterol The main dietary factors associated with elevated blood LDL cholesterol are high saturated fat and high *trans* fat intakes.*[9] LDL cholesterol indicates a risk of heart disease because high LDL concentrations promote the uptake of cholesterol in the blood vessel walls.

Fats from animal sources are the main contributors of saturated fats in most people's diets. (✚) Some vegetable fats (coconut oil, palm kernel oil, and palm oil) and hydrogenated fats such as shortening or stick margarine provide smaller amounts of saturated fats. To minimize intake of saturated fat, most people need to eat less meat. When eating meat, choose the leanest cuts, and trim away the visible fat.[10] Selecting fat-free milk and using nonhydrogenated margarine and unsaturated cooking oil such as olive oil, safflower oil, or canola oil are other simple changes that can dramatically lower saturated fat intake and heart disease risk. (✚)

Trans-Fatty Acids and Blood Cholesterol Consuming fats with *trans*-fatty acids poses a risk to the health of the heart and arteries by raising LDL and lowering HDL cholesterol, and by producing inflammation.[11] When news of *trans*-fatty acids' effects on heart health was first emerging, some people hastily switched from using margarine back to butter, believing oversimplified reports that margarine provided no heart health advantage over butter. It is true that hard margarines and virtually all shortenings are made from mostly hydrogenated fats and therefore contain substantial *trans*-fatty acids. (✚) Since the requirement that *trans* fats be listed on the Nutrition Facts panel of food labels took effect in 2006, however, margarine makers have reformulated their products to contain much less *trans* fat.[12] Soft or liquid varieties are made from unhydrogenated oils, which are mostly unsaturated and so are less likely to elevate blood cholesterol than the saturated fats of butter. Some margarines contain olive oil, omega-3 fatty acids, or plant sterols (mentioned earlier), making these products preferable to butter and other margarines for the heart.†

With more than 50 types of margarines and spreads on the market in sticks, tubs, sprays, and liquids, consumers must educate themselves, read labels, and select margarines that provide the preferred flavor with the least saturated and *trans* fat. When oils (but not hydrogenated oils) are the first ingredient listed on a margarine label, that margarine is probably low in both *trans*-fatty acids and saturated fat. In general, margarine contributes less *trans* fat to the average diet than do other contributors such as processed foods.

Simply adding margarine that contains plant sterols, olive oil, or omega-3 fatty acids to a high-fat diet is unlikely to bring benefits. These substances cannot undo the damage from a diet consistently high in saturated fats. Margarines with plant sterols have drawbacks, too. They cost three or four times more than regular margarine, they equal regular margarine in kcalories, and they are not proven safe for use by certain populations, such as growing children.

Many foods other than margarine also contribute *trans*-fatty acids. (✚) Fast foods, chips, baked goods, and other commercially prepared foods are high in fats containing up to 50 percent *trans*-fatty acids. The 2006 labeling requirement to list *trans* fat on packaged food has prompted many food manufacturers to eliminate or greatly reduce *trans* fats in foods. Many restaurants have also taken steps to eliminate or reduce *trans* fats from their menu items.[13] The average daily intake of *trans*-fatty acids in the United States is about 6 grams per day—mostly from products that have been hydrogenated.

Dietary Cholesterol and Blood Cholesterol Dietary cholesterol has also been implicated in raising blood cholesterol and increasing the risk of heart disease, although its effect is not as strong as that of saturated fat or *trans* fat. Still, health experts advise limiting cholesterol intake.

---

* It should be noted that not all saturated fatty acids have the same cholesterol-raising effect. Stearic acid, an 18-carbon fatty acid, does not seem to raise blood cholesterol.
† Two brand names of margarines with plant sterols currently on the market are *Benecol* and *Take Control*.

✚ Major sources of saturated fats:
- Whole milk (and even reduced-fat milk), cheese, butter, cream, cream cheese, sour cream, and ice cream
- Fatty cuts of beef and pork, and processed meats such as bacon, sausage, and hot dogs
- Tropical oils (coconut, palm, and palm kernel) and products that contain them such as cakes, cookies, doughnuts, and pastries
- Shortening and lard

✚ Nutrition in Practice 4 examines various types of fats and their roles in supporting or harming heart health.

✚ The words *hydrogenated vegetable oil or shortening* in an ingredients list indicate *trans*-fatty acids in the product.

✚ Major food sources of *trans* fats:
- Cakes, cookies, pies, doughnuts, and crackers
- Meat and dairy products
- Hard margarine
- Fried potatoes and other commercial fried foods such as chicken
- Potato chips and corn chips
- Shortening

Grilling or broiling fish, instead of frying them, preserves their beneficial omega-3 fatty acids while adding little or no saturated fat.

© FoodCollection/Stockfood America

Recall that cholesterol is found primarily in foods derived from animals. Consequently, eating less fat from meats, eggs, and milk products helps lower dietary cholesterol intake (as well as total and saturated fat intakes). (+)

Monounsaturated Fatty Acids and Blood

Cholesterol Replacing saturated and *trans* fats with monounsaturated fat such as olive oil may be an effective dietary strategy to prevent heart disease.(+) The lower rates of heart disease among people in the Mediterranean region of the world are often attributed to their liberal use of olive oil, a rich source of monounsaturated fatty acids.[14] Olive oil also delivers valuable phytochemicals that help to protect against heart disease.[15] Nutrition in Practice 4 examines the role of olive oil and other fats in supporting or harming heart health.

Polyunsaturated Fatty Acids, Blood Cholesterol, and Heart Disease Risk

Polyunsaturated fatty acids (PUFA) of the omega-6 and omega-3 families are potent protectors against heart disease. The primary omega-6 fatty acid, linoleic acid, which is found in vegetable oils such as corn and sunflower oil, exerts most of its beneficial effect by lowering both total blood cholesterol and LDL cholesterol.[16] (+)

The omega-3 fatty acids EPA and DHA, which are found mainly in fatty fish, exert their beneficial effects by influencing the function of both the heart and blood vessels. Specifically, EPA and DHA protect heart health by:[17]

- Lowering blood triglycerides.
- Preventing blood clots.
- Protecting against irregular heartbeats.
- Lowering blood pressure.
- Defending against inflammation.

The primary member of the omega-3 family, linolenic acid, may benefit heart health as well, but evidence for this effect is much less certain than for EPA and DHA. Table 4-3 provides sources of omega-6 and omega-3 fatty acids.

Balance Omega-6 and Omega-3 Intakes

The U.S. diet is high in omega-6 fatty acids (due to the increased production and use of vegetable cooking oils such as corn and cottonseed oils) and low in omega-3 fatty acids. Experts recommend a more balanced intake. The best way for people to increase their intakes of omega-3 fatty acids is to follow the advice of the American Heart Association: eat at least two servings of fatty fish (see Table NP4-1 on p. 114) each week.[18] Even one fish meal per week has been associated with a reduced risk of heart disease.[19]

Greater heart health benefits can be expected when fish is grilled, baked, or broiled, partly because the varieties prepared this way often contain more EPA and DHA than species used for fried fish in fast-food restaurants and frozen products. Additionally, benefits are attained by avoiding commercial frying fats, which are often laden with *trans* fat and saturated fat. Further benefits arise when fish replaces high-fat meats or other foods rich in saturated fats in several meals each week.

Some species of fish and shellfish, however, may contain significant levels of mercury or other environmental contaminants. Most healthy people can safely consume most species of ocean fish several times a week, but some people face greater risks. Women who may become pregnant, pregnant and lactating women, and children are more sensitive to contaminants than others, but even they can benefit from safer fish varieties within recommended limits (see Chapter 10 for details).

For everyone, consuming a variety of different types of fish is a good idea to minimize exposure to any single toxin that may accumulate in a favored species. The margin lists the species most heavily contaminated with mercury and those that are low in mercury. (+) As for freshwater fish in some areas, consumers should check local advisories about the safety of fish caught by family and friends.

Omega-3 Supplements

Fish, not fish oil supplements, is the preferred source of omega-3 fatty acids, except for persons with cardiovascular disease who cannot obtain enough EPA and DHA from fish, and then only under a physician's supervision.[20] Supplements of 2 grams a day of EPA or more than 3 grams of fish oil

TABLE 4-3	Food Sources of Omega-6 and Omega-3 Fatty Acids	
Omega-6		
Linoleic acid	Leafy vegetables, seeds, nuts, grains, vegetable oils (corn, cottonseed, safflower, sesame, soybean, sunflower), poultry fat	
Omega-3		
Linolenic acid[a]	Oils (canola, flaxseed, soybean, walnut, wheat germ; liquid or soft margarine made from canola or soybean oil)	
	Nuts and seeds (flaxseeds, walnuts, soybeans)	
	Vegetables (soybeans)	
EPA and DHA	Human milk	
	Fatty coldwater fish and other seafood (see Table NP4-1)	

[a] Alpha-linolenic acid. Also found in the seed oil of the herb *evening primrose*.

interfere with blood clotting and cause prolonged bleeding times.[21] Supplements also lack the *other* beneficial nutrients that fish provides. Some fish oil supplements also taste fishy, and people often complain of a lingering or repeating taste for hours after taking them.

Finally, fish oil supplements are made from fish skins and livers, which can accumulate toxic concentrations of dioxins and other industrial contaminants from polluted waters.[‡22] As stated earlier, mercury contamination is also a problem in the flesh of both freshwater and saltwater species. For supplements, newer processing methods can rid fish oil of most contaminants but not all supplements are refined in this way. In addition to contamination, fish liver oil naturally contains high levels of the two most potentially toxic vitamins, A and D. Lastly, supplements of fish oil are expensive—they must be purchased in addition to food, while fatty fish replaces other protein foods that would have been purchased instead.

RECOMMENDATIONS

Some fat in the diet is essential for good health, but too much fat, especially saturated fat and *trans* fat, increases the risks of chronic diseases. Defining the exact amount of fat, saturated fat, or cholesterol that benefits health or begins to harm health, however, is not possible. For this reason, no RDA or Upper Level has been set.[23] Instead, the DRI and *Dietary Guidelines* suggest a diet that is low in saturated fat, *trans* fat, and cholesterol and provides 20 to 35 percent of the daily energy intake from fat. (✚) These recommendations recognize that diets with up to 35 percent of kcalories from fat can be compatible with good health if energy intake is reasonable and saturated and *trans* fat intakes are low. When total fat intake exceeds 35 percent of kcalories, saturated fat intakes increase to unhealthy levels.[24] Fat and oil intakes below 20 percent of kcalories increase the risk of inadequate essential fatty acid intakes. The FDA established Daily Values on food labels using 30 percent of energy intake as the guideline for fat. (✚)

Part of the allowance for total fat should provide for the essential fatty acids—linoleic acid and linolenic acid. Recommendations suggest that linoleic acid provide 5 to 10 percent of the daily energy intake and linolenic acid, 0.6 to 1.2 percent. (✚)

Saturated fats, *trans* fats, and cholesterol increase total blood cholesterol and LDL cholesterol and, therefore, the risk of heart disease. Even low intakes of each may elevate heart disease risk.[25] Thus, recommendations urge people to eat diets that are low in

 DRI for fat:
- 20 to 35 percent of energy intake

Dietary Guidelines for Americans:
- Keep total fat intake between 20 and 35 percent of kcalories, with most fats coming from sources of polyunsaturated and monounsaturated fatty acids, such as fish, nuts, and vegetable oils.

✚ Daily Value:
- 65 g fat (based on 30 percent of 2000 kcal diet)

✚ Linoleic acid (omega-6) AI:
- 5 to 10 percent of energy intake

Men:
- 19–50 yr: 17 g/day
- 51+ yr: 14 g/day

Women:
- 19–50 yr: 12 g/day
- 51+ yr: 11 g/day

Linolenic acid (omega-3) AI:
- 0.6 to 1.2 percent of energy intake
- Men: 1.6 g/day
- Women: 1.1 g/day

‡ Contaminants include organically bound arsenic, organochlorines, polychlorinated biphenyls (PCBs), and others.

saturated fat, *trans* fat, and cholesterol. (✚) Specifically, consume less than 10 percent of kcalories from saturated fat, keep *trans* fat intakes as low as possible, and consume less than 300 milligrams of cholesterol each day. (✚)[26] To help consumers meet these goals, the FDA established Daily Values on food labels using 10 percent of energy intake for saturated fat; the Daily Value for cholesterol is 300 milligrams, regardless of energy intake. (✚) There is no Daily Value for *trans* fat.

Nutrition in Practice 4 suggests substituting monounsaturated or polyunsaturated fats for harmful saturated fats. No beneficial change in blood lipids occurs when monounsaturated or polyunsaturated fat is *added* to a diet rich in saturated or *trans* fat, however. The best diet for heart health is also rich in fruits, vegetables, nuts, and whole grains that offer many health advantages by supplying abundant nutrients, fiber, and phytochemicals.

Review Notes

- High intakes of saturated or *trans* fats contribute to heart disease, obesity, and other health problems.
- High blood cholesterol, specifically, poses a risk of heart disease, and high intakes of saturated fat contribute most to high blood cholesterol. High intakes of *trans*-fatty acids also appear to raise blood cholesterol. Cholesterol in foods presents less of a risk.
- Polyunsaturated fatty acids of the omega-6 and omega-3 families protect against heart disease.
- When monounsaturated fat such as olive oil replaces saturated and *trans* fats in the diet, the risk of heart disease may be lessened.
- Though some fat in the diet is necessary, health authorities recommend a diet moderate in total fat and low in saturated fat, *trans* fat, and cholesterol.

Fats in Foods

Fats are important in foods as well as in the body. Many of the compounds that give foods their flavors and aromas are found in fats and oils. The delicious aromas associated with bacon, ham, and other meats, as well as with onions being sautéed, come from fats. Fats also influence the texture of many foods, enhancing smoothness, creaminess, moistness, or crispness. In addition, four vitamins—A, D, E, and K—are soluble in fat. When the fat is removed from a food, many fat-soluble compounds, including these vitamins, are also removed. Table 4-4 summarizes the roles of fats in foods.

Fats are also an important part of most people's ethnic or national cuisines. Each culture has its own favorite food sources of fats and oils. In Canada, canola oil (also known as rapeseed oil) is widely used. In the Mediterranean area, Greeks, Italians, and Spaniards rely heavily on olive oil. Both canola oil and olive oil are rich sources of monounsaturated fatty acids. Asians use the polyunsaturated oil of soybeans. Jewish people traditionally employ chicken fat. Everywhere in North America, butter and margarine are widely used.

FINDING THE FATS IN FOODS

The remainder of this chapter and the Nutrition in Practice show you how to choose fats wisely with the goals of providing optimal health and pleasure in eating. To achieve such goals, you need to know which foods offer unsaturated fats that provide the essential fatty acids and which offer harmful saturated and *trans* fats. Perhaps most important for many people

TABLE 4-4	The Functions of Fats in Foods

Fats in foods:

- *Nutrient.* Fats provide essential fatty acids.
- *Energy.* Fats provide a concentrated energy source in foods.
- *Transport.* Fats carry fat-soluble vitamins A, D, E, and K along with some phytochemicals and assist in their absorption.
- *Sensory appeal.* Fats contribute to the taste and smell of foods.
- *Appetite.* Fats stimulate the appetite.
- *Satiety.* Fats contribute to feelings of fullness.
- *Texture.* Fats help make foods tender.

is learning to control portion sizes, particularly portions of fatty foods that can pack hundreds of kcalories into just a few bites.

The *Dietary Guidelines for Americans* urge that, beyond a healthy minimum, people should limit their fat intakes in order to limit intakes of saturated fat, *trans* fat, and kcalories. To do this requires consistently making nutrient-dense choices, such as fat-free milk, fat-free cheese, and the leanest meats, and refraining from adding solid fats, such as butter, hard margarine, or shortening, to foods during preparation or at the table. Higher-fat foods may be included in the diet, but the fat kcalories they provide must fit within a person's discretionary kcalorie allowance. Exceptions are the fats of fatty fish, nuts, and vegetable oils: they provide EPA and DHA, linoleic acid and linolenic acid, and vitamin E needed for a healthful diet. (✚) Within kcalorie limits, the kcalories these fats provide are necessary, not discretionary. Many people, especially sedentary people, have few or no discretionary kcalories to spend on high-fat foods. (✚)

Added Fats in Foods A dollop of dessert topping, a spread of butter on bread, oil or shortening in a recipe, dressing on a salad—all of these are examples of *added* fats. Indeed, all sorts of fats can be added to foods during commercial or home preparation or at the table. The following amounts of these fats contain about 5 grams of pure fat, providing 45 kcalories and negligible protein and carbohydrate:

- 1 teaspoon of oil or shortening
- 1½ teaspoons of mayonnaise, butter, or margarine
- 1 tablespoon of regular salad dressing, cream cheese, or heavy cream
- 1½ tablespoons of sour cream

The majority of added fats in the diet are invisible. They are the hidden fats of fried foods and baked goods, sauces and mixed dishes, and dips and spreads. Other invisible fats include the fats in the marbling of meat and the fat ground into lunch meats and hamburger.

Milk, Yogurt, and Cheese The fat in whole milk is about 63 percent saturated fat; the cholesterol content is 24 milligrams per cup for whole milk or 5 milligrams for fat-free milk. (✚) Thus, choosing fat-free in place of whole milk reduces your intake of cholesterol as well as of saturated fat.

Note that cream and butter do not appear in the milk group. Milk and yogurt are rich in calcium and protein, but cream and butter are not. Cream and butter are fats, as are whipped cream, sour cream, and cream cheese, so they are grouped together with the solid fats. That is why the food group that includes milk is carefully labeled the "milk, yogurt, and cheese group," not the "dairy group." Cheeses are major contributors of saturated fat in people's diets.

Meat, Poultry, Fish, Legumes, Eggs, and Nuts Meats conceal a good deal of the fat—and much of the saturated fat—that people consume. To help "see" the fat in meats, it is useful to think of them in four categories according to their fat contents: very lean, lean, medium-fat, and high-fat meats, as the exchange lists do in Appendix C. Meats in all four categories contain about equal amounts of protein, but their fat contents differ, and their saturated fat and kcalorie amounts vary significantly. Table 1-12 on pp. 27–28 in Chapter 1 provided some definitions concerning the fat contents of meats.

The USDA Food Guide suggests that most adults limit a day's intake of meats or equivalents to about 5 to 7 ounces. For comparison, the smallest fast-food hamburger weighs about 3 ounces. A steak served in a restaurant often runs 8, 12, or 16 ounces, more than a whole day's meat allowance. You may have to weigh a serving or two of meat to see how much you are eating.

People think of meat as protein food, but calculation of its nutrient content reveals a surprising fact. A big (4-ounce), fast-food hamburger sandwich contains 23 grams of protein and 20 grams of fat. Because protein offers 4 kcalories per gram and fat offers 9, the sandwich provides 92 kcalories from protein and about twice that amount from fat. The kcalorie total, counting carbohydrates from the bun and condiments, is more than 400 kcalories, with more than 50 percent of them from fat. Hot dogs, fried chicken

✚ Table 1-7 of Chapter 1 specifies how much oil is required to meet nutrient needs at several kcalorie levels.

✚ The concept of discretionary kcalories was discussed in Chapter 1.

✚ 1 c whole milk:
- 8 g fat
- 5 g saturated fat
- 24 mg cholesterol

1 c reduced-fat milk:
- 5 g fat
- 2 g saturated fat
- 20 mg cholesterol

1 c low-fat milk:
- 2 g fat
- 1.5 g saturated fat
- 10 mg cholesterol

1 c fat-free milk:
- 0 g fat
- 0 g saturated fat
- 5 mg cholesterol

sandwiches, and fried fish sandwiches are also high-fat choices. Because so much of the energy in a meat eater's diet is hidden from view, people can easily overeat on high-fat food, making weight control difficult.

When choosing beef or pork, look for lean cuts named *loin* or *round* from which the fat can be trimmed. Eat small portions, too. As for chicken and turkey, these meats are naturally lean, but commercial processing and frying add fats, especially in "patties," "nuggets," "fingers," or "wings." Chicken wings are mostly skin, and a chicken stores most of its fat just under its skin. The tastiest wing snacks have also been fried in cooking fat (often a hydrogenated, saturated type with *trans*-fatty acids); smothered with a buttery, spicy sauce; and then dipped in blue cheese dressing, making wings an extraordinarily high-fat snack. People who snack on wings may want to plan on eating low-fat foods at several other meals to balance them out.

Vegetables, Fruits, and Grains

Choosing vegetables, fruits, whole grains, and legumes also helps lower the saturated fat, cholesterol, and total fat content of the diet. Most vegetables and fruits naturally contain little or no fat; avocados and olives are exceptions, but most of their fat is unsaturated, which is not harmful to heart health. Most grains contain only small amounts of fat. Some grain *products* such as fried taco shells, croissants, and biscuits are high in saturated fat, so consumers need to read food labels. Similarly, many people add butter, margarine, or cheese sauce to grains and vegetables, which raises their saturated and *trans* fat contents. Because fruits are often eaten without added fat, a diet that includes several servings of fruit daily can help a person meet the dietary recommendations for fat.

A diet rich in vegetables, fruits, whole grains, and legumes offers abundant vitamin C, folate, vitamin A, vitamin E, and dietary fiber—all important in supporting health. Consequently, such a diet protects against disease by both reducing saturated fat, cholesterol, and total fat and by increasing nutrients. It also provides valuable phytochemicals that help defend against heart disease.

CUTTING FAT INTAKE AND CHOOSING UNSATURATED FATS

Knowing which foods contain the most fat is the first step toward meeting the recommendation to limit dietary fat in general and saturated fat in particular. As a general rule, a person who eats meat and wishes to reduce both saturated fat and cholesterol intake can eat fewer high-fat meats and dairy foods; fewer eggs; and more poultry (without the skin), fish, and fat-free dairy products. A vegetarian who eats dairy products and eggs can shift to fat-free milk and fat-free cheeses and limit butter and egg intake. Vegetarians who omit animal-derived foods generally eat less saturated fat and little or no cholesterol because plant foods do not contain significant amounts of cholesterol. The "How to" (p. 106) offers strategies for making heart-healthy choices, food group by food group.

Fats and kCalories

Removing fat from food also removes energy, as Figure 4-5 shows. A pork chop with the fat trimmed to within a half-inch of the lean provides 340 kcalories; with the fat trimmed off completely, it supplies 230 kcalories. A baked potato with butter and sour cream (1 tablespoon each) has 350 kcalories; a plain baked potato has 220 kcalories. The single most effective step you can take to reduce the energy value of a food is to eat it with less fat.

Choosing Unsaturated Fats

When a person does eat fats, those to choose are the unsaturated ones. Remember, the softer a fat is, the more unsaturated it is. Generally speaking, vegetable and fish oils are rich in polyunsaturates, olive oil and canola oil are rich in monounsaturates, and the harder fats—animal fats—are more saturated (see Figure 4-6 on p. 107).

Don't Overdo Fat Restriction

Some people actually manage to eat too *little* fat—to their detriment. Among them are young women and men with

At room temperature, unsaturated fats (such as those found in oil), are usually liquid, whereas saturated fats (such as those found in butter) are solid.

Lipids

FIGURE
4-5
Cutting Fat Cuts kCalories—and Saturated Fat

Pork chop with fat (340 kcal, 19 g fat, 7 g saturated fat)

Potato with 1 tbs butter and 1 tbs sour cream (350 kcal, 14 g fat, 10 g saturated fat)

Whole milk, 1 c (150 kcal, 8 g fat, 5 g saturated fat)

Pork chop with fat trimmed off (230 kcal, 9 g fat, 3 g saturated fat)

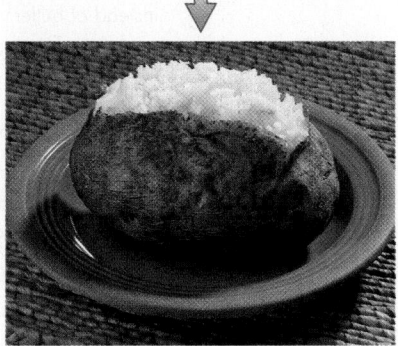

Plain potato (220 kcal, <1 g fat, 0 g saturated fat)

Fat-free milk, 1 c (90 kcal, <1 g fat, <1 g saturated fat)

eating disorders, described in Nutrition in Practice 7. As a practical guideline, it is wise to include the equivalent of at least a teaspoon of fat in every meal.

Cautions People who wish to make choices consistent with current recommendations need to learn how to read food labels, limit fat in general, and seek out the polyunsaturated and monounsaturated fats in preference to the saturated ones. Remember, however, that vegetable fat or vegetable oil doesn't always mean unsaturated fat. Both coconut oil and palm oil, for example, which are often used in nondairy creamers, are saturated fats, and both raise blood cholesterol.

Fat Replacers Today, consumers can choose from thousands of fat-reduced products. Many bakery goods, lunch meats, cheeses, spreads, frozen desserts, and other products made with **fat replacers** offer less than half a gram of fat, saturated fat, and *trans* fat in a serving. Some of these products contain **artificial fats**, and others use conventional ingredients in unconventional ways to reduce fats and kcalories. Among the latter, manufacturers can:

- Add water or whip air into foods.
- Add fat-free milk to creamy foods.
- Use lean meats and soy protein to replace high-fat meats.
- Bake foods instead of frying them.

Common food ingredients such as fibers, sugars, or proteins can also take the place of fats in some foods. In particular, fat replacers made from oats or barley not only cut down on fats in foods but also introduce beneficial viscous fibers, while imparting desirable tastes and textures associated with real fats.[27] Products made from sugars or proteins still provide kcalories but far fewer kcalories from fats. Manufactured fat replacers consist of chemical derivatives of carbohydrate, protein, or fat, or modified versions of foods rich in those constituents.

fat replacers: ingredients that replace some or all of the functions of fat in foods and may or may not provide energy.

artificial fats: zero-energy fat replacers that are chemically synthesized to mimic the sensory and cooking qualities of naturally occurring fats but are totally or partially resistant to digestion.

HOW TO | Make Heart-Healthy Choices—by Food Group

Breads and Cereals

- Select breads, cereals, and crackers that are low in saturated and *trans* fat (for example, bagels instead of croissants).

- Prepare pasta with a tomato sauce instead of a cheese or cream sauce.

Vegetables and Fruits

- Enjoy the natural flavor of steamed vegetables (without butter) for dinner and fruits for dessert.

- Eat at least two vegetables (in addition to a salad) with dinner.

- Snack on raw vegetables or fruits instead of high-fat items like potato chips.

- Buy frozen vegetables without sauce.

Milk and Milk Products

- Switch from whole milk to reduced-fat, from reduced-fat to low-fat, and from low-fat to fat-free (nonfat).

- Use fat-free and low-fat cheeses (such as part-skim ricotta and low-fat mozzarella) instead of regular cheeses.

- Use fat-free or low-fat yogurt or sour cream instead of regular sour cream.

- Use evaporated fat-free milk instead of cream.

- Enjoy fat-free frozen yogurt, sherbet, or ice milk instead of ice cream.

Meat and Legumes

- Fat adds up quickly, even with lean meat; limit intake to about 6 ounces (cooked weight) daily.

- Eat at least two servings of fish per week (particularly fish such as mackerel, lake trout, herring, sardines, and salmon).

- Choose fish, poultry, or lean cuts of pork or beef; look for unmarbled cuts named *round* or *loin* (eye of round, top round, bottom round, round tip, tenderloin, sirloin, center loin, and top loin).

- Choose processed meats such as lunch meats and hot dogs that are low in saturated fat and cholesterol.

- Trim the fat from pork and beef; remove the skin from poultry.

- Grill, roast, broil, bake, stir-fry, stew, or braise meats; don't fry. When possible, place food on a rack so that fat can drain.

- Use lean ground turkey or lean ground beef in recipes; brown ground meats without added fat, then drain off fat.

- Select tuna, sardines, and other canned meats packed in water; rinse oil-packed items with hot water to remove much of the fat.

- Fill kabob skewers with lots of vegetables and slivers of meat; create main dishes and casseroles by combining a little meat, fish, or poultry with a lot of pasta, rice, or vegetables.

- Use legumes often.

- Eat a meatless meal or two daily.

- Use egg substitutes in recipes instead of whole eggs or use two egg whites in place of each whole egg.

Fats and Oils

- Use butter or stick margarine sparingly; select soft margarines instead of hard margarines.

- Use fruit butters, reduced-kcalorie margarines, or butter replacers instead of butter.

- Use low-fat or fat-free mayonnaise and salad dressing instead of regular.

- Limit use of lard and meat fat.

- Limit use of products made with coconut oil, palm kernel oil, and palm oil (read labels on bakery goods, processed foods, popcorn oils, and nondairy creamers).

- Reduce use of hydrogenated shortenings and stick margarines and products that contain them (read labels on crackers, cookies, and other commercially prepared baked goods); use vegetable oils instead.

Miscellaneous

- Use a nonstick pan, or coat the pan lightly with vegetable oil.

- Refrigerate soups and stews; when the fat solidifies, remove it before reheating.

- Use wine; lemon, orange, or tomato juice; herbs; spices; fruits; or broth instead of butter or margarine when cooking.

- Stir-fry in a small amount of oil; add moisture and flavor with broth, tomato juice, or wine.

- Use variety to enhance enjoyment of the meal: vary colors, textures, and temperatures—hot cooked versus cool raw foods—and use garnishes to complement food.

- Omit high-fat meat gravies and cheese sauces.

- Order pizzas with lots of vegetables, a little lean meat, and half the cheese.

SOURCE: Adapted from Expert Panel on Detection, Evaluation, and Treatment of High Blood Cholesterol in Adults (Adult Treatment Panel III), Third Report of the National Cholesterol Education Program (NCEP), NIH publication no. 02-5215 (Bethesda, MD: National Heart, Lung, and Blood Institute, 2002), pp. V-25–V-27.

A familiar example of an artificial fat that has been approved for use in snack foods such as potato chips, crackers, and tortilla chips is **olestra**. Olestra's chemical structure is similar to that of a regular fat (a triglyceride) but with important differences. A triglyceride is composed of a glycerol molecule with three fatty acids attached, whereas olestra is made of a sucrose molecule with six to eight fatty acids attached. Enzymes in the digestive tract cannot break the bonds of olestra, so unlike sucrose or fatty acids, olestra passes through the system unabsorbed.

olestra: a synthetic fat made from sucrose and fatty acids that provides zero kcalories per gram; also known as *sucrose polyester.*

FIGURE
4-6
Comparison of Dietary Fats

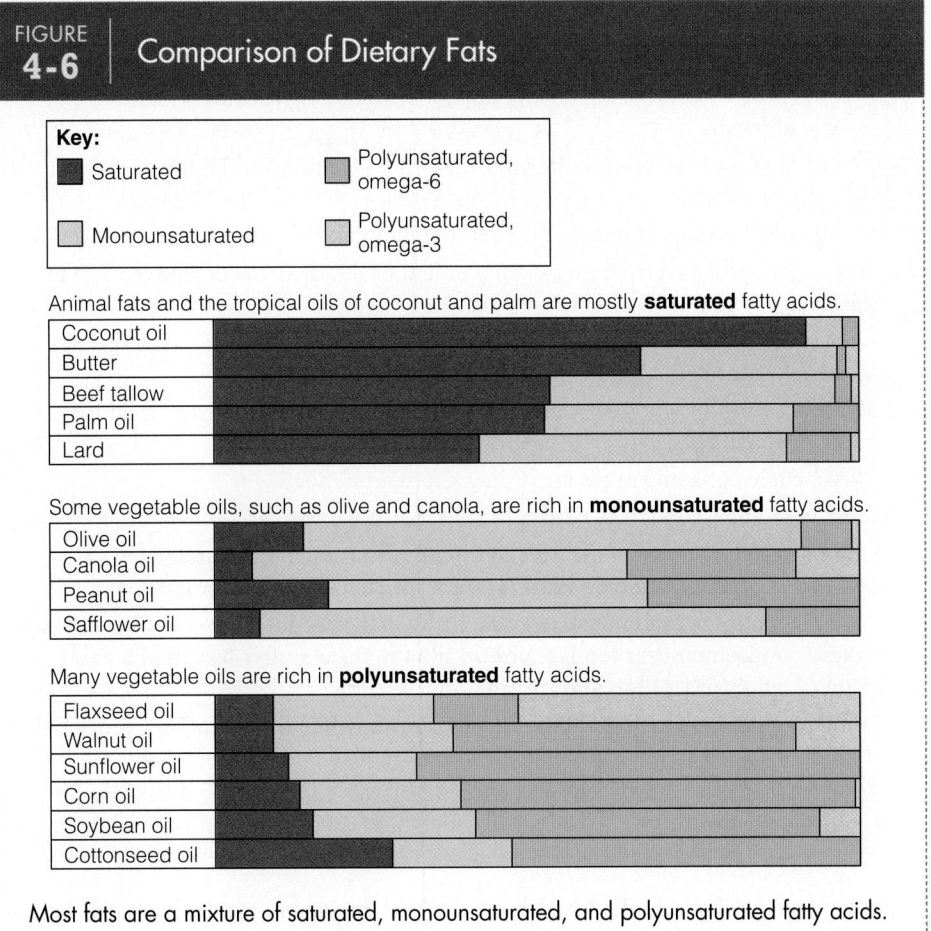

Key:

- ■ Saturated
- ▨ Polyunsaturated, omega-6
- ▢ Monounsaturated
- ▢ Polyunsaturated, omega-3

Animal fats and the tropical oils of coconut and palm are mostly **saturated** fatty acids.

- Coconut oil
- Butter
- Beef tallow
- Palm oil
- Lard

Some vegetable oils, such as olive and canola, are rich in **monounsaturated** fatty acids.

- Olive oil
- Canola oil
- Peanut oil
- Safflower oil

Many vegetable oils are rich in **polyunsaturated** fatty acids.

- Flaxseed oil
- Walnut oil
- Sunflower oil
- Corn oil
- Soybean oil
- Cottonseed oil

Most fats are a mixture of saturated, monounsaturated, and polyunsaturated fatty acids.

The FDA's evaluation of olestra's safety addressed two questions. First, is olestra toxic? Research on both animals and humans supports the safety of olestra as a partial replacement for dietary fats and oils, with no reports of cancer or birth defects. Second, does olestra affect either nutrient absorption or the health of the digestive tract? When olestra passes through the digestive tract unabsorbed, it binds with the fat-soluble vitamins A, D, E, and K and carries them out of the body, robbing the person of these valuable nutrients. To compensate for these losses, the FDA requires the manufacturer to fortify olestra with vitamins A, D, E, and K. Saturating olestra with these vitamins does not make the product a good source of vitamins, but it does block olestra's ability to bind with the vitamins from other foods. An asterisk in the ingredients list informs consumers that these added vitamins are "dietarily insignificant."

Some consumers experience digestive distress with olestra consumption: cramps, gas, bloating, and diarrhea. The FDA initially required a label warning stating that "olestra may cause abdominal cramping and loose stools" and that it "inhibits the absorption of some vitamins and other nutrients," but the FDA recently concluded that such a statement is no longer warranted.

Consumers need to keep in mind that low-fat and fat-free foods still deliver kcalories. Decades ago, consumers hailed the arrival of artificial sweeteners as a weight-loss wonder, but in reality, kcalories saved by using artificial sweeteners were readily replaced by kcalories from other foods. Alternatives to fat can help to lower energy intake and support weight loss only when they actually *replace* fat and energy in the diet.

Read Food Labels

Labels list total fat, saturated fat, *trans* fat, and cholesterol contents of foods in addition to fat kcalories, per serving. Because each package provides information for a single serving and serving sizes are standardized, consumers can easily compare similar products.

Review Notes

- Fats in foods contribute to sensory appeal—enhancing the flavor, aroma, and texture of foods.
- Fats in foods deliver fat-soluble vitamins, energy, and essential fatty acids.
- While some fat in the diet is necessary, the *Dietary Guidelines for Americans* recommend limiting fat intakes in order to limit intakes of saturated fat and *trans* fat.
- Fats added to foods during preparation or at the table are a major source of fat in the diet.
- The choice between whole and fat-free milk products can make a big difference to the fat, saturated fat, and cholesterol content of a diet.
- Meats account for a large proportion of the hidden fat and saturated fat in many people's diets.
- Most people consume more meat than is recommended.
- Most vegetables and fruits naturally contain little or no fat.
- Grain products such as croissants and biscuits can be high in saturated fat, so consumers need to read food labels to learn which foods in this group contain fats.
- Consumers today can choose from an array of fat-reduced products, and many bakery goods and other foods made with fat replacers offer less than a half a gram of fat, saturated fat, and *trans* fat in a serving.
- Some products use artificial fats such as olestra, while others use conventional ingredients such as water or fat-free milk to reduce fat and kcalories.
- Food labels list total fat, saturated fat, cholesterol, and *trans* fat, as well as fat kcalories per serving.

Chapters 3 and 4 have looked briefly at the two major energy fuels in the body—carbohydrate and fat. When used for energy, each has desirable characteristics. The glucose derived from carbohydrate is needed by the brain and nerve tissues and is easily used for energy in other cells. Fat is a particularly useful fuel because the body stores it efficiently and in generous amounts. Chapter 5 looks at protein, a nutrient that can be used as fuel, but whose primary role is to provide machinery for getting things done.

Self Check

1. • Three classes of lipids in the body are:
   a. triglycerides, fatty acids, and cholesterol.
   b. triglycerides, phospholipids, and sterols.
   c. fatty acids, phospholipids, and cholesterol.
   d. glycerol, fatty acids, and triglycerides.

2. • A triglyceride consists of:
   a. three glycerols attached to a lipid.
   b. three fatty acids attached to a glucose.
   c. three fatty acids attached to a glycerol.
   d. three phospholipids attached to a cholesterol.

3. • A fatty acid that has the maximum possible number of hydrogen atoms is known as a(n):
   a. saturated fatty acid.
   b. monounsaturated fatty acid.

   c. PUFA.
   d. essential fatty acid.

4. • The difference between *cis*- and *trans*-fatty acids is:
   a. the number of double bonds.
   b. the length of their carbon chains.
   c. the location of the first double bond.
   d. the configuration around the double bond.

5. • Essential fatty acids:
   a. are used to make substances that regulate blood pressure, among other functions.
   b. can be made from carbohydrates.
   c. include lecithin and cholesterol.
   d. cannot be found in commonly eaten foods.

Lipids

6 • Lecithins and other phospholipids in the body function as:
   a. emulsifiers.
   b. enzymes.
   c. temperature regulators.
   d. shock absorbers.

7 • To minimize saturated fat intake and lower the risk of heart disease, most people need to:
   a. eat less meat.
   b. select fat-free milk.
   c. use nonhydrogenated margarines and cooking oils such as olive oil or canola oil.
   d. all of the above.

8 • To include omega-3 fatty acids in the diet, the American Heart Association recommends eating:
   a. cholesterol-free margarine.
   b. fish oil supplements.
   c. hydrogenated margarine.
   d. at least two fish meals per week.

9 • Some examples of foods with hidden fats are:
   a. cheese, lettuce, and fruit juices.
   b. fried foods, sauces, dips, and lunch meats.
   c. fish, rice, and potatoes.
   d. baked potatoes, vegetables, and fruits.

10 • Generally speaking, vegetable and fish oils are rich in:
   a. polyunsaturated fat.
   b. saturated fat.
   c. cholesterol.
   d. *trans*-fatty acids.

Answers to these questions are found in Appendix H.

Clinical Applications

1 • The connection between the overconsumption of fats, especially saturated and *trans* fat, and chronic diseases (obesity, diabetes, cancer, and cardiovascular disease) underscores the importance of being alert to a client's fat intake. What advice would you offer a client who reports the following?

   • Eats two or more 6-ounce servings of meat each day.
   • Drinks whole milk and eats regular cheddar cheese each day.
   • Eats four to five servings of breads and cereals each day, including a bagel with cream cheese for breakfast, a bologna sandwich on white bread for lunch, and biscuits or cornbread with butter to accompany dinner.
   • Eats one serving of fruit each day and eats vegetables only on occasion.

2 • Make a list of foods, beverages, and seasonings that your client can substitute for foods high in saturated fat.

Nutrition on the Net

For further study of the topics in this chapter, access these websites.

• Find updates and quick links to these and other nutrition-related sites at our website: www.cengage.com/nutrition/whitney/nhhc4e
• Search for cholesterol and dietary fat at the U.S. government health information site: www.healthfinder.gov

• Search for "fat" at the International Food Information Council site: www.ific.org

Notes

1. G. Govindarajan, M. A. Alpert, and L. Tejwani, Endocrine and metabolic effects of fat: Cardiovascular implications, *American Journal of Medicine* 121 (2008): 366–370; T. Yamauchi and T. Kadowaki, Physiological and pathophysiological roles of adiponectin and adiponectin receptors in the integrated regulation of metabolic and cardiovascular diseases, *International Journal of Obesity* 32 (2008): S13–S18; T. Yamada and H. Katagiri, Avenues of communication between the brain and tissues/organs involved in energy homeostasis, *Endocrine Journal* 54 (2007): 497–505.

2. W. S. Harris and coauthors, Omega-6 fatty acids and risk for cardiovascular disease, A science advisory from the American Heart Association Nutrition Subcommittee of the Council on Nutrition, Physical Activity, and Metabolism; Council on Cardiovascular Nursing; and Council on Epidemiology and Prevention, *Circulation* 119 (2009): 902–907; P. C. Calder, n-3 Polyunsaturated fatty acids, inflammation, and inflammatory diseases, *American Journal of Clinical Nutrition* 83 (2006): 1505S–1519S.

3. S. M. Innis, Dietary (n-3) fatty acids and brain development, *Journal of Nutrition* 137 (2007): 855–859.

4. C. Agostoni, Role of long-chain polyunsaturated fatty acids in the first year of life, *Journal of Pediatric Gastroenterology and Nutrition* 47 (2008): S41–S44; E. E. Birch and coauthors, Visual acuity and cognitive outcomes at 4 years of age in a double-blind, randomized trial of long-chain polyunsaturated fatty acid-supplemented infant formula, *Early Human Development* 83 (2007): 279–284.

5. P. J. Smith and coauthors, Association between n-3 fatty acid consumption and ventricular ectopy after myocardial infarction, *American Journal of Clinical Nutrition* 89 (2009): 1315–1320; J. K. Virtanen and coauthors, Fish consumption and risk of major chronic disease in men, *American Journal of Clinical Nutrition* 88 (2008): 1618–1625; J. M. Norris and coauthors, Omega-3 polyunsaturated fatty acid intake and islet autoimmunity in children at increased risk for type 1 diabetes, *Journal of the American Medical Association* 298 (2007): 1420–1428; J. Shannon and coauthors, Erythrocyte fatty acids and breast cancer risk: A case-control study in Shanghai, China, *American Journal of Clinical Nutrition* 85 (2007): 1090–1097; H. E. Theobald and coauthors, Low-dose docosahexaenoic acid lowers diastolic blood pressure in middle-aged men and women, *Journal of Nutrition* 137 (2007): 973–978; W. C. Willett, The role of dietary n-6 fatty acids in the prevention of cardiovascular disease, *Journal of Cardiovascular Medicine* 8 (2007): S42–S45; C. Chrysohoou and coauthors, Long-term fish consumption is associated with protection against arrhythmia in healthy persons in a Mediterranean region—the ATTICA study, *American Journal of Clinical Nutrition* 85 (2007): 1385–1391; J. L. Breslow, n-3 fatty acids and cardiovascular disease, *American Journal of Clinical Nutrition* 83 (2006): 1477S–1482S.

6. S. B. Racette and coauthors, Dose effects of dietary phytosterols on cholesterol metabolism: A controlled feeding study, *American Journal of Clinical Nutrition* 91 (2010): 32–38; S. Klingberg and coauthors, Inverse relation between dietary intake of naturally occurring plant sterols and serum cholesterol in northern Sweden, *American Journal of Clinical Nutrition* 87 (2008): 993–1001.

7. S. Sieri and coauthors, Dietary fat and breast cancer risk in the European Prospective Investigation into Cancer and Nutrition, *American Journal of Clinical Nutrition* 88 (2008): 1304–1312; A. C. Thiébaut and coauthors, Dietary fat and postmenopausal invasive breast cancer in the National Institutes of Health—AARP Diet and Health Study cohort, *Journal of the National Cancer Institute* 99 (2007): 451–462; R. Prentice and coauthors, Low-fat dietary pattern and cancer incidence in the Women's Health Initiative Dietary Modification Randomized Controlled Trial, *Journal of the National Cancer Institute* 99 (2007): 1534–1543.

8. J. Shannon and coauthors, Erythrocyte fatty acids and breast cancer risk: A case-control study in Shanghai, China, *American Journal of Clinical Nutrition* 85 (2007): 1090–1097; E. Theodoratou and coauthors, Dietary fatty acids and colorectal cancer: A case-control study, *American Journal of Epidemiology* 166 (2007): 181–195; R. S. Chapkin, D. N. McMurray, and J. R. Lupton, Colon cancer, fatty acids and anti-inflammatory compounds, *Current Opinion in Gastroenterology* 23 (2007): 48–54.

9. L. Van Horn and coauthors, The evidence for dietary prevention and treatment of cardiovascular disease, *Journal of the American Dietetic Association* 108 (2008): 287–331; Position of the American Dietetic Association and Dietitians of Canada: Dietary fatty acids, *Journal of the American Dietetic Association* 107 (2007): 1599–1611.

10. Standing Committee on the Scientific Evaluation of Dietary Reference Intakes, Food and Nutrition Board, Institute of Medicine, *Dietary Reference Intakes for Energy, Carbohydrate, Fiber, Fat, Fatty Acids, Cholesterol, Protein, and Amino Acids* (Washington, D.C.: National Academies Press, 2005), pp. 835–836.

11. S. K. Wallace and D. Mozaffarian, Trans-fatty acids and nonlipid risk factors, *Current Atherosclerosis Reports* 11 (2009): 423–433; D. Mozaffarian, A. Aro, and W. C. Willett, Health effects of trans-fatty acids: Experimental and observational evidence, *European Journal of Clinical Nutrition* 63 (2009): S5–S21; Standing Committee on the Scientific Evaluation of Dietary Reference Intakes, 2005, pp. 494–505.

12. D. B. Haytowitz, P. R. Pehrsson, and J. M. Holden, The National Food and Nutrient Analysis Program: A decade of progress, *Journal of Food Composition and Analysis* 21 (2008): S94–S102; M. J. Albers and coauthors, 2006 marketplace survey of *trans*-fatty acid content of margarines and butters, cookies and snack cakes, and savory snacks, *Journal of the American Dietetic Association* 108 (2008): 367–370.

13. S. Borra and coauthors, An update of *trans*-fat reduction in the American diet, *Journal of the American Dietetic Association* 107 (2007): 2048–2050.

14. S. Cicerale and coauthors, Chemistry and health of olive oil phenolics, *Critical Reviews in Food Science and Nutrition* 49 (2009): 218–236; F. Visioli and coauthors, Virgin Olive Oil Study (VOLOS): Vasoprotective potential of extra virgin olive oil in mildly dislipidemic patients, *European Journal of Nutrition* 44 (2005): 121–127.

15. Cicerale and coauthors, 2009; J. Ruano and coauthors, Intake of phenol-rich virgin olive oil improves the postprandial prothrombotic profile in hypercholesterolemic patients, *American Journal of Clinical Nutrition* 86 (2007): 341–346; M. I. Covas and coauthors, The effect of polyphenols in olive oil on heart disease risk factors, *Annals of Internal Medicine* 145 (2006): 333–341; Visioli and coauthors, 2005.

16. Harris and coauthors, 2009.

17. N. D. Riediger and coauthors, A systemic review of the roles of n-3 fatty acids in health and disease, *Journal of the American Dietetic Association* 109 (2009): 668–679; P. P. Dimitrow and M. Jawien Pleiotropic, Cardioprotective effects of omega-3 polyunsaturated fatty acids, *Mini Reviews in Medicinal Chemistry* 9 (2009): 1030–1039; Van Horn and coauthors, 2008; Breslow, 2006.

18. A. H. Lichtenstein and coauthors, Diet and lifestyle recommendations revision 2006: A scientific statement from the American Heart Association Nutrition Committee, *Circulation* 114 (2006): 82–96.

19. Breslow, 2006.

20. P. M. Kris-Etherton and A. M. Hill, n-3 Fatty acids: Foods or supplements? *American Dietetic Association* 108 (2008): 1125–1130; Lichtenstein and coauthors, 2006.

21. Fish and Omega-3 Fatty Acids 2009, a document available at www.americanheart.org; R. Emsley and coauthors, Safety of the omega-3 fatty acid, eicosapentaenoic acid (EPAP in psychiatric patients: results from a randomized, placebo controlled trial, *Psychiatry Research* 161 (2008): 284–291.

22. Riediger and coauthors, 2009.

23. Standing Committee on the Scientific Evaluation of Dietary Reference Intakes, 2005, pp. 769–770.

24. Standing Committee on the Scientific Evaluation of Dietary Reference Intakes, 2005, pp. 797–802.

25. Standing Committee on the Scientific Evaluation of Dietary Reference Intakes, 2005, pp. 835–836.

26. U.S. Department of Agriculture and U.S. Department of Health and Human Services, *Dietary Guidelines for Americans 2005*, 6th ed., available online at www.healthierus.gov.

27. Position of the American Dietetic Association: Fat replacers, *Journal of the American Dietetic Association* 105 (2005): 266–275.

NUTRITION IN PRACTICE

Figuring Out Fats

To consumers, advice about dietary fat appears to change almost daily. "Eat less fat." "Eat more fatty fish." "Give up butter—use margarine instead." "Give up margarine—replace it with olive oil." "Steer clear of saturated fats." "Seek out omega-3." "Stay away from *trans* fats." "Stick with mono- and polyunsaturated fats." No wonder people feel confused about dietary fat. This Nutrition in Practice begins with a look at the dietary guidelines for fat intake. It continues by identifying which foods provide which fats. It closes with strategies to help consumers choose the right amounts of the right kinds of fats for a healthy diet.

Why do today's fat messages seem to change constantly and become more confusing?

The confusion stems in part from the complexities of fat and in part from the nature of recommendations. As Chapter 4 explained, "dietary fat" refers to several kinds of fats; some fats support health whereas others damage it, and foods typically provide a mixture of fats in varying proportions. It has taken researchers decades to sort through the relationships among the various kinds of fat and their roles in supporting or harming health. Translating these research findings into dietary recommendations is a challenging process. Too little information can mislead consumers, but too much detail can overwhelm them. As scientific understanding has grown, recommendations have evolved to become less general and more specific. Recommendations may seem to "change constantly and become more confusing," but in fact they are becoming more meaningful.

How exactly have dietary recommendations for fat changed to become more meaningful for consumers?

Dietary recommendations for fat have changed by shifting the emphasis from lowering total fat, in general, to limiting saturated and *trans* fat, specifically. For decades, health experts urged consumers to limit total fat intake to 30 percent or less of energy intake. This advice was straightforward—cut the fat, improve your health. Health experts recognized that saturated fats and *trans* fats were the ones that raise blood cholesterol, but they reasoned that when total fat was limited, saturated and *trans* fat intake would

decline as well. People were simply advised to cut back on all fat so that they would cut back on saturated and *trans* fat. Such advice may have oversimplified the message and unnecessarily restricted total fat.

But low-fat diets have been recommended for years to help people manage weight and reduce the risk of heart disease. Are you saying that low-fat diets are no longer recommended?

Low-fat diets remain a key recommendation in treatment plans for people with elevated blood lipids or heart disease and therefore are important in nutrition.[1] As for healthy people, evidence from around the world has led researchers to change population-wide recommendations from a "low-fat" to a "wise-fat" approach. Several problems accompany low-fat diets. For one, many people find low-fat diets difficult to maintain over time. For another, low-fat diets are not necessarily low-kcalorie diets; if energy intake exceeds energy needs, weight gain follows, and obesity brings a host of health problems, including heart disease. For another, diets high in refined carbohydrates, even if low in fat, can cause blood triglycerides to rise and HDL to fall, a deleterious combination for heart health.[2] Finally, taken to the extreme, a low-fat diet may exclude fatty fish, nuts, seeds, and vegetable oils—all valuable sources of many essential fatty acids, phytochemicals, vitamins, and minerals. Importantly, the fats from these sources protect against heart disease, as later sections explain.

How have today's recommendations for fat been revised?

Today, health experts have revised dietary recommendations to acknowledge that not all fats have damaging health consequences.[3] In fact, higher intakes of some kinds of fats (for example, the omega-3 fatty acids) support good health. Instead of urging people to cut back on all fats, current recommendations suggest carefully replacing the "bad" saturated and *trans* fats with the "good" unsaturated fats and enjoying these fats within kcalorie limits.[4] The goal is to create a diet moderate in kcalories that provides enough of the fats that support good health, but not too much of those that harm health. (Turn to pp. 98–102 for a review of the health consequences of each type of fat.)

With these findings and goals in mind, the DRI committee concluded that a diet containing 20 to 35 percent of energy intake from fat, but reduced in saturated fat and *trans* fat and moderate in energy, is compatible with low rates of heart disease, diabetes, obesity, and cancer.[5] The *Dietary Guidelines for Americans* make clear that the human body has no need of dietary saturated fat or *trans* fat, so the less consumed the better, as long as the diet is adequate in nutrients, including the essential fatty acids.[6]

How can people distinguish between the fats in foods that support health and those that might harm it?

Asking consumers to limit their total fat intake was less than perfect advice, but it was straightforward—find the fat and cut back. Asking consumers to keep their intakes of saturated fats, *trans* fats, and cholesterol low and to use monounsaturated and polyunsaturated fats instead may be more on target with heart health, but it also makes diet planning more complicated. To make appropriate selections, consumers must first learn which foods contain which fats. For example, avocados, bacon, walnuts, potato chips, and mackerel are all high-fat foods, yet some of these foods have detrimental effects on heart health when consumed in excess, and others seem neutral or even beneficial.

Is there evidence to clarify why some high-fat foods are compatible with a heart-healthy diet and others are not?

Yes. The traditional diets of Greece and other countries in the Mediterranean region are exemplary in their use of "good" fats, especially olives and olive oil. A classic study of the world's people, the Seven Countries Study, found that death rates from heart disease were strongly associated with diets high in saturated fats, but only weakly linked with total fat.[7] In fact, the two countries with the highest fat intakes, Finland and the Greek island of Crete, had the highest (Finland) and lowest (Crete) rates of heart disease deaths. In both countries, the people consumed 40 percent or more of their kcalories from fat. Clearly, a high-fat diet was not the primary problem, so researchers refocused their attention on the type of fat. They found that the Cretes ate diets high in olive oil but low in saturated fat (less than 10 percent of kcalories), a pattern they linked with relatively low disease risks. Many studies that followed yielded similar results—people who eat "Mediterranean-type" diets have low rates of heart disease, some cancers, and

other chronic diseases, and their life expectancy is high.[8] Unfortunately, many busy Mediterranean people today, especially the young, are trading labor-intensive traditional diets for convenient and fast Western-style foods. At the same time, their health advantages are rapidly disappearing.[9]

When olive oil replaces saturated fats, such as those of butter, coconut oil or palm oil, hydrogenated stick margarine, lard, or shortening, it may offer numerous health benefits.[10] Olive oil helps to protect against heart disease by:

- Lowering total and LDL cholesterol and not lowering HDL cholesterol or raising triglycerides.[11]
- Reducing LDL cholesterol's susceptibility to oxidation.[12]
- Lowering blood-clotting factors.[13]
- Providing phytochemicals that act as antioxidants (see Nutrition in Practice 8).[14]
- Lowering blood pressure.[15]
- Interfering with the inflammatory response.[16]

The labels of olive oil and foods containing it are allowed to state the following qualified health claim: "limited and not conclusive scientific evidence suggests that eating 2 tablespoons of olive oil daily may reduce the risk of coronary heart disease due to the monounsaturated fat in olive oil. To achieve this possible benefit, olive oil is to replace a similar amount of saturated fat and not increase the total number of kcalories you eat in a day. One serving of this product contains X grams of olive oil."

When compared with other fats, olive oil seems to be a wise choice, but controlled clinical trials are too scarce to support population-wide recommendations to switch to a high-fat diet rich in olive oil. Importantly, olive oil is not

Matthew Farruggio

Olives and their oil may benefit heart health.

a magic potion; drizzling it on foods does not make them healthier. Like other fats, olive oil delivers 9 kcalories per gram, which can contribute to weight gain in people who fail to balance their energy intake with their energy output. Its role in a healthy diet is to *replace* the saturated fats. When choosing olive oils, select the darker "extra virgin" kind because it contains the highest levels of potentially beneficial phytochemicals.

Other vegetable oils, such as canola oil or safflower oil, in their liquid unhydrogenated states are also generally low in saturated fats and high in unsaturated fats. Such oils, when they replace solid, saturated fats in the diet, preserve heart health.

Good, olive oil may help protect against heart disease; are there other food fats that may also be protective?

Possibly so. People who eat a 1-ounce serving of nuts on five or more days a week have lower LDL cholesterol and a reduced risk of heart disease compared with people who consume no nuts.[17] Even in women with diabetes, whose risks are high, nuts (5 ounces per week) or peanut butter (5 tbs per week) were associated with reduced heart disease risk.[18]

The nuts under study are those commonly eaten in the United States: almonds, Brazil nuts, cashews, hazelnuts, macadamia nuts, pecans, pistachios, walnuts, even peanuts, and, as mentioned, peanut butter.[19] On average, these nuts contain mostly monounsaturated fat (59 percent), some polyunsaturated fat (27 percent), and little saturated fat (14 percent).

Research has shown a benefit from walnuts and almonds in particular. In study after study, walnuts, when substituted for other fats in the diet, produce favorable effects on blood lipids—even in people with elevated total and LDL cholesterol.[20] Results are similar for almonds.[21]

Studies on peanuts, macadamia nuts, pecans, and pistachios follow suit, indicating that including nuts may be a wise strategy against heart disease. Nuts may protect against heart disease because they provide:

- Monounsaturated and polyunsaturated fats in abundance but few saturated fats.
- Fiber, vegetable protein, and other valuable nutrients, including the antioxidant vitamin E.
- Phytochemicals that act as antioxidants (see Nutrition in Practice 8).
- Plant sterols.

In addition to their heart benefits, nuts may also benefit other body organs—people who frequently consume nuts and other healthy fats suffer fewer gallbladder problems.[22]

Stay mindful of kcalories when snacking on nuts.

Tree nuts and peanuts once had no place in a low-fat or low-kcalorie diet—and for good reason. Nuts provide up to 80 percent of their kcalories from fat, and a quarter cup (about an ounce) of mixed nuts provides more than 200 kcalories. Nuts provide substantially more kcalories per bite than whole-grain pretzels or crunchy raw vegetables, for example. However, today's research does not support greater weight gain in those who consume nuts, so even dieters may choose to include a few nuts each day for their potential health benefits.[23]

What about fish? I have a friend whose doctor told her that eating fish is good for the heart. Is this true?

Yes. The preceding chapter made clear that fish oils hold the potential to improve health, and particularly the health of the heart. Research studies have provided strong evidence that increasing omega-3 fatty acids in the diet supports heart health and lowers the risk of death from heart disease.[24] For this reason, the American Heart Association and other authorities recommend including two fatty fish servings a week in a heart-healthy diet. People who eat some fish each week can lower their risks of heart attack and stroke.[25] Table NP4-1 (p. 114) ranks commonly eaten fish by their omega-3 fatty acid content.

Fish is the best source of EPA and DHA in the diet, but it is also a major source of mercury and other environmental contaminants. Most fish contain at least trace amounts of mercury, but tilefish, swordfish, king mackerel, marlin, and shark have especially high levels. Freshwater fish may contain PCBs and other pollutants, so local advisories warn sport fishers of species that can pose problems. The chapter listed safer species of fish. To minimize risks while obtaining fish benefits, vary your choices among fatty fish species often.

TABLE NP4-1	Omega-3 Fatty Acid Content of Commonly Eaten Fish		
	>500 mg per 3.5 oz serving	150–500 mg per 3.5 oz serving	<150 mg per 3.5 oz serving
	Bronzini	Black bass	Cod (Pacific)
	Herring (Atlantic and Pacific)	Catfish (wild and farmed)	Corvina
	Mackerel	Clam	Grouper
	Oyster (Pacific)	Cod (Atlantic)	Lobster
	Salmon (chinook, coho, Copper River, farmed, pink, sockeye, wild Atlantic)	Crab (Alaskan king)	Mahi-mahi
	Sardines	Croakers	Monkfish
	Toothfish	Escolar	Red snapper
	Trout (wild and farmed)	Flounder	Skate
		Haddock	Triggerfish
		Hake	Tuna
		Halibut	Wahoo
		Oyster (eastern and farmed)	
		Perch	
		Scallop	
		Shrimp (mixed varieties)	
		Sole	
		Swordfish	
		Tilapia (farmed)	

SOURCE: K. L. Weaver and coauthors, The content of favorable and unfavorable polyunsaturated fatty acids found in commonly eaten fish, *Journal of the American Dietetic Association* 108 (2008): 1178–1185; P. M. Kris-Etherton, W. S. Harris, and L. J. Appel, Fish consumption, fish oil, omega-3 fatty acids, and cardiovascular disease, *Circulation* 106 (2002): 2747–2757.

Fish is a good source of the omega-3 fatty acids.

© www.comstock.com

If olive oil, nuts, and fatty fish are protective against heart disease, which fats are harmful?

The number one dietary determinant of LDL cholesterol is saturated fat. Figure NP4-1 shows that each 1 percent increase in energy from saturated fatty acids in the diet may produce a 2 percent jump in heart disease risk by elevating blood LDL cholesterol. Conversely, reducing saturated fat intake by 1 percent can be expected to produce a 2 percent drop in heart disease risk by the same mechanism. Even a 2 percent drop in LDL represents a significant improvement for the health of the heart.[26] Like saturated fats, *trans* fats also raise heart disease risk by elevating LDL cholesterol. A heart-healthy diet limits foods rich in these two types of fat.

Which foods are highest in saturated and *trans* fats?

The major sources of saturated fats in the U.S. diet are fatty meats, whole-milk products, tropical oils, and products made from any of these foods. To limit saturated fat intake, consumers must choose carefully among

FIGURE NP4-1 | Potential Relationships among Saturated Fat Intakes, LDL Cholesterol, and Heart Disease Risk

[a]Percentage of change in total dietary energy from saturated fatty acids.
[b]Percentage of change in blood LDL cholesterol.
[c]Percentage of change in an individual's risk of heart disease; the percentage of change in risk may increase when blood lipid changes are sustained over time.

SOURCE: *Third Report of the National Cholesterol Education Program (NCEP) Expert Panel on Detection, Evaluation, and Treatment of High Blood Cholesterol in Adults (Adult Treatment Panel III)*, NIH publication no. 02-5215 (Bethesda, Md.: National Heart, Lung, and Blood Institute, 2002), pp. V-8 and II-4.

these high-fat foods. More than a third of the fat in most meats is saturated. Similarly, more than half of the fat is saturated in whole milk and other high-fat dairy products, such as cheese, butter, cream, half-and-half, cream cheese, sour cream, and ice cream. Consumers rarely use the tropical oils of palm, palm kernel, and coconut in the kitchen, but these oils are used heavily by food manufacturers and so are commonly found in many commercially prepared foods.

When choosing meats, milk products, and commercially prepared foods, look for those lowest in saturated fat. Labels provide a useful guide for comparing products in this regard, and Appendix A lists the saturated fat in several thousand foods.

Even with careful selections, a nutritionally adequate diet will provide some saturated fat. Zero saturated fat is not possible even when experts design menus with the mission to keep saturated fat as low as possible.[27] Diets based on fruits, vegetables, legumes, nuts, soy products, and whole grains can, and often do, deliver less saturated fat than diets that depend heavily on animal-derived foods, however.

As for *trans* fats, Chapter 4 explained that solid shortening and margarine are made from vegetable oil that has been hardened through hydrogenation. This process both saturates some of the unsaturated fatty acids and introduces *trans*-fatty acids. Many convenience foods contain *trans* fats. Table NP4-2 (p. 116) summarizes which foods provide which fats. Substituting unsaturated fats for saturated fats at each meal and snack can help protect against heart disease. Table NP4-3 (p. 117) provides several examples and shows how such substitutions can lower saturated fat and raise unsaturated fat—even when total fat and kcalories remain unchanged.

So it seems that some fats are "good" and others are "bad" from the body's point of view. Is that right?

The saturated and *trans* fats do indeed seem mostly bad for the health of the heart. Aside from providing energy, which unsaturated fats can do equally well, saturated and *trans* fats bring no indispensable benefits to the body. Furthermore, no harm can come from consuming diets low in them.

In contrast, the unsaturated fats are mostly good for the health of the heart when consumed in moderation. To date, their one proven fault seems to be that they, like all fats, provide abundant energy to the body and so may promote obesity if they drive kcalorie intakes higher than energy needs.[28] Obesity, in turn, often begets many body ills, as Chapter 6 makes clear.

When judging foods by their fatty acids, keep in mind that the fat in foods is a mixture of "good" and "bad," providing both saturated and unsaturated fatty acids. Even predominantly monounsaturated olive oil delivers some saturated fat. Consequently, even when a person chooses foods with mostly unsaturated fats, saturated fat can still add up if total fat is high. For this reason, fat must be kept below 35 percent of total kcalories if the diet is to be moderate in saturated fat.

Additionally, food manufacturers may come to the assistance of consumers wishing to avoid the health threats from saturated and *trans* fats. Some companies now make margarine without *trans* fats, and many snack manufacturers have reduced the saturated and *trans* fats in some products and offer snack foods in 100-kcalorie packages. Other companies are likely to follow if consumers respond favorably.

Healthful Fatty Acids		
Monounsaturated	*Omega-6 polyunsaturated*	*Omega-3 polyunsaturated*
Avocado Oils (canola, olive, peanut, safflower, sesame) Nuts (almonds, cashews, filberts, hazelnuts, macadamia nuts, peanuts, pecans, pistachios) Olives Peanut butter Seeds (sesame)	Margarine (nonhydrogenated) Oils (corn, cottonseed, soybean) Nuts (pine nuts, walnuts) Mayonnaise Salad dressing Seeds (pumpkin, sunflower)	Fatty fish (herring, mackerel, salmon, tuna) Flaxseed Nuts (walnuts)

Harmful Fatty Acids	
Saturated	*Trans*
Bacon Butter Chocolate Coconut Cream cheese Cream, half-and-half Lard Meat Milk and milk products (whole) Oils (coconut, palm, palm kernel) Shortening Sour cream	Fried foods (hydrogenated shortening) Margarine (hydrogenated or partially hydrogenated) Nondairy creamers Many fast foods Shortening Commercial baked goods (including doughnuts, cakes, cookies) Many snack foods (including microwave popcorn, chips, crackers)

NOTE: Keep in mind that foods contain a mixture of fatty acids.

Basing one's diet on vegetables, fruits, and legumes as part of a balanced daily diet is a good idea, as is *replacing* saturated fats such as butter, shortening, and meat fat with unsaturated fats like olive oil and the oils from nuts and fish. These foods provide vitamins, minerals, and phytochemicals—all valuable in protecting the body's health. To further protect health, you may want to reduce fats from convenience foods and fast foods; choose small portions of meats, fish, and poultry; and include fresh foods from all the groups each day. Take care to select portion sizes that will best meet your energy needs. Also, be physically active each day.

TABLE NP4-3 | Choosing Unsaturated Fat Instead of Saturated Fat

Examples of ways to replace saturated fats with unsaturated fats include sautéing foods in olive oil instead of butter, garnishing salads with sunflower seeds instead of bacon, snacking on mixed nuts instead of potato chips, using avocado instead of cheese on a sandwich, and eating salmon instead of steak. Portion sizes have been adjusted so that each of these foods provides approximately 100 kcalories. Notice that, for a similar number of kcalories and grams of fat, the first choices offer less saturated fat and more unsaturated fat.

Foods (100 kcal portions)	Saturated Fat (g)	Unsaturated Fat (g)	Total Fat (g)
Olive oil 1 tbs vs. butter 1 tbs	2 vs. 7	9 vs. 4	11 vs. 11
Sunflower seeds 2 tbs vs. bacon 2 slices	1 vs. 3	7 vs. 6	8 vs. 9
Mixed nuts 2 tbs vs. potato chips 10 chips	1 vs. 2	8 vs. 5	9 vs. 7
Avocado 6 slices vs. cheese 1 slice	2 vs. 4	8 vs. 4	10 vs. 8
Salmon 2 oz vs. steak 1 oz	1 vs. 2	3 vs. 3	4 vs. 5
Totals	7 vs. 18	35 vs. 22	42 vs. 40

Notes

1. A. H. Lichtenstein and coauthors, Diet and lifestyle recommendations revision 2006: A scientific statement from the American Heart Association Nutrition Committee, *Circulation* 114 (2006): 82–96.
2. A. H. Lichtenstein, Dietary fat, carbohydrate, and protein: Effects on plasma lipoprotein patterns, *Journal of Lipid Research* 47 (2006): 1661–1667.
3. S. S. Gidding and coauthors, Implementing American Heart Association Pediatric and Adult Nutrition Guidelines: A scientific statement from the American Heart Association Nutrition Committee of the Council on Nutrition, Physical Activity and Metabolism, Council on Cardiovascular Disease in the Young, Council on Arteriosclerosis, Thrombosis and Vascular biology, Council on Cardiovascular Nursing, Council on Epidemiology and Prevention, and Council for High Blood Pressure Research, *Circulation* 119 (2009): 1161–1175; M. U. Jakobsen and coauthors, Major types of dietary fat and risk of coronary heart disease: A pooled analysis of 11 cohort studies, *American Journal of Clinical Nutrition* 89 (2009): 1425–1432; L. Van Horn and coauthors, The evidence for dietary prevention and treatment of cardiovascular disease, *Journal of the American Dietetic Association* 108 (2008): 287–331.
4. Lichtenstein and coauthors, 2006; U.S. Department of Agriculture and U.S. Department of Health and Human Services, *Dietary Guidelines for Americans 2005*, 6th ed., available online at www.heathierus.gov; Standing Committee on the Scientific Evaluation of Dietary Reference Intakes, Food and Nutrition Board, Institute of Medicine, *Dietary Reference Intakes for Energy, Carbohydrate, Fiber, Fat, Fatty Acids, Cholesterol, Protein, and Amino Acids* (Washington, D.C.: National Academies Press, 2005).
5. Standing Committee on the Scientific Evaluation of Dietary Reference Intakes, 2005, pp. 769–770.
6. U.S. Department of Agriculture and U.S. Department of Health and Human Services, 2005.
7. A. Keys, *Seven Countries: A Multivariate Analysis of Death and Coronary Heart Disease* (Cambridge, MA: Harvard University Press, 1980).
8. A. Trichopoulou, C. Bamia, and D. Trichopoulos, Anatomy of health effects of Mediterranean diet: Greek EPIC prospective cohort study, *British Medical Journal* 338 (2009), doi:10.1136/bmj.b2337; F. Sofi, The Mediterranean diet revisited: Evidence of its effectiveness grows, *Current Opinion in Cardiology* 24 (2009): 442–446; M. C. Sparling and J. J. B. Anderson, The Mediterranean diet and cardiovascular diseases, *Nutrition Today* 44 (2009): 124–133.
9. F. Bellisle, Infrequently asked questions about the Mediterranean diet, *Public Health Nutrition* 12 (2009): 1644–1647; P. A. Gilbert and S. Khokhar, Changing dietary habits of ethnic groups in Europe and implications for health, *Nutrition Reviews* 66 (2008): 203–215.
10. S. Cicerale and coauthors, Chemistry and health of olive oil phenolics, *Critical Reviews in Food Science and Nutrition* 49 (2009): 218–236; F. Visioli and coauthors, Virgin Olive Oil Study (VOLOS): Vasoprotective potential of extra virgin olive oil in mildly dislipidemic patients, *European Journal of Nutrition* 44 (2005): 121–127.
11. E. Waterman and B. Lockwood, Active components and clinical applications of olive oil, *Alternative Medicine Review* 12 (2007): 331–342; M. I. Covas and coauthors, The effect of polyphenols in olive oil on heart disease risk factors, *Annals of Internal Medicine* 145 (2006): 333–341.
12. M. Fitó and coauthors, Effect of a traditional Mediterranean diet on lipoprotein oxidation, *Archives of Internal Medicine* 167 (2007): 1195–1203.
13. J. López-Miranda, Monounsaturated fat and cardiovascular risk, *Nutrition Reviews* 64 (2006): S2–S12.
14. Cicerale and coauthors, 2009; J. Ruano and coauthors, Intake of phenol-rich virgin olive oil improves the postprandial prothrombotic profile in hypercholesterolemic patients, *American Journal of Clinical Nutrition* 86 (2007): 341–346; Covas and coauthors, 2006; Visioli and coauthors, 2005;
15. Waterman and Lockwood, 2007; B. M. Rasmussen and coauthors, Effects of dietary saturated, monounsaturated, and n-3 fatty acids on blood pressure in healthy subjects, *American Journal of Clinical Nutrition* 83 (2006): 221–226.
16. F. Pérez-Jiménez and coauthors, The influence of olive oil on human health: Not a question of fat alone, *Molecular Nutrition and Food Research* 51 (2007): 1199–1208.
17. A. E. Griel and P. M. Kris-Etherton, Tree nuts and the lipid profile: A review of clinical studies, *British Journal of Nutrition* 96 (2006): S68–S78; J. H. Kelly and J. Sabaté, Nuts and coronary heart disease: An epidemiological perspective, *British Journal of Nutrition* 96 (2006): S61–S67.
18. T. Y. Li and coauthors, Regular consumption of nuts is associated with a lower risk of cardiovascular disease in women with type 2 diabetes, *Journal of Nutrition* 139 (2009): 1333–1338.
19. J. Sabaté and Y. Ang, Nuts and health outcomes: New epidemiologic evidence, *American Journal of Clinical Nutrition* 89 (2009): 1643S–1648S; S. K. Gebauer

and coauthors, Effects of pistachios on cardiovascular disease risk factors and potential mechanisms of action: A dose-response study, *American Journal of Clinical Nutrition* 88 (2008): 651–659.

20. S. Rajaram and coauthors, Walnuts and fatty fish influence different serum lipid fractions in normal to mildly hyperlipidemic individuals: A randomized controlled study, *American Journal of Clinical Nutrition* 89 (2009): 1657S–1663S; D. K. Banel and F. B. Hu, Effects of walnut consumption on blood lipids and other cardiovascular risk factors: A meta-analysis and systematic review, *American Journal of Clinical Nutrition* 90 (2009): 56–63.

21. P. M. Kris-Etherton, W. Karmally, and R. Ramakrishnan, Almonds lower LDL cholesterol, *Journal of the American Dietetic Association* 109 (2009): 1521–1522; O. J. Phung and coauthors, Almonds have a neutral effect on serum lipid profile: A meta-analysis of randomized trials, *Journal of the American Dietetic Association* 109 (2009): 865–873; S. Rajaram, K. M. Connell, and J. Sabaté, Effect of almond-enriched high-monounsaturated fat diet on selected markers of inflammation: A randomized, controlled, crossover study, *British Journal of Nutrition,* October 29, 2009, e-pub ahead of print.

22. Sabaté and Ang, 2009.

23. M. Bes-Rastrollo and coauthors, Prospective study of nut consumption, long-term weight change, and obesity risk in women, *American Journal of Clinical Nutrition* 89 (2009): 1913–1919; Sabaté and Ang, 2009; S. Rajaram and J. Sabaté, Nuts, body weight and insulin resistance, *British Journal of Nutrition* 96 (2006): S79–S86.

24. N. D. Riediger and coauthors, A systemic review of the roles of n-3 fatty acids in health and disease, *Journal of the American Dietetic Association* 109

(2009): 668–679; J. K. Virtanen and coauthors, Fish consumption and risk of major chronic disease in men, *American Journal of Clinical Nutrition* 88 (2008): 1618–1625; M. K. Duda and coauthors, Fish oil, but not flaxseed oil, decreases inflammation and prevents pressure overload-induced cardiac dysfunction, *Cardiovascular Research* 81 (2009): 319–327; C. Chrysohoou and coauthors, Long-term fish consumption is associated with protection against arrhythmia in healthy persons in Mediterranean region—the ATTICA study, *American Journal of Clinical Nutrition* 85 (2007): 1385–1391; D. S. Kelley and coauthors, Docosahexaenoic acid supplementation improves fasting and postprandial lipid profiles in hypertriglyceridemic men, *American Journal of Clinical Nutrition* 86 (2007): 324–333; J. L. Breslow, n-3 fatty acids and cardiovascular disease, *American Journal of Clinical Nutrition* 86 (2006): 1477S–1482S.

25. T. L. Psota, S. K. Gebauer, and P. Kris-Etherton, Dietary omega-3 fatty acid intake and cardiovascular risk, *American Journal of Cardiology* 98 (2006): 3i–18i; D. Mozaffarian, R. N. Lemaitre, and L. H. Kuller, Fish consumption and stroke risk in elderly individuals, *Archives of Internal Medicine* 165 (2005): 200–206.

26. *Third Report of the National Cholesterol Education Program (NCEP) Expert Panel on Detection, Evaluation, and Treatment of High Blood Cholesterol in Adults (Adult Treatment Panel III)*, NIH publication no. 025215 (Bethesda, MD.: National Heart, Lung, and Blood Institute, 2002), p. V-8.

27. Standing Committee on the Scientific Evaluation of Dietary Reference Intakes, 2005, p. 835.

28. Standing Committee on the Scientific Evaluation of Dietary Reference Intakes, 2005, pp. 796–797.

CHAPTER 5 | Protein

Copyright Polara Studios Inc.

CONTENTS

PEOPLE THINK OF PROTEINS AS BODYBUILDING NUTRIENTS, THE MATE-rial of strong muscles, and rightly so. No new living tissue can be built without them. Some proteins form structures such as muscle, bone, skin, and other tissues. Other proteins do the cells' work. The energy to fuel that work comes primarily from carbohydrates and fats.

The Chemist's View of Proteins

Proteins are chemical compounds that contain the same atoms as carbohydrates and lipids—carbon (C), hydrogen (H), and oxygen (O)—but proteins are different in that they also contain nitrogen (N) atoms. These nitrogen atoms give the name *amino* (nitrogen containing) to the amino acids that form the links in the chains we call proteins.

THE STRUCTURE OF PROTEINS

About 20 different **amino acids** may appear in proteins.* All amino acids share a common chemical "backbone," and it is these backbones that are linked together to form proteins. Each amino acid also carries a side group, which varies from one amino acid to another (see Figure 5-1). The side group makes the amino acids differ in size, shape, and electrical charge. The side groups on amino acids are what make proteins so varied in comparison with either carbohydrates or lipids.

Protein Chains The 20 amino acids can be linked end-to-end in a virtually infinite variety of sequences to form proteins. When two amino acids bond together, the resulting structure is known as a **dipeptide**. Three amino acids bonded together form a **tripeptide**. As additional amino acids join the chain, the structure becomes a **polypeptide**. Most proteins are a few dozen to several hundred amino acids long.

Protein Shapes Polypeptide chains twist into complex shapes. Each amino acid has special characteristics that attract it to, or repel it from, the surrounding fluids and other amino acids. Because of these interactions, polypeptide chains fold and intertwine into intricate coils (see Figure 5-2) and other shapes. The amino acid sequence of a protein determines the specific way the chain will fold.

Protein Functions The dramatically different shapes of proteins enable them to perform different tasks in the body. Some, such as hemoglobin in the blood (see Figure 5-3), are globular in shape; some are hollow balls that can carry and store materials within them; and some, such as those that form tendons, are more than 10 times as long as they are wide, forming stiff, sturdy, rodlike structures.

FIGURE 5-1 | Amino Acid Structure and Examples of Amino Acids

Side group varies

Amino group   Acid group

Backbone

Valine   Leucine   Tyrosine

All amino acids have a "backbone" made of an amino acid group (which contains nitrogen) and an acid group. The side group varies from one amino acid to the next.

Note that the side group is a unique structure that differentiates one amino acid from another.

*Besides the 20 common amino acids, which can all be components of proteins, others occur individually (for example, ornithine).

FIGURE
5-2

The Coiling and Folding of a Protein Molecule

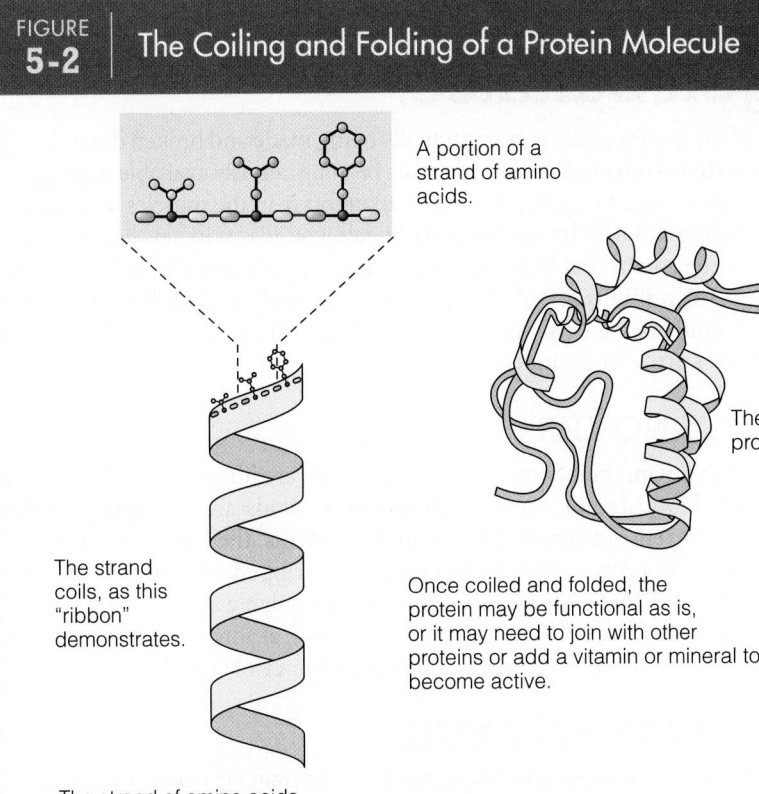

A portion of a strand of amino acids.

The strand coils, as this "ribbon" demonstrates.

The completed protein.

Once coiled and folded, the protein may be functional as is, or it may need to join with other proteins or add a vitamin or mineral to become active.

The strand of amino acids takes on a spring-like shape as their side groups variously attract and repel each other.

+ Some researchers refer to essential amino acids as *indispensable* and to nonessential amino acids as *dispensable*.

nonessential amino acids: amino acids that the body can synthesize.

essential amino acids: amino acids that the body cannot synthesize in amounts sufficient to meet physiological need. Nine amino acids are known to be essential for human adults:

- *histidine* (HISS-tuh-deen)
- *isoleucine* (eye-so-LOO-seen)
- *leucine* (LOO-seen)
- *lysine* (LYE-seen)
- *methionine* (meh-THIGH-oh-neen)
- *phenylalanine* (fen-il-AL-uh-neen)
- *threonine* (THREE-oh-neen)
- *tryptophan* (TRIP-toe-fane, TRIP-toe-fan)
- *valine* (VAY-leen)

conditionally essential amino acid: an amino acid that is normally nonessential but must be supplied by the diet in special circumstances when the need for it becomes greater than the body's ability to produce it.

ESSENTIAL AMINO ACIDS

Proteins in foods do not provide body proteins directly, but rather they supply the amino acids from which the body makes its own proteins. More than half of the amino acids are **nonessential**, meaning that the body can make them for itself. Proteins in foods usually deliver these amino acids, but it is not essential that they do so. There are other amino acids that the body cannot make at all, however, and some that it cannot make fast enough to meet its needs. The proteins in foods must supply these nine amino acids to the body; they are therefore called **essential amino acids. (+)**

Under special circumstances, a nonessential amino acid can become essential. For example, the body normally makes tyrosine (a nonessential amino acid) from the essential amino acid phenylalanine. If the diet fails to supply enough phenylalanine or if the body cannot make the conversion for some reason (as happens in the inherited disease phenylketonuria), then tyrosine becomes a **conditionally essential amino acid.**

FIGURE
5-3

The Structure of Hemoglobin

Four highly folded polypeptide chains form the globular hemoglobin protein.

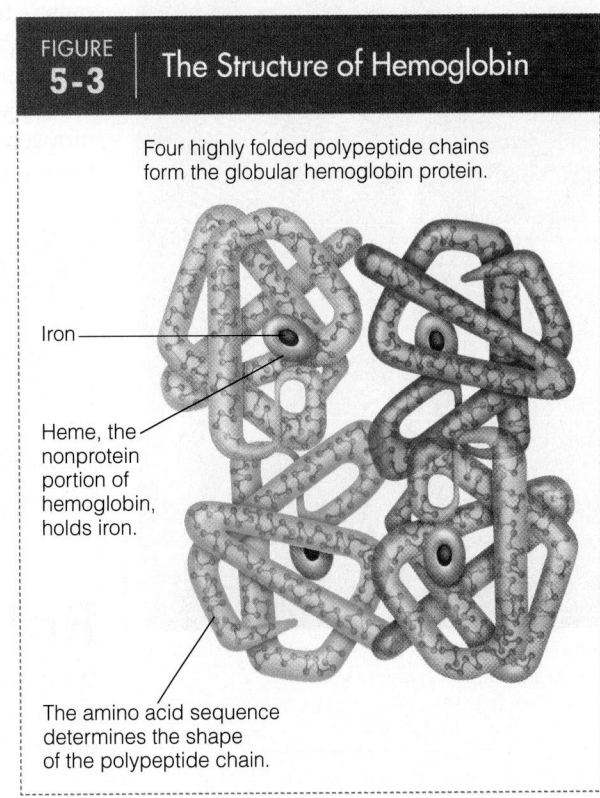

Iron

Heme, the nonprotein portion of hemoglobin, holds iron.

The amino acid sequence determines the shape of the polypeptide chain.

Review Notes

- Chemically speaking, proteins are more complex than carbohydrates or lipids; proteins are made of some 20 different amino acids, 9 of which the body cannot make (they are essential).
- Each amino acid contains a central carbon atom with an amino group, an acid group, a hydrogen atom, and a unique side group attached to it.
- The distinctive sequence of amino acids in each protein determines its shape and function.

protein turnover: the continuous breakdown and synthesis of body proteins involving the recycling of amino acids.

nitrogen balance: the amount of nitrogen consumed (N in) as compared with the amount of nitrogen excreted (N out) in a given period of time. The laboratory scientist can estimate the protein in a sample of food, body tissue, or excreta by measuring the nitrogen in it.

Protein Turnover and Nitrogen Balance

Within each cell of the body, proteins are continually being made and broken down, a process known as **protein turnover**. Amino acids must be continuously available to build the proteins of new tissues. The new tissues may be in an embryo, in the muscles of an athlete in training, in a growing child, in the scar tissue that heals wounds, or in new hair and nails.

Less obvious is the protein that helps replace worn-out cells and internal cell structures. For example, the millions of cells that line the intestinal tract live for three to five days; they are constantly being shed and must be replaced. The cells of the skin die and rub off, and new ones grow from underneath.

PROTEIN TURNOVER

When proteins break down, their component amino acids are liberated within the cells or released into the bloodstream. Some of these amino acids are promptly recycled into other proteins. By reusing amino acids to build proteins, the body conserves and recycles a valuable commodity. Other amino acids are stripped of their nitrogen and used for energy. Each day, about a quarter of the body's available amino acids are irretrievably broken down and used for energy. For this reason, amino acids from food are needed each day to support the new growth and maintenance of cells.

NITROGEN BALANCE

Researchers use **nitrogen balance** studies to estimate protein requirements. (**+**) In healthy adults, protein synthesis balances with protein degradation, and nitrogen intake from protein in food balances with nitrogen excretion in the urine, feces, and sweat. When nitrogen intake equals nitrogen output, a person is in nitrogen equilibrium, or zero nitrogen balance.

If the body synthesizes more than it degrades and adds protein, nitrogen status becomes positive. Nitrogen status is positive in growing infants, children, and adolescents; pregnant women; and people recovering from protein deficiency or illness; their nitrogen intake exceeds their nitrogen output. They are retaining protein in new tissues as they add blood, bone, skin, and muscle to their bodies.

If the body degrades more than it synthesizes and loses protein, nitrogen status becomes negative. Nitrogen status is negative in people who are starving or suffering other severe stresses such as burns, injuries, infections, and fever; their nitrogen output exceeds their nitrogen intake. During these times, the body loses nitrogen as it breaks down muscle and other body proteins for energy.

Review Notes

- The process by which proteins are continually being made and broken down is known as protein turnover.
- The body needs dietary amino acids to grow new cells and to replace worn-out ones.
- When nitrogen intake equals nitrogen output, a person is in nitrogen equilibrium, or zero nitrogen balance.

© Jupiterimages

Growing children end each day with more bone, blood, muscle, and skin cells than they had at the beginning of the day.

Roles of Body Proteins

What distinguishes you chemically from any other human being are minute differences in your particular body proteins (enzymes, antibodies, and others). These differences are determined by your proteins' amino acid sequences, which are written into the genes you inherited from your parents and ancestors. The genes direct the making of all the body's proteins.

The human body contains an estimated 30,000 or more different kinds of proteins. The roles of more than 3000 of these proteins are now known, although the number is growing rapidly with the recent surge in knowledge gained from sequencing the human genome.(➕) Only a few of the many roles proteins play are described here, but these should serve to illustrate proteins' versatility, uniqueness, and importance.

➕ The *human genome* is the full set of chromosomes, including all of the genes and associated DNA. Nutrition genomics is the topic of Nutrition in Practice 13.

enzymes: protein catalysts. A catalyst is a compound that facilitates chemical reactions without itself being changed in the process.

AS STRUCTURAL COMPONENTS

A great deal of the body's protein exists in muscle tissue, which allows the body to move. The amino acids of muscle protein can also be released when the need is dire, as in starvation. These amino acids are integral parts of the muscle structure, and their loss exacts a cost of functional protein, as a later section makes clear.

Other structural proteins confer shape and strength on bones, teeth, tendons, cartilage, blood vessels, and other tissues. These proteins exist in a stable form and are more resistant to breakdown than are the proteins of muscles.

AS ENZYMES

Enzymes are catalysts that are essential to all life processes. Enzymes in the cells of plants or animals put together the pairs of sugars that make disaccharides and the long strands of sugars that make starch, cellulose, and glycogen. Enzymes also dismantle these compounds to free their constituent parts and release energy. Enzymes also assemble and disassemble lipids, assemble all other compounds that the body makes, and disassemble all compounds that the body can use for building tissue and other metabolic work. As Figure 5-4 shows, enzymes themselves are not altered by the reactions they facilitate. All enzymes are proteins, and when amino acids have to be put together to make proteins, it is enzymes that put them together, too. In other words, these proteins can even make other proteins.

The protein story moves in a circle. To follow the circle in nutrition, start with a person eating food proteins. The food proteins are broken down by digestive enzymes, proteins themselves, into amino acids. The amino acids enter the cells of the body, where other proteins (enzymes) put the amino acids together in long chains whose sequences are specified by the genes. The chains fold and twist back on themselves to form proteins, and some of these proteins become enzymes themselves. Some of these enzymes break apart compounds; others put compounds together. Day by day, in billions of reactions, these processes repeat themselves, and life goes on. Only living systems can achieve such self-renewal. A toaster cannot produce another toaster; a car cannot fix a broken-down car. Only living creatures and the parts they are composed of—the cells—can duplicate and repair themselves.

FIGURE 5-4 | Enzyme Action

The separate compounds, A and B, are attracted to the enzyme's active site, making a reaction likely.

The enzyme forms a complex with A and B.

The enzyme is unchanged, but A and B have formed a new compound, AB.

Each enzyme facilitates a specific chemical reaction. In this diagram, an enzyme enables two compounds to make a more complex structure, but the enzyme itself remains unchanged.

FIGURE 5-5 | One Cell and Its Associated Fluids

Fluid between the cells (intercellular or interstitial)

Cell membrane

Nucleus

Fluid within the cell (intracellular)

Fluid within the blood vessels (intravascular)

Blood vessel

➕ Minerals are helper nutrients. The attraction of protein and mineral particles to water is due to osmotic pressure (see Chapter 9).

fluid and electrolyte balance: maintenance of the necessary amounts and types of fluid and minerals in each compartment of the body fluids.

edema (eh-DEEM-uh): the swelling of body tissue caused by leakage of fluid from the blood vessels and accumulation of the fluid in the interstitial spaces.

acids: compounds that release hydrogen ions in a solution.

bases: compounds that accept hydrogen ions in a solution.

acid-base balance: the balance maintained between acid and base concentrations in the blood and body fluids.

pH: the concentration of hydrogen ions. The lower the pH, the stronger the acid. Thus, pH 2 is a strong acid; pH 6 is a weak acid; pH 7 is neutral; and a pH above 7 is alkaline.

denaturation (dee-nay-cher-AY-shun): the change in a protein's shape brought about by heat, acid, or other agents. Past a certain point, denaturation is irreversible.

AS TRANSPORTERS

A large group of proteins specialize in transporting other substances, such as lipids, vitamins, and minerals, around the body. To do their jobs, those substances must move from place to place within the blood, into and out of cells, or around the cellular interiors. Two familiar examples: the protein hemoglobin carries oxygen from the lungs to the cells, and the lipoproteins transport lipids in the watery blood.

AS REGULATORS OF FLUID AND ELECTROLYTE BALANCE

Proteins help maintain the body's **fluid and electrolyte balance**. As Figure 5-5 shows, the body's fluids are contained in three major body compartments: (1) the spaces inside the blood vessels; (2) the spaces within the cells; and (3) the spaces between the cells (the interstitial spaces outside the blood vessels). Fluids flow back and forth between these compartments, and proteins in the fluids, together with minerals, (➕) help to maintain the needed distribution of these fluids.

Proteins are able to help determine the distribution of fluids in living systems for two reasons: first, proteins cannot pass freely across the membranes that separate the body compartments, and second, they are attracted to water. A cell that "wants" a certain amount of water in its interior space cannot move the water around directly, but it can manufacture proteins, and these proteins will hold water. Thus, the cell can use proteins to help regulate the distribution of water indirectly. Similarly, the body makes proteins for the blood and the interstitial (intercellular) spaces. These proteins help maintain the fluid volume in those spaces. Excess fluid accumulation in the interstitial spaces is called **edema**.

Not only is the quantity of the body fluids vital to life, but so is their composition. Special transport proteins in the membranes of cells continuously transfer substances into and out of cells to maintain balance. For example, sodium is concentrated outside the cells, and potassium is concentrated inside. The balance of these two minerals is critical to nerve transmission and muscle contraction. Any disturbance in this balance triggers a major medical emergency. Such imbalances can cause irregular heartbeats, kidney failure, muscular weakness, and even death.

AS REGULATORS OF ACID-BASE BALANCE

Proteins also help maintain the balance between **acids** and **bases** within the body's fluids. Normal body processes continually produce acids and bases, which must be carried by the blood to the kidneys and lungs for excretion. The blood must do this without upsetting its own **acid-base balance**. Blood **pH** is one of the most tightly controlled conditions in the body. If the blood becomes too acidic, vital proteins may undergo **denaturation**, losing their shape and ability to function. A similar situation arises when there is an excess of base. These imbalances are known as **acidosis** and **alkalosis**, respectively, and both can be fatal. Figure 5-6 shows the normal and abnormal pH ranges of body fluids, as well as the pHs of some common substances.

Proteins such as albumin in blood help to prevent acid-base imbalances. In a sense, the proteins protect one another by gathering up extra acid (hydrogen) ions when there are too many in the surrounding medium and by releasing them when there are too few. By accepting and releasing hydrogen ions, proteins act as **buffers**, maintaining the acid-base balance of the blood and body fluids.

AS ANTIBODIES

Other proteins in the blood—the **antibodies**—defend against viruses, bacteria, and other disease agents. The antibodies work so efficiently that if a million bacterial cells are injected into the skin of a healthy person, fewer than 10 are likely to survive for five hours, which explains why most diseases never have a chance to get started. Without sufficient protein, however, the body cannot maintain its resistance to disease.

FIGURE
5-6 | The pH Scale

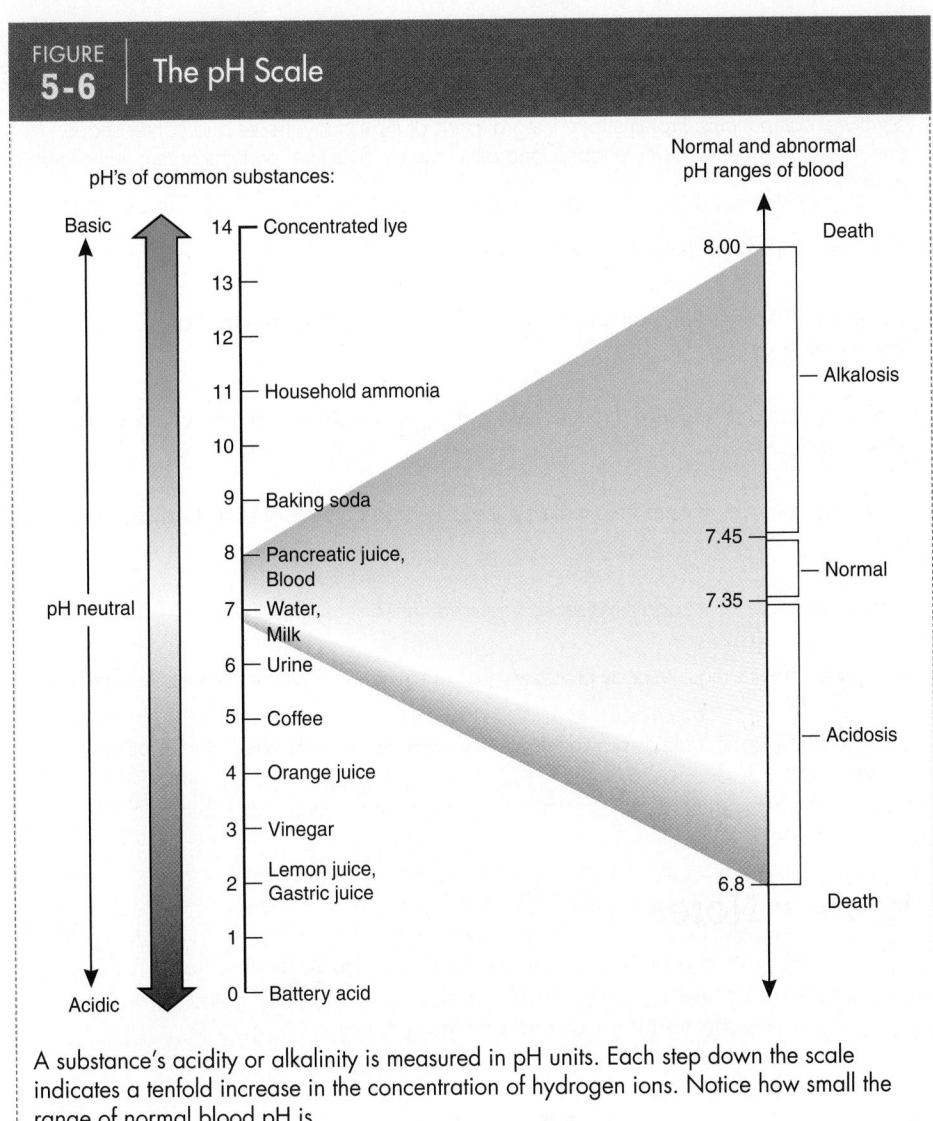

pH's of common substances:

Basic

14 — Concentrated lye

13

12

11 — Household ammonia

10

9 — Baking soda

8 — Pancreatic juice, Blood

pH neutral

7 — Water, Milk

6 — Urine

5 — Coffee

4 — Orange juice

3 — Vinegar

2 — Lemon juice, Gastric juice

1

Acidic

0 — Battery acid

Normal and abnormal pH ranges of blood

8.00 — Death

Alkalosis

7.45 — Normal

7.35

Acidosis

6.8 — Death

A substance's acidity or alkalinity is measured in pH units. Each step down the scale indicates a tenfold increase in the concentration of hydrogen ions. Notice how small the range of normal blood pH is.

AS HORMONES

The blood also carries messenger molecules known as **hormones**, and *some* hormones are proteins. (Recall that some hormones are sterols, members of the lipid family.) Among the proteins that act as hormones are glucagon and insulin. Hormones have many profound effects, which will become evident in subsequent chapters.

AS A SOURCE OF ENERGY AND GLUCOSE

Without energy, cells die; without glucose, the brain and nervous system falter. Even though amino acids are needed to do the work that only they can perform—build vital proteins—they will be sacrificed to provide energy and glucose during times of starvation or insufficient carbohydrate intake.[1] When glucose or fatty acids are limited, cells are forced to use amino acids for energy and glucose. The body does not make a specialized storage form of protein as it does for carbohydrate and fat. Glucose is stored as glycogen in the liver and muscles, fat as triglycerides in the adipose tissue, but body protein is available only as the working and structural components of the tissues. When the need arises, the body dismantles its tissue proteins and uses them for energy. Thus, over time, energy deprivation (starvation) always incurs wasting of lean body tissue as well as fat loss.

acidosis: acid accumulation in the blood and body fluids; depresses the central nervous system and can lead to disorientation and, eventually, coma.

alkalosis: excessive base in the blood and body fluids.

buffers: compounds that can reversibly combine with hydrogen ions to help keep a solution's acidity or alkalinity constant.

antibodies: large proteins of the blood and body fluids, produced in response to invasion of the body by unfamiliar molecules (mostly proteins) called antigens. Antibodies inactivate the invaders and so protect the body. *anti* = against

hormones: chemical messengers. Hormones are secreted by a variety of glands in the body in response to altered conditions. Each travels to one or more target tissues or organs and elicits specific responses to restore normal conditions.

TABLE
5-1 | Summary of Functions of Proteins

Structural components. Proteins form integral parts of most body tissues and confer shape and strength on bones, skin, tendons, and other tissues. Structural proteins of muscles allow movement.

Enzymes. Proteins facilitate chemical reactions.

Transporters. Proteins transport substance such as lipids, vitamins, minerals, and oxygen around the body.

Fluid and electrolyte balance. Proteins help to maintain the distribution and composition of various body fluids.

Acid-base balance. Proteins help maintain the acid-base balance of body fluids by acting as buffers.

Antibodies. Proteins act against disease agents to fight diseases.

Hormones. Proteins regulate body processes. Some, but not all, hormones are made of protein.

Energy and glucose. Proteins provide some fuel, and glucose if needed, for the body's energy needs.

Review Notes

- The list of protein functions discussed here and summarized in Table 5-1 is by no means exhaustive. Nevertheless, it does give some sense of the immense variety of proteins and their importance in the body.

Protein and Health

During the time that scientists have been studying nutrition, no nutrient has been more intensely scrutinized than protein. As you know by now, it is indispensable to life. And it should come as no surprise that protein deficiency can have devastating effects on people's health. But, as with the other nutrients, protein in excess can be harmful, too, so this section also discusses the consequences of protein excess.

PROTEIN-ENERGY MALNUTRITION

When people are deprived of food and suffer an energy deficiency, they degrade their own body protein for energy and indirectly suffer a protein deficiency as well. This combination—**protein-energy malnutrition (PEM)**—is the most widespread form of malnutrition in the world today. PEM is prevalent in Africa, Central America, South America, the Middle East, and East and Southeast Asia, but developed countries including the United States are not immune to it. PEM is common among some population groups in the United States: impoverished people living in inner cities and in rural areas; many elderly people; homeless children; and those suffering from the eating disorder anorexia nervosa. (✚)

Of all population groups, children are most seriously affected by malnutrition. Worldwide, three-fourths of those who die each year from starvation and related illnesses are children.[2] Children who are thin for their heights may have recently developed PEM, whereas children who are short for their ages may have experienced PEM for extended periods of time. Stunted growth due to PEM is easy to overlook because a small child

✚ PEM can be a consequence of many different conditions. PEM has been recognized in people with many chronic diseases such as cancer and AIDS and in those who have severe stresses such as burns or extensive infections (see Chapter 16). The consequences of PEM as a world malnutrition problem are considered here; the problems associated with PEM and illness are described throughout later chapters.

protein-energy malnutrition (PEM): a deficiency of protein and food energy; the world's most widespread malnutrition problem, including both marasmus and kwashiorkor.
mal = bad, poor

may look quite normal, but it may be the most common sign of malnutrition in the developing countries. PEM takes two different forms, with some cases exhibiting a combination of the two. In one form, the person is shriveled and emaciated—this disease is called **marasmus**. In the second, a swollen belly and skin rash are present, and the disease is named **kwashiorkor**. In the combination, some features of each type are present. Marasmus reflects a severe deprivation of food over a long time (chronic PEM). Put simply, the person is starving and suffering from an inadequate energy *and* protein intake (and inadequate essential fatty acids, vitamins, and minerals as well). Kwashiorkor may result from severe acute malnutrition, with too little protein to support body functions.

Marasmus Marasmus commonly occurs in children from 6 to 18 months of age in all the overpopulated and impoverished areas of the world. Children in impoverished nations subsist on a weak cereal drink that supplies scant energy and protein of low quality: such food can barely sustain life, much less support growth. Consequently, marasmic children look like little old people—just skin and bones.

Without adequate nutrition, muscles, including the heart muscle, waste and weaken. Because the brain normally grows to almost its full adult size within the first two years of life, marasmus impairs brain development and learning ability. Reduced synthesis of key hormones leads to a metabolism so slow that body temperature drops below normal. There is little or no fat under the skin to insulate against cold. Some hospital workers find that the primary need of marasmic children is to be clothed, covered, and kept warm.

The starving child faces this threat to life by engaging in as little activity as possible—not even crying for food. The body gathers all its forces to meet the crisis, so it cuts down on any expenditure of energy not needed for the heart, lungs, and brain to function. Growth ceases; the child is no larger at age four than at age two. Digestive enzymes are in short supply, the digestive tract lining deteriorates, and absorption fails. The child cannot assimilate what little food is eaten.

Blood proteins, including hemoglobin, are no longer synthesized. Antibodies to fight off invading bacteria are degraded to provide amino acids for other uses, rendering the child vulnerable to infection. Then **dysentery**, an infection of the digestive tract, causes diarrhea, further depleting the body of nutrients. In the marasmic child, once infection has set in, kwashiorkor often follows and the immune response weakens further. The infection that occurs with malnutrition (✚) is responsible for two-thirds of the deaths of young children in developing countries.

If the condition is caught in time, the life of a starving child may be saved with rehydration and nutrition intervention.[3] In severe cases, children with diarrhea will have incurred dramatic fluid and mineral losses that need to be replaced during the first 24 to

✚ When two variables interact so that each increases the other, the interaction is known as *synergism* (SIN-er-jiz-um). Malnutrition and infection are a deadly combination because they work in this way.
syn = with, together
ergism = work

marasmus (ma-RAZZ-mus): the most common form of severe PEM before one year of age. Marasmus is characterized by generalized muscle wasting associated with extreme deprivation, or impaired absorption, of energy, protein, vitamins, and minerals.

kwashiorkor (kwash-ee-OR-core or kwash-ee-or-CORE): a severe form of PEM that occurs more frequently after 18 months of age. Kwashiorkor is characterized by failure to grow and develop, changes in the pigmentation of the hair and skin, edema, and fatty liver. Kwashiorkor is associated with inadequate protein intake and infections.

dysentery (DIS-en-terry): an infection of the gastrointestinal tract caused by an amoeba or bacterium that gives rise to severe diarrhea.
dys = bad
entery = intestine

FAO/13670/G. Kent

FAO/13670/G. Kent

In the photo on the left, the extreme loss of muscle and fat characteristic of marasmus is apparent in the child's matchstick arms and legs. In contrast, the edema and enlarged liver characteristic of kwashiorkor are apparent in the swollen bellies of the children in the photo on the right.

48 hours to help raise the blood pressure and strengthen the heartbeat. After that, protein and energy may be given in *small* quantities several times a day, with intakes *gradually* increased as tolerated.[4] Years after PEM is corrected, however, a child may still experience deficits in thinking and achievement in school compared with well-nourished peers.

Kwashiorkor Kwashiorkor typically reflects a sudden and recent deprivation of food (acute PEM). *Kwashiorkor* is a Ghanaian word meaning a "sickness that infects the first child when the second child is born." If you consider how kwashiorkor often develops, you can easily see how the Ghanaians arrived at this name for the disease. When a mother who has been nursing her first child bears a second child, she weans the first child and puts the second one on the breast. The first child, suddenly switched from nutrient-dense, protein-rich breast milk to a starchy, protein-poor gruel, soon begins to sicken and die. Kwashiorkor typically sets in between 18 months and 2 years. Kwashiorkor usually develops rapidly as a result of protein deficiency or, more commonly, is precipitated by an illness such as measles or other infection.[5]

Some symptoms of kwashiorkor resemble those of marasmus (see Table 5-2). Proteins and hormones that previously maintained fluid balance diminish, and fluid leaks into the interstitial spaces. The child's limbs and belly become swollen with edema, a distinguishing feature of kwashiorkor; a **fatty liver** develops due to a lack of the protein carriers that transport fat out of the liver. The child's hair loses its color; the skin becomes patchy and scaly, sometimes with ulcers and sores that fail to heal.

fatty liver: an accumulation of fat in the liver. In PEM, fat accumulates in the liver because no protein is available to form the lipoproteins that normally escort fat molecules in the blood (see Chapter 19).

TABLE 5-2	Features of Marasmus and Kwashiorkor in Children

Separating PEM into two classifications oversimplifies the condition, but at the extremes, marasmus and kwashiorkor exhibit marked differences. Marasmus-kwashiorkor mix presents symptoms common to both marasmus and kwashiorkor. In all cases, children are likely to develop diarrhea, infections, and multiple nutrient deficiencies.

Marasmus	Kwashiorkor
Infancy (less than 2 yr)	Older infants and young children (1 to 3 yr)
Severe deprivation, or impaired absorption, of protein, energy, vitamins, and minerals	Inadequate protein intake or, more commonly, infections
Develops slowly; chronic PEM	Rapid onset; acute PEM
Severe weight loss	Some weight loss
Severe muscle wasting, with no body fat	Some muscle wasting, with retention of some body fat
Growth: <60% weight-for-age	Growth: 60 to 80% weight-for-age
No detectable edema	Edema
No fatty liver	Enlarged fatty liver
Anxiety, apathy	Apathy, misery, irritability, sadness
Good appetite possible	Loss of appetite
Hair is sparse, thin, and dry; easily pulled out	Hair is dry and brittle; easily pulled out; changes color; becomes straight
Skin is dry, thin, and easily wrinkles	Skin develops lesions

Clearly, preventing marasmus and kwashiorkor from developing in the first place is more desirable than attempting to treat the conditions after they have set in. Experts assure us that we possess the knowledge, technology, and resources to end the hunger that leads to PEM. Programs that have involved the local people in the process of identifying the problem and devising its solution have met with some success. But until those who have the food, technology, and resources make fighting hunger a priority, the war on hunger will not be won.

PROTEIN EXCESS

While many of the world's people struggle to obtain enough food and enough protein to survive, in the developed nations protein is so abundant that problems of protein excess are observed. Overconsumption of protein offers no benefits and may pose health risks for the heart, weakened kidneys, and the bones.[6] Selecting too many protein-rich foods, such as red meats and fat-containing milk products, adds saturated fat and crowds out fruits, vegetables, and whole grains, a problem from the standpoint of chronic disease risks.

Heart Disease Foods rich in animal protein can also be rich in saturated fats. Consequently, it is not surprising that people who take in a great deal of animal protein (red meats and dairy products) have a greater risk of heart disease.[7] In the United States, meat consumption often accompanies higher energy (kcalorie) intakes and increased abdominal body fatness, and excess abdominal fat raises the risk for heart disease.[8] As the Nutrition in Practice points out, people who substitute vegetable protein for animal protein lower their risk of dying from heart disease.[9]

Kidney Disease Excretion of the end products of protein metabolism depends, in part, on an adequate fluid intake and healthy kidneys. A high protein intake increases the work of the kidneys but does not appear to damage healthy kidneys or cause kidney disease.[10] A high-protein diet does worsen existing kidney disease and may accelerate a decline in only mildly impaired kidneys.[11] One of the most effective ways to slow the progression of kidney disease is to restrict dietary protein.

Adult Bone Loss When human subjects are given increasing doses of purified protein, they release larger and larger amounts of calcium from the body into the urine. This fact raises concerns that a high-protein diet may cause or worsen adult bone loss. In a recent study, however, researchers concluded that, unlike intakes of purified protein, high protein intakes from whole food sources, such as meat or milk products, do not appear to increase calcium losses.[12] Other factors, such as low intakes of vitamin D and bone minerals, ultimately harm bone health to a greater degree than high intakes of protein.[13]

Conversely, too little dietary protein almost certainly weakens the bones, both during childhood years of bone development and in malnourished elderly individuals; protein deficiency and hip fractures often occur together, and restoring dietary protein along with calcium and vitamin D supplements improves bone status.[14*] In establishing protein recommendations, the DRI committee considered protein's effect on bone health but did not find sufficient evidence to set a Tolerable Upper Intake Level.[15]

Review Notes

- Protein deficiencies arise from both energy-poor and protein-poor diets and lead to the devastating diseases of marasmus and kwashiorkor.
- Together, these diseases are known as protein-energy malnutrition (PEM), a major form of malnutrition causing death in children worldwide.
- Excesses of protein offer no advantage; in fact, overconsumption of protein-rich foods may cause health problems as well.

---

*The calcium supplement was citrate malate.

PROTEIN AND AMINO ACID SUPPLEMENTS

Why do people take protein or amino acid supplements? Athletes often take them when trying to build muscle. Dieters may take them to spare their bodies' protein while losing weight. Some women take them to strengthen their fingernails. People take individual amino acid supplements too—to cure herpes, to make themselves sleep better, to lose weight, and to relieve pain and depression. Do protein and amino acid supplements really do these things? Probably not. Are they safe? Not always.

Protein Supplements Though protein supplements are popular with athletes, well-fed athletes do not need them. Dietary protein is necessary for building muscle tissue, and consuming protein in conjunction with resistance exercise helps muscles build new proteins.[16] Protein supplements, however, do not improve athletic performance beyond the gains from well-timed meals of ordinary foods. And, if supplements create a surplus of protein or certain amino acids, the excess must be metabolized, placing a burden on the kidneys to excrete excess nitrogen.

Weight-loss dieters may benefit from consistently consuming protein-rich foods because protein often satisfies the appetite, while insufficient protein may increase it.[17] However, extra protein from powders, pills, or beverages is unlikely to dampen the appetite further, although it contributes unneeded kcalories—the wrong effect for weight loss. Evidence does not support taking protein supplements for weight loss, and common sense opposes it.

Amino Acid Supplements Enthusiastic popular reports have led to widespread use of individual amino acids. One such amino acid is lysine, promoted to prevent or relieve the infections that cause herpes sores on the mouth or genital organs. Lysine does not cure herpes infections. Whether it reduces outbreaks or even whether it is safe is unknown because scientific studies are lacking.

Tryptophan supplements are advertised to relieve pain, depression, and insomnia. Tryptophan plays a role as a precursor for the brain neurotransmitter serotonin, an important regulator of sleep, appetite, mood, and sensory perception. The DRI committee concludes that high doses of tryptophan may induce sleepiness, but they may also cause side effects, such as nausea and skin disorders. A serious blood disorder, EMS, probably caused by contaminants, once threatened takers of tryptophan supplements, but improved regulations have reduced this risk.[18]*

The body is designed to handle whole proteins best. It breaks them into manageable pieces (dipeptides and tripeptides), then splits these, a few at a time, simultaneously releasing them into the blood. This slow bit-by-bit assimilation is ideal because groups of chemically similar amino acids compete for the carriers that absorb them into the blood. An excess of one amino acid can produce such a demand for a carrier that it limits the absorption of another amino acid, creating a temporary imbalance.[19]

Many supplement takers experience digestive disturbances. Amino acids in concentrated supplements cause excess water to flow into the digestive tract, causing diarrhea.[20]

The DRI committee reviewed the available research on amino acids, but with next to no safety research in existence, the committee was unable to set Tolerable Upper Intake Levels for supplemental doses. Until research becomes available, no level of amino acid supplementation can be assumed to be safe for all people. Growth or altered metabolism makes the following groups of people especially likely to suffer harm from amino acid supplements:

- All women of childbearing age
- Pregnant or lactating women
- Infants, children, and adolescents
- Elderly people
- People with inborn errors of metabolism that affect their bodies' handling of amino acids
- Smokers
- People on low-protein diets
- People with chronic or acute mental or physical illnesses who take amino acids without medical supervision

*EMS is short for *eosinophilia-myalgia syndrome*.

Anyone considering taking amino acid supplements should be cautious not to exceed levels normally found in foods.[21]

PROTEIN RECOMMENDATIONS AND INTAKES

The committee that established the RDA states that a generous daily protein allowance for a healthy adult is 0.8 gram per kilogram (2.2 pounds) of healthy body weight. (✚) The RDA covers the needs for replacing worn-out tissue, so it increases for larger people; it also covers the needs for building new tissue during growth, so is slightly higher for infants, children, and pregnant and lactating women.

In setting the RDA, the committee assumes that the protein eaten will be of good quality, that it will be consumed together with adequate energy from carbohydrate and fat, and that other nutrients in the diet will be adequate. The committee also assumes that the RDA will be applied only to healthy individuals with no unusual alteration of protein metabolism.

Most people assume that Americans eat too much protein. Research demonstrates that a median protein intake for U.S. adult males is about 16 percent of total kcalories, an amount that falls directly within the DRI suggested range of between 10 and 35 percent of kcalories.[22] Women, children, and some elderly people may typically take in less protein—13 to 15 percent. A small percentage of adolescent girls and elderly women consume insufficient protein or barely enough to meet their needs.[23]

Review Notes

- Normal, healthy people do not need amino acid or protein supplements.
- Optimally, an adult's diet will be adequate in energy from carbohydrate and fat and will deliver at least 0.8 grams of protein per kilogram of healthy body weight each day.

Protein in Foods

In the United States and Canada, where nutritious foods are abundant, most people easily obtain enough protein to receive all the amino acids that they need. In countries where food is scarce and the people eat only marginal amounts of protein-rich foods, however, the *quality* of the protein becomes crucial.

PROTEIN QUALITY

The protein quality of the diet determines, in large part, how well children grow and how well adults maintain their health. Put simply, **high-quality proteins** provide enough of all the essential amino acids needed to support the body's work, and low-quality proteins don't. Two factors influence protein quality—the protein's digestibility and its amino acid composition.

Digestibility As explained earlier, proteins must be digested before they can provide amino acids. **Protein digestibility** depends on such factors as the protein's source and the other foods eaten with it. The digestibility of most animal proteins is high (90 to 99 percent); plant proteins are less digestible (70 to 90 percent for most, but more than 90 percent for soy).

Amino Acid Composition To make proteins, cells must have all the needed amino acids available simultaneously. The liver can produce any nonessential amino acid that may be in short supply so that the cells can continue linking amino acids into protein strands. If an essential amino acid is missing, however, a cell must dismantle its

✚ RDA for protein (adult) = 0.8 g/kg
- 10 to 35 percent of energy intake

To calculate your protein need:

1. Find your body weight in pounds (or kilograms).
2. Convert pounds to kilograms, if necessary (pounds divided by 2.2).
3. Multiply kilograms by 0.8 to find total grams of protein recommended.

For example:

1. Weight = 150 lb
2. 150 lb ÷ 2.2 lb/kg = 68 kg
3. 68 kg × 0.8 g/kg = 54 g

high-quality proteins: dietary proteins containing all the essential amino acids in relatively the same amounts that human beings require. They may also contain nonessential amino acids.

protein digestibility: a measure of the amount of amino acids absorbed from a given protein intake.

Vegetarians obtain their protein from whole grains, legumes, nuts, vegetables, and, in some cases, eggs and milk products.

© Polara Studios, Inc

own proteins to obtain it. Therefore, to prevent protein breakdown, dietary protein must supply at least the nine essential amino acids plus enough nitrogen-containing amino groups and energy for the synthesis of the others. If the diet supplies too little of any essential amino acid, protein synthesis will be limited. The body makes whole proteins only; if one amino acid is missing, the others cannot form a "partial" protein. An essential amino acid that is available in the shortest supply relative to the amount needed to support protein synthesis is called a **limiting amino acid**.

High-Quality Proteins A high-quality protein contains all the essential amino acids in amounts adequate for human use; it may or may not contain all the others. Generally, proteins derived from animal foods (meats, fish, poultry, cheese, eggs, yogurt, and milk) are high quality, although gelatin is an exception. Proteins derived from plant foods (legumes, grains, and vegetables) tend to be limiting in one or more essential amino acids. Some plant proteins are notoriously low quality—for example, corn protein. Others are high quality—for example, soy protein. As discussed in Nutrition in Practice 5, the educated vegetarian can design a diet that is adequate in protein by choosing a variety of legumes, whole grains, nuts, and vegetables. Table 5-3 lists the protein contents of foods based on the

limiting amino acid: an essential amino acid that is present in dietary protein in the shortest supply relative to the amount needed for protein synthesis in the body.

TABLE 5-3 | Protein-Containing Foods

Milk, Yogurt, and Cheese

Each of the following provides about 8 grams of protein:
- 1 c milk, buttermilk, or yogurt (choose low fat or fat free)
- 1 oz regular cheese (for example, cheddar or Swiss; choose low fat)
- ¼ c cottage cheese (choose low fat or fat free)

Meat, Poultry, Fish, Legumes, Eggs, and Nuts

Each of the following provides about 7 grams of protein:
- 1 oz meat, poultry, or fish (choose lean meats to limit saturated fat intake)
- ½ c legumes (navy beans, pinto beans, black beans, lentils, soybeans, and other dried beans and peas)
- 1 egg
- ½ c tofu (soybean curd)
- 2 tbs peanut butter
- 1 to 2 oz nuts or seeds

Grains

Each of the following provides about 3 grams of protein:
- 1 slice of bread
- ½ c cooked rice, pasta, cereals, or other grain foods

Vegetables

Each of the following provides about 2 grams of protein:
- ½ c cooked vegetables
- 1 c raw vegetables

food groups of the USDA Food Guide in Chapter 1. Fruits are not included in Table 5-3 because they contribute only small amounts of protein.

Complementary Proteins If the body does not receive all the essential amino acids it needs, the supply of essential amino acids will dwindle until body organs are compromised. Obtaining enough essential amino acids presents no problem to people who regularly eat high-quality proteins, such as those of meat, fish, poultry, cheese, eggs, milk, and many soybean products. The proteins of these foods contain ample amounts of all the essential amino acids. An equally sound choice is to eat two different protein foods from plants so that each supplies the amino acids missing in the other. In this strategy, the two protein-rich foods are combined to yield **complementary proteins** (see Figure 5-7)—proteins containing all the essential amino acids in amounts sufficient to support health. The two proteins need not even be eaten together, as long as the day's meals supply them both, and the diet provides enough energy and total protein from a variety of sources.

FIGURE 5-7	Complementary Proteins			
	Ile	Lys	Met	Trp
Legumes	✓	✓		
Grains			✓	✓
Together	✓	✓	✓	✓

In general, legumes provide plenty of isoleucine (Ile) and lysine (Lys) but fall short in methionine (Met) and tryptophan (Trp). Grains have the opposite strengths and weaknesses, making them a perfect match for legumes.

PROTEIN SPARING

Dietary protein—no matter how high the quality—will not be used efficiently and will not support growth when energy from carbohydrate and fat is lacking. The body assigns top priority to meeting its energy need and, if necessary, will break down protein to meet this need. After stripping off and excreting the nitrogen from the amino acids, the body will use the remaining carbon skeletons in much the same way it uses those from glucose or fat. A major reason why people must have ample carbohydrate and fat in the diet is to prevent this wasting of protein. (✚)

PROTEIN ON FOOD LABELS

All food labels must state the *quantity* of protein in grams. The "percent Daily Value" for protein is not mandatory on all labels, but it is required whenever a food makes a protein claim or is intended for consumption by children under four years old. (✚)* Whenever the Daily Value percentage is declared, researchers must determine the *quality* of the protein. Thus, when a % Daily Value is stated for protein, it reflects both quantity and quality.

Review Notes

- A diet inadequate in any of the essential amino acids limits protein synthesis.
- The best guarantee of amino acid adequacy is to eat foods containing high-quality proteins or combinations of foods containing complementary proteins so that each can supply the amino acids missing in the other.
- Vegetarians who consume no foods of animal origin can meet their protein needs by eating a variety of whole grains, legumes, seeds, nuts, and vegetables.
- Ample carbohydrate and fat in the diet allow amino acids to be used to build body proteins.
- All food labels must state the quantity of protein in grams.

✚ Reminder: Carbohydrate and fat allow amino acids to be used to build body proteins. This is known as the *protein-sparing effect* of carbohydrate and fat.

✚ Daily Value:
• 50 g protein (based on 10 percent of 2000-kcal diet)

complementary proteins: two or more proteins whose amino acid assortments complement each other in such a way that the essential amino acids missing from one are supplied by the other.

---

* For labeling purposes, the Daily Values for protein are as follows: for infants, 14 grams; for children under age four, 16 grams; for older children and adults, 50 grams; for pregnant women, 60 grams; and for lactating women, 65 grams.

Self Check

1 • Proteins are chemically different from carbohydrates and fats because they also contain:

    a. iron.

    b. sodium.

    c. nitrogen.

    d. phosphorus.

2 • The basic building blocks for protein are:

    a. side groups.

    b. amino acids.

    c. glucose units.

    d. saturated bonds.

3 • Enzymes are proteins that, among other things:

    a. defend the body against disease.

    b. regulate fluid and electrolyte balance.

    c. facilitate chemical reactions by changing themselves.

    d. help assemble disaccharides into starch, cellulose, or glycogen.

4 • Functions of proteins in the body include:

    a. supplying omega-3 fatty acids for growth, lowering serum cholesterol, and helping with weight control.

    b. supplying fiber to aid digestion, digesting cellulose, and providing the main fuel source for muscles.

    c. protecting organs against shock, helping the body use carbohydrate efficiently, and providing triglycerides.

    d. serving as structural components, supplying hormones to regulate body processes, and maintaining fluid and electrolyte balance.

5 • The swelling of body tissue caused by the leakage of fluid from the blood vessels into the interstitial spaces is called:

    b. edema.

    c. anemia.

    d. acidosis.

    e. sickle-cell anemia.

6 • Major proteins in the blood that protect against bacteria and other disease agents are called:

    a. acids.

    b. buffers.

    c. antigens.

    d. antibodies.

7 • Marasmus can be distinguished from kwashiorkor because in marasmus:

    a. only adults are victims.

    b. the cause is usually an infection.

    c. severe wasting of body fat and muscle occurs.

    d. the limbs and face swell with edema, and the belly bulges with a fatty liver.

8 • The RDA for protein for a healthy adult is _____ gram(s) per kilogram of appropriate or average body weight for height.

    a. 0.5

    b. 0.8

    c. 1.1

    d. 1.4

9 • Generally speaking, from which of the following foods are complete proteins derived?

    a. Milk, gelatin, and soy

    b. Rice, potatoes, and eggs

    c. Meats, fish, and poultry

    d. Vegetables, grains, and fruits

10 • An incomplete protein lacks one or more:

    a. hydrogen bonds.

    b. essential fatty acids.

    c. saturated fatty acids.

    d. essential amino acids.

Answers to these questions can be found in Appendix H.

Clinical Applications

1 • Considering the health effects of too little dietary protein, what suggestions would you have for a teenage girl who reports the following information about her food intake:

    • She never eats any meat or other animal-derived foods because she is a vegan. On a typical day, she consumes toast and juice for breakfast; chips, a soft drink, and a piece of fruit for lunch; and a small serving of plain pasta with tomato sauce or steamed vegetables for dinner, along with a glass of water or tea.

    • She takes amino acid supplements because a friend told her that the only way to get amino acids if she doesn't eat meat is to take them as supplements.

2 • Considering the health effects of excess dietary protein, what advice would you have for a college athlete who tells you he wants to bulk up his muscles and reports the following information about his food intake:

- He eats large servings of meat (usually red meat) at least twice a day. He drinks whole milk two or three times a day and eats eggs and bacon for breakfast almost every day.

- He avoids breads, cereals, and pasta in order to save room for protein-rich foods such as meat, milk, and eggs.

- He eats a piece of fruit once in a while but seldom eats vegetables because they are too time consuming to prepare.

Nutrition on the Net

For further study of the topics of this chapter, access these websites.

- Find updates and quick links to these and other nutrition-related sites at our website: www.cengage.com/nutrition/whitney/nhhc4e
- To learn more about protein in foods, visit the American Dietetic Association (ADA) site: www.eatright.org
- For more on vegetarian diets, search the Food and Drug Administration (FDA) site for foods: www.fda.gov

- Search among thousands of current scientific and medical abstracts for any topic related to protein at: www.ncbi.nlm.nih.gov/PubMed/
- Learn more about protein-energy malnutrition and world hunger from the World Health Organization's Nutrition Programme: www.who.int

Notes

1. Standing Committee on the Scientific Evaluation of Dietary Reference Intakes, Food and Nutrition Board, Institute of Medicine, *Dietary Reference Intakes for Energy, Carbohydrate, Fiber, Fat, Fatty Acids, Cholesterol, Protein, and Amino Acids* (Washington, D.C.: National Academies Press, 2005), p. 605.
2. Food and Agriculture Organization of the United Nations, *The State of Food Insecurity in the World, 2009*, Food Security Statistics, available from www.fao.org.
3. J. F. Desjeux, Recent issues in energy-protein malnutrition in children, *Nestle Nutrition Workshop Series: Pediatric Program* 58 (2006): 177–184.
4. D. R. Brewster, Critical appraisal of the management of severe malnutrition: 2. Dietary management, *Journal of Paediatrics and Child Health* 42 (2006): 575–582; A. A. Jackson, A. Ashworth, and S. Khanum, Improving child survival: Malnutrition Task Force and the paediatrician's responsibility, *Archives of Diseases in Childhood* 91 (2006): 706–710.
5. N. S. Scrimshaw, Fifty-five-year personal experience with human nutrition worldwide, *Annual Review of Nutrition* 27 (2007): 1–18.
6. H. Frank and coauthors, Effect of short-term high-protein compared with normal-protein diets on renal hemodynamics and associated variables in health young men, *American Journal of Clinical Nutrition* 90 (2009): 1509–1516; Standing Committee on the Scientific Evaluation of Dietary Reference Intakes, 2005, p. 694.
7. L. E. Kelemen and coauthors, Associations of dietary protein with disease and mortality in a prospective study of postmenopausal women, *American Journal of Epidemiology* 161 (2005): 239–249.
8. Y. Wang and M. A. Beydoun, Meat consumption is associated with obesity and central obesity among US adults, *International Journal of Obesity* 33 (2009): 621–628.
9. N. R. Matthan and coauthors, Effect of soy protein from differently processed products on cardiovascular disease risk factors and vascular endothelial function in hypercholesterolemic subjects, *American Journal of Clinical Nutrition* 85 (2007): 960–966; B. L. McVeigh and coauthors, Effect of soy protein varying in isoflavone content on serum lipids in healthy young men, *American Journal of Clinical Nutrition* 83 (2006): 244–251.
10. R. Pecoits-Filho, Dietary protein intake and kidney disease in Western diet, *Contributions to Nephrology* 155 (2007): 102–112.
11. A. M. Bernstein, L. Treyzon, and Z. Li, Are high-protein, vegetable-based diets safe for kidney function? A review of the literature, *Journal of the American Dietetic Association* 107 (2007): 644–650.

12. A. L. Darling and coauthors, Dietary protein and bone health: A systematic review and meta-analysis, *American Journal of Clinical Nutrition* (90): 1674–1692. K. Rafferty and R. P. Heaney, Nutrient effects on the calcium economy: Emphasizing the potassium controversy, *Journal of Nutrition* 138 (2008): 166S–171S.
13. Rafferty and Heaney, 2008.
14. R. Rizzoli, Nutrition: Its role in bone health, *Best Practice and Research: Clinical Endocrinology and Metabolism* 22 (2008): 813-829; A. D. Conigrave, E. M. Brown, and R. Rizzoli, Dietary protein and bone health: Roles of amino acid-sensing receptors in the control of calcium metabolism and bone homeostasis, *Annual Review of Nutrition* 28 (2008): 131–155; S. Boonen and coauthors, Addressing the musculoskeletal components of fracture risk with calcium and vitamin D: A review of the evidence, *Calcified Tissue International* 78 (2006): 257–270.
15. Standing Committee on the Scientific Evaluation of Dietary Reference Intakes, 2005, p. 694.
16. M. K. C. Hesselink, R. Minnaard, and P. Schrauwen, Eat the meat or feed the meat: Protein turnover in remodeling muscle, *Current Opinion in Clinical Nutrition and Metabolic Care* 9 (2006): 672–676; R. R. Wolfe, Skeletal muscle protein metabolism and resistance exercise, *Journal of Nutrition* 136 (2006): 525S–528S.
17. J. W. Apolzan and coauthors, Inadequate dietary protein increases hunger and desire to eat in younger and older men, *Journal of Nutrition* 137 (2007): 1478–1482.
18. U.S. Food and Drug Administration, Final rule promotes safe use of dietary supplements, *FDA Consumer Health Information*, June 22, 2007, available at www.fda.gov/consumer/updates/dietarysupps062207.html.
19. G. Wu, Amino acids: Metabolism, functions, and nutrition, *Amino Acids*, 37 (2009): 1–17.
20. G. K. Grimble, Adverse gastrointestinal effects of arginine and related amino acids, *Journal of Nutrition* 137 (2007): 1693S–1701S.
21. *Dietary Reference Intakes—The Essential Guide to Nutrient Requirements* (Washington, D.C.: National Academies Press, 2006), p. 152.
22. V. L. Fulgoni III, Current protein intake in America: Analysis of the National Health and Nutrition Examination survey, 2003-2004, *American Journal of Clinical Nutrition* 87 (2008): 1554S–1557S.
23. Fulgoni III, 2008.

Vegetarian Diets

Eating patterns all along the continuum of dietary choices—from one end, where people eat no foods of animal origin, to the other end, where they eat generous quantities of meat every day—can support or compromise nutritional health. The quality of the diet depends not on whether it consists of all plant foods or centers on meat, but on whether the eater's food choices are based on sound nutrition principles: adequacy of nutrient intakes, balance and variety of foods chosen, appropriate energy intake, and moderation in intakes of substances such as saturated fat, *trans* fat, added sugars, sodium, and alcohol that are harmful when consumed in excess. As mentioned in Chapter 5, however, because vegetarian diets exclude at least some animal-derived foods, they are usually lower in saturated fat and cholesterol than many meat-based diets.

People choose to exclude meat and other animal-derived foods from their diets for various reasons—concern for animal welfare, beliefs about health, religious convictions, or convenience. Some believe that vegetarianism is better for the environment; some, that it is healthier; and some, that it is less costly than the meat-eating alternative. Some just like it better. Whatever the reasons, vegetarians and health professionals who work with them should be aware of the nutrition and health implications of vegetarian diets.

Because vegetarian diets vary in both the types and the amounts of animal-derived foods they include, these differences must be considered when evaluating the health status of vegetarians. The accompanying glossary defines the various kinds of vegetarian diets.

Are vegetarian diets nutritionally sound?

The American Dietetic Association takes the position that well-planned vegetarian diets offer nutrition and health benefits to adults in general.[1] Research suggests that meat-eating adults who switch to vegetarian diets reduce their risks of heart disease, hypertension, diabetes, some types of cancer, and obesity.[2]

What should be my main concerns when planning a nutritionally sound vegetarian diet?

A vegetarian diet planner faces the same task as other diet planners—obtaining a variety of foods that provide all the needed nutrients within an energy allowance that maintains a healthy body weight. The challenge is to do so using at least one less food group. Because all vegetarians omit meat and some omit other animal-derived foods, protein, the nutrient that meat is famous for, merits some discussion here.

Isn't protein a problem in vegetarian diets?

No, protein is not the problem it was once thought to be in vegetarian diets. People who include animal-derived foods such as milk and eggs in their diets need not worry at all about protein deficiency. Even for **vegans**—those who eat only plant-based foods—protein intakes are usually satisfactory as long as energy intakes are adequate and protein sources are varied.[3] A mixture of proteins from whole grains, legumes, seeds, nuts, and vegetables can provide adequate amounts of high-quality protein. An advantage of many vegetarian sources of protein is that they are generally lower in saturated fat than meat and are often high in fiber and richer in some vitamins and minerals.

Some vegetarians may use meat replacements made of textured vegetable protein (soy protein). These foods are formulated to look and taste like meat, fish, or poultry. Many of these products are fortified to provide the

Glossary

lacto-ovo vegetarians: people who include milk or milk products and eggs but exclude meat, fish, shellfish, and poultry from their diets.

lacto-vegetarians: people who include milk or milk products but exclude meat, poultry, fish, shellfish, and eggs from their diets.

ovo-vegetarians: people who include eggs, vegetables, grains, legumes, fruits, and nuts but exclude flesh, seafood, and milk products.

partial vegetarians: people who include some, but not all, groups of animal-derived foods in their diets; they usually exclude meat and may occasionally include poultry, fish, and shellfish.

vegans: people who exclude all animal-derived foods (including meat, poultry, fish, shellfish, eggs, cheese, and milk) from their diets; also called *strict vegetarians* or *total vegetarians*.

vegetarians: people who include plant-based foods and eliminate some or all animal-derived foods.

vitamins and minerals found in animal sources of protein. Some products, however, may fall short of providing the nutrients of meat, and they may be high in salt, sugar, or other additives. Labels list all of the ingredients in such foods. A wise vegetarian learns to use a variety of whole, unrefined foods often and commercially prepared foods less frequently. Vegetarians may also use soybeans in other forms, such as plain tofu (soybean curd), edamame (cooked green soybeans), or soy flour, to bolster protein intake without consuming unwanted salt, sugar, or other additives.

What sorts of food energy intakes do vegetarian diets provide?

Researchers find that vegetarians as a group are closer to a healthy body weight than nonvegetarians.[4] Because obesity impairs health in a number of ways, vegetarians therefore have a health advantage. Vegetarian diets tend to be high in starch- and fiber-rich carbohydrates and low in saturated fat, characteristics that are consistent with current dietary recommendations aimed at reducing the incidence of obesity and other chronic diseases in this country.

Not all vegetarians fit the average pattern, though. Obesity does threaten vegetarians who include milk, eggs, and cheese in their diets. They can easily consume excess saturated fat and food energy and so must be careful to select fat-free and low-fat dairy foods and to avoid relying too heavily on these foods in general.

In contrast, people who exclude all animal-derived foods (vegans) may have trouble obtaining *enough* food energy. This is especially true for children. Vegan diets can fail to provide food energy sufficient to support the growth of a child within a bulk of food small enough for the child to eat. Frequent meals of fortified breads, cereals, or pastas with legumes, nuts, nut butters, and sources of unsaturated fats can help to meet protein and energy needs in a smaller volume at each sitting.[5] The MyPyramid resources, introduced in Chapter 1, include tips for planning vegetarian diets using the USDA Food Guide. In addition, several food guides have been developed specifically for vegetarian diets. They all address the particular nutrition concerns of vegetarians but differ slightly. Figure NP5-1 presents one version.

How can vegetarians and health professionals who plan vegetarian meals best utilize the vegetarian food pyramid?

The vegetarian food pyramid is flexible enough that a variety of people can use it: people who have adopted various vegetarian diets, those who want to make the transition to a vegetarian diet, and those who simply want to include more plant-based meals in their diets. When selecting from the vegetable and fruit groups, vegetarians should emphasize particularly good sources of calcium and iron, respectively. Green leafy vegetables, for example, provide almost five times as much calcium per serving as other vegetables. Similarly, dried fruits deserve special notice in the fruit group because they deliver six times as much iron as other fruits. The milk group features fortified soy milks for those who do not use milk, cheese, or yogurt. The meat group is called "proteins" and includes legumes, soy products, nuts, and seeds. A group for oils encourages the use of vegetable oils, nuts, and seeds rich in unsaturated fats and omega-3

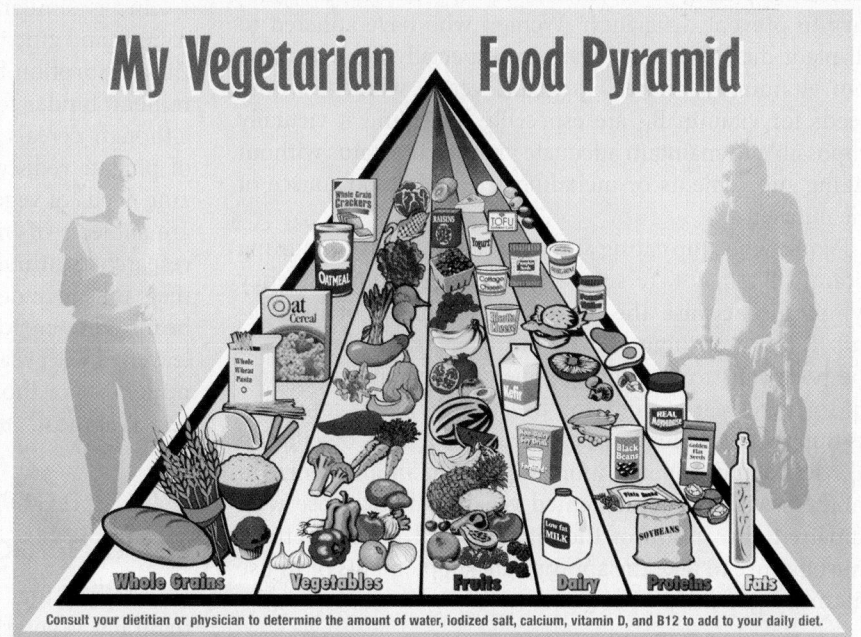

FIGURE NP5-1 An Example of a Vegetarian Food Pyramid

Review Figure 1-4 and Table 1-7 of Chapter 1 to find the recommended daily amounts from each food group, serving size equivalents, examples of foods within each group and the most notable nutrients for each group. Tips for planning a vegetarian diet can be found at MyPyramid.gov.

Source: Reprinted from V. Messina, et al, A New Food Guide for North American Vegetarians, Journal of the American Dietetic Assn., 103(2003): 771–775. Copyright 2003 with permission from Elsevier.

fatty acids. To ensure adequate intakes of vitamin B_{12}, vitamin D, and calcium, vegetarians need to select fortified foods or use supplements daily. Like MyPyramid, the vegetarian food pyramid in Figure NP5-1 also encourages physical activity.

Most vegetarians easily obtain large quantities of the nutrients that are abundant in plant foods: carbohydrate, fiber, thiamin, folate, vitamin B_6, vitamin C, vitamin A, and vitamin E. Vegetarian food guides help to ensure adequate intakes of the main nutrients vegetarian diets might otherwise lack: protein, iron, zinc, calcium, vitamin B_{12}, vitamin D, and omega-3 fatty acids. Table NP5-1 presents good vegetarian sources of these key nutrients.

Tell me about vitamins and minerals. Does a person eating a vegetarian diet need to take vitamin supplements?

That depends on the kind of vegetarian diet. The diet of **lacto-ovo vegetarians** can be complete in all vitamins, but for vegans, several vitamins may be a problem. One such vitamin is B_{12}. Because vitamin B_{12} occurs only in animal-derived foods, regular use of vitamin B_{12}-fortified foods, such as fortified soy and rice beverages, some breakfast cereals, and meat replacements, or supplements, is necessary to prevent deficiency.[6] Women who have adhered to all-plant diets for many years are especially likely to have low vitamin B_{12} stores. Pregnant vegan women, whose needs for vitamin B_{12} are especially high, find it virtually impossible to maintain adequate vitamin B_{12} status without taking supplements or including a reliable food source of the nutrient.

People who stop eating animal-derived foods containing vitamin B_{12} may take several years to develop deficiency symptoms because the body recycles much of its vitamin B_{12}, reabsorbing it over and over again. Even when the body fails to absorb vitamin B_{12}, deficiency may take up to three years to develop because the body conserves its supply. Neurological degeneration, a sign of vitamin B_{12} deficiency, appears more rapidly in infants born to mothers with unsupplemented vegan diets or those with impaired absorption of the vitamin.[7] All vegan mothers must be sure to take the appropriate supplements or to use vitamin B_{12}-fortified products.

Because vegans do not drink vitamin D–fortified cow's milk, do they get enough vitamin D?

Overall, vegetarians are similar to nonvegetarians in their vitamin D status; factors such as taking supplements, skin color, and sun exposure have a greater influence on vitamin D than diet.[8] People who do not use vitamin D–fortified foods and do not receive enough exposure to sunlight to synthesize adequate vitamin D may need supplements to fend off bone loss. Of particular concern are infants, children, and older adults in northern climates during winter months.

So, on a vegan diet, vitamin B_{12} and vitamin D can be problems if a person is not careful. What about minerals?

For *all* vegetarians, not just the vegan, two minerals may be of concern—iron and zinc. The iron in plant foods such as legumes, dark green leafy vegetables, iron-fortified cereals, and whole-grain breads and cereals is not as absorbable as that in meat. For this reason, the iron recommendation for adult vegetarian men, premenopausal women, and adolescent girls is almost double the recommendation for meat eaters of the same gender and age.[9]

Fortunately, the body seems to adapt to a vegetarian diet by absorbing iron more efficiently. Furthermore, iron absorption is enhanced by vitamin C, and vegetarians typically eat many vitamin C–rich fruits and vegetables. Consequently, vegetarians suffer no more iron deficiency than other people do.

Zinc is similar to iron in that meat is its richest food source, and zinc from plant sources is not as well absorbed. Zinc absorption from plant foods is hindered by phytate, a mineral binder found in grains, legumes, and seeds. Thus, although cereals and legumes contain zinc, the presence of phytate reduces zinc absorption from these foods. The zinc needs of vegetarians and the effects of mineral binders are subjects of intensive study at the present time. While research continues, vegetarians are advised to eat varied diets that include legumes such as navy beans and kidney beans, zinc-enriched cereals, and whole-grain breads well leavened with yeast, which improves the availability of their minerals. For those who include seafood in their diets, oysters, crabmeat, and shrimp are rich in zinc.

What about calcium for the vegan?

Good thinking. Yes, calcium is of concern. The milk-drinking vegetarian is protected from deficiency, but the vegan must find other sources of calcium. Some good calcium sources are regular and ample servings of dark green leafy vegetables such as kale and collard; legumes; calcium-fortified foods such as breakfast cereals, soy milk, and orange juice; some nuts such as almonds; and certain seeds such as sesame seeds. The choices should be varied because binders in some of these foods may hinder

TABLE NP5-1 | Vegetarian Sources of Key Nutrients

Nutrients	Food Groups					
	Grains	Vegetables	Fruits	Legumes and Other Protein-Rich Foods	Milk or Soymilk	Oils
Protein	Whole grains[1]			Legumes, seeds, nuts, soy products (tempeh, tofu, veggie burgers) Eggs (for ovo-vegetarians)	Milk, cheese, yogurt (for lacto vegetarians) Soymilk, soy yogurt, soy cheeses	
Iron	Fortified cereals, enriched and whole grains	Dark green leafy vegetables (spinach, turnip greens)	Dried fruits (apricots, prunes, raisins)	Legumes (blackeyed peas, kidney beans, lentils), soy products		
Zinc	Fortified cereals, whole grains			Legumes (garbanzo beans, kidney beans, navy beans), nuts, seeds (pumpkin seeds)	Milk, cheese, yogurt (for lacto vegetarians) Soymilk, soy yogurt, soy cheeses	
Calcium	Fortified cereals	Dark green leafy vegetables (bok choy, broccoli, collard greens, kale, mustard greens, turnip greens, watercress)	Fortified juices, figs	Fortified soy products, nuts (almonds), seeds (sesame seeds)	Milk, cheese, yogurt (for lacto vegetarians) Fortified soy milk, fortified soy yogurt, fortified soy cheese	
Vitamin B₁₂	Fortified cereals			Eggs (for ovo-vegetarians) Fortified soy products	Milk, cheese, yogurt (for lacto vegetarians) Fortified soy milk, fortified soy yogurt, fortified soy cheese	
Vitamin D	Fortified cereals				Milk, cheese, yogurt (for lacto vegetarians) Fortified soy milk, fortified soy yogurt, fortified soy cheese	
Omega-3 Fatty Acids		Marine algae and its oils		Flaxseed, walnuts, soybeans Fortified margarine Fortified eggs (for ovo-vegetarians)		Flaxseed oil, walnut oil, soybean oil

[a]As Chapter 5 explains, many plant proteins do not contain all the essential amino acids in the amounts and proportions needed by human beings. To improve protein quality, vegetarians can eat grains and legumes together, for example, although it is not necessary if protein intake is varied and energy intake is sufficient.

Source: Reprinted from V. Messina, et al, A New Food Guide for North American Vegetarians, *Journal of the American Dietetic Assn.,* 103(2003): 771–775. Copyright 2003 with permission from Elsevier.

calcium absorption. The vegan is urged to use calcium-fortified soy milk in ample quantities regularly. This is especially important for children. Infant formula based on soy is fortified with calcium and can easily be used in food preparation, even for adults.

Do vegetarian diets provide adequate amounts of the essential fatty acids?

Vegetarian diets typically provide enough of the essential fatty acids linoleic acid and linolenic acid, but they lack a dietary source of EPA and DHA.[10] Fatty fish and DHA-fortified eggs and other fortified products can provide EPA and DHA, but all of these sources ultimately derive from fish, an unacceptable food for vegans. Alternatively, certain marine algae and their oils provide DHA and more foods are being fortified with such oils, which are listed among the ingredients on a food's label.[11] A vegetarian's daily diet should include small amounts of flaxseed, walnuts, and their oils, as well as soybeans and canola oil to provide essential fatty acids.

Are there any other health advantages to the vegetarian diet?

Yes. Vegetarian protein foods are often higher in fiber, richer in certain vitamins and minerals, and lower in fat—especially saturated fat—than meats. Vegetarians can enjoy a nutritious diet low in saturated fat provided that they limit foods such as butter, cream cheese, and sour cream. If vegetarians follow the guidelines presented here and plan carefully, they can support their health as well as, or perhaps better than, nonvegetarians.

Abundant evidence supports the idea that vegetarians may actually be healthier than meat eaters. Informed vegetarians are not only more likely to be at the desired weights for their heights, but they are also more likely to have lower blood cholesterol levels, lower rates of certain kinds of cancer, better digestive function, and more. Even among people who are health conscious, generally vegetarians experience fewer deaths from cardiovascular disease than meat eaters do. Because many vegetarians also abstain from smoking and the consumption of alcohol, dietary practices alone probably do not account for all the aspects of improved health. Clearly, however, they contribute significantly to it.

Notes

1. Position of the American Dietetic Association, Vegetarian diets, *Journal of the American Dietetic Association* 109 (2009): 1266–1282.
2. G. E. Fraser, Vegetarian diets: What do we know of their effects on common chronic diseases? *American Journal of Clinical Nutrition* 89 (2009): 1607S–1612S; N. D. Barnard and coauthors, A low-fat vegan diet and a conventional diabetes diet in the treatment of type 2 diabetes: A randomized, controlled, 74-wk clinical trial, *American Journal of Clinical Nutrition* 89 (2009): 1588S–1596S; W. J. Craig, Health effects of vegan diets, *American Journal of Clinical Nutrition* 89 (2009): 1627S–1633S; T. J. Key, P. N. Appleby, and M. S. Rosell, Health effects of vegetarian and vegan diets, *Proceedings of the Nutrition Society* 65 (2006): 35–41.
3. Position of the American Dietetic Association, 2009.
4. Fraser, 2009; R. Robinson-O'Brien and coauthors, Adolescent and young adult vegetarianism: Better dietary intake and weight outcomes but increased risk of disordered eating behaviors, *Journal of the American Dietetic Association* 109 (2009): 648–655; S. E. Berkow and N. Barnard, Vegetarian diets and weight status, *Nutrition Reviews* 64 (2006): 175–188; M. Rosell and coauthors, Weight gain over 5 years in 21,966 meat-eating, fish-eating, vegetarian, and vegan men and women in EPIC-Oxford, *International Journal of Obesity* 30 (2006): 1389–1396.
5. Position of the American Dietetic Association, 2009.
6. Position of the American Dietetic Association, 2009.
7. D. K. Dror and L. H. Allen, Effect of vitamin B_{12} deficiency on neurodevelopment in infants: Current knowledge and possible mechanisms, *Nutrition Reviews* 66 (2008): 250–255.
8. J. Chan, K. Jaceldo-Siegl, and Gary E. Fraser, Serum 25-hydroxyvitamin D status of vegetarians, partial vegetarians, and nonvegetarians: The Adventist Health Study, *American Journal of Clinical Nutrition* 89 (2009): 1686S–1692S.
9. Standing Committee on the Scientific Evaluation of Dietary Reference Intakes, Food and Nutrition Board, Institute of Medicine, *Dietary Reference Intakes for Vitamin A, Vitamin K, Arsenic, Boron, Chromium, Copper, Iodine, Iron, Manganese, Molybdenum, Nickel, Silicon, Vanadium, and Zinc* (Washington, D.C.: National Academy Press, 2001), pp. 9–45.
10. I. Mangat, Do vegetarians have to eat fish for optimal cardiovascular protection? *American Journal of Clinical Nutrition* 89 (2009): 1597–1601.
11. J. Whelan and C. Rust, Innovative dietary sources of n-3 fatty acids, *Annual Review of Nutrition* 26 (2006): 75–103.

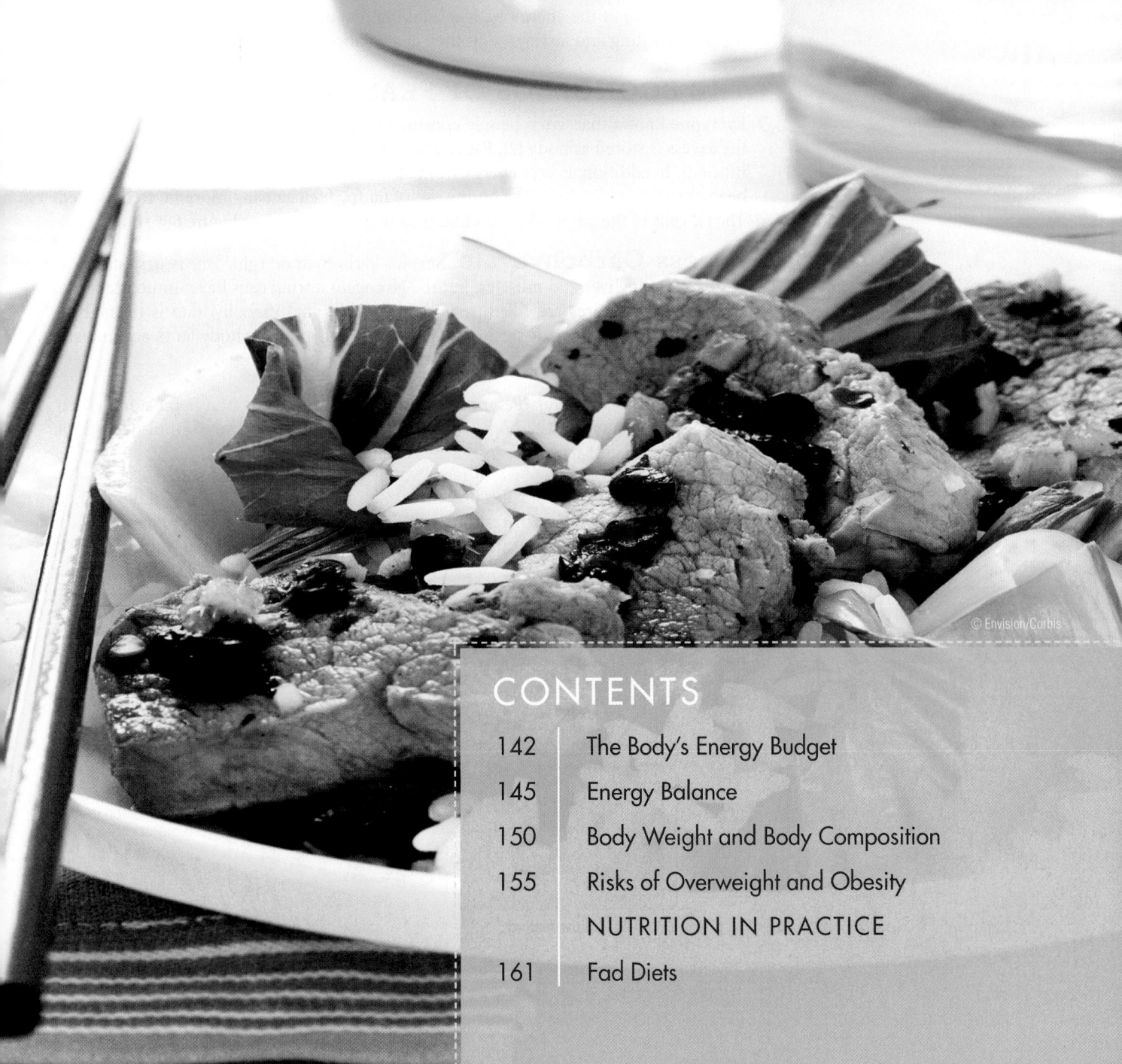

CHAPTER 6 | Energy Balance and Body Composition

CONTENTS

THE BODY MANAGES ITS ENERGY SUPPLY WITH AMAZING PRECISION. Consider that most people maintain their weight within about a 10- to 20-pound range throughout their lives. How do they do this? How does the body manage excess energy? And how does it manage to do without food for prolonged periods—as when someone is starving or fasting? The answers to these questions lie in understanding how the body adapts to energy imbalances, the focus of the first part of this chapter. The chapter then describes energy balance, body composition, and the health risks associated with too much body fat. The next chapter offers strategies toward solving the problems of too much or too little body fat.

The Body's Energy Budget

The average person takes in and expends close to a million kcalories a year while maintaining a stable weight for years on end. In other words, the body's energy budget is balanced. Many people, however, eat too much or exercise too little and get fat; others eat too little or exercise too much and get thin. This section examines metabolism from the perspective of the energy budget, looking first at the two forms of an unbalanced budget—feasting and fasting—and then at a balanced budget.

THE ECONOMICS OF FEASTING

Everyone knows that when people consume more energy than they expend, much of the excess is stored as body fat. Fat can be made from an excess of any energy-yielding nutrient. In addition, excess energy from alcohol is also stored as fat.[1] Alcohol has also been shown to slow down the body's use of fat for fuel, causing more fat to be stored. The fat cells of the adipose tissue enlarge as they fill with fat, as Figure 6-1 shows.

Excess Carbohydrate Surplus carbohydrate (glucose) is first stored as glycogen in the liver and muscles, but the glycogen-storing cells have limited capacity. Once glycogen stores are filled, most of the additional carbohydrate is burned for energy, displacing the body's use of fat for energy and allowing body fat to accumulate. Thus, excess carbohydrate can contribute to obesity.

Excess Fat Surplus dietary fat contributes easily to the body's fat stores. After a meal, fat is routed to the body's adipose tissue, where it is stored until needed for energy. Thus, excess fat from food easily adds to body fat.

Excess Protein Surplus protein may also contribute to body fat. If not needed to build body protein (as in response to physical activity) or to meet energy needs, amino acids will lose their nitrogens and be converted, through intermediates, to

FIGURE 6-1 | Fat Cell Enlargement

Skin

Fat cells

Muscle

Before overeating

Skin

Fat cells enlarge when a person eats too much of any energy-yielding nutrient—carbohydrate, fat, or protein.

Muscle

After overeating

FIGURE
6-2 | Feasting

When a person overeats (feasting):

Food component:	Is broken down in the body to:	And then ends up as:
Carbohydrate	Glucose	Liver and muscle glycogen stores
Fat	Fatty acids	Body fat stores
Protein	Amino acids (first used to replace body proteins)	Nitrogen lost in urine

When people overeat, they store energy.

triglycerides. These, too, swell the fat cells and add to body weight. Figure 6-2 shows the metabolic events of feasting.

Review Notes

- Too little physical activity encourages body fat accumulation.
- Any food can make you fat if you eat too much of it. A net excess of energy is almost all stored in the body as fat in adipose (fat) tissue.
- Alcohol both delivers kcalories and encourages storage of body fat.
- Fat from food is particularly easy for the body to store as adipose tissue.
- If not needed to build body protein or to meet energy needs, excess protein can be converted to fat.
- In short, excess energy intake from carbohydrate, fat, protein, and alcohol leads to storage of body fat.

THE ECONOMICS OF FASTING

The body expends energy all the time. Even when a person is asleep and totally relaxed, the cells of many organs are hard at work. In fact, this cellular work, which maintains all life processes, represents about two-thirds of the total energy a sedentary person expends in a day. (The other one-third is the work that a person's muscles do voluntarily during waking hours.)

Energy Deficit The body's top priority is to meet the energy needs for this ongoing cellular activity. Its normal way of doing so is by periodic refueling, that is, by eating several times a day. When food is not available, the body uses fuel reserves from its own tissues. If people voluntarily choose not to eat, we say they are fasting; if they have no choice (as in a famine), we say they are starving. The body, however, makes no distinction between the two—metabolically, fasting and starvation are identical. In either case, the body is forced to switch to a wasting metabolism, drawing on its stores of carbohydrate and fat and, within a day or so, on its vital protein tissues as well.

Glycogen Used First

As fasting begins, glucose from the liver's glycogen stores and fatty acids from the body's adipose tissue flow into the cells to fuel their work. Within a day, liver glycogen is exhausted, and most of the glucose is used up. Low blood glucose concentrations serve as a signal to promote further fat breakdown.

Glucose Needed for the Brain

At this point, a few hours into a fast, most of the cells depend on fatty acids to continue providing fuel. But the nervous system (brain and nerves) and red blood cells cannot use fatty acids; they still need glucose. Even if other energy sources are available, glucose has to be present to permit the brain's energy-metabolizing machinery to work. (✚) Normally, the nervous system consumes a little more than half of the total glucose used each day—about 400 to 600 kcalories' worth.

Protein Breakdown and Ketosis

Because fat stores cannot provide the glucose needed by the brain and nerves, body protein tissues (such as liver and muscle) always break down to some extent during fasting. In the first few days of a fast, body protein provides about 90 percent of the needed glucose, and glycerol provides about 10 percent.* If body protein losses were to continue at this rate, death would ensue within about three weeks. As the fast continues, however, the body finds a way to use its fat to fuel the brain. It adapts by condensing together fragments derived from fatty acids to produce ketone bodies, (✚) which can serve as fuel for some brain cells. Ketone body production rises until, after several weeks of fasting, it is meeting much of the nervous system's energy needs. Still, many areas of the brain rely exclusively on glucose, and body protein continues to be sacrificed to produce it. (✚) Figure 6-3 shows the metabolic events that occur during fasting.

Slowed Metabolism

As fasting continues and the nervous system shifts to partial dependence on ketone bodies for energy, the body simultaneously reduces its energy output (metabolic rate) and conserves both fat and lean tissue. Because of the slowed metabolism, energy use falls to a bare minimum.

Hazards of Fasting

The body's adaptations to fasting are sufficient to maintain life for a long period. Mental alertness need not be diminished. Even physical energy may remain unimpaired for a surprisingly long time. Still, fasting is not without its hazards. Among the many changes that take place in the body are:

- Wasting of lean tissues.
- Impairment of disease resistance.
- Lowering of body temperature.
- Disturbances of the body's fluid and electrolyte balances.

For the person who wants to lose weight, fasting is not the best way to go. The body's lean tissue continues to be degraded, sometimes amounting to as much as 50 percent of the weight lost over the first week. Over the long term, a diet only moderately restricted in energy promotes primarily *fat* loss and the retention of more lean tissue than a severely restricted fast.

✚ Reminder: The liver releases glucose, and the fat cells release fat to fuel the body's cells, but the brain can use only glucose.

✚ Reminder: *Ketone bodies* are acidic, fat-related compounds formed from the incomplete breakdown of fat when carbohydrate is not available. Small amounts of ketone bodies are normally produced during energy metabolism, but when their blood concentration rises, they spill into the urine. The combination of a high blood concentration of ketone bodies (*ketonemia*) and ketone bodies in the urine (*ketonuria*) is called *ketosis*.

✚ In fasting, muscle and lean tissues give up protein to supply amino acids for conversion to glucose. This glucose, with ketone bodies produced from fat, fuels the brain's activities.

Review Notes

- When fasting, the body makes a number of adaptations: increasing the breakdown of fat to provide energy for most of the cells, using glycerol and amino acids to make glucose for the red blood cells and central nervous system, producing ketones to fuel the brain, and slowing metabolism.
- All of these measures conserve energy and minimize losses.
- Over the long term, a diet moderately restricted in energy promotes primarily fat loss and the retention of lean tissue.

*The small glycerol portion of a triglyceride can yield glucose, but glycerol represents only about 5 percent of the weight of a triglyceride molecule. Thus, fat is an inefficient source of glucose. About 95 percent of a triglyceride (the fatty acids attached to the glycerol) cannot be converted to glucose.

FIGURE
6-3 | Fasting

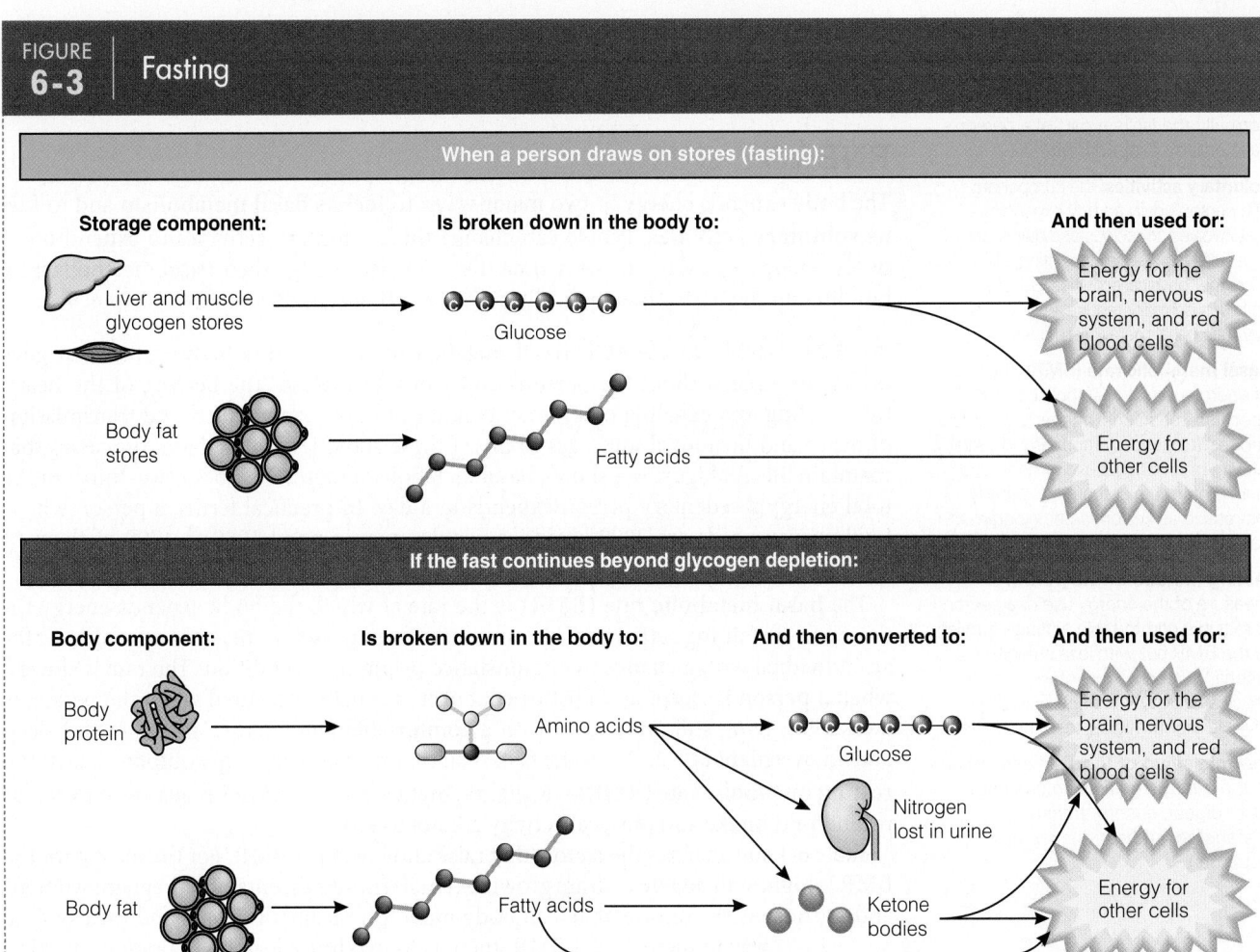

When a person draws on stores (fasting):

Storage component: → **Is broken down in the body to:** → **And then used for:**

Liver and muscle glycogen stores → Glucose → Energy for the brain, nervous system, and red blood cells

Body fat stores → Fatty acids → Energy for other cells

If the fast continues beyond glycogen depletion:

Body component: → **Is broken down in the body to:** → **And then converted to:** → **And then used for:**

Body protein → Amino acids → Glucose → Energy for the brain, nervous system, and red blood cells

Amino acids → Nitrogen lost in urine

Body fat → Fatty acids → Ketone bodies → Energy for other cells

When people are fasting, they draw on stored energy.

Energy Balance

If a person maintains a healthy weight over time, the person is in energy balance. Food energy intake equals energy expenditure: deposits of fat made at one time have been compensated for by withdrawals made at another. In other words, the body uses fat as a savings account for energy. But, unlike money, having more fat is not better; there is an optimum.

A day's energy balance can be stated like this: change in energy stores equals the food energy taken in (kcalories) minus the energy spent on metabolism and physical activities (kcalories). More simply:

Change in energy stores = energy in (kcalories) – energy out (kcalories).

ENERGY IN

The energy in food and beverages is the only contributor to the "energy in" side of the energy balance equation. Before you can decide how much food will supply the energy you or one of your clients needs in a day, you must first become familiar with the amounts of energy in foods and beverages. One way to do so is to look up the kcalories provided by various foods and beverages in the Table of Food Composition (Appendix A). Alternatively, computer programs can readily provide this information for those with computer access.

Food composition data would reveal that an apple provides about 70 kcalories from carbohydrate and a candy bar supplies about 250 kcalories, mostly from fat and carbohydrate. You may already know that for each 3500 kcalories you eat in excess of expenditures, you store approximately 1 pound of body fat. (➕) Similarly, a pound

➕ 1 lb body fat = 3500 kcal. Body fat, or adipose tissue, is composed of a mixture of mostly fat, some protein, and water. A pound of body fat (454 g) is approximately 87 percent fat, or 395 g (454 × 0.87); 395 g × 9 kcal/g = 3555 kcal.

of fat is lost for each 3500 kcalories expended beyond those consumed. The fat stores of even a healthy-weight adult represent an ample reserve of energy—50,000 to 200,000 kcalories.

ENERGY OUT

The body expends energy in two major ways: to fuel its **basal metabolism** and to fuel its **voluntary activities**. People can change their voluntary activities to expend more or less energy in a day, and over time they can also change their basal metabolism by building up the body's metabolically active lean tissue, as explained in Chapter 7.

Basal Metabolism Basal metabolism supports the body's work that goes on all the time without the person's conscious awareness. The beating of the heart, the inhaling and exhaling of air, maintenance of body temperature, and transmission of nerve and hormonal messages to direct these activities are the basal processes that maintain life. As Figure 6-4 shows, basal metabolism represents about two-thirds of the total energy a sedentary person expends in a day. In practical terms, a person whose total energy needs are 2000 kcalories per day may expend 1000 to 1300 of them to support basal metabolism.

The **basal metabolic rate (BMR)** is the rate at which the body expends energy for these life-sustaining activities. This rate varies from person to person and may vary for an individual with a change in circumstance or physical condition. The rate is slowest when a person is sleeping undisturbed, but it is usually measured when the person is awake, but lying still, in a room with a comfortable temperature after a restful sleep and an overnight (12- to 14-hour) fast. A similar measure of energy output—called the **resting metabolic rate (RMR)**—is slightly higher than the BMR because its criteria for recent food intake and physical activity are not as strict.

Table 6-1 summarizes the factors that raise and lower the BMR. For the most part, the BMR is highest in people who are growing (children, adolescents, and pregnant women) and in those with considerable lean body mass (physically fit people and males). One way to increase the BMR, then, is to maximize lean body tissue by participating regularly in endurance and strength-building activities. The BMR is also fast in people who are tall and so have a large surface area for their weight, in people with fever or under stress, in people taking certain medications, and in people with highly active thyroid glands. The BMR slows down with a loss of lean body mass and during fasting and malnutrition.

Energy for Physical Activities The number of kcalories spent on voluntary activities depends on three factors: muscle mass, body weight, and activity. The larger the muscle mass required for the activity and the heavier the weight of the body part being moved, the more kcalories are spent. The activity's duration, frequency, and intensity also influence energy costs: the longer, the more frequent, and the more intense the activity, the more kcalories expended. Table 6-2 (pp.148–149) gives average energy expenditures for people of different body weights engaged in various activities and shows that a heavy person usually uses more energy per minute than a light person does in the same activity.

Energy to Manage Food When food is taken into the body, many cells that have been dormant become active. The muscles that move the food through the intestinal tract speed up their rhythmic contractions, and the cells that manufacture and secrete digestive juices begin their tasks. All these and other cells need extra energy as they participate in the digestion, absorption, and metabolism of food. This cellular activity produces heat and is known as the **thermic effect of food**. The thermic effect of food is generally thought to represent about 10 percent of the total food energy taken in. For purposes of rough estimates, though, the thermic effect of food is not always included.

| FIGURE 6-4 | Components of Energy Expenditure |

The amount of energy spent in a day differs for each individual, but in general, basal metabolism is the largest component of energy expenditure, and the thermic effect of food is the smallest. The amount spent in voluntary physical activities has the greatest variability, depending on a person's activity patterns. For a sedentary person, physical activities may account for less than half as much energy as basal metabolism, whereas an extremely active person may expand as much on activity as for basal metabolism.

30–50% Physical activities

10% Thermic effect of food

50–65% Basal metabolism

TABLE 6-1 | Factors That Affect the BMR

Factor	Effect on BMR
Age	Lean body mass diminishes with age, slowing the BMR.[a]
Height	In tall, thin people, the BMR is higher.[b]
Growth	In children and pregnant women, the BMR is higher.
Body composition (gender)	The more lean tissue, the higher the BMR (which is why males usually have a higher BMR than females). The more fat tissue, the lower the BMR.
Fever	Fever raises the BMR.[c]
Stresses	Stresses (including many diseases and certain drugs) raise the BMR.
Environmental temperature	Both heat and cold raise the BMR.
Fasting/starvation	Fasting/starvation lowers the BMR.[d]
Malnutrition	Malnutrition lowers the BMR.
Hormones (gender)	The thyroid hormone thyroxin, for example, can speed up or slow down the BMR.[e] Premenstrual hormones slightly raise the BMR.
Smoking	Nicotine increases energy expenditure.
Caffeine	Caffeine increases energy expenditure.
Sleep	BMR is lowest when sleeping.

[a]The BMR begins to decrease in early adulthood (after growth and development cease) at a rate of about 2 percent a decade. A reduction in voluntary activity as well brings the total decline in energy expenditure to 5 percent a decade.

[b]If two people weigh the same, the taller, thinner person will have the faster metabolic rate, reflecting the greater skin surface, through which heat is lost by radiation, in proportion to the body's volume.

[c]Fever raises the BMR by 7 percent for each degree Fahrenheit.

[d]Prolonged starvation reduces the total amount of metabolically active lean tissue in the body, although the decline occurs sooner and to a greater extent than body losses alone can explain. More likely, the neural and hormonal changes that accompany fasting are responsible for changes in the BMR.

[e]The thyroid gland releases hormones that travel to the cells and influence cellular metabolism. Thyroid hormone activity can speed up or slow down the rate of metabolism by as much as 50 percent.

ESTIMATING ENERGY REQUIREMENTS

In estimating energy requirements, the DRI committee developed equations that consider how the following factors influence energy expenditure: (✚)

- *Gender.* In general, women have a lower BMR than men, in large part because men typically have more lean body mass. In addition, menstrual hormones influence the BMR in women, raising it just prior to menstruation. Two sets of energy equations—one for men and one for women—were developed to accommodate the influence of gender on energy expenditure.
- *Growth.* The BMR is high in people who are growing. For this reason, pregnant and lactating women, infants, children, and adolescents have their own sets of energy equations.
- *Age.* The BMR declines during adulthood as lean body mass diminishes. Physical activities tend to decline as well, bringing the average reduction in energy

✚ Note that Table 6-1 listed these factors among those that influence BMR and, consequently, energy expenditure.

TABLE
6-2 | Energy Spent on Various Activities

The values listed in this table reflect both the energy spent in physical activity and the amount used for BMR.

Activity	kcal/lb/min[a]	kCalories per Minute at Different Body Weights				
		110 lb	125 lb	150 lb	175 lb	200 lb
Aerobic dance (vigorous)	.062	6.8	7.8	9.3	10.9	12.4
Basketball (vigorous, full court)	.097	10.7	12.1	14.6	17.0	19.4
Bicycling						
13 mph	.045	5.0	5.6	6.8	7.9	9.0
15 mph	.049	5.4	6.1	7.4	8.6	9.8
17 mph	.057	6.3	7.1	8.6	10.0	11.4
19 mph	.076	8.4	9.5	11.4	13.3	15.2
21 mph	.090	9.9	11.3	13.5	15.8	18.0
23 mph	.109	12.0	13.6	16.4	19.0	21.8
25 mph	.139	15.3	17.4	20.9	24.3	27.8
Canoeing, flat water, moderate pace	.045	5.0	5.6	6.8	7.9	9.0
Cross-country skiing						
8 mph	.104	11.4	13.0	15.6	18.2	20.8
Golf (carrying clubs)	.045	5.0	5.6	6.8	7.9	9.0
Handball	.078	8.6	9.8	11.7	13.7	15.6
Horseback riding (trot)	.052	5.7	6.5	7.8	9.1	10.4
Rowing (vigorous)	.097	10.7	12.1	14.6	17.0	19.4
Running						
5 mph	.061	6.7	7.6	9.2	10.7	12.2
6 mph	.074	8.1	9.2	11.1	13.0	14.8
7.5 mph	.094	10.3	11.8	14.1	16.4	18.8
9 mph	.103	11.3	12.9	15.5	18.0	20.6
10 mph	.114	12.5	14.3	17.1	20.0	22.9
11 mph	.131	14.4	16.4	19.7	22.9	26.2
Soccer (vigorous)	.097	10.7	12.1	14.6	17.0	19.4
Studying	.011	1.2	1.4	1.7	1.9	2.2
Swimming						
20 yd/min	.032	3.5	4.0	4.8	5.6	6.4
45 yd/min	.058	6.4	7.3	8.7	10.2	11.6
50 yd/min	.070	7.7	8.8	10.5	12.3	14.0
Table tennis (skilled)	.045	5.0	5.6	6.8	7.9	9.0

Activity	kcal/lb/min[a]	kCalories per Minute at Different Body Weights				
		110 lb	125 lb	150 lb	175 lb	200 lb
Tennis (beginner)	.032	3.5	4.0	4.8	5.6	6.4
Walking (brisk pace)						
3.5 mph	.035	3.9	4.4	5.2	6.1	7.0
4.5 mph	.048	5.3	6.0	7.2	8.4	9.6
Weight lifting						
light-to-moderate effort	.024	2.6	3.0	3.6	4.2	4.8
vigorous effort	.048	5.2	6.0	7.2	8.4	9.6
Wheelchair basketball	.084	9.2	10.5	12.6	14.7	16.8
Wheeling self in wheelchair	.030	3.3	3.8	4.5	5.3	6.0

[a]To calculate kcalories spent per minute of activity for your own body weight, multiply kcal/lb/min by your exact weight and then multiply that number by the number of minutes spent in the activity. For example, if you weigh 142 pound and you want to know how many kcalories you spent doing 30 minutes of vigorous aerobic dance: 0.062 × 142 = 8.8 kcalories per minute; 8.8 × 30 (minutes) = 264 total kcalories spent.

expenditure to about 5 percent per decade. The decline in the BMR that occurs when a person becomes less active reflects the loss of lean body mass and may be prevented with ongoing physical activity. Because age influences energy expenditure, it is also factored into the energy equations.

- *Physical activity.* Using individual values for various physical activities (as in Table 6-2) is time consuming and impractical for estimating the energy needs of a population. Instead, various activities are clustered according to the typical intensity of a day's efforts. Energy equations include a physical activity factor for various levels of intensity for each gender.
- *Body composition and body size.* The BMR is high in people who are tall and so have a large surface area. Similarly, the more a person weighs, the more energy is expended on basal metabolism. For these reasons, the energy equations include a factor for both height and weight.

As just explained, energy needs vary among individuals depending on such factors as gender, growth, age, physical activity, and body composition. Even when two people are similarly matched, however, their energy needs will still differ because of genetic differences. Perhaps one day genetic research will reveal how to estimate requirements for each individual. For now, the "How to" (p. 150) provides instructions on calculating estimated energy requirements using the DRI equations and physical activity factors. (✚)

Appendix D presents tables that provide a shortcut to estimating total energy expenditure and instructions to help you determine the appropriate physical activity factor to use in the equations.

Physical activity expends energy and benefits health in many ways.

Review Notes

- A person takes in energy from food and, on average, expends most of it on basal metabolic activities, some of it on physical activities, and about 10 percent on the thermic effect of food.
- Because energy requirements vary from person to person, such factors as age, gender, and weight must be considered when calculating energy expended on basal metabolism, and the intensity and duration of the activity must be taken into account when calculating expenditures on physical activities.

To determine your estimated energy requirements (EER), use the appropriate equation (of the two options below), inserting your age in years, weight (wt) in kilograms, height (ht) in meters, and physical activity (PA) factor from the accompanying table. (To convert pounds to kilograms, divide by 2.2; to convert inches to meters, divide by 39.37.)

- For men 19 years and older:
  $EER = [662 - (9.53 \times age)] + PA \times [(15.91 \times wt) + (539.6 \times ht)]$

- For women 19 years and older:
  $EER = [354 - (6.91 \times age)] + PA \times [(9.36 \times wt) + (726 \times ht)]$

For example, consider an active 30-year-old male who is 5 feet 11 inches tall and weighs 178 pounds. First, he converts his weight from pounds to kilograms and his height from inches to meters, if necessary:

$$178 \text{ lb} \div 2.2 = 80.9 \text{ kg}$$

$$71 \text{ in} \div 39.37 = 1.8 \text{ m}$$

Next, he considers his level of daily physical activity and selects the appropriate PA factor from the accompanying table (in this example, 1.25 for an active male). Then, he inserts his age, PA factor, weight, and height into the appropriate equation:

$$EER = [662 - (9.53 \times 30)] + 1.25 \times [(15.91 \times 80.9) + (539.6 \times 1.8)]$$

(A reminder: do calculations within the parentheses first, and multiply before adding or subtracting.) He calculates:

$$EER = [662 - (9.53 \times 30)] + 1.25 \times (1287 + 971)$$

$$EER = [662 - (9.53 \times 30)] + (1.25 \times 2258)$$

$$EER = 662 - 286 + 2823$$

$$EER = 3199$$

The estimated energy requirement for an active 30-year-old male who is 5 feet 11 inches tall and weighs 178 pounds is about 3200 kcalories/day. His actual requirement probably falls within a range of 200 kcalories above and below this estimate.

Physical Activity (PA) Factors for EER Equations

	Men	Women	Physical Activity
Sedentary	1.0	1.0	Typical daily living activities
Low active	1.11	1.12	Plus 30 to 60 minutes moderate activity
Active	1.25	1.27	Plus ≥ 60 minutes moderate activity
Very active	1.48	1.45	Plus ≥ 60 minutes moderate activity and 60 minutes vigorous activity or 120 minutes moderate activity

Note: Moderate activity is equivalent to walking at 3½ to 4½ miles per hour.

Body Weight and Body Composition

The body's weight reflects its composition—the proportions of its bone, muscle, fat, fluid, and other tissue. All of these body components can vary in quantity and quality: the bones can be dense or porous, the muscles can be well developed or underdeveloped, fat can be abundant or scarce, and so on. By far the most variable tissue, though, is body fat. For health's sake, weight management efforts should focus on eating and activity habits to improve body composition.

DEFINING HEALTHY BODY WEIGHT

How much should a person weigh? How can a person know if her weight is appropriate for her height and age? How can a person know if his weight is jeopardizing his health? Questions such as these seem so simple, yet the answers can be complex—and different depending on whom you ask.

The Criterion of Fashion In asking what is ideal, people often mistakenly turn to fashion for the answer and judge body weight by appearances. No doubt our society sets unrealistic ideals for body weight, especially for women. Magazines, movies, and television all convey the message that to be thin is to be beautiful and happy. As a result, the media have a great influence on the weight concerns and dieting patterns of people of all ages but most tragically on young, impressionable children and adolescents.[2]

Importantly, perceived body image has little to do with actual body weight or size. People of all shapes, sizes, and ages—including extremely thin fashion models with anorexia nervosa and fitness instructors with ideal body composition—have learned to be unhappy with their "overweight" bodies. Such dissatisfaction can lead to damaging behaviors, such as starvation diets, diet pill abuse, and failure to seek health care.[3] The first step toward making healthy changes may be self-acceptance. Keep in mind that fashion is fickle; body shapes that our society values change with time. Furthermore, body shapes that our society values differ from those valued by other societies. The standards defining "ideal" are subjective and frequently have little in common with health. Table 6-3 offers some tips for adopting health as an ideal, rather than society's misconceived image of beauty.

The Criterion of Health
Even if our society were to accept fat as beautiful, **obesity** would still be a major risk factor for several life-threatening diseases as discussed later in the chapter. For this reason, the most important criterion for determining how much a person should weigh and how much body fat a person needs is not appearance but good health and longevity. A range of healthy body weights has been identified using a common measure of weight and height—the body mass index.

Body Mass Index
The **body mass index (BMI)** describes relative weight for height: (✚)

$$BMI = \frac{weight\ (kg)}{height\ (m)^2} \quad or \quad \frac{weight\ (lb)}{height\ (in)^2} \times 703$$

The BMI table on the inside back cover shows weights for various heights, and defines underweight, healthy weight, overweight, and obesity. As the BMI table shows, healthy weight falls between a BMI of 18.5 and 24.9. Most people with a BMI within this range have few of the health risks typically associated with too-low or too-high body weight.

TABLE 6-3	Tips for Accepting a Healthy Body Weight

- Value yourself and others for human attributes other than body weight. Realize that prejudging people by weight is as harmful as prejudging them by race, religion, or gender.

- Use positive, nonjudgmental descriptions of your body.

- Accept positive comments from others.

- Focus on your whole self including your intelligence, social grace, and professional and scholastic achievements.

- Accept that no magic diet exists.

- Stop dieting to lose weight. Adopt a lifestyle of healthy eating and physical activity permanently.

- Follow the USDA Food Guide. Never restrict food intake below the minimum levels that meet nutrient needs.

- Become physically active, not because it will help you get thin but because it will make you feel good and enhance your health.

- Seek support from loved ones. Tell them of your plan for a healthy life in the body you have been given.

- Seek professional counseling, *not* from a weight-loss counselor but from someone who can help you make gains in self-esteem without weight as a factor.

✚
- To convert pounds to kilograms, divide by 2.2.
- To convert inches to meters, divide by 39.37.

obesity: overweight with adverse health effects; BMI 30 or higher.

body mass index (BMI): an index of a person's weight in relation to height; determined by dividing the weight (in kilograms) by the square of the height (in meters).

FIGURE
6-5

Body Mass Index and Mortality

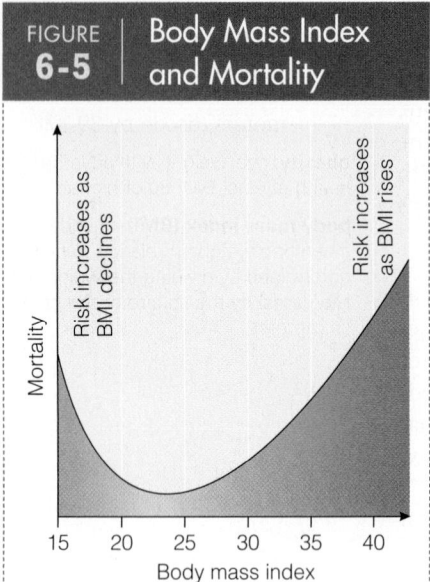

Risk increases as BMI declines

Risk increases as BMI rises

Mortality

Body mass index

15 20 25 30 35 40

This J-shaped curve describes the relationship between body mass index (BMI) and mortality and shows that both underweight and overweight present risks of a premature death.

Risks increase as BMI falls below 18.5 or rises above 24.9 (see Figure 6-5), reflecting the reality that both **underweight** and **overweight** impair health status. Figure 6-6 presents body shapes associated with various BMI values.

The BMI values are most accurate in assessing degrees of obesity and are less useful for evaluating nonobese people's body fatness. BMI values fail to reveal two valuable pieces of information in assessing disease risk: they don't reveal how much of the weight is fat, and they don't indicate where the fat is located. For this knowledge, measures of body composition are needed.

BODY COMPOSITION

For many people, being overweight compared with the standard means that they are over*fat*. This is not the case, though, for athletes with dense bones and well-developed muscles; they may be over*weight* but carry little body fat. Conversely, inactive people may seem to have acceptable weights but still carry too much body fat. In addition, the distribution of fat on the body may be even more critical than overfatness alone.

Central Obesity The distribution of fat on the body may be more critical than the total amount of fat alone. Fat that collects deep within the central abdominal area of the body, called **visceral fat**, may be especially likely to lead to diabetes, stroke, hypertension, and coronary artery disease (see Figure 6-7).[4] The risk of death from all causes may be higher for those with **central obesity** than for those whose fat accumulates elsewhere in the body.[5]

One possible explanation for why fat in the abdomen increases the risk of disease involves **adipokines**, hormones released by visceral adipose tissue. Adipokines help to regulate **inflammation** (✚) and energy metabolism in the tissues.[6]

✚ The inflammatory response is described in detail in Chapter 16.

underweight: body weight below some standard of acceptable weight that is usually defined in relation to height (such as BMI); BMI below 18.5.

overweight: body weight above some standard of acceptable weight that is usually defined in relation to height (such as BMI); BMI 25.0 to 29.9.

visceral fat: fat stored within the abdominal cavity in association with the internal abdominal organs, as opposed to fat stored directly under the skin (subcutaneous fat); also called *intra-abdominal fat*.

central obesity: excess fat around the trunk of the body; also called *abdominal fat* or *upper-body fat*.

adipokines (AD-ih-poh-kynz): protein hormones made and released by adipose tissue (fat) cells.

inflammation: an immunological response to cellular injury characterized by an increase in white blood cells.

FIGURE
6-6

Silhouettes and BMI (Actual BMI Shown)

Women

17   18   20   22.5   24   32   35

Men

18   21   23.5   24.5   26.5   31.5   37

Source: Reprinted from "The Body Test" (1988). Copyright Dietitians of Canada.

FIGURE
6-7 | Abdominal Fat

In healthy-weight people, some fat is stored around the organs of the abdomen.

In overweight people, excess abdominal fat increases the risks of diseases.

Insulin resistance is a central feature of the metabolic syndrome, which is discussed in Nutrition in Practice 20.

subcutaneous fat: fat stored directly under the skin.

- *sub* = beneath
- *cutaneous* = skin

waist circumference: a measurement used to assess a person's abdominal fat.

In central obesity, a shift occurs in the balance of adipokines, favoring those that increase both inflammation and insulin resistance of tissues.[7] The resulting chronic inflammation and insulin resistance contribute to diabetes, atherosclerosis (a cause of heart disease), and other chronic diseases.[8] (✚) With weight loss, the adipokine balance is restored, and inflammation and insulin resistance are relieved.[9] Chronic disease risks drop in response.

Abdominal fat creates the "apple" profile of central obesity. **Subcutaneous fat** around the hips and thighs creates more of a "pear" profile (see Figure 6-8). Abdominal fat is common in women past menopause and even more common in men. Even when total body fat is similar, men have more abdominal fat than either premenopausal or postmenopausal women. For those women with abdominal fat, the risks of cardiovascular disease and mortality are increased, just as they are for men. Interestingly, smokers tend to have more visceral fat than nonsmokers even though they typically have a lower BMI.[10] Two other factors that may affect body fat distribution are intakes of alcohol and physical activity. Moderate-to-high alcohol consumption may favor central obesity.[11] In contrast, regular physical activity seems to prevent abdominal fat accumulation.[12]

Waist Circumference

A person's **waist circumference** is a good indicator of fat distribution and central obesity (see Figure 6-9 on p. 154).[13] In general, women with a waist circumference greater than 35 inches and men with a waist circumference greater than 40 inches have a high risk of central obesity–related health problems.

FIGURE
6-8 | "Apple" and "Pear" Body Shapes Compared

Upper-body fat is more common in men than in women and is closely associated with heart disease, stroke, diabetes, hypertension, and some types of cancer.

Lower-body fat is more common in women than in men and is not usually associated with chronic diseases.

Popular articles sometimes call bodies with upper-body fat "apples" and those with lower-body fat, "pears."

Measuring Waist Circumference

Using a nonstretching tape measure, measure around the body near the belly button. (The skeleton shows the tape position relative to the hip bone.) Take the measure at the end of a normal expiration. A healthy waist circumference for men is no larger than 102 centimeters (40 inches); for women, no larger than 88 centimeters (35 inches).

At 6 feet 4 inches tall and 250 pounds, this runner would be considered overweight by most standards. Yet he is clearly not overfat.

Skinfold Measures Skinfold measurements provide an accurate estimate of total body fat and a fair assessment of the fat's location. About half of the fat in the body lies directly beneath the skin, so the thickness of this subcutaneous fat is assumed to reflect total body fat. Measures taken from central-body sites (around the abdomen) better reflect changes in fatness than those taken from upper sites (arm and back). A skilled assessor can obtain an accurate **skinfold measure** and then compare the measurement with standards (see Appendix E).

HOW MUCH BODY FAT IS TOO MUCH?

People often ask exactly how much fat is too fat for health. Ideally, a person has enough fat to meet basic needs but not so much as to incur health risks. The ideal amount of body fat depends partly on the person. A man with a BMI within the recommended range may have between 13 and 21 percent body fat; a woman, because of her greater quantity of indispensable fat, 23 to 31 percent.

Many athletes have a lower percentage of body fat—just enough fat to provide fuel, insulate and protect the body, assist in nerve impulse transmissions, and support normal hormone activity, but not so much as to burden the muscles. For athletes, then, body fat might be 5 to 10 percent for men and 15 to 20 percent for women.

For an Alaskan fisherman, a higher-than-average percentage of body fat is probably beneficial because fat helps prevent heat loss in cold weather. A woman starting a pregnancy needs sufficient body fat to support conception and fetal growth. Below a certain threshold for body fat, individuals may become infertile, develop depression, experience abnormal hunger regulation, or be unable to keep warm. These thresholds differ for each function and for each individual; much remains to be learned about them.

Review Notes

- Clearly, the most important criterion of appropriate fatness is health.
- Current standards for body weight are based on the body mass index (BMI), which describes a person's weight in relation to height.
- Health risks increase with a BMI below 18.5 or above 24.9.
- Central obesity, in which excess fat is distributed around the trunk of the body, presents greater health risks than excess fat distributed on the lower body.
- Researchers use a number of techniques to assess body composition including waist circumference and skinfold measures.

Risks of Overweight and Obesity

Despite our nation's preoccupation with body image and weight loss, the prevalence of overweight and obesity continues to rise dramatically (see Figure 6-10 on p. 156).[14] During the previous three decades, obesity increased in every state, in both genders, and across all ages, races, and education levels. Today, 68 percent of U.S. adults are overweight (BMI of 25 or greater), or dangerously obese (BMI of 30 or greater).[15] Even severe obesity increased alarmingly, although some recent news reports a slowdown in the rate of increase.[†16] Among children and adolescents, an estimated 32 percent are overweight and 17 percent are obese.[17] The prevalence of overweight is especially high among women, the poor, and some ethnic groups. The problem reaches around the globe, in urban and rural areas alike.[18] In short, obesity is a major public health problem that is becoming more and more prevalent.

HEALTH RISKS OF OBESITY

The growing prevalence of overweight and obesity is a matter of concern because both conditions present risks to health. Indeed, the health risks of obesity are so many that it has been declared a disease. For example, excess weight contributes to more than half of all cases of hypertension, thereby increasing the risk of heart attack and stroke.[19] Obesity raises blood pressure in part by altering kidney function and promoting fluid retention.[20] Often weight loss alone can normalize the blood pressure of an overweight or obese person.

Excess body weight also increases the risk of type 2 diabetes. Most adults with type 2 diabetes are overweight or obese, and obesity itself can directly cause some degree of **insulin resistance**.[21] Diabetes (type 2) is three times more likely to develop in an obese person than in a nonobese person. Furthermore, the person with type 2 diabetes often has central obesity. Central-body fat cells appear to be larger and more insulin resistant than lower-body fat cells.[22]

insulin resistance: the condition in which a normal amount of insulin produces a subnormal effect in muscle, adipose, and liver cells, resulting in an elevated fasting glucose; a metabolic consequence of obesity that precedes type 2 diabetes.

---

† Defined as more than 100 pounds overweight.

FIGURE
6-10

The Increasing Prevalence of Obesity among U.S. Adults by State

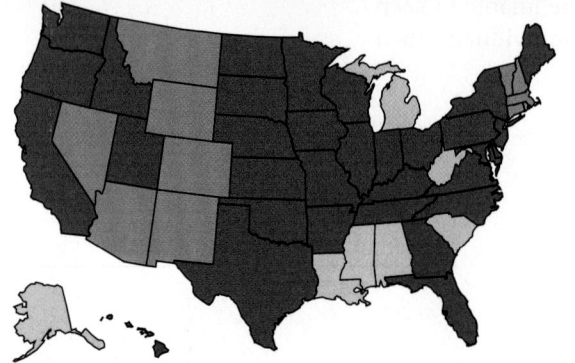

1998: Most states had prevalence rates less than 20 percent.

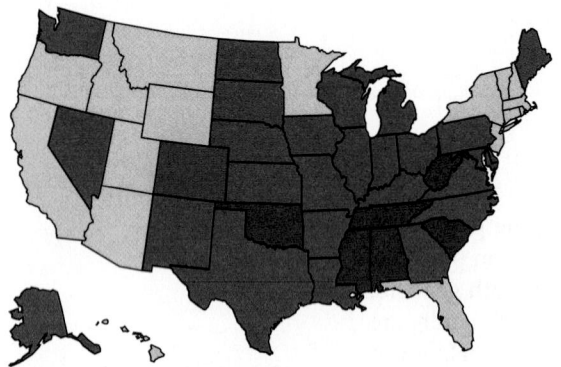

2008: Most states had prevalence rates greater than 25 percent, with six states reporting prevalence rates greater than or equal to 30 percent.

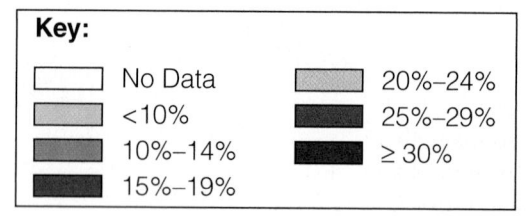

Key:

☐ No Data	▨ 20%–24%
▨ <10%	▨ 25%–29%
▨ 10%–14%	■ ≥ 30%
▨ 15%–19%	

Source: www.cdc.nccdphp/dnpa/obesity/trend/maps/index.htm

Besides diabetes and hypertension, other risks threaten obese adults. Among them are high blood lipids, cardiovascular disease, sleep apnea (abnormal ceasing of breathing during sleep), osteoarthritis, abdominal hernias, some cancers, varicose veins, gout, gallbladder disease, kidney stones, respiratory problems (including Pickwickian syndrome, a breathing blockage linked with sudden death), nonalcoholic fatty liver disease, complications in pregnancy and surgery, flat feet, and even a high accident rate.[23] Each year these obesity-related illnesses cost our nation billions of dollars. The cost in terms of lives is also great. People with lifelong obesity are twice as likely to die prematurely as others. In the United States, obesity is second only to tobacco use as the most significant cause of preventable death.

The precise level at which excess weight begins to present risks has not been established. Some evidence indicates that being even moderately overweight aggravates the risk of heart disease, assuming that the excess weight is fat, not muscle.[24] Some overweight people, however, remain healthy and live long lives despite their body fatness. Genetic inheritance, smoking habits, and level of physical activity may help to explain why some overweight individuals stay well while others become ill.[25] Some research suggests that physical fitness, despite body fatness, may protect against early death from disease.[26] A recent study of more than 1700 men, however, seems to refute the idea that people can be overweight and yet still be healthy. Researchers found that overweight men with normal metabolic profiles (healthy blood pressure, normal cholesterol and blood glucose levels) at age 50 had a 52 percent greater risk of developing heart disease within 30 years compared with men who were normal weight and had similar metabolic profiles.[27] In other words, excess weight, even with a healthy metabolic profile, still presents an increased risk of heart disease. To help in identifying those most at risk, obesity experts have developed guidelines, described next.

NATIONAL GUIDELINES FOR IDENTIFYING THOSE AT RISK FROM OBESITY

The U.S. guidelines for identifying and evaluating the risks to health from overweight and obesity rely on three indicators. The first indicator is a person's BMI. As a general guideline, overweight for adults is defined as BMI of 25.0 through 29.9, and obesity is defined as BMI equal to or greater than 30.

The second indicator is waist circumference, which, as discussed earlier, reflects the degree of abdominal fatness in proportion to body fatness. Women with a waist circumference greater than 35 inches and men with a waist circumference greater than 40 inches are at greater risk of type 2 diabetes, hypertension, and cardiovascular disease than women or men with waist circumferences equal to or below these measures. In other words, waist circumference is an independent predictor of disease risk.

The third indicator is the person's disease risk profile. The disease risk profile takes into account life-threatening diseases, family history, and common risk factors for

Energy Balance and Body Composition

chronic diseases (such as blood lipid profile). The higher the BMI, the greater the waist circumference, and the more risk factors—the greater the urgency to treat obesity. People who have one or more of the diseases listed in the margin, (✚) or three or more of the cardiovascular disease risk factors listed, have a very high risk for disease complications and mortality that requires aggressive treatment to manage the disease or modify the risk factors.

OTHER RISKS OF OBESITY

Although some obese people seem to escape health problems, few in our society can avoid the social and economic handicaps. Our society places enormous value on thinness. Obese people are less sought after for romance, less often hired, and less often admitted to college.[28] They pay higher insurance premiums, and they pay more for clothing. This is especially true for women. In contrast, people with other chronic conditions such as asthma, diabetes, and epilepsy do not differ socially or economically from nonoverweight people.

Prejudice defines people by their appearance rather than by their abilities and characters. Obese people suffer emotional pain when others treat them with insensitivity, hostility, and contempt, and they may internalize a sense of guilt and self-deprecation. Health-care professionals, even dietitians, can be among the offenders without realizing it.[29] To free our society of its obsession with body fatness and prejudice against obese people, activists are promoting respect for individuals of all body weights.

✚ The National Heart, Lung, and Blood Institute states that aggressive treatment is urgently needed for a clinically obese person (BMI ≥30) who also has any of the following:
- Heart disease
- Diabetes (type 2)
- Sleep apnea, including temporary stopping of breathing

The same urgency for treatment exists for an obese person with any *three* of the following CVD risk factors:
- Hypertension
- Cigarette smoking
- High LDL cholesterol
- Low HDL cholesterol
- Impaired glucose tolerance
- Age older than 45 years (men) or 55 years (women)
- Heart disease of an immediate family member before age 55 (male) or 65 (female)

Source: National Heart, Lung, and Blood Institute, National Institutes of Health, *The Practical Guide: Identification, Evaluation, and Treatment of Overweight and Obesity in Adults,* NIH publication no. 00-4084 (Washington, D.C.: Government Printing Office, 2000).

Review Notes

- The health risks of obesity are many and serious.
- Guidelines for identifying the health risks of overweight and obesity are based on a person's BMI, waist circumference, and disease risk profile.
- Obesity also incurs social, economic, and psychological risks.

Self Check

1 • As carbohydrate and fat stores are depleted during fasting or starvation, the body then uses ___ as its fuel source.
   a. alcohol
   b. protein
   c. glucose
   d. triglycerides

2 • When carbohydrate is not available to provide energy for the brain, as in starvation, the body produces ketone bodies from:
   a. glucose.
   b. glycerol.
   c. fatty acid fragments.
   d. amino acids.

3 • Three hazards of fasting are:
   a. water weight loss, decrease in mental alertness, and wasting of lean tissue.
   b. water weight gain, impairment of disease resistance, and lowering of body temperature.
   c. water weight gain, decrease in mental alertness, and impairment of disease resistance.
   d. wasting of lean tissue, impairment of disease resistance, and disturbances of the body's salt and water balance.

4 • Two activities that contribute to the basal metabolic rate are:
   a. walking and running.
   b. maintenance of heartbeat and running.
   c. maintenance of body temperature and walking.
   d. maintenance of heartbeat and body temperature.

5 • Three factors that affect the body's basal metabolic rate are:
   a. height, weight, and energy intake.
   b. age, body composition, and height.
   c. fever, body composition, and altitude.
   d. weight, fever, and environmental temperature.

6 • The largest component of energy expenditure is:
   a. basal metabolism.
   b. physical activity.
   c. indirect calorimetry.
   d. thermic effect of food.

7 • Which of the following reflects height and weight?
   a. Body mass index
   b. Central obesity
   c. Waist circumference
   d. Body composition

8 • The BMI range that correlates with the fewest health risks is:
   a. 16.5 to 20.9.
   b. 18.5 to 24.9.
   c. 25.5 to 30.9.
   d. 30.5 to 34.9.

9 • The profile of central obesity is sometimes referred to as a(an):
   a. beer.
   b. pear.
   c. apple.
   d. potato.

10 • Which of the following health risks is **not** associated with being overweight?
   a. Hypertension
   b. Heart disease
   c. Type 1 diabetes
   d. Gallbladder disease

Answers to these questions can be found in Appendix H.

Clinical Applications

1 • Compare the energy a person might spend on various physical activities. Refer to Table 6-2 on pp. 148–149, and compute how much energy a person who weighs 142 pounds would spend doing each of the following activities. An example using aerobic dance has been provided for you. You may want to compare various activities based on your own weight.
   30 minutes of vigorous aerobic dance:
   0.062 kcal/lb/min × 142 lb = 8.8 kcal/min.
   8.8 kcal/min × 30 min = 264 kcal.

   a. 2 hours of golf, carrying clubs.
   b. 20 minutes running at 9 mph.
   c. 45 minutes of swimming at 20 yd/min.
   d. 1 hour of walking at 3.5 mph.

2 • Using the "How to" on p. 150 as a guide, determine your estimated energy requirements (EER).

Answers

1. (a) 0.045 kcal/lb/min × 142 lb = 6.4 kcal/min, 6.4 kcal/min × 120 min = 768 kcal; (b) 0.103 kcal/lb/min × 142 lb = 14.6 kcal/min, 14.6 kcal/min × 20 min = 292 kcal; (c) 0.032 kcal/lb/min × 142 lb = 4.5 kcal/min, 4.5 kcal/min × 45 = 202.5 kcal; (d) 0.035 kcal/lb/min × 142 lb = 5 kcal/min, 5 kcal/min × 60 min = 300 kcal.

Nutrition on the Net

For further study of the topics in this chapter, access these websites.

- Find updates and quick links to these and other nutrition-related sites at our website:
  www.cengage.com/nutrition/whitney/nhhc4e
- Obtain food composition data from the USDA Nutrient Data Laboratory:
  www.ars.usda.gov/ba/bhnrc/ndl
- Search for "obesity" and "weight control" at the U.S. government health information site:
  www.healthfinder.gov
- Review the Clinical Guidelines on the Identification, Evaluation, and Treatment of Overweight and Obesity in Adults:
  www.nhlbi.nih.gov/guidelines/obesity/ob_home.htm
- Learn about the 10,000 Steps Program at Shape Up America:
  www.shapeup.org

- Visit the special web pages and interactive applications for Healthy Weight:
  www.nhlbi.nih.gov/health/prof/heart/index.htm#obesity
- Find helpful information on achieving and maintaining a healthy weight from the Calorie Control Council:
  www.caloriecontrol.org
- Learn how to end size discrimination and improve the quality of life for fat people from the National Association to Advance Fat Acceptance:
  www.naafaonline.com/dev2/
- Consider ways to live a healthy life at any weight:
  www.bodypositive.com

Notes

1. S. G. Wannamethee, A. G. Shaper, and P. H. Whincup, Alcohol and adiposity: Effects of quantity and type of drink and time relation with meals, *International Journal of Obesity and Related Metabolic Disorders* 29 (2005): 1436–1444; R. A. Breslow and B. A. Smothers, Drinking patterns and body mass index in never smokers, *American Journal of Epidemiology* 161 (2005): 368–376.

2. M. J. Hogan and V. C. Strasburger, Body image, eating disorders, and the media, *Adolescent Medicine: State of the Art Reviews* 19 (2009): 521–546; A. J. Hill, Motivation for eating behavior in adolescent girls: The body beautiful, *Proceedings of the Nutrition Society* 65 (2006): 376–384.

3. C. A. Drury and M. Louis, Exploring the association between body weight, stigma of obesity, and health care avoidance, *Journal of the American Academy of Nurse Practitioners* 14 (2002): 554–561.

4. S. S. Dhaliwal and T. A. Welborn, Central obesity and multivariable cardiovascular risk as assessed by the Framingham Prediction Scores, *American Journal of Cardiology* 103 (2009): 1403–1407; G. A. Bray and coauthors, Relation of central adiposity and body mass index to the development of diabetes in the Diabetes Prevention Program, *American Journal of Clinical Nutrition* 87 (2008): 1212–1218; C. S. Fox and coauthors, Abdominal visceral and subcutaneous adipose tissue compartments: Association with metabolic risk factors in the Framingham Heart Study, *Circulation* 116 (2007): 39–48; A. Tchernof, Visceral adipocytes and the Metabolic Syndrome, *Nutrition Reviews* 65 (2007): S24–S29; C. D. Lee and coauthors, Abdominal obesity and coronary artery calcification in young adults: The Coronary Artery Risk Development in Young Adults (CARDIA) Study, *American Journal of Clinical Nutrition* 86 (2007): 48–54; S. B. Votruba and M. D. Jensen, Regional fat deposition as a factor in FFA metabolism, *Annual Review of Nutrition* 27 (2007): 149–163.

5. J. P. Reis and coauthors, Overall obesity and abdominal adiposity as predictors of mortality in U. S. white and black adults, *Annals of Epidemiology* 19 (2009): 134–142.

6. G. Govindarajan, M. A. Alpert, and L. Tejwani, Endocrine and metabolic effects of fat: Cardiovascular implications, *American Journal of Medicine* 121 (2008): 366–370; G. Fantuzzi and T. Mazzone, Adipose tissue and atherosclerosis: Exploring the connection, *Arteriosclerosis, Thrombosis, and Vascular Biology* 27 (2007): 996–1003; P. Trayhurn, C. Bing, and I. S. Wood, Adipose tissue and adipokines—Energy regulation from the human perspective, *Journal of Nutrition* 136 (2006): 1935S–1939S; C. Bulcão and coauthors, The new adipose tissue and adipocytokines, *Current Diabetes Reviews* 2 (2006): 19–28; T. J. Guzik, D. Mangalat, and R. Korbut, Adipocytokines—Novel link between inflammation and vascular function? *Journal of Physiology and Pharmacology* 57 (2006): 505–528.

7. W. V. Brown and coauthors, Obesity: Why be concerned? *American Journal of Medicine* 122 (2009): S4–S11; J. Korner, S. C. Woods, and K. A. Woodworth, Regulation of energy homeostasis and health consequences in obesity, *American Journal of Medicine* 122 (2009): S12–S18; W. L. Holland and coauthors, Lipid mediators of insulin resistance, *Nutrition Reviews* 65 (2007): S39–S46; R. Weiss, Fat distribution and storage: How much, where, and how? *European Journal of Endocrinology* 157 (2007): S39–S45; P. Trayhurn, C. Bing, and I. S. Wood, Adipose tissue and adipokines—Energy regulation from the human perspective, *Journal of Nutrition* 136 (2006): 1935S–1939S.

8. Brown and coauthors, 2009; V. Z. Rocha and P. Libby, The multiple facets of the fat tissue, *Thyroid* 18 (2008): 175–183; P. Calabro and E. T. Yeh, Intra-abdominal adiposity, inflammation, and cardiovascular risk: New insight into global cardiometabolic risk, *Current Hypertension Reports* 10 (2008): 32–38; D. C. W. Lau and coauthors, Adipokines: Molecular links between obesity and atherosclerosis, *American Journal of Physiology—Heart and Circulatory Physiology* 288 (2005): H2031–H2041.

9. J. P. Bastard and coauthors, Recent advances in the relationship between obesity, inflammation, and insulin resistance, *European Cytokine Network* 17 (2006): 4–12.

10. E. W. Demerath, Causes and consequences of human variation in visceral adiposity, *American Journal of Clinical Nutrition* 91 (2010): 1–2; E. A. Molenaar and coauthors, Association of lifestyle factors with abdominal subcutaneous and visceral adiposity: The Framingham Heart Study, *Diabetes Care* 32 (2009): 505–510; D. Canoy and coauthors, Cigarette smoking and fat distribution in 21,828 British men and women: A population-based study, *Obesity Research* 13 (2005): 1466–1475.

11. Molenaar and coauthors, 2009; Wannamethee, Shaper, and Whincup, 2005.

12. B. J. Arsenault and coauthors, Physical inactivity, abdominal obesity and risk of coronary heart disease in apparently healthy men and women, *International Journal of Obesity* 34 (2010): 340–347; Y. Kim and S. Lee, Physical activity and abdominal obesity in youth, *Applied Physiology, Nutrition and Metabolism* 34 (2009): 571–581.

13. J. P. Després and coauthors, Abdominal obesity and the metabolic syndrome: Contribution to global cardiometabolic risk, *Arteriosclerosis, Thrombosis, and Vascular Biology* 28 (2008): 1039–1049; S. Klein and coauthors, Waist circumference and cardiometabolic risk: A consensus statement from Shaping America's Health: Association for Weight Management and Obesity Prevention; NAASO, The Obesity Society; The American Society for Nutrition; and the American Diabetes Association, *American Journal of Clinical Nutrition* 85 (2007): 1197–1202.

14. C. M. Apovian, The causes, prevalence, and treatment of obesity revisited in 2009: What have we learned so far? *American Journal of Clinical Nutrition* 91 (2010): 277S–279S; C. L. Ogden and coauthors, Prevalence of overweight and obesity in the United States, 1999–2004, *Journal of the American Medical Association* 295 (2006): 1549–1555.

15. K. M. Flegal and coauthors, Prevalence and trends in obesity among U.S. adults, 1999-2008, *Journal of the American Medical Association* 303 (2010): 235-241.

16. C. L. Ogden and coauthors, Obesity among adults in the United States—No statistically significant change since 2003–2004, HCHS Data Brief November 2007, pp.1–6; R. Sturm, Increases in morbid obesity in the USA: 2000–2005, *Public Health* 121 (2007): 492–496.

17. C. L. Ogden, and coauthors, Prevalence of high body mass index in children and adolescents, 2007-2008, *Journal of the American Medical Association* 303 (2010): 242-249.

18. B. M. Popkin, Recent dynamics suggest selected countries catching up to U.S. obesity, *American Journal of Clinical Nutrition* 91 (2010): 284S–288S.

19. G. Hu and coauthors, Body mass index, waist circumference, and waist-hip ratio on the risk of total and type-specific stroke, *Archives of Internal Medicine* 167 (2007): 1420–1427.

20. J. Redon and coauthors, Mechanisms of hypertension in the cardiometabolic syndrome, *Journal of Hypertension* 27 (2009): 441–451; F. W. Visser and coauthors, Rise in extracellular fluid volume during high sodium depends on BMI in healthy men, *Obesity (Silver Spring)* 17 (2009): 1684–1688.

21. American Diabetes Association, Diagnosis and classification of diabetes mellitus, *Diabetes Care* 32 (2009): S62–S67.

22. E. H. Livingston, Lower body subcutaneous fat accumulation and diabetes mellitus risk, *Surgery for Obesity and Related Diseases* 2 (2006): 362–368.

23. L. W. York, S. Puthalapattu, and G. Y. Wu, Nonalcoholic fatty liver disease and low-carbohydrate diets, *Annual Review of Nutrition* 29 (2009): 365–379; G. Whitlock and coauthors, Body-mass index and cause-specific mortality in 900,000 adults: Collaborative analyses of 57 prospective studies, *Lancet* 373 (2009): 1083–1096; C. J. Lavie, R. V. Milani, and H. O. Ventura, Obesity and cardiovascular disease: Risk factor, paradox, and impact of weight loss, *Journal of the American College of Cardiology* 53 (2009): 1925–1932;

A. G. Renehan and coauthors, Body-mass index and incidence of cancer: A systematic review and meta-analysis of prospective observational studies, *Lancet* 371 (2008): 569–578; K. F. Adams and coauthors, Body mass and colorectal cancer risk in the NIH-AARP cohort, *American Journal of Epidemiology* 166 (2007): 36–45; S. R. Patel and coauthors, Association between reduced sleep and weight gain in women, *American Journal of Epidemiology* 164 (2006): 947–954.

24. D. P. Guh and coauthors, The incidence of co-morbidities related to obesity and overweight: A systematic review and meta-analysis, *BMC Public Health* 9 (2009): 88; R. P. Bogers and coauthors, Association of overweight with increased risk of coronary heart disease partly independent of blood pressure and cholesterol levels: A meta-analysis of 21 cohort studies including more than 300,000 persons, *Archives of Internal Medicine* 167 (2009): 1720–1728.

25. N. Stefan and coauthors, Identification and characterization of metabolically benign obesity in humans, *Archives of Internal Medicine* 168 (2008): 1609–1616; R. P. Wildman and coauthors, The obese without cardiometabolic risk factor clustering and the normal weight with cardiometabolic risk factor clustering, *Archives of Internal Medicine* 168 (2008): 1617–1624; P. T. Williams, Maintaining vigorous activity attenuates 7-yr weight gain in 8340 runners, *Medicine & Science in Sports & Exercise* 39 (2007): 801–809.

26. V. Hainer, H. Toplak, and V. Stich, Fat or fit: What is more important? *Diabetes Care* 32 (2009): S392–S397.

27. J. Arnlöv and coauthors, Impact of body mass index and the metabolic syndrome on the risk of cardiovascular disease and death in middle-aged men, *Circulation* 121 (2010): 230–236.

28. M. S. Argugete, J. L. Edman, and A. Yates, Romantic interest in obese college students, *Eating Behaviors* 10 (2009): 143–145.

29. D. E. Berryman and coauthors, Dietetics students possess negative attitudes toward obesity similar to nondietetics students, *Journal of the American Dietetic Association* 106 (2006): 1678–1682.

Fad Diets

To paraphrase William Shakespeare, "a fad diet by any other name would still be a fad diet." And the names are legion: the Atkins Diet, the Cheater's Diet, the South Beach Diet, the Zone Diet*. Year after year, "new and improved" diets appear on bookstore shelves and circulate among friends. Sometimes fad diets seem to work for a while, but more often than not, their success is short-lived. Then another fad diet takes the spotlight. Here's how Dr. K. Brownell, an obesity researcher at Yale University, describes this phenomenon: "When I get calls about the latest diet fad, I imagine a trick birthday cake candle that keeps lighting up and we have to keep blowing it out."

Why don't health professionals speak out against the relentless promotion of fad diets?

Realizing that many fad diets do not offer a safe and effective plan for weight loss, health professionals speak out, but they never get the candle blown out permanently. New fad diets can keep making outrageous claims because no one requires their advocates to prove what they say. Fad diet gurus do not have to conduct credible research on the benefits or dangers of their diets. They can simply make

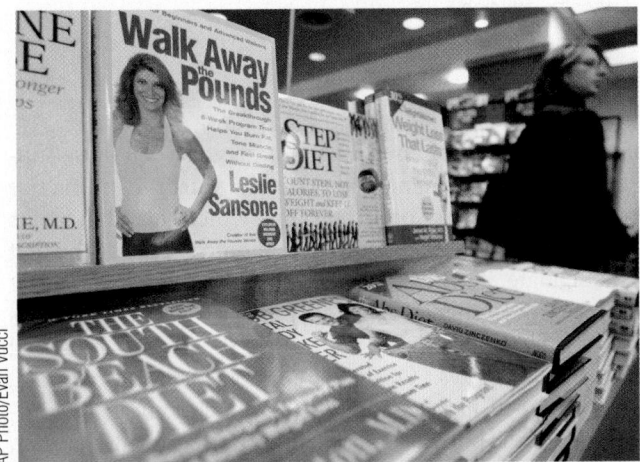

AP Photo/Evan Vucci

*The following sources offer comparisons and evaluations of various fad diets for your review: New diet winners, *Consumer Reports,* June 2007, pp. 12–17; Battle of the diet books II, *Nutrition Action Healthletter,* July/August 2006, pp. 10–11; B. Liebman, Weighing the diet books, *Nutrition Action Healthletter,* January/February 2004, pp. 1–8.

recommendations and then later, if questioned, search for bits and pieces of research that support the conclusions they have already reached. That's backwards. Diet and health recommendations should *follow* years of sound research that has been reviewed by panels of scientists *before* being offered to the public.

How can the promoters of fad diets get away with exaggerated claims?

Because anyone can publish anything—in books or on the Internet—peddlers of fad diets can make unsubstantiated statements that fall far short of the truth, but sound impressive to the uninformed. They often offer distorted bits of legitimate research. They may start with one or more actual facts, but then leap from one erroneous conclusion to the next. Anyone who wants to believe these claims has to wonder how the thousands of scientists working on obesity research over the past century could possibly have missed such obvious connections. Table NP6-1 (p. 162) presents some of the claims and truths of fad diets.

Each popular diet features a unique way to make losing weight fast and easy. Which one works best?

Fad diets come in almost as many shapes and sizes as the people who search them out. Some restrict fats or carbohydrates, some limit portion sizes, some focus on food combinations, and some claim that a person's genetic type or blood type determines the foods best suited to manage weight and prevent disease. Despite claims that each new diet is "unique" in its approach to weight loss, most fad diets are designed to ensure a low energy intake. The "magic feature" that best supports weight loss is to limit energy intake to less than energy expenditure. Most of the sample menu plans, especially in the early stages, deliver an average of 1200 kcalories per day. Total kcalories tend to be low simply because food intake is so limited. Table NP6-2 (pp. 163–164) compares some of today's more popular diets.

What is the appeal of fad diets?

Probably the greatest appeal of fad diets is that they tend to ignore current diet recommendations. Foods such as meats and milk products that need to be selected carefully to limit saturated fat can now be eaten with abandon. Whole grains, legumes, vegetables, and fruits that should be eaten

TABLE NP6-1 | The Claims and Truths of Fad Diets

The Claim: You can lose weight "easily."

The Truth: Most fad diet plans have complicated rules that require you to calculate protein requirements, count carbohydrate grams, combine certain foods, time meal intervals, purchase special products, plan daily menus, and measure serving sizes.

The Claim: You can lose weight by eating a specific ratio of carbohydrate, protein, and fat.

The Truth: Weight loss depends on expending more energy than you take in, not on the proportion of energy nutrients.

The Claim: This "revolutionary diet" can "reset your genetic code."

The Truth: You inherited your genes and cannot alter your genetic code.

The Claim: High-protein diets are popular, selling more than 20 million books, because they work.

The Truth: Weight-loss books are popular because people grasp for quick fixes and simple solutions to their weight problems. If book sales were an indication of weight-loss success, we would be a lean nation—but they're not, and neither are we.

The Claim: People gain weight on low-fat diets.

The Truth: People can gain weight on low-fat diets if they overindulge in carbohydrates and proteins while cutting fat; low-fat diets are not necessarily low-kcalorie diets. But people can also lose weight on low-fat diets if they cut kcalories as well as fat.

The Claim: High-protein diets energize the brain.

The Truth: The brain depends on glucose for its energy; the primary dietary source of glucose is carbohydrate, not protein.

The Claim: Thousands of people have been successful with this plan.

The Truth: Authors of fad diets have not published their research findings in scientific journals. Success stories are anecdotal, and failures are not reported.

The Claim: Carbohydrates raise blood glucose levels, triggering insulin production and fat storage.

The Truth: Insulin promotes fat storage when energy intake exceeds energy needs. Furthermore, insulin is only one of many hormones involved in the complex processes of maintaining the body's energy balance and health.

The Claim: Eat protein and lose weight.

The Truth: For every complicated problem, there is a simple—and wrong—solution.

---

in abundance can now be bypassed. For some people, this is a dream come true: steaks without the potatoes, ribs without the coleslaw, and meatballs without the pasta. Who can resist the promise of weight loss while eating freely from a list of favorite foods?

Dieters are also lured into fad diets by sophisticated—yet often erroneous—explanations of the metabolic consequences of eating certain foods. Terms such as *eicosanoids* or *adipokines* are scattered about, often intimidating readers into believing that the authors must be right given their brilliance in understanding the body.

Are fad diets adequate?

When food choices are limited, nutrient intakes may be inadequate. To help shore up some of these inadequacies, fad diets often recommend a dietary supplement. Conveniently,

many of the companies selling fad diets also sell these supplements, often at an inflated price. As Nutrition in Practice 9 explains, however, foods offer many more health benefits than any supplement can provide.[1] Quite simply, if the diet is inadequate, it needs to be improved, not supplemented.

When researchers evaluated popular weight-loss plans against dietary standards for health, they found most fell short in some ways.[2] Of the eight popular plans examined, Ornish ranked highest and Atkins, which famously eliminates most carbohydrate-containing foods from the diet, ranked lowest.

Are the diets effective?

If fad diets were entirely ineffective, consumers would eventually stop pursuing them. Obviously, this is not the case. Similarly, if the diets were especially effective,

Diet	Major Premise Promoted	Strong Point(s)	Weak Point(s)
Atkins Diet	• People are overweight or obese because they have metabolic imbalances caused by eating too many carbohydrates; by restricting carbohydrates, these imbalances can be corrected. • You can lose weight without lowering kcalorie intake.	• Quick, short-term weight loss is achieved.	• Restricts carbohydrates to a level that induces ketosis. • Ketosis can cause nausea, lightheadedness, and fatigue. • Ketosis can worsen existing medical problems such as kidney disease. • A diet high in fat such as Atkins can increase the risk of heart disease and some cancers.
Cheater's Diet	• Successful weight loss depends on eliminating boredom and allowing indulgences. • Cheating on weekends "stokes your metabolism."	• Meals are proportioned one-half fruit or vegetables, one-fourth lean protein, and one-fourth whole grains. • Encourages as much exercise as possible.	• No scientific data on cheating to boost metabolism or support weight loss.
Eat Right 4 Your Type	• Your blood type determines which foods you should eat or not eat.	None	• Food groups or individual foods are excluded, depending on blood type. • No scientific data on the relationship between blood type and food choices.
Glucose Revolution	• Low-glycemic index foods satisfy hunger, control blood glucose, and promote weight loss.	• Emphasizes fiber-rich vegetables, legumes, fruits, and whole grains. • Minimizes saturated fat intake.	• Difficult to know the glycemic index of some foods.
Ornish Diet	• By strictly limiting fat (both animal and vegetable), you eat fewer kcalories without eating less food.	• High-fiber, low-fat foods in this plan can lower blood cholesterol and blood pressure.	• So little fat that essential fatty acids may be lacking. • Limits fish, nuts, and olive oil, which may protect against heart disease.
Pritikin Program	• By eating low-fat, mainly plant-based foods, you can eat more food and still feel satisfied.	• No food group is completely eliminated in this high-fiber, low-fat diet program. • Some use of foods rich in omega-3 fatty acids is encouraged.	• For some people, very low-fat diets may be unsatisfying and therefore difficult to adhere to.
Sonoma Diet	• Enjoying portion-controlled Mediterranean-style foods supports weight loss and promotes good health.	• Emphasizes nutrient-dense foods.	• Initial phase restricts fruits and limits milk products.

(Continued)

Diet	Major Premise Promoted	Strong Point(s)	Weak Point(s)
South Beach Diet	• Eating "good carbohydrates" such as vegetables, whole-wheat pastas, and brown rice will maintain satiety and resist cravings for "bad carbohydrates" such as white rice and potatoes.	• Encourages consumption of vegetables, lean meats, and fish, and the use of unsaturated oils when cooking. • Restricts fatty meats and cheeses as well as sweets.	• Starchy carbohydrates and all fruits are completely excluded during the first two weeks.
Ultimate Weight Solution Diet	• Foods that require great effort to prepare and eat are nutrient dense; eating these kinds of foods (raw vegetables, vegetable soups, whole grains, beans, meats, poultry, and fish) will lead to weight loss. • Foods that take little effort to prepare and eat provide excess kcalories relative to nutrients; eating these kinds of foods (fast foods, puddings, high-kcalorie convenience foods, processed foods) leads to uncontrolled eating and weight gain.	• Encourages consumption of lean meats and fish; whole grains; vegetables; fruit; and low-fat milk, yogurt, and cheese. • Restricts fatty meats and cheeses as well as sweets. • Encourages exercise.	• Confusing as to exactly what to eat or how much.
Zone Diet	• Eating the correct proportions of carbohydrates, fat, and protein leads to hormonal balance, weight loss, disease prevention, and increased vitality.	• Promotes weight loss because it is a low-kcalorie diet.	• The diet is rigid, restrictive, and complicated, making it difficult for most people to follow accurately. • The overblown health claims of the diet's proponents are based on misinterpreted science and remain unsubstantiated.

then consumers who tried them would lose weight and the obesity problem would be solved. Clearly, this is not happening either. As mentioned earlier, most fad diets succeed in contriving ways to limit kcalorie intakes, and so produce weight loss (at least in the short term). Simple kcalorie deficit, as it turns out, is the key to weight loss; an emphasis on protein, carbohydrate, or fat, or any other gimmick does not improve weight loss.[3]

With over half of our nation's adults overweight and many more concerned about their weight, weight-loss books and products are a $33 billion-a-year business. Even a plan that offers only minimal weight-loss success easily attracts a following.

Many people seem confused about what kinds of dietary changes they need to make to lose weight. Isn't it helpful to follow a plan?

Yes. Most people need specific instructions and examples to make dietary changes. Popular diets offer dieters a plan. The user doesn't have to decide what foods to eat, how to prepare them, or how much to eat. Unfortunately, these instructions serve short-term weight-loss needs only. Over the long run, people tire of the monotony of diet plans and most revert to their previous patterns.

By now you can see that the major drawback of most fad weight-loss schemes is that they fail to create lifestyle changes needed to support long-term weight maintenance and improve health.[4] For that, people must do the hard work of learning the facts about nutrition and weight loss, setting their own realistic goals, and then devising a lifestyle plan that can achieve them. A balanced, kcalorie-restricted diet with sufficient physical activity to support it may not be the shortcut that most people wish for, but it assures nutrient adequacy and provides the best chance of long-term success.[5] Table NP6-3 offers guidelines for identifying fad diets and other weight-loss scams; it includes the hallmarks of healthy weight-loss programs as well. Chapter 7 includes reasonable approaches to weight management and concludes that the ideal diet is one you can live with for the rest of your life. Keep that criterion in mind when you evaluate the next "latest and greatest weight-loss diet" that comes along.

TABLE NP6-3	Guidelines for Identifying Fad Diets and Other Weight-Loss Scams	
Fad Diets and Weight-Loss Scams	**Healthy Diet Guidelines**
1. They promise dramatic, rapid weight loss.	1. Weight loss should be gradual and not exceed 2 pounds per week.
2. They promote diets that are nutritionally unbalanced or extremely low in kcalories.	2. Diets should provide: • A reasonable number of kcalories (not fewer than 1200 kcalories per day) • Enough, but not too much, protein (between the RDA and twice the RDA) • Enough, but not too much, fat (between 20 and 35 percent of daily energy intake from fat) • Enough carbohydrates to spare protein and prevent ketosis (at least 100 grams per day) and 20 to 30 grams of fiber from food sources • A balanced assortment of vitamins and minerals from a variety of foods from each of the food groups • At least 1 liter (about 1 quart) of water daily or 1 milliliter per kcalorie daily—whichever is more
3. They use liquid formulas rather than foods.	3. Foods should accommodate a person's ethnic background, taste preferences, and financial means.
4. They attempt to make clients dependent upon special foods or devices.	4. Programs should teach clients how to make good choices from the conventional food supply.
5. They fail to encourage permanent, realistic lifestyle changes.	5. Programs should teach physical activity plans that involve expending at least 300 kcalories a day and behavior-modification strategies that help to correct poor eating habits.
6. They misrepresent salespeople as "counselors" supposedly qualified to give guidance in nutrition and/or general health.	6. Even if adequately trained, such "counselors" would still be objectionable because of the obvious conflict of interest that exists when providers profit directly from products they recommend and sell.
7. They collect large sums of money at the start or require that clients sign contracts for expensive, long-term programs.	7. Programs should be reasonably priced and run on a pay-as-you-go basis.

(Continued)

Fad Diets and Weight-Loss Scams	Healthy Diet Guidelines
8. They fail to inform clients of the risks associated with weight loss in general or the specific program being promoted.	8. They should provide information about dropout rates, the long-term success of their clients, and possible diet side effects.
9. They promote unproven or spurious weight-loss aids such as human chorionic gonadotropin hormone (HCG), starch blockers, diuretics, sauna belts, body wraps, passive exercise, ear stapling, acupuncture, electric muscle-stimulating (EMS) devices, spirulina, amino acid supplements (e.g., arginine, ornithine), glucomannan, methylcellulose (a "bulking agent"), "unique" ingredients, and so forth.	9. They should focus on nutrient-rich foods and regular exercise.
10. They fail to provide for weight maintenance after the program ends.	10. They should provide a plan for weight maintenance after successful weight loss.

Sources: Adapted from National Heart, Lung, and Blood Institute, National Institutes of Health, *The Practical Guide: Identification, Evaluation, and Treatment of Overweight and Obesity in Adults,* NIH publication no. 00-4084 (Washington, D.C.: Government Printing Office, 2000), pp. 25–33; American College of Sports Medicine, *ACSM's Guidelines for Exercise Testing and Prescription* (Baltimore: Lippincott Williams & Wilkins, 2006), pp. 133–173.

Notes

1. D. R. Jacobs, M. D. Gross, and L. C. Tapsell, Food Synergy: An operational concept for understanding nutrition, *American Journal of Clinical Nutrition* 89 (2009): 1543S-1548S.
2. Y. Ma and coauthors, A dietary quality comparison of popular weight-loss plans, *Journal of the American Dietetic Association* 107 (2007): 1786-1791.
3. F. M. Sacks and coauthors, Comparison of weight-loss diets with different compositions of fat, protein, and carbohydrates, *New England Journal of Medicine* 360 (2009): 859-873.
4. I. Shai and M. J. Stampfer, Weight-loss diets—can you keep it off? *American Journal of Clinical Nutrition* 88 (2008): 1185-1186.
5. I. Shai and M. J. Stampfer, 2008; B. Strasser, A. Spreitzer, and P. Haber, Fat loss depends on energy deficit only, independently of the method for weight loss, *Annals of Nutrition and Metabolism* 51 (2007): 428-432.

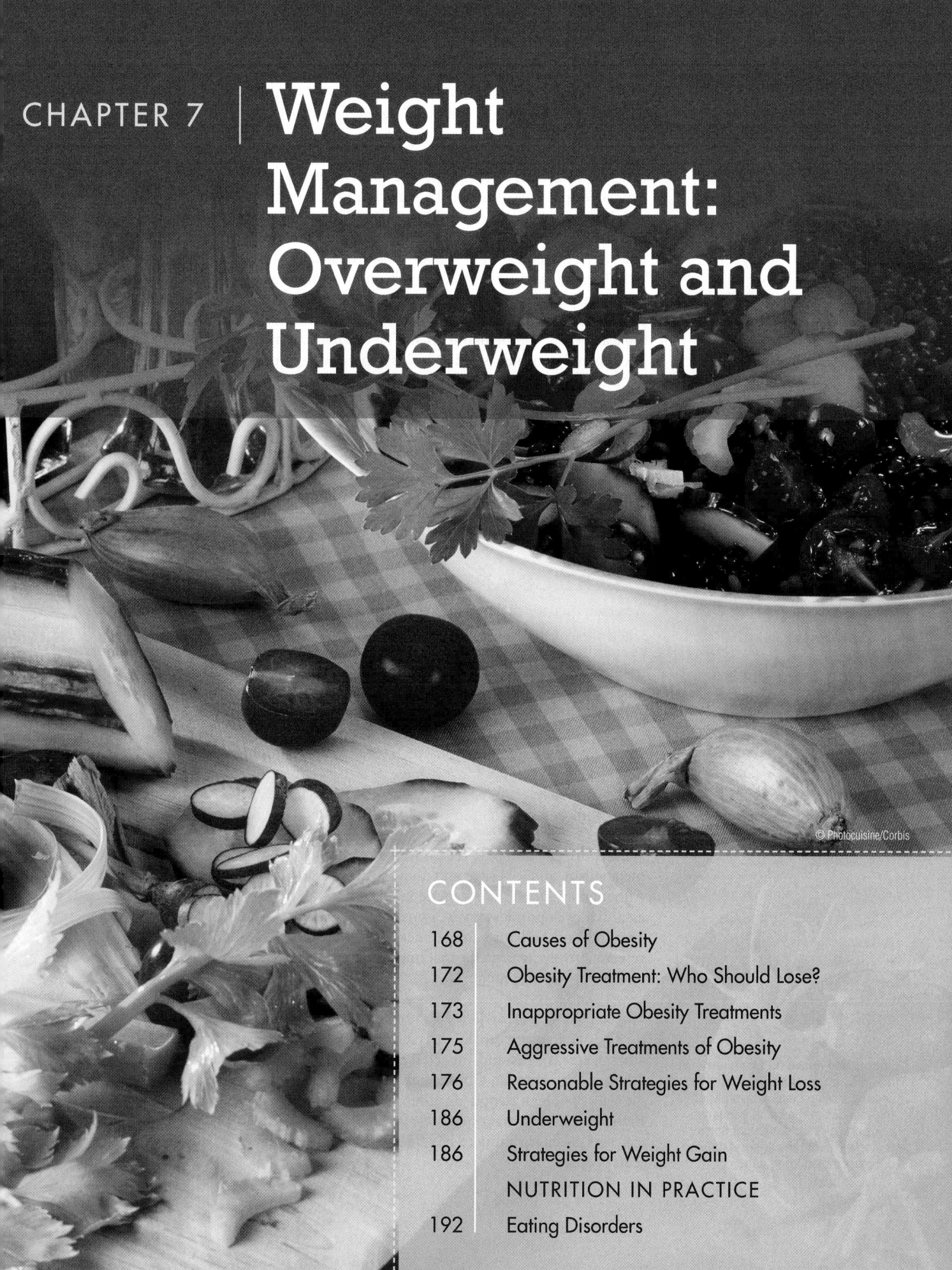

CHAPTER 7 | Weight Management: Overweight and Underweight

© Photocuisine/Corbis

CONTENTS

ARE YOU PLEASED WITH YOUR BODY WEIGHT? IF YOU ANSWERED YES, YOU are a rare individual. Nearly all people in our society think they should weigh more or less (mostly less) than they do. Usually, their primary reason is appearance, but they often perceive, correctly, that their weight is also related to physical health. Chapter 6 addressed the health risks of being overweight. As discussed in a later section of this chapter, health risks also accompany underweight.

Overweight and underweight both result from energy imbalance. The simple picture is as follows. Overweight people have consumed more food energy than they have expended and have banked the surplus in their body fat. To reduce body fat, overweight people need to expend more energy than they take in from food. In contrast, underweight people have consumed too little food energy to support their activities and so have depleted their bodies' fat stores and possibly some of their lean tissues as well. To gain weight, they need to take in more food energy than they expend.

This chapter's missions are to present strategies toward solving the problems of excessive and deficient body fatness and to point out how appropriate body composition, once achieved, can be maintained. The chapter emphasizes overweight because it has been more intensively studied and is a more widespread health problem in the developed countries.

Causes of Obesity

Henceforth, this chapter will use the term *obesity* to refer to excess body fat. Excess body fat accumulates when people take in more food energy than they expend. Why do they do this? Is it genetic? Metabolic? Psychological? Behavioral? All of these? Most likely, obesity has many interrelated causes.

GENETICS AND WEIGHT

A person's genetic makeup influences the body's tendency to consume or store too much energy or to expend too little.[1] Evidence that genes influence eating behavior and body composition comes from family, twin, and adoption studies.[2] Adopted children tend to be more similar in weight to their biological parents than to their adoptive parents.[3] Studies of twins yield similar findings: compared with fraternal twins, identical twins are twice as likely to weigh the same.[4] Genes clearly influence a person's tendency to gain weight or stay lean. The risk of obesity is two to three times higher for a person with a family history of obesity than for a person without such history.[5] Despite such findings, however, only 1 to 5 percent of obesity cases can be explained by a single gene mutation.[6] Furthermore, although genomics researchers have identified hundreds of genes with possible roles in obesity development, they have not yet identified genetic causes of common obesity.[7]

Exceptionally complex relationships exist among the many genes related to energy metabolism and obesity, and they each interact with environmental factors, too. Although an individual's genetic inheritance may make obesity likely, it will not necessarily develop unless given a push by environmental factors that encourage energy consumption and discourage energy expenditure.[8] The following sections describe research involving proteins that might help explain appetite control, energy regulation, and obesity development.

Lipoprotein Lipase Some of the research investigating genetic influence on obesity focuses on the enzyme **lipoprotein lipase (LPL)**, which promotes fat storage in fat cells and muscle cells. People with high LPL activity are especially efficient at storing fat. Obese people generally have much more LPL activity in their fat cells than lean people do (their muscle cell LPL activity is similar, though). This high LPL activity makes fat storage especially efficient. Consequently, even modest excesses in energy intake have a more dramatic impact on obese people than on lean people.

lipoprotein lipase (LPL): an enzyme mounted on the surface of fat cells (and other cells). It hydrolyzes triglycerides in the blood into fatty acids and glycerol for absorption into the cells. There they are metabolized or reassembled for storage.

Leptin Researchers have discovered a gene in humans called the obesity *(ob)* gene. The obesity gene codes for the protein **leptin**. (✚) Leptin is a hormone primarily produced and secreted by the fat cells in proportion to the amount of fat stored.[9] A gain in body fatness stimulates the production of leptin, which, by way of the hypothalamus, suppresses the appetite, increases energy expenditure, and produces fat loss.[10] Fat loss produces the opposite effect—suppression of leptin production, increased appetite, and decreased energy expenditure. As the accompanying photo shows, mice with a defective obesity gene do not produce leptin and can weigh up to three times as much as normal mice. When injected with leptin, the mice lose weight. (Because leptin is a protein, it would be destroyed during digestion if given orally; consequently, it must be given by injection.)

Although it is extremely rare, researchers have identified a genetic deficiency of leptin in human beings as well.[11] An error in the gene that codes for leptin was discovered in two extremely obese children whose blood levels of leptin were barely detectable. Without leptin, the children had little appetite control; they were constantly hungry and ate considerably more than their siblings or peers. Given daily injections of leptin, these children lost a substantial amount of weight, confirming leptin's role in regulating appetite and body weight.

Most obese people do not have leptin deficiency, however. In fact, most obese people produce plenty of leptin, but they fail to respond to it, a condition called *leptin resistance*.[12] Researchers speculate that blood leptin rises in an effort to suppress appetite and inhibit fat storage when fat cells are ample. Obese people with elevated leptin concentrations may be resistant to its satiating effect. The absence of or resistance to leptin in obesity parallels the scenario of insulin in diabetes: some people have an insulin deficiency (type 1), whereas many others have elevated insulin but are resistant to its glucose-storing effect (type 2).

Adiponectin In addition to leptin, adipose tissue secretes another protein known as **adiponectin**. Unlike leptin, however, adiponectin correlates inversely with body fat: lean people have higher amounts than obese people—which helps to explain some of the relationships between obesity and diseases.[13] Adiponectin seems to have the beneficial effects of inhibiting inflammation and protecting against insulin resistance, type 2 diabetes, and cardiovascular disease.[14] Researchers are hopeful that, if they can find ways to raise adiponectin levels or enhance its activity, they will be able to reduce the disease risks associated with obesity.[15]

Ghrelin Another protein known as **ghrelin** works in the opposite direction of leptin. Ghrelin is synthesized and secreted primarily by the stomach cells and promotes a positive energy balance by stimulating appetite and promoting efficient energy storage.[16] The role ghrelin plays in regulating food intake and body weight is the subject of much intense research.[17] Pharmaceutical companies are eager to develop products that mimic ghrelin to treat wasting conditions, as well as products that oppose ghrelin's actions to treat obesity.

Ghrelin powerfully triggers the desire to eat. Blood levels of ghrelin typically rise before and fall after a meal in proportion to the kcalories ingested—reflecting the hunger and satiety that precede and follow eating. In general, fasting blood levels correlate inversely with body weight: lean people have high ghrelin levels and obese people have low levels.[18]

Ghrelin fights to maintain a stable body weight. On average, ghrelin levels are high whenever the body is in negative energy balance, as occurs during low-kcalorie diets, for example. This response may help explain why weight loss is so difficult to maintain. Ghrelin levels decline again whenever the body is in positive energy balance, as occurs with weight gains.

Courtesy Amgen, Inc. Photo © John Sholtis/The Rockefeller University

The mouse on the left is genetically obese—it lacks the gene for producing leptin. The mouse on the right is *also* genetically obese, but because it receives leptin, it eats less, expends more energy, and is less obese than it would be had it not received the leptin.

✚ Genes instruct cells to make proteins, and each protein performs a unique function.

leptin: a hormone produced by fat cells under the direction of the *(ob)* gene. It decreases appetite and increases energy expenditure.
leptos = thin

adiponectin: a protein produced by the fat cells that inhibits inflammation and protects against insulin resistance, type 2 diabetes, and cardiovascular disease.

ghrelin (GRELL-in): a hormone produced primarily by the stomach cells. It signals the hypothalamus of the brain to stimulate appetite and food intake.

FIGURE
7-1 | Fat Cell Development

During growth, fat cells increase in number.

When energy intake exceeds expenditure, fat cells increase in size.

When fat cells have enlarged and energy intake continues to exceed energy expenditure, fat cells increase in number again.

With fat loss, the size of the fat cells shrinks, but not the number.

Fat cells are capable of increasing their size by 20-fold and their number by several thousandfold.

Fat Cell Development Another cause of obesity may be the development of excess fat cells during childhood. The amount of fat on a person's body reflects both fat cell *number* and fat cell *size*. The number of fat cells increases most rapidly during the growing years of late childhood and early puberty. Fat cell numbers increase more rapidly in obese children than in lean children, and obese children entering their teen years may already have as many fat cells as do adults of normal weight.

Fat cells can also expand in size. After they reach their maximum size, more cells can develop to store more fat. Thus, obesity develops when a person's fat cells increase in number, in size, or quite often both. Figure 7-1 illustrates fat cell development.

With fat loss, the size of the fat cells shrinks, but their number cannot. For this reason, people with extra fat cells may tend to regain lost weight rapidly. Prevention of obesity, then, is most critical during the growing years when fat cell numbers are increasing.

Set-Point Theory One popular theory of why a person may store too much fat is the **set-point theory**. The set-point theory proposes that body weight, like body temperature, is physiologically regulated. Researchers have noted that many people who lose weight, quickly regain all their lost weight. This suggests that somehow the body chooses a preferred weight and defends that weight by regulating eating behaviors and hormonal actions. Research confirms that the body adjusts its metabolism whenever it gains or loses weight—in the direction that returns to the initial body weight: energy expenditure increases with weight gain and decreases with weight loss. These changes in energy expenditure are greater than those predicted based on body composition and help to explain why it is so difficult for an obese person to maintain weight losses.[19] An individual's set point for body weight may be adjustable, shifting over the life span in response to physiological changes and to genetic, dietary, and other factors.

ENVIRONMENTAL STIMULI

As discussed earlier, genetic factors play a partial role in determining a person's susceptibility to obesity, but they do not fully explain obesity. Obesity rates have risen dramatically during recent decades, but the human gene pool has remained unchanged. The environment must therefore play a role as well. Obesity reflects the interaction between genes and the environment.[20] The *environment* includes all of the circumstances that people encounter daily that push them toward fatness or thinness. Over the past four decades, the demand for physical activity has decreased as the abundance of food has increased.[21]

set-point theory: the theory that the body tends to maintain a certain weight by means of its own internal controls.

Overeating

People may overeat in response to stimuli in their surroundings—primarily, the availability of many delectable foods. Most people in the United States find high-kcalorie foods readily available, relatively inexpensive, heavily advertised, and reasonably tasty. Food is available everywhere, all the time—thanks largely to fast food. Our highways are lined with fast-food restaurants, and convenience stores and service stations offer fast food as well. Fast food is available in malls, airports, and even schools. Fast food is convenient, and it's available morning, noon, and night—and all times in between.

Most alarming are the extraordinarily large serving sizes and ready-to-go meals offered in supersize combinations.[22] People buy the large sizes and combinations, perceiving them to be a good value, but then they eat more than they need. Research shows that people eat more if they're served more.[23] "Portion distortion" is a term used to describe the perception that large portions are the appropriate amounts to eat at a single sitting.[24] And portion sizes of virtually all foods and beverages (and even plates, glasses, and utensils) have increased markedly in the past several decades, most notably at fast-food restaurants.[25] The increase in portion sizes parallels the growing prevalence of the overweight and the obese in the United States, beginning in the 1970s, rising sharply in the 1980s and 1990s, and continuing today.

Research suggests that fast-food consumption contributes significantly to the development of obesity.[26] Fast food is often energy-dense food, which increases energy intake, BMI, and body fatness.[27] The combination of large portions and energy-dense foods strikes a double blow.[28] Reducing portion sizes is helpful, but the real kcalorie savings come from lowering the energy density.[29] Satisfying portions of foods with low energy density such as fruits and vegetables can help with weight loss.[30] Unfortunately, low-energy-dense foods tend to be more expensive and less convenient than energy-dense foods.[31] The financial interests of the food industry do not always align with consumer health goals.[32] Consumers' health would benefit from restaurants providing appropriate portion sizes and offering more fruits, vegetables, legumes, and whole grains.

Learned Behavior

Psychological stimuli also trigger inappropriate eating behaviors in some people. Appropriate eating behavior is a response to **hunger**. Hunger is a drive programmed into people by their heredity. **Appetite**, in contrast, is learned and can lead people to ignore hunger or to over-respond to it. Hunger is physiological, whereas appetite is psychological, and the two do not always coincide.

Food behavior is also intimately connected to deep emotional needs such as the primitive fear of starvation. Yearnings, cravings, and addictions with profound psychological significance can express themselves in people's eating behavior. An emotionally insecure person might eat rather than call a friend and risk rejection. Another person might eat to relieve boredom or to ward off depression.

Physical Inactivity

The possible causes of obesity mentioned so far all relate to the input side of the energy equation. What about output? People may be obese, not because they eat too much, but because they move too little. Obese people observed closely are often seen to eat less than lean people, but they are sometimes so extraordinarily inactive that they still manage to accumulate an energy surplus. Reducing their food intake further would jeopardize health and incur nutrient deficiencies. Physical activity, then, is a necessary component of nutritional health. People must be physically active if they are to eat enough food to deliver all the nutrients needed without unhealthy weight gain.

Our environment, however, fosters inactivity. In turn, inactivity contributes to obesity and poor health.[33] Television and sedentary video and computer entertainment have all but replaced outdoor activity for many people.[34] In addition, most people work at sedentary jobs. One hundred years ago, 30 percent of the energy used in farm and factory work came from muscle power; today, only 1 percent does. Modern technology has replaced physical activity at home, at work, at school,

© Stockbyte/Jupiter Images

Lack of physical activity fosters obesity.

and in transportation. The more time spent sitting still, the higher the risk of dying from heart disease and other causes.[35]

Health experts urge people to "take the stairs instead of the elevator" or "walk or bike to work." These are excellent suggestions: climbing stairs provides an impromptu workout, and people who walk or ride a bicycle for transportation most often meet their needs for physical activity.[36]

Some aspects of the **built environment**, including buildings, sidewalks, and transportation opportunities, can discourage physical activity. For example, most stairwells of modern buildings are inconvenient, isolated, and unsafe. Roadways often lack sidewalks, crosswalks, or lanes marked for bicycles. The air on roadways can be dangerously high in carbon monoxide gas and other pollutants from gasoline engine emissions. Hot and cold weather also poses hazards for outdoor commuters. In contrast, those with access to health-promoting foods and built environments more easily make healthy choices.[37] Safe, affordable biking and walking areas and public exercise facilities help maintain health and body leanness. Physical activity strategies for weight loss and weight maintenance are offered in a later section of this chapter.

Review Notes

- Genetics, fat cell development, set point, and overeating all offer possible, but still incomplete, explanations of obesity.
- Most likely, obesity has not one cause but different causes and combinations of causes in different people.
- Some causes may be within a person's control, and some may be beyond it.
- Like all the other "causes" of obesity, inactivity alone fails to explain it fully.

Obesity Treatment: Who Should Lose?

Millions of U.S. adults are trying to lose weight at any given time. Some of these people do not even need to lose weight. Others may benefit from weight loss but are not successful. Relatively few people succeed in losing weight, and even fewer succeed permanently.

Many people assume that every overweight person can achieve slenderness and should pursue that goal. Consider, however, that most overweight people cannot become slender. People vary in their weight tendencies just as they vary in their potentials for height and degrees of health. The question of whether a person should lose weight depends on many factors: the extent of overweight, age, health, and genetics, to name a few. Weight-loss advice, then, does not apply equally to all overweight people. Some people may risk more in the process of losing weight than in remaining overweight. Others may reap significant health benefits with just modest weight loss.

Review Notes

- Weight-loss advice does not apply equally to all overweight people.
- Some people may risk more through misguided efforts to lose weight than by remaining overweight, whereas others may benefit from just a modest weight loss.

built environment: the buildings, roads, utilities, homes, fixtures, parks, and all other manufactured entities that form the physical characteristics of a community.

Inappropriate Obesity Treatments

The risks people incur in attempting to lose weight often depend on how they go about it. Weight-loss plans and obesity treatments abound—some are adequate, but many are ineffective and possibly dangerous. Fad diets are the topic of Nutrition in Practice 6. This section addresses other inappropriate obesity interventions. Aggressive approaches to obesity for those obese people who face high risks of medical problems and must lose weight rapidly are discussed in the next section. Reasonable approaches to overweight for those seeking safe, gradual weight losses are saved for the last part of the obesity treatment discussion.

OVER-THE-COUNTER WEIGHT-LOSS SUPPLEMENTS AND DRUGS

Millions of people in the United States use nonprescription weight-loss products, believing them to be safe. Most of the people who use such products are women, especially young overweight women, but almost 10 percent are of normal weight.[38] Promoters and marketers of weight-loss products make all kinds of claims for their products with only one intention—profit. Such claims as "eat all you want and lose weight," "take three pills before bedtime and watch the fat disappear," "blocks carbs," "blocks fat," and many more lure people into believing that maybe this time a product will really work.

In an investigation of over-the-counter weight-loss pills, powders, and other "dietary supplements," the FDA found an alarming number of products to illegally contain prescription medications. Strong diuretics, unproven experimental drugs, psychotropic drugs used to treat mental illnesses, and even drugs deemed unsafe and so banned from U.S. markets were among those discovered, and all pose serious health risks.[39] The FDA recently approved the first nonprescription weight-loss drug for use in the United States. The drug is a low-dose version of the prescription drug orlistat, discussed in the next section.

HERBAL PRODUCTS AND DIETARY SUPPLEMENTS

In their search for weight-loss magic, some consumers turn to "natural" herbal products and dietary supplements, even though few have proved to be effective.[40] People falsely believe that "natural" herbs are not harmful to the body, but many herbs contain toxins. Belladonna and hemlock are infamous examples, but many lesser-known herbs, such as sassafras, contain toxins as well. Furthermore, because herbs are marketed as "dietary supplements," manufacturers need not present scientific evidence of their safety or effectiveness to the FDA before marketing them. Evidence about their safety is gathered only through reports of consumers who sicken or die after using the remedies.

A now familiar example is ephedra (also called ma huang), an herb that showed promise as a weight-loss drug in preliminary studies. Immediately, ephedra-containing products for dieters and athletes flooded the market. Many consumers of these products reported ill effects including cardiac arrest, abnormal heartbeats, hypertension, strokes, and seizures; the supplements have been linked to some deaths as well. For this reason, the FDA has banned the sale of dietary supplements containing ephedra and its active constituent, ephedrine.* (✚) Table 7-1 (p. 174) presents the claims and the dangers behind ephedrine and several other weight-loss supplements.

Herbal laxatives containing senna, aloe, rhubarb root, cascara, castor oil, and buckthorn (or various combinations) are commonly sold as "dieter's tea." Such concoctions cause nausea, vomiting, diarrhea, cramping, and fainting and may have contributed to the deaths of four women who had drastically reduced their food intakes. Consumers mistakenly believe that laxatives will diminish nutrient

✚ Ephedrine is an amphetamine-like substance extracted from the Chinese herb ma huang.

---

*Ma huang (ephedrine) is illegal in Canada.

Product	Claims	Research Findings	Risks
Bitter orange[a] (Citrus aurantium, a natural flavoring that contains synephrine, a compound structurally similar to epinephrine)	Stimulates weight loss; provides an alternative to ephedra	Little evidence available	May increase blood pressure; may interact with drugs
Chitosan[b] (pronounced KITE-oh-san; derived from chitin, the substance that forms the hard shells of lobsters, crabs, and other crustaceans)	Binds to dietary fat, preventing digestion and absorption	Ineffective	Impaired absorption of fat-soluble vitamins
Chromium (trace mineral)	Eliminates body fat	Ineffective; weight gain reported when not accompanied by exercise	Headaches, sleep disturbances, and mood swings; hexavalent form is toxic and carcinogenic
Conjugated linoleic acid (CLA; a group of fatty acids related to linoleic acid but with different cis- and trans-configurations)	Reduces body fat and suppresses appetite	Some evidence in animal studies, modest fat loss in human studies	None known
Ephedrine[c] (amphetamine-like substance derived from the Chinese ephedra herb ma huang)	Speeds body's metabolism	Short-term weight loss and dangerous side effects	Insomnia, tremors, heart attacks, strokes, and death; FDA has banned the sale of these products
Fucoxanthin[d] (derived from seaweed)	Speeds metabolism; burns fat	No evidence available	None known
Hoodia (derived from cactus)	Suppresses appetite	Little evidence available	None known
Hydroxycitric acid[e] (active ingredient derived from the rind of the tropical fruit Garcinia cambogia)	Inhibits the enzyme that converts citric acid to fat; suppresses appetite	Ineffective	Toxicity symptoms reported in animal studies; headaches, respiratory and gastrointestinal distress in humans
Pyruvate[f] (3-carbon compound produced during glycolysis)	Speeds body's metabolism	Modest weight loss with high doses	GI distress
Yohimbine (derived from the bark of a West African tree)	Promotes weight loss	Ineffective	Nervousness, insomnia, anxiety, dizziness, tremors, headaches, nausea, vomiting, hypertension

[a] Marketed under the trade names Xenadrine EFX, Metabolife Ultra, and NOW Diet Support.

[b] Marketed under the trade names Chitorich, Exofat, Fat Breaker, Fat Blocker, Fat Magnet, Fat Trapper, and Fatsorb.

[c] Marketed under the trade names Diet Fuel, Metabolife, and Nature's Nutrition Formula One.

[d] Marketed under the trade name FucoThin.

[e] Marketed under the trade names Ultra Burn, Citralean, CitriMax, Citrin, Slim Life, Brindleslim, Medislim, and Beer Belly Busters.

[f] Marketed under the trade names Exercise in a Bottle, Pyruvate Punch, Pyruvate-c, and Provate.

Note: The FDA has not approved the use of any of these products; most products are used in conjunction with a 1000- to 1800-kcalorie diet.

absorption and reduce kcalorie intake, but remember that absorption occurs primarily in the upper small intestine and these laxatives act on the lower large intestine. Nutrition in Practice 14 explores the possible benefits and potential dangers of herbal products and other alternative therapies. Anyone using dietary supplements for weight loss should first consult a physician.

OTHER GIMMICKS

Other gimmicks don't help with weight loss either. Hot baths do not speed up metabolism so that pounds can be lost in hours. Steam and sauna baths do not melt the fat off the body, although they may dehydrate people so that they lose water weight. Brushes, sponges, wraps, creams, and massages intended to move, burn, or break up **"cellulite"** do nothing of the kind, because there is no such thing as cellulite.

Review Notes

- When pursued via unwise weight-loss techniques, such as over-the-counter supplements and herbal products, weight-loss efforts can be physically and psychologically damaging.

Aggressive Treatments of Obesity

For some obese people, the medical problems caused by their obesity demand treatment approaches that may, themselves, incur some risks. The health benefits to be gained by weight loss, however, may make these risks worth taking.

OBESITY DRUGS

Several prescription medications for weight loss have been tried over the years. When used as part of a long-term, comprehensive weight-loss program, medications can help with modest weight loss. (✚) Because weight regain commonly occurs with the discontinuation of drug therapy, treatment is long term—and the long-term use of medications poses risks. Medical experts do not yet know whether a person would benefit more from maintaining a 50-pound excess or from taking a medication for a decade to keep the 50 pounds off.

The challenge, then, is to develop an effective drug—or more likely, a combination of drugs—that can be used over time without adverse side effects or the potential for abuse.[41] The FDA has approved two drugs for long-term treatment of obesity: sibutramine and orlistat.

Sibutramine   Sibutramine is an appetite suppressant that works on the brain's neurotransmitters.* The drug is most effective when used in combination with a reduced-kcalorie diet and increased physical activity. Side effects include dry mouth, rapid heart rate, insomnia, headache, and high blood pressure. The FDA warns those with heart failure, hypertension, irregular heart beats, and other heart problems not to use sibutramine and advises others to monitor their blood pressure. As more information becomes known about the molecular chemistry of appetite control, safer appetite suppressants may be developed.

Orlistat   Orlistat takes a different approach to weight loss.† Not an appetite suppressant, orlistat inhibits the action of fat-digesting enzymes in the GI tract and so reduces fat digestion and absorption by about 30 percent.[42] As a result of absorbing less fat, people

✚ Drugs may be an option for people with all of the following conditions:
- Unable to achieve adequate weight loss with diet and exercise
- BMI ≥30, or BMI ≥27 with weight-related health problems
- No medical contraindications

cellulite (SELL-you-light or SELL-you-leet): supposedly, a lumpy form of fat; actually, a fraud. Fatty areas of the body may appear lumpy when the strands of connective tissue that attach the skin to underlying muscles pull tight where the fat is thick. The fat itself is the same as fat anywhere else in the body. If the fat in these areas is lost, the lumpy appearance disappears.

*Sibutramine's trade name is Meridia.

†Orlistat's trade name is Xenical.

often lose weight. The drug is taken with meals and is most effective when accompanied by a reduced-kcalorie, low-fat diet. Side effects include gas, frequent bowel movements, and reduced absorption of fat-soluble vitamins. As mentioned earlier, an over-the-counter, low-dose version of orlistat is also available.*

Phentermine Phentermine reduces appetite and is a widely prescribed weight-loss drug. However, phentermine use is approved by the FDA for no longer than three months.[43] Side effects include dry mouth, insomnia, and constipation.

SURGERY

Surgery as an approach to weight loss is justified in some specific cases of **clinically severe obesity**. Two procedures, **gastric bypass** and **gastric banding**, have gained wide acceptance. Both procedures limit food intake by effectively reducing the capacity of the stomach and suppressing hunger by reducing the production of ghrelin.[44] The results are significant: depending on the type of surgery, initial weight loss is 20 to 32 percent of body weight and 14 to 25 percent after 10 years.[45] Research shows that weight-loss surgery also helps to improve blood lipids, diabetes, sleep apnea, and hypertension.[46]

Laparoscopic weight-loss surgery techniques are now used to perform gastric bypass and other weight loss surgeries. Laparoscopic weight-loss surgery produces significant, long-term weight loss, shortens recovery, and is less invasive than open surgery.[47]

The long-term safety and effectiveness of gastric surgery depend, in large part, on compliance with dietary instructions. Common immediate postsurgical complications include infections, nausea, vomiting, and dehydration; in the long term, vitamin and mineral deficiencies and psychological problems are common. Lifelong medical supervision is necessary for those who choose the surgical route, but in suitable candidates, the health benefits of weight loss may prove worth the risks.[48]

Review Notes

- Obese people with high risks of medical problems may need aggressive treatment, including drugs or surgery.

clinically severe obesity: a BMI of 40 or greater, or a BMI of 35 or greater with one or more serious conditions such as hypertension. Another term used to describe the same condition is *morbid obesity*.

gastric bypass: surgery that restricts stomach size and reroutes food from the stomach to the lower part of the small intestine; creates a chronic, lifelong state of malabsorption by preventing normal digestion and absorption of nutrients.

gastric banding: a surgical means of producing weight loss by restricting stomach size with a constricting band; used in people whose severe obesity brings extreme health risks.

laparoscopic weight-loss surgery: a procedure in which surgeons gain access to the abdomen via several small incisions. A tiny video camera is inserted through one of the incisions and surgical instruments through the others. The surgeons watch their work on a large-screen monitor.

Reasonable Strategies for Weight Loss

Successful weight-loss strategies embrace small changes, moderate losses, and reasonable goals.[49] People who lose 10 to 20 pounds in a year by consistently choosing nutrient-dense foods and engaging in regular physical activity are much more likely to maintain the loss and reap health benefits than if they were to lose more weight in less time by adopting the latest fad diet. In keeping with this philosophy, the *Dietary Guidelines for Americans* advise that those who need to lose weight should "aim for a slow, steady weight loss by decreasing kcalorie intake while maintaining an adequate nutrient intake and increasing physical activity." Modest weight loss, even when a person is still overweight, can improve control of diabetes and reduce the risks of heart disease by lowering blood pressure and blood cholesterol, especially for those with abdominal fat.[50]

Of course, the same eating and activity habits that improve health often lead to a healthier body weight and composition as well. Successful weight loss, then, is defined not by pounds lost but by health gained. People less concerned with disease risks may prefer to set goals for personal fitness, such as being able to play with children or climb stairs without becoming short of breath.

---

*The low-dose, over-the-counter version of orlistat is marketed under the trade name Alli (AL-eye).

Whether the goal is health or fitness, weight-loss expectations need to be reasonable. Unreachable targets ensure frustration and failure. Setting reasonable goals helps to achieve the desired result in managing weight. For example, obese people who must reduce their weight to lower their disease risks might set three broad goals:

1. Reduce body weight by about 10 percent over half a year's time.
2. Maintain a lower body weight over the long term.
3. At a minimum, prevent further weight gain.

Such goals may be achieved or even exceeded, providing a sense of accomplishment instead of disappointment.

Courtesy of the author

A healthy body contains enough lean tissue to support health and the right amount of fat to meet body needs.

A HEALTHFUL EATING PLAN

Contrary to the claims of many fad diets, no particular eating plan is magical, and no specific food must be either included or avoided for weight management. You are the one who will have to live with the plan, so you had better be involved in the planning. The diet is successful only if you can maintain a healthy weight. Think of it as an eating plan that you will adopt for life. It must consist of foods that you like, that are available to you, and that are within your means.

A Realistic Energy Intake The main characteristic of a weight-loss diet is that it provides less energy than the person needs to maintain present body weight. If food energy is restricted too severely, dieters may not receive sufficient nutrients and may lose lean tissue. Rapid weight loss usually means excessive loss of lean tissue, a lower BMR, and a rapid weight gain to follow. Restrictive eating may also set in motion the unhealthy behaviors of eating disorders (described in Nutrition in Practice 7).

Table 7-2 (p. 178) outlines the recommendations of a weight-loss diet. Energy intake should provide nutritional adequacy without excess—that is, somewhere between deprivation and complete freedom to eat whatever, whenever. A reasonable suggestion is that an adult needs to increase activity and reduce food intake to create a deficit of 500 to 1000 kcalories per day. (✚) Such a deficit produces a weight loss of 1 to 2 pounds per week—a rate that supports the loss of fat efficiently while retaining lean tissue.[51] In general, weight-loss diets provide about 1200 kcalories per day for women and 1600 kcalories per day for men.[52] Table 7-3 (p. 179) suggests daily food amounts from which to build balanced 1200- to 1600-kcalorie diets.

Some people skip meals, typically breakfast, in an effort to reduce energy intake, but research suggests such a strategy may be counterproductive. Breakfast frequency is inversely associated with obesity—that is, people who frequently eat breakfast have lower BMI than those who tend to skip breakfast.[53] Furthermore, when people eat breakfast, overall diet quality is better and daily energy density is lower—two factors that support healthy body weight.[54]

Nutritional Adequacy Nutritional adequacy is difficult to achieve on fewer than 1200 kcalories a day, and most healthy adults need never consume any less than that. A plan that provides an adequate intake supports a healthier and more successful weight loss than a restrictive plan that creates feelings of starvation and deprivation, which can lead to an irresistible urge to binge.

Take a look at the 1200-kcalorie diet in Table 7-3. Such an intake would allow most people to lose weight and still meet their nutrient needs with careful, nutrient-dense food selections. (Women might need calcium or iron supplements.) Keep in mind that well-balanced diets that emphasize fruits, vegetables, whole grains, lean meats or meat alternatives, and low-fat or fat-free milk products offer many health rewards even when

✚ 1 lb body fat = 3500 kcal. To lose a pound a week, cut 500 kcal/day.

TABLE 7-2	Recommendations for a Weight-Loss Diet	
Nutrient	**Recommended Intake**	
kcalories for people with BMI ≥35	Approximately 500 to 1000 kcalories per day reduction from usual intake	
For people with BMI between 27 and 35	Approximately 300 to 500 kcalories per day reduction from usual intake	
Total fat	30% or less of total kcalories	
Saturated fatty acids[a]	8 to 10% of total kcalories	
Monounsaturated fatty acids	Up to 15% of total kcalories	
Polyunsaturated fatty acids	Up to 10% of total kcalories	
Cholesterol[a]	<300 mg per day	
Protein[b]	Approximately 15% of total kcalories	
Carbohydrate[c]	55% or more of total kcalories	
Sodium chloride[d]	No more than 2300 mg of sodium or approximately 6 g of sodium chloride (salt) per day	
Calcium	1000 to 1500 mg per day	
Fiber[c]	20 to 30 g per day	

[a] People with high blood cholesterol should aim for less than 7 percent kcalories from saturated fat and 200 milligrams cholesterol per day.

[b] Protein should be derived from plant sources and lean sources of animal protein.

[c] Carbohydrates and fiber should be derived from vegetables, fruits, and whole grains.

[d] Value from the *Dietary Guidelines for Americans 2005*; the Tolerable Upper Intake Level for sodium is 2300 milligrams.

Source: National Heart, Lung, and Blood Institute, National Institutes of Health, *The Practical Guide: Identification, Evaluation, and Treatment of Overweight and Obesity in Adults,* NIH publication no. 00-4084 (Washington, D.C.: Government Printing Office, 2000), p. 27.

they don't result in weight loss.[55] A dietary supplement providing vitamins and minerals at or below 100 percent of the Daily Values can help people following low-kcalorie diets to achieve nutrient adequacy.

Small Portions As mentioned earlier, large portion sizes increase energy intakes, and the huge helpings served by restaurants and sold in packages are the enemy of people striving to manage their weight.[56] Similarly, big bowls, plates, utensils, and drinking glasses encourage people to take and consume larger portions. Small plates and bowls, tall and thin drinking glasses, and luncheon-sized plates have the opposite effect.[57]

For health's sake, overweight people may need to learn to eat less food at each meal—one piece of chicken for dinner instead of two, a teaspoon of butter on the vegetables instead of a tablespoon, and one cookie for dessert instead of six. Chew foods slowly and thoroughly. The goal is to eat enough food for energy, nutrients, and pleasure, but not more. This amount should leave a person feeling satisfied—not necessarily full.

Food Group	1200 kCalories	1400 kCalories	1600 kCalories
Fruit	1 c	1 ½ c	1 ½ c
Vegetables	1 ½ c	1 ½ c	2 c
Grains	4 oz	5 oz	5 oz
Meat and legumes	3 oz	4 oz	5 oz
Milk	3 c	3 c	3 c
Oils	3 tsp	3 tsp	4 tsp

TABLE 7-3 | Daily Amounts from Each Food Group for 1200- to 1600-kCalorie Diets

Note: The USDA Food Guide patterns for 1200 and 1400 kcalories were designed for children and provided 2 cups milk. They were modified here to include an additional cup of milk, as 3 cups per day is recommended for all adults. The discretionary kcalorie allowance for these patterns is about 100 kcalories.

Keep in mind that even fat-free and low-fat foods can deliver a lot of kcalories when a person eats large quantities.

Balancing Carbohydrates, Fats, and Protein Healthy diets based on abundant fresh fruits and vegetables; low-fat milk products; legumes; lean meats, fish, poultry, or meat alternatives; and whole grains are high in carbohydrates, adequate in fiber and protein, and low in the kinds of fats associated with diseases. They are also best for managing weight. As earlier chapters described, each of the energy-yielding nutrients is important to health. Therefore, diets for weight management should provide all three within the ranges recommended by the DRI committee (see the margin). (✚)

Wholesome, high-fiber, unprocessed or lightly processed foods offer bulk and satiety for fewer kcalories than smooth, quickly consumed refined foods. Thus, choosing whole grains and fiber-rich vegetables in place of most refined grains and added fats and sugars benefits both weight and nutrition. Choose fats sensibly by avoiding sources of saturated and *trans* fats and including enough of the health-supporting fats (details in Nutrition in Practice 4) to provide satiety but not so much as to oversupply kcalories. Nuts provide fat and protein, and including a moderate amount in the diet may assist in controlling body weight.[58] Lean meats or other low-fat protein sources also provide satiety. Limit these foods, but don't eliminate them.

Lower Energy Density As discussed earlier, to lower energy intake, people can choose smaller portion sizes, or they can reduce the energy density of the foods they eat. Research shows that eating satisfying portions of foods that are low in energy density (such as fruits, vegetables, and broth-based soups) maintains satiety while reducing energy intake.[59] Foods containing substantial water or fiber and those low in fat help to lower a meal's energy density (see Figure 7-2 on p. 180). The Clinical Applications feature at the end of this chapter describes how to calculate the energy density of foods.

Sugar and Alcohol A person trying to achieve or maintain a healthy weight needs to pay attention to sugar and alcohol, as well as fat. Using them for pleasure on occasion is compatible with health as long as most daily choices are of nutrient-dense foods.

✚ The DRI committee recommends:
- 45 to 65 percent kcalories from carbohydrate
- 20 to 35 percent kcalories from fat
- 10 to 35 percent kcalories from protein

FIGURE
7-2 | Energy Density

Matthew Farruggio (all)

Selecting grapes with their high water content instead of raisins increases the volume and cuts the energy intake in half.

Even at the same weight and similar serving sizes, the fiber-rich broccoli delivers twice the fiber of the potatoes for about one-fourth the energy.

By selecting the water-packed tuna (on the right) instead of the oil-packed tuna, a person can enjoy the same amount for fewer kcalories.

Decreasing the energy density (kcal/g) of foods allows a person to eat satisfying portions while still reducing energy intake. To lower energy density, select foods high in water or fiber and low in fat.

Meal Spacing Three meals a day is standard in our society, but no law says you can't have four or five—just be sure they are smaller, of course. People who eat small, frequent meals can be as successful at weight loss and maintenance as those who eat three.[60] Make sure that mild hunger, not appetite, is prompting you to eat. Eat regularly, and eat before you become extremely hungry.

Adequate Water Learn to satisfy thirst with water. Water helps with weight management in several ways. For one, foods with high water content (such as broth-based soups) increase fullness, reduce hunger, and consequently reduce energy intake.[61] For another, drinking a large glass of water before a meal may ease hunger, fill the stomach, and reduce energy intake.[62] Importantly, water adds no kcalories. The average U.S. diet delivers an estimated 75 to 150 kcalories a day from sweetened beverages.[63] Consuming large portions of kcalorie-containing beverages increases energy intake.[64] Simply replacing nutrient-poor, energy-dense beverages with water could save a person up to 15 pounds a year. Water also helps the GI tract adapt to a high-fiber diet.

PHYSICAL ACTIVITY

The best approach to weight management includes physical activity.[65] Either energy restriction or physical activity alone can produce some weight loss. Clearly, however, the combination is most effective.[66] People who combine diet and physical activity are more likely to lose more fat, retain more muscle, and regain less weight than those who only diet.[67] Table 1-5 in Chapter 1 presented the *Physical Activity Guidelines for Americans, 2008*, which specify the minimum amount of physical activity people need to gain general *health* benefits. Table 7-4 presents physical activity strategies from the American College of Sports Medicine developed specifically to prevent weight gain and promote at least modest weight loss.[68]

Even without weight loss, physical activity may also help counteract some of the negative effects of excess body weight on health.[69] For example, physical activity reduces abdominal obesity, and this change improves blood pressure, insulin resistance, and fitness of the heart and lungs, even without weight loss.[70]

Energy Expenditure Physical activity directly increases energy output by the muscles and cardiovascular system. Table 6-2 in Chapter 6 (pp. 148–149) shows how much energy each of several activities uses. The number of kcalories spent in an activity depends on body weight, intensity, and duration. For example, a 150-pound person who walks 3.5 miles in 60 minutes expends about 315 kcalories. That same

TABLE 7-4	Physical Activity Strategies for Weight Management

A negative energy balance incurred through physical activity will result in weight loss, and the larger the negative energy balance, the greater the weight loss.

- Weight gain prevention and augmented weight loss occur with at least 2 hours and 30 minutes (150 minutes) per week of at least moderate-intensity physical activity.

- Greater weight loss and improved weight maintenance after weight loss occur with more than 4 hours and 10 minutes (>250 minutes) per week of at least moderate-intensity physical activity.

- Both aerobic (endurance) and muscle-strengthening (resistance) physical activities are beneficial, but kcalorie restriction must accompany resistance training to achieve weight loss.

Source: Adapted from American College of Sports Medicine, Position stand: Appropriate physical activity intervention strategies for weight loss and prevention of weight regain for adults, Medicine and Science in Sports and Exercise 41(2009): 459–471.

Benefits of physical activity in a weight-management program:
- Improved body composition
- Favorable effects on disease risks
- Short-term increase in energy expenditure (from exercise and from a slight rise in BMR)
- Long-term increase (slight) in BMR
- Appetite control
- Stress reduction and control of stress eating
- Physical, and therefore psychological, well-being
- Improved self-esteem

person running 3 miles in 30 minutes uses a similar amount. By comparison, a 200-pound person running 3 miles in 30 minutes expends an additional 125 kcalories or so (about 444 kcalories total). The goal is to expend as much energy as time allows. The greater the energy deficit created by physical activity, the greater the fat loss. A word of caution, however: people who reward themselves with high-kcalorie foods for "good behavior" can easily negate any kcalorie deficits incurred with physical activity.[71]

BMR Activity also contributes to energy output in an indirect way—by speeding up basal metabolism. It does this both immediately and over the long term. On any given day, basal metabolism remains slightly elevated for several hours after intense and prolonged exercise.[72] Over the long term, a person who engages in daily vigorous activity gradually develops more lean tissue, which is more active metabolically than fat tissue. Metabolic rate rises accordingly, and this makes a contribution toward continued weight loss or maintenance.

Appetite Control Physical activity also helps to control appetite. People think that exercising will make them want to eat, but this is not entirely true. Active people do have healthy appetites, but appetite is suppressed immediately following a workout and satiation during meals is heightened.[73] The reasons are unclear, but physical activity may help to control appetite by altering the levels of appetite-regulating hormones.[74]

Psychological Benefits Physical activity helps especially to curb the inappropriate appetite that prompts a person to eat when bored, anxious, or depressed. Weight-management programs encourage people to go out and be active when they're tempted to eat but are not really hungry.

Physical activity also helps to reduce stress. Because stress itself is a cue to inappropriate eating behavior for many people, activity can help here, too.

Activity offers still more psychological advantages. The fit person looks and feels healthy, and high self-esteem accompanies these benefits. High self-esteem tends to support a person's resolve to persist in a weight-control effort, rounding out a beneficial cycle. (+)

© Joe Sampson, Courtesy of Jennifer Portnick

Being active—even if overweight—is healthier than being sedentary. Weight loss itself, however, best reduces disease risks.

Choosing Activities What kind of physical activity is best? For health, a combination of moderate-to-vigorous aerobic physical activity along with **resistance training** at a safe level provides benefits. However, any physical activity is better than being sedentary.[75]

People seeking to lose weight should choose activities that they enjoy and are willing to do regularly. Health care professionals frequently advise people who want to manage their body weight and lose fat to engage in activities of low-to-moderate intensity for a long duration, such as an hour-long fast-paced walk. The reasoning behind such advice is that people exercising at low-to-moderate intensity are likely to stick with their activity for longer times and are less likely to injure themselves. People who regularly engage in more *vigorous* physical activities (fast bicycling or endurance running, for example), however, have less body fat than those who engage in moderately intense activities. The conditioned body that is adapted to strenuous and prolonged aerobic activity uses more fat all day long, not just during activity. The bottom line on physical activity and weight and/or fat loss seems to be that total energy expenditure is the main factor, regardless of how a person does it.

In addition to activities such as walking or cycling, there are hundreds of ways to incorporate energy-expending activities into daily routines: take the stairs instead of the elevator, walk to the neighbor's apartment instead of making a phone call, and rake the leaves instead of using a blower. These activities burn only a few kcalories each, but over a year's time they become significant.

Spot Reducing People sometimes ask about "spot reducing." Unfortunately, no one part of the body gives up fat in preference to another. Fat cells all over the body release fat in response to demand, and the fat is then used by whatever muscles are active. No exercise can remove the fat from any one particular area—and, incidentally, neither can a massage machine that claims to break up fat on trouble spots.

Physical activity can help with trouble spots in another way, though. Strengthening muscles in a trouble area can help to improve their tone; stretching to gain flexibility can help with posture problems. Thus, cardiorespiratory endurance, strength, and flexibility workouts all have a place in fitness programs.

BEHAVIOR AND ATTITUDE

Behavior-modification therapy provides ways to overcome barriers to making dietary changes and increasing physical activity. Behavior-modification therapy does more than help people decide which behaviors to change: it also teaches them how to change.[76] Behavior and attitude are important supporting factors in achieving and maintaining appropriate body weight and composition. Changing the behaviors of overeating and underexercising that lead to, and perpetuate, obesity requires time and effort. A person must commit to take action.

Becoming Aware of Behaviors A person who is aware of all the behaviors that create a problem has a head start on developing a solution. First, the person needs to establish a baseline (a record of present eating and physical activity behaviors) against which to measure future progress. It is best to keep a diary (see Figure 7-3) that includes the time and place of meals and snacks, the type and amount of foods eaten, the persons present when food is eaten, and a description of the individual's feelings when eating. The diary should also record physical activities: the kind, the intensity level, the duration, and the person's feelings about them. These entries will help the individual identify possible behaviors to change.

Making Small Changes Behavior modification strategies focus on learning desired eating and exercise behaviors and eliminating unwanted behaviors. With so many possible behavior changes, a person can feel overwhelmed. Start with small time-specific goals for each behavior—for example, "I'm going to take a 30-minute walk after dinner every evening" instead of "I'm going to run a marathon someday." Practice desired behaviors until they become routine. Using a reward system

resistance training: the use of free weights or weight machines to provide resistance for developing muscle strength, power, and endurance; also called *weight training*. A person's own body weight may also be used to provide resistance as when a person does push-ups, pull-ups, or abdominal crunches.

behavior modification: the changing of behavior by the manipulation of *antecedents* (cues or environmental factors that trigger behavior), the behavior itself, and *consequences* (the penalties or rewards attached to behavior).

Weight Management: Overweight and Underweight

FIGURE
7-3
Food and Activity Diary

Time	Place	Activity or food eaten	People present	Mood
10:30–10:40	School vending machine	6 peanut butter crackers and 12 oz. cola	by myself	Starved
12:15–12:30	Restaurant	Sub sandwich and 12 oz. cola	friends	relaxed & friendly
3:00–3:45	Gym	Weight training	work out partner	tired
4:00–4:10	Snack bar	Small frozen yogurt	by myself	OK

The entries in a food and activity diary should include the times and places of meals and snacks, the types and amounts of foods eaten, and a description of the individual's feelings when eating. The diary should also record physical activities: the kind, the intensity level, the duration, and the person's feelings about them.

seems to effectively support weight-loss efforts.[77] The "How to" (p. 184) describes behavioral strategies to support weight management. A particularly attractive feature of these strategies is that they do not involve blaming oneself or putting oneself down—an important element in fostering self-esteem.

Cognitive Skills Behavior therapists often teach **cognitive skills**, or new ways of thinking, to help overweight people solve problems and correct false thinking that can undermine healthy eating behaviors.[78] Thinking habits are as important as eating and activity habits to achieve a healthy body weight, and thinking habits can be changed.* A paradox of making a change is that it takes belief in oneself and honoring of oneself to lay the foundation for changing that self. That is, self-acceptance predicts success, while self-loathing predicts failure. "Positive self-talk" is a concept worth cultivating—many people succeed because their mental dialogue supports, rather than degrades, their efforts. Negative thoughts ("I'm not getting thin anyway, so what is the use of continuing?") should be viewed in light of empirical evidence ("my starting weight: 174 pounds; today's weight: 163 pounds").

Take credit for new behaviors; be aware of any physical improvements, too, such as lower blood pressure, or less painful knees, even without a noticeable change in pant size. Finally, remember to enjoy your emerging fit and healthy self.

Personal Attitude For many people, overeating and being overweight may have become an integral part of their identity. Changing diet and activity behaviors without attention to a person's self-concept invites failure.

Many people overeat to cope with the stresses of life. To break out of that pattern, they must first identify the particular stressors that trigger their urges to overeat. Then, when faced with these situations, they must learn to practice problem-solving skills. When the problems that trigger the urge to overeat are dealt with in alternative ways, people may find that they eat less. The message is that sound emotional health supports the ability to take care of health in all ways—including nutrition, weight management, and fitness.

---

*Psychologists have a term for changing thinking habits: *cognitive restructuring*.

cognitive skills: as taught in behavior therapy, changes to conscious thoughts with the goal of improving adherence to lifestyle modifications; examples are problem-solving skills or the correction of false negative thoughts, termed *cognitive restructuring*.

1. Eliminate inappropriate cues:
   - Do not buy problem foods.
   - Eat only in one room at the designated time.
   - Shop when not hungry.
   - Avoid vending machines, fast-food restaurants, and convenience stores.
   - Turn off television, video games, and computers.

2. Suppress the cues you cannot eliminate:
   - Serve individual plates; do not serve "family style."
   - Make small portions look large by spreading them over the plate.
   - Create obstacles to consuming problem foods—wrap them and freeze them, making them less quickly accessible.
   - Control deprivation; plan and eat regular meals.
   - Plan the time spent in sedentary activities, such as watching television or using a computer—do not use these activities just to fill time.

3. Strengthen cues to appropriate behaviors:
   - Share appropriate foods with others.
   - Store appropriate foods in convenient spots in the refrigerator.
   - Learn appropriate portion sizes.
   - Plan appropriate snacks.
   - Keep sports and play equipment by the door.

4. Repeat desired behaviors:
   - Slow down eating—put down utensils between bites.
   - Always use utensils.
   - Leave some food on your plate.
   - Move more—shake a leg, pace, stretch often.
   - Join groups of active people and participate.

5. Arrange negative consequences for negative behavior:
   - Ask that others respond neutrally to your deviations (make no comments—even negative attention is a reward).
   - If you slip, do not punish yourself.

6. Reward yourself personally and immediately for positive behaviors:
   - Buy tickets to sports events, movies, concerts, or other nonfood amusement.
   - Indulge in a new small purchase.
   - Get a massage; buy some flowers.
   - Take a hot bath; read a good book.
   - Treat yourself to a lesson in a new active pursuit such as horseback riding, handball, or tennis.
   - Praise yourself; visit friends.
   - Nap; relax.

Weight Maintenance Finally, be aware that it can be hard to maintain weight loss. Millions of people have experienced the frustration of achieving a desired change in weight only to see their hard work visibly slip away in a seemingly never-ending cycle of weight loss and weight regain. Disappointment, frustration, and self-condemnation are common in people who have slipped back to their original weight or even higher. Some hints for successful long-term weight loss can be gleaned from data of the National Weight Control Registry, a self-selected population of 6,000 people who lost at least 30 pounds and kept it off for at least a year.[79]

A key to weight maintenance is accepting it as a lifelong endeavor and not a goal to be achieved and then forgotten. People who maintain their weight loss continue to employ the behaviors that reduced their weight in the first place. They cultivate habits of people who maintain a healthy weight, such as eating low-kcalorie meals (averaging 1800 kcalories per day) and being physically active. They must also control susceptibility to overeating regardless of the initial weight-loss method.[80] Those who maintain weight losses over time also generally:

- Believe they have the ability to control their weight, an attribute known as **self-efficacy**.
- Eat breakfast every day.
- Average about one hour of physical activity per day.
- Monitor body weight about once a week.
- Maintain consistent lower-kcalorie eating patterns.
- Quickly address small **lapses** to prevent small gains from turning into major ones.
- Watch less than 10 hours of television per week.
- Eat high-fiber food, particularly whole grains, vegetables, and fruit, and consume sufficient water each day.[81]
- Cultivate and honor realistic expectations regarding body size and shape.

self-efficacy: a person's belief in his or her ability to succeed in an undertaking.

lapses: periods of returning to old habits.

Review Notes

- A person who adopts a lifelong "eating plan for good health" rather than a "diet for weight loss" will be more likely to keep the lost weight off. Table 7-5 offers several tips for successful weight management.
- Physical activity should be an integral part of a weight-management program.
- Physical activity can increase energy expenditure, improve body composition, help control appetite, reduce stress and stress eating, and enhance physical and psychological well-being.
- Behavior modification provides ways to overcome barriers to successful weight management.

TABLE 7-5	Weight-Management Strategies

In General

- Focus on healthy eating and activity habits, not on weight losses or gains.
- Adopt reasonable expectations about health and fitness goals and about how long it will take to achieve them.
- Make nutritional adequacy a high priority.
- Learn, practice, and follow a healthful eating plan for the rest of your life.
- Participate in some form of physical activity regularly.
- Adopt permanent lifestyle changes to achieve and maintain a healthy weight.

For Weight Loss

- Energy out should exceed energy in by about 500 kcalories/day. Increase your physical activity enough to spend more energy than you consume from foods.
- Emphasize foods with a low energy density and a high nutrient density.
- Eat small portions. Share a restaurant meal with a friend or take home half for lunch tomorrow.
- Eat slowly.
- Limit high-fat foods. Make legumes, whole grains, vegetables, and fruits central to your diet plan.
- Limit low-fat treats to the serving size on the label.
- Limit concentrated sweets and alcoholic beverages.
- Drink a glass of water before you begin to eat and another while you eat. Drink plenty of water throughout the day (eight glasses or more per day).
- Keep a record of diet and exercise habits; it reveals problem areas, the first step toward improving behaviors.
- Learn alternative ways to deal with emotions and stresses.
- Attend support groups regularly or develop supportive relationships with others.

For Weight Gain

- Energy in should exceed energy out by at least 500 kcalories/day. Increase your food intake enough to store more energy than you spend in exercise. Exercise and eat to build muscles.
- Expect weight gain to take time (1 pound per month would be reasonable).
- Emphasize energy-dense foods.
- Eat at least three meals per day.
- Eat large portions of foods and expect to feel full.
- Eat snacks between meals.
- Drink plenty of juice and milk.

Underweight

Underweight is far less prevalent than overweight, affecting no more than 5 percent of U.S. adults. Whether the underweight person needs to gain weight is a question of health and, like weight loss, a highly individual matter. People who are healthy at their present weight may stay there; there are no compelling reasons to try to gain weight. Those who are thin because of malnourishment or illness, however, might benefit from a diet that supports weight gain. Medical advice can help make the distinction.

An extreme underweight condition known as anorexia nervosa is sometimes seen in young people who exercise unreasonable self-denial in order to control their weight. They go to such extremes that they become severely undernourished and underweight. The distinguishing feature of a person with anorexia nervosa, as opposed to other thin people, is that the starvation is intentional. Anorexia nervosa is a major eating disorder seen in our society today. Another is bulimia nervosa—compulsive overeating, usually with purging. Eating disorders are the subject of the Nutrition in Practice that follows this chapter.

Review Notes

- Both the incidence of underweight and the health problems associated with it are less prevalent than overweight and its associated problems.

Strategies for Weight Gain

Some people are unalterably thin by reasons of genetics or early physical influences. Those who wish to gain weight for appearance's sake or to improve athletic performance should be aware that a healthful weight can be achieved only through physical activity, particularly strength training, combined with a high energy intake. Eating many high-kcalorie foods can bring about weight gain, but it will be mostly fat, and this can be as detrimental to health as being slightly underweight. In an athlete, such a weight gain can impair performance. Therefore, in weight gain, as in weight loss, physical activity and energy intake are essential components of a sound plan.

PHYSICAL ACTIVITY TO BUILD MUSCLES

The person who wants to gain weight should use resistance training primarily. As activity is increased, energy intake must be increased to support that activity. Eating extra food will then support a gain of both muscle and fat.

ENERGY-DENSE FOODS

Energy-dense foods (the very ones eliminated from a successful weight-loss diet) hold the key to weight gain. Pick the highest-kcalorie items from each food group—that is, milk shakes instead of fat-free milk, peanut butter instead of lean meat, avocados instead of cucumbers, and whole-wheat muffins instead of whole-wheat bread. Because fat contains more than twice as many kcalories per teaspoon as sugar does, fat adds kcalories without adding much bulk.

Be aware that health experts recommend a moderate-fat diet for the general U.S. population because the general population is overweight and at risk for heart disease. Consumption of excessive fat is not healthy for most people, of course, but may be essential for an underweight individual who needs to gain weight. An underweight person who is physically active and eating a nutritionally adequate diet can afford a few extra kcalories from fat. For health's sake, it is wise to select foods with monounsaturated and polyunsaturated fats instead of those with saturated or *trans* fats: for example, sautéing vegetables in olive oil instead of butter or hydrogenated margarine.

THREE MEALS DAILY

People wanting to gain weight should eat at least three hearty meals a day. Many people who are underweight have simply been too busy (sometimes for months) to eat enough to gain or maintain weight. Therefore, they need to make meals a priority and plan them in advance. Taking time to prepare and eat each meal can help, as can learning to eat more food within the first 20 minutes of a meal before you begin to feel full. Another suggestion is to eat meaty appetizers or the main course first and leave the soup or salad until later.

LARGE PORTIONS

It is also important for the underweight person to learn to eat more food at each meal: have two sandwiches for lunch instead of one, drink milk from a larger glass, and eat cereal from a larger bowl. Expect to feel full. Most underweight individuals are accustomed to small quantities of food. When they begin eating significantly more, they feel uncomfortable. This is normal and passes over time.

EXTRA SNACKS

Because a substantially higher energy intake is needed each day, in addition to eating more food at each meal, it is necessary to eat more frequently. Between-meal snacking offers a solution. For example, a student might make three sandwiches in the morning and eat them between classes in addition to the day's three regular meals.

JUICE AND MILK

Beverages provide an easy way to increase energy intake. Consider that 6 cups of cranberry juice add almost 1000 kcalories to the day's intake. kCalories can be added to milk by mixing in powdered milk or packets of instant breakfast.

For people who are underweight due to illness, concentrated liquid formulas are often recommended because a weak person can swallow them easily. A registered dietitian can recommend high-protein, high-kcalorie formulas to help the underweight person maintain or gain weight. Used in addition to regular meals, these formulas can help considerably.

> ## Review Notes
>
> - To gain weight, a person must train physically and increase energy intake by selecting energy-dense foods, eating regular meals, taking larger portions, and consuming extra snacks and beverages. Review the tips for weight gain in Table 7-5.

Self Check

1. Two causes of obesity in humans are:
   a. set-point theory and BMI.
   b. genetics and physical inactivity.
   c. genetics and low-carbohydrate diets.
   d. mineral imbalances and fat cell imbalance.

2. The protein produced by the fat cells under the direction of the *ob* gene is called:
   a. leptin.
   b. orlistat.
   c. sibutramine.
   d. lipoprotein lipase.

3. All of the following describe the behavior of fat cells *except:*
   a. the number decreases when fat is lost from the body.
   b. the storage capacity for fat depends on both cell number and cell size.
   c. the size is larger in obese people than in normal-weight people.
   d. the number increases several-fold during the growth years and tapers off when adult status is reached.

4. The obesity theory that suggests the body chooses to be at a specific weight is the:
   a. fat cell theory.
   b. enzyme theory.
   c. set-point theory.
   d. external cue theory.

5. The biggest problem associated with the use of prescription drugs in the treatment of obesity is:
   a. cost.
   b. the necessity for long-term dosage.
   c. ineffectiveness.
   d. adverse side effects.

6. A nutritionally sound weight-loss diet might restrict daily energy intake to create a:
   a. 1000-kcalorie-per-month deficit.
   b. 500-kcalorie-per-month deficit.
   c. 500-kcalorie-per-day deficit.
   d. 3500-kcalorie-per-day deficit.

7. What is the best approach to weight loss?
   a. Avoid foods containing carbohydrates.
   b. Eliminate all fats from the diet and decrease water intake.
   c. Greatly increase protein intake to prevent body protein loss.
   d. Reduce daily energy intake and increase energy expenditure.

8. Physical activity does *not* help a person to:
   a. lose weight.
   b. lose fat in trouble spots.
   c. retain muscle.
   d. maintain weight loss.

9. Suggestions to change behaviors for successful weight control include:
   a. shop only when hungry.
   b. eat in front of the television for distraction.
   c. learn appropriate portion sizes.
   d. eat quickly.

10. Which strategy would *not* help an underweight person to gain weight?
    a. Exercise.
    b. Drink plenty of water.
    c. Eat snacks between meals.
    d. Eat large portions of foods.

Answers to these questions can be found in Appendix H.

Clinical Applications

1. Chapter 1 discussed the nutrient density of foods—their nutrient contribution per kcalorie. Another way to evaluate foods is to consider their energy density—their energy contribution per gram:
   - A carrot weighing 72 grams delivers 31 kcalories.
   - To calculate the energy density, divide kcalories by grams: 31 kcalories divided by 72 grams = 0.43 kcalories per gram.

2. Do the same for french fries weighing 50 grams and contributing 167 kcalories: 167 kcalories divided by 50 grams = _____ kcalories per gram.
   - The more kcalories per gram, the greater the energy density.
   - Which food is more energy dense? The conclusion is no surprise, but understanding the mathematics may offer valuable insight into the concept of energy density.

Matthew Farruggio

- French fries are more energy dense, providing 3.34 kcalories per gram. They provide more energy per gram—and per bite.

3 • Considering a food's energy density is especially useful in planning diets for weight management. Foods with a high energy density can help with weight gain, whereas those with a low energy density can help with weight loss. Give some examples of foods that you might suggest for a client who wants to gain weight and some that might be appropriate for a client who is trying to lose weight.

Nutrition on the Net

For further study of the topics in this chapter, access these websites.

- Find updates and quick links to these and other nutrition-related sites at our website: www.cengage.com/nutrition/whitney/nhhc4e
- Information on a variety of obesity topics is available at the Obesity Society website: www.obesity.org/
- Search for obesity at: www.eatright.org/
- Explore the Weight Management section of the U.S. government site: www.nutrition.gov
- Learn about weight control and the WIN program from the Weight-Control Information Network: www.win.niddk.nih.gov
- Learn about the drugs used for weight loss from the Center for Drug Evaluation and Research: www.fda.gov/cder

- Visit weight-loss support groups, such as Take Off Pounds Sensibly (TOPS), Overeaters Anonymous (OA), and Weight Watchers: www.tops.org, www.oa.org, and www.weightwatchers.com
- Read the latest materials on obesity diagnosis and treatment here: www.nhlbi.nih.gov/guidelines/obesity/ob_home.htm
- Find helpful information on achieving and maintaining a healthy weight from the Calorie Control Council: www.caloriecontrol.org

Notes

1. M. de Krom and coauthors, Genetic variation and effects on human eating behavior, *Annual Review of Nutrition* 29 (2009): 283–304; T. Rankinen and C. Bouchard, Genetics of food intake and eating behavior phenotypes in humans, *Annual Review of Nutrition* 26 (2006): 413–434.
2. J. Hebebrand and A. Hinney, Environmental and genetic risk factors in obesity, *Child and Adolescent Psychiatric Clinics of North America* 18 (2009): 83–94.
3. K. Silventhoinen and coauthors, The genetic and environment influences on childhood obesity: A systematic review of twin and adoption studies, *International Journal of Obesity* 34 (2010): 29–40.
4. J. Wardle and coauthors, Evidence for a strong genetic influence on childhood adiposity despite the force of the obesogenic environment, *American Journal of Clinical Nutrition* 87 (2008): 398–404.
5. A. Newell and coauthors, Addressing the obesity epidemic: A genomics perspective, *Preventing Chronic Disease* [CDC serial online] April 2007, available at www.cdc.gov/pcd/issues/2007/apr/06_0068.htm.
6. C. Bouchard, Defining the genetic architecture of the predisposition to obesity: A challenging but not insurmountable task, *American Journal of Clinical Nutrition* 91 (2010): 5–6; Newell and coauthors, 2007.
7. Li Shengxu and coauthors, Cumulative effects and predictive value of common obesity-susceptibility variants identified by genome-wide association studies, *American Journal of Clinical Nutrition* 91 (2010): 184–190.
8. I. Romao and J. Roth, Genetic and environmental interactions in obesity and type 2 diabetes, *Journal of the American Dietetic Association* 108 (2008): S24–S28.
9. S. C. Woods, R. J. Seeley, and D. Cota, Regulation of food intake through hypothalamic signaling networks involving mTOR, *Annual Review of Nutrition* 28 (2008): 295–311.
10. J. M. Friedman, Leptin at 14 y of age: An ongoing story, *American Journal of Clinical Nutrition* 89 (2009): 973S–979S.
11. I. S. Farooqi and S. O'Rahilly, Leptin: A pivotal regulator of human homeostasis, *American Journal of Clinical Nutrition* 89 (2009): 980S–984S.
12. Friedman, 2009.
13. J. Beltowski, A. Jamroz-Wisniewska, and S. Widomska, Adiponectin and its role in cardiovascular disease, *Cardiovascular & Hematological Disorders Drug Targets* 8 (2008): 7–46.
14. S. Li and coauthors, Adiponectin levels and risk of type 2 diabetes: A systematic review and meta-analysis, *Journal of the American Medical Association* 302 (2009): 179–188; G. Wolf, New insights into thiol-mediated regulation of adiponectin secretion, *Nutrition Reviews* 66 (2008): 642–645; M. Garaulet and coauthors, Adiponectin, the controversial hormone, *Public Health Nutrition* 10 (2007): 1145–1150; Y. Takemura, K. Walsh, N. Ouchi, Adiponectin and cardiovascular inflammatory responses, *Current Atherosclerosis Report* 9 (2007): 238–243.
15. M. Guerre-Millo, Adiponectin: An update, *Diabetes & Metabolism* 34 (2008): 12–18.
16. D. E. Cummings, K. E. Foster-Schubert, and J. Overduin, Ghrelin and energy balance: Focus on current controversies, *Current Drug Targets* 6 (2005): 153–169.
17. T. R. Castaneda and coauthors, Ghrelin in the regulation of body weight and metabolism, *Frontiers in Neuroendocrinology* 31 (2010): 44–60; Cummings, Foster-Schubert, and Overduin, 2005.
18. V. Monti and coauthors, Relationship of ghrelin and leptin hormones with body mass index and waist circumference in a random sample of adults, *Journal of the American Dietetic Association* 106 (2006): 822–828.
19. G. C. Major and coauthors, Clinical significance of adaptive thermogenesis, *International Journal of Obesity* 31 (2007): 204–212.

20. D. Heber, An integrative view of obesity, *American Journal of Clinical Nutrition;* 91 (2010): 280S–283S; L. Qi and Y. A. Cho, Gene-environment interaction and obesity, *Nutrition Reviews* 66 (2008): 684–694; Newell and coauthors, 2007.

21. W. P. James, The fundamental drivers of the obesity epidemic, *Obesity Reviews* 9 (2008): S6–S13.

22. B. Wansink and K. Van Ittersum, Portion size me: Downsizing our consumption, *Journal of the American Dietetic Association* 107 (2007): 1103–1106.

23. B. J. Rolls, Plenary Lecture 1: Dietary strategies for the prevention and treatment of obesity, *Proceedings of the Nutrition Society* 69 (2010): 70–79; I. H. Steenhuis and W. M. Vermeer, Portion size: Review and framework for interventions, *International Journal of Behavioral Nutrition and Physical Activity* 6 (2009): 58.

24. Position of the American Dietetic Association: Weight management, *Journal of the American Dietetic Association* 109 (2009): 330–346.

25. Wansink and Van Ittersum, 2007; L. R. Young and M. Nestle, Portion sizes and obesity: Responses of fast-food companies, *Journal of Public Health Policy* 28 (2007): 238–248.

26. K. J. Duffey and coauthors, Regular consumption from fast food establishments relative to other restaurants is differentially associated with metabolic outcomes in young adults, *Journal of Nutrition* 139 (2009): 2113–2118; R. Rosenheck, Fast food consumption and increased caloric intake: A systematic review of a trajectory towards weight gain and obesity risk, *Obesity Reviews* 9 (2008): 535–547; M. A. Pereira and coauthors, Fast-food habits, weight gain, and insulin resistance (the CARDIA Study): 15-year prospective analysis, *Lancet* 365 (2005): 36–42.

27. L. Johnson and coauthors, Energy-dense, low-fiber, high-fat dietary pattern is associated with increased fatness in childhood, *American Journal of Clinical Nutrition* 87 (2008): 846–854; N. C. Howarth and coauthors, Dietary energy density is associated with overweight status among 5 ethnic groups in the Multiethnic Cohort Study, *Journal of Nutrition* 136 (2006): 2243–2248.

28. B. J. Rolls, L. S. Roe, and J. S. Meengs, Reductions in portion size and energy density of foods are additive and lead to sustained decreases in energy intake, *American Journal of Clinical Nutrition* 83 (2006): 11–17.

29. B. J. Rolls, A. Drewnowski, and J. H. Ledikwe, Changing the energy density of diet as a strategy for weight management, *Journal of the American Dietetic Association* 105 (2005): 98S–103S.

30. J. A. Ello-Martin, J. H. Ledikwe, and B. J. Rolls, The Influence of food portion size and energy density on energy intake: Implications for weight management, *American Journal of Clinical Nutrition* 82 (2005): 236S–241S.

31. A. Drewnowski and P. Eichelsdoefer, Can low-income Americans afford a healthy diet? *Nutrition Today* 44 (2009): 246–249; P. Monsivais and A. Drewnowski, The rising cost of low-energy-density foods, *Journal of the American Dietetic Association* 107 (2007): 2071–2076; L. H. Epstein and coauthors, Price and maternal obesity influence purchasing of low- and high-energy-dense foods, *American Journal of Clinical Nutrition* 86 (2007): 914–922.

32. D. S. Ludwig and M. Nestle, Can the food industry play a constructive role in the obesity epidemic? *Journal of the American Medical Association* 300 (2008): 1808–1811.

33. P. T. Katzmarzyk and coauthors, Sitting time and mortality from all causes, cardiovascular disease, and cancer, *Medicine and Science in Sports and Exercise* 41 (2009): 998–1005; S. Mandic and coauthors, Characterizing differences in mortality at the low end of the fitness spectrum, *Medicine and Science in Sports and Exercise* 41 (2009): 1573–1579; American College of Sports Medicine, Position stand: Appropriate physical activity intervention strategies for weight loss and prevention of weight regain for adults, *Medicine and Science in Sports and Exercise* 41 (2009): 459–471; P. Gordon-Larsen and coauthors, Fifteen-year longitudinal trends in walking patterns and their impact on weight change, *American Journal of Clinical Nutrition* 89 (2009): 19–26.

34. B. Swinburn and A. Shelly, Effects of TV time and other sedentary pursuits, *International Journal of Obesity* 32 (2008): S132–S136; D. A. Raynor and coauthors, Television viewing and long-term maintenance: Results from the National Weight Control Registry, *Obesity* 14 (2006): 1816–1824.

35. Katzmarzyk and coauthors, 2009.

36. D. Berrigan and coauthors, Active transportation increases adherence to activity recommendations, *American Journal of Preventive Medicine* 31 (2006): 210–216.

37. S. K. Kumanyika and coauthors, Population-based prevention of obesity: The need for comprehensive promotion of healthful eating, physical activity, and energy balance. A scientific statement from the American Heart Association Council on Epidemiology and Prevention, Interdisciplinary Committee for Prevention, *Circulation* 118 (2008): 428–464.

38. J. L. Pilletteri and coauthors, Use of dietary supplements for weight loss in the United States: Results of a national survey, *Obesity (Silver Springs)* 16 (2008): 790–796.

39. U.S. Food and Drug Administration, Questions and answers about FDA's initiative against contaminated weight loss products, April 30, 2009, available at http://www.fda.gov/Drugs/ResourcesForYou/Consumers/QuestionsAnswers/ucm136187.htm.

40. Ethics opinion: Weight loss products and medications, *Journal of the American Dietetic Association* 108 (2008): 2109–2113; H. M. Blanck and coauthors, Use of nonprescription dietary supplements for weight loss is common among Americans, *Journal of the American Dietetic Association* 107 (2007): 441–447.

41. R. F. Kushner, Anti-obesity drugs, *Expert Opinion on Pharmacotherapy* 9 (2008): 1339–1350.

42. Position of the American Dietetic Association, 2009.

43. Position of the American Dietetic Association, 2009.

44. Cummings, Foster-Schubert, and Overduin, 2005.

45. L. Sjostrom and coauthors, Effects of bariatric surgery on mortality in Swedish obese subjects, *New England Journal of Medicine* 357 (2007): 741–752; G. L. Blackburn, Solutions in weight control: Lessons from gastric surgery, *American Journal of Clinical Nutrition* 82 (2005): 248S–252S.

46. J. B. Dixon and coauthors, Adjustable gastric banding and conventional therapy for type 2 diabetes: A randomized controlled trial, *Journal of the American Medical Association* 299 (2008): 316–323; E. N. Hansen, A. Torquati, and N. N. Abumrad, Results of bariatric surgery, *Annual Review of Nutrition* 26 (2006): 481–511.

47. Blackburn, 2005.

48. M. K. Robinson, Surgical Treatment of obesity—weighing the facts, *New England Journal of Medicine* 361 (2009): 520–521; B. R. Smith, P. Schauer, and N. T. Nguyen, surgical approaches to the treatment of obesity: Bariatric surgery, *Endocrinology Metabolism Clinics of North America* 37 (2008): 943–964; J. A. Vogel and coauthors, Reduction in predicted coronary heart disease risk after substantial weight reduction after bariatric surgery, *American Journal of Cardiology* 99 (2007): 222–226.

49. Position of the American Dietetic Association, 2009; J. O. Hill, Can a small-changes approach help address the obesity epidemic? A report of the Joint Task Force of the American Society for Nutrition, Institute of Food Technologists, and International Food Information Council, *American Journal of Clinical Nutrition* 89 (2009): 477–484.

50. D. R. Jacobs and coauthors, Association of 1-y change in diet pattern with cardiovascular disease risk factors and adipokines: Results from the 1-y randomized Oslo Diet and Exercise Study, *American Journal of Clinical Nutrition* 89 (2009): 509–517; M. L. Fernandez, The metabolic syndrome, *Nutrition Reviews* 65 (2007): S30–S34; C. Galani and H. Schneider, Prevention and treatment of obesity with lifestyle interventions: Review and meta-analysis, *International Journal of Public Health* 52 (2007): 348–359.

51. Position of the American Dietetic Association, 2009; National Heart, Lung, and Blood Institute, National Institutes of Health, *The Practical Guide: Identification, Evaluation, and Treatment of Overweight and Obesity in Adults,* NIH publication no. 00-4084 (Washington, D.C.: Government Printing Office, 2000), p. 23.

52. National Heart, Lung, and Blood Institute, National Institutes of Health, 2000, pp. 26–27.

53. M. T. Timlin and coauthors, Breakfast eating and weight change in a 5-year prospective analysis of adolescents: Project EAT (Eating Among Teens), *Pediatrics* 121 (2008): e638; M. T. Timlin and M. A. Pereira, Breakfast frequency and quality in the etiology of adult obesity and chronic diseases, *Nutrition Reviews* 65 (2007): 268–281.

54. A. K. Kant and coauthors, Association of breakfast energy density with diet quality and body mass index in American adults: National Health and Nutrition Examination Surveys, 1999–2004, *American Journal of Clinical Nutrition* 88 (2008): 1396–1404.

55. M. Bulló and coauthors, Inflammation, obesity and comorbidities: The role of diet, *Public Health Nutrition* 10 (2007): 1164–1172.

56. Rolls, Roe, and Meengs, 2006.

57. K. Van Ittersum and B. Wansink, Do children really prefer large portions? Visual illusions bias their estimates and intake, *Journal of the American Dietetic Association* 107 (2007): 1107–1110; B. Wansink, K. Van Ittersum, and J. E. Painter, Ice cream illusions: Bowls, spoons, and self-served portion sizes, *American Journal of Preventive Medicine* 31 (2006): 240–243.

58. M. Bes-Rastrollo and coauthors, Prospective study of nut consumption, long-term weight change, and obesity risk in women, *American Journal of Clinical Nutrition* 89 (2009): 1913–1919.

59. M. C. de Oliveira, R. Sichieri, and R. V. Mozzer, A low-energy-dense diet adding fruit reduces weight and energy intake in women, *Appetite* 51 (2008): 291–295; J. A. Ello-Martin, and coauthors, dietary energy density

in the treatment of obesity: A year-long trial comparing 2 weight-loss diets, *American Journal of Clinical Nutrition* 85 (2007): 1465–1477.

60. M. A. Palmer, S. Capra, and S. K. Baines, Association between eating frequency, weight, and health, *Nutrition Reviews* 67 (2009): 379–390.

61. J. E. Flood and B. J. Rolls, Soup preloads in a variety of forms reduce meal energy intake, *Appetite* 49 (2007): 626–634.

62. B. M. Davy and coauthors, Water consumption reduces energy intake at a breakfast meal in obese older adults, *Journal of the American Dietetic Association* 108 (2008): 1236–1239; E. L. Van Walleghen and coauthors, Pre-meal water consumption reduces meal energy intake in older but not younger subjects, *Obesity* 15 (2007): 93–99.

63. B. M. Popkin and coauthors, A new proposed guidance system for beverage consumption in the United States, *American Journal of Clinical Nutrition* 83 (2006): 529–542.

64. J. E. Flood and coauthors, The effect of increased beverage portion size on energy intake at a meal, *Journal of the American Dietetic Association* 106 (2006): 1984–1990.

65. D. E. Larson-Meyer and coauthors, Caloric restriction with or without exercise: The fitness versus fatness debate, *Medicine and Science in Sports and Exercise* 42 (2010): 152–159; American College of Sports Medicine, 2009; Position of the American Dietetic Association, 2009.

66. A. E. Field and coauthors, Weight control behaviors and subsequent weight change among adolescents and young adult females, *American Journal of Clinical Nutrition* 91 (2010): 147–153; American College of Sports Medicine, 2009.

67. B. J. Nicklas and coauthors, Effect of exercise intensity on abdominal fat loss during calorie restriction in overweight and obese postmenopausal women: A randomized, controlled trial, *American Journal of Clinical Nutrition* 89 (2009): 1043–1052; American College of Sports Medicine, 2009; S. J. Elder and S. B. Roberts, The effects of exercise on food intake and body fatness: A summary of published studies, *Nutrition Reviews* 65 (2007): 1–19.

68. American College of Sports Medicine, 2009.

69. Larson-Meyer and coauthors, Management of the Metabolic Syndrome and type 2 diabetes through lifestyle modification, *Annual Review of Nutrition* 29 (2009): 223–256; F. Magkos and coauthors, 2010.

70. M. Hamer and G. O'Donovan, Cardiorespiratory fitness and metabolic risk factors in obesity, *Current Opinion in Lipidology* 21 (2010): 1–7; B. A. Irving and coauthors, Effect of exercise training intensity on abdominal visceral fat and body composition, *Medicine and Science in Sports and Exercise* 40 (2008): 1863–1872; M. Fogelhom, How physical activity can work? *International Journal of Pediatric Obesity* 3 (2008): 10–14.

71. N. A. King and coauthors, Individual variability following 12 weeks of supervised exercise: Identification and characterization of compensation for exercise-induced weight loss, *International Journal of Obesity (London)* (2008): 177–184.

72. K. Ohkawara and coauthors, Twenty-four-hour analysis of elevated energy expenditure after physical activity in a metabolic chamber: Models of daily total energy expenditure, *American Journal of Clinical Nutrition* 87 (2008): 1268–1276.

73. N. A. King and coauthors, Dual process action of exercise on appetite control: Increase in orexigenic drive but improvement in meal-induced satiety, *American Journal of Clinical Nutrition* 90 (2009): 921–927; C. Martins and coauthors, effects of exercise on gut peptides, energy intake and appetite, *Journal of Endocrinology* 193 (2007): 251–258.

74. C. Martins, L. Morgan, and H. Truby, A review of the effects of exercise on appetite regulation: An obesity perspective, *International Journal of Obesity* 32 (2008): 1337–1347; D. R. Broom and coauthors, Exercise-induced suppression of acylated ghrelin in humans, *Journal of Applied Physiology* 102 (2007): 2165–2171; R. R. Kraemer and V. D. Castracane, Exercise and humoral mediators of peripheral energy balance: Ghrelin and adiponectin, *Experimental Biology and Medicine (Maywood)*: 232 (2007): 184–194.

75. U.S. Department of Agriculture and U.S. Department of Health and Human Services, *2008 Physical Activity Guidelines for Americans,* available at. www.health.gov/paguidelines/default.aspx.

76. B. Van Dorsten and E. M. Lindley, Cognitive and behavioral approaches in the treatment of obesity, *Endocrinology and Metabolism Clinics of North America* 37 (2008): 905–922; M. D. Tsiros and coauthors, cognitive behavioral therapy improves diet and body composition in overweight and obese adolescents, *American Journal of Clinical Nutrition* 87 (2008): 1134–1140.

77. K. G. Volpp and coauthors, Financial incentive-based approaches for weight loss: A randomized trial, *Journal of the American Medical Association* 300 (2008): 2631–2637.

78. A. N. Fabricatore, Behavior therapy and cognitive-behavioral therapy for obesity: Is there a difference? *Journal of the American Dietetic Association* 107 (2007): 92–99.

79. R. Wing, Secrets of successful losers, *Nutrition Action Health Letter,* January/February, 2008, p. 8.

80. D. S. Bond, Weight-loss maintenance in successful weight losers: Surgical vs non-surgical methods, *International Journal of Obesity (London)* 33 (2009): 173–180.

81. J. N. Davis and coauthors, Normal-weight adults consume more fiber and fruit than their age- and height-matched overweight/obese counterparts, *Journal of the American Dietetic Association* 106 (2006): 833–840.

Eating Disorders

The exact number of people in the United States afflicted with some form of an **eating disorder** (see the accompanying glossary for the relevant terms) is unknown because many cases never get reported.[1] An estimated 6 percent of females and 3 percent of males have **anorexia nervosa**, **bulimia nervosa**, or **binge eating disorder**.[2] Many more suffer from other related conditions that do not meet the strict criteria for anorexia nervosa, bulimia nervosa, or binge eating disorder but still imperil a person's well-being. Characteristics of disordered eating such as restrained eating, binge eating, purging, fear of fatness, and distortion of body image are common, especially among young middle-class girls. In most other societies, these behaviors and attitudes are much less prevalent.

Why do so many young people in our society suffer from eating disorders?

Most experts agree that the causes are multifactorial: sociocultural, psychological, and probably also neuro-chemical.[3] Excessive pressure to be thin is at least partly to blame. When low body weight becomes an important goal, people begin to view normal, healthy body weight as too fat. Healthy people then take unhealthy actions to lose weight. Severe restriction of food intake may create intense hunger that leads to binges. Research confirms this theory, showing that unhealthy or dangerous diets often precede binge eating in adolescent girls.[4] Energy restriction followed by bingeing can set in motion a pattern of **weight cycling**, which may make weight loss and maintenance more difficult over time.

People who attempt extreme weight loss are dissatisfied with their bodies to begin with; they may also be depressed or suffer social anxiety.[5] As weight loss becomes more and more difficult, psychological problems worsen, and the likelihood of developing full-blown eating disorders intensifies.

People with anorexia nervosa suffer from an extreme preoccupation with weight loss that seriously endangers their health and even their lives. People with bulimia engage in episodes of binge eating alternating with periods of severe dieting or self-starvation. Some bulimics also follow binge eating with self-induced vomiting, laxative abuse, or diuretic abuse to "undo the damage."

Glossary

amenorrhea (ay-MEN-oh-REE-ah): the absence of or cessation of menstruation. **Primary amenorrhea** is menarche delayed beyond 16 years of age. **Secondary amenorrhea** is the absence of three to six consecutive menstrual cycles.

anorexia nervosa: an eating disorder characterized by a refusal to maintain a minimally normal body weight, self-starvation to the extreme, and a disturbed perception of body weight and shape; seen (usually) in adolescent girls and young women.

> *anorexia* = without appetite
> *nervosa* = of nervous origin

binge eating disorder: an eating disorder whose criteria are similar to those of bulimia nervosa, excluding purging or other compensatory behaviors.

bulimia (byoo-LEEM-ee-uh) **nervosa:** recurring episodes of binge eating combined with a morbid fear of becoming fat, usually followed by self-induced vomiting or purging.

cathartic: a strong laxative.

cognitive therapy: psychological therapy aimed at changing undesirable behaviors by changing underlying thought processes contributing to these behaviors. In anorexia nervosa, a goal is to replace false beliefs about body weight, eating, and self-worth with health-promoting beliefs.

eating disorder: a disturbance in eating behavior that jeopardizes a person's physical and psychological health.

emetic (em-ETT-ic): an agent that causes vomiting.

female athlete triad: a potentially fatal triad of medical problems: disordered eating, amenorrhea, and osteoporosis.

stress fractures: bone damage or breaks caused by stress on bone surfaces during exercise.

weight cycling: repeated rounds of weight loss and subsequent regain, with reduced ability to lose weight with each attempt; also called *yo-yo dieting*.

Are there other groups, besides girls and young women, who are vulnerable to anorexia nervosa and bulimia nervosa?

Yes. Athletes who participate in sports that emphasize leanness are at special risk for developing eating disorders.[6] Athletes must often meet stringent weight requirements to compete in their sport. Many athletes report that they engage in behaviors that are typical of people with eating disorders. Female athletes are most vulnerable, but males—especially dancers, wrestlers, skaters, jockeys, and gymnasts—suffer from eating disorders, too, and their numbers may be increasing.[7] These athletes may engage in extreme weight-loss practices such as overtraining, prolonged fasting, vomiting, taking diet pills, and using steam baths and saunas to induce sweating.

Wrestlers, for example, are required to "make weight" to compete in the lowest weight class to face the smallest possible opponents. To that end, wrestlers starve themselves, don rubber suits, sweat in steam rooms, and take diuretics to shed water weight before weighing in for competition. Athletes engaging in these practices actually compromise their athletic abilities. The diminished anaerobic strength, reduced endurance, decreased oxygen capacity, and general weakness caused by food deprivation and dehydration can impair performance, an effect lasting days after food and water are replenished.

Even among athletes, however, women are most susceptible to developing eating disorders. Many female athletes appear healthy but in fact may develop the three interrelated components of the **female athlete triad**: disordered eating, **amenorrhea** (the absence of three or more consecutive menstrual cycles), and osteoporosis (see Figure NP7-1).

How does the female athlete triad develop?

Many athletic women engage in self-destructive eating behaviors (disordered eating) because they and their coaches have adopted unsuitable weight standards. An athlete's body must be heavier for height than a nonathlete's body because the athlete's bones and muscles are denser. Weight standards that may be appropriate for others are inappropriate for athletes. Techniques such as skinfold measures yield more useful information about body composition.

Many young female athletes severely restrict energy intakes to improve performance, enhance the aesthetic appeal of their performance, or meet the weight guidelines of their specific sports. They fail to realize that the loss of lean tissue that accompanies energy restriction actually impairs their physical performance. Risk factors for the female athlete triad include the following:

- Young age (adolescence)
- Pressure to excel at a chosen physical activity
- Focus on achieving or maintaining an "ideal" body weight or body fat percentage
- Participation in sports or competitions that judge performance on aesthetic appeal such as gymnastics, figure skating, or dance
- Weight-loss dieting at an early age
- Unsupervised dieting

As for amenorrhea, its prevalence among premenopausal women in the United States is about 2 to 5 percent overall, but among female athletes it may be as high as 66 percent. Contrary to previous notions, amenorrhea is *not* a normal adaptation to strenuous physical training: it is a symptom of something going wrong. Amenorrhea is characterized by low blood estrogen, infertility, and often bone mineral losses.

In general, weight-bearing physical activity, dietary calcium, and the hormone estrogen protect against the bone loss of osteoporosis, but in women with disordered eating and amenorrhea, strenuous activity may impair bone health.[8] Vigorous training combined with low food energy intakes disrupts metabolic and hormonal balances. These disturbances compromise bone health, greatly increasing the risks of **stress fractures**.[9] Stress fractures, a serious form of bone injury, commonly occur among dancers and other competitive athletes with amenorrhea, low calcium intakes, and disordered eating. Many underweight young athletes have bones like those of postmenopausal women, and they may never recover their lost bone even after diagnosis and treatment—which makes prevention critical. Young athletes should be encouraged to consume at least 1300 milligrams of calcium each day, to eat nutrient-dense foods, and to obtain enough food energy to support weight gain and the energy expended in physical activity. Nutrition is critical to bone recovery.[10]

What can be done to prevent eating disorders in athletes and dancers?

To prevent eating disorders in athletes and dancers, both the performers and their coaches must be educated about links between inappropriate body weight ideals, improper

FIGURE NP7-1 | The Female Athlete Triad

Eating Disorder
- Restrictive dieting (inadequate energy and nutrient intake)
- Overexercising
- Weight loss
- Lack of body fat

Osteoporosis
- Loss of calcium from bones

Amenorrhea
- Diminished hormones

TABLE NP7-1	Strategies to Combat Eating Disorders

The following guidelines may be useful in combating eating disorders:

- Never restrict food intakes to below the amounts suggested for adequacy by the USDA Food Guide.

- Eat frequently. People often do not eat frequent meals because of time constraints, but eating can be incorporated into other activities, such as snacking while studying or commuting. The person who eats frequently never gets so hungry as to allow hunger to dictate food choices.

- If not at a healthy weight, establish a reasonable weight goal based on a healthy body composition.

- Allow a reasonable time to achieve the goal. A reasonable loss of excess fat can be achieved at the rate of about 1 percent of body weight per week.

- Learn to recognize media image biases, and reject ultra-thin standards for beauty. Shift focus to health, competencies, and human interactions; bring behaviors in line with those beliefs.

Specific guidelines for athletes and dancers:

- Replace weight-based goals with performance-based goals.

- Remember that eating disorders impair physical performance. Seek confidential help in obtaining treatment if needed.

- Restrict weight-loss activities to the off-season.

- Focus on proper nutrition as an important facet of your training—as important as proper technique.

weight-loss techniques, eating disorder development, adequate nutrition, and safe weight-control methods. Coaches and dance instructors should never encourage unhealthy weight loss to qualify for competition or to conform with distorted artistic ideals. Frequent weighings can push young people who are striving to lose weight into a cycle of starving to confront the scale and then bingeing uncontrollably afterward. The erosion of self-esteem that accompanies these events can interfere with the normal psychological development of the teen years and set the stage for serious problems later on.

Table NP7-1 provides some suggestions to help athletes and dancers protect themselves against developing eating disorders. The next sections describe eating disorders that anyone, athlete or nonathlete, may experience.

What are the characteristics of anorexia nervosa?

Most anorexia nervosa victims are females who come from middle- or upper-class families. The person with anorexia nervosa is often a perfectionist who works hard to please her parents. She may identify so strongly with her parents' ideals and goals for her that she sometimes feels she has no identity of her own. She is respectful of authority but sometimes feels like a robot, and she may act that way, too: polite but controlled, rigid, and unspontaneous. She earnestly

desires to control her own destiny, but she feels controlled by others. When she does not eat, she gains control.

How does a person know when dieting is going too far?

When a person loses weight to well below the average for her height and is no longer slim, but too slim, and still doesn't stop, she has gone too far. Regardless of how thin she is, she looks in the mirror and sees herself as fat. Central to the diagnosis of anorexia nervosa is a distorted body image that overestimates body fatness. Table NP7-2 shows the criteria that professionals use to diagnose anorexia nervosa. Anorexia nervosa resembles an addiction. The characteristic behavior is obsessive and compulsive. Before drawing conclusions about someone who is extremely thin or who eats very little, remember that diagnosis of anorexia nervosa requires professional assessment.

What is the harm in being very thin?

Anorexia nervosa damages the body much as starvation does. In young people, growth ceases, and normal development falters. They lose so much lean tissue that basal metabolic rate slows. Additionally, the heart pumps inefficiently and irregularly, the heart muscle becomes weak and thin, the heart chambers

A person with anorexia nervosa demonstrates the following:

A. Refusal to maintain body weight at or above a minimal normal weight for age and height, for example, weight loss leading to maintenance of body weight less than 85 percent of that expected; or failure to make expected weight gain during period of growth, leading to body weight less than 85 percent of that expected.

B. Intense fear of gaining weight or becoming fat, even though underweight.

C. Disturbance in the way in which one's body weight or shape is experienced; undue influence of body weight or shape on self-evaluation, or denial of the seriousness of the current low body weight.

D. In females past puberty, amenorrhea, that is, the absence of at least three consecutive menstrual cycles. (A woman is considered to have amenorrhea if her periods occur only following hormone administration, e.g., estrogen.)

Two types:

• **Restricting type:** During the episode of anorexia nervosa, the person does not regularly engage in binge eating or purging behavior (i.e., self-induced vomiting or the misuse of laxatives, diuretics, or enemas).

• **Binge eating/purging type:** During the episode of anorexia nervosa, the person regularly engages in binge eating or purging behavior (i.e., self-induced vomiting or the misuse of laxatives, diuretics, or enemas).

Source: Reprinted with permission from the *Diagnostic and Statistical Manual of Mental Disorders*, 4th ed., Text Revision, American Psychiatric Association, 2000.

People with anorexia nervosa see themselves as fat, even when they are dangerously underweight.

© David Young-Wolff/PhotoEdit

diminish in size, and the blood pressure falls. Minerals that help to regulate the heartbeat become unbalanced. Many deaths in people with anorexia nervosa are due to heart failure. Kidneys often fail as well.[11]

Starvation brings other physical consequences as well: loss of brain tissue, impaired immune response, anemia, and a loss of digestive function that worsens malnutrition.[12] Digestive functioning becomes sluggish, the stomach empties slowly, and the lining of the intestinal tract shrinks. The ailing digestive tract fails to sufficiently digest any food the victim may eat. The pancreas slows its production of digestive enzymes. The person may suffer from diarrhea, further worsening malnutrition.

What kind of treatment helps people with anorexia nervosa?

Treatment of anorexia nervosa requires a multidisciplinary approach that addresses two sets of issues and behaviors: those relating to food and weight, and those involving relationships with oneself and others. Teams of physicians, nurses, psychiatrists, family therapists, and dietitians work together to treat people with anorexia nervosa. The expertise of a registered dietitian is essential because an appropriate, individually crafted diet is crucial for normalizing body weight, and nutrition counseling is indispensable.[13] Seldom are clients willing to eat for themselves, but if they are, chances are they can recover without other interventions.

Professionals classify clients based on the risks posed by the degree of malnutrition present.* Clients with low risks may benefit from family counseling, **cognitive therapy**, behavior modification, and nutrition guidance; those with greater risks may also need other forms of psychotherapy and supplemental formulas to provide extra nutrients and energy.

Sometimes, intensive behavior management treatment in a live-in facility can help to normalize food intake and exercise.[14] When starvation leads to severe underweight (less than 75 percent of ideal body weight), high medical risks ensue and patients require hospitalization. They must be stabilized and carefully fed to forestall death.[15] However, involuntary feeding through a tube can cause psychological trauma and may not be necessary in all cases.[16] Antidepressant and other drugs are commonly prescribed but are often ineffective in anorexia nervosa.[17]

Stopping weight loss is a first goal; establishing regular eating patterns is next. Because body weight is low and fear of weight gain is high, initial food intake may be small— 1200 calories per day can be an achievement.[18] A variety of high-energy foods and beverages can help deliver needed kcalories and nutrients.[19] Even after recovery, however, energy intakes and eating behaviors may not fully return to normal.

Almost half of women who are treated can successfully maintain their body weight at just below a healthy weight; at that weight, many of them begin menstruating again. The other half have poor or fair treatment outcomes, relapse into abnormal eating behaviors, or die. Anorexia nervosa has one of the highest mortality rates among psychiatric disorders.[20] An estimated 1000 women die each year of anorexia nervosa—most commonly from cardiac complications due to malnutrition or from suicide.

How does bulimia nervosa differ from anorexia nervosa?

Bulimia nervosa is distinct from anorexia nervosa and is more prevalent. More men suffer from bulimia nervosa than from anorexia, but bulimia is still more common in women. The secretive nature of bulimic behaviors makes recognition of the problem difficult, but once it is recognized, diagnosis is based on the criteria listed in Table NP7-3.

The typical person with bulimia is well educated, in her early twenties, and close to ideal body weight. She is a high

*Indicators of malnutrition include a low percentage of body fat, low blood proteins, and impaired immune response.

TABLE NP7-3	Criteria for Diagnosis of Bulimia Nervosa

A person with bulimia nervosa demonstrates the following:

A. Recurrent episodes of binge eating. An episode of binge eating is characterized by both of the following:

  1. Eating, in a discrete period of time (e.g., within any two-hour period), an amount of food that is definitely larger than most people would eat during a similar period of time and under similar circumstances

  2. A sense of lack of control over eating during the episode (e.g., a feeling that one cannot stop eating or control what or how much one is eating)

B. Recurrent inappropriate compensatory behavior in order to prevent weight gain, such as self-induced vomiting; misuse of laxatives, diuretics, enemas, or other medications; fasting; or excessive exercise.

C. Binge eating and inappropriate compensatory behaviors that both occur, on average, at least twice a week for three months.

D. Self-evaluation unduly influenced by body shape and weight.

E. The disturbance does not occur exclusively during episodes of anorexia nervosa.

Two types:

- **Purging type:** The person regularly engages in self-induced vomiting or the misuse of laxatives, diuretics, or enemas.

- **Nonpurging type:** The person uses other inappropriate compensatory behaviors, such as fasting or excessive exercise, but does not regularly engage in self-induced vomiting or the misuse of laxatives, diuretics, or enemas.

Source: Reprinted with permission from the *Diagnostic and Statistical Manual of Mental Disorders*, 4th ed., Text Revision, American Psychiatric Association, 2000.

Weight Management: Overweight and Underweight

achiever but emotionally insecure. She experiences considerable social anxiety and has difficulty establishing personal relationships. She is sometimes depressed and often exhibits impulsive behavior.

Like the person with anorexia nervosa, the person with bulimia spends much time thinking about her body weight and food. Her preoccupation with food manifests itself in secretive binge eating episodes followed by self-induced vomiting, fasting, or the use of laxatives or diuretics. Such behaviors typically begin in late adolescence after a long series of various unsuccessful weight-reduction diets. People with bulimia commonly follow a pattern of restrictive dieting interspersed with bulimic behaviors and experience weight fluctuations of more than 10 pounds up and down over short periods of time.

Unlike the person with anorexia nervosa, the person with bulimia is aware of the consequences of her behavior, feels that it is abnormal, and is deeply ashamed of it. She feels inadequate and unable to control her eating, so she tends to be passive and to look to others for confirmation of her sense of self-worth. When she is rejected, either in reality or in her imagination, her bulimia becomes worse. If her depression deepens, she may seek solace in drug or alcohol abuse or other addictive behaviors. Clinical depression is common in people with bulimia nervosa, and the rates of substance abuse are high.

What exactly is binge eating?

Binge eating is unlike normal eating, and the food is not consumed for its nutritional value. The binge eater has a compulsion to eat. A typical binge occurs periodically, is done in secret, usually at night, and lasts an hour or more. A binge frequently follows a period of rigid dieting, so the binge eating is accelerated by hunger. During a binge, the person with bulimia may consume a thousand kcalories or more. The food typically contains little fiber or water, has a smooth texture, and is high in sugar and fat, so it is easy to consume vast amounts rapidly with little chewing.

What are the consequences of binge eating?

After a binge, the person may use a **cathartic**—a strong laxative that can injure the lower intestinal tract. Or the person may induce vomiting, using an **emetic**—a drug intended as first aid for poisoning.

On first glance, purging seems to offer a quick and easy solution to the problems of unwanted kcalories and body weight. Many people perceive such behavior as neutral or even positive, when, in fact, bingeing and purging have serious physical consequences. Fluid and electrolyte imbalances caused by vomiting or diarrhea can lead to abnormal heart rhythms and injury to the kidneys. Vomiting causes

irritation and infection of the pharynx, esophagus, and salivary glands; erosion of the teeth; and dental caries. The esophagus may rupture or tear, as may the stomach. Overuse of emetics depletes potassium concentrations and can lead to death by heart failure.

What is the treatment for bulimia nervosa?

As for people with anorexia nervosa, a team approach provides the most effective treatment for people with bulimia nervosa. Bulimia nervosa is easier to treat than anorexia nervosa in many respects because it seems to be more of a chosen behavior. People with bulimia know that their behavior is abnormal, and many are willing to try to cooperate.

The goal of the dietary plan to treat bulimia is to help the client gain control, establish regular eating patterns, and restore nutritional health. Energy intake should not be severely restricted—hunger can be a trigger for a binge.[21] The person needs to learn to eat a quantity of nutritious food sufficient to nourish her body and to satisfy hunger (at least 1600 kcalories a day). Table NP7-4 (p. 198) offers some ways to begin correcting bulimia nervosa. Most people diagnosed with bulimia nervosa recover within 5 to 10 years, with or without treatment, but treatment probably speeds the recovery process.

Anorexia nervosa and bulimia nervosa are distinct eating disorders, yet they sometimes overlap. Anorexia victims may purge, and victims of both conditions share an over-concern with body weight and the tendency to drastically undereat. The two disorders can also appear in the same person, or one can lead to the other. Other people have eating disorders that fall short of anorexia nervosa or bulimia nervosa but share some of their features, such as fear of body fatness. One such condition is binge eating disorder (defined earlier in the glossary).

How does binge eating disorder differ from bulimia nervosa?

Up to half of all people who restrict eating to lose weight periodically binge without purging, including about one-third of obese people who regularly engage in binge eating. Obesity itself, however, does not constitute an eating disorder. Table NP7-5 (p. 198) lists the official diagnostic criteria for binge eating disorder.

Clinicians note differences between people with bulimia nervosa and those with binge eating disorder. People with binge eating disorder consume less during a binge, rarely purge, and exert less restraint during times of dieting. Similarities also exist, including feeling out of control, disgusted, depressed, embarrassed, guilty, or distressed because of their self-perceived gluttony. Binge eating

TABLE NP7-4 | Strategies to Combat Bulimia Nervosa

Planning Principles

- Plan meals and snacks; record plans in a food diary prior to eating.
- Plan meals and snacks that require eating at the table and using utensils.
- Refrain from finger foods.
- Refrain from "dieting" or skipping meals.

Nutrition Principles

- Eat a well-balanced diet and regularly timed meals consisting of a variety of foods.
- Include raw vegetables, salad, or raw fruit at meals to prolong eating times.
- Choose whole-grain, high-fiber breads, pasta, rice, and cereals to increase bulk.
- Consume adequate fluid, particularly water.

Other Tips

- Choose foods that provide protein and fat for satiety and bulky, fiber-rich carbohydrates for immediate feelings of fullness.
- Try including soups and other water-rich foods for satiety.
- Choose portions that meet the definition of "a serving" according to the USDA Food Guide (pp. 18–19).
- For convenience (and to reduce temptation) select foods that naturally divide into portions. Select one potato, rather than rice or pasta that can be overloaded onto the plate; purchase yogurt and cottage cheese in individual containers; look for small packages of precut steak or chicken; choose frozen dinners with measured portions.
- Include 30 minutes of physical activity every day—exercise may be an important tool in defeating bulimia.

behavior responds more readily to treatment than other eating disorders, and resolving such behaviors can be a first step to authentic weight control. Successful treatment also improves physical health, mental health, and the chances of breaking the cycle of rapid weight losses and gains.

Chapter 6 describes how our society sets unrealistic ideals for body weight, especially in women, and devalues those who do not conform to them. Anorexia nervosa and bulimia nervosa are not a form of rebellion against these unreasonable expectations but rather the exaggerated acceptance of them. Body dissatisfaction is a primary factor in the development of eating disorders. Perhaps a person's best defense against these disorders is to learn to appreciate his or her own uniqueness.

TABLE NP7-5 | Criteria for Diagnosis of Binge Eating Disorder

A person with a binge eating disorder demonstrates the following:

A. Recurrent episodes of binge eating. An episode of binge eating is characterized by both of the following:

   1. Eating, in a discrete period of time (e.g., within any two-hour period), an amount of food that is definitely larger than most people would eat in a similar period of time under similar circumstances.

   2. A sense of lack of control over eating during the episode (e.g., a feeling that one cannot stop eating or control what or how much one is eating).

B. Binge eating episodes are associated with at least three of the following:

   1. Eating much more rapidly than normal.
   2. Eating until feeling uncomfortably full.
   3. Eating large amounts of food when not feeling physically hungry.
   4. Eating alone because of being embarrassed by how much one is eating.
   5. Feeling disgusted with oneself, depressed, or very guilty after overeating.

Weight Management: Overweight and Underweight

C. The binge eating causes marked distress.

D. The binge eating occurs, on average, at least twice a week for six months.

E. The binge eating is not associated with the regular use of inappropriate compensatory behaviors (e.g., purging, fasting, excessive exercise) and does not occur exclusively during the course of anorexia nervosa or bulimia nervosa.

Source: Reprinted with permission from the *Diagnostic and Statistical Manual of Mental Disorders*, 4th ed., Text Revision, American Psychiatric Association, 2000.

Notes

1. Position of the American Dietetic Association: Nutrition intervention in the treatment of anorexia nervosa, bulimia nervosa, and other eating disorders, *Journal of the American Dietetic Association* 106 (2006): 2073–2082.
2. J. L. Hudson and coauthors, the prevalence and correlates of eating disorders in the National Comorbidity Survey Replication, *Biological Psychiatry* 61 (2007): 348–358.
3. S. E. Mazzeo and C. M. Bulik, Environmental and genetic risk factors for eating disorders: What the clinician needs to know, *Child and Adolescent Psychiatric Clinics of North America* 18 (2009): 67–82; S. S. O'Sullivan, A. H. Evans, and A. J. Lees, Dopamine dysregulation syndrome: An overview of its epidemiology, mechanisms, and management, *CNS Drugs* 23 (2009): 157–170; T. D. Müller and coauthors, Leptin-mediated neuroendocrine alterations in anorexia nervosa: Somatic and behavioral implications, *Child and Adolescent Psychiatric Clinics of North America* 18 (2009): 117–129.
4. D. Neumark-Sztainer and coauthors, Obesity, disordered eating, and eating disorders in a longitudinal study of adolescents: How do dieters fare 5 years later? *Journal of the American Dietetic Association* 106 (2006): 559–568; B. A. Spear, does dieting increase the risk for obesity and eating disorders? *Journal of the American Dietetic Association* 106 (2006): 523–525.
5. B. Blaine, Does depression cause obesity? A meta-analysis of longitudinal studies of depression and weight control, *Journal of Health Psychology* 13 (2008): 1190–1197; S. E. Anderson and coauthors, Association of depression and anxiety disorders with weight change in a prospective community-based study of children followed up into adulthood, *Archives of Pediatric and Adolescent Medicine* 160 (2006): 285–291.
6. M. Vertalino and coauthors, Participation in weight-related sports is associated with higher use of unhealthful weight-control behaviors and steroid use, *Journal of the American Dietetic Association* 107 (2007): 434–440; American College of Sports Medicine, Position stand: The female athlete triad, *Medicine and Science in Sports and Exercise* 39 (2007): 1867–1882.
7. J. L. Glazer, Eating disorders among male athletes, *Current Sports Medicine Reports* 7 (2008): 332–337.
8. M. T. Barrack and coauthors, Dietary restraint and low bone mass in female adolescent endurance runners, *American Journal of Clinical Nutrition* 87 (2008): 36–43; D. L. Nichols, C. F. Sanborn, and E. V. Essery, Bone density and young athletic women, *Sports Medicine* 37 (2007): 1001–1014.
9. J. L. Kelsey and coauthors, Risk factors for stress fracture among young female cross-country runners, *Medicine and Science in Sports and Exercise* 39 (2007): 1457–1463.
10. J. Dominguez and coauthors, Treatment of anorexia nervosa is associated with increases in bone mineral density, and recovery is a biphasic process involving both nutrition and return of menses, *American Journal of Clinical Nutrition* 86 (2007): 92–99.
11. J. M. Torpy, Anorexia nervosa, JAMA patient page, *Journal of the American Medical Association* 295 (2006): 2684.
12. J. Yager and A. E. Andersen, Anorexia nervosa, *New England Journal of Medicine* 353 (2005): 1481–1488.
13. Position of the American Dietetic Association, 2006.
14. E. Attia and B. T. Walsh, Behavioral management for anorexia nervosa, *New England Journal of Medicine* 360 (2009): 500–506.
15. Position of the American Dietetic Association, 2006.
16. C. Theils, Forced treatment of patients with anorexia, *Current Opinion in Psychiatry* 21 (2008): 495–498.
17. B. T. Walsh and coauthors, Fluoxetine after weight restoration in anorexia nervosa: A randomized controlled trial, *Journal of the American Medical Association* 295 (2006): 2605–2612.
18. Yager and Andersen, 2005.
19. J. E. Schebendach and coauthors, Dietary energy density and diet variety as predictors of outcome in anorexia nervosa, *American Journal of Clinical Nutrition* 87 (2008): 810–816.
20. J. M. Holm-Denoma and coauthors, Deaths by suicide among individuals with anorexia as arbiters between competing explanations of the anorexia-suicide link, *Journal of Affective Disorders* 107 (2008): 231–236; G. Murialdo and coauthors, Alterations in the autonomic control of heart rate variability in patients with anorexia or bulimia nervosa: Correlations between sympathovagal activity, clinical features, and leptin levels, *Journal of Endocrinological Investigation* 30 (2007): 356–362; D. Casiero and W. H. Frishman, Cardiovascular complications of eating disorders, *Cardiology in Review* 14 (2006): 227–231; M. Pompili and coauthors, Suicide and attempted suicide in eating disorders, obesity and weight-image concern, *Eating Behaviors* 7 (2006): 384–394.
21. Position of the American Dietetic Association, 2006.

CHAPTER 8 | The Vitamins

CONTENTS

© Royalty-Free/Corbis

EARLIER CHAPTERS FOCUSED PRIMARILY ON THE ENERGY-YIELDING nutrients—carbohydrate, fat, and protein. This chapter and the next one discuss the nutrients everyone thinks of when nutrition is mentioned—the vitamins and minerals.

The Vitamins—An Overview

The **vitamins** occur in foods in much smaller quantities than do the energy-yielding nutrients, and they themselves contribute no energy to the body. Instead, they serve mostly as facilitators of body processes. They are a powerful group of substances, as their absence attests: Vitamin A deficiency can cause blindness, a lack of niacin can cause dementia, and a lack of vitamin D can retard bone growth. The consequences of deficiencies are so dire and the effects of restoring the needed nutrients so dramatic that people spend billions of dollars each year on **dietary supplements** to cure many different ailments. Vitamins certainly contribute to sound nutritional health, but supplements do not cure all ills. Actually, a vitamin can cure only the disease caused by a deficiency of that vitamin. The vitamins' roles in supporting optimal health extend far beyond preventing deficiency diseases, however. Emerging evidence points to relationships between low intakes of vitamins and chronic diseases such as cancer and heart disease.

A child once defined vitamins as "what, if you don't eat, you get sick." The description is both insightful and accurate. A more prosaic definition is that vitamins are potent, essential, nonkcaloric, organic nutrients needed from foods in trace amounts to perform specific functions that promote growth, reproduction, and the maintenance of health and life. Two characteristics distinguish vitamins from energy nutrients:

- Vitamins do not yield energy when broken down, but rather they assist the enzymes that release energy from carbohydrate, fat, and protein.
- The amounts of vitamins people ingest daily from foods and the amounts they require are measured in *micrograms* (µg) or *milligrams* (mg), rather than grams (g).

The vitamins are similar to the energy-yielding nutrients, though, in that they are vital to life, organic, and available from foods.

As the individual vitamins were discovered, they were named or given letters, numbers, or both. This led to the confusion that still exists today. This chapter uses the names shown in Table 8-1; alternative names are given in Tables 8-3 and 8-4, which appear later in the chapter.

BIOAVAILABILITY

The amount of vitamins available from foods depends on two factors: the quantity provided by a food and the amount absorbed and used by the body (the vitamin's **bioavailability**). Researchers analyze foods to determine their vitamin contents and publish the results in tables of food composition such as Appendix A. Determining the bioavailability of a vitamin is more difficult because it depends on many factors, including:

- The efficiency of digestion and time of transit through the GI tract.
- A person's previous nutrient intake and nutrition status.
- Other foods eaten at the same time.
- The method of food preparation (raw or cooked, for example).
- The source of the nutrient (naturally occurring, synthetic, or fortified).

This chapter and the next describe factors that inhibit or enhance the absorption of individual vitamins and minerals. Experts consider these factors when estimating recommended intakes.

PRECURSORS

Some of the vitamins are available from foods in inactive forms known as **precursors**, or provitamins. Once inside the body, the precursor is converted to the active form of the vitamin. Thus, in measuring a person's vitamin intake, it is important to count both the amount of the actual vitamin and the potential amount available from its precursors.

TABLE 8-1	Vitamin Names
Fat-Soluble Vitamins	
Vitamin A	
Vitamin D	
Vitamin E	
Vitamin K	
Water-Soluble Vitamins	
B vitamins	
Thiamin	
Riboflavin	
Niacin	
Pantothenic acid	
Biotin	
Vitamin B_6	
Folate	
Vitamin B_{12}	
Vitamin C	

vitamins: essential, nonkcaloric, organic nutrients needed in tiny amounts in the diet.

dietary supplements: products that are added to the diet and contain any of the following ingredients: a vitamin; a mineral; an herb or other botanical; an amino acid; a metabolite; a constituent; or an extract.

bioavailability: the rate and extent to which a nutrient is absorbed and used.

precursors: compounds that can be converted into other compounds; with regard to vitamins, compounds that can be converted into active vitamins; also known as **provitamins**.

TABLE 8-2	Minimizing Nutrient Losses

Each of these tactics saves a small percentage of the vitamins in foods, but repeated each day this can add up to significant amounts in a year's time.

Prevent enzymatic destruction:
- Refrigerate most fruits, vegetables, and juices to slow breakdown of vitamins.

Protect from light and air:
- Store milk and enriched grain products in opaque containers to protect riboflavin.
- Store cut fruits and vegetables in the refrigerator in airtight wrappers; reseal opened juice containers before refrigerating.

Prevent heat destruction or losses in water:
- Wash intact fruits and vegetables before cutting or peeling to prevent vitamin losses during washing.
- Cook fruits and vegetables in a microwave oven, or quickly stir fry, or steam them over a small amount of water to preserve heat-sensitive vitamins and to prevent vitamin loss in cooking water. Recapture dissolved vitamins by using cooking water for soups, stews, or gravies.
- Avoid high temperatures and long cooking times.

ORGANIC NATURE

Being organic, (✚) vitamins can be destroyed and left unable to function. Therefore, they must be handled with care during storage and in cooking. Prolonged heating may destroy much of the thiamin in food. Because riboflavin can be destroyed by the ultraviolet rays of the sun or by fluorescent light, foods stored in transparent glass containers are most likely to lose riboflavin. Oxygen destroys vitamin C, so losses occur when foods are cut, processed, and stored. Table 8-2 summarizes ways to minimize nutrient losses in the kitchen.

SOLUBILITY

Vitamins fall naturally into two classes—fat soluble and water soluble. The solubility of a vitamin confers on it many characteristics and determines how it is absorbed, transported, stored, and excreted. This discussion of vitamins begins with the fat-soluble vitamins.

Review Notes

- Vitamins are essential, nonkcaloric nutrients that are needed in trace amounts in the diet to help facilitate body processes.

The Fat-Soluble Vitamins

The fat-soluble vitamins—A, D, E, and K—usually occur together in the fats and oils of foods, and the body absorbs them in the same way it absorbs lipids. Therefore, any condition that interferes with fat absorption can precipitate a deficiency of the fat-soluble vitamins. Once absorbed, fat-soluble vitamins are stored in the liver and fatty tissues until the body needs them. They are not readily excreted, and, unlike most of the water-soluble vitamins, they can build up to toxic concentrations. Excesses of vitamins A and D from supplements can reach toxic levels especially easily.

The capacity to store fat-soluble vitamins affords a person some flexibility in dietary intake. When blood concentrations begin to decline, the body can retrieve the vitamins from storage. Thus, a person need not eat a day's allowance of each fat-soluble vitamin every day but need only make sure that, over time, average daily intakes approximate recommended intakes. In contrast, most water-soluble vitamins must be consumed more regularly because the body does not store them to any great extent.

✚ Organic nutrients contain carbon.

VITAMIN A AND BETA-CAROTENE

Vitamin A has the distinction of being the first fat-soluble vitamin to be recognized. A century later, vitamin A and its plant-derived precursor, **beta-carotene**, continue to intrigue researchers with their diverse roles and profound effects on health.

Vitamin A is a versatile vitamin, with roles in gene expression, vision, cell differentiation (thereby maintaining the health of body linings and skin), immunity, and reproduction and growth.[1] Three different forms of vitamin A are active in the body: retinol, retinal, and retinoic acid. Each form of vitamin A performs specific tasks. Retinol supports reproduction and is the major transport and storage form of the vitamin; the cells convert retinol to retinal or retinoic acid as needed. Retinal is active in vision, and retinoic acid acts as a hormone, regulating cell differentiation, growth, and embryonic development. A special transport protein, **retinol-binding protein (RBP)**, picks up retinol from the liver, where it is stored, and carries it in the blood. (✚)

Vitamin A's Role in Gene Expression

Vitamin A exerts considerable influence on body functions through its regulation of the activities of the genes.[2] Genes direct the synthesis of proteins, including enzymes, and enzymes perform the metabolic work of the tissues (see Chapter 5). Hence, factors that influence gene expression also affect the metabolic activities of the tissues and the health of the body. Hundreds of genes have been suggested as regulatory targets of the retinoic acid form of vitamin A.[3]

Researchers have long known that simply possessing the genetic equipment needed to make a particular protein does not guarantee that the protein will be produced, any more than owning a car guarantees you a trip across town. To get the car rolling, you must also use the right key to trigger the events that start up its engine or turn it off at the appropriate time. Some dietary components, including the retinoic acid form of vitamin A, are now known to be such keys—they help to activate or deactivate certain genes and thus affect the production of specific proteins.[4]

Vitamin A's Role in Vision

Vitamin A plays two indispensable roles in the eye. It helps maintain a healthy, crystal-clear outer window, the **cornea**; and it participates in the events of light detection at the **retina**. Some of the photosensitive cells (✚) of the retina contain **pigment** molecules called **rhodopsin**; each rhodopsin molecule is composed of a protein called **opsin** bonded to a molecule of the retinal form of vitamin A. When light passes through the cornea of the eye and strikes the retina, rhodopsin responds by changing shape and becoming bleached. In turn, this initiates the signal that conveys the sensation of sight to the optic center in the brain. Figure 8-1 shows vitamin A's site of action inside the eye.

When vitamin A is lacking, the eye has difficulty adapting to changing light levels. At night, after the eye has adapted to darkness, a lag occurs before the eye can see again after a flash of bright light. This lag in the recovery of night vision is known as **night blindness**. Because night blindness is easy to test, it aids in the diagnosis of vitamin A deficiency. Night blindness is only a symptom, however, and may indicate a condition other than vitamin A deficiency.

Vitamin A's Role in Protein Synthesis and Cell Differentiation

The role that vitamin A plays in vision is undeniably important, but only one-thousandth of the body's vitamin A is in the retina. Much more is in the skin and the linings of organs, where it works behind the scenes at the genetic level to promote protein synthesis and cell **differentiation**. The process of cell differentiation allows each type of cell to mature so that it is capable of performing a specific function.

✚ Measurement of the blood concentration of RBP is a sensitive test of vitamin A status.

✚ Photosensitive cells of the retina:
- Rods contain the rhodopsin pigment and respond to faint light.
- Cones contain the iodopsin pigment and function in color vision.

vitamin A: a fat-soluble vitamin. Its three chemical forms are *retinol* (the alcohol form), *retinal* (the aldehyde form), and *retinoic acid* (the acid form).

beta-carotene: a vitamin A precursor made by plants and stored in human fat tissue; an orange pigment.

retinol-binding protein (RBP): the specific protein responsible for transporting retinol.

cornea (KOR-nee-uh): the hard, transparent membrane covering the outside of the eye.

retina (RET-in-uh): the layer of light-sensitive nerve cells lining the back of the inside of the eye; consists of rods and cones.

pigment: a molecule capable of absorbing certain wavelengths of light so that it reflects only those that we perceive as a certain color.

rhodopsin (ro-DOP-sin): a light-sensitive pigment of the retina; contains the retinal form of vitamin A and the protein opsin.
hod = red (pigment)
opsin = visual protein

FIGURE 8-1 Vitamin A's Role in Vision

As light enters the eye, pigments within the cells of the retina absorb the light.

Retina cells (rods and cones)

Light energy

Cornea

Eye   Nerve impulses to the brain

+ Nutrition during pregnancy is discussed in Chapter 10.

+ A placebo is an inactive substance used in research studies.

+ Reminder: *Phytochemicals* are compounds in plants that confer color, taste, and other characteristics. Some phytochemicals are bioactive food components in functional foods. Phytochemicals and functional foods are the topic of Nutrition in Practice 8.

opsin: (OP-sin): the protein portion of the visual pigment molecule.

night blindness: the slow recovery of vision after exposure to flashes of bright light at night; an early symptom of vitamin A deficiency.

differentiation: the development of specific functions different from those of the original.

epithelial (ep-i-THEE-lee-ul) cells: cells on the surface of the skin and mucous membranes.

epithelial tissue: tissue composing the layers of the body that serve as selective barriers between the body's interior and the environment (examples are the cornea, the skin, the respiratory lining, and the lining of the digestive tract).

mucous membrane: membrane composed of mucus-secreting cells that lines the surfaces of body tissues. (Reminder: *Mucus* is the smooth, slippery substance secreted by these cells.)

antioxidant (anti-OX-ih-dant): a compound that protects other compounds from oxygen by itself reacting with oxygen. *Oxidation* is a potentially damaging effect of normal cell chemistry involving oxygen.
anti = against
oxy = oxygen

free radicals: highly reactive chemical forms that can cause destructive changes in nearby compounds, sometimes setting up a chain reaction.

dietary antioxidants: compounds typically found in plant foods that significantly decrease the adverse effects of oxidation on living tissues. The major antioxidant vitamins are vitamin E, vitamin C, and beta-carotene.

All body surfaces, both inside and out, are covered by layers of cells known as **epithelial cells**. The **epithelial tissue** on the outside of the body is, of course, the skin. The epithelial tissues inside the body include the linings of the mouth, stomach, and intestines; the linings of the lungs and the passages leading to them; the lining of the bladder; the linings of the uterus and vagina; and the linings of the eyelids and sinus passageways. The epithelial tissues on the inside of the body must be kept smooth. To ensure that they are, the epithelial cells on their surfaces secrete a smooth, slippery substance (mucus) that coats the tissues and protects them from invasive microorganisms and other harmful particles. The **mucous membrane** that lines the stomach also shields its cells from digestion by gastric juices. Vitamin A, by way of its role in cell differentiation, helps to maintain the integrity of the epithelial cells.

Vitamin A's Role in Immunity
Vitamin A has gained a reputation as an "anti-infective" vitamin because so many of the body's defenses against infection depend on an adequate supply.[5] Much research supports the need for vitamin A in the regulation of the genes involved in immunity. Without sufficient vitamin A, these genetic interactions produce an altered response to infection that weakens the body's defenses.

Vitamin A's Role in Reproduction, Growth, and Development
Vitamin A is crucial to normal reproduction and growth. In men, vitamin A participates in sperm development, and, in women, vitamin A promotes normal fetal growth and development.[6] During pregnancy, vitamin A is transferred to the fetus and is essential to the development of the nervous system, lungs, heart, kidneys, skeleton, eyes, and ears. (+)

Beta-Carotene's Role as an Antioxidant
For many years scientists believed beta-carotene to be of interest solely as a vitamin A precursor. Eventually, though, researchers began to recognize that beta-carotene is an extremely effective **antioxidant** in the body. Antioxidants are compounds that protect other compounds (such as lipids in cell membranes) from attack by oxygen. Oxygen triggers the formation of compounds known as **free radicals** that can start chain reactions in cell membranes. If left uncontrolled, these chain reactions can damage cell structures and impair cell functions. Oxidative and free-radical damage to cells is suspected of instigating some early stages of cancer and heart disease.[7] Research has identified links between oxidative damage and the development of many other diseases, including age-related blindness, Alzheimer's disease, arthritis, cataracts, diabetes, and kidney disease.[8]

Studies of populations suggest that people whose diets are low in foods rich in beta-carotene have higher incidences of certain types of cancer than those whose diets contain generous amounts of such foods. Based on findings that beta-carotene in foods may protect against cancer, researchers designed a study to determine the effects of beta-carotene *supplements* on the incidence of lung cancer among smokers. The researchers expected to see a beneficial effect, but instead they found that smokers taking the beta-carotene supplements suffered a *greater* incidence of lung cancer than those taking placebos. (+) Beta-carotene is one of many **dietary antioxidants** present in foods—others include vitamin E, vitamin C, the mineral selenium, and many phytochemicals. (+) Dietary antioxidants are just one class of a complex array of constituents in whole foods that seem to benefit health synergistically.[9] Until more is known, eating beta-carotene–rich foods, not supplements, is in the best interests of health. Based on research so far, the DRI committee has not established a recommended intake value for beta-carotene.

Vitamin A Deficiency
Up to a year's supply of vitamin A can be stored in the body, 90 percent of it in the liver. If a healthy adult were to stop eating vitamin A–rich foods, deficiency symptoms would not begin to appear until after stores were depleted, which would take one to two years. Then, however, the consequences would be profound and severe.[10] Table 8-3, later in this chapter, lists some of them.

In vitamin A deficiency, cell differentiation and maturation are impaired. The epithelial cells flatten and begin to produce **keratin**—the hard, inflexible protein of hair and nails. In the eye, this process leads to drying and hardening of the cornea, which may progress to permanent blindness. (✚) (✚) Vitamin A deficiency is the major cause of preventable blindness in children worldwide, causing as many as half a million children to lose their sight every year.[11] As many as 250 million children worldwide endure less severe forms of vitamin A deficiency, making them vulnerable to infectious diseases. Routine vitamin A supplementation and food fortification can be life-saving interventions.[12]

All body surfaces, both inside and out, maintain their integrity with the help of vitamin A. When vitamin A is lacking, cells of the skin harden and flatten, making it dry, rough, scaly, and hard. An accumulation of keratin makes a lump around each hair **follicle** (keratinization). (✚)

In the mouth, a vitamin A deficiency results in drying and hardening of the salivary glands, making them susceptible to infection. Secretions of mucus in the stomach and intestines are reduced, hindering normal digestion and absorption of nutrients. Infections of other mucous membranes also become likely.

Vitamin A's role in maintaining the body's defensive barriers may partially explain the relationship between vitamin A deficiency and susceptibility to infection. In developing countries around the world, measles is a devastating infectious disease, killing 450 children each day.[13] Deaths are usually due to related infections such as pneumonia and severe diarrhea. Providing large doses of vitamin A reduces the risk of dying from these infections.

The evidence that vitamin A reduces the severity of measles and measles-related infections and diarrhea has prompted the World Health Organization (WHO) and the United Nations International Children's Emergency Fund (UNICEF) to make control of vitamin A deficiency a major goal in their quest to improve child survival throughout the developing world. They recommend routine vitamin A supplementation for all children with measles in areas where vitamin A deficiency is a problem or where the measles death rate is high. The American Academy of Pediatrics recommends vitamin A supplementation for certain groups of measles-infected infants and children in the United States.

Vitamin A Toxicity

Vitamin A toxicity is a real possibility when people consume concentrated amounts of **preformed vitamin A** in foods derived from animals, fortified foods, or supplements.[14] Plant foods contain the vitamin only as beta-carotene, its inactive precursor form. The precursor does not convert to active vitamin A rapidly enough to cause toxicity.

Overdoses of vitamin A damage the same body systems that exhibit symptoms in vitamin A deficiency (see Table 8-3 later in the chapter). Children are most vulnerable to vitamin A toxicity because they need less vitamin A and are more sensitive to overdoses. The availability of breakfast cereals, instant meals, fortified milk, and chewable candy-like vitamins, each containing 100 percent or more of the recommended daily intake of vitamin A, makes it possible for a well-meaning parent to provide several times the daily allowance of the vitamin to a child within a few hours.[15] Serious toxicity is seen in infants and young children when they are given more than 10 times the recommended amount every day for weeks at a time.

Excessive vitamin A also poses a **teratogenic** risk.[16] Excessive vitamin A during pregnancy can injure the spinal cord of the developing fetus, increasing the risk of birth defects.[17] The Tolerable Upper Intake Level of 3000 micrograms for women of childbearing age is based on the teratogenic effect of vitamin A.[18]

Excessive amounts of vitamin A over the years may weaken the bones and contribute to fractures and osteoporosis (see the later discussion of vitamin D for more on osteoporosis).[19] More research is needed to clarify the relationship between vitamin A intake and bone health, but such findings suggest that most people should not take vitamin A supplements. Even multivitamin supplements provide more vitamin A than most people need. (✚)

Certain vitamin A relatives are available by prescription as acne treatments. When applied directly to the skin surface, these preparations help relieve the symptoms of acne. Taking massive doses of vitamin A internally will *not* cure acne, however, and may

✚ The progressive blindness caused by vitamin A deficiency is called *xerophthalmia* (zer-off-THAL-mee-uh).
xero = dry
ophthalm = eye

✚ An early sign of xerophthalmia is *xerosis* (drying of the cornea); the last and most severe stage is *keratomalacia* (kerr-uh-to-mal-AY-shuh), or total blindness.
malacia = softening, weakening

✚ The accumulation of the hard material keratin around each hair follicle is *follicular hyperkeratosis*.

✚ Multivitamin supplements typically provide:
- 750 µg (2500 IU).
- 1500 µg (5000 IU).

For perspective, the RDA for vitamin A is 700 µg for women and 900 µg for men. The IU (*international unit*) was once used to express the amount of vitamins in foods and is still used on supplement labels.

keratin (KERR-uh-tin): a water-insoluble protein; the normal protein of hair and nails. Keratin-producing cells may replace mucus-producing cells in vitamin A deficiency.

follicle (FOLL-i-cul): a group of cells in the skin from which a hair grows.

preformed vitamin A: vitamin A in its active form.

teratogenic (ter-AT-oh-jen-ik): causing abnormal fetal development and birth defects.
terato = monster
genic = to produce

FIGURE 8-2 | Symptom of Beta-Carotene Excess—Discoloration of the Skin

The hand on the right shows the skin discoloration that occurs from excess beta-carotene. (The hand on the left belongs to someone else and is shown for comparison.)

✚ 1 μg RAE = 1 μg retinol
= 12 μg beta-carotene from food

retinol activity equivalents (RAE): a measure of vitamin A activity; the amount of retinol that the body will derive from a food containing preformed retinol or its precursor beta-carotene.

cause the symptoms itemized in Table 8-3. In most cases, foods are a better choice than supplements for needed nutrients. The best way to ensure a safe vitamin A intake is to eat generous servings of vitamin A–rich foods.

Beta-Carotene Conversion and Toxicity Nutrition scientists do not use micrograms to specify the quantity of beta-carotene in foods. Instead, they use a value known as **retinol activity equivalents (RAE),** (✚) which express the amount of retinol the body actually derives from a plant food after conversion. The body can make one unit of retinol from about 12 units of beta-carotene.

As mentioned earlier, beta-carotene from plant foods is not converted to the active form of vitamin A rapidly enough to be hazardous. It has, however, been known to turn people bright yellow if they eat too much. (✚) Beta-carotene builds up in the fat just beneath the skin and imparts a yellowish cast (see Figure 8-2). As discussed earlier, however, overconsumption of beta-carotene from *supplements* may be harmful, especially to smokers.[20]

Vitamin A in Foods Preformed vitamin A is found only in foods of animal origin. The richest sources of vitamin A are liver and fish oil, but milk, cheese, and fortified cereals are also good sources. Healthy people can eat vitamin A–rich foods in large amounts without risking toxicity with the possible exception of liver. Eating liver once every week or so is enough. Butter and eggs also provide some vitamin A to the diet.

Because vitamin A is fat soluble, it is lost when milk is skimmed. To compensate, reduced-fat, low-fat, and fat-free milks are often fortified with vitamin A. Margarine is also usually fortified so as to provide the same amount of vitamin A as butter. Snapshot 8-1 shows a sampling of the richest food sources of both preformed vitamin A and beta-carotene.

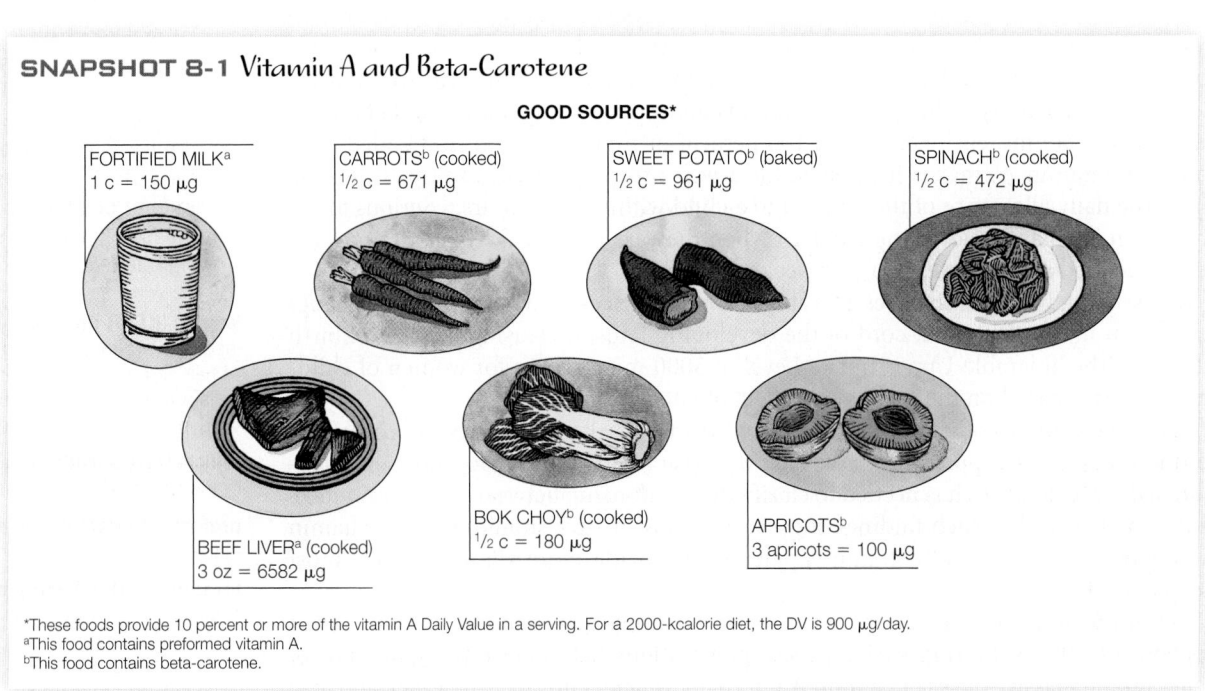

SNAPSHOT 8-1 *Vitamin A and Beta-Carotene*

GOOD SOURCES*

FORTIFIED MILK[a]
1 c = 150 μg

CARROTS[b] (cooked)
½ c = 671 μg

SWEET POTATO[b] (baked)
½ c = 961 μg

SPINACH[b] (cooked)
½ c = 472 μg

BEEF LIVER[a] (cooked)
3 oz = 6582 μg

BOK CHOY[b] (cooked)
½ c = 180 μg

APRICOTS[b]
3 apricots = 100 μg

*These foods provide 10 percent or more of the vitamin A Daily Value in a serving. For a 2000-kcalorie diet, the DV is 900 μg/day.
[a]This food contains preformed vitamin A.
[b]This food contains beta-carotene.

Fast-food meals often lack vitamin A. When fast-food restaurants offer salads with cheese, carrots, and other vitamin A–rich foods, the nutritional quality of their meals greatly improves.

Beta-Carotene in Foods Many foods from plants contain beta-carotene, the orange pigment responsible for the bold colors of many fruits and vegetables. Carrots, sweet potatoes, pumpkins, cantaloupe, and apricots are all rich sources, and their bright orange color enhances the eye appeal of the plate. Another colorful group, *dark* green vegetables, such as spinach, other greens, and broccoli, owe their color to both chlorophyll and beta-carotene. The orange and green pigments together impart a deep, murky green color to the vegetables. Other colorful vegetables, such as iceberg lettuce, beets, and sweet corn, can fool you into thinking they contain beta-carotene, but these foods derive their color from other pigments and are poor sources of beta-carotene. As for "white" plant foods such as rice and potatoes, they have little or none. Recommendations to eat *dark* green or *deep* orange vegetables and fruits at least every other day help people to meet their vitamin A needs.

VITAMIN D

Vitamin D (✚) is different from all the other nutrients in that the body can synthesize it in significant quantities with the help of sunlight. Therefore, in a sense, vitamin D is not an essential nutrient. Given enough sun, people need no vitamin D from foods.

Vitamin D's Metabolic Conversions The liver manufactures a vitamin D precursor, (✚) which migrates to the skin, where it is converted to a second precursor with the help of the sun's ultraviolet rays. Next, the liver and then the kidneys alter the second precursor to produce the active vitamin. (✚) Whether made from sunlight or obtained from food, vitamin D requires the same two conversions by the liver and kidneys to become active.[21] The biological activity of the active vitamin is 500- to 1000-fold greater than that of its precursor. Diseases that affect either the liver or the kidneys may impair the transformations of precursor vitamin D to active vitamin D and therefore produce symptoms of vitamin D deficiency.

Vitamin D's Actions Although known as a vitamin, vitamin D is actually a hormone—a compound manufactured by one organ of the body that has effects on another. The best-known vitamin D target organs are the small intestine, the kidneys, and the bones, but scientists have discovered more than 30 other vitamin D target tissues, including the brain, the pancreas, the skin, the reproductive organs, and cells of the immune system.[22] In many cases, vitamin D enhances or suppresses the activity of genes that regulate cell growth.[23] As such, it may be valuable in treating a number of diseases.[24]

Research suggests that a deficit of vitamin D is associated with an increased risk of high blood pressure; cardiovascular diseases; some common cancers; infections such as tuberculosis; inflammatory conditions; autoimmune diseases such as type 1 diabetes, rheumatoid arthritis, and multiple sclerosis; and even premature death.[25] The well-established vitamin D roles, however, concern calcium balance and the bones during growth and throughout life.

Vitamin D's Roles in Bone Growth Vitamin D is a member of a large, cooperative bone-making and maintenance team composed of nutrients and other compounds, including vitamins A, C, and K; the hormones parathormone (parathyroid hormone) and calcitonin; the protein collagen; and the minerals calcium, phosphorus, magnesium, and fluoride. (✚) Many of these interactions take place at the genetic level in ways that are under investigation.[26] Vitamin D's special role in bone health is to assist in the absorption of calcium and phosphorus, thus helping to maintain blood concentrations of these minerals.[27] The bones grow denser and stronger as they absorb and deposit these minerals. Details of calcium balance and mineral deposition appear in Chapter 9.

Sunlight promotes vitamin D synthesis in the skin. Exposure to the sun should be moderate, however; excessive exposure may cause skin cancer.

✚ Yellowing of the skin caused by excess carotene in the blood is known as *carotenemia* (KAR-oh-teh-NEE-me-ah). Carotenemia can be distinguished from jaundice because the mucous membranes lining the eyelids do not turn yellow as they do in jaundice.

✚ Vitamin D comes in many forms, but the two most important in the diet are a plant version called vitamin D$_2$, or *ergocalciferol* (ER-go-kal-SIF-er-ol), and an animal version called vitamin D$_3$, or *cholecalciferol* (KO-lee-kal-SIF-er-ol).

✚ The precursor of vitamin D made in the liver is 7-dehydrocholesterol, which is made from cholesterol. This is one of the body's many "good" uses for cholesterol.

✚ The final, active vitamin is calcitriol (1-25 dihydroxyvitamin D).

✚ Key bone nutrients:
- Vitamin D, vitamin K, vitamin A
- Calcium, phosphorus, magnesium, fluoride

Vitamin D raises blood concentrations of bone minerals in three ways. When the diet is sufficient, vitamin D enhances their absorption from the GI tract. When the diet is insufficient, vitamin D provides the needed minerals from other sources: reabsorption by the kidneys and mobilization from the bones into the blood.[28] The vitamin may work alone, as it does in the GI tract, or in combination with parathyroid hormone, as it does in the bones and kidneys.[29]

Vitamin D Deficiency Overt signs of vitamin D deficiency are relatively rare, but vitamin D insufficiency is remarkably common.[30] According to one estimate, two-thirds of U.S. residents over one year of age take in too little vitamin D.[31] Factors that contribute to vitamin D deficiency include dark skin, breastfeeding without supplementation, lack of sunlight, and not using fortified milk.

Worldwide, the prevalence of the vitamin D–deficiency disease **rickets** is extremely high, affecting more than half of the children in countries such as Mongolia, Tibet, and the Netherlands.[32] In the United States, more than 58 million children are reported to be vitamin D deficient or insufficient, but rickets itself is uncommon.[33] When it occurs, black children and adolescents—especially females and overweight teens—are the ones most likely to be affected.[34] To prevent rickets, the American Academy of Pediatrics recommends a minimum daily intake of 400 IU vitamin D for all infants, children, and adolescents.[35] (✚) In rickets, the bones fail to calcify normally, causing growth retardation and skeletal abnormalities. The bones become so weak that they bend when they have to support the body's weight (see Figure 8-3). A child with rickets who is old enough to walk characteristically develops bowed legs, often the most obvious sign of the disease. Another sign is the beaded ribs that result from the poorly formed attachments of the bones to the cartilage.

Adolescents, who often abandon vitamin D–fortified milk in favor of soft drinks, may also prefer indoor pastimes such as computer games to outdoor activities during daylight hours. Such teens often lack vitamin D and so fail to develop the bone density needed to prevent bone loss in later life.[36]

| FIGURE 8-3 | Vitamin D–Deficiency Symptoms—Bowed Legs and Beaded Ribs of Rickets |

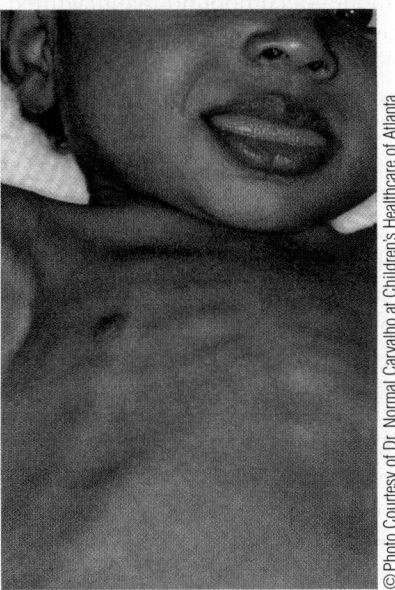

Bowed legs. In rickets, the poorly formed long bones of the legs bend outward as weight-bearing activities such as walking begin.

Beaded ribs. In rickets, a series of "beads" develop where the cartilages and bones attach.

© Biophoto Associates/Photo Researchers, Inc.

© Photo Courtesy of Dr. Normal Carvalho at Children's Healthcare of Atlanta

✚ For perspective, 1 cup of fortified milk provides about 50 IU vitamin D.

rickets: the vitamin D–deficiency disease in children.

osteomalacia (os-tee-oh-mal-AY-shuh): a bone disease characterized by softening of the bones. Symptoms include bending of the spine and bowing of the legs. The disease occurs most often in adults with renal failure or malabsorption disorders.
    osteo = bone
    mal = bad (soft)

In adults, the poor mineralization of bone results in the painful bone disease **osteomalacia**. Any failure to synthesize adequate vitamin D or obtain enough from foods sets the stage for a loss of calcium from the bones, which can result in fractures secondary to **osteoporosis** (reduced bone density). The simple act of taking a combined vitamin D and calcium supplement could easily save the life of an elderly person who might otherwise suffer dangerous bone fractures and falls.[37]

Vitamin D Toxicity Whereas vitamin D deficiency depresses calcium absorption, blood calcium, and bone mineralization, an excess of vitamin D does the opposite. It enhances calcium absorption, produces high blood calcium, and promotes return of bone calcium into the blood. The excess calcium then tends to precipitate in the soft tissues, forming stones, including kidney stones.[38] Calcification may also harden the blood vessels and is especially dangerous in the major arteries of the brain, heart, and lungs, where it can cause death.

Vitamin D in excess is the most toxic of all the vitamins. The amounts of vitamin D in foods available in the United States and Canada are well within safe limits, but supplements containing the vitamin in concentrated form are not. Adults should use caution when taking vitamin D supplements and keep them out of the reach of children. The DRI committee has set a Tolerable Upper Intake Level for vitamin D at 50 micrograms per day (2000 IU on supplement labels).

Vitamin D from the Sun Most of the world's population relies on natural exposure to sunlight to maintain adequate vitamin D nutrition. The sun imposes no risk of vitamin D toxicity. Prolonged exposure to sunlight degrades the vitamin D precursor in the skin, preventing its conversion to the active vitamin. Even lifeguards on southern beaches are safe from vitamin D toxicity from the sun.

Prolonged exposure to sunlight has other undesirable consequences, however, such as premature wrinkling of the skin and skin cancers. UV radiation from the sun, including UVB that promotes vitamin D synthesis, is carcinogenic, contributing to about a million skin cancers per year in the United States.[39] Sunscreens help reduce the risks of premature wrinkling and skin cancers, but sunscreens with sun protection factors (SPF) of 8 and above also retard vitamin D synthesis. Still, even with an SPF 15–30 sunscreen, sufficient vitamin D synthesis can be obtained in 10 to 20 minutes of sun exposure.[40] A strategy to avoid this dilemma is to apply sunscreen after enough time has elapsed to provide sufficient vitamin D. For most people, exposing hands, face, and arms on a clear summer day for 5 to 10 minutes, a few times a week, should be sufficient to maintain vitamin D nutrition. Dark-skinned people require longer exposure than light-skinned people, but by three hours, vitamin D synthesis in heavily pigmented skin arrives at the same plateau as in fair skin after 30 minutes.

Latitude, season, and time of day also have dramatic effects on vitamin D synthesis and status.[41] (✛) Heavy clouds, smoke, or smog block the ultraviolet (UV) rays of the sun that promote vitamin D synthesis. Differences in skin pigmentation, latitude, and smog may account for the finding that African American people, especially those in northern, smoggy cities, are most likely to be vitamin D deficient and develop rickets. Vitamin D deficiency is especially prevalent in the winter.[42] To ensure an adequate vitamin D status, supplements may be needed. The body's vitamin D supplies from summer synthesis alone are insufficient to meet winter needs.[43]

The ultraviolet rays from tanning lamps and tanning booths may also stimulate vitamin D synthesis, but the hazards outweigh any possible benefits. The Food and Drug Administration (FDA) warns that, if the lamps are not properly filtered, people using tanning booths risk burns, damage to the eyes and blood vessels, and skin cancer.

Vitamin D in Foods Only a few animal foods, notably, eggs, liver, butter, some fatty fish, and fortified milk, supply significant amounts of vitamin D. For those who use margarine in place of butter, fortified margarine is a significant source. Infant formulas are fortified with vitamin D in amounts adequate for daily intake as long as infants consume at least one liter (1000 milliliters) or one quart (32 ounces) of formula. Breast milk is low in vitamin D, so vitamin D supplements (10 micrograms daily)

✛ Factors that may limit sun exposure and, therefore, vitamin D synthesis:
- Geographic location
- Season of the year
- Time of day
- Air pollution
- Clothing
- Tall buildings
- Indoor living
- Sunscreens

osteoporosis: (os-tee-oh-pore-OH-sis): literally, porous bones; reduced density of the bones, also known as *adult bone loss*.

are recommended for infants who are breastfed exclusively and for those who do not receive at least 1000 milliliters of vitamin D–fortified formula per day.[44] These sources, plus any exposure to the sun, provide infants with more than enough of this vitamin.

The fortification of milk with vitamin D is the best guarantee that children will meet their vitamin D needs and underscores the importance of milk in children's diets. Vitamin D supplements (10 micrograms daily) are recommended for children and adolescents who do not obtain 10 micrograms of vitamin D per day by drinking vitamin D–fortified milk and eating fortified foods such as dry cereals.[45] Unlike milk, cheese and yogurt are not fortified with vitamin D. Vegans, and especially their children, may have low vitamin D intakes because few fortified plant sources exist. Exceptions include margarine and some soy milks. In the United States, breakfast cereals may be fortified with vitamin D, as their labels indicate.

Vitamin D Recommendations In setting dietary recommendations, the DRI Committee assumed that no vitamin D was available from skin synthesis. Advancing age increases the risk of vitamin D deficiency, so intake recommendations increase with age (see the margin). (✚) Current recommendations may be insufficient, however, given research showing numerous health benefits and safety of higher intakes.[46] To achieve optimal blood levels, some research suggests that vitamin D intake should be between 40 and 125 micrograms per day.[47]

VITAMIN E

More than 80 years ago, researchers discovered a compound in vegetable oils necessary for reproduction in rats. The compound was named **tocopherol**, which means "offspring." Eventually, the compound was named vitamin E. When chemists isolated four tocopherol compounds, they designated them by the first four letters of the Greek alphabet: alpha, beta, gamma, and delta. Of these, alpha-tocopherol is the gold standard for vitamin E activity; recommended intakes are based on it. Table 8-3 later in the chapter summarizes important information about vitamin E.

Vitamin E as an Antioxidant Like beta-carotene, vitamin E is a fat-soluble antioxidant. It protects other substances from oxidation (✚) by being oxidized itself. If there is plenty of vitamin E in the membranes of cells exposed to an oxidant, chances are this vitamin will take the brunt of any oxidative attack, protecting the lipids and other vulnerable components of the membranes. Vitamin E is especially effective in preventing the oxidation of the polyunsaturated fatty acids (PUFA), but it protects all other lipids (for example, vitamin A) as well.

Vitamin E exerts an especially important antioxidant effect in the lungs, where the cells are exposed to high concentrations of oxygen. Vitamin E also protects the lungs from air pollutants that are strong oxidants.

Some evidence suggests that vitamin E may also offer protection against heart disease by protecting low-density lipoproteins (LDL) from oxidation and reducing inflammation.[48] The oxidation of LDL encourages the development of atherosclerosis. Despite this theoretical understanding of how vitamin E may exert protection against heart disease, the results of controlled clinical studies in which human beings were given vitamin E supplements have been disappointing.[49] Several leading vitamin E researchers point out that clinical trials of vitamin E supplementation differ in many important ways, such as the selection of subjects, the source of the vitamin, the dose of the vitamin, and the outcomes studied. Such differences may partly explain the inconsistent findings.

Further research that addresses such issues may clarify the relationship between vitamin E and heart disease. In the meantime, the American Heart Association supports the consumption of antioxidant-rich fruits and vegetables, as well as whole grains and nuts, to reduce the risk of heart disease.[50]

Vitamin E Deficiency When blood concentrations of vitamin E fall below a certain critical level, the red blood cells tend to break open and spill their contents, probably because the PUFA in their membranes oxidize. This classic vitamin E–deficiency symptom, known as **erythrocyte hemolysis**, is seen in premature infants

✚ Vitamin D AI:
- Adults (19–50 yr): 5 µg/day
- Adults (51–70 yr): 10µg/day
- Adults (>70 yr): 15µg/day

✚ Reminder: *Oxidation* is a type of chemical reaction, so named because oxygen is one of the agents that often brings it about.

tocopherol (tuh-KOFF-er-ol): a general term for several chemically related compounds, one of which has vitamin E activity.

erythrocyte (er-REETH-ro-cite) hemolysis (he-MOLL-uh-sis): rupture of the red blood cells, caused by vitamin E deficiency.
erythro = red
cyte = cell
hemo = blood
lysis = breaking

born before the transfer of vitamin E from the mother to the fetus that takes place in the last weeks of pregnancy. Vitamin E treatment corrects **hemolytic anemia**.

The few symptoms of vitamin E deficiency that have been observed in adults include loss of muscle coordination and reflexes with impaired movement, vision, and speech. Vitamin E treatment corrects all of these symptoms.

In adults, vitamin E deficiency is usually associated with diseases, notably those that cause malabsorption of fat. These include diseases of the liver, gallbladder, and pancreas, as well as various hereditary diseases involving digestion and use of nutrients. (✚)

On rare occasions, vitamin E deficiencies develop in people without diseases. Most likely, such deficiencies occur after years of eating diets extremely low in fat; using fat substitutes, such as diet margarines and salad dressings, as the only sources of fat; or consuming diets composed of highly processed or "convenience" foods. Extensive heating in the processing of foods destroys vitamin E.

Vitamin E Toxicity

Vitamin E in foods is safe to consume. Reports of vitamin E toxicity symptoms are rare across a broad range of intakes.[51] Vitamin E supplement use has increased in recent years, however, as its antioxidant action against disease has been recognized. As a result, signs of toxicity are now known or suspected, although vitamin E toxicity is not nearly as common, and its effects are not as serious, as vitamin A or vitamin D toxicity. Extremely high doses of vitamin E interfere with the blood-clotting action of vitamin K and enhance the action of anticoagulant medications, leading to hemorrhage.

Recently, the pooled results from 67 experiments involving almost a quarter-million people suggested that taking vitamin E supplements may slightly increase mortality in both healthy and sick people.[52] Other studies find no effect or a slight decrease in mortality among certain groups.[53] To err on the safe side, until more is known about the safety of vitamin E supplements, intakes should probably be kept low, and they certainly should not exceed the UL of 1000 milligrams of alpha-tocopherol per day. The UL for vitamin E is more than 65 times greater than the recommended intake for adults (15 milligrams).

Vitamin E in Foods

Vitamin E is widespread in foods. Much of the vitamin E in the diet comes from vegetable oils and the products made from them, such as margarine, salad dressings, and shortenings. Wheat germ oil is especially rich in vitamin E. Other sources of the vitamin include whole grains, fruits, vegetables, and nuts. Because vitamin E is readily destroyed by heat processing and oxidation, fresh or lightly processed foods are the best sources of this vitamin.

Prior to 2000, values of the vitamin E in food reflected all of the different tocopherols and were expressed in "milligrams of tocopherol equivalents." These measures overestimated the amount of alpha-tocopherol. To estimate the alpha-tocopherol content of foods stated in tocopherol equivalents, multiply by 0.8.

VITAMIN K

Vitamin K has long been known for its role in blood clotting, (✚) where its presence can make the difference between life and death. The vitamin also participates in the synthesis of several bone proteins. Without vitamin K, the bones produce an abnormal protein that cannot bind to the minerals that normally form bones, resulting in low bone density.[54] An adequate intake of vitamin K helps to decrease bone turnover and protect against fractures.[55] People who consume abundant vitamin K, often in the form of green leafy vegetables, suffer fewer hip fractures than those with lower intakes. Vitamin K supplements seem ineffective against bone loss, however.[56] Vitamin K is also under investigation for roles in heart disease prevention.[57]

Blood Clotting

At least 13 different proteins and the mineral calcium are involved in making blood clot. Vitamin K is essential for the activation of several of these proteins, among them prothrombin, the precursor of the enzyme thrombin (see Figure 8-4 on p. 212). When any of the blood-clotting factors is lacking, **hemorrhagic disease** results. If an artery or vein is cut or broken, bleeding goes unchecked. Of course, this is not to say that hemorrhaging is always caused by a vitamin K deficiency.

✚ Nutrition and upper GI disorders are discussed in Chapter 17.
Nutrition and lower GI disorders are discussed in Chapter 18.
Nutrition and liver disorders are discussed in Chapter 19.

✚ K stands for the Danish word *koagulation* (coagulation, or "clotting").

hemolytic (HE-moh-LIT-ick) anemia: the condition of having too few red blood cells as a result of erythrocyte hemolysis.

hemorrhagic (hem-oh-RAJ-ik) disease: the vitamin K–deficiency disease in which blood fails to clot.

Vegetable oils, some nuts and seeds such as almonds and sunflower seeds, and wheat germ are rich in vitamin E.

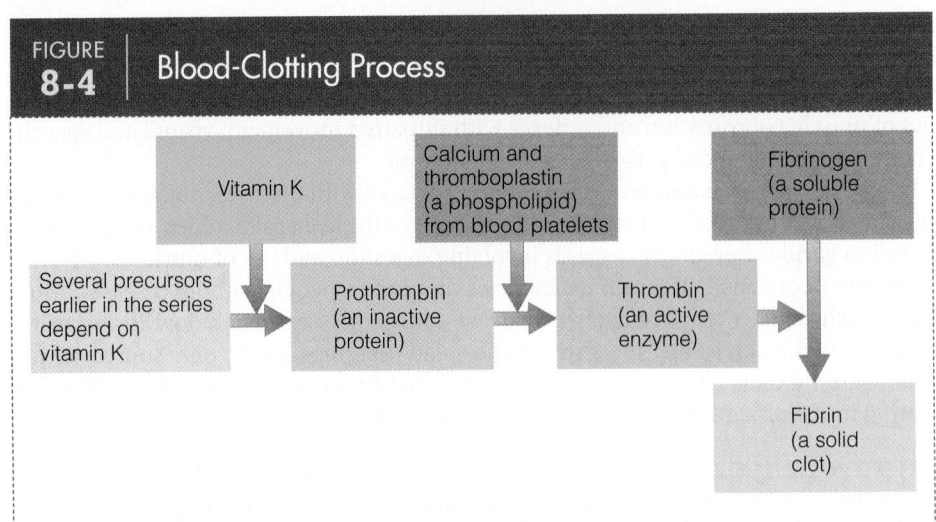

FIGURE 8-4 | Blood-Clotting Process

Several precursors earlier in the series depend on vitamin K

Vitamin K → Prothrombin (an inactive protein)

Calcium and thromboplastin (a phospholipid) from blood platelets → Thrombin (an active enzyme)

Fibrinogen (a soluble protein) → Fibrin (a solid clot)

When blood is exposed to air, foreign substances, or secretions from injured tissues, platelets (small, cell-like structures in the blood) release a phospholipid known as thromboplastin. Thromboplastin catalyzes the conversion of the inactive protein prothrombin to the active enzyme thrombin. Thrombin then catalyzes the conversion of the precursor protein fibrinogen to the active protein fibrin that forms the clot.

Intestinal Synthesis Like vitamin D, vitamin K can be obtained from a nonfood source. Bacteria in the intestinal tract (➕) synthesize vitamin K that the body can absorb, but people cannot depend on this source alone for their vitamin K.

Vitamin K Deficiency Vitamin K deficiency is rare, but it may occur in two circumstances. First, it may arise in conditions of fat malabsorption. Second, some medications interfere with vitamin K's synthesis and action in the body: antibiotics kill the vitamin K–producing bacteria in the intestine, and anticoagulant medications interfere with vitamin K metabolism and activity. When vitamin K deficiency does occur, it can be fatal.

Vitamin K for Newborns Newborn infants present a unique case of vitamin K nutrition. An infant is born with a **sterile** digestive tract, and some weeks pass before the vitamin K–producing bacteria become fully established in the infant's intestines. At the same time, plasma prothrombin concentrations are low (this helps prevent blood clotting during the stress of birth, which might otherwise be fatal). A single dose of vitamin K, usually in a water-soluble form, is recommended at birth to prevent hemorrhagic disease in the newborn.

Vitamin K Toxicity Vitamin K toxicity is rare, and no adverse effects have been reported with high intakes. Therefore, a Tolerable Upper Intake Level has not been established. High doses of vitamin K can reduce the effectiveness of anticoagulant medications used to prevent blood clotting. People taking these medications should eat vitamin K–rich foods in moderation and keep their intakes consistent from day to day.

Vitamin K in Foods Many foods contain ample amounts of vitamin K, notably, green leafy vegetables, members of the cabbage family, and some vegetable oils. Other vegetables such as iceberg lettuce and green beans provide smaller amounts.

© Matthew Farruggio

Notable food sources of vitamin K include green vegetables such as collards, spinach, bib lettuce, brussels sprouts, and cabbage and vegetable oils such as soybean oil and canola oil.

Review Notes
• The fat-soluble vitamins are vitamins A, D, E, and K.
• Vitamin A is essential to gene expression, vision, cell differentiation and integrity of epithelial tissues, immunity, and reproduction and growth.

- Vitamin A deficiency can cause blindness, sickness, and death and is a major problem worldwide.
- Overdoses of vitamin A are possible and dangerous.
- Vitamin D raises calcium and phosphorus levels in the blood. A deficiency can cause rickets in children or osteomalacia in adults.
- Vitamin D is the most toxic of all the vitamins.
- People exposed to the sun make vitamin D in their skin; fortified milk is an important food source.
- Vitamin E acts as an antioxidant in cell membranes and is especially important in the lungs where cells are exposed to high concentrations of oxygen.
- Vitamin E may protect against heart disease, but the evidence is not conclusive yet.
- Vitamin E deficiency is rare in healthy human beings. The vitamin is widely distributed in plant foods.
- Vitamin K is necessary for blood to clot and for bone health.
- The bacterial inhabitants of the digestive tract produce vitamin K, but people need vitamin K from foods as well.
- Dark green, leafy vegetables are good sources of vitamin K.
- Table 8-3 offers a complete summary of the fat-soluble vitamins.

TABLE 8-3	The Fat-Soluble Vitamins—A Summary			
Vitamin Name	Chief Functions	Deficiency Symptoms	Toxicity Symptoms	Significant Sources
Vitamin A (Retinol, retinal, retinoic acid; main precursor is beta-carotene)	Vision, maintenance of cornea, epithelial cells, mucous membranes, skin; bone and tooth growth; reproduction; regulation of gene expression; immunity	Infectious diseases, night blindness, blindness (xerophthalmia), keratinization	Reduced bone mineral density, liver abnormalities, birth defects	Retinol: milk and milk products; eggs; liver Beta-carotene: spinach and other dark, leafy greens; broccoli; deep orange fruits (apricots, cantaloupe) and vegetables (carrots, winter squashes, sweet potatoes, pumpkin)
Vitamin D (Calciferol, cholecalciferol, dihydroxy vitamin D; precursor is cholesterol)	Mineralization of bones (raises blood calcium and phosphorus by increasing absorption from digestive tract, withdrawing calcium from bones, stimulating retention by kidneys)	Rickets, osteomalacia	Calcium imbalance (calcification of soft tissues and formation of stones)	Synthesized in the body with the help of sunshine; fortified milk, margarine, butter, and cereals; eggs; liver; fatty fish (salmon, sardines)
Vitamin E (Alpha-tocopherol, tocopherol)	Antioxidant (stabilization of cell membranes, regulation of oxidation reactions, protection of polyunsaturated fatty acids [PUFA] and vitamin A)	Erythrocyte hemolysis, nerve damage	Hemorrhagic effects	Polyunsaturated plant oils (margarine, salad dressings, shortenings), green and leafy vegetables, wheat germ, whole-grain products, nuts, seeds
Vitamin K (Phylloquinone, menaquinone, naphthoquinone)	Synthesis of blood-clotting proteins and bone proteins	Hemorrhage	None known	Synthesized in the body by GI bacteria; green, leafy vegetables; cabbage-type vegetables; vegetable oils

The Water-Soluble Vitamins

The B vitamins and vitamin C are the water-soluble vitamins. These vitamins, found in the watery compartments of foods, are distributed into water-filled compartments of the body. They are easily absorbed into the bloodstream and are just as easily excreted if their blood concentrations rise too high. Thus, the water-soluble vitamins are less likely to reach toxic concentrations in the body than are the fat-soluble vitamins. Foods never deliver excessive amounts of the water-soluble vitamins, but the large doses concentrated in vitamin supplements can reach toxic levels.

THE B VITAMINS

Despite advertisements that claim otherwise, the B vitamins do not give people energy. Carbohydrate, fat, and protein—the *energy-yielding* nutrients—supply the fuel for energy. The B vitamins *help* the body use that fuel but do not serve as fuel themselves.

Coenzymes The eight B vitamins were listed in Table 8-1. Each is part of an enzyme helper known as a **coenzyme**. Some B vitamins have other important functions in the body as well, but the roles these vitamins play as parts of coenzymes are the best understood. A coenzyme is a small molecule that combines with an enzyme to make it active. With the coenzyme in place, a substance is attracted to the enzyme, and the reaction proceeds instantaneously. Figure 8-5 illustrates coenzyme action.

Active forms of five of the B vitamins—thiamin, riboflavin, niacin, pantothenic acid, and biotin—participate in the release of energy from carbohydrate, fat, and protein. A coenzyme containing vitamin B_6 assists enzymes that metabolize amino acids. Folate and vitamin B_{12} help cells to multiply. Among these cells are the red blood cells and the cells lining the GI tract—cells that deliver energy to all the others.

The eight B vitamins play many specific roles in helping the enzymes to perform thousands of different molecular conversions in the body. They must be present in every cell continuously for the cells to function as they should. As for vitamin C, its primary role, discussed later, is as an antioxidant.

B Vitamin Deficiencies In academic and clinical discussions of the vitamins, different sets of deficiency symptoms are ascribed to each individual vitamin. Such clear-cut symptoms, however, are found only in laboratory animals that have been fed contrived diets that lack just one nutrient. In reality, a deficiency of any single B vitamin seldom shows up in isolation because people do not eat nutrients one by one; they eat foods containing mixtures of many nutrients. If a major class of foods is missing from the diet, all of the nutrients delivered by those foods will be lacking to various extents.

In only two cases have dietary deficiencies associated with single B vitamins been observed on a large scale in human populations. Diseases have been named for these deficiency states. One of them, **beriberi**, was first observed in Southeast Asia when the custom of polishing rice became widespread. Rice contributed 80 percent of the energy intake of the people in these areas, and rice bran was their principal source of thiamin. When the bran was removed to make the rice whiter, beriberi spread like wildfire.

The niacin-deficiency disease, **pellagra**, became widespread in the southern United States in the early part of the 20th century among people who subsisted on a low-protein diet with a staple grain of corn. This diet was unusual in that it supplied neither enough niacin nor enough tryptophan, its amino acid precursor, to make the niacin intake adequate.

Even in the cases of beriberi and pellagra, the deficiencies were probably not pure. When foods were provided containing the one vitamin known to be needed, other vitamins that may have been in short supply came as part of the package.

---

coenzyme (co-EN-zime): a small molecule that works with an enzyme to promote the enzyme's activity. Many coenzymes have B vitamins as part of their structure.

co = with

beriberi: the thiamin-deficiency disease; characterized by loss of sensation in the hands and feet, muscular weakness, advancing paralysis, and abnormal heart action.

pellagra (pell-AY-gra): the niacin-deficiency disease. Symptoms include the "4 Ds": diarrhea, dermatitis, dementia, and, ultimately, death.

pellis = skin
agra = seizure

| FIGURE 8-5 | Coenzyme Action |

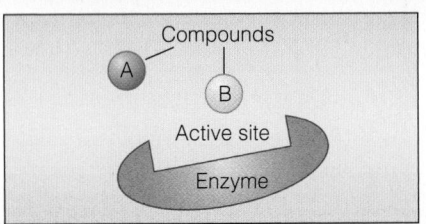

Without the coenzyme, compounds A and B do not respond to the enzyme.

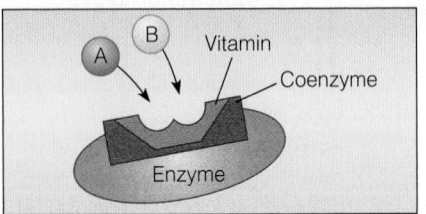

With the coenzyme in place, compounds A and B are attracted to the active site on the enzyme, and they react.

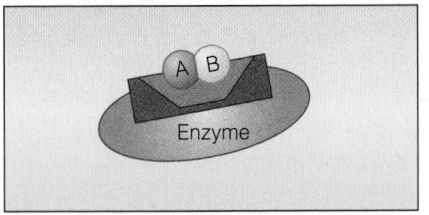

The reaction is completed with the formation of a new product. In this case the product is AB.

The product AB is released.

Major deficiency diseases such as pellagra and beriberi no longer occur in the United States and Canada, but more subtle deficiencies of nutrients, including the B vitamins, are sometimes observed. When they do occur, it is usually in people whose food choices are poor because of poverty, ignorance, illness, or poor health habits such as alcohol abuse.

Interdependent Systems Table 8-4, at the end of this chapter, sums up a few of the better-established facts about B vitamin deficiencies. A look at the table will make another generalization possible. Different body systems depend on these vitamins to different extents. Processes in nerves and in their responding tissues, the muscles, depend heavily on glucose metabolism and hence on thiamin, so paralysis sets in when this vitamin is lacking. But thiamin is important in all cells, not just in nerves and muscles. Similarly, because the red blood cells and GI tract cells divide the most rapidly, two of the first symptoms of a deficiency of folate are a type of anemia and GI tract deterioration—but again, all systems depend on folate, not just these. The list of symptoms in Table 8-4 is far from complete.

B Vitamin Enrichment of Foods If the staple food of a region is made from **refined grain**, vitamin B deficiencies are especially likely. One way to protect people from deficiencies is to add nutrients to their staple food, a process known as **fortification** or **enrichment**. (✚) The enrichment of refined breads and cereals has drastically reduced the incidence of iron and B vitamin deficiencies.

The preceding discussion has shown both the great importance of the B vitamins in promoting normal, healthy functioning of all body systems and the severe consequences of deficiency. Now you may want to know how to be sure you and your clients are getting enough of these vital nutrients. The next sections present information on each B vitamin. While reading further, keep in mind that *foods* can provide all the needed nutrients and that supplements are a poor second choice. Some supplements are absurdly costly, but even if they are inexpensive, most people don't need them. Nutrition in Practice 9 discusses uses and choices of supplements in more detail.

THIAMIN

All cells use thiamin, which plays a critical role in their energy metabolism. Thiamin also occupies a special site on nerve cell membranes. Consequently, as mentioned earlier, thiamin is critical to the normal functioning of the nerves and muscles.

Thiamin Need As long as people consume enough food to meet their energy needs—and obtain that energy from nutritious foods—thiamin needs will be met. People who derive a large proportion of their energy from empty-kcalorie items, like sugar or alcohol, however, risk thiamin deficiency, a condition that seems to be reappearing as the population of malnourished and homeless people rises. A person who is fasting or who has adopted a very low-kcalorie diet needs as much thiamin as when eating enough to meet energy needs.

In developed countries today, abuse of alcohol may lead to a severe form of thiamin deficiency, Wernicke-Korsakoff syndrome.[58] Alcohol contributes energy but carries almost no nutrients with it and often displaces food. In addition, alcohol impairs absorption of thiamin from the digestive tract and hastens its excretion in urine, tripling the risk of deficiency. Wernicke-Korsakoff syndrome is characterized by symptoms that are almost indistinguishable from alcohol abuse itself: mental confusion, disorientation, loss of memory, jerky eye movements, and staggering gait. Unlike alcohol toxicity, the syndrome responds quickly to an injection of thiamin, and some experts recommend a precautionary dose for any patients suspected of having the syndrome.

Thiamin in Foods Thiamin occurs in small quantities in virtually all nutritious foods, but it is concentrated in only a few foods, of which pork is the most commonly eaten. A useful guideline for meeting thiamin needs is to keep empty-kcalorie foods to a minimum and to include 10 or more different servings of nutritious foods each

✚ Note: The terms *fortified* and *enriched* may be used interchangeably.

refined grain: a product from which the bran, germ, and husk have been removed, leaving only the endosperm.

fortification: the addition to a food of nutrients that were either not originally present or present in insignificant amounts. Fortification can be used to correct or prevent a widespread nutrient deficiency, to balance the total nutrient profile of a food, or to restore nutrients lost in processing.

enrichment: the addition to a food of nutrients to meet a specified standard. In the case of refined bread or cereal, five nutrients have been added: thiamin, riboflavin, niacin, and folate in amounts approximately equivalent to, or higher than, those originally present and iron in amounts to alleviate the prevalence of iron-deficiency anemia.

Nutritious foods such as pork, legumes, sunflower seeds, and enriched and whole-grain breads are valuable sources of thiamin.

© Polara Studios, Inc.

Milk and milk products supply much (about 50 percent) of the riboflavin in people's diets, but meats, eggs, green vegetables, and enriched and whole-grain breads and cereals are good sources, too.

+ Thiamin RDA:
- Men: 1.2 mg/day
- Women: 1.1 mg/day

+ Riboflavin RDA:
- Men: 1.3 mg/day
- Women: 1.1 mg/day

niacin equivalents (NE): the amount of niacin present in food, including the niacin that can theoretically be made from tryptophan, its precursor, present in the food.

Niacin-rich foods include meat, fish, poultry, and peanut butter, as well as enriched breads and cereals and a few vegetables.

day, assuming that each serving will contribute, on the average, about 10 percent of needs. (**+**) Foods chosen from the bread and cereal group should be either whole grain or enriched. Thiamin is not stored in the body to any great extent, so daily intake is important.

RIBOFLAVIN

Like thiamin, riboflavin facilitates energy metabolism in the body. The needs of infants, children, and pregnant women rise rapidly during periods of active growth.

Riboflavin Deficiency and Toxicity
When thiamin is deficient, riboflavin may be lacking too, but its deficiency symptoms, such as cracks at the corners of the mouth and sore throat, may go undetected because those of thiamin are more severe. A diet that remedies riboflavin deficiency invariably contains some thiamin and so clears up both deficiencies. Excesses of riboflavin appear to cause no harm, and no UL has been established.

Riboflavin in Foods
Unlike thiamin, riboflavin is not evenly distributed among the food groups. (**+**) The major contributors of riboflavin to people's diets are milk and milk products, followed by enriched breads, cereals, and other grain products. Green vegetables (broccoli, turnip greens, asparagus, and spinach) and meats are also contributors. The riboflavin richness of milk and milk products is a good reason to include these foods in every day's meals. No other commonly eaten food can make such a substantial contribution. People who omit milk and milk products from their diets can substitute generous servings of dark green, leafy vegetables. Among the meats, liver and heart are the richest sources, but all lean meats, as well as eggs, offer some riboflavin.

Effects of Light
Riboflavin is light sensitive; the ultraviolet rays of the sun or of fluorescent lamps can destroy it, as can irradiation. For this reason, milk is often sold in cardboard or opaque plastic containers to protect the riboflavin in the milk from light. In contrast, riboflavin is heat stable, so ordinary cooking does not destroy it.

NIACIN

Like thiamin and riboflavin, niacin participates in the energy metabolism of every body cell. Niacin is unique among the B vitamins in that the body can make it from protein. The amino acid tryptophan can be converted to niacin in the body: 60 milligrams of tryptophan yield 1 milligram of niacin. Recommended intakes are therefore stated in **niacin equivalents (NE)**, (**+**) reflecting the body's ability to convert tryptophan to niacin. (**+**)

Naturally occurring niacin from foods causes no harm. Certain forms of niacin supplements taken in doses three to four times the dietary recommendation or larger cause "niacin flush," a dilation of the capillaries of the skin with perceptible tingling that, if intense, can be painful. The Tolerable Upper Intake Level (35 milligrams NE) is based on flushing as the critical adverse effect.

Niacin Used as a Medication
Physicians sometimes use diet and large doses of a form of niacin (nicotinic acid) to lower blood cholesterol in the treatment of atherosclerosis. (**+**) When used this way, niacin leaves the realm of nutrition to become a pharmacological agent, a drug. As with any medication, self-dosing with niacin is ill advised; large doses may injure the liver and produce some symptoms of diabetes.[59]

Niacin in Foods
Meat, poultry, fish, legumes, and enriched and whole grains contribute about half the niacin equivalents most people consume. Among the vegetables, mushrooms, asparagus, and potatoes are the richest niacin sources. Niacin is less vulnerable to losses during food preparation and storage than other water-soluble vitamins. Being fairly heat resistant, niacin can withstand reasonable cooking times, but like other water-soluble vitamins, it will leach into cooking water.

PANTOTHENIC ACID AND BIOTIN

Two other B vitamins—pantothenic acid and biotin—are also important in energy metabolism. Pantothenic acid was first recognized as a substance that stimulates growth. It is a component of a key enzyme that makes possible the release of energy from the energy nutrients. Pantothenic acid is involved in more than 100 different steps in the synthesis of lipids, neurotransmitters, steroid hormones, and hemoglobin. Biotin plays an important role in metabolism as a coenzyme that carries carbon dioxide. Emerging evidence indicates that biotin participates in other processes such as gene expression and cell signaling and in the structure of DNA-binding proteins in the cell nucleus.[60]

Pantothenic Acid and Biotin in Foods Both pantothenic acid (✚) and biotin (✚) are more widespread in foods than the other vitamins discussed so far. There seems to be no danger that people who consume a variety of foods will suffer deficiencies. Claims that pantothenic acid and biotin are needed in pill form to prevent or cure disease conditions are at best unfounded and at worst intentionally misleading.

Biotin Deficiency Biotin deficiencies are rare but have been reported in adults fed artificially by vein without biotin supplementation. Researchers can induce biotin deficiency in animals or human beings by feeding them raw egg whites, which contain a protein that binds biotin and prevents its absorption. (✚)

VITAMIN B$_6$

A surge of recent research interest in vitamin B$_6$ has not only revealed new knowledge but has also raised new questions. For example, unlike the other water-soluble vitamins, vitamin B$_6$ is stored extensively in muscle tissue. Most recently, research interest has centered on a possible role for vitamin B$_6$ in the treatment of disease.[61]

Metabolic Roles of Vitamin B$_6$ Vitamin B$_6$ has long been known to play roles in protein and amino acid metabolism. In the cells, vitamin B$_6$ helps convert one kind of amino acid, which the cells have in abundance, to other nonessential amino acids that the cells lack. It also aids in the conversion of the amino acid tryptophan to niacin and plays important roles in the synthesis of hemoglobin and neurotransmitters, the communication molecules of the brain. Vitamin B$_6$ also assists in releasing stored glucose from glycogen and thus contributes to the regulation of blood glucose. Research suggests roles for vitamin B$_6$ in immune function, cognitive performance, and hormone response.[62] The association between vitamin B$_6$ and immune function is related to the critical role the vitamin plays in protein metabolism. Vitamin B$_6$ deficiency can significantly impair the immune response, perhaps by way of impaired antibody production.

Vitamin B$_6$ status may be related to cardiovascular disease risk. Elevated blood levels of the amino acid homocysteine correlate with a high incidence of heart disease.[63] Evidence suggests that low blood concentrations of vitamin B$_6$, vitamin B$_{12}$, and folate are associated with elevated homocysteine concentrations.[64] The missing link, however, is how, or even whether, a deficiency of B vitamins or elevated homocysteine directly affects processes leading to heart disease.[65]

Vitamin B$_6$ Deficiency Besides a weakening immune response, vitamin B$_6$ deficiency is expressed in general symptoms, such as weakness, depression, confusion, and irritability. Other symptoms include a greasy, flaky dermatitis; anemia; and, in advanced cases, convulsions.

Vitamin B$_6$ Toxicity For years it was believed that vitamin B$_6$, like other water-soluble vitamins, could not reach toxic concentrations in the body. Toxic effects of vitamin B$_6$ became known when a physician reported them in women who had been taking more than 2 *grams* of vitamin B$_6$ daily (20 times the current UL of 100 *milligrams*) for two months or more, attempting to cure premenstrual syndrome. The first symptom of toxicity was numb feet; then the women lost sensation in their hands; then they became unable to walk. The women recovered after they discontinued the supplements.

✚ A food containing 1 mg of niacin and 60 mg of tryptophan contains the niacin equivalent of 2 mg, or 2 mg NE.

✚ Niacin RDA:
- Men: 16 mg NE/day
- Women: 14 mg NE/day

✚ When a normal dose of a nutrient clears up a deficiency condition, the effect is a *physiological* one. When a large dose of a nutrient overwhelms a body system and acts like a drug, the effect is a *pharmacological* one.

✚ Pantothenic acid AI:
- Adults: 5 mg/day

✚ Biotin AI:
- Adults: 30 µg/day

✚ The protein *avidin* in egg whites binds biotin.

Most protein-rich foods such as meat, fish, and poultry provide ample vitamin B$_6$; some vegetables and fruits are good sources too.

Vitamin B$_6$ Recommendations Because vitamin B$_6$ coenzymes play many roles in amino acid metabolism, previous RDA were expressed in terms of protein intakes; the current RDA (✚) for vitamin B$_6$, however, is not. Research does not support claims that large doses of vitamin B$_6$ enhance muscle strength or physical endurance.

Vitamin B$_6$ in Foods The richest food sources of vitamin B$_6$ are protein-rich meat, fish, and poultry. Potatoes, a few other vegetables, and some fruits are good sources, too. Foods lose vitamin B$_6$ when heated.

FOLATE

The B vitamin folate is active in cell division. During periods of rapid growth and cell division, such as pregnancy and adolescence, folate needs increase, and deficiency is especially likely. When a deficiency occurs, the replacement of the rapidly dividing cells of the blood and the GI tract falters. Not surprisingly, then, two of the first symptoms of a folate deficiency are a type of anemia and GI tract deterioration (see Table 8-4).

Folate, Alcohol, and Drugs Of all the vitamins, folate appears to be the most vulnerable to interactions with alcohol and other drugs.[66] As Nutrition in Practice 19 describes, alcohol-addicted people risk folate deficiency because alcohol impairs folate's absorption and increases its excretion. Furthermore, as people's alcohol intakes rise, their folate intakes decline. Many medications, including aspirin, oral contraceptives, and anticonvulsants, also impair folate status. Smoking exerts a negative effect on folate status as well.

Folate and Neural Tube Defects Research studies confirm the importance of folate in preventing **neural tube defects (NTD)**. (✚) The brain and spinal cord develop from the neural tube, and defects in its orderly formation during the early weeks of pregnancy may result in various central nervous system disorders and death. Folate supplements taken before conception and continued throughout the first trimester of pregnancy can prevent NTD. For this reason, all women of childbearing age who are capable of becoming pregnant should consume 400 micrograms (0.4 milligrams) of folate daily from supplements, fortified foods, or both, *in addition* to eating folate-rich foods.

Folate status improves more with supplementation or fortification than with a dietary intake that meets recommendations. (✚) Neural tube defects arise early in pregnancy before most women realize they are pregnant, and most women eat too few fruits and vegetables to supply even half the folate needed to prevent NTD.[67] For these reasons, the FDA mandated that enriched grain products (flour, cornmeal, pasta, and rice) be fortified with an especially absorbable synthetic form of folate, folic acid. (✚)

Fortification has improved folate status in women of childbearing age and lowered the number of neural tube defects that occur each year.[68] Folate fortification also raises safety concerns, however. High doses of folate can complicate the diagnosis of vitamin B$_{12}$ deficiency, as discussed later. Other suspected but unconfirmed potential harms from high blood folic acid levels include suppression of normal immune functioning and increased cancer risks.[69] The DRI committee set a Tolerable Upper Intake Level of 1000 micrograms per day from fortified foods or supplements. Except for individuals who take supplements with more than 400 micrograms of folic acid, few people (less than 3 percent of the U.S. population) exceed the Tolerable Upper Intake Level for folic acid.[70] Thus, researchers conclude that the current level of fortification of the food supply appears to be safe.

Folate in Foods As Snapshot 8-2 shows, the best food sources of folate are liver, legumes, beets, and leafy green vegetables (the vitamin's name suggests the word *foliage*). Among the fruits, oranges, orange juice, and cantaloupe are the best sources. With fortification, grain products are good sources of folate, too. Heat and oxidation during cooking and storage can destroy up to half of the folate in foods.

✚ Vitamin B$_6$ RDA:
• Adults (19–50): 1.3 mg/day

✚ The two main types of neural tube defects are *spina bifida* (literally, "split spine") and *anencephaly* ("no brain"). Chapter 10 includes a figure of a neural tube defect and a discussion.

✚ Folate RDA:
• Adults: 400 µg/day

✚ Bread products, flour, corn grits, and pasta must be fortified with 140 µg per 100 g of food (about ½ c cooked food or 1 slice of bread).

neural tube defects (NTD): malformations of the brain, spinal cord, or both that occur during embryonic development.

Folate is expressed in terms of dietary folate equivalents (DFE) because synthetic folate from supplements and fortified foods is absorbed at almost twice (1.7 times) the rate of naturally occurring folate from other foods. Use the following equation to calculate:

$$DFE = \mu g \text{ food folate} + (1.7 \times \mu g \text{ synthetic folate})$$

Consider, for example, a pregnant woman who takes a supplement and eats a bowl of fortified corn flakes, two slices of fortified bread, and one cup of fortified pasta. From the supplement and fortified foods, she obtains synthetic folate:

Supplement	100 µg folate
Fortified corn flakes	100 µg folate
Fortified bread	40 µg folate
Fortified pasta	60 µg folate
	300 µg folate

To calculate the DFE, multiply the amount of synthetic folate by 1.7:

$$300 \text{ µg} \times 1.7 = 510 \text{ µg DFE}$$

Now add the naturally occurring folate from the other foods in her diet—in this example, another 90 micrograms of folate.

$$510 \text{ µg DFE} + 90 \text{ µg} = 600 \text{ µg DFE}$$

Notice that if we had not converted synthetic folate from supplements and fortified foods to DFE, this woman's intake would appear to fall short of the 600 micrograms recommended for pregnancy (300 µg + 90 µg = 390 µg). But as this example shows, her intake does meet the recommendation. At this time, supplement and fortified food labels list folate in micrograms only, not micrograms DFE, making such calculations necessary.

The difference in absorption between naturally occurring food folate and synthetic folate that enriches foods and is added to supplements necessitated a new unit of measurement for folate: the **dietary folate equivalents**, or **DFE**. The DFE convert all forms of folate into units that are equivalent to the folate in foods. Most food labels and tables of food composition express folate values in micrograms, however, so the accompanying "How to" describes how to estimate dietary folate equivalents.

dietary folate equivalents (DFE): the amount of folate available to the body from naturally occurring sources, fortified foods, and supplements, accounting for differences in bioavailability from each source.

VITAMIN B$_{12}$

Vitamin B$_{12}$ and folate share a special relationship: vitamin B$_{12}$ assists folate in cell division. Their roles intertwine, but each performs a specific task that the other cannot accomplish.

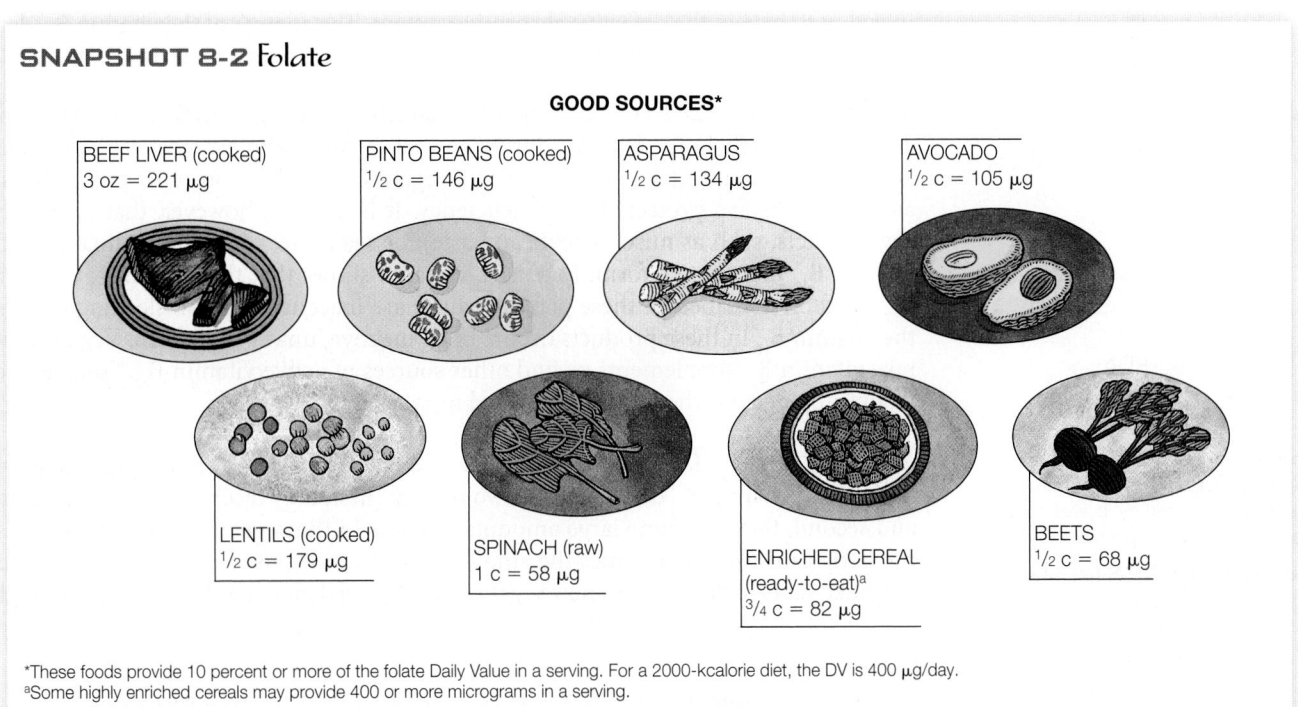

SNAPSHOT 8-2 Folate

GOOD SOURCES*

BEEF LIVER (cooked)
3 oz = 221 µg

PINTO BEANS (cooked)
½ c = 146 µg

ASPARAGUS
½ c = 134 µg

AVOCADO
½ c = 105 µg

LENTILS (cooked)
½ c = 179 µg

SPINACH (raw)
1 c = 58 µg

ENRICHED CEREAL
(ready-to-eat)[a]
¾ c = 82 µg

BEETS
½ c = 68 µg

*These foods provide 10 percent or more of the folate Daily Value in a serving. For a 2000-kcalorie diet, the DV is 400 µg/day.
[a]Some highly enriched cereals may provide 400 or more micrograms in a serving.

Vitamin B$_{12}$, Folate, and Cell Division

Vitamin B$_{12}$ (in coenzyme form) stands by to accept carbon groups from folate as folate removes them from other compounds. The passing of these carbon groups from folate to vitamin B$_{12}$ regenerates the active form of folate so that it can continue its dismantling tasks. In the absence of vitamin B$_{12}$, folate is trapped in its inactive, metabolically useless form, unable to do its job. When folate is either trapped due to a vitamin B$_{12}$ deficiency or unavailable due to a deficiency of folate itself, cells that are growing most rapidly—notably, the blood cells—are the first to be affected. Thus, a deficiency of either nutrient—vitamin B$_{12}$ or folate—impairs maturation of the blood cells and produces anemia. The anemia is identifiable by microscopic examination of the blood, which reveals many large, immature red blood cells. (✚) Either vitamin B$_{12}$ or folate will clear up the anemia.

Vitamin B$_{12}$ and the Nervous System

Although either vitamin will clear up the anemia caused by vitamin B$_{12}$ deficiency, if folate is given when vitamin B$_{12}$ is needed, the result is disastrous, not to the blood but to the nervous system. The reason: vitamin B$_{12}$ also helps maintain nerve fibers. A vitamin B$_{12}$ deficiency can ultimately result in devastating neurological symptoms, undetectable by a blood test. A deceptive folate "cure" of the anemia in vitamin B$_{12}$ deficiency allows the nerve deterioration to progress, leading to paralysis and permanent nerve damage. This interaction between folate and vitamin B$_{12}$ raises safety concerns about the use of folate supplements and fortification of foods.[71] In an effort to prevent excessive folate intakes that could mask symptoms of a vitamin B$_{12}$ deficiency, the FDA specifies the exact amounts of folic acid that can be added to enriched foods.

The way folate masks vitamin B$_{12}$ deficiency underlines a point already made several times: it takes a skilled diagnostician to make a correct diagnosis. A person who self-diagnoses on the basis of a single observed symptom takes a serious risk.

Vitamin B$_{12}$ Absorption

Absorption of vitamin B$_{12}$ requires an **intrinsic factor**, a compound made by the stomach with instructions from the genes. With the help of the stomach's acid to liberate vitamin B$_{12}$ from the food proteins that bind it, intrinsic factor attaches to the vitamin and the complex is absorbed into the bloodstream.

A few people have an inherited defect in the gene for intrinsic factor, which makes vitamin B$_{12}$ absorption abnormal, beginning in mid-adulthood. In later years, many others lose the ability to produce enough stomach acid and intrinsic factor to allow efficient absorption of vitamin B$_{12}$.[72] * In these cases, vitamin B$_{12}$ must be supplied by injection to bypass the defective absorptive system. The anemia of the vitamin B$_{12}$ deficiency caused by lack of intrinsic factor is known as **pernicious anemia**.

Vitamin B$_{12}$ in Foods

A unique characteristic of vitamin B$_{12}$ is that it is found almost exclusively in foods derived from animals. People who eat meat are guaranteed an adequate intake, (✚) and lacto-ovo vegetarians (who consume milk, cheese, and eggs) are also protected from deficiency. It is a myth, however, that fermented soy products, such as miso (a soybean paste), or sea algae, such as spirulina, provide vitamin B$_{12}$ in its active form. Extensive research shows that the amounts of vitamin B$_{12}$ listed on the labels of these plant products are inaccurate and misleading because the vitamin B$_{12}$ in these products occurs in an inactive, unavailable form. Vegans must take vitamin B$_{12}$ supplements or find other sources of active vitamin B$_{12}$. Some loss of vitamin B$_{12}$ occurs when foods are heated in microwave ovens.

Vitamin B$_{12}$ Deficiency in Vegans

Vegans are at special risk for undetected vitamin B$_{12}$ deficiency for two reasons: first, they receive none in their diets, and second, they consume large amounts of folate in the vegetables they eat. Because the body can store many times the amount of vitamin B$_{12}$ used each day, a deficiency may take years to develop in a new vegetarian. When a deficiency does develop, though,

---

✚ Large-cell anemia is known as *macrocytic* or *megaloblastic* anemia.

> *macro* = large
> *cyte* = cell
> *mega* = large
> *blast* = immature cell

✚ Vitamin B$_{12}$ RDA:
• Adults: 2.4 μg/day

intrinsic factor: inside the system. Anemia that reflects a vitamin B$_{12}$ deficiency caused by lack of intrinsic factor is known as *pernicious anemia.*

pernicious (per-NISH-us) anemia: a vitamin B$_{12}$–deficiency disease caused by lack of intrinsic factor and characterized by large, immature red blood cells and damage to the nervous system (*pernicious* means "highly injurious or destructive").

---

*The condition is atrophic gastritis (a-TROH-fik gas-TRY-tis), a chronic inflammation of the stomach accompanied by a diminished size and functioning of the stomach's mucous membrane and glands.

it may progress to a dangerous extreme because the deficiency of vitamin B$_{12}$ may be masked by the high folate intake.

Worldwide, vitamin B$_{12}$ deficiency among vegetarians is a growing problem.[73] A pregnant or lactating vegetarian woman who eats no foods of animal origin should be aware that her infant can develop a vitamin B$_{12}$ deficiency, even if the mother appears healthy. Breastfed infants born to vegan mothers with low concentrations of vitamin B$_{12}$ in their breast milk can develop severe neurological symptoms such as seizures and cognitive problems.[74]

NON–B VITAMINS

Other compounds are sometimes inappropriately called B vitamins because, like the true B vitamins, they serve as coenzymes in metabolism. Even if they were essential, however, supplements would be unnecessary because these compounds are abundant in foods.

Inositol, Choline, and Carnitine
Among the non–B vitamins are a trio of substances known as inositol, choline, and carnitine. Researchers are exploring the possibility that these substances may be essential. Thus far, only choline has been assigned an Adequate Intake value. ()

Other Non–B Vitamins
Other substances have also been mistaken for essential nutrients. They include para-aminobenzoic acid (PABA), bioflavonoids (vitamin P or hesperidin), and ubiquinone. Other names you may hear are "vitamin B$_{15}$" (a hoax) and "vitamin B$_{17}$" (laetrile, a fake cancer-curing drug and not a vitamin by any stretch of the imagination). There is, however, one other water-soluble vitamin of great interest and importance—vitamin C.

VITAMIN C

Three hundred and sixty years ago, any man who joined the crew of a seagoing ship knew he had only half a chance of returning alive—not because he might be slain by pirates or die in a storm, but because he might contract the dread disease **scurvy**. Then, a physician with the British navy found that citrus fruits could cure the disease, and thereafter, all ships were required to carry lime juice for every sailor. (This is why British sailors are still called "limeys" today.) In the 1930s, the antiscurvy factor in citrus fruits was isolated from lemon juice and named **ascorbic acid**. Today, hundreds of millions of vitamin C pills are produced in pharmaceutical laboratories.

Metabolic Roles of Vitamin C
Vitamin C's action defies a simple, tidy description. It plays many important roles in the body, and its modes of action differ in different situations.

Vitamin C's Role in Collagen Formation
The best-understood action of vitamin C is its role in helping to form **collagen**, the single most important protein of connective tissue. Collagen serves as the matrix on which bone is formed, the material of scars, and an important part of the "glue" that attaches one cell to another. This latter function is especially important in the artery walls, which must expand and contract with each beat of the heart, and in the walls of the capillaries, which are thin and fragile. Vitamin C also plays a role in the production of carnitine, important for transporting fatty acids within cells.

Vitamin C as an Antioxidant
Vitamin C is also an important antioxidant. Recall that the antioxidants beta-carotene and vitamin E protect fat-soluble substances from oxidizing agents; vitamin C protects water-soluble substances the same way. By being oxidized itself, vitamin C regenerates already-oxidized substances such as iron and copper to their original, active form. In the intestines, it protects iron from oxidation and so enhances iron absorption. In the cells and body fluids, it helps to protect other molecules, including the fat-soluble compounds vitamin A, vitamin E, and the polyunsaturated fatty acids.

Choline AI:
- Men: 550 mg/day
- Women: 425 mg/day

scurvy: the vitamin C–deficiency disease.

ascorbic acid: one of the two active forms of vitamin C. Many people refer to vitamin C by this name.
a = without
scorbic = having scurvy

collagen: the characteristic protein of connective tissue.
kolla = glue
gennan = produce

Vitamin C in Amino Acid Metabolism

Vitamin C is also involved in the metabolism of several amino acids. Some of these amino acids end up being used to make substances of great importance in body functioning, among them the neurotransmitter norepinephrine and the hormone thyroxine.

Role of Stress

During stress, the adrenal glands release large quantities of vitamin C together with the stress hormones epinephrine and norepinephrine. The vitamin's exact role in the stress reaction remains unclear, but physical stresses (described in a later section) raise vitamin C needs.

Vitamin C as a Possible Antihistamine

Newspaper headlines touting vitamin C as a cure for colds and cancer have appeared frequently over the years. Some research suggests that vitamin C (2 grams per day for two weeks) may reduce the severity and duration of cold and allergy symptoms by reducing blood histamine concentrations. In other words, vitamin C acts as an antihistamine. If further research confirms vitamin C's antihistamine effect, its use may permit people to rely less heavily on antihistamine drugs when suffering from cold and allergy symptoms.

Vitamin C's Role in Cancer Prevention and Treatment

The role of vitamin C in the prevention and treatment of cancer is still being studied. Evidence to date indicates that foods containing vitamin C probably protect against cancer of the esophagus.[75] The correlation may reflect not just an association with vitamin C but the broader benefits of a diet rich in fruits and vegetables and low in fat. It does not support the taking of vitamin C supplements to prevent or treat cancer.

Vitamin C Deficiency

When intake of vitamin C is inadequate, the body's vitamin C pool dwindles, and **latent** scurvy appears. The blood vessels show the first deficiency signs. The gums around the teeth begin to bleed easily, and capillaries under the skin break spontaneously, producing pinpoint hemorrhages. Then the symptoms of **overt** scurvy appear. Muscles, including the heart muscle, may degenerate. The skin becomes rough, brown, scaly, and dry. Wounds fail to heal because scar tissue will not form without collagen. Bone rebuilding falters; the ends of the long bones become softened, malformed, and painful; and fractures occur. The teeth may become loose in the jawbone and fall out. Anemia and infections are common. Sudden death is likely, perhaps because of massive bleeding into the joints and body cavities.

It takes only 10 or so milligrams of vitamin C a day to prevent overt scurvy, and not much more than that to cure it. Once diagnosed, scurvy is readily reversible with moderate doses, in the neighborhood of 100 milligrams per day. Such an intake is easily achieved by including vitamin C–rich foods in the diet.

Vitamin C Toxicity

The easy availability of vitamin C in pill form and the publication of books recommending vitamin C to prevent everything from the common cold to life-threatening cancer have led thousands of people to take megadoses of vitamin C. (✚) Not surprisingly, instances of vitamin C causing harm have surfaced.

Some of the suspected toxic effects of vitamin C megadoses have not been confirmed, but others have been seen often enough to warrant concern. Nausea, abdominal cramps, and diarrhea are often reported. Several instances of interference with medical regimens are known. Large amounts of vitamin C excreted in the urine obscure the results of tests used to detect diabetes. People taking anticoagulants (✚) may unwittingly counteract the effect of these medications if they also take massive doses of vitamin C. Vitamin C megadoses can also enhance iron absorption too much, resulting in iron overload (see Chapter 9).

People with sickle-cell anemia may be especially vulnerable to megadoses of vitamin C. Those who have a tendency toward **gout**, as well as those who have a genetic abnormality that alters the way they metabolize vitamin C, are more prone to forming kidney stones if they take megadoses of vitamin C.

✚ Doses of 10 to 30 or more times the recommended intake of a nutrient are termed *megadoses*. In the case of vitamin C, current recommendations are 75 mg/day for women and 90 mg/day for men. The Tolerable Upper Intake Level for vitamin C is 2000 mg/day.

✚ The anticoagulants with which vitamin C interferes are warfarin and dicumarol.

latent: the period in the course of a disease when the condition is present but the symptoms have not begun to appear.
latens = lying hidden

overt: out in the open, full blown.
ouvrire = to open

gout (GOWT): a metabolic disease in which crystals of uric acid precipitate in the joints.

Recommended Intakes of Vitamin C The vitamin C RDA is 90 milligrams for men and 75 milligrams for women. These amounts are far higher than the 10 milligrams per day needed to prevent the symptoms of scurvy. In fact, they are close to the amount at which the body's pool of vitamin C is full to overflowing: about 100 milligrams per day.

Special Needs for Vitamin C As is true of all nutrients, unusual circumstances may raise vitamin C needs. Among the stresses known to do so are infections; burns; surgery; extremely high or low temperatures; toxic doses of heavy metals, such as lead, mercury, and cadmium; and the chronic use of certain medications, including aspirin, barbiturates, and oral contraceptives. Smoking, too, has adverse effects on vitamin C status. Cigarette smoke contains oxidants, which deplete this potent antioxidant. Accordingly, the vitamin C recommendation for smokers is set high, at 125 milligrams for men and 105 milligrams for women.

Safe Limits Few instances warrant the taking of more than 100 to 300 milligrams of vitamin C a day. The risks may not be great for adults who dose themselves with 1 to 2 grams a day, but those taking more than 2 grams, and especially those taking above 3 grams per day, should be aware of the distinct possibility of harm.[76]

Vitamin C in Foods The inclusion of intelligently selected fruits and vegetables in the daily diet guarantees a generous intake of vitamin C. Even those who wish to ingest amounts well above the RDA can easily meet their goals by eating certain foods (see Snapshot 8-3). Citrus fruits are rightly famous for their vitamin C contents. Certain other fruits and vegetables are also rich sources: cantaloupe, strawberries, broccoli, and brussels sprouts. No animal foods other than organ meats, such as chicken liver and kidneys, contain vitamin C. The humble potato is an important source of vitamin C in Western countries, where potatoes are eaten so frequently that they make substantial vitamin C contributions overall. They provide about 20 percent of all the vitamin C in the average diet. Vitamin C in foods is easily oxidized, so store cut produce and juices in airtight containers.

SNAPSHOT 8-3 *Vitamin C*

GOOD SOURCES*

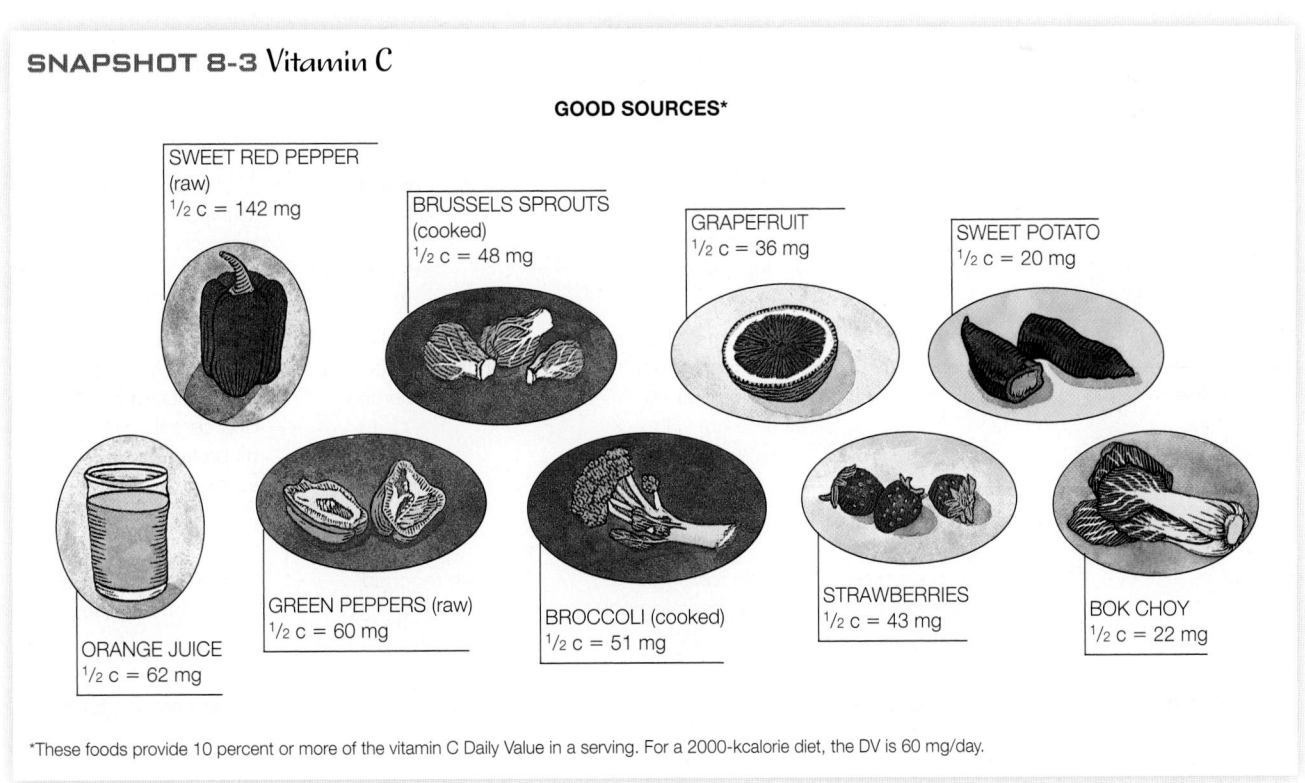

SWEET RED PEPPER (raw)
1/2 c = 142 mg

BRUSSELS SPROUTS (cooked)
1/2 c = 48 mg

GRAPEFRUIT
1/2 c = 36 mg

SWEET POTATO
1/2 c = 20 mg

ORANGE JUICE
1/2 c = 62 mg

GREEN PEPPERS (raw)
1/2 c = 60 mg

BROCCOLI (cooked)
1/2 c = 51 mg

STRAWBERRIES
1/2 c = 43 mg

BOK CHOY
1/2 c = 22 mg

*These foods provide 10 percent or more of the vitamin C Daily Value in a serving. For a 2000-kcalorie diet, the DV is 60 mg/day.

Iron is discussed in Chapter 9.

Vitamin C and Iron Absorption Eating foods containing vitamin C at the same meal with foods containing iron can double or triple the absorption of iron from those foods. (✚) This strategy is highly recommended for women and children, whose energy intakes are not large enough to guarantee that they will get enough iron from the foods they eat.

Review Notes

- The B vitamins and vitamin C are the water-soluble vitamins.
- Each B vitamin is part of an enzyme helper known as a coenzyme.
- As parts of coenzymes, the B vitamins assist in the release of energy from glucose, amino acids, and fats and help in many other body processes.
- Folate and vitamin B_{12} are important in cell division.
- Vitamin C's primary role is as an antioxidant.
- Historically, famous B vitamin–deficiency diseases are beriberi (thiamin) and pellagra (niacin). The vitamin C–deficiency disease is known as scurvy.

Table 8-4 summarizes functions, deficiency and toxicity symptoms, and food sources of the water-soluble vitamins.

TABLE 8-4 | The Water-Soluble Vitamins—A Summary

Vitamin Name	Chief Functions	Deficiency Symptoms	Toxicity Symptoms	Significant Sources
Thiamin (Vitamin B_1)	Part of a coenzyme used in energy metabolism	Beriberi (edema or muscle wasting), anorexia and weight loss, neurological disturbances, muscular weakness, heart enlargement and failure	None reported	Enriched, fortified, or whole-grain products; pork
Riboflavin (Vitamin B_2)	Part of coenzymes used in energy metabolism	Inflammation of the mouth, skin, and eyelids; sensitivity to light; sore throat	None reported	Milk products; enriched, fortified, or whole-grain products; liver
Niacin (Nicotinic acid, nicotinamide, niacinamide, vitamin B_3; precursor is dietary tryptophan, an amino acid)	Part of coenzymes used in energy metabolism	Pellagra (diarrhea, dermatitis, and dementia)	Niacin flush, liver damage, impaired glucose tolerance	Milk, eggs, meat, poultry, fish, whole-grain and enriched breads and cereals, nuts, and all protein-containing foods
Biotin	Part of a coenzyme used in energy metabolism	Skin rash, hair loss, neurological disturbances	None reported	Widespread in foods; GI bacteria synthesis
Pantothenic acid	Part of a coenzyme used in energy metabolism	Digestive and neurological disturbances	None reported	Widespread in foods

Vitamin	Chief Functions	Deficiency Symptoms	Toxicity Symptoms	Significant Sources
Vitamin B₆ (Pyridoxine, pyridoxal, pyridoxamine)	Part of coenzymes used in amino acid and fatty acid metabolism	Scaly dermatitis, depression, confusion, convulsions, anemia	Nerve degeneration, skin lesions	Meats, fish, poultry, potatoes, legumes, noncitrus fruits, fortified cereals, liver, soy products
Folate (Folic acid, folacin, pteroylglutamic acid)	Activates vitamin B₁₂; helps synthesize DNA for new cell growth	Anemia; smooth, red tongue; mental confusion; elevated homocysteine	Masks vitamin B₁₂ deficiency	Fortified grains, leafy green vegetables, legumes, seeds, liver
Vitamin B₁₂ (Cobalamin)	Activates folate; helps synthesize DNA for new cell growth; protects nerve cells	Anemia; nerve damage and paralysis	None reported	Foods derived from animals (meat, fish, poultry, shellfish, milk, cheese, eggs), fortified cereals
Vitamin C (Ascorbic acid)	Synthesis of collagen, carnitine, hormones, neurotransmitters; antioxidant	Scurvy (bleeding gums, pinpoint hemorrhages, abnormal bone growth, and joint pain)	Diarrhea, GI distress	Citrus fruits, cabbage-type vegetables, dark green vegetables (such as bell peppers and broccoli), cantaloupe, strawberries, lettuce, tomatoes, potatoes, papayas, mangoes

Self Check

1 • Which of the following vitamins are fat soluble?
   a. Vitamins B, C, and E
   b. Vitamins B, C, D, and E
   c. Vitamins A, C, E, and K
   d. Vitamins A, D, E, and K.

2 • Which of the following describes fat-soluble vitamins?
   a. They include thiamin, vitamin A, and vitamin K.
   b. They cannot be stored to any great extent and so must be consumed daily.
   c. Toxic levels can be reached by consuming citrus fruits and vegetables.
   d. They can be stored in the liver and fatty tissues and can build up toxic concentrations.

3 • Night blindness and susceptibility to infection are the result of a deficiency of which vitamin?
   a. Niacin
   b. Vitamin C
   c. Vitamin A
   d. Vitamin K

4 • Good sources of vitamin D include:
   a. eggs, fortified milk, and sunlight.
   b. citrus fruits, sweet potatoes, and spinach.
   c. leafy, green vegetables; cabbage; and liver.
   d. breast milk, polyunsaturated plant oils, and citrus fruits.

5 • Which of the following describes water-soluble vitamins?
   a. They include vitamins D and E.
   b. They are frequently toxic.
   c. They are stored extensively in tissues.
   d. They are easily absorbed and excreted.

6 • A coenzyme is:
   a. a fat-soluble vitamin.
   b. an energy-yielding nutrient.
   c. a source of vitamin K.
   d. a molecule that combines with an enzyme to make it active.

7 • Good food sources of folate include:
   a. citrus fruits, dairy products, and eggs.
   b. liver; legumes; and leafy, green vegetables.
   c. dark green vegetables, corn, and cabbage.
   d. potatoes, broccoli, and whole-wheat bread.

8 • Which vitamin is present only in foods of animal origin?

    a. Riboflavin

    b. Pantothenic acid

    c. Vitamin B_{12}

    d. The inactive form of vitamin A

9 • Which of the following nutrients is an antioxidant that protects water-soluble substances from oxidizing agents?

    a. Beta-carotene

    b. Thiamin

    c. Vitamin C

    d. Vitamin D

10 • Eating foods containing vitamin C at the same meal can increase the absorption of which mineral?

    a. Iron

    b. Calcium

    c. Magnesium

    d. Folate

Answers to these questions appear in Appendix H.

Clinical Applications

1 • How might a vitamin deficiency weaken a client's resistance to disease?

2 • Pull together information from Chapter 1 about the different food groups and the significant sources of vitamins shown in the photos and snapshots throughout this chapter. Consider which vitamins might be lacking in the diet of a client who reports the following:

- Dislikes leafy, green vegetables
- Never uses milk, milk products, or cheese
- Follows a very low-fat diet
- Eats a fruit or vegetable once a day

What additional information would help you pinpoint problems with vitamin intake?

Nutrition on the Net

For further study of the topics in this chapter, access these websites. Be aware that many websites on the Internet are peddling vitamin supplements, not accurate information.

- Find updates and quick links to these and other nutrition-related sites at our website: www.cengage.com/nutrition/whitney/nhhc4e

- Search for "vitamins" at the American Dietetic Association: www.eatright.org

- Visit the World Health Organization to learn about "vitamin deficiencies" around the world: www.who.int

- Search for "vitamins" at the U.S. government health information site: www.healthfinder.gov

- Learn more about neural tube defects from the Spina Bifida Association of America: www.sbaa.org

- Read about Dr. Joseph Goldberger and his groundbreaking discovery linking pellagra to diet by searching for his name at: www.nih.gov or www.pbs.org

- Learn how fruits and vegetables support a healthy diet rich in vitamins from the Fruits & Veggies: More Matters program: www.fruitsandveggiesmorematters.gov

Notes

1. S. M. Ahmad and coauthors, Markers of innate immune function are associated with vitamin A stores in men, *Journal of Nutrition* 139 (2009): 377–385; M. A. Marzinke and coauthors, Calmin expression in embryos and the adult brain, and its regulation by all-trans retinoic acid, *Developmental Dynamics* 239 (2009): 610–619; M. A. Muhit and coauthors, Causes of severe visual impairment and blindness in Bangladesh: A study of 1935 children, *British Journal of* *Ophthalmology* 91 (2007): 1000–1004; A. C. Ross, Vitamin A and carotenoids, in M. E. Shils and coeditors, *Modern Nutrition in Health and Disease*, 10th ed. (Philadelphia: Lippincott, Williams, & Wilkins, 2006), pp. 351–375.

2. R. Blomhoff and H. K. Blomhoff, Overview of retinoid metabolism and function, *Journal of Neurobiology* 66 (2006): 606–630.

3. Blomhoff and Blomhoff, 2006.

4. G. Wolf, Retinoic acid as cause of cell proliferation or cell growth inhibition depending on activation of one of two different nuclear receptors, *Nutrition Reviews* 66 (2008): 55–59.

5. Ahmad and coauthors, 2009; C. Trottier and coauthors, Retinoids inhibit measles virus through a type I IFN-dependent bystander effect, *FASEB Journal* 23 (2009): 3203–3212; K. Z. Long and coauthors, Impact of vitamin A on selected gastrointestinal pathogen infections and associated diarrheal episodes among children in Mexico City, Mexico, *Journal of Infectious Diseases* 194 (2006): 1217–1225.

6. C. Debier and Y. Larondelle, Vitamins A and E: Metabolism, roles, and transfer to offspring, *British Journal of Nutrition* 93 (2005): 153–174.

7. E. Herrera and coauthors, Aspects of antioxidant foods and supplements in health and disease, *Nutrition Reviews* 67 (2009): S140–S144; L. C. Yong and coauthors, High dietary antioxidant intakes are associated with decreased chromosome translocation frequency in airline pilots, *American Journal of Clinical Nutrition* 90 (2009): 1402–1410.

8. Herrera and coauthors, 2009; J. K. Shen and coauthors, Oxidative damage in age-related macular degeneration, *Histology and Histopathology* 12 (2007): 1301–1308.

9. D. R. Jacobs, M. D. Gross, and L. C. Tapsell, Food synergy: An operational concept for understanding nutrition, *American Journal of Clinical Nutrition* 89 (2009): 1543S–1548S.

10. A. Sommer, Vitamin A deficiency and clinical disease: An historical overview, *Journal of Nutrition* 138 (2008): 1835–1839.

11. World Health Organization, Micronutrient deficiencies: Vitamin A deficiency, available at www.who.int/topics/vat/en, accessed February 3, 2010; Standing Committee on the Scientific Evaluation of Dietary Reference Intakes, *Dietary Reference Intakes for Vitamin A, Vitamin D, Arsenic, Boron, Chromium, Copper, Iodine, Iron, Manganese, Molybdenum, Nickel, Silicon, Vanadium, and Zinc* (Washington, D.C.: National Academy Press, 2001), pp. 95–97.

12. S. A. Abrams and D. C. Hilmers, Postnatal vitamin A supplementation in developing countries: An intervention whose time has come? *Pediatrics* 122 (2008): 180–181; K. Kraemer and coauthors, Are low tolerable upper intake levels for vitamin A undermining effective food fortification efforts? *Nutrition Reviews* 66 (2008): 517–525.

13. World Health Organization, Measles, available at www.who.int/mediacentre/factsheets, accessed February 3, 2010.

14. A. Sheth, R. Khurana, and V. Khurana, Potential liver damage associated with over-the-counter vitamin supplements, *Journal of the American Dietetic Association* 108 (2008): 1536–1537; K. L. Penniston and S. A. Tanumihardjo, The acute and chronic toxic effects of vitamin A, *American Journal of Clinical Nutrition* 83 (2006): 191–201.

15. H. S. Lam and coauthors, Risk of vitamin A toxicity from candy-like chewable vitamin supplements for children, *Pediatrics* 118 (2006): 820–824.

16. Standing Committee on the Scientific Evaluation of Dietary Reference Intakes, 2001, pp. 128–129.

17. J. Zhao and coauthors, Retinoic acid downregulates microRNAs to induce abnormal development of spinal cord in spina bifida rat model, *Child's Nervous System* 24 (2008): 485–492.

18. Standing Committee on the Scientific Evaluation of Dietary Reference Intakes, 2001, pp. 126–133.

19. J. D. Ribaya-Mercado and J. B. Blumberg, Vitamin A: Is it a risk factor for osteoporosis and bone fracture? *Nutrition Reviews* 65 (2007): 425–438; Penniston and Tanumihardjo, 2006.

20. T. Tanvetyanon and G. Bepler, Beta-carotene in multivitamins and the possible risk of lung cancer among smokers versus former smokers: A meta-analysis and evaluation of national brands, *Cancer* 113 (2008): 150–157.

21. A. W. Norman, From vitamin D to hormone D: Fundamentals of the vitamin D endocrine system essential for good health, *American Journal of Clinical Nutrition* 88 (2008): 491S–499S.

22. Norman, 2008.

23. S. Samual and M. D. Sitrin, Vitamin D's role in cell proliferation and differentiation, *Nutrition Reviews* 66 (2008): S116–S124.

24. E. van Etten and coauthors, Regulation of vitamin D homeostasis: Implications for the immune system, *Nutrition Reviews* 66 (2008): S125–S134.

25. S. Cheng and coauthors, Adiposity, Cardiometabolic risk, and vitamin status: The Framingham heart study, *Diabetes* 59 (2010): 242–248; A. Kilkkinen and coauthors, Vitamin D status and the risk of cardiovascular death, *American Journal of Epidemiology* 170 (2009): 1032–1039; C. F. Garland and coauthors, Vitamin D for cancer prevention: Global perspective, *Annals of Epidemiology* 19 (2009): 468–483; A. Zitterman, J. Gummert, and J. Börgermann, Vitamin D deficiency and mortality, *Current Opinion in Clinical Nutrition and Metabolic Care* 12 (2009): 634–639; R. P. Heaney, Vitamin D and calcium interactions: Functional outcomes, *American Journal of Clinical Nutrition* 88 (2008): 541S–544S; M. T. Cantorna, Vitamin D and multiple sclerosis: An update, *Nutrition Reviews* 66 (2008): S135–S138; M. F. Holick, Vitamin D: A d-lightful health perspective, *Nutrition Reviews* 66 (2008): S182–S194; S. E. Judd and coauthors, Optimal vitamin D status attenuates the age-associated increase in systolic blood pressure in white Americans: Results from the third National Health and Nutrition Examination Survey, *American Journal of Clinical Nutrition* 87 (2008): 136–141; J. M. Lappe and coauthors, Vitamin D and calcium supplementation reduces cancer risk: Results of a randomized trial, *American Journal of Clinical Nutrition* 85 (2007): 1586–1591; J. Lin and coauthors, Intakes of calcium and vitamin D and breast cancer risk in women, *Archives of Internal Medicine* 167 (2007): 1050–1059; G. E. Mullin and A. Dobs, Vitamin D and its role in cancer and immunity: A prescription for sunlight, *Nutrition in Clinical Practice* 22 (2007): 305–322; Y. Cui and T. E. Rohan, Vitamin D, calcium, and breast cancer risk: A review, *Cancer Epidemiological, Biomarkers and Prevention* 15 (2006): 1427–1437; A. F. Gombart, Q. T. Luong, and H. P. Koeffler, Vitamin D compounds: Activity against microbes and cancer, *Anticancer Research* 26 (2006): 2531–2542; P. T. Liu and coauthors, Toll-like receptor triggering of a vitamin D-mediated human antimicrobial response, *Science* 311 (2006): 1770–1773; L. A. Martini and R. J. Wood, Vitamin D status and the metabolic syndrome, *Nutrition Reviews* 64 (2006): 479–486; K. L. Munger and coauthors, Serum 25-hydroxyvitamin D levels and risk of multiple sclerosis, *Journal of the American Medical Association* 296 (2006): 2832–2838; S. S. Schleithoff and coauthors, Vitamin D supplementation improves cytokine profiles in patients with congestive heart failure: A double-blind, randomized, placebo-controlled trial, *American Journal of Clinical Nutrition* 83 (2006): 754–759.

26. R. P Heaney, Vitamin D and calcium interactions: Functional outcomes, *American Journal of Clinical Nutrition* 88 (2008): 541S–544S.

27. Heaney, 2008.

28. H. F. Deluca, Evolution of our understanding of vitamin D, *Nutrition Reviews* 66 (2008): S73–S87; M. R. Haussler and coauthors, Vitamin D receptor: Molecular signaling and actions of nutritional ligands in disease prevention, *Nutrition Reviews* 66 (2008): S98–S112.

29. R. C. Khanal and I. Nemere, Regulation of intestinal calcium transport, *Annual Review of Nutrition* 28 (2008): 179–196.

30. A. C. Looker and coauthors, Serum 25-hydroxyvitamin D status of the US population: 1988–1994 compared with 2000–2004, *American Journal of Clinical Nutrition* 88 (2008): 1519–1527; S. A. Bowden and coauthors, Prevalence of vitamin D deficiency and insufficiency in children with osteopenia or osteoporosis referred to a pediatric metabolic bone clinic, *Pediatrics* 121 (2008): e1585–e1590; M. L. Neuhouser and coauthors, Vitamin D insufficiency in a multiethnic cohort of breast cancer survivors, *American Journal of Clinical Nutrition* 88 (2008): 133–139.

31. A. Moshfegh and coauthors, *What We Eat in America, NHANES 2005–2006: Usual Nutrient Intakes from Food and Water Compared to 1997 Dietary Reference Intakes for Vitamin D, Calcium, Phosphorus, and Magnesium,* (Beltsville, MD: USDA 2009), available at www.ars.usda.gov/ba/bhnrc/fsrg.

32. A. Prentice, Vitamin D deficiency: A global perspective, *Nutrition Reviews* 66 (2008): S153–S164.

33. J. Kumar and coauthors, Prevalence and associations of 25-hydroxyvitamin D deficiency in US children: NHANES 2001–2004, *Pediatrics* 124 (2009): e362–e370.

34. S. Saintonge, H. Bang, and L. M. Gerber, Implications of a new definition of vitamin D deficiency in a multiracial U.S. adolescent population: The National Health and Nutrition Examination Survey III, *Pediatrics* 123 (2009): 797–803; F. R. Greer, 25-Hydroxyvitamin D: Functional outcome in infants and young children, *American Journal of Clinical Nutrition* (2008): 529S–533S; S. Y. Huh and C. M. Gordon, Vitamin D deficiency in children and adolescents: Epidemiology, impact and treatment, *Reviews in Endocrine and Metabolic Disorders* 9 (2008): 161–170; M. Misra and coauthors, Vitamin D deficiency in children and its management: Review of current knowledge and recommendations, *Pediatrics* 122 (2008): 398–417.

35. C. L. Wagner, F. R. Greer, and the Section on Breastfeeding and Committee on Nutrition, Prevention of rickets and vitamin D deficiency in infants, children, and adolescents, *Pediatrics* 122 (2008): 1142–1152.

36. K. D. Cashman and coauthors, Low vitamin D status adversely affects bone health parameters in adolescents, *American Journal of Clinical Nutrition* 87 (2008): 1039–1044.

37. H. A. Bischoff-Ferrari and coauthors, Prevention of nonvertebral fractures with oral vitamin D and dose dependency: A meta-analysis of randomized controlled trials, *Archives of Internal Medicine* 169 (2009): 551–561; G. Buhr and C. W. Bales, Nutritional supplements for older adults: Review and recommendations—part I, *Journal of Nutrition for the Elderly* 28 (2009): 5–29; A. Avenell and coauthors, Vitamin D and vitamin D analogues for preventing fractures associated with involutional and post-menopausal osteoporosis, *Cochrane Database of Systematic Reviews* 2 (2009), CD000227; B. Dawson-Hughes, Serum 25-hydroxyvitamin D and

functional outcomes in the elderly, *American Journal of Clinical Nutrition* 88 (2008): 537S–540S; S. A. Talwar and coauthors, Dose response to vitamin D supplementation among postmenopausal African American women, *American Journal of Clinical Nutrition* 86 (2007): 1657–1662.

38. R. P. Heaney, Vitamin D: Criteria for safety and efficacy, *Nutrition Reviews* 66 (2008): S178–S181.

39. F. Ghissassi and coauthors, A review of human carcinogens—Part D: Radiation, *The Lancet* 10 (2009): 751–752; B. A. Gilchrest, Sun exposure and vitamin D sufficiency, *American Journal of Clinical Nutrition* 88 (2008): 570S–577S.

40. Gilchrest, 2008.

41. A. Prentice, F. R. Goldberg, and I. Schoenmakers, Vitamin D across the lifecycle: Physiology and biomarkers, *American Journal of Clinical Nutrition* 88 (2008): 500S–506S; M. J. Bolland and coauthors, The effects of seasonal variation of 25-hydroxyvitamin D and fat mass on a diagnosis of vitamin D sufficiency, *American Journal of Clinical Nutrition* 86 (2007): 959–964.

42. E. Hyppönen and C. Power, Hypovitaminosis D in British adults at age 45 y: Nationwide cohort study of dietary and lifestyle predictors, *American Journal of Clinical Nutrition* 85 (2007): 860–868; F. L. Weng and coauthors, Risk factors for low serum 25-hydroxyvitamin D concentrations in otherwise healthy children and adolescents, *American Journal of Clinical Nutrition* 86 (2007): 150–158.

43. K. D. Cashman and coauthors, Estimation of the dietary requirement for vitamin D in healthy adults, *American Journal of Clinical Nutrition* 88 (2008): 1535–1542.

44. Wagner, Greer, and the Section on Breastfeeding and Committee on Nutrition, 2008.

45. Wagner, Greer, and the Section on Breastfeeding and Committee on Nutrition, 2008.

46. R. P. Heaney, Vitamin D: Criteria for safety and efficacy, *Nutrition Reviews* 66 (2008): S178–S181; L. Mosekilde, Vitamin D requirement and setting recommendation levels: Long-term perspectives, *Nutrition Reviews* 66 (2008): S170–S177; R. Vieth and coauthors, The urgent need to recommend an intake of vitamin D that is effective, *American Journal of Clinical Nutrition* 85 (2007): 649–650; H. A. Bischoff-Ferrari and coauthors, Estimation of optimal serum concentrations of 25-hydroxyvitamin D for multiple health outcomes, *American Journal of Clinical Nutrition* 84 (2006): 18–28.

47. Cashman and coauthors, Estimation of the dietary requirement for vitamin D in healthy adults, 2008; J. F. Aloia and coauthors, Vitamin D intake to attain a desired serum 25-hydroxyvitamin D concentration, *American Journal of Clinical Nutrition* 87 (2008): 1952–1958.

48. D. L. Rainwater and coauthors, Vitamin E dietary supplementation significantly affects multiple risk factors for cardiovascular disease in baboons, *American Journal of Clinical Nutrition* 86 (2007): 597–603; U. Singh, S. Devaraj, and I. Jialal, Vitamin E, oxidative stress, and inflammation, *Annual Review of Nutrition* 25 (2005): 151–174.

49. B. J. Wilcox, J. D. Curb, and B. L. Rodriguez, Antioxidants in cardiovascular health and disease: Key lessons from epidemiologic studies, *American Journal of Cardiology* 101 (2009): 75D–86D.

50. A. H. Lichtenstein and coauthors, Diet and lifestyle recommendations revision 2006, A scientific statement from the American Heart Association Nutrition Committee, *Circulation* 114 (2006): 82–96.

51. J. N. Hathcock and coauthors, Vitamins E and C are safe across a broad range of intakes, *American Journal of Clinical Nutrition* 81 (2005): 736–745.

52. G. Bjelakovic and coauthors, Antioxidant supplements for prevention of mortality in healthy participants and patients with various diseases, *Cochrane Database of Systematic Reviews* April 16, 2008: CD007176.

53. G. Pocobelli and coauthors, Use of supplements of multivitamins, vitamin C and vitamin E in relation to mortality, *American Journal of Epidemiology* 170 (2009): 472–483.

54. H. M. MacDonald and coauthors, Vitamin K₁ intake is associated with higher bone mineral density and reduced bone resorption in early postmenopausal Scottish women: No evidence of gene-nutrient interaction with apolipoprotein E polymorphisms, *American Journal of Clinical Nutrition* 87 (2008): 1513–1520; S. Cockayne and coauthors, Vitamin K and the prevention of fractures: Systematic review and meta-analysis of randomized controlled trials, *Archives of Internal Medicine* 166 (2006): 1256–1261.

55. Cockayne and coauthors, 2006; J. Iwamoto, T. Takeda, and Y. Sato, Menatetrenone (vitamin K₂) and bone quality in the treatment of postmenopausal osteoporosis, *Nutrition Reviews* 64 (2006): 509–517; K. D. Cashman, Vitamin K status may be an important determinant of childhood bone health, *Nutrition Reviews* 63 (2005): 284–293.

56. K. D. Cashman and E. O'Connor, Does high vitamin K₁ intake protect against bone loss in later life? *Nutrition Reviews* 66 (2008): 532–538; M. K. Shea and S. L. Booth, Update on the role of vitamin K in skeletal health, *Nutrition Reviews* 66 (2008): 549–557.

57. M. K. Shea and coauthors, Vitamin K supplementation and progression of coronary artery calcium in older men and women, *American Journal of Clinical Nutrition* 89 (2009): 1799–1807.

58. R. F. Butterworth, Thiamin, in M. E. Shils and coeditors, *Modern Nutrition in Health and Disease*, 10th ed., (Philadelphia: Lippincott, Williams, & Wilkins, 2006), pp. 426–433.

59. C. Bourgeois, D. Cercantes-Laurean, and J. Moss, Niacin, in M. E. Shils and coeditors, *Modern Nutrition in Health and Disease*, 10th ed. (Philadelphia: Lippincott, Williams, & Wilkins, 2006), pp. 426–433.

60. Y. L. Hassan and J. Zempleni, A novel, enigmatic histone modification: Biotinylation of histones by holocarboxylase synthetase, *Nutrition Reviews* 66 (2008): 721–725; J. Zempleni, Uptake, localization, and noncarboxylase roles of biotin, *Annual Review of Nutrition* 25 (2005): 175–196.

61. J. Shen and coauthors, Association of vitamin B-6 status with inflammation, oxidative stress, and chronic inflammatory conditions: The Boston Puerto Rican Health Study, *American Journal of Clinical Nutrition* 91 (2010): 337–342.

62. E. S. Wintergerst, S. Maggini, and D. H. Hornig, Contribution of selected vitamins and trace elements to immune function, *Annals of Nutrition and Metabolism* 51 (2007): 301–323; A. D. Mackey, S. R. Davis, and J. F. Gregory, Vitamin B₆, in M. E. Shils and coeditors, *Modern Nutrition in Health and Disease*, 10th ed. (Philadelphia: Lippincott, Williams, & Wilkins, 2006), pp. 452–461.

63. L. L. Humphrey and coauthors, Homocysteine level and coronary heart disease incidence: A systematic review and meta-analysis, *Mayo Clinic Proceedings* 83 (2008): 3–16.

64. K. Woolf and M. M. Manore, Elevated plasma homocysteine and low vitamin B-6 status in nonsupplementing older women with rheumatoid arthritis, *Journal of the American Dietetic Association* 108 (2008): 443–453; J. Selhub, Public health significance of elevated homocysteine, *Food and Nutrition Bulletin* 29 (2008): S116–S125.

65. J. H. Page and coauthors, Plasma B(6) and risk of myocardial infarction in women, *Circulation* 120 (2009): 649–655; A. J. Marti-Carvajal and coauthors, Homocysteine lowering interventions for preventing cardiovascular events, *Cochrane Database of Systematic Reviews* October 7, 2009: CD006612; M. Ebbing and coauthors, Mortality and cardiovascular events in patients treated with homocysteine-lowering B vitamins after coronary angiography: A randomized controlled trial, *Journal of the American Medical Association* 300 (2008): 795–804.

66. R. Carmel, Folic acid, in M. E. Shils and coeditors, *Modern Nutrition in Health and Disease*, 10th ed. (Philadelphia: Lippincott, Williams, & Wilkins, 2006), pp. 470–481.

67. R. L. Bailey and coauthors, Total folate and folic acid intake from foods and dietary supplements in the United States: 2003–2006, *American Journal of Clinical Nutrition* 91 (2010): 231–237.

68. P. D. Wals and coauthors, Reduction in neural-tube defects after folic acid fortification in Canada, *New England Journal of Medicine* 357 (2007): 135–142.

69. M. Ebbing and coauthors, Cancer incidence and mortality after treatment with folic acid and vitamin B₁₂, *Journal of the American Medical Association* 302 (2009): 2119–2126; U. C. Ericson and coauthors, Increased breast cancer risk at high plasma folate concentrations among women with the MTHFR 677T allele, *American Journal of Clinical Nutrition* 90 (2009): 1380–1389; A. M. Troen and coauthors, Unmetabolized folic acid in plasma is associated with reduced natural killer cell cytotoxicity among postmenopausal women, *Journal of Nutrition* 136 (2006): 189–194.

70. Bailey and coauthors, 2010; Q. Yang and coauthors, Folic acid source, usual intake, and folate and vitamin B-12 status in US adults: National Health and Nutrition Examination Survey (NHANES) 2003–2006, *American Journal of Clinical Nutrition* 91 (2010): 64–72.

71. J. W. Miller and coauthors, Metabolic evidence of vitamin B-12 deficiency, including high homocysteine and methylmalonic acid and low holotranscobalamin, is more pronounced in older adults with elevated plasma folate, *American Journal of Clinical Nutrition* 90 (2009): 1586–1592.

72. S. Park and M. A. Johnson, What is an adequate dose of oral vitamin B₁₂ in older people with poor vitamin B₁₂ status? *Nutrition Reviews* 64 (2006): 383–388.

73. I. Elmadfa and I. Singer, Vitamin B-12 and homocysteine status among vegetarians, *American Journal of Clinical Nutrition* 89 (2009): 1693S–1698S.

74. Carmel, 2006.

75. World Cancer Research Fund and American Institute for Cancer Research, *Food, Nutrition, Physical Activity, and the Prevention of Cancer: A Global Perspective* (Washington, D.C.: American Institute for Cancer Research, 2007), pp. 253–258.

76. Standing Committee on the Scientific Evaluation of Dietary Reference Intakes, *Dietary Reference Intakes for Vitamin C, Vitamin E, Selenium, and Carotenoids* (Washington, D.C.: National Academy Press, 2000, p. 155.

Phytochemicals and Functional Foods

The wisdom of the familiar advice, "Eat your vegetables; they're good for you," stands on firmer scientific ground today than ever before as population studies around the world suggest that diets rich in vegetables and fruits protect against heart disease, cancer, and other chronic diseases.[1] We now know that the "goodness" of vegetables, fruits, and other whole foods such as legumes and grains comes not only from the nutrients they contain but also from the **phytochemicals** that they offer.[2] Phytochemicals often act as **bioactive food components**, food constituents with the ability to alter body processes. (Terms are defined in Table NP8-1 on p. 230.)

Vegetables, fruits, and other whole foods are the simplest examples of foods now known as **functional foods**. Functional foods provide health benefits beyond basic nutrition by altering one or more physiological processes. Modified foods, such as those that have been fortified, enriched, or enhanced with nutrients, phytochemicals, herbs, or other food components, also are functional foods.[3] Functional foods that fit this description include orange juice fortified with calcium, folate-enriched cereal, beverages with herbal additives, and margarine enhanced with **phytosterols**. This Nutrition in Practice begins with a look at the evidence concerning the effectiveness and safety of a few selected phytochemicals in the simplest of functional foods—vegetables, fruits, and other whole foods. Then, the discussion turns to examine the most controversial of functional foods—novel foods to which phytochemicals have been added to promote health. How these foods fit into a healthy diet is still unclear.[4]

What are phytochemicals, and what do they do?

Phytochemicals are bioactive compounds found in plants. In foods, phytochemicals impart tastes, aromas, colors, and other characteristics. They give hot peppers their burning sensation, garlic and onions their pungent flavor, chocolate its bitter tang, and tomatoes their dark red color. In the body, phytochemicals can have profound physiological effects—acting as antioxidants, mimicking hormones, stimulating or inhibiting enzymes, interfering with DNA replication, destroying bacteria, and binding physically to cell walls. Any of these actions may suppress the development of diseases.[5] Notably, cancer and heart disease are linked to processes involving oxygen compounds in the body, and **antioxidants** are thought to oppose these actions. Table NP8-2 (pp. 231–232) introduces the names, possible physiological effects, and food sources of some of the better-known phytochemicals.

Why are phytochemicals receiving so much attention these days, and what are some examples of those in the spotlight?

Diets rich in whole grains, legumes, vegetables, and fruits seem to be protective against heart disease and cancer, but identifying *the* specific foods or components of foods that are responsible is difficult. Scientists are conducting extensive research studies to discover phytochemical connections to disease prevention, but, so far, solid evidence is generally lacking. Some of the likeliest candidates include **flavonoids** and **carotenoids** (including **lycopene**).

What are flavonoids, and in which foods are they found?

Flavonoids, a large group of phytochemicals known for their health-promoting qualities, are found in whole grains, soy, vegetables, fruits, herbs, spices, teas, chocolate, nuts, olive oil, and red wine. Flavonoids are powerful antioxidants that may help to protect LDL against oxidation, minimize inflammation, and reduce blood platelet stickiness, thereby slowing the progression of atherosclerosis and making blood clots less likely.[6] Whereas an abundance of flavonoid-containing *foods* in the diet may lower the risks of chronic diseases, no claims can be made for flavonoids themselves as the protective factor, particularly when they are extracted from foods and sold as supplements.

Flavonoids impart a bitter taste to foods, so manufacturers often refine away the natural flavonoids to please consumers, who usually prefer milder flavors. For example, the hearty taste of whole-wheat foods vanishes when whole wheat is refined into white flour by removing the tough brown parts that contain flavonoids. For white grape juice or white wine, manufacturers remove the red, flavonoid-rich grape skins to lighten the flavor and color of the product, while greatly reducing its beneficial flavonoid content. For example, one flavonoid in purple grape juice and red wine, **resveratrol**, seems to hold promise as a disease fighter, but the amount present in wine or a serving of grape juice may be too small to benefit human health.[7]

antioxidants (anti-OX-ih-dants): compounds that protect other compounds from damaging reactions involving oxygen by themselves reacting with oxygen (*anti* means "against"; *oxy* means "oxygen"); *oxidation* is a potentially damaging effect of normal cell chemistry involving oxygen.

bioactive food components: compounds in foods, either nutrients or phytochemicals, that alter physiological processes in the body. Also defined in Chapter 1.

carotenoids (Kah-ROT-eh-noyds): pigments commonly found in plants and animals, some of which have vitamin A activity. The carotenoid with the greatest vitamin A activity is beta-carotene.

flavonoids (FLAY-von-oyds): yellow pigments in foods; phytochemicals that may exert physiological effects on the body. *Flavus* means "yellow."

flaxseed: small brown seed of the flax plant; valued in nutrition as a source of fiber, lignans, and the omega-3 fatty acid linolenic acid.

functional foods: whole or modified foods that contain bioactive food components believed to provide health benefits, such as reduced disease risks, beyond the benefits that their nutrients contribute. All whole foods are functional in some ways because they provide at least some needed substances, but certain foods stand out as rich sources of bioactive food components. Also defined in Chapter 1.

genistein (GEN-ih-steen): a phytoestrogen found primarily in soybeans that both mimics and blocks the action of estrogen in the body.

lignans: phytochemicals present in flaxseed, but not flaxseed oil, that are converted to phytoestrogens by intestinal bacteria and are under study as possible anticancer agents.

lutein (LOO-teen): a plant pigment of yellow hue; a phytochemical believed to play roles in eye functioning and health.

lycopene (LYE-koh-peen): a pigment responsible for the red color of tomatoes and other red-hued vegetables; a phytochemical that may act as an antioxidant in the body.

organosulfur compounds: a large group of phytochemicals containing the mineral sulfur. Organosulfur phytochemicals are responsible for the pungent flavors and aromas of foods belonging to the onion, leek, chive, shallot, and garlic family and are thought to stimulate cancer defenses in the body.

phytochemicals (FIGH-toe-CHEM-ih-cals): compounds in plants that confer color, taste, and other characteristics. Some phytochemicals are bioactive food components in functional foods. Also defined in Chapter 1.

phytoestrogens (FIGHT-toe-ESS-troh-gens): phytochemicals structurally similar to human estrogen. Phytoestrogens weakly mimic or modulate estrogen in the body.

phytosterols: phytochemicals that resemble cholesterol in structure but that lower blood cholesterol by interfering with cholesterol absorption in the intestine. Phytosterols include sterol esters and stanol esters.

resveratrol (rez-VER-ah-trol): a flavonoid of grapes under study for potential health benefits.

tofu: white curd made of soybeans, popular in Asian cuisines, and considered to be a functional food.

Chemical Name	Possible Effects	Food Sources
Alkylresorcinols (phenolic lipids)	May contribute to the protective effect of grains in reducing the risks of diabetes, heart disease, and some cancers	Whole-grain wheat and rye
Allicin (organosulfur compound)	Antimicrobial that may reduce ulcers; may lower blood cholesterol	Chives, garlic, leeks, onions
Capsaicin	Modulates blood clotting, possibly reducing the risk of fatal clots in heart and artery disease	Hot peppers
Carotenoids (include beta-carotene, lycopene, lutein, and hundreds of related compounds)	Act as antioxidants, possibly reducing risks of cancer and other diseases	Deeply pigmented fruits and vegetables (apricots, broccoli, cantaloupe, carrots, pumpkin, spinach, sweet potatoes, tomatoes)
Curcumin	Acts as an antioxidant and anti-inflammatory agent; may reduce blood clot formation; may inhibit enzymes that activate carcinogens	Tumeric, a yellow-colored spice
Flavonoids (include flavones, flavonols, isoflavones, catechins, and others)	Act as antioxidants; scavenge carcinogens; bind to nitrates in the stomach, preventing conversion to nitrosamines; inhibit cell proliferation	Berries, black tea, celery, citrus fruits, green tea, olives, onions, oregano, purple grapes, purple grape juice, soybeans and soy products, vegetables, whole wheat, wine
Genistein and daidzein (isoflavones)	Phytoestrogens that inhibit cell replication in GI tract; may reduce or elevate risk of breast, colon, ovarian, prostate, and other estrogen-sensitive cancers; may reduce cancer cell survival; may reduce risk of osteoporosis	Soybeans, soy flour, soy milk, tofu, textured vegetable protein, other legume products
Indoles (organosulfur compound)	May trigger production of enzymes that block DNA damage from carcinogens; may inhibit estrogen action	Cruciferous vegetables such as broccoli, brussels sprouts, cabbage, cauliflower; horseradish, mustard greens, kale
Isothiocyanates (organosulfur compounds that include sulforaphane)	Act as antioxidants; inhibit enzymes that activate carcinogens; activate enzymes that detoxify carcinogens; may reduce risk of breast cancer, prostate cancer	Cruciferous vegetables such as broccoli, brussels sprouts, cabbage, cauliflower; horseradish, mustard greens, kale
Lignans	Phytoestrogens that block estrogen activity in cells, possibly reducing the risk of cancer of the breast, colon, ovaries, and prostate	Flaxseed and its oil, whole grains
Monoterpenes (including limonene)	May trigger enzyme production to detoxify carcinogens; inhibit cancer promotion and cell proliferation	Citrus fruit peels and oils
Phenolic acids	May trigger enzyme production to make carcinogens water soluble, facilitating excretion	Coffee beans, fruits (apples, blueberries, cherries, grapes, oranges, pears, prunes), oats, potatoes, soybeans
Phytic acid	Binds to minerals, preventing free-radical formation, possibly reducing cancer risk	Whole grains

(Continued)

Chemical Name	Possible Effects	Food Sources
Resveratrol	Acts as antioxidant; may inhibit cancer growth; reduces inflammation, LDL oxidation, and blood clot formation	Red wine, peanuts, grapes, raspberries
Saponins (glucosides)	May interfere with DNA replication, preventing cancer cells from multiplying; stimulate immune response	Alfalfa sprouts, other sprouts, green vegetables, potatoes, tomatoes
Tannins	Act as antioxidants; may inhibit carcinogen activation and cancer promotion	Black-eyed peas, grapes, lentils, red and white wine, tea

What about carotenoids?

In addition to flavonoids, fruits and vegetables are rich in carotenoids—the red and yellow pigments of plants. Some carotenoids, such as beta-carotene, are vitamin A precursors. Some research suggests that a diet rich in carotenoids is associated with a lower risk of heart disease.[8] Among the carotenoids that may defend against heart disease is lycopene. Lycopene may also protect against certain types of cancer.

What is lycopene, and what foods contain it?

Lycopene is a red pigment with powerful antioxidant activity found in guava, papaya, pink grapefruit, tomatoes (especially cooked tomatoes and tomato products), and watermelon. More than 80 percent of the lycopene consumed in the United States comes from tomato products such as tomato sauce, tomato juice, and catsup. Around the world, people who eat five or more tomato-containing meals per week are less likely to suffer from cancers of the esophagus, prostate, or stomach than those who avoid tomatoes. Lycopene is a leading candidate for this protective effect.

Theoretically, the potent antioxidant capability of lycopene plays a role in its action against cancer, but, so far, research does not support the idea.[9] Tomatoes contain many other phytochemicals and nutrients that may contribute to the beneficial health effects of eating tomatoes and tomato products. An evidence-based review by the FDA concluded that little or no credible evidence exists to support an association between lycopene or tomato consumption and reduced cancer rates.[10]

Do foods contain other phytochemicals that may help to protect people from cancer or other diseases?

Foods contain thousands of different phytochemicals, and so far only a few have been researched at all. There are still many questions about the phytochemicals that have been studied and only tentative answers about their roles in human health. For example, compared with people in the West, Asians living in Asia suffer less frequently from cancers, especially of the breast, colon, and prostate; heart disease; and osteoporosis (adult bone loss). Among many differences between the diets of the two regions, Asians consume far more soybeans and soy products such as **tofu** than do Westerners.

Soybeans are rich sources of phytochemicals known as **phytoestrogens**. Researchers suspect that the phytoestrogens of soy foods, their protein content, or a combination of these factors may be responsible for health effects in soy-eating peoples. Nevertheless, research, though ongoing, is limited. So far, we know with certainty that phytoestrogens are plant-derived chemical relatives of the human hormone estrogen and that they weakly mimic or modulate the hormone's effects on some body tissues. With regard to cancer, concerns about breast cancer, colon cancer, and prostate cancer involve estrogen-sensitive varieties—cancers that grow when exposed to estrogen. The age of the person eating soy affects the results: a high soy intake during childhood and adolescence seems to reduce breast cancer risk in women before menopause; soy intake by adults may or may not reduce this risk, but more research is needed to clarify these relationships.[11] With regard to the biological activity of soy, scientific understanding is incomplete.[12]

Low doses of one soy phytoestrogen, **genistein**, appear to speed up division of breast cancer cells in laboratory cultures and in mice, whereas high doses seemed to do the opposite.[13] Still under study is whether dietary soy phytoestrogens have similar effects on cancer cells in living people, but it seems unlikely that moderate intakes of soy foods would do so.[14] If they did, soy-eating cultures would have higher, not lower, incidences of these cancers.

The opposing actions of phytoestrogens should raise a red flag against taking supplements, especially by people who have had cancer or whose close relatives have developed cancer. The American Cancer Society recommends that breast cancer survivors and those under treatment for breast cancer should consume only moderate amounts of soy foods as part of a healthy plant-based diet and should not intentionally ingest very high levels of soy products.

Other foods under study for potential health benefits include **flaxseed** and its oil. Flaxseed is found as a whole seed or ground meal, or as flaxseed oil. Flaxseed is of interest for its possible benefits to heart health because it is a good source of soluble fiber, and it is the richest known source of both the omega-3 fatty acid linolenic acid and **lignans**, compounds converted into biologically active phytoestrogens by bacteria that normally reside in the human intestine.[15] Flaxseed oil, though rich in linolenic acid, does not contain fiber or lignans. Large quantities of flaxseed can cause digestive distress, and severe allergic reactions to flaxseed have been reported.

What about other phytochemical supplements?

Even when people don't eat in the best interest of health, taking supplements of purified phytochemicals is not the way to go. Phytochemicals can alter body functions, sometimes powerfully. Researchers are just beginning to understand how a handful of phytochemicals work, and what is current today may change tomorrow. Foods deliver thousands of bioactive food components, all within a food matrix that maximizes their availability and effectiveness.[16] The body is equipped to handle phytochemicals in diluted form, mixed with all of the other constituents of foods, but it does not adapt well to phytochemicals in concentrated form. The best way to reap the benefits of phytochemicals is by eating foods, not taking supplements (see Figure NP8-1 on p. 234).

How do whole foods compare with processed foods that have been enriched with phytochemicals?

Good question. The American food supply is being transformed by a proliferation of functional foods—foods claimed to provide health benefits beyond those of the traditional nutrients. Virtually all whole foods have some special value in supporting health and are therefore functional foods. Cranberries may protect against urinary tract infections because cranberries contain a phytochemical that dislodges bacteria from the tract.[17] Cooked tomatoes, as mentioned, provide lycopene, along with **lutein** (an antioxidant associated with healthy eye function), vitamin C (an antioxidant vitamin), and many other healthful attributes. This has not stopped food manufacturers from trying to create functional foods as well. As consumer demand for healthful foods continues to grow, so will the development of functional foods.[18]

What are some examples of manufactured functional foods?

Many processed foods become functional foods when they are fortified with nutrients (calcium-fortified orange juice to support bone health, for example). In other cases, processed foods are enhanced with bioactive food components (margarine blended with a phytosterol to lower cholesterol, for example). The creation of some novel manufactured functional foods raises the question—is it a food or a drug?[19]

Isn't the distinction between a food and a drug pretty clear?

Not too long ago, most of us could agree on what was a food and what was a drug. Today, functional foods blur the distinctions. They have characteristics similar to both foods and drugs but do not fit neatly into either category. Consider the margarine example above.

Eating nonhydrogenated margarine sparingly instead of butter generously may lower blood cholesterol slightly over several months and clearly falls into the food category. Taking a statin drug, on the other hand, lowers blood cholesterol significantly within weeks and clearly falls into the drug category. But margarine enhanced with a phytosterol that lowers blood cholesterol is in a gray area between the two.* The margarine looks and tastes like a food, but it acts like a drug.

The use of functional foods as drugs creates a whole new set of diet-planning problems. Not only must foods provide an adequate intake of all the nutrients to support good health, but they must also deliver druglike ingredients to protect against disease. Like drugs used to treat chronic diseases, functional foods may need to be eaten several times a day for several months or years to have a beneficial effect. Sporadic users may be disappointed in the results. Margarine enhanced with 2 to 3 grams of phytosterols may reduce cholesterol by up to 15 percent, much more than regular margarine does, but not nearly as much as the more than 30 percent reduction seen with cholesterol-lowering drugs.[20] For this reason, functional foods may be more useful for prevention and mild cases of disease than for intervention and more severe cases.

How do the costs of functional foods compare with those of conventional foods?

Foods and drugs differ dramatically in cost. Functional foods such as fruits and vegetables incur no added costs, of course, but foods that have been manufactured with added phytochemicals can be expensive, costing up to six times as

---

*Margarine products that lower blood cholesterol contain either sterol esters—from vegetable oils, soybeans, and corn—or stanol esters from wood pulp.

Broccoli and broccoli sprouts contain an abundance of the cancer-fighting phytochemical sulforaphane.

An apple a day—rich in flavonoids—may protect against lung cancer.

The phytoestrogens of soybeans seem to starve cancer cells and inhibit tumor growth; the phytosterols may lower blood cholesterol and protect cardiac arteries.

Garlic, with its abundant organosulfur compounds, may lower blood cholesterol and protect against stomach cancer.

The phytochemical resveratrol found in grapes (and nuts) protects against cancer by inhibiting cell growth and against heart disease by limiting clot formation and inflammation.

The ellagic acid of strawberries may inhibit certain types of cancer.

The monoterpenes of citrus fruits (and cherries) may inhibit cancer growth.

The flavonoids in black tea may protect against heart disease, whereas those in green tea may defend against cancer.

The flavonoids in cocoa and chocolate defend against oxidation and reduce the tendency of blood to clot.

Tomatoes, with their abundant lycopene, may defend against cancer by protecting DNA from oxidative damage.

Spinach and other colorful vegetables contain the carotenoids lutein and zeaxanthin, which help protect the eyes against macular degeneration.

Flaxseed, the richest source of lignans, may prevent the spread of cancer.

Blueberries, a rich source of flavonoids, improve memory in animals.

Garlic, Citrus fruits, © EyeWire, Inc.; Flaxseed, Courtesy of Flax Council of Canada; Broccoli, Courtesy of Brassica Protection Products. Apples, Strawberries, Tomatoes, Blueberries, Black Tea, Soybeans, Grapes, Digital Imagery © 2001 PhotoDisc, Inc., Orange, Spinach, Cocoa by Matthew Farruggio

much as their conventional counterparts. The price of functional foods typically falls between that of traditional foods and medicines.

What about using sterol-enhanced margarines to lower cholesterol or other manufactured functional foods to help prevent cancer?

To achieve a desired health effect, which is the better choice: to eat a food designed to affect some body function or simply to adjust the diet? Does it make more sense to use a margarine enhanced with a phytosterol that lowers blood cholesterol or simply to limit the amount of butter eaten? Is it smarter to eat eggs enriched with omega-3 fatty acids or to restrict egg consumption? Might functional foods offer a sensible solution for improving our nation's health—if done correctly? Perhaps so—but there is a problem with functional foods: the food industry is moving too fast for either scientists or the Food and Drug Administration (FDA) to keep up. Consumers were able to buy soup with St. John's wort that claimed to enhance mood and fruit juice with echinacea that was supposed to fight colds while scientists were still conducting their studies on these ingredients. Research to determine the safety and effectiveness of these substances is still in progress. Until this work is complete, consumers are on their own in finding the answers to the following questions:

- *Does it work?* Research is generally lacking, and findings are often inconclusive.
- *How much does it contain?* Food labels are not required to list the quantities of added phytochemicals. Even if they were, consumers have no standard for comparison and cannot deduce whether the amounts listed are a little or a lot. Most importantly, until research is complete, food manufacturers do not know what amounts (if any) are most effective—or most toxic.
- *Is it safe?* Functional foods can act like drugs. They contain ingredients that can alter body functions and cause allergies, drug interactions, drowsiness, and other side effects. Yet, unlike drug labels, food labels do not provide instructions for the dosage, frequency, or duration of treatment.
- *Has the FDA issued warnings about any of the ingredients?* Check the FDA's website (www.fda.gov) to find out.
- *Is it healthy?* Adding phytochemicals to a food does not magically make it a healthy choice. A candy bar may be fortified with phytochemicals, but it is still made mostly of sugar and fat.

Critics suggest that the designation "functional foods" may be nothing more than a marketing tool. After all, even the most experienced researchers cannot yet identify the perfect combination of nutrients and phytochemicals to support optimal health. Yet manufacturers are freely experimenting with various concoctions as if they possessed that knowledge. Is it okay for them to sprinkle phytochemicals on fried snack foods and label them "functional," thus implying health benefits? Do we want our children receiving their nourishment from fortified caramel candies and chocolate cakes?

What is the final word regarding phytochemicals and functional foods?

Nature has elegantly designed foods to provide us with a complex array of dozens of nutrients and thousands of additional compounds that may benefit health—most

Functional foods currently on the market promise to "enhance mood," "promote relaxation and good karma," "increase alertness," and "improve memory," among other claims.

of which we have yet to identify or understand. Over the years, we have taken those foods and first deconstructed them and then reconstructed them in an effort to "improve" them. With new scientific understandings of how nutrients—and the myriad of other compounds in foods—interact with genes, we may someday be able to design foods to meet the *exact* health needs of *each* individual. Indeed, our knowledge of the human genome and of human nutrition may well merge to allow specific recommendations for individuals based on their predisposition to diet-related diseases.

If the present trend continues, then someday physicians may be able to prescribe the perfect foods to enhance a person's health, and farmers will be able to grow them. In the meantime, however, it seems clear that a moderate approach to phytochemicals and functional foods is warranted. People who eat the recommended amounts of a variety of fruits and vegetables may cut their risk of many diseases by as much as half. Replacing some meat with soy foods and other legumes may also lower heart disease and cancer risks. Beneficial constituents are widespread among foods. Take a no-nonsense approach where your health is concerned: choose a wide variety of whole grains, legumes, fruits, and vegetables in the context of an adequate, balanced, and varied diet, and receive all of the health benefits that these foods offer.

Notes

1. S. S. Gidding and coauthors, Implementing American Heart Association pediatric and adult nutrition guidelines: A scientific statement from the American Heart Association Nutrition Committee of the Council on Nutrition, Physical Activity and Metabolism, Council on Cardiovascular Disease in the Young, Council on Arteriosclerosis, Thrombosis, and Vascular Biology, Council on Cardiovascular Nursing, Council on Epidemiology and Prevention, and Council for High Blood Pressure Research, *Circulation* 119 (2009): 1161–11745; F. Sofi, The Mediterranean diet revisited: Evidence of its effectiveness grows, *Current Opinion in Cardiology* 24 (2009): 442–446; J. A. Nettleton and coauthors, Dietary patterns and incident cardiovascular disease in the Multi-Ethnic Study of Atherosclerosis, *American Journal of Clinical Nutrition* 90 (2009): 647–654; F. J. B. van Duijnhoven and coauthors, Fruit, vegetables, and

colorectal cancer risk: The European Prospective Investigation into Cancer and Nutrition, *American Journal of Clinical Nutrition* 89 (2009): 1441–1452; C. La Vecchia, Association between Mediterranean dietary patterns and cancer risk, *Nutrition Reviews* 67 (2009): S126–S129.

2. N. Khan, F. Afaq, and H. Mukhtar, Cancer chemoprevention through dietary antioxidants: Progress and promise, *Antioxidants and Resox Signaling* 10 (2008): 475–510; M. Rhone and A. Basu, Phytochemicals and age-related eye diseases, *Nutrition Reviews* 66 (2008): 465–472; C. C. Udenigwe and coauthors, Potential of resveratrol in anticancer and anti-inflammatory therapy, *Nutrition Reviews* 66 (2008): 445–454; D. R. Jacobs, L. F. Andersen, and R. Blomhoff, Whole-grain consumption is associated with a reduced risk of noncardiovascular, noncancer death attributed to inflammatory diseases in the Iowa Women's Health Study, *American Journal of Clinical Nutrition* 85 (2007): 1606–1614; D. F. Birt, Phytochemicals and cancer prevention: From epidemiology to mechanism of action, *Journal of the American Dietetic Association* 106 (2006): 20–21.

3. Position of the American Dietetic Association: Functional foods, *Journal of the American Dietetic Association* 109 (2009): 735–746.

4. G. Williamson and coauthors, Functional foods for health promotion: State-of-the-science on dietary flavonoids. Extended abstracts from the 12th Annual Conference on Functional Foods for Health Promotion, April, 2009, *Nutrition Reviews* 67 (2009): 736–743; L. R. Ferguson, Nutrigenomics approaches to functional foods, *Journal of the American Dietetic Association* 109 (2009): 452–458.

5. S. Jew, S. S. AbuMweis, and P. J. Jones, Evolution of the human diet: Linking our ancestral diet to modern functional foods as a means of chronic disease prevention, *Journal of Medicinal Foods* 12 (2009): 925–934; M. Kaur, C. Agarwal, and R. Agarwal, Anticancer and cancer chemopreventive potential of grape seed extract and other grape-based products, *Journal of Nutrition* 139 (2009): 1806S–1812S; G. Riccioni and coauthors, Protective effect of lycopene in cardiovascular disease, *European Review for Medical and Pharmacological* Sciences 12 (2008): 183–190.

6. Williamson and coauthors, 2009; M. Monagas and coauthors, Effect of cocoa powder on the modulation of inflammatory biomarkers in patients at high risk of cardiovascular disease, *American Journal of Clinical Nutrition* 90 (2009): 1144–1150; R. di Giuseppe and coauthors, Regular consumption of dark chocolate is associated with low serum concentrations of C-reactive protein in a healthy Italian population, *Journal of Nutrition* 138 (2008): 1939–1945; I. Erlund and coauthors, Favorable effects of berry consumption on platelet function, blood pressure, and HDL cholesterol, *American Journal of Clinical Nutrition* 87 (2008): 323–331; L. Hooper and coauthors, Flavonoids, flavonoid-rich foods, and cardiovascular risk: A meta-analysis of randomized controlled trials, *American Journal of Clinical Nutrition* 88 (2008): 38–50; W. M. Loke and coauthors, Pure dietary flavonoids quercetin and (–)-epicatechin augment nitric oxide products and reduce endothelin-1 acutely in healthy men, *American Journal of Clinical Nutrition* 88 (2008): 1018–1025.

7. M. D. Knutson and C. Leeuwenburgh, Resveratrol and novel potent activators of SIRT1: Effects on aging and age-related diseases, *Nutrition Reviews* 66 (2008): 591–596.

8. A. Hozawa and coauthors, Circulating carotenoid concentrations and incident hypertension: The Coronary Artery Risk Development in Young Adults

(CARDIA) Study, *Journal of Hypertension* 27 (2009): 237–242; G. Riccioni, Carotenoids and cardiovascular disease, *Current Atherosclerosis Reports* 11 (2009): 434–439; G. Riccioni and coauthors, Protective effect of lycopene in cardiovascular disease, *European Review for Medical and Pharmacological Sciences* 12 (2008): 183–190; S. Voutilainen and coauthors, Carotenoids and cardiovascular health, *American Journal of Clinical Nutrition* 83 (2006): 1265–1271.

9. J. R. Mein, F. Lian, and X-D Wang, Biological activity of lycopene metabolites: Implications for cancer prevention, *Nutrition Reviews* 66 (2008): 667–683; U. Peters and coauthors, Serum lycopene, other carotenoids, and prostate cancer risk: A nested case-control study in the Prostate, Lung, Colorectal, and Ovarian Cancer Screening Trial, *Cancer Epidemiology Biomarkers and Prevention* 16 (2007): 962–968.

10. C. J. Kavanaugh, P. R. Trumbo, and K. E. Ellwood, The U.S. Food and Drug Administration's evidence-based review for qualified health claims: Tomatoes, lycopene, and cancer, *Journal of the National Cancer Institute* 99 (2007): 1047–1085.

11. S-A. Lee and coauthors, Adolescent and adult soy food intake and breast cancer risk: Results from the Shanghai Women's Health Study, *American Journal of Clinical Nutrition* 89 (2009): 1920–1926; M. Messina and A. H. Wu, Perspectives on the soy–breast cancer relation, *American Journal of Clinical Nutrition* 89 (2009): 1673S–1679S; A. Warri and coauthors, The role of early life genistein exposures in modifying breast cancer risk, *British Journal of Cancer* 98 (2008): 1485–1493.

12. J. W. Lampe, Is equol the key to the efficacy of soy foods? *American Journal of Clinical Nutrition* 89 (2009): 1664S–1667S.

13. Y. Zhang, and coauthors, Soy isoflavones and their bone protective effects, *Inflammopharmacology* 16 (2008): 213–215.

14. C. K. Taylor and coauthors, The effect of genistein aglycone on cancer and cancer risk: A review of in vitro, preclinical, and clinical studies, *Nutrition Reviews* 67 (2009): 398–415.

15. A. Pan and coauthors, Meta-analysis of the effects of flaxseed interventions on blood lipids, *American Journal of Clinical Nutrition* 90 (2009): 288–297.

16. D. R. Jacobs, M. D. Gross, and L. C. Tapsell, Food synergy: An operational concept for understanding nutrition, *American Journal of Clinical Nutrition* 89 (2009): 1543S–1548S.

17. D. R. Guay, Cranberry and urinary tract infections, *Drugs* 69 (2009): 775–807; J. Jass and G. Reid, Effect of cranberry drink on bacterial adhesion in vitro and vaginal microbiota in healthy females, *Canadian Journal of Urology* 16 (2009): 4901–4907.

18. Position of the American Dietetic Association, 2009.

19. P. J. Jones and K. A. Varady, Are functional foods redefining nutritional requirements? *Applied Physiology, Nutrition, and Metabolism* 33 (2008): 118–123.

20. K. G. Moruisi, W. Oosthuizen, and A. M. Opperman, Phytosterols/stanols lower cholesterol concentrations in familial hypercholesterolemic subjects: A systematic review with meta-analysis, *Journal of the American College of Nutrition* 25 (2006): 41–48; C. S. Patch, L. C. Tapsell, and P. G. Williams, Plant sterol/stanol prescription is an effective treatment strategy for managing hypercholesterolemia in outpatient clinical practice, *Journal of the American Dietetic Association* 105 (2005): 46–52.

CHAPTER 9 | Water and the Minerals

CONTENTS

Water is the most indispensable nutrient of all.

THE BODY'S WATER CANNOT BE CONSIDERED SEPARATELY FROM THE minerals dissolved in it. A person can drink pure water, but in the body, water mingles with minerals to become fluids in which all life processes take place. This chapter begins by discussing the body's fluids and their chief minerals. The focus then shifts to other functions of the minerals.

Water and Body Fluids

Water constitutes about 60 percent of an adult's body weight and a higher percentage of a child's. Every cell in the body is bathed in a fluid of the exact composition that is best for that cell. The body fluids bring to each cell the ingredients it requires and carry away the end products of the life-sustaining reactions that take place within the cell's boundaries. The water in the body fluids:

- Carries nutrients and waste products throughout the body.
- Maintains the structure of large molecules such as proteins and glycogen.
- Participates in metabolic reactions.
- Serves as the solvent for minerals, vitamins, amino acids, glucose, and many other small molecules.
- Maintains blood volume.
- Aids in the regulation of normal body temperature, as the evaporation of sweat from the skin removes excess heat from the body.
- Acts as a lubricant and cushion around joints and inside the eyes, spinal cord, and amniotic sac surrounding a fetus in the womb.

To support these and other vital functions, the body actively regulates its **water balance**.

WATER BALANCE

The cells themselves regulate the composition and amounts of fluids within and surrounding them. The entire system of cells and fluids remains in a delicate but firmly maintained state of dynamic equilibrium. Imbalances such as **dehydration** (see Table 9-1) and **water intoxication** can occur, but the body quickly restores the balance to normal if it can. The body controls both water intake and water excretion to maintain water equilibrium.

Water Intake Regulation The body can survive for only a few days without water. In healthy people, thirst and satiety govern water intake.[1] Thirst is finely adjusted to ensure a water intake that meets the body's needs. When the blood becomes too concentrated (having lost water but not salt and other dissolved substances), the mouth becomes dry, and the brain center known as the **hypothalamus** initiates drinking behavior.

Thirst lags behind the lack of water. A water deficiency that develops slowly can switch on drinking behavior in time to prevent serious dehydration, but a deficiency that develops quickly may not. Also, thirst itself does not remedy a water deficiency; a person must pay attention to the thirst signal and take the time to get a drink. With aging, thirst sensations may diminish. Dehydration can threaten elderly people who do not develop the habit of drinking water regularly.

Water intoxication, on the other hand, is rare but can occur with excessive water consumption and kidney disorders that reduce urine production. The symptoms may include severe headache, confusion, convulsions, and even death in extreme cases. Excessive water ingestion (several gallons) within a few hours dilutes the sodium concentration of the blood and contributes to a dangerous condition known as **hyponatremia**.

Water Excretion Regulation Water excretion is regulated by the brain and the kidneys. The cells of the brain's hypothalamus, which monitor blood salts, stimulate the **pituitary gland** to release **antidiuretic hormone (ADH)** whenever the salts are too concentrated, or the blood volume or blood pressure is too low. ADH stimulates the kidneys to reabsorb water rather than excrete it. Thus, the more water you need, the less you excrete.

water balance: the balance between water intake and water excretion that keeps the body's water content constant.

dehydration: the loss of water from the body that occurs when water output exceeds water input. The symptoms progress rapidly from thirst, to weakness, to exhaustion and delirium, and end in death if not corrected.

water intoxication: the rare condition in which body water contents are too high. The symptoms may include confusion, convulsion, coma, and even death in extreme cases.

hypothalamus (high-poh-THALL-uh-mus): a part of the brain that helps regulate many body balances, including fluid balance.

hyponatremia (HIGH-po-na-TREE-me-ah): a decreased concentration of sodium in the blood.

pituitary (pit-TOO-ih-tary) gland: in the brain, the "king gland" that regulates the operation of many other glands.

antidiuretic hormone (ADH): a hormone released by the pituitary gland in response to high salt concentrations in the blood. The kidneys respond by reabsorbing water.

TABLE 9-1	Signs of Mild and Severe Dehydration	
Mild Dehydration **(Loss of <5% Body Weight)**		**Severe Dehydration** **(Loss of >5% Body Weight)**
Thirst		Pale skin
Sudden weight loss		Bluish lips and fingertips
Rough, dry skin		Confusion; disorientation
Dry mouth, throat, body linings		Rapid, shallow breathing
Rapid pulse		Weak, rapid, irregular pulse
Low blood pressure		Thickening of blood
Lack of energy; weakness		Shock; seizures
Impaired kidney function		Coma; death
Reduced quantity of urine; concentrated urine		
Decreased mental functioning		
Decreased muscular work and athletic performance		
Fever or increased internal temperature		
Fainting		

Source: Adapted from Standing Committee on the Scientific Evaluation of Dietary Reference Intakes, Food and Nutrition Board, Institute of Medicine, Dietary Reference Intakes: Water, Potassium, Sodium, Chloride, and Sulfate (Washington, DC: National Academies Press, 2005), pp. 90–122.

If too much water is lost from the body, blood volume and blood pressure fall. Cells in the kidneys respond to the low blood pressure by releasing an enzyme. (✚) Through a complex series of events involving the hormone **aldosterone**, this enzyme also causes the kidneys to retain more water. Again, the effect is that, when more water is needed, less is excreted.

Minimum Water Needed
These mechanisms can maintain water balance only if a person drinks enough water. The body must excrete a minimum of about 500 milliliters (✚) each day as urine—enough to carry away the waste products generated by a day's metabolic activities. Above this amount, excretion adjusts to balance intake, so the more a person drinks, the more dilute the urine becomes. In addition to urine, some water is lost from the lungs as vapor, some is excreted in feces, and some evaporates from the skin. A person's water losses from all of these routes total about 2½ liters (about 2½ quarts) a day on the average. Table 9-2 (p. 240) shows how fluid intake and output naturally balance out.

Water Recommendations and Sources
Water needs vary greatly depending on the foods a person eats, the environmental temperature and humidity,

✚ The enzyme renin (REN-in), released by the kidneys in response to low blood pressure, aids the kidneys in retaining water through the renin-angiotensin mechanism.

✚ 500 mL = about ½ qt

aldosterone (al-DOS-ter-own): a hormone secreted by the adrenal glands that stimulates the reabsorption of sodium by the kidneys; also regulates chloride and potassium concentrations.

TABLE 9-2	Water Balance		
Water Sources	Amount (mL)	Water Losses	Amount (mL)
Liquids	550 to 1500	Kidneys (urine)	500 to 1400
Foods	700 to 1000	Skin (sweat)	450 to 900
Metabolic water	200 to 300	Lungs (breath)	350
		GI tract (feces)	150
Total	1450 to 2800	Total	1450 to 2800

the person's activity level, and other factors. Accordingly, a general water requirement is difficult to establish. In the past, recommendations for adults were expressed in proportion to the amount of energy expended under normal environmental conditions. For the person who expends about 2000 kcalories a day, this works out to 2 to 3 liters, or about 8 to 12 cups. This recommendation is in line with the Adequate Intake (AI) for *total* water (✚) set by the DRI committee. Total water includes not only drinking water but also water in other beverages and in foods as well.[2]

Because a wide range of water intakes will prevent dehydration and its harmful consequences, the AI is based on average intakes. Strenuous physical activity and heat stress can increase water needs considerably, however.[3] In general, you can tell from the color of the urine whether a person needs more water. Pale yellow urine reflects appropriate dilution.[4]

The obvious dietary sources of water are water itself and other beverages, but nearly all foods also contain water. Water constitutes up to 95 percent of the volume of most fruits and vegetables and at least 50 percent of many meats and cheeses (see Table 9-3). The energy nutrients in foods also give up water during metabolism.

Which beverages are best? Any beverage can readily meet the body's fluid needs, but those with few or no kcalories do so without contributing to weight gain. Given that obesity is a major health problem and that beverages contribute more than 20 percent of the total energy intake in the United States, water is the best choice for most people.[5] Other choices include tea, coffee, nonfat and low-fat milk and soy milk, artificially sweetened beverages, fruit and vegetable juices, sports drinks, and, lastly, sweetened nutrient-poor beverages. By far, carbonated soft drinks are chosen most often, but this choice often crowds more nutritious beverages out of the diet, and the regular sugar-sweetened varieties provide a great deal of added sugar to the day's discretionary kcalorie intake.[6]

People often ask whether caffeine-containing beverages such as coffee, tea, or soda can help to meet water needs. When people who normally abstain from caffeine drink a caffeine-containing beverage, their urine output increases somewhat more than it would for a similar amount of water. This occurs because caffeine acts as a mild diuretic. Research is mixed on whether any but the highest caffeine intakes (four or five cups of coffee) cause a net water deficit in the body; most people make up for small water losses by drinking additional fluid later. The DRI committee considered such findings in making its recommendations for water intake and concluded that "caffeinated beverages contribute to the daily total water intake similar to that contributed by non-caffeinated beverages."[7] In other words, it doesn't seem to matter whether people rely on caffeine-containing beverages or other beverages to meet their fluid needs.

In contrast, alcohol should probably not be used to meet fluid needs. As Nutrition in Practice 19 explains, alcohol acts as a diuretic, and it has many adverse effects on health and nutrition status.

✚ AI for *total* water:
- Men: 3.7 L/day
- Women: 2.7 L/day

TABLE 9-3	Percentage of Water in Selected Foods
100%	Water, diet soft drinks, seltzer (unflavored), plain tea
90–99%	Fat-free milk, black coffee, Gatorade, gelatin dessert, strawberries, watermelon, grapefruit, tomato, lettuce, cabbage, celery, spinach, broccoli, cucumber, summer squash, clear broth
80–89%	Fruit juice, sugar-sweetened soft drinks, whole milk, yogurt, low-fat cottage cheese, apples, grapes, oranges, carrots, egg white, cooked oatmeal
70–79%	Shrimp, bananas, instant pudding, corn, potatoes, avocados, ricotta cheese
60–69%	Pasta, macaroni and cheese, cooked rice, legumes, salmon, lean steak, chicken breast, ice cream, low-kcalorie mayonnaise
50–59%	Ground beef, pork chop, pork sausage, hot dogs, feta cheese
40–49%	Pizza, cheeseburger
30–39%	Cheddar cheese, bagels, bread
20–29%	Pepperoni sausage, cake, biscuits
10–19%	Butter, margarine, raisins, regular mayonnaise
1–9%	Crackers, ready-to-eat cereals, pretzels, taco shells, peanut butter, nuts
0%	Oils, white sugar, meat fats, shortening

➕ Exceptions: A compound in which the positive ions are hydrogen ions (H^+) is an acid (example: hydrochloric acid, or H^+Cl^-); a compound in which the negative ions are hydroxyl ions (OH^-) is a base (example: potassium hydroxide, or K^+OH^-).

➕ The simple statement that water follows salt describes the force that chemists call *osmosis*.

salts: compounds composed of charged particles (ions). An example of a salt is potassium chloride (K^+Cl^-).

electrolyte: a salt that dissolves in water and dissociates into charged particles called ions.

electrolyte solutions: solutions that can conduct electricity.

FLUID AND ELECTROLYTE BALANCE

When mineral **salts** dissolve in water, they separate (dissociate) into charged particles known as ions, which can conduct electricity. For this reason, a salt that dissociates in water is known as an **electrolyte**. (➕) The body fluids, which contain water and partly dissociated salts, are **electrolyte solutions**.

The body's electrolytes are vital to the life of the cells and therefore must be closely regulated to help maintain the appropriate distribution of body fluids. The major minerals form salts that dissolve in the body fluids; the cells direct where these salts go; and the movement of the salts determines where the fluids flow because water follows salt. (➕) Cells use this force to move fluids back and forth across their membranes. Thanks to the electrolytes, water can be held in compartments where it is needed.

Proteins in the cell membranes move ions into or out of the cells. These protein pumps tend to concentrate sodium and chloride outside cells and potassium and other ions inside. By maintaining specific amounts of sodium outside and potassium inside, cells can regulate the exact amounts of water inside and outside their boundaries.

Healthy kidneys regulate the body's sodium, as well as its water, with remarkable precision. The intestinal tract absorbs sodium readily, and it travels freely in the blood, but the kidneys excrete unneeded amounts. The kidneys actually filter all of the sodium out of the blood; then, they return to the bloodstream the exact amount the body needs to retain.

© Craig M. Moore

Water follows salt. Notice the beads of "sweat," formed on the right-hand slices of eggplant, which were sprinkled with salt. Cellular water moves across each cell's membrane (water-permeable divider) toward the higher concentration of salt (dissolved particles) on the surface.

The body's responses to severe stress and trauma are discussed in Chapter 16.

buffers: compounds that can reversibly combine with hydrogen ions to help keep a solution's acidity or alkalinity constant. Also defined in Chapter 5.

major minerals: essential mineral nutrients required in the adult diet in amounts greater than 100 milligrams per day.

trace minerals: essential mineral nutrients required in the adult diet in amounts less than 100 milligrams per day.

Thus, the body's total electrolytes remain constant, while the urinary electrolytes fluctuate according to what is eaten.

In some cases, the body's mechanisms for maintaining fluid and electrolyte balances cannot compensate for a sudden loss of large amounts of fluid and electrolytes. Vomiting, diarrhea, heavy sweating, fever, burns, wounds, and the like may incur great fluid and electrolyte losses, precipitating an emergency that demands medical intervention. (✚)

ACID–BASE BALANCE

The body uses ions not only to help maintain water balance but also to regulate the acidity (pH) of its fluids. Like proteins, electrolyte mixtures in the body fluids protect the body against changes in acidity by acting as **buffers**—substances that can accommodate excess acids or bases.

The body's buffer systems serve as a first line of defense against changes in the fluids' acid–base balance. The lungs, skin, gastrointestinal (GI) tract, and kidneys provide other defenses. Of these organ systems, the kidneys play the primary role in maintaining acid–base balance. Thus, disorders of the kidneys impair the body's ability to regulate its acid–base balance, as well as its fluid and electrolyte balances.

TABLE 9-4	The Major and Trace Minerals
Major Minerals	**Trace Minerals**
Calcium	Arsenic
Chloride	Boron
Magnesium	Chromium
Phosphorus	Cobalt
Potassium	Copper
Sodium	Fluoride
Sulfur	Iodine
	Iron
	Manganese
	Molybdenum
	Nickel
	Selenium
	Silicon
	Vanadium
	Zinc

Review Notes

- Water makes up about 60 percent of the body's weight.
- Water helps transport nutrients and waste products throughout the body, participates in metabolic reactions, acts as a solvent, assists in maintaining blood volume and body temperature, acts as a lubricant and cushion around joints, and serves as a shock absorber.
- To maintain water balance, intake from liquids, foods, and metabolism must equal losses from kidneys, skin, lungs, and feces.
- Electrolytes help maintain the appropriate distribution of body fluids and help to maintain acid–base balance as well.

The Major Minerals

Table 9-4 lists the major and trace minerals in the body, and Figure 9-1 shows the amounts found in the body. As you can see, the most prevalent minerals are calcium and phosphorus, the chief minerals of bone. The distinction between the **major minerals** and the **trace minerals** does not mean that one group is more important than the other. A deficiency of the few micrograms of iodine needed daily is just as serious as a deficiency of the several hundred milligrams of calcium. The major minerals are so named because they are present, and needed, in larger amounts in the body than the trace minerals.

Although all the major minerals influence the body's fluid balance, sodium, chloride, and potassium are most noted for that role. For this reason, these three minerals are discussed first. Each major mineral also plays other specific roles in the body. Sodium, potassium, calcium, and magnesium are critical to nerve transmission and muscle contractions. Phosphorus and magnesium are involved in energy metabolism. Calcium, phosphorus, and magnesium contribute to the structure of the bones. Sulfur helps determine the shape of proteins. Table 9-7, shown later in the chapter, provides a summary of information about the major minerals.

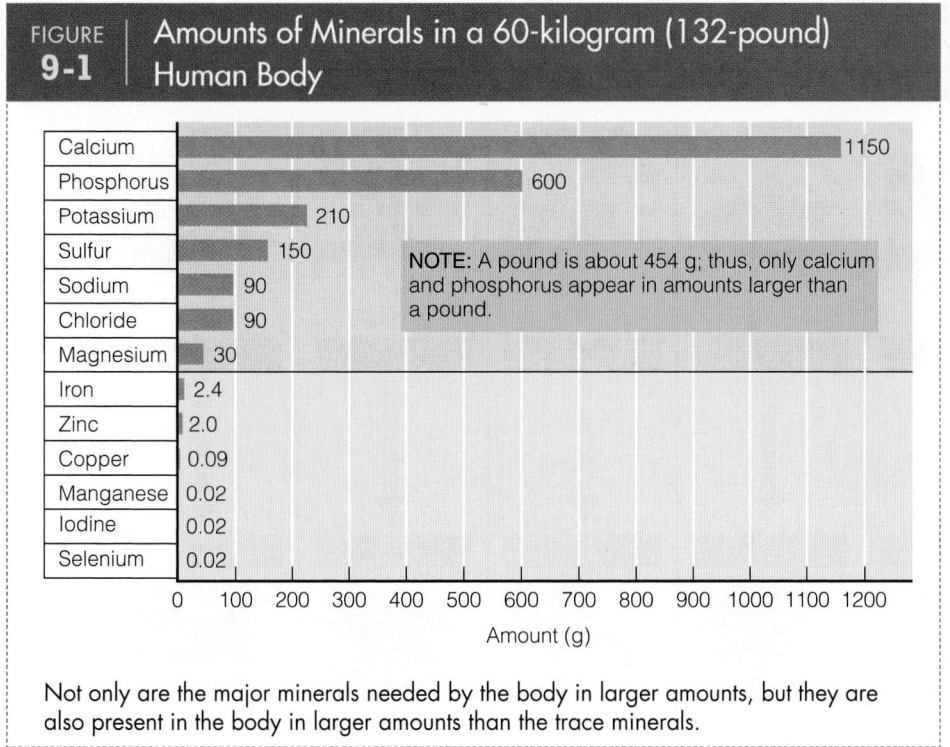

FIGURE 9-1 | Amounts of Minerals in a 60-kilogram (132-pound) Human Body

Mineral	Amount (g)
Calcium	1150
Phosphorus	600
Potassium	210
Sulfur	150
Sodium	90
Chloride	90
Magnesium	30
Iron	2.4
Zinc	2.0
Copper	0.09
Manganese	0.02
Iodine	0.02
Selenium	0.02

NOTE: A pound is about 454 g; thus, only calcium and phosphorus appear in amounts larger than a pound.

Not only are the major minerals needed by the body in larger amounts, but they are also present in the body in larger amounts than the trace minerals.

SODIUM

Sodium is the principal electrolyte in the **extracellular fluid** (the fluid outside the cells) and the primary regulator of the extracellular fluid volume. When the blood concentration of sodium rises, as when a person eats salted foods, thirst prompts the person to drink water until the appropriate sodium-to-water ratio is restored. Sodium also helps maintain acid–base balance and is essential to muscle contraction and nerve transmission. Too much sodium, however, can contribute to high blood pressure.

Sodium Recommendations and Food Sources Diets rarely lack sodium, and even when intakes are low, the body adapts by reducing sodium losses in urine and sweat, thus making deficiencies unlikely. Sodium recommendations (✚) are set low enough to protect against high blood pressure but high enough to allow an adequate intake of other nutrients. Because high sodium intakes correlate with high blood pressure, the Tolerable Upper Intake Level (UL) for adults is set at 2300 milligrams per day, slightly lower than the Daily Value used on food labels (2400 milligrams). The UL corresponds to about 1 teaspoon of salt (sodium chloride). (✚)

Today, the average U.S. sodium intake is more than 3400 mg per day, an amount that far exceeds the UL.[8] Three groups of people encompassing about 70 percent of U.S. adults—persons with hypertension, all middle-aged and older adults, and all African Americans—are urged to limit their sodium intakes (to no more than 1500 milligrams of sodium per day) for the sake of their blood pressure and heart health.[9]

Sodium intakes also vary widely. People who eat mostly processed and fast foods have the highest sodium intakes, whereas those who eat mostly whole, unprocessed foods, such as fresh fruits and vegetables, have the lowest intakes. In fact, about three-fourths of the sodium in people's diets comes from salt added to foods by manufacturers. Figure 9-2 (p. 244) shows that processed foods contain not only more sodium but also less potassium than their less processed counterparts.

Sodium and Blood Pressure High intakes of salt among the world's people correlate with high rates of **hypertension**, heart disease, and cerebral

✚ Sodium AI:
- 1500 mg/day (19–50 yr)
- 1300 mg/day (51–70 yr)
- 1200 mg/day (>70 yr)

✚ Salt (sodium chloride) is about 40 percent sodium.
1 g salt contributes 400 mg sodium.
6 g salt = 1 tsp.
1 tsp salt contributes about 2300 mg sodium.

extracellular fluid: fluid residing outside the cells; includes the fluid between the cells (*interstitial fluid*), plasma, and the water of structures such as the skin and bones. Extracellular fluid accounts for about one-third of the body's water.

hypertension: high blood pressure.

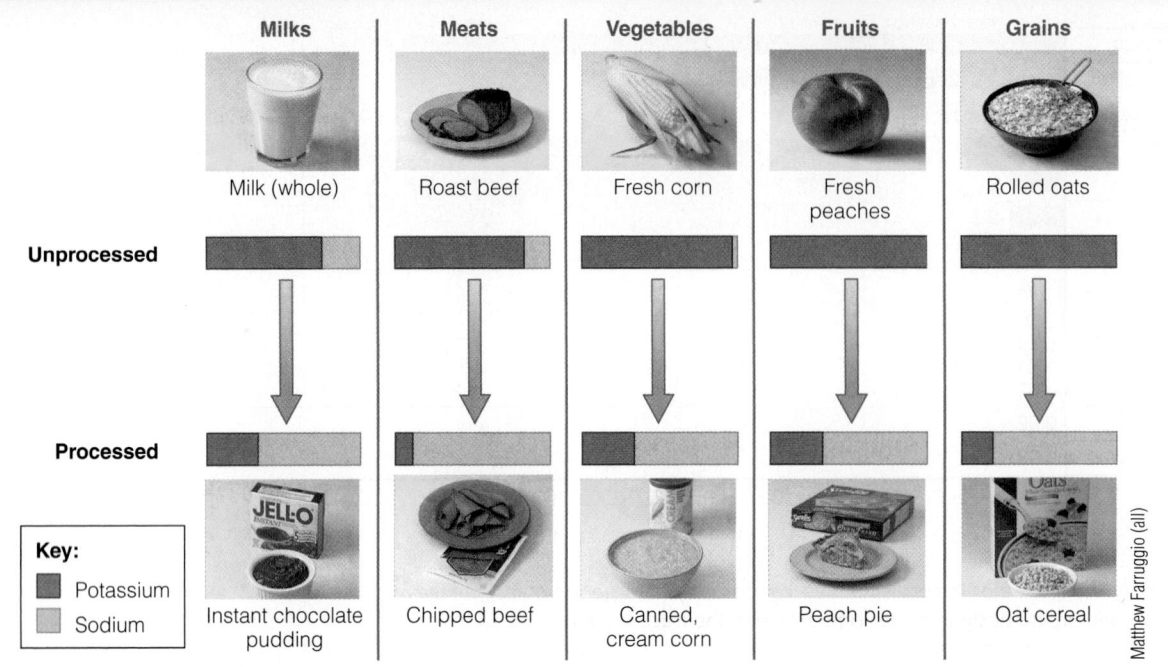

Key:
- ■ Potassium
- ■ Sodium

People who eat foods high in salt often happen to be eating fewer potassium-containing foods at the same time. Notice how potassium is lost and sodium is gained as foods become more processed, causing the potassium-to-sodium ratio to fall dramatically. Even when potassium is not lost, the addition of sodium still lowers the potassium-to-sodium ratio.

hemorrhage, a hypertension-related stroke.[10] An estimated 29 percent of U.S. adults have hypertension (that is, high blood pressure), and another 28 percent have **prehypertension**.[11] (✚)

In many people, the relationship between salt intake and blood pressure is immediate and direct—as sodium intakes increase, blood pressure rises with them in a stepwise fashion within just days or weeks of exposure.[12] And with high blood pressure, the heart becomes damaged and risks of death from stroke and heart disease climb steeply.[13] In a large 15-year intervention study, when people with prehypertension reduced their sodium intakes, they reduced their risk of developing heart disease or dying from it by 25 to 30 percent.[14]

In fact, a salt-restricted diet lowers blood pressure in people without hypertension as well. Because reducing salt intake causes no harm and diminishes the risk of hypertension and heart disease, the *Dietary Guidelines for Americans* advise limiting daily *sodium* intakes to less than 2300 milligrams (approximately 1 teaspoon of *salt*). Higher intakes seem to be well tolerated in most healthy people, however. The accompanying "How to" offers strategies for cutting salt (and, therefore, sodium) intake.

One diet plan known as the DASH (Dietary Approaches to Stop Hypertension) diet also lowers blood pressure.[15] The DASH approach emphasizes fruits, vegetables, and low-fat dairy products; includes whole grains, nuts, poultry, and fish; and calls for reduced intakes of red meat, butter, and other high-fat foods. The DASH diet in combination with a reduced sodium intake is even more effective at lowering blood pressure than either strategy alone. Chapter 21 offers a complete discussion of hypertension and the dietary recommendations for its prevention and treatment.

✚ Chapter 21 presents more details about blood pressure and lists standard ranges for blood pressure readings.

prehypertension: blood pressure values that predict hypertension.

CHLORIDE

The chloride ion is the major negative ion of the extracellular fluids, where it occurs primarily in association with sodium. Like sodium, chloride is critical to maintaining

Most people eat more salt (and, therefore, sodium) than they need. Some people can lower their blood pressure by avoiding highly salted foods and removing the saltshaker from the table. Foods eaten without salt may seem less tasty at first, but with repetition, people can learn to enjoy the natural flavors of many unsalted foods. Strategies to cut salt intake include:

- Select fresh, unprocessed foods.
- Cook with little or no added salt.
- Prepare foods with sodium-free spices such as basil, bay leaves, curry, garlic, ginger, mint, oregano, pepper, rosemary, and thyme; lemon juice; vinegar; or wine.
- Add little or no salt at the table; taste foods before adding salt.
- Read labels with an eye open for sodium. (See the Glossary on pp. 27–28 for terms used to describe the sodium contents of foods on labels.)
- Select low-salt or salt-free products when available.

Use these foods sparingly:

- Foods prepared in brine, such as pickles, olives, and sauerkraut.
- Salty or smoked meats, such as bologna, corned or chipped beef, bacon, frankfurters, ham, lunch meats, salt pork, sausage, and smoked tongue.
- Salty or smoked fish, such as anchovies, caviar, salted and dried cod, herring, sardines, and smoked salmon.
- Snack items such as potato chips, pretzels, salted popcorn, salted nuts, and crackers.
- Condiments such as bouillon cubes; seasoned salts; MSG; soy, teriyaki, Worcestershire, and barbeque sauces; prepared horseradish, catsup, and mustard.
- Cheeses, especially processed types.
- Canned and instant soups.

fluid, electrolyte, and acid–base balances in the body. In the stomach, the chloride ion is part of hydrochloric acid, which maintains the strong acidity of the gastric fluids.

Salt is a major food source of chloride, and, as with sodium, processed foods are a major contributor of this mineral to people's diets. Because salt contains a higher proportion of chloride (by weight) than sodium, chloride recommendations () are slightly higher than, but still equivalent to, those of sodium. In other words, ¾ teaspoon of salt will deliver some sodium, more chloride, and still meet the AI for both.

POTASSIUM

Potassium is the principal positively charged ion inside the body cells. It plays a major role in maintaining fluid and electrolyte balance and cell integrity. Potassium is also critical to keeping the heartbeat steady. The sudden deaths that occur in severe diarrhea and in children with kwashiorkor or people with eating disorders are likely due to heart failure caused by potassium loss.

Potassium Deficiency and Toxicity Potassium deficiency is characterized by an increase in blood pressure, salt sensitivity, kidney stones, and bone turnover. As deficiency progresses, symptoms include irregular heartbeats, muscle weakness, and glucose intolerance. Potassium deficiency results more often from excessive losses than from deficient intakes. Deficiency arises in abnormal conditions such as diabetic acidosis, dehydration, or prolonged vomiting or diarrhea; potassium deficiency can also result from the regular use of certain medications, including **diuretics**, **steroids**, and **cathartics**. One of the earliest symptoms of deficiency is muscle weakness. Inadequate potassium intakes are possible with diets low in fresh fruits and vegetables, but out-and-out deficiencies of potassium are unlikely in healthy people.

Potassium toxicity does not result from overeating foods high in potassium; therefore, a Tolerable Upper Intake Level was not set. Toxicity can result from overconsumption of potassium salts or supplements and from certain diseases or medications.[16] Given more potassium than the body needs, the kidneys accelerate their excretion. If the GI tract is bypassed, however, and potassium is injected directly into a vein, it can stop the heart.

Potassium Recommendations and Food Sources In healthy people, almost any reasonable diet provides enough potassium to prevent the dangerously low blood potassium that indicates a severe deficiency. Potassium

 Chloride AI:
- 2300 mg/day (19–50 yr)
- 2000 mg/day (51–70 yr)
- 1800 mg/day (>70 yr)

diuretics (dye-yoo-RET-ics): medications that promote the excretion of water through the kidneys. Not all diuretics increase the urinary loss of potassium. Some, called potassium-sparing diuretics, are less likely to result in a potassium deficiency (see Chapter 21).

steroids (STARE-oids): medications used to reduce tissue inflammation, to suppress the immune response, or to replace certain steroid hormones in people who cannot synthesize them.

cathartics (ca-THART-ics): strong laxatives.

Fresh fruits and vegetables provide potassium in abundance.

Potassium AI:
• Adults: 4700 mg

is abundant inside all living cells, both plant and animal, and because cells remain intact until foods are processed, the richest sources of potassium are *fresh* foods of all kinds—especially fruits and vegetables. A typical U.S. diet, however, with its low intakes of fruits and vegetables, provides only about half the recommended intake.[17] (✚) Although blood potassium may remain normal on such a diet, chronic diseases are more likely to occur.

CALCIUM

Calcium occupies more space in this chapter than any other major mineral. Other minerals are revisited later in this book, where their key roles in heart disease and kidney disease are discussed. Calcium, though, deserves emphasis here in the normal nutrition part of the book because an adequate intake of calcium early in life helps grow a healthy skeleton and prevent bone disease in later life.

Calcium Roles in the Body
Calcium owns the distinction of being the most abundant mineral in the body. Ninety-nine percent of the body's calcium is stored in the bones, where it plays two important roles. First, it is an integral part of bone structure. Second, it serves as a calcium bank available to the body fluids should a drop in blood calcium occur.

Calcium in Bone
As bones begin to form, calcium salts form crystals on a matrix of the protein collagen. As the crystals become denser, they give strength and rigidity to the maturing bones. As a result, the long leg bones of children can support their weight by the time they have learned to walk. Figure 9-3 shows the lacy network of calcium-containing crystals in the bone.

Many people have the idea that bones are inert, like rocks. Not so. Bones continuously gain and lose minerals in an ongoing process of remodeling. Growing children gain more bone than they lose, and healthy adults maintain a reasonable balance. When withdrawals substantially exceed deposits, however, problems such as osteoporosis develop.

From birth to approximately age 20, the bones are actively growing by modifying their length, width, and shape (see Figure 9-4). This rapid growth phase overlaps with the next period of peak bone mass development, which occurs between the ages of 12 and 30. During this period, skeletal mass increases. Bones grow thicker and denser by remodeling, a maintenance and repair process involving the loss of existing bone and the deposition of new bone. In the final phase, which begins between 30 and 40 years of age and continues throughout the remainder of life, bone loss exceeds new bone formation.

FIGURE 9-3 | Cross Section of Bone

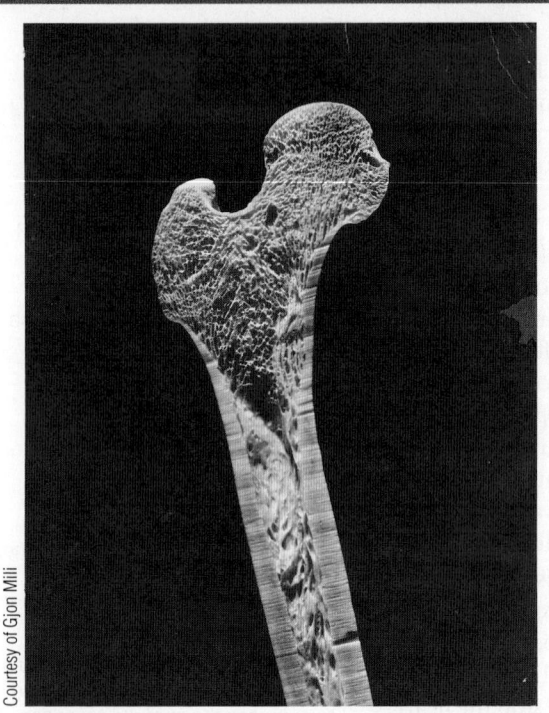

The lacy structural elements are *trabeculae* (tra-BECK-you-lee), which can be drawn on to replenish blood calcium.

Calcium in Body Fluids
The 1 percent of the body's calcium that circulates in the fluids as ionized calcium is vital to life. It plays these major roles:

- Regulates the transport of ions across cell membranes and is particularly important in nerve transmission
- Helps maintain normal blood pressure
- Plays an essential role in the clotting of blood
- Is essential for muscle contraction and therefore for the heartbeat
- Allows secretion of hormones, digestive enzymes, and neurotransmitters
- Activates cellular enzymes that regulate many processes

Because of its importance, blood calcium is tightly controlled.

Calcium Balance
Blood calcium concentration is tightly controlled.[18] Whenever blood calcium rises too high, a system of

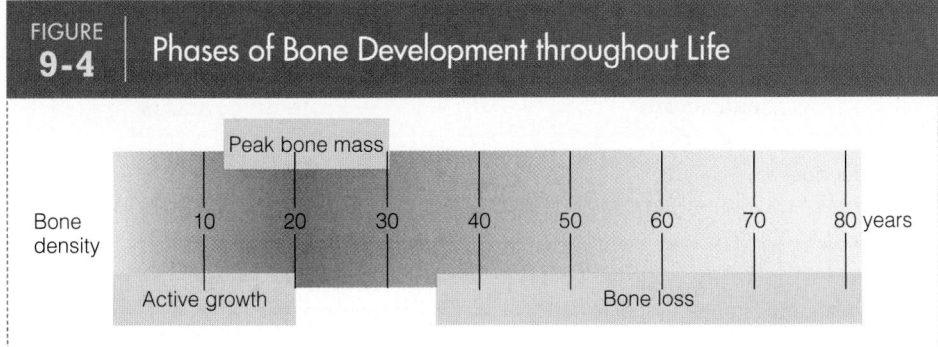

FIGURE 9-4 | Phases of Bone Development throughout Life

Peak bone mass

Bone density

10   20   30   40   50   60   70   80 years

Active growth   Bone loss

The active growth phase occurs from birth to approximately age 20. The next phase of peak bone mass development occurs between the ages of 12 and 30. The final phase, when bone resorption exceeds formation, begins between the ages of 30 and 40 and continues through the remainder of life.

hormones and vitamin D promotes its deposit into bone. Whenever blood calcium falls too low, the regulatory system (✚) acts in three locations to raise it:

1. The small intestine absorbs more calcium.
2. The bones release more calcium into the blood.
3. The kidneys excrete less calcium.

Thus, blood calcium rises to normal.

The calcium stored in bone provides a nearly inexhaustible source of calcium for the blood. Even in a calcium deficiency, blood calcium remains normal. Blood calcium changes only in response to abnormal regulatory control, not to diet. Blood calcium above normal causes **calcium rigor**: the muscles contract and cannot relax. Blood calcium below normal causes **calcium tetany**—also characterized by uncontrolled muscle contraction. These conditions are caused by a lack of vitamin D or by abnormal concentrations of the hormones that regulate calcium homeostasis.

Although a chronic *dietary* deficiency of calcium or a chronic deficiency due to poor absorption does not change blood calcium, it does deplete the calcium in the bones. Because this is an important concept, we repeat: it is the bones, not the blood, that are robbed by calcium deficiency.

Calcium and Osteoporosis As mentioned earlier, bone mass peaks at the time of skeletal maturity (about age 30), and a high peak bone mass is the best protection against later age-related bone loss and fracture. Adequate calcium nutrition during the growing years is essential to achieving optimal peak bone mass.[19] Following menopause, women lose about 15 percent of their bone mass, as do middle-aged and older men. When bone loss has reached such an extreme that bones fracture under even common, everyday stresses, the condition is known as osteoporosis. (✚) Osteoporosis afflicts more than 40 million people, mostly women 50 years of age or older.[20] Men, however, are not immune to osteoporosis. Each year, more than 2 million people—30 percent of them men—suffer broken hips, pelvises, legs, arms, hands, and ankles attributable to osteoporosis.

Both genetic and environmental factors contribute to osteoporosis. Table 9-5 (p. 248) summarizes risk and protective factors for osteoporosis. Osteoporosis is more prevalent in women than men for several reasons. First, women consume less dietary calcium than men do. Second, at all ages, women's bone mass is lower than men's because women generally have smaller bodies. Finally, bone loss accelerates after menopause and exceeds men's losses for up to 10 years.

In addition to calcium, many other minerals and vitamins, including phosphorus, magnesium, fluoride, and vitamin D, help to form and stabilize the structure of bones. Any or all of these elements are needed to prevent bone loss. The first, most obvious lines of defense, however, are to maintain a lifelong adequate intake of calcium and to "exercise it into place." Active bones are denser than sedentary bones.[21] Weight-bearing

✚ The regulators are hormones from the thyroid and parathyroid glands, as well as vitamin D. One hormone, parathormone, raises blood calcium. Another hormone, calcitonin, lowers blood calcium by inhibiting release of calcium from bone. The hormonelike vitamin D raises blood calcium by acting at the three sites listed.

✚ Reminder: *Osteoporosis* is a condition characterized by reduced density of the bones. The bones become porous and fragile and fracture easily.

calcium rigor: hardness or stiffness of the muscles caused by high blood calcium.

calcium tetany: intermittent spasms of the extremities due to nervous and muscular excitability caused by low blood calcium.

TABLE 9-5	Risk Factors and Protective Factors for Osteoporosis	
	Risk Factors	**Protective Factors**
	• Older age	• Younger age
	• Low BMI	• High BMI
	• Caucasian, Asian, or Hispanic heritage	• African American heritage
	• Cigarette smoking	• No smoking
	• Alcohol consumption in excess	• Alcohol consumption in moderation
	• Sedentary lifestyle	• Regular weight-bearing exercise
	• Use of glucocorticoids or anticonvulsants	• Use of diuretics
	• Female gender	• Male gender
	• Maternal history of osteoporosis fracture or personal history of fracture	• Bone density assessment and treatment (if necessary)
	• Estrogen deficiency in women (amenorrhea or menopause, especially early or surgically induced); testosterone deficiency in men	• Use of estrogen therapy
	• Lifetime diet inadequate in calcium and vitamin D	• Lifetime diet rich in calcium and vitamin D

physical activity, such as walking, running, dancing, and weight training, prompts the bones to deposit minerals. It has long been known that, when people are confined to bed, both their muscles and their bones lose strength. Muscle strength and bone strength go together: when muscles work, they pull on the bones, and both are stimulated to grow stronger.

Calcium and Disease Prevention Calcium may protect against hypertension, although research results are inconsistent and inconclusive.[22] Considering the success of the DASH diet in lowering blood pressure, restricting sodium to treat hypertension may be narrow advice. The DASH diet is not particularly low in sodium, but it is rich in calcium, as well as in potassium and magnesium. As mentioned earlier, the DASH diet, together with a reduced sodium intake, is more effective at lowering blood pressure than either strategy alone. Some research also suggests protective relationships between calcium and blood cholesterol, diabetes, and colon and rectal cancers.[23] Calcium from low-fat milk and milk products (but not from supplements) has been linked with having a healthy body weight in some, but not all, studies.[24] Large, well-designed clinical studies are needed to clarify any effects of dietary calcium on body weight.[25]

Calcium Recommendations As mentioned earlier, blood calcium concentration does not reflect calcium status. Calcium recommendations (✚) are therefore based on balance studies, which measure daily intake and excretion. An optimal calcium intake reflects the amount needed to retain the most calcium. The more calcium retained, the greater the bone density (within genetic limits) and, potentially, the lower the risk of osteoporosis. Calcium recommendations during adolescence are

✚ Calcium AI:
• Adults (19–50 yr): 1000 mg/day
• Adults (51 and older): 1200 mg/day

set high (1300 milligrams) to help ensure that the skeleton will be strong and dense. Between the ages of 19 and 50, recommendations are lowered to 1000 milligrams a day. For those over 50, recommendations are raised again, to 1200 milligrams, to minimize bone loss. Some authorities advocate calcium recommendations as high as 1500 milligrams per day for women over 50. Many people in the United States have calcium intakes below current recommendations.[26] High intakes of calcium from supplements may have adverse effects, such as kidney stone formation. For this reason, a UL has been established (see inside front cover).

Calcium in Foods

Calcium is found most abundantly in a single food group—milk and milk products. For this reason, dietary recommendations advise daily consumption of low-fat or fat-free milk products. A cup of milk offers about 300 milligrams of calcium, so an adult who drinks 3 cups of milk a day (or eats the equivalent in yogurt) is well on the way to meeting daily calcium needs (see Table 9-6). The other dairy food that contains comparable amounts of calcium is cheese. One slice of cheese (1 ounce) contains about two-thirds as much calcium as a cup of milk. Cottage cheese, however, contains much less. Snapshot 9-1 shows foods that are rich in calcium, and the "How to" (p. 250) suggests ways of adding calcium to meals.

Some foods offer large amounts of calcium because of fortification. Calcium-fortified juice, high-calcium milk (milk with extra calcium added), and calcium-fortified cereals are examples. Some calcium-rich mineral waters provide as much as 500 milligrams of calcium per liter, offering a convenient way to meet both calcium and water needs.[27]

Among the vegetables, mustard greens, kale, parsley, watercress, and broccoli are good sources of available calcium. Some dark green, leafy vegetables—notably, spinach and Swiss chard—appear to be calcium rich but actually provide very little, if any, calcium to the body. These foods contain **binders** that prevent calcium absorption.

Aided by vitamin D, the body is able to regulate its absorption of calcium by altering its production of the calcium-binding protein. More of this protein is made if more calcium is needed. Infants and children absorb up to 60 percent of the calcium they

TABLE 9-6	Suggested Minimum Daily Fluid Milk Intakes	
Young children (2 to 8 years of age)		2 cups
Older children and adolescents		3 cups
Adults		3 cups
Pregnant or lactating women		3 cups
Women past menopause		3 cups

binders: chemical compounds in foods that combine with nutrients (especially minerals) to form complexes the body cannot absorb. Examples include *phytates* and *oxalates*.

SNAPSHOT 9-1 *Calcium*

GOOD SOURCES*

SARDINES (with bones)
3 oz = 325 mg

MILK
1 c = 300 mg

TOFU (calcium set)
½ c = 275 mg

CHEDDAR CHEESE
1½ oz = 288 mg

TURNIP GREENS (cooked)
1 c = 198 mg

WAFFLE (whole grain)
1 waffle = 196 mg

BROCCOLI[a] (cooked)
1½ c = 93 mg

* These foods provide 10 percent or more of the calcium Daily Value in a serving. For a 2000-kcalorie diet, the DV is 1000 mg/day.
[a] Broccoli, kale, and some other cooked green leafy vegetables are also important sources of bioavailable calcium. Almonds also supply calcium. Other greens, such as spinach and chard, contain calcium in an unabsorbable form. Some calcium-rich mineral waters may also be good sources.

For those who tolerate milk, many cooks slip extra calcium into meals by sprinkling a tablespoon or two of fat-free dry milk into almost everything. The added kcalorie value is small, and changes to the taste and texture of the dish are practically nil. Yet each 2 tablespoons adds about 100 extra milligrams of calcium and moves people closer to meeting the recommendation to obtain 3 cups of milk each day. Here are some more tips for including calcium-rich foods in your meals.

At Breakfast

- Choose calcium-fortified orange or vegetable juice.
- Serve tea or coffee, hot or iced, with milk.
- Choose cereals, hot or cold, with milk.
- Cook hot cereals with milk instead of water; then mix in 2 tablespoons of fat-free dry milk.
- Make muffins or quick breads with milk and extra fat-free powdered milk.
- Add milk to scrambled eggs.
- Moisten cereals with flavored yogurt.

At Lunch

- Add low-fat cheeses to sandwiches, burgers, or salads.
- Use a variety of green vegetables, such as watercress or kale, in salads and on sandwiches.
- Drink fat-free milk or calcium-fortified soy milk as a beverage or in a smoothie.

- Drink calcium-rich mineral water as a beverage (studies suggest significant calcium absorption).
- Marinate cabbage shreds or broccoli spears in low-fat Italian dressing for an interesting salad that provides calcium.
- Choose coleslaw over potato and macaroni salads.
- Mix the mashed bones of canned salmon into salmon salad or patties.
- Eat sardines with their bones.
- Stuff potatoes with broccoli and low-fat cheese.
- Try pasta such as ravioli stuffed with low-fat ricotta cheese instead of meat.
- Sprinkle Parmesan cheese on pasta salads.

At Supper

- Toss a handful of thinly sliced green vegetables, such as kale or young turnip greens, with hot pasta; the greens wilt pleasingly in the steam of the freshly cooked pasta.
- Serve a green vegetable every night and try new ones—how about kohlrabi? It tastes delicious when cooked like broccoli.
- Learn to stir-fry Chinese cabbage and other Asian foods.
- Try tofu (the calcium-set kind); this versatile food has inspired whole cookbooks devoted to creative uses.
- Add fat-free powdered milk to almost anything—meatloaf, sauces, gravies, soups, stuffings, casseroles, blended beverages, puddings, quick breads, cookies, brownies. Be creative.
- Choose frozen yogurt, ice milk, or custards for dessert.

ingest, and pregnant women, about 50 percent. Other adults, who are not growing, absorb about 25 percent.

People may think that taking a calcium supplement is preferable to getting calcium from food, but foods offer important fringe benefits. For example, drinking 3 cups of milk fortified with vitamins A and D will supply substantial amounts of other nutrients. Furthermore, the vitamin D and possibly other nutrients in the milk enhance calcium absorption. Some people absorb calcium better from milk and milk products than from even the most absorbable supplements. The National Institutes of Health concludes that foods are the best sources of calcium and recommends supplements only when intake from food is insufficient.

PHOSPHORUS

Phosphorus is the second most abundant mineral in the body. About 85 percent of it is found combined with calcium in the crystals of the bones and teeth. As part of one of the body's buffer systems (phosphoric acid), phosphorus is also found in all body tissues. Phosphorus is a part of DNA and RNA, the genetic material present in every cell. Thus, phosphorus is necessary for all growth. Phosphorus also plays many key roles in the transfer of energy that occurs during cellular metabolism. Phosphorus-containing lipids (phospholipids) help transport other lipids in the blood. Phospholipids are also principal components of cell membranes.

Animal protein is the best source of phosphorus because the mineral is so abundant in the cells of animals. Diets that provide adequate energy and protein also supply adequate phosphorus. (✚) Dietary deficiencies are rare. A summary of facts about phosphorus appears in Table 9-7 later in the chapter.

✚ Phosphorus RDA:
- Adults: 700 mg/day

MAGNESIUM

Magnesium barely qualifies as a major mineral. Only about 1 ounce of magnesium is present in the body of a 130-pound person, more than half of it in the bones.[28] Most of the rest is in the muscles, heart, liver, and other soft tissues, with only 1 percent in the body fluids. Bone magnesium seems to be a reservoir to ensure that some will be on hand for vital reactions regardless of recent dietary intake.

Magnesium is critical to the operation of hundreds of enzymes. It acts in all the cells of the soft tissues, where it forms part of the protein-making machinery and is necessary for the release of energy. Magnesium also helps muscles to relax after contraction.

Magnesium Deficiency
Magnesium deficiency can result from vomiting, diarrhea, alcohol abuse, or protein malnutrition; in people who have been fed incomplete fluids intravenously for too long after surgery; or in people using diuretics. A severe magnesium deficiency causes tetany, an extreme and prolonged contraction of the muscles similar to the calcium tetany described earlier. Magnesium deficiency is thought to cause the hallucinations commonly experienced during withdrawal from alcohol intoxication.

Magnesium Toxicity
Magnesium toxicity is rare, but it can be fatal. Toxicity occurs only with high intakes from nonfood sources such as supplements or magnesium salts. Accidental poisonings may occur in children with access to medicine cabinets and in older adults who abuse magnesium-containing laxatives, antacids, and other medications. The consequences include diarrhea, abdominal cramps, and, in severe cases, acid–base imbalance and potassium depletion.[29]

Magnesium Intakes and Food Sources
Although almost half the U.S. population has magnesium intakes below those recommended, deficiency symptoms are rare in healthy people.[30] (✚) In various parts of the country, the water contains both calcium and magnesium. Known as "hard" water, this water can contribute significantly to magnesium intakes.

Magnesium-rich food sources include dark green, leafy vegetables; nuts; legumes; whole-grain breads and cereals; seafood; chocolate; and cocoa (see Snapshot 9-2). Magnesium is easily lost from foods during processing, so unprocessed foods are the best choices.

✚ Magnesium RDA:
- Men (19–30 yr): 400 mg/day
  (31 and older): 420 mg/day
- Women (19–30 yr):
  310 mg/day
  (31 and older): 320 mg/day

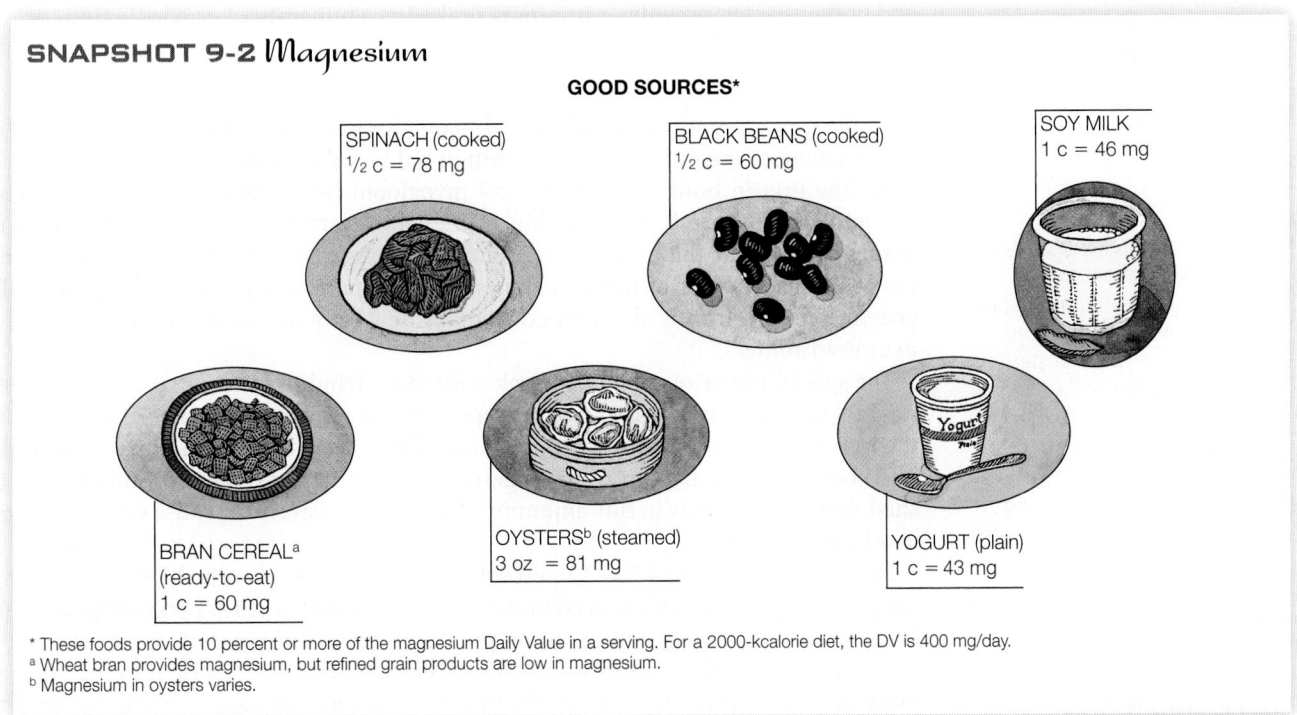

SNAPSHOT 9-2 *Magnesium*

GOOD SOURCES*

SPINACH (cooked)
1/2 c = 78 mg

BLACK BEANS (cooked)
1/2 c = 60 mg

SOY MILK
1 c = 46 mg

BRAN CEREAL[a]
(ready-to-eat)
1 c = 60 mg

OYSTERS[b] (steamed)
3 oz = 81 mg

YOGURT (plain)
1 c = 43 mg

* These foods provide 10 percent or more of the magnesium Daily Value in a serving. For a 2000-kcalorie diet, the DV is 400 mg/day.
[a] Wheat bran provides magnesium, but refined grain products are low in magnesium.
[b] Magnesium in oysters varies.

SULFATE

Sulfate is the oxidized form of sulfur as it exists in food and water. The body requires sulfate for the synthesis of many important sulfur-containing compounds. Sulfur-containing amino acids play an important role in helping to shape strands of protein. (✚) The particular shape of a protein enables it to do its specific job, such as enzyme work. Skin, hair, and nails contain some of the body's more rigid proteins, which have high sulfur contents.

There is no recommended intake for sulfur, and no deficiencies are known. Only a person who lacks protein to the point of severe deficiency will lack the sulfur-containing amino acids.

Review Notes

- All of the major minerals influence the body's fluid balance, but sodium, chloride, and potassium are most noted for this role.
- Excess sodium in the diet contributes to high blood pressure.
- Most of the body's calcium is in the bones, where it provides a rigid structure and a reservoir of calcium for the blood.
- Table 9-7 offers a summary of the major minerals and their functions.

The Trace Minerals

Figure 9-1, earlier in this chapter, shows how tiny the quantities of trace minerals in the human body are. If you could remove all of them from your body, you would have only a bit of dust, hardly enough to fill a teaspoon. Yet each of the trace minerals performs some vital role for which no substitute will do. A deficiency of any of them can be fatal, and an excess of many can be equally deadly.

Recommendations have been established for nine of the trace minerals. Others are recognized as essential nutrients for some animals but have not been proved to be required for human beings (see Table 9-8 on p. 254). Still others are under study to determine whether they, too, perform indispensable roles in the body. Table 9-9, at the end of the chapter, provides a summary of the trace minerals.

IRON

Every living cell—both plant and animal—contains iron. Most of the iron in the body is a component of the proteins **hemoglobin** in red blood cells and **myoglobin** in muscle cells. The iron in both hemoglobin and myoglobin helps them carry and hold oxygen and then release it. Hemoglobin in the blood carries oxygen from the lungs to tissues throughout the body. Myoglobin holds oxygen for the muscles to use when they contract. As part of many enzymes, iron is vital to the processes by which cells generate energy. Iron is also needed to make new cells, amino acids, hormones, and neurotransmitters.

The special provisions the body makes for iron's handling show that it is a precious mineral to be tightly hoarded. For example, when a red blood cell dies, the liver saves the iron and returns it to the bone marrow, which uses it to build new red blood cells. The body does lose iron from the digestive tract, in nail and hair trimmings, and in shed skin cells, but only in tiny amounts.[31] Bleeding, however, can cause significant iron loss from the body.

Normally, only about 10 to 15 percent of dietary iron is absorbed, but if the body's supply is diminished or if the need increases for any reason (such as pregnancy), absorption increases. The body makes several provisions for absorbing iron. A special protein in the intestinal cells captures iron and holds it in reserve for release into the body as needed; another protein transfers the iron to a special iron carrier in the blood. The blood protein (**transferrin**) carries the iron to tissues throughout the body. When more

✚ The sulfur-containing amino acids are methionine and cysteine. Cysteine in one part of a protein chain can bind to cysteine in another part of the chain by way of a sulfur-sulfur bridge, thus helping to stabilize the protein structure.

hemoglobin: the oxygen-carrying protein of the red blood cells.
hemo = blood
globin = globular protein

myoglobin: the oxygen-carrying protein of the muscle cells.
myo = muscle

transferrin (trans-FERR-in): the body's iron-carrying protein.

TABLE
9-7 | The Major Minerals—A Summary

Mineral Name	Chief Functions in the Body	Deficiency Symptoms	Toxicity Symptoms	Significant Sources
Sodium	With chloride and potassium (electrolytes), maintains cells' normal fluid balance and acid–base balance in the body. Also critical to nerve impulse transmission and muscle contraction.	Muscle cramps, mental apathy, loss of appetite	Hypertension	Salt, soy sauce, processed foods
Chloride	Part of the hydrochloric acid found in the stomach and necessary for proper digestion.	Does not occur under normal circumstances	Normally harmless (the gas chlorine is a poison but evaporates from water); can cause vomiting	Salt, soy sauce; moderate quantities in whole, unprocessed foods; large amounts in processed foods
Potassium	Facilitates reactions, including the making of protein; the maintenance of fluid and electrolyte balance; the support of cell integrity; the transmission of nerve impulses; and the contraction of muscles, including the heart.	Moderate deficiency: elevated blood pressure, increased salt sensitivity, increased risk of kidney stones, increased bone turnover. Severe deficiency: cardiac arrhythmias, muscle weakness, glucose intolerance.	Causes muscular weakness; triggers vomiting; if given into a vein, can stop the heart	All whole foods: meats, milk, fruits, vegetables, grains, legumes
Calcium	The principal mineral of bones and teeth. Also acts in normal muscle contraction and relaxation, nerve functioning, blood clotting, blood pressure, and immune defenses.	Stunted growth in children; adult bone loss (osteoporosis)	Constipation; increased risk of urinary stone formation and kidney dysfunction; interference with absorption of other minerals	Milk and milk products, oysters, small fish (with bones), tofu (bean curd), greens, legumes
Phosphorus	Involved in the mineralization of bones and teeth. Important in cells' genetic material, in cell membranes as phospholipids, in energy transfer, and in buffering systems.	Phosphorus deficiency unknown	Calcification of nonskeletal tissues, particularly the kidneys	Foods from animal sources (meat, fish, poultry, eggs, milk)
Magnesium	Another factor involved in bone mineralization, the building of protein, enzyme action, normal muscular contraction, and transmission of nerve impulses.	Weakness; confusion; if extreme, convulsions, bizarre movements (especially of eyes and face), hallucinations, and difficulty in swallowing; in children, growth failure[a]	From nonfood sources only; diarrhea; acid–base imbalance; potassium depletion	Nuts, legumes, whole grains, dark green vegetables, seafoods, chocolate, cocoa
Sulfate	A component of certain amino acids; part of the vitamins biotin and thiamin and the hormone insulin; stabilizes protein shape by forming sulfur-sulfur bridges.	None known; protein deficiency would occur first.	Would occur only if sulfur amino acids were eaten in excess; this (in animals) depresses growth	All protein-containing foods (meats, fish, poultry, eggs, milk, legumes, nuts)

[a] A still more severe deficiency causes tetany, an extreme, prolonged contraction of the muscles similar to that caused by low blood calcium.

TABLE 9-8	Trace Minerals

RDA

Copper

Iodine

Iron

Molybdenum

Selenium

Zinc

Adequate Intake (AI)

Chromium

Fluoride

Manganese

Known Essential for Animals; Human Requirements under Study

Arsenic

Boron

Nickel

Silicon

Vanadium

Known Essential for Some Animals; No Evidence That Intake by Humans Is Ever Limiting; No Recommendation Necessary

Cobalt

Note: The evidence for requirements and essentiality is weak for the trace minerals cadmium, lead, lithium, and tin.

✚ The storage proteins are ferritin (FERR-i-tin) and hemosiderin (heem-oh-SID-er-in).

✚ Stages of iron deficiency:
• Iron stores diminish.
• Transport iron decreases.
• Hemoglobin production declines.

iron deficiency: the condition of having depleted iron stores.

iron-deficiency anemia: a blood iron deficiency characterized by small, pale red blood cells; also called **microcytic hypochromic anemia**.
micro = small
cytic = cells
hypo = too little
chrom = color

iron is needed, more of these special proteins are produced so that more than the usual amount of iron can be absorbed and carried. If there is a surplus of iron, special storage proteins (✚) in the liver, bone marrow, and other organs store it.

Researchers are discovering genes that participate in the regulation of the body's iron at an extraordinary pace.[32] Along the way, new information about how the body controls the uptake, storage, and distribution of iron is emerging. For example, it has long been known that the liver is the main site of iron storage in the body, but only recently has research revealed that the hormone hepcidin, produced by the liver, is central to the regulation of iron balance.[33] Hepcidin helps to maintain blood iron within the normal range by limiting absorption from the small intestine and controlling release from the liver, spleen, and bone marrow.

Iron Deficiency
Worldwide, **iron deficiency** is the most common nutrient deficiency, with **iron-deficiency anemia** affecting more than 1.6 billion people—almost half preschool children and pregnant women.[34] In the United States, iron deficiency is less prevalent, but it still affects about 14 percent of toddlers and 10 percent of adolescent girls and women of childbearing age.[35] Iron deficiency is also more prevalent among overweight children and adolescents compared with those who are normal weight.[36] The association between iron deficiency and obesity has yet to be explained, but researchers are currently examining the relationships between the inflammation that develops with excess body fat and reduced iron absorption.[37]

Women are especially prone to iron deficiency during their reproductive years because of blood losses during menstruation. Pregnancy places further iron demands on women: iron is needed to support the added blood volume, the growth of the fetus, and blood loss during childbirth. Infants (six months or older) and young children receive little iron from their high-milk diets, yet they need extra iron to support their rapid growth and brain development.[38] The rapid growth of adolescence, especially for males, and the blood losses of menstruation for females also demand extra iron that a typical teen diet may not provide.

Causes of Iron Deficiency
The cause of iron deficiency is usually inadequate intake from an ignorance of which foods to choose, from sheer lack of food altogether, or from high consumption of iron-poor foods. In the Western world, high sugar and fat intakes are often associated with low iron intakes. Blood loss is the primary nonnutritional cause, especially in poor regions of the world where parasitic infections of the GI tract may lead to blood loss.

Assessment of Iron Deficiency
Iron deficiency develops in stages. (✚) This section provides a brief overview of how to detect these stages, and Appendix E provides more details. In the first stage of iron deficiency, iron stores diminish, as do levels of ferritin, an iron-storing protein. Measures of serum ferritin (in the blood) reflect iron stores and are most valuable in assessing iron status at this earliest stage.[39]

The second stage of iron deficiency is characterized by a decrease in transport iron: levels of serum iron fall, and the levels of iron-carrying protein transferrin *increase* (an adaptation that enhances iron absorption). Together, these two measures can determine the severity of the deficiency—the more transferrin and the less iron in the blood, the more advanced the deficiency is. Transferrin saturation—the percentage of transferrin that is saturated with iron—decreases as iron stores decline.

The third stage of iron deficiency occurs when the lack of iron limits hemoglobin production. Now the hemoglobin precursor, **erythrocyte protoporphyrin**, begins to accumulate as hemoglobin and **hematocrit** values decline.

Hemoglobin and hematocrit tests are easy, quick, and inexpensive, so they are the tests most commonly used in evaluating iron status. Their usefulness is limited, however, because they are late indicators of iron deficiency. Furthermore, other nutrient deficiencies and medical conditions can influence their values.

FIGURE
9-5 | Normal and Anemic Blood Cells

 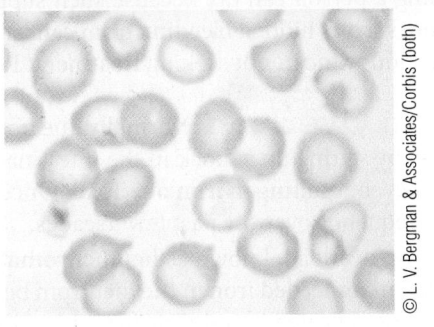

© L. V. Bergman & Associates/Corbis (both)

Normal red blood cells. Both size and color are normal.

Blood cells in iron-deficiency anemia. These cells are small and pale because they contain less hemoglobin.

Iron Deficiency and Anemia

Iron deficiency and iron-deficiency anemia are not the same: people may be iron deficient without being anemic. The term *iron deficiency* refers to depleted body iron stores without regard to the degree of depletion or to the presence of anemia. The term *iron-deficiency anemia* refers to the severe depletion of iron stores that results in a low hemoglobin concentration. In iron-deficiency anemia, red blood cells are pale and small (see Figure 9-5). They can't carry enough oxygen from the lungs to the tissues. Without adequate iron, energy metabolism in the cells falters. The result is fatigue, weakness, headaches, apathy, pallor, and poor resistance to cold temperatures. Because hemoglobin is the bright red pigment of the blood, the skin of a fair person who is anemic may become noticeably pale. In a dark-skinned person, the tongue and eye lining, normally pink, will be very pale.

The fatigue that accompanies iron-deficiency anemia differs from the tiredness a person experiences from a simple lack of sleep. People with anemia feel fatigue only when they exert themselves. Iron supplementation can, over time, relieve the fatigue and improve the body's response to physical activity.

Less severe iron deficiency produces symptoms, too. Long before the red blood cells are affected and anemia is diagnosed, a developing iron deficiency affects behavior.[40] Even at slightly lowered iron levels, energy metabolism is impaired and neurotransmitter synthesis is altered, reducing physical work capacity and mental productivity. Without the physical energy and mental alertness to work, plan, think, play, sing, or learn, people simply do these things less. They have no obvious deficiency signs; they just appear unmotivated, apathetic, and less physically fit. Children deprived of iron become irritable, restless, and unable to pay attention. (➕) These symptoms are among the first to appear when the body's iron begins to fall and among the first to disappear when iron status is restored.

➕ The effects of iron deficiency on children's behavior are revisited in Chapter 11.

Iron Deficiency and Pica

A curious behavior seen in some iron-deficient people, especially in women and children of low-income groups, is **pica**—the craving for and consumption of ice, chalk, starch, and other nonfood substances. These substances contain no iron and cannot remedy a deficiency; in fact, clay actually inhibits iron absorption, which may explain the iron deficiency that accompanies such behavior. Pica is poorly understood. Its cause is unknown, but researchers hypothesize that it may be motivated by hunger, nutrient deficiencies, or an attempt to protect against toxins or microbes.[41]

Caution on Self-Diagnosis

Low hemoglobin may reflect an inadequate iron intake, and, if it does, the physician may prescribe iron supplements. Any nutrient deficiency, disease, or agent that interferes with hemoglobin synthesis, disrupts hemoglobin function, or causes a loss of red blood cells can precipitate anemia, however.

erythrocyte protoporphyrin (PRO-toh-PORE-fe-rin): a precursor to hemoglobin.

hematocrit (hee-MAT-oh-crit): measurement of the volume of the red blood cells packed by centrifuge in a given volume of blood.

pica (PIE-ka): a craving for nonfood substances; also known as *geophagia* (jee-oh-FAY-jee-uh) when referring to clay-eating behavior.

   picus = woodpecker or magpie
   geo = earth
   phagein = to eat

Feeling fatigued, weak, and apathetic is thus a sign that something is wrong, but it does not indicate that a person should take iron supplements; it means that the person should consult a physician. In fact, taking iron supplements may be the worst possible thing a person can do, because such supplements can mask a serious medical condition, such as hidden bleeding from cancer or an ulcer. Furthermore, a person can waste precious time in not seeking treatment. Remember, don't self-diagnose.

Iron Overload

Normally, the body protects itself against absorbing too much iron by setting up a block in the intestinal cells. (✚) The system can be overwhelmed, however, resulting in **iron overload**. Once considered rare, iron overload has increased in frequency over the past few decades.

Iron overload, known as **hemochromatosis**, is usually caused by a genetic failure to prevent unneeded iron in the diet from being absorbed.[42] Other causes of iron overload include repeated blood transfusions, massive doses of supplementary iron, and other rare metabolic disorders.

Some of the signs and symptoms of iron overload are similar to those of iron deficiency: apathy, lethargy, and fatigue. Therefore, taking iron supplements before assessing iron status is clearly unwise; hemoglobin tests alone would fail to make the distinction because excess iron accumulates in storage. Iron overload assessment tests measure transferrin saturation and serum ferritin.

Iron overload is characterized by tissue damage, especially in iron-storing organs such as the liver. Infections are likely because bacteria thrive on iron-rich blood.[43] Symptoms are most severe in alcohol abusers because alcohol damages the intestine, further impairing its defenses against absorbing excess iron. Untreated hemochromatosis aggravates the risk of diabetes, liver cancer, heart disease, and arthritis.

Iron overload is much more common in men than in women and is twice as prevalent among men as iron deficiency.[44] The widespread fortification of foods with iron makes it difficult for people with hemochromatosis to follow an iron-restricted diet.

Iron Poisoning

The rapid ingestion of massive amounts of iron can cause sudden death. Iron-containing supplements can easily cause accidental poisonings in young children.[45] As few as five iron tablets have caused death in a child. Keep iron-containing supplements out of children's reach. If you suspect iron poisoning, call the nearest poison center or a physician immediately.

Iron Recommendations

The average diet in the United States provides only about 6 to 7 milligrams of iron for every 1000 kcalories. (✚) Men need 8 milligrams of iron each day; most men easily take in more than 2000 kcalories, so a man can meet his iron needs without special effort. The recommendation for women during childbearing years, however, is 18 milligrams. Because women have higher iron needs and typically consume fewer than 2000 kcalories per day, they have trouble achieving appropriate iron intakes. On the average, women receive only 12 to 13 milligrams of iron per day, not enough until after menopause. To meet their iron needs from foods, premenopausal women need to select iron-rich foods at every meal. Vegetarians, because vegetable sources of iron are poorly absorbed, should aim for 1.8 times the normal requirement. (✚) Vegetarian diets are the topic of Nutrition in Practice 5.

Iron in Foods

Iron occurs in two forms in foods, one of which is up to 10 times more absorbable than the other. The most absorbable form is heme iron, which is bound into the iron-carrying proteins hemoglobin and myoglobin in meat, poultry, and fish. (✚) Heme iron contributes a small portion of the iron consumed by most people, but it is absorbed at a fairly constant rate of about 23 percent. The less absorbable form is nonheme iron, found in meats and also in plant foods. People absorb nonheme iron at a lower rate (2 to 20 percent); its absorption depends on several dietary factors and iron stores. Most of the iron people consume is nonheme iron from vegetables, grains, eggs, meat, fish, and poultry. Snapshot 9-3 shows the iron amounts found in usual serving sizes of different foods.

✚ Binding proteins in the intestinal cells (*mucosal ferritin* and *mucosal transferrin*) capture and hold unneeded iron to be shed with the cells, thereby forming a mucosal block to iron absorption.

✚ Iron RDA:
- Men (19 and older): 8 mg/day
- Women (19–50 yr): 18 mg/day
- Women (>50 yr): 8 mg/day

✚ To calculate the RDA for vegetarians, multiply by 1.8:
- 8 mg × 1.8 = 14 mg/day (vegetarian men)
- 18 mg × 1.8 = 32 mg/day (vegetarian women, 19 to 50 yr)

✚ About 40 percent of the iron in meat, fish, and poultry is bound into molecules of heme (HEEM), the iron-holding part of the hemoglobin and myoglobin proteins. This heme iron is much more absorbable than nonheme iron.

iron overload: toxicity from excess iron.

hemochromatosis (heem-oh-crome-a-TOH-sis): iron overload characterized by deposits of iron-containing pigment in many tissues, with tissue damage. Hemochromatosis is usually caused by a hereditary defect in iron absorption.

tannins: compounds in tea (especially black tea) and coffee that bind iron.

Water and the Minerals

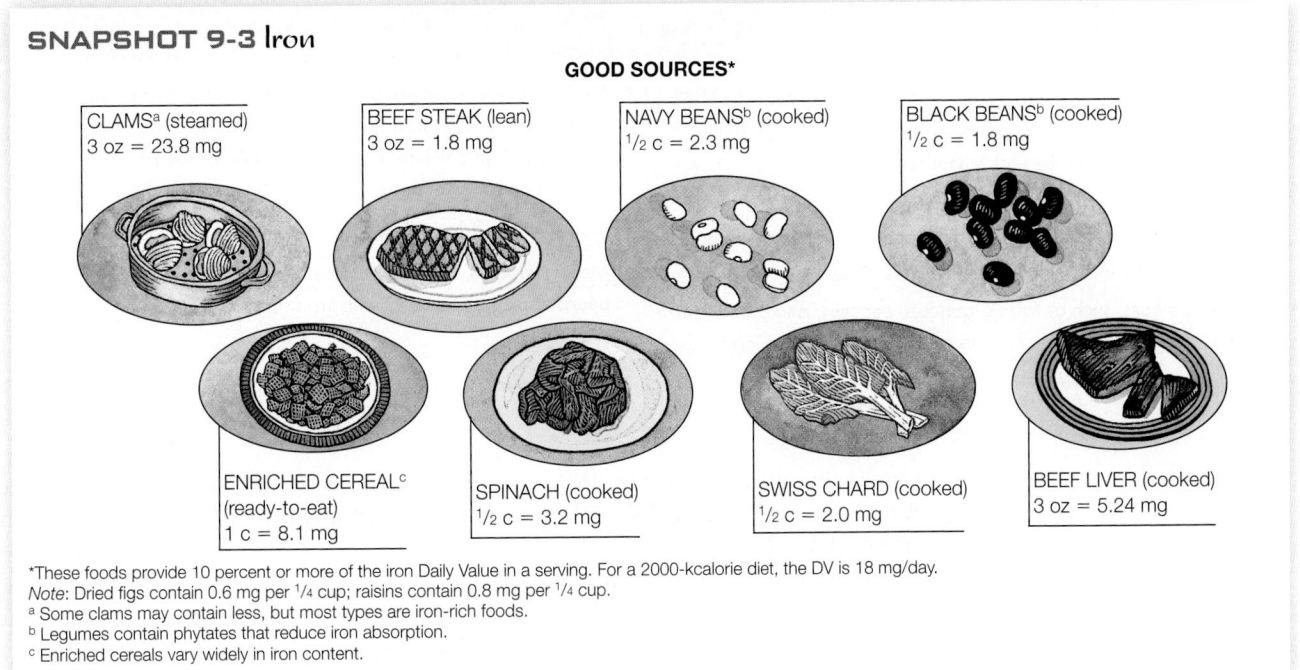

SNAPSHOT 9-3 Iron

GOOD SOURCES*

CLAMS^a (steamed)
3 oz = 23.8 mg

BEEF STEAK (lean)
3 oz = 1.8 mg

NAVY BEANS^b (cooked)
½ c = 2.3 mg

BLACK BEANS^b (cooked)
½ c = 1.8 mg

ENRICHED CEREAL^c
(ready-to-eat)
1 c = 8.1 mg

SPINACH (cooked)
½ c = 3.2 mg

SWISS CHARD (cooked)
½ c = 2.0 mg

BEEF LIVER (cooked)
3 oz = 5.24 mg

*These foods provide 10 percent or more of the iron Daily Value in a serving. For a 2000-kcalorie diet, the DV is 18 mg/day.
Note: Dried figs contain 0.6 mg per ¼ cup; raisins contain 0.8 mg per ¼ cup.
^a Some clams may contain less, but most types are iron-rich foods.
^b Legumes contain phytates that reduce iron absorption.
^c Enriched cereals vary widely in iron content.

Iron absorption from foods can be maximized by two substances that enhance iron absorption: MFP factor and vitamin C. Meat, fish, and poultry contain a factor (MFP factor) other than heme that promotes the absorption of iron. MFP factor even enhances the absorption of nonheme iron from other foods eaten at the same time. Vitamin C eaten in the same meal also doubles or triples nonheme iron absorption. Additionally, cooking with iron skillets can contribute iron to the diet. Some substances impair iron absorption; they include the **tannins** of tea and coffee, the calcium in milk, and the **phytates** that accompany fiber in legumes and whole-grain cereals.[46] The "How to" (p. 258) offers suggestions on obtaining adequate iron.

ZINC

Zinc is a versatile trace mineral required as a cofactor by more than 100 enzymes. These zinc-requiring enzymes perform tasks in the eyes, liver, kidneys, muscles, skin, bones, and male reproductive organs. Zinc works with the enzymes that make genetic material; manufacture heme; digest food; metabolize carbohydrate, protein, and fat; liberate vitamin A from storage in the liver; and dispose of damaging free radicals.[47] Zinc also interacts with platelets in blood clotting, affects thyroid hormone function, assists in immune function, and affects behavior and learning performance.[48] Zinc is needed to produce the active form of vitamin A in visual pigments and is essential to wound healing, taste perception, the making of sperm, and fetal development. When zinc deficiency occurs, it impairs all these and other functions.

The body's handling of zinc differs from that of iron but with some interesting similarities. For example, like iron, extra zinc that enters the body is held within the intestinal cells, and only the amount needed is released into the bloodstream. As with iron, zinc status influences the percentage of zinc absorbed from the diet; if more is needed, more is absorbed.

Zinc's main transport vehicle in the blood is the protein albumin. This may account for observations that serum zinc concentrations decline in conditions that lower plasma albumin concentrations—for example, pregnancy and malnutrition.

Zinc Deficiency Zinc deficiency in human beings was first reported in the 1960s from studies of growing children and male adolescents in Egypt, Iran, and Turkey. Their diets were typically low in zinc and high in fiber and phytates (which

phytates: nonnutrient components of grains, legumes, and seeds. Phytates can bind minerals such as iron, zinc, calcium, and magnesium in insoluble complexes in the intestine, and the body excretes them unused.

This chili dinner provides iron and MFP factor from meat, iron from legumes, and vitamin C from tomatoes. The combination of heme iron, nonheme iron, MFP factor, and vitamin C helps to achieve maximum iron absorption.

© Tim Hill/Alamy

The following set of guidelines can be used for planning an iron-rich diet:

- *Breads and cereals.* Use only whole-grain, enriched, and fortified products (iron is one of the enrichment nutrients).

- *Vegetables.* The dark green, leafy vegetables are good sources of vitamin C and iron. Eat vitamin C–rich vegetables often to enhance absorption of the iron from foods eaten with them.

- *Fruits.* Dried fruits, such as raisins, apricots, peaches, and prunes, are high in iron. Eat vitamin C–rich fruits often with iron-containing foods.

- *Milk and cheese.* Do not overdo foods from the milk group; they are poor sources of iron. But do not omit them either because they are rich in calcium. Drink fat-free milk to free kcalories to be invested in iron-rich foods.

- *Meats.* Meat, fish, and poultry are excellent iron sources.

- *Meat alternates.* Include legumes frequently. One cup of peas or beans can supply up to 7 milligrams of iron.

impair zinc absorption). The zinc deficiency was marked by dwarfism, or severe growth retardation, and arrested sexual maturation—symptoms that were responsive to zinc supplementation.

Since that time, zinc deficiency has been recognized elsewhere and is known to affect more than growth. It drastically impairs immune function, causes loss of appetite, and, during pregnancy, may lead to growth and developmental disorders.[49] Zinc deficiency is a substantial contributor to illness throughout the developing world and is responsible for almost half a million deaths each year.[50] A detailed list of symptoms of zinc deficiency is presented later in Table 9-9. Conditions other than poor diet that contribute to the development of zinc deficiency include loss of blood due to parasitic infections, climates that increase sweat losses, and the practice of clay eating. (✚)

Pronounced zinc deficiency is not widespread in developed countries, but deficiencies do occur in the most vulnerable groups of the U.S. population—pregnant women, young children, the elderly, and the poor.[51] Even mild zinc deficiency can result in metabolic changes such as impaired immune response, abnormal taste, and abnormal dark adaptation (zinc is required to produce the active form of vitamin A, retinal, in visual pigments).[52]

Some people are at greater risk of zinc deficiency than others. Pregnant teenagers need zinc for their own growth as well as for the developing fetus. Vegetarians whose diets emphasize whole grains, legumes, and other plant foods may also be at risk. These foods, though rich in zinc, also contain phytate, a potent inhibitor of zinc absorption.[53] Protein enhances zinc absorption, but most plant-protein foods also contain phytate. The DRI committee suggests that the dietary zinc requirement for vegetarians who exclude all animal-derived foods may be as much as 50 percent greater than the RDA, but so far evidence is insufficient to establish zinc recommendations based on the presence of other food components or nutrients.[54] Vegetarians who include cheese, eggs, or other animal protein in their diet absorb more zinc than those who exclude these foods.

Zinc Toxicity

Zinc can be toxic if consumed in large enough quantities. A high zinc intake is known to produce copper-deficiency anemia by inducing the intestinal cells to synthesize large amounts of a protein (metallothionein) that captures copper in a nonabsorbable form. Accidental consumption of high levels of zinc can cause vomiting, diarrhea, headaches, exhaustion, and other symptoms (see Table 9-9, later in the chapter). Large doses can even be fatal. The Tolerable Upper Intake Level for zinc for adults is 40 milligrams per day.

Zinc Recommendations and Food Sources

Most people in the United States have zinc intakes that approximate recommendations.[55] (✚)

Zinc is most abundant in foods high in protein, such as shellfish (especially oysters), meats, and poultry. In general, two ordinary servings a day of animal protein provide most of the zinc a healthy person needs. Milk, eggs, and whole-grain products are good sources of zinc if eaten in large quantities. For infants, breast milk is a good source of zinc, which is more efficiently absorbed from human milk than from cow's milk. Commercial infant formulas are fortified with zinc, of course. Snapshot 9-4 shows zinc-rich foods.

✚ Clay eating is a form of pica (see p. 255).

✚ Zinc RDA:
- Men: 11 mg/day
- Women: 8 mg/day

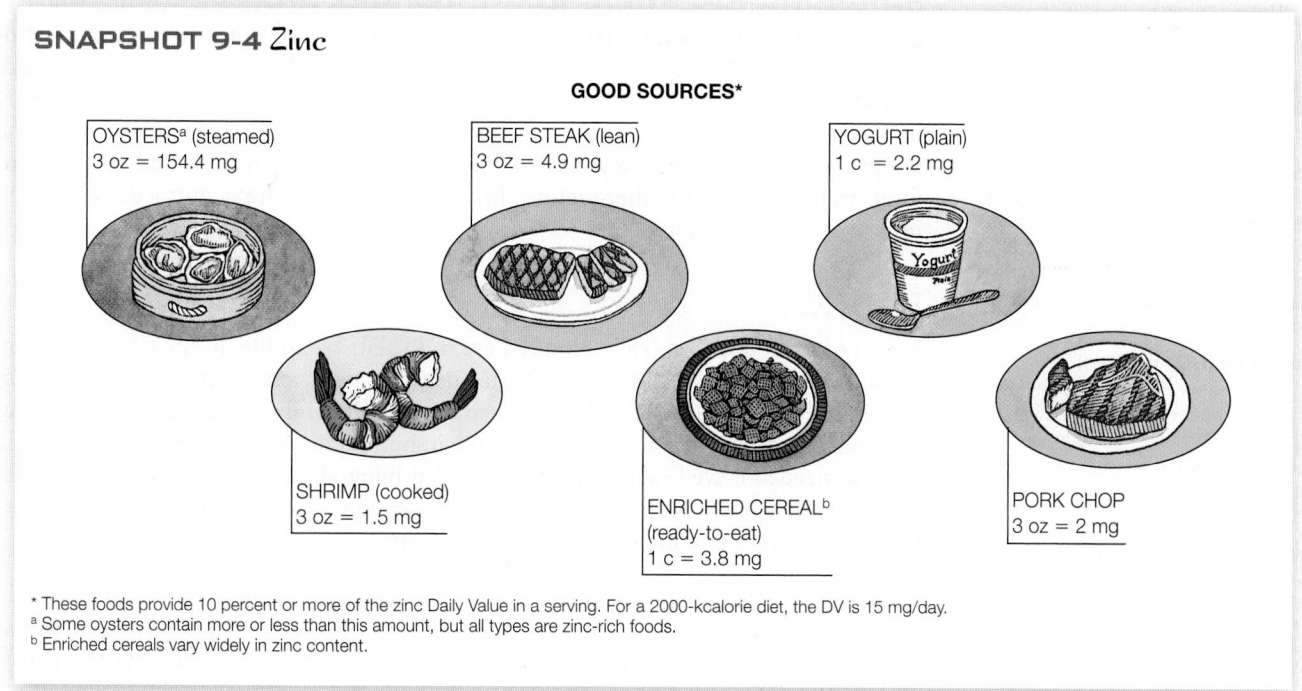

SNAPSHOT 9-4 *Zinc*

GOOD SOURCES*

OYSTERS[a] (steamed)
3 oz = 154.4 mg

BEEF STEAK (lean)
3 oz = 4.9 mg

YOGURT (plain)
1 c = 2.2 mg

SHRIMP (cooked)
3 oz = 1.5 mg

ENRICHED CEREAL[b]
(ready-to-eat)
1 c = 3.8 mg

PORK CHOP
3 oz = 2 mg

* These foods provide 10 percent or more of the zinc Daily Value in a serving. For a 2000-kcalorie diet, the DV is 15 mg/day.
[a] Some oysters contain more or less than this amount, but all types are zinc-rich foods.
[b] Enriched cereals vary widely in zinc content.

Zinc supplements are not recommended except for an accurately diagnosed zinc deficiency or when needed for use as a medication to displace other ions in unusual medical circumstances. Normally, it should be possible to obtain enough zinc from the diet.

The use of zinc lozenges and nasal sprays or gels to treat the common cold has been controversial and inconclusive, with some studies finding them effective and others not.[56] Zinc from cold-relief lozenges, sprays, and gels may or may not relieve a cold, but these products contribute zinc to the body, and the FDA has reported permanent loss of the sense of smell in people who used nasal zinc products.[57]

SELENIUM

Selenium is an essential trace mineral that functions as an antioxidant nutrient, working primarily as a part of proteins—most notably, the enzyme glutathione peroxidase.[58] Glutathione peroxidase and vitamin E work in tandem. Glutathione peroxidase prevents free-radical formation, thus blocking the damaging chain reaction before it begins; if free radicals do form, and a chain reaction starts, vitamin E halts it. Selenium-containing enzymes are necessary for the proper functioning of the iodine-containing thyroid hormones that regulate metabolism.[59]

Selenium and Cancer The question of whether selenium protects against the development of some cancers, particularly prostate cancer, is under investigation.[60] Given the potential for harm and the lack of additional evidence, recommendations to take selenium supplements to prevent cancer would be premature.

Selenium Deficiency Selenium deficiency is associated with a heart disease in children and young women living in regions of China where the soil and foods lack selenium. Although the primary cause of this heart disease is probably a virus, selenium deficiency appears to predispose people to it, and adequate selenium seems to prevent it. The heart disease is named *Keshan disease* for one of the provinces of China where it was studied.

Selenium Toxicity Because high doses of selenium are toxic, a UL has been set (see inside front cover). Selenium toxicity causes vomiting, diarrhea, loss of hair and nails, and lesions of the skin and nervous system.[61]

goiter (GOY-ter): an enlargement of the thyroid gland due to an iodine deficiency, malfunction of the gland, or overconsumption of a thyroid antagonist. Goiter caused by iodine deficiency is sometimes called *simple goiter.*

goitrogen (GOY-troh-jen): a substance that enlarges the thyroid gland and causes *toxic goiter.* Goitrogens occur naturally in such foods as cabbage, kale, brussels sprouts, cauliflower, broccoli, and kohlrabi.

cretinism (CREE-tin-ism): an iodine-deficiency disease characterized by mental and physical retardation.

In iodine deficiency, the thyroid gland enlarges—a condition known as simple goiter.

Selenium Recommendations and Intakes Anyone who eats a normal diet composed mostly of unprocessed foods need not worry about meeting selenium recommendations. (✚) Selenium is widely distributed in foods such as meats and shellfish and in vegetables and grains grown on selenium-rich soil. Some regions in the United States and Canada produce crops on selenium-poor soil, but people are protected from deficiency because they eat selenium-rich meat and supermarket foods transported from other regions. Eating as few as two Brazil nuts a day effectively improves selenium status.[62]

IODINE

Traces of the iodine ion (called iodide) are indispensible to life. In the GI tract, iodine from foods becomes iodide. This chapter uses the term *iodine* when referring to the nutrient in foods, and *iodide* when referring to it in the body. Iodide occurs in the body in minuscule amounts, but its principal role in human nutrition is well known, and the amount needed is well established. Iodide is an integral part of the thyroid hormones, which regulate body temperature, metabolic rate, reproduction, growth, the making of blood cells, nerve and muscle function, and more.

Iodine Deficiency When the iodide concentration in the blood is low, the cells of the thyroid gland enlarge in an attempt to trap as many particles of iodide as possible. If the gland enlarges until it is visible, the swelling is called a **goiter**. People with iodine deficiency this severe become sluggish and may gain weight. Goiter afflicts about 200 million people the world over, many of them in South America, Asia, and Africa. In most cases of goiter, the cause is iodine deficiency, but some people have goiter because they overconsume foods of the cabbage family and others that contain an antithyroid substance (**goitrogen**) whose effect is not counteracted by dietary iodine.

Goiter may be the earliest and most obvious sign of iodine deficiency, but the most tragic and prevalent damage occurs in the brain. Iodine deficiency is the most common cause of *preventable* mental retardation and brain damage in the world. Children with even a mild iodine deficiency typically have goiters and perform poorly in school. With sustained treatment, however, mental performance in the classroom as well as thyroid function improves.

A severe iodine deficiency during pregnancy causes the extreme and irreversible mental and physical retardation known as **cretinism**. A child with cretinism may have an IQ as low as 20 (100 is normal) and a face and body with many abnormalities. Cretinism can be averted if the pregnant woman's deficiency is detected and treated in time.[63]

Iodine Toxicity Excessive intakes of iodine can enlarge the thyroid gland, just as deficiencies can. Intakes in the United States are slightly above the recommended intake of 150 micrograms (✚) but still below the Tolerable Upper Intake Level of 1100 micrograms per day for an adult.[64]

Iodine Sources The ocean is the world's major source of iodine. In coastal areas, seafood, water, and even iodine-containing sea mist are important iodine sources. Further inland, the amount of iodine in the diet is variable and generally reflects the amount present in the soil in which plants are grown or on which animals graze. In the United States and Canada, the use of iodized salt has largely wiped out the iodine deficiency that once was widespread. In the United States, you have to read the label to find out whether salt is iodized; in Canada, all table salt is iodized.

COPPER

The body contains about 100 milligrams of copper. About one-fourth is in the muscles; one-fourth is in the liver, brain, and blood; and the rest is in the bones, kidneys, and other tissues. The primary function of copper in the body is to serve as a constituent of enzymes.[65] The copper-containing enzymes have diverse metabolic roles: they catalyze the formation of hemoglobin, help manufacture the protein collagen, assist in the healing of wounds, and help maintain the sheaths around nerve fibers. One of copper's most vital roles is to help cells use iron. Like iron, copper is needed in many reactions related to respiration and energy metabolism.

Copper Deficiency Copper deficiency is rare but not unknown. It has been seen in premature infants and malnourished infants. High intakes of zinc interfere with copper absorption and can lead to deficiency.

Copper Toxicity Some genetic disorders create a copper toxicity. Copper toxicity from foods, however, is unlikely. The Tolerable Upper Intake Level for copper is set at 10,000 micrograms per day.

Copper Recommendations and Food Sources The RDA for copper is 900 micrograms per day, (✚) which is slightly below the average intake for adults in the United States.[66] The best food sources of copper are legumes, whole grains, seafood, nuts, and seeds.

MANGANESE

The human body contains a tiny 20 milligrams of manganese, mostly in the bones and metabolically active organs such as the liver, kidneys, and pancreas. Manganese is a cofactor for many enzymes, helping to facilitate dozens of different metabolic processes. Deficiencies of manganese have not been noted in people, but toxicity may be severe. Miners who inhale large quantities of manganese dust on the job over prolonged periods show many symptoms of a brain disease, along with abnormalities in appearance and behavior. The Tolerable Upper Intake Level for manganese is 11 milligrams per day.

Manganese requirements are low, (✚) and plant foods such as nuts, whole grains, and leafy green vegetables contain significant amounts of this trace mineral. Deficiencies are therefore unlikely.

FLUORIDE

Only a trace of fluoride occurs in the human body, but research demonstrates that where diets are high in fluoride during the growing years, crystalline deposits in bones and teeth are larger and harder. When bones and teeth become mineralized, first a crystal called hydroxyapatite forms from calcium and phosphorus. Then fluoride replaces the hydroxy portion of hydroxyapatite, forming **fluorapatite**, which makes the bones stronger and the teeth more resistant to decay. Once the teeth have erupted, the topical application of fluoride by way of toothpaste or mouth rinse continues to exert a caries-reducing effect.

Fluoride Deficiency Where fluoride is lacking in the water supply, the incidence of dental decay is high. Fluoridation of water to raise its fluoride concentration to 1 part per million is recommended as an important public health measure. Those fortunate enough to have had sufficient fluoride during the tooth-forming years of infancy and childhood are protected throughout life from dental decay. Dental problems are of great concern because they can lead to a multitude of other health problems affecting the whole body. Based on the accumulated evidence of its beneficial effects, water fluoridation has been endorsed by nearly 100 national and international organizations including the National Institute of Dental Health, the American Dietetic Association, the American Medical Association, the National Cancer Institute, and the Centers for Disease Control and Prevention (CDC).[67] In fact, the CDC named water fluoridation as one of the 10 most important public health measures of the 20th century.[68] About 70 percent of the U.S. population served by public water systems receives optimal levels of fluoride (see Figure 9-6 on p. 262).[69] Most bottled waters lack fluoride.

Fluoride Sources All normal diets include some fluoride, but drinking water; processed soft drinks and fruit juice made with fluoridated water; and fluoride toothpastes, gels, and oral rinses are the most common fluoride sources in the United States. (✚) Fish and tea may supply substantial amounts as well.

✚ Copper RDA:
- Adults: 900 µg/day

✚ Manganese AI:
- Men: 2.3 mg/day
- Women: 1.6 mg/day

✚ Fluoride AI:
- Men: 4 mg/day
- Women: 3 mg/day

✚ Fluoride Tolerable Upper Intake Level:
- Adults: 10 mg/day

✚ To prevent fluorosis:
- Monitor the fluoride content of the local water supply.
- Supervise children younger than six when they brush their teeth (to ensure that they don't swallow the toothpaste), and use only a pea-size amount of toothpaste.
- Use fluoride supplements only as prescribed by a physician.

fluorapatite (floor-APP-uh-tite): the stabilized form of bone and tooth crystal, in which fluoride has replaced the hydroxy portion of hydroxyapatite.

FIGURE 9-6 | U.S. Population with Access to Fluoridated Water through Public Water Systems

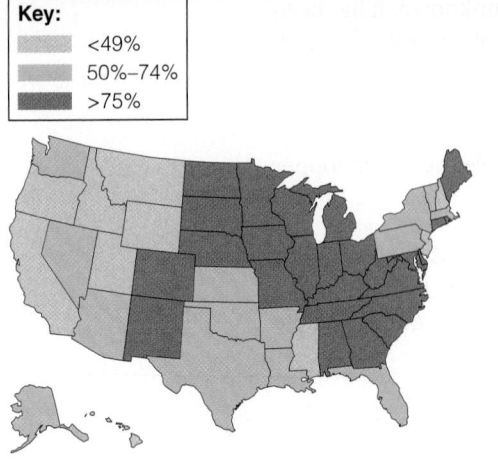

Key:
- ☐ <49%
- ☐ 50%–74%
- ■ >75%

Source: Centers for Disease Control and Prevention, Recommendations for using fluoride to prevent and control dental caries in the United States, *Morbidity and Mortality Weekly Report* (supplement), August 17, 2001, p. 10.

✚ Small organic compounds that enhance insulin's activity are called glucose tolerance factors (GTF). Some glucose tolerance factors contain chromium.

✚ Chromium AI:
- Men (19–50 yr): 35 µg/day (51 and older): 30 µg/day
- Women (19–50 yr): 25 µg/day (51 and older): 20 µg/day

✚ Molybdenum RDA: 45 µg/day

fluorosis (floor-OH-sis): mottling of the tooth enamel from ingestion of too much fluoride during tooth development.

molybdenum (mo-LIB-duh-num): a trace element.

In some areas, the natural fluoride concentration in water is high, and too much fluoride can damage teeth, causing **fluorosis**. For this reason, a Tolerable Upper Intake Level (✚) has been established. In mild cases, the teeth develop small white specks; in severe cases, the enamel becomes pitted and permanently stained (see Figure 9-7). Fluorosis occurs only during tooth development and cannot be reversed, making its prevention a high priority. (✚)

CHROMIUM

Chromium is an essential mineral that participates in carbohydrate and lipid metabolism. Chromium enhances the activity of the hormone insulin.[70] (✚) When chromium is lacking, a diabetes-like condition may develop with elevated blood glucose and impaired glucose tolerance, insulin response, and glucagon response. Some research findings suggest that chromium supplements improve glucose or insulin responses in diabetes, but these relationships are uncertain.[71]

Chromium deficiency is unlikely, given the small amount of chromium required (✚) and its presence in a variety of foods. The more refined foods people eat, however, the less chromium they obtain from their diets. Unrefined foods such as liver, brewer's yeast, whole grains, nuts, and cheeses are the best sources.

OTHER TRACE MINERALS

An RDA has been established for one other trace mineral, molybdenum. (✚) **Molybdenum** functions as a working part of several metal-containing enzymes, some of which are giant proteins. Deficiencies or toxicities of molybdenum are unknown.

Several other trace minerals are known or suspected to contribute to the health of the body. Nickel is recognized as important for the health of many body tissues. Nickel deficiencies harm the liver and other organs. Silicon is involved in the formation of bones and collagen. Cobalt is found in the large vitamin B$_{12}$ molecule. Boron influences the activity of many enzymes and may play a key role in bone health, brain activities, and immune response.[72] The future may reveal that other trace minerals also play key roles. Even arsenic—famous as the deadly poison in many murder mysteries and known to be a carcinogen—may turn out to be an essential nutrient in tiny quantities.

FIGURE 9-7 | Fluoride Toxicity Symptom— The Mottled Teeth of Fluorosis

© Dr. P. Marrazi/Science Photo Library/ Photo Researchs Inc.

Review Notes

- The body requires trace minerals in tiny amounts, and they function in similar ways—assisting enzymes all over the body.
- Eating a diet that consists of a variety of foods is the best way to ensure an adequate intake of these important nutrients.
- Many dietary factors, including the trace minerals themselves, affect the absorption and availability of these nutrients.
- Table 9-9 offers a summary of facts about trace minerals in the body.

TABLE
9-9 | The Trace Minerals—A Summary

Mineral Name	Chief Functions in the Body	Deficiency Symptoms	Toxicity Symptoms	Significant Sources
Iron	Part of the protein hemoglobin, which carries oxygen in the blood; part of the protein myoglobin in muscles, which makes oxygen available for muscle contraction; necessary for the utilization of energy	Anemia: weakness, pallor, headaches, reduced work productivity, inability to concentrate, impaired cognitive function (children), lowered cold tolerance	Iron overload: infections, liver injury, possible increased risk of heart attack, acidosis, bloody stools, shock	Red meats, fish, poultry, shellfish, eggs, legumes, dried fruits
Zinc	Part of the hormone insulin and many enzymes; involved in making genetic material and proteins, immune reactions, transport of vitamin A, taste perception, wound healing, the making of sperm, and normal fetal development	Growth retardation, delayed sexual maturation, impaired immune function, loss of taste, poor wound healing, eye and skin lesions	Loss of appetite, impaired immunity, low HDL, nausea, vomiting, diarrhea, headaches, copper and iron deficiencies	Protein-containing foods: meats, fish, shellfish, poultry, grains, vegetables
Selenium	Assists a group of enzymes that break down reactive chemicals that harm cells	Predisposition to heart disease characterized by cardiac tissue becoming fibrous (uncommon)	Nausea, abdominal pain, nail and hair changes, nerve damage	Seafoods, organ meats, other meats, whole grains and vegetables (depending on soil content)
Iodine	A component of two thyroid hormones, which help to regulate growth, development, and metabolic rate	Goiter, cretinism	Depressed thyroid activity; goiterlike thyroid enlargement	Iodized salt; seafood; bread; plants grown in most parts of the country and animals fed those plants
Copper	Necessary for the absorption and use of iron in the formation of hemoglobin; part of several enzymes	Anemia, bone abnormalities	Vomiting, diarrhea, liver damage	Organ meats, seafood, nuts, seeds, whole grains, drinking water
Manganese	Facilitator, with enzymes, of many cell processes; bone formation	Rare	Nervous system disorders	Nuts, whole grains, leafy vegetables, tea
Fluoride	An element involved in the formation of bones and teeth; helps to make teeth resistant to decay	Susceptibility to tooth decay	Fluorosis (pitting and discoloration of teeth)	Drinking water (if fluoride containing or fluoridated), tea, seafood
Chromium	Enhances insulin action and may improve glucose tolerance	Diabetes-like condition marked by an inability to use glucose normally	None reported	Meats, whole grains

Self Check

1. Which of the following body structures helps to regulate thirst?
   a. Brain stem
   b. Cerebellum
   c. Optic nerve
   d. Hypothalamus

2. Which of the following is *not* a function of water in the body?
   a. Lubricant
   b. Source of energy
   c. Maintains protein structure
   d. Participant in chemical reactions

3. Two situations in which a person may experience fluid and electrolyte imbalances are:
   a. vomiting and burns.
   b. diarrhea and cuts.
   c. broken bones and fever.
   d. heavy sweating and excessive carbohydrate intake.

4. Three-fourths of the sodium in people's diets comes from:
   a. fresh meats.
   b. home-cooked foods.
   c. frozen vegetables and meats.
   d. salt added to food by manufacturers.

5. Which mineral is critical to keeping the heartbeat steady and plays a major role in maintaining fluid and electrolyte balance?
   a. Sodium
   b. Calcium
   c. Potassium
   d. Magnesium

6. The two best ways to prevent age-related bone loss and fracture are to:
   a. take calcium supplements and estrogen.
   b. participate in aerobic activity and drink 8 glasses of milk daily.
   c. eat a diet low in fat and salt and refrain from smoking.
   d. maintain a lifelong adequate calcium intake and engage in weight-bearing physical activity.

7. Three good food sources of calcium are:
   a. milk, sardines, and broccoli.
   b. spinach, yogurt, and sardines.
   c. cottage cheese, spinach, and tofu.
   d. Swiss chard, mustard greens, and broccoli.

8. Foods high in iron that help prevent or treat anemia include:
   a. green peas and cheese.
   b. dairy foods and fresh fruits.
   c. homemade breads and most fresh vegetables.
   d. meat and dark green, leafy vegetables.

9. Two groups of people who are especially at risk for zinc deficiency are:
   a. Asians and children.
   b. infants and teenagers.
   c. smokers and athletes.
   d. pregnant adolescents and vegetarians.

10. A deficiency of ___ is one of the world's most common preventable causes of mental retardation.
    a. zinc
    b. iodine
    c. selenium
    d. magnesium

Answers to these questions appear in Appendix H.

Clinical Applications

1. Pull together information from Chapter 1 about the different food groups and the significant sources of minerals shown or discussed in this chapter. Consider which minerals might be lacking (or excessive) in the diet of a client who reports the following:

   - Relies on highly processed foods, snack foods, and fast foods as mainstays of the diet.
   - Never uses milk, milk products, or cheese.
   - Dislikes leafy green vegetables.
   - Never eats meat, fish, poultry, or even meat alternates such as legumes.

   What additional information would help you pinpoint problems with mineral intake?

Nutrition on the Net

For further study of the topics in this chapter, access these websites.

- Find updates and quick links to these and other nutrition-related sites at our website:
  http://www.cengage.com/nutrition/whitney/nhhc4e
- Find information about mineral supplements:
  http://dietary-supplements.info.nih.gov
- Search for "minerals" at the American Dietetic Association site:
  www.eatright.org
- Find tips and recipes for including more milk in the diet:
  www.whymilk.com

- Learn about the benefits of calcium from the National Dairy Council: www.nationaldairycouncil.org
- Search for the individual minerals by name at the U.S. government health information site: www.healthfinder.org
- Learn more about iron overload from the Iron Overload Diseases Association: www.ironoverload.org
- Learn more about iodine deficiency and thyroid disease from the American Thyroid Association: www.thyroid.org

Notes

1. A. K. Johnson, The sensory psychobiology of thirst and salt appetite, *Medicine and Science in Sports and Exercise* 39 (2007): 1388–1400.
2. Standing Committee on the Scientific Evaluation of Dietary Reference Intakes, Food Nutrition Board, Institute of Medicine, *Dietary Reference Intakes for Water, Potassium, Sodium, Chloride, and Sulfate* (Washington, D.C.: National Academies Press, 2005), p. 73.
3. K. M. Kolasa, C. J. Lackey, and A. C. Grandjean, Hydration and health promotion, *Nutrition Today* 44 (2009): 190–201; American College of Sports Medicine, Position stand: Exercise and fluid replacement, *Medicine and Science in Sports and Exercise* 39 (2007): 377–390.
4. L. E. Armstrong, Assessing hydration status: The elusive gold standard, *Journal of the American College of Nutrition* 26 (2007): 575S–584S.
5. B. M. Popkin and coauthors, A new proposed guidance system for beverage consumption in the United States, *American Journal of Clinical Nutrition* 83 (2006): 529–542.
6. L. R. Vartanian, M. B. Schwartz, and K. D. Brownell, Effects of soft drink consumption on nutrition and health: A systematic review and meta-analysis, *American Journal of Public Health* 97 (2007): 667–675.
7. Standing Committee on the Scientific Evaluation of Dietary Reference Intakes, 2005, pp. 133–134.
8. Centers for Disease Control and Prevention, Application of Lower Sodium Intake Recommendations to Adults—United States, 1999–2006, *Morbidity and Mortality Weekly Report* 58 (2009): 281–283.
9. Centers for Disease Control and Prevention, 2009.
10. R. Takachi and coauthors, Consumption of sodium and salted foods in relation to cancer and cardiovascular disease: The Japan Public Health Center-based prospective study, *American Journal of Clinical Nutrition* 91 (2010): 456–464; F. J. He and G. A. MacGregor, A comprehensive review on salt and health and current experience of worldwide salt reduction programmes, *Journal of Human Hypertension* 23 (2009): 363–384; H. J. Androgue' and N. E. Madias, Sodium and potassium in the pathogenesis of hypertension, *New England Journal of Medicine* 356 (2007): 1966–1978.
11. Centers for Disease Control and Prevention, 2009.
12. B. N. Van Vliet and J.-P. Montani, The time course of salt-induced hypertension, and why it matters, *International Journal of Obesity* 32 (2008): S35–S47; Standing Committee on the Scientific Evaluation of Dietary Reference Intakes, 2005, pp. 269–272.
13. U.S. Department of Agriculture and U.S. Department of Health and Human Services, *2005 Dietary Guidelines Committee Report, 2005,* available online at www.health.gov/dietaryguidelines/dga2005/report/.
14. N. R. Cook and coauthors, Long-term effects of dietary sodium reduction on cardiovascular disease outcomes: Observational follow-up of the trials of hypertension prevention (TOHP), *British Medical Journal* 334 (2007): 885–888.
15. J. A. Blumenthal and coauthors, Effects of the DASH diet alone and in combination with exercise and weight loss on blood pressure and cardiovascular biomarkers in men and women with high blood pressure: The ENCORE study, *Archives of Internal Medicine* 170 (2010): 126–135.
16. M. S. Oh and J. Uribarri, Electrolytes, water, and acid-base balance, in M. E. Shils and coeditors, *Modern Nutrition in Health and Disease*, 10th ed. (Philadelphia: Lippincott, Williams, & Wilkins, 2006), pp. 149–193.
17. Standing Committee on the Scientific Evaluation of Dietary Reference Intakes, 2005, pp. 186–268.
18. R. C. Khanal and I. Nemere, Regulation of intestinal calcium transport, *Annual Review of Nutrition* 28 (2008): 179–196.
19. L. L. Moore and coauthors, Effects of average childhood dairy intake on adolescent bone health, *Journal of Pediatrics* 153 (2008): 667–673; K. S. Ondrak and D. W. Morgan, Physical activity, calcium intake and bone health in children and adolescents, *Sports Medicine* 37 (2007): 587–600; R. P. Heaney, Bone biology in health and disease, in M. E. Shils and coeditors, *Modern Nutrition in Health and Disease*, 10th ed. (Philadelphia: Lippincott, Williams, & Wilkins, 2006), pp. 1314–1325.
20. National Osteoporosis Foundation, *Osteoporosis: Fast facts* (2008), available at www.nof.org/osteoporosis/diseasefacts.htm.
21. A. Guadalupe-Grau and coauthors, Exercise and bone mass in adults, *Sports Medicine* 39 (2009): 439–468; D. C. Wilks, S. F. Gilliver, and J. Rittweger, Forearm and tibial bone measures of distance- and sprint-trained master cyclists, *Medicine and Science in Sports and Exercise* 41 (2009): 566–573; American College of Sports Medicine, Position Stand: Physical activity and bone health, *Medicine and Science in Sports and Exercise* 36 (2004): 1985–1996.
22. V. Centeno and coauthors, Molecular mechanisms triggered by low-calcium diets, *Nutrition Research Reviews* 22 (2009): 163–174; P. R. Trumbo and K. C. Ellwood, supplemental calcium and risk reduction of hypertension, pregnancy-induced hypertension, and preeclampsia: An evidence-based review by the US Food and Drug Administration, *Nutrition Reviews* 65 (2007): 78–87.
23. Y. Park and coauthors, Dairy food, calcium, and risk of cancer in the NIH-AARP Diet and Health Study, *Archives of Internal Medicine* 169 (2009): 391–401; J. Ishihara and coauthors, Dietary calcium, vitamin D, and the risk of colorectal cancer, *American Journal of Clinical Nutrition* 88 (2008): 1576–1583; C. S. Guerreiro and coauthors, The *D1822V APC* polymorphism interacts with fat, calcium, and fiber intakes in modulating the risk of colorectal cancer in Portuguese persons, *American Journal of Clinical Nutrition* 85 (2007): 1592–1597; M. E. Martínez and E. T. Jacobs, Calcium supplementation and prevention of colorectal neoplasia: Lessons from clinical trials, *Journal of the National Cancer Institute* 99 (2007): 99–100; S. C. Larsson and coauthors, Calcium and dairy food intakes are inversely associated with colorectal cancer risk in the Cohort of Swedish Men, *American Journal of Clinical Nutrition* 83 (2006): 667–673.
24. R. P. Heaney and K. Rafferty, Preponderance of the evidence: An example from the issue of calcium intake and body composition, *Nutrition Reviews* 67 (2009): 32–39; G. C. Major and coauthors, Recent developments in calcium-related obesity research, *Obesity Reviews* 9 (2008): 428–445; M. B. Snijder and coauthors, Is higher dairy consumption associated with lower body weight and fewer metabolic disturbances? The Hoorn Study, *American Journal of Clinical Nutrition* 85 (2007): 989–995; G. Barba and P. Russo, Dairy foods, dietary calcium and obesity: A short review of the evidence, *Nutrition, Metabolism, and Cardiovascular Diseases* 16 (2006): 445–451.
25. M. Bortolotti and coauthors, Dairy calcium supplementation in overweight or obese persons: Its effect on markers of fat metabolism, *American Journal of Clinical Nutrition* 88 (2008): 877–885; S. N. Rajpathak and coauthors, Calcium and dairy intakes in relation to long-term weight gain in U.S. men, *American Journal of Clinical Nutrition* 83 (2006): 559–566.
26. A. Moshfegh and coauthors, *What We Eat in America, NHANES 2005–2006: Usual Nutrient Intakes from Food and Water Compared to 1997 Dietary Reference Intakes for Vitamin D, Calcium, Phosphorus, and Magnesium* (Beltsville, MD: USDA, 2009); J. Ma, R. A. Johns, and R. S. Stafford, Americans are not meeting current calcium recommendations, *American Journal of Clinical Nutrition* 85 (2007): 1361–1366.

27. R. P. Heaney, Absorbability and utility of calcium in mineral water, *American Journal of Clinical Nutrition* 84 (2006): 371–374.

28. R. K. Rude and M. E. Shils, Magnesium, in M. E. Shils and coeditors, *Modern Nutrition in Health and Disease*, 10th ed. (Philadelphia: Lippincott, Williams, & Wilkins, 2006), pp. 223–247.

29. *Dietary Reference Intakes: The Essential Guide to Nutrient Requirements*, eds., J. J. Otten, J. P. Hellwig, and L. D. Meyers (Washington, D.C.: National Academies Press, 2006), pp. 341–349.

30. Moshfegh and coauthors, 2009.

31. J. R. Hunt, C. A. Zito, and L. K. Johnson, Body iron excretion by healthy men and women, *American Journal of Clinical Nutrition* 89 (2009): 1792–1798.

32. M. U. Muckenthaler, B. Galy, and M. W. Hentze, Systemic iron homeostasis and the iron-responsive element/iron-regulatory protein (IRE/IRP) regulatory network, *Annual Review of Nutrition* 28 (2008): 197–213.

33. M. D. Knutson, Into the matrix: Regulation of the iron regulatory hormone hepcidin by matriptase-2, *Nutrition Reviews* 67 (2009): 284–288; M. F. Young and coauthors, Serum hepcidin is significantly associated with iron absorption from food and supplemental sources in healthy young women, *American Journal of Clinical Nutrition* 89 (2009): 533–538; Muckenthaler, Galy, and Hentze, 2008; E. Nemeth and T. Ganz, Regulation of iron metabolism by hepcidin, *Annual Review of Nutrition* 26 (2006): 323–342.

34. *Worldwide prevalence of anaemia 1993–2005: WHO Global Database on Anaemia*, published 2008, available at www.who.org.

35. M. E. Cogswell and coauthors, Assessment of iron deficiency in US preschool children and nonpregnant females of childbearing age: National Health and Nutrition Examination survey 2003–2006, *American Journal of Clinical Nutrition* 89 (2009): 1334–1342.

36. L. M. Tussing-Humphreys and coauthors, Excess adiposity, inflammations, and iron-deficiency in female adolescents, *Journal of the American Dietetic Association* 109 (2009): 297–302.

37. J. P. McClung and J. P. Karl, Iron deficiency and obesity: The contribution of inflammation and diminished iron absorption, *Nutrition Reviews* 67 (2009): 100–104; E. M. del Giudice and coauthors, Hepcidin in obese children as a potential mediator of the association between obesity and iron deficiency, *Journal of Endocrinology and Metabolism* 94 (2009): 5102–5107.

38. J. L. Beard, Why iron deficiency is important in infant development, *Journal of Nutrition* 138 (2008): 2534–2536.

39. Z. Yang and coauthors, Comparison of plasma ferritin concentration with the ratio of plasma transferrin receptor to ferritin in estimating body iron stores: Results of 4 intervention trials, *American Journal of Clinical Nutrition* 87 (2008): 1892–1898.

40. J. C. McCann and B. N. Ames, An overview of evidence for a causal relation between iron deficiency during development and deficits in cognitive or behavioral function, *American Journal of Clinical Nutrition* 85 (2007): 931–945.

41. S. L. Young and coauthors, Toward a comprehensive approach to the collection and analysis of pica substances, with emphasis on geophagic materials, *PloS ONE* 3 (2008): e3147.

42. A. Pietrangelo, Hereditary hemochromatosis, *Annual Review of Nutrition* 26 (2006): 251–270.

43. H. Drakesmith and A. Prentice, Viral infection and iron metabolism, *Nature Reviews: Microbiology* 6 (2008): 541–552; A. M. Prentice, Iron metabolism, malaria, and other infections: What is all the fuss about? *Journal of Nutrition* 138 (2008): 2537–2541; C. Ratledge, Iron metabolism and infection, *Food and Nutrition Bulletin* 28 (2007): S515–S523.

44. K. J. Allen and coauthors, Iron-overload—Related disease in *HFE* hereditary hemochromatosis, *New England Journal of Medicine* 358 (2008): 221–230.

45. M. Carlsson and coauthors, Severe iron intoxication treated with exchange transfusion, *Archives of Disease in Childhood* 93 (2008): 321–322; M. D. Aldridge, Acute iron poisoning: What every pediatric intensive care unit nurse should know, *Dimensions in Critical Care Nursing* 26 (2007): 43–48.

46. Standing Committee on the Scientific Evaluation of Dietary Reference Intakes, Food and Nutrition Board, National Institute of Health, *Dietary Reference Intakes for Vitamin A, Vitamin K, Arsenic, Boron, Chromium, Copper, Iodine, Iron, Manganese, Molybdenum, Nickel, Silicon, Vanadium, and Zinc* (Washington, D.C.: National Academy Press, 2001), pp. 311–316.

47. S. G. Bell and B. L. Vallee, The metallothionein/thionein system: An oxidoreductive metabolic zinc link, *ChemBioChem* 10 (2009): 55–62; Y. Song and coauthors, Zinc deficiency affects DNA damage, oxidative stress, antioxidant defenses, and DNA repair in rats, *Journal of Nutrition* 139 (2009): 1626–1631.

48. H. Haase and L. Rink, Functional significance of zinc-related signaling pathways in immune cells, *Annual Review of Nutrition* 29 (2009): 133–152; G. A. Kandhro and coauthors, Effect of zinc supplementation on the zinc level in serum and urine and their relation to thyroid hormone profile in male and female goitrous patients, *Clinical Nutrition* 28 (2009): 162–168; C. Maxwell and S. L. Volpe, Effect of zinc supplementation on thyroid hormone function: A case study of two college females, *Annals of Nutrition and Metabolism* 51 (2007): 188–194.

49. S. Y. Hess and J. C. King, Effects of maternal zinc supplementation on pregnancy and lactation outcomes, *Food and Nutrition Bulletin* 30 (2009): S60–S78.

50. C. L. Fischer Walker, M. Ezzati, and R. E. Black, Global and regional child mortality and burden of disease attributable to zinc deficiency, *European Journal of Clinical Nutrition* 63 (2009): 591–597.

51. S. N. Meydani and coauthors, Serum zinc and pneumonia in nursing home elderly, *American Journal of Clinical Nutrition* 86 (2007): 1167–1173; J. M. Schneider and coauthors, The prevalence of low serum zinc and copper levels and dietary habits associated with serum zinc and copper in 12- to 36-month-old children from low-income families at risk for iron deficiency, *Journal of the American Dietetic Association* 107 (2007): 1924–1929.

52. J. C. King and R. J. Cousins, Zinc, in M. E. Shils and coeditors, *Modern Nutrition in Health and Disease*, 10th ed. (Philadelphia: Lippincott, Williams, & Wilkins, 2006), pp. 271–285.

53. J. R. Hunt, J. M. Beiseigel, and L. K. Johnsosn, Adaptation in human zinc absorption as influenced by dietary zinc and bioavailability, *American Journal of Clinical Nutrition* 87 (2008): 1336–1345.

54. Standing Committee on the Scientific Evaluation of Dietary Reference Intakes, 2001, pp. 479–480.

55. Standing Committee on the Scientific Evaluation of Dietary Reference Intakes, 2001, p. 442.

56. T. J. Caruso, C. G. Prober, and J. M. Gwaltney, Treatment of naturally acquired common colds with zinc: A structured review, *Clinical Infectious Diseases* 45 (2007): 569–574.

57. FDA, Warnings on three Zicam intranasal zinc products, *For Consumers*, June 2009, available at www.fda.gov/forconsumers/ConsumerUpdates/ucm166931.htm.

58. X. G. Lei, W. Cheng, and J. P. McClung, Metabolic regulation and function of glutathione peroxidase-1, *Annual Review of Nutrition* 27 (2007): 41–61; F. P. Bellinger and coauthors, Regulation and function of selenoproteins in human disease, *Biochemical Journal* 422 (2009): 11–22.

59. D. L. St. Germain, V. A. Galton, and A. Hernandez, Minireview: Defining the roles of the iodothyronine deiodinases: Current concepts and challenges, *Endocrinology* 150 (2009): 1097–1107.

60. S. M. Lippman and coauthors, Effect of selenium and vitamin E on risk of prostate cancer and other cancers: The Selenium and Vitamin E Cancer Prevention Trial (SELECT), *Journal of the American Medical Association* 301 (2009): 39–51; N. Facompre and K. El-Bayoumy, Potential stages for prostate cancer prevention with selenium: Implications for cancer survivors, *Cancer Research* 69 (2009): 2699–2703; J. R. Marshall and coauthors, Design and progress of a trial of selenium to prevent prostate cancer among men with high-grade prostatic intraepithelial neoplasia, *Cancer Epidemiology Biomarkers and Prevention* 15 (2006): 1479–1484.

61. R. F. Burk and O. A. Levander, Selenium, in M. E. Shils and coeditors, *Modern Nutrition in Health and Disease*, 10th ed. (Philadelphia: Lippincott, Williams, & Wilkins, 2006), pp. 312–325.

62. C. D. Thomson and coauthors, Brazil nuts: An effective way to improve selenium status, *American Journal of Clinical Nutrition* 87 (2008): 379–384.

63. M. B. Zimmermann, Iodine deficiency in pregnancy and the effects of maternal iodine supplementation on the offspring: A review, *American Journal of Clinical Nutrition* 89 (2009): 668S–672S.

64. Standing Committee on the Scientific Evaluation of Dietary Reference Intakes, 2001, pp. 278–282.

65. J. R. Turnlund, Copper, in M. E. Shils and coeditors, *Modern Nutrition in Health and Disease*, 10th ed. (Philadelphia: Lippincott, Williams, & Wilkins, 2006), pp. 286–299.

66. Standing Committee on the Scientific Evaluation of Dietary Reference Intakes, 2001, pp. 224–257.

67. Position of the American Dietetic Association: The impact of fluoride on health, *Journal of the American Dietetic Association* 105 (2005): 1620–1628.

68. D. P. DePaola and coauthors, Nutrition and dental medicine, in M. E. Shils and coeditors, *Modern Nutrition in Health and Disease*, 10th ed. (Philadelphia: Lippincott, Williams, & Wilkins, 2006), pp. 1152–1178; Position of the American Dietetic Association, 2005.

69. Populations receiving optimally fluoridated public drinking water: United States, 1992–2006, *Morbidity and Mortality Weekly Report* 57 (2008): 737–741.

70. Standing Committee on the Scientific Evaluation of Dietary Reference Intakes, 2001, pp. 197–223.

71. E. M. Balk and coauthors, Effect of chromium supplementation on glucose metabolism and lipids: A systematic review of randomized controlled trials, *Diabetes Care* 30 (2007): 2154–2163; C. L. Broadhurst and P. Domenico, Clinical studies on chromium picolinate supplementation in diabetes mellitus—A review, *Diabetes Technology and Therapeutics* 8 (2006): 677–687; P. R. Trumbo and K. C. Ellwood, Chromium picolinate intake and risk of type 2 diabetes: An evidence-based review by the United States Food and Drug Administration, *Nutrition Reviews* 64 (2006): 357–363.

72. F. H. Nielsen, Is boron nutritionally relevant? *Nutrition Reviews* 66 (2008): 183–191.

Vitamin and Mineral Supplements

At least half of U.S. adults collectively spend tens of *billions* of dollars a year on dietary supplements.[1] This trend is accelerating as scientists discover more and more links between nutrition and disease prevention. Most people take a daily multivitamin and mineral pill to make up for dietary shortfalls; others take single nutrient supplements in an attempt to ward off diseases.[2] In many cases, taking supplements is a costly but harmless practice; sometimes, it is both costly and harmful to health. The main message of this Nutrition in Practice is that most healthy people can get the nutrients they need from foods. Supplements cannot substitute for a healthy diet. For some people, however, certain nutrient supplements may be desirable. In some cases, they can correct deficiencies; in others, they can reduce the risks of disease.

Do foods really contain enough vitamins and minerals to supply all that most people need?

Emphatically, yes, for both healthy adults and children who choose a variety of foods. The USDA Food Guide described in Chapter 1 is the guide to follow to achieve adequate intakes. People who meet their nutrient needs from foods, rather than supplements, have little risk of deficiency or toxicity.

© Tom Carter/PhotoEdit

Do some people need supplements?

Yes, some people may suffer marginal nutrient deficiencies due to illness, alcohol or drug addiction, or other conditions that limit food intake.[3] People who may benefit from nutrient supplements in amounts consistent with the RDA include:

- People with specific nutrient deficiencies need specific nutrient supplements.
- People whose energy intakes are particularly low (fewer than 1600 kcalories per day) need multivitamin and mineral supplements.
- Vegetarians who eat all-plant diets (vegans) and older adults with atrophic gastritis need vitamin B_{12}.
- People who have lactose intolerance or milk allergies or who otherwise do not consume enough milk products to forestall extensive bone loss need calcium.
- People in certain stages of the life cycle who have increased nutrient requirements need specific nutrient supplements. For example, infants need iron and fluoride, women of childbearing age and pregnant women need folate and iron, and the elderly need vitamins B_{12} and D.
- People who have inadequate milk intakes, limited sun exposure, or heavily pigmented skin need vitamin D.
- People who have diseases, infections, or injuries or who have undergone surgery that interferes with the intake, absorption, metabolism, or excretion of nutrients may need specific nutrient supplements. (The increased metabolic needs associated with these severe stresses are discussed in Chapter 16.)
- People taking medications that interfere with the body's use of specific nutrients may need specific nutrient supplements.

Except for people in these circumstances, most adults can normally get all the nutrients they need by eating a varied diet of nutrient-dense foods. Whenever a health care professional finds a person's diet inadequate, the right corrective step is to improve the person's food choices and eating patterns, not to begin supplementation.

Why do so many people take supplements?

People frequently take supplements for mistaken reasons, such as "They give me energy" or "They make me strong." Other invalid reasons why people may take supplements include:

- Their feeling of insecurity about the nutrient content of the food supply.
- Their belief that extra vitamins and minerals will help them cope with stress.

- Their belief that supplements can enhance athletic performance or build lean body tissue without physical work.
- Their desire to prevent, treat, or cure symptoms or diseases ranging from the common cold to cancer.[4]

Ironically, many supplement users eat more nutrient-dense diets than nonusers and therefore need supplements less.[5] In addition, little relationship exists between the nutrients people need and the ones they take in supplements. In fact, an argument against supplements is that they may lull people into a false sense of security. A person might eat irresponsibly, thinking, "My supplement will cover my needs."

Are there other arguments against taking supplements?

Yes, there are several arguments against taking supplements. First, foods rarely cause nutrient imbalances or toxicities, but supplements can. The higher the dose, the greater the risk of harm. People's tolerances for high doses of nutrients vary, just as their risks of deficiencies do. Amounts that some can tolerate may be harmful for others, and no one knows who falls where along the spectrum. The Tolerable Upper Intake Levels of the DRI (see inside front cover) answer the question "How much is too much?" by defining the highest amount that appears safe for most healthy people.

Second, supplement users are more likely to have excessive intakes of certain nutrients—notably iron, zinc, vitamin A, and niacin.[6] The true extent of supplement toxicity in this country is unknown, but many adverse effects are reported each year from vitamins, minerals, essential oils, herbs, and other supplements.[7] Only a few alert health care professionals can recognize toxicity, even when it is acute. When it is chronic, with the effects developing subtly and progressing slowly, it often goes unrecognized. In view of the potential hazards, some authorities believe supplements should bear warning labels, advising consumers that large doses may be toxic.

Toxic overdoses of vitamins and minerals in children are more readily recognized and, unfortunately, fairly common. Fruit-flavored, chewable vitamins shaped like cartoon characters entice young children to eat them like candy in amounts that can cause poisoning. High-potency iron supplements (30 milligrams of iron or more per tablet) are especially toxic and are the leading cause of accidental ingestion fatalities among children.

Third, the U.S. Food and Drug Administration recently identified more than 140 dietary supplements sold on the U.S. market that were contaminated with pharmaceutical drugs, such as steroid hormones and stimulants. Toxic plant material, toxic heavy metals, bacteria, and other substances have also shown up in a wide variety of dietary supplements. Even some children's chewable vitamins have contained appreciable lead, a destructive heavy metal for young children.[8] While hazardous products are quickly removed from the market upon discovery, many others remain on store shelves because current regulations make the supplement market difficult to monitor and control.[9] Plain multivitamin and mineral supplements from reputable sources, without herbs or add-ons, often test free from contamination.

A fourth argument against taking supplements arises when people who are ill come to believe that high doses of vitamins or minerals can be therapeutic. Not only can high doses be toxic, but the person may take them instead of seeking medical help.

A final argument against taking supplements is that the body absorbs nutrients best from foods that dilute and disperse them among other substances to facilitate their absorption and use by the body.[10] Taken in pure, concentrated form, nutrients are likely to interfere with one another's absorption or with the absorption of other nutrients from foods eaten at the same time. Such effects are particularly well known among the minerals. For example, zinc hinders copper and calcium absorption, iron hinders zinc absorption, and calcium hinders magnesium and iron absorption. Among vitamins, vitamin C supplements *enhance* iron absorption, making iron overload likely in susceptible people. These and other interactions present drawbacks to supplement use.

Do antioxidant supplements prevent cancer?

Again, it is better advice to eat a very nutritious diet. Convincing evidence exists linking high intakes of antioxidant-rich fruits and vegetables with good health and disease prevention.[11] More than 200 population studies have examined the effects of fruits and vegetables on cancer risk, and many show that people who eat more of these foods are less likely to develop certain cancers. Findings from other types of studies, such as intervention studies and clinical trials, however, show weaker associations between fruit and vegetable intake and reduced risk of cancer. Some researchers speculate that fruit and vegetable intake may play a smaller role in total cancer protection than previously thought, but fruits and vegetables do contain protective factors for specific cancers. For example, research suggests dietary fiber protects against colorectal cancer.[12] When research combines many different fruits and vegetables, specific protective factors may not stand out. Many experts agree that the antioxidant vitamins in these foods are probably important protective factors, but they also note that other constituents of fruits and vegetables (see Table NP8-2 on p. 231–232) certainly have not been ruled out as contributing factors.

The way to apply this information is to eat nutritious foods. Before supplementation is recommended as a strategy to prevent cancer or other diseases, researchers must determine the optimal doses to reduce risk and the potential adverse effects of long-term supplementation.

When a person needs a vitamin-mineral supplement, what kind should be used?

Take your health care professional's advice, if it is offered. If you are selecting a supplement yourself, a single, balanced vitamin-mineral supplement with no added extras such as herbs should suffice. Choose the kind that provides all the nutrients in amounts less than, equal to, or very close to the RDA (remember, you get some nutrients from foods). For those who require a higher dose, such as young women who need supplemental folate in the childbearing years, choose a supplement with just the needed nutrient or in combination with a reasonable dose of others. Avoid any preparations that, in a daily dose, provide more than the recommended intake of vitamin A, vitamin D, or any mineral or more than the Tolerable Upper Intake Level for any nutrient. In addition, avoid the following:

- High doses of iron (more than 10 milligrams per day), except for menstruating women. People who menstruate need more iron, but people who don't, don't.
- "Organic" or "natural" preparations with added substances. They are no better than standard types, but they cost more.
- "High-potency" or "therapeutic dose" supplements. More is not better.
- Items not needed in human nutrition such as inositol and carnitine. These particular items won't harm you, but they reveal a marketing strategy that makes the whole mix suspect.

As for price, be aware that local or store brands may be just as good as or better than nationally advertised brands. If they are less expensive, it may be because the price does not have to cover the cost of national advertising. Finally, be aware that if you see a USP symbol on the label, it means that the manufacturer has voluntarily paid an independent laboratory to test the product and affirm that it contains the ingredients listed and that it will dissolve or disintegrate in the digestive tract to make the ingredients available for absorption. The symbol does not imply that the supplement has been tested for safety or effectiveness with regard to health, however.

This symbol means that a supplement contains the nutrients stated and that it will dissolve in the digestive system—the symbol does not guarantee safety or health advantages.

Can supplement labels help consumers make informed choices?

Yes, to some extent. To enable consumers to make more informed choices about nutrient supplements, the Food and Drug Administration (FDA), with the encouragement of the American Dietetic Association (ADA), published labeling regulations for supplements. The Dietary Supplement Health and Education Act subjects supplements to the same general labeling requirements that apply to foods. Specifically:

- Nutrition labeling for dietary supplements is required. The nutrition panel on supplements is called "Supplement Facts" (see Figure NP9-1). The Supplement Facts

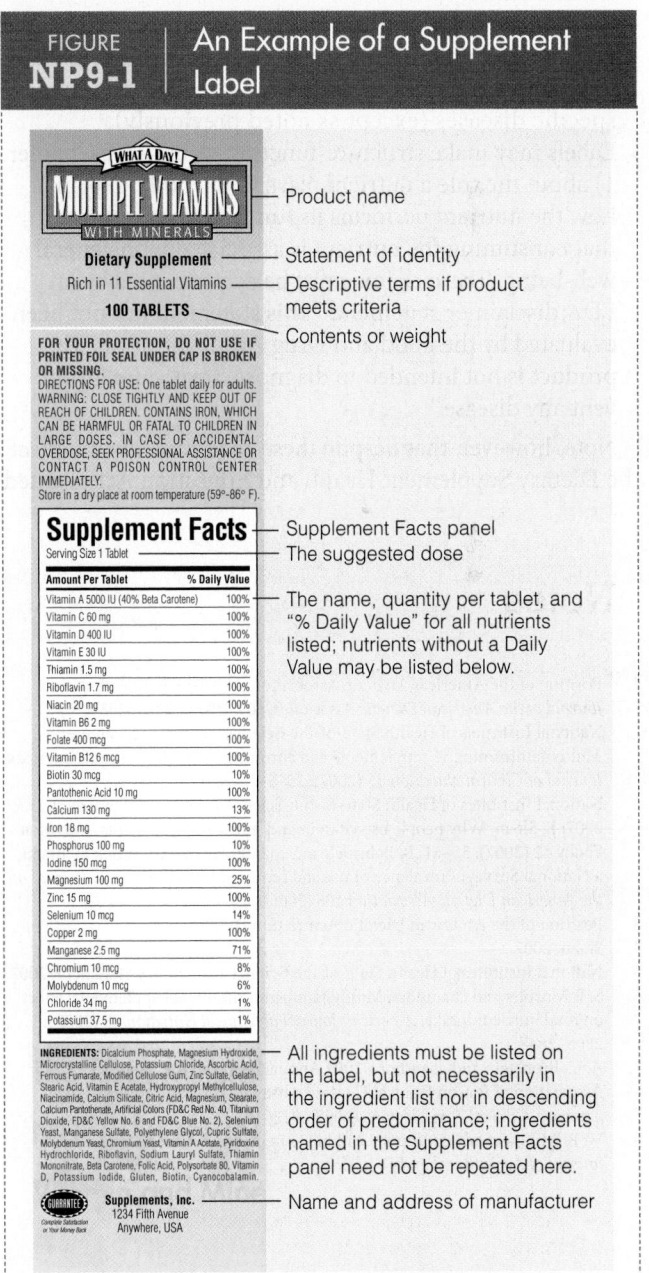

FIGURE NP9-1 | An Example of a Supplement Label

panel lists the quantity and the percentage of the Daily Value for each nutrient in the supplement. Ingredients that have no Daily Value—for example, sugars and gelatin—appear in a list below the Supplement Facts panel.

- Labels may make nutrient claims (as "high" or "low") according to specific criteria (for example, "an excellent source of vitamin C").
- Labels may make health claims that are supported by significant scientific agreement and are not brand specific (for example, "folate protects against neural tube defects").
- Labels may claim that the lack of a nutrient can cause a deficiency disease, but if they do, they must also include the prevalence of that deficiency disease in the United States.
- Labels may claim to diagnose, treat, cure, or relieve common complaints such as menstrual cramps or memory loss, but they may *not* make claims about specific diseases (except as noted previously).
- Labels may make structure-function claims (see Chapter 1) about the role a nutrient plays in the body, explain how the nutrient performs its function, and indicate that consuming the nutrient is associated with general well-being. These claims must be accompanied by an FDA disclaimer statement: "This statement has not been evaluated by the Food and Drug Administration. This product is not intended to diagnose, treat, cure, or prevent any disease."

Note, however, that despite these requirements, in effect, the Dietary Supplement Health and Education Act resulted in the deregulation of the supplement industry. Under current law, FDA is responsible only for taking action against unsafe dietary supplements already on the market. No advance registration or approval by the FDA is needed before a manufacturer can put a supplement on store shelves.[13] To act against unsafe supplements, FDA must receive manufacturers' reports concerning serious adverse health effects reported to them by consumers.[14] Manufacturers do list contact information on supplement labels for this purpose, but many symptoms of adverse reactions are easily mistaken for something else—stomach flu or headache or fatigue. Consumers can also report adverse reactions from supplements directly to the FDA via its hotline or website, but most people are unaware of these options (see the note on this page).*

People in developed nations are far more likely to suffer from *overnutrition* and poor lifestyle choices than from nutrient deficiencies. People wish that swallowing vitamin pills would boost their health. The truth—that they need to improve their eating and exercise habits—is harder to swallow.

Don't waste time and money trying to single out a few nutrients to take as supplements. Invest energy in eating a wide variety of fruits and vegetables in generous quantities, along with the recommended daily amounts of whole grains, lean meats, and milk products every day, and take supplements only when they are truly needed.

---

*Consumers should report suspected harm from dietary supplements to their health providers or to the FDA's MedWatch program at (800) FDA-1088 or on the Internet at www.fda.gov/medwatch/.

Notes

1. Position of the American Dietetic Association: Nutrient Supplementation, *Journal of the American Dietetic Association* 109 (2009): 2073–2085; National Institutes of Health State-of-the-Science Conference Statement: Multivitamin/mineral supplements and chronic disease prevention, *American Journal of Clinical Nutrition* 85 (2007): 257S–264S.
2. National Institutes of Health State-of-the-Science Conference Statement, 2007; E. Sloan, Why people use vitamin and mineral supplements, *Nutrition Today* 42 (2007): 55–61; B. Babgaleh and coauthors, Dietary supplements in a National Survey: Prevalence of use and reports of adverse events, *Journal of the American Dietetic Association* 106 (2006): 1966–1974.
3. Position of the American Dietetic Association, 2009.
4. Sloan, 2007.
5. National Institutes of Health State-of-the-Science Conference Statement, 2007.
6. S. P. Murphy and coauthors, Multivitamin-multimineral supplements' effect on total nutrient intake, *American Journal of Clinical Nutrition* 85 (2007): 280S–284S.
7. A. C. Bronstein and coauthors, 2007 Annual report of the American Association of Poison Control Centers' national poisoning and exposure database, *Clinical Toxicology* 46 (2008): 927–1057.
8. W. R. Mindak and coauthors, Lead in women's and children's vitamins, *Journal of Agricultural and Food Chemistry* 56 (2008): 6892–6896;

J. F. Kaufman and coauthors, Lead in pharmaceutical products and dietary supplements, *Regulatory Toxicology and Pharmacology* 48 (2007): 128–134.
9. P. A. Cohen, American roulette—contaminated dietary supplements, *New England Journal of Medicine* 361 (2009): 1523–1525.
10. D. R. Jacobs, M. D. Gross, and L. C. Tapsell, Food synergy: An operational concept for understanding nutrition, *American Journal of Clinical Nutrition* 89 (2009): 1543S–1548S.
11. L. Djousse, J. A. Driver, and J. M. Gazianao, Relation between modifiable lifestyle factors and lifetime risk of heart failure, *Journal of the American Medical Association* 302 (2009): 394–400; F. J. B. van Duijnhoven and coauthors, Fruit, vegetables, and colorectal cancer risk: The European Prospective Investigation into Cancer and Nutrition, *American Journal of Clinical Nutrition* 89 (2009): 1441–1452; World Cancer Research Fund/American Institute for Cancer Research, *Food, Nutrition, Physical Activity and the Prevention of Cancer: A Global Perspective* (Washington, D.C.: AICR, 2007), pp. 75–115.
12. World Cancer Research Fund/American Institute for Cancer Research, 2007, pp. 280–288.
13. U.S. Food and Drug Administration, Center for Food Safety and Applied Nutrition, *Dietary Supplements,* available at www.cfsan.fda.gov.
14. DSHEA slightly strengthened, *Consumer Health Digest,* January 30, 2007, available at www.quackwatch.org.

CHAPTER 10 | # Nutrition through the Life Span: Pregnancy and Infancy

© Betsie Van Der Meer/Getty Images

CONTENTS

fertility: the capacity of a woman to produce a normal ovum periodically and of a man to produce normal sperm; the ability to reproduce.

low birthweight (LBW): a birthweight less than 5½ lb (2500 g); indicates probable poor health in the newborn and poor nutrition status of the mother during pregnancy. Optimal birthweight for a full-term infant is 6.8 to 7.9 lb (about 3100 to 3600 g).

Low-birthweight infants are of two different types. Some are **premature**; they are born early and are of a weight **appropriate for gestational age (AGA)**. Others have suffered growth failure in the uterus; they may or may not be born early, but they are **small for gestational age (SGA)**.

ALL PEOPLE NEED THE SAME NUTRIENTS, BUT THE AMOUNTS THEY need vary depending on their stage of life. This chapter focuses on nutrition in preparation for, and support of, pregnancy, lactation, and infancy. The next two chapters address the needs of children, adolescents, and older adults.

Pregnancy: The Impact of Nutrition on the Future

The woman who enters pregnancy with full nutrient stores, sound eating habits, and a healthy body weight has done much to ensure an optimal pregnancy. Then, if she eats a variety of nutrient-dense foods during pregnancy, her own and her infant's health will benefit further.

NUTRITION PRIOR TO PREGNANCY

A discussion on nutrition prior to pregnancy must, by its nature, focus mainly on women. A man's nutrition may affect his **fertility** and possibly the genetic contributions he makes to his children, but nutrition exerts its primary influence through the woman. Her body provides the environment for the growth and development of a new human being. Full nutrient stores *before* pregnancy are essential both to conception and to healthy infant development during pregnancy. In the early weeks of pregnancy, before many women are even aware that they are pregnant, significant developmental changes occur that depend on a woman's nutrient stores. In preparation for a healthy pregnancy, a woman can establish the following habits:[1]

- *Achieve and maintain a healthy body weight.* Both underweight and overweight women, and their newborns, face increased risks of complications.
- *Choose an adequate and balanced diet.* Malnutrition reduces fertility and impairs the early development of an infant should a woman become pregnant.
- *Be physically active.* A woman who wants to be physically active *when* she is pregnant needs to become physically active *beforehand*.
- *Receive regular medical care.* Regular health care visits can help ensure a healthy start to pregnancy.
- *Avoid harmful influences.* Both maternal and paternal ingestion of harmful substances (such as cigarettes, alcohol, drugs, or environmental contaminants) can cause miscarriage or abnormalities, alter genes or their expression, and interfere with fertility.

Young adults who nourish and protect their bodies do so not only for their own sakes but also for future generations.

Both parents can prepare in advance for a healthy pregnancy.

PREPREGNANCY WEIGHT

Appropriate weight prior to pregnancy benefits pregnancy outcome. Being either underweight or overweight (see p. 283) presents medical risks during pregnancy and childbirth. Underweight women are therefore advised to gain weight before becoming pregnant, and overweight women to lose excess weight.

Underweight Infant birthweight correlates with prepregnancy weight and weight gain during pregnancy and is the most potent single predictor of the infant's future health and survival. An underweight woman has a high risk of having a **low-birthweight** infant, especially if she is unable to gain sufficient weight during pregnancy.[2] Compared with normal-weight infants, low-birthweight infants are more likely to contract diseases and nearly 40 times more likely to die in the first month of life. Impaired growth and development during pregnancy may have long-term health effects as well. Research suggests that, when nutrient supplies fail to meet demands, permanent adaptations take place that may make obesity or chronic diseases such as heart disease and hypertension more likely in later life (see Nutrition in Practice 11).[3] Other potential problems of low birthweight may include lower adult IQ and other brain impairments, short stature, and educational disadvantages.[4] Underweight women are therefore advised to gain weight before becoming pregnant and to strive to gain adequately during pregnancy.

Nutritional deficiency, coupled with low birthweight, is the underlying cause of more than half of all the deaths worldwide of children under five years of age. In the United States, the infant mortality rate in 2005 was 6.8 deaths per 1000 live births.[5] This rate, though higher than that of some other developed countries, has seen a significant steady decline over the past two decades and stands as a tribute to public health efforts aimed at reducing infant deaths (see Figure 10-1).

Not all cases of low birthweight reflect poor nutrition. Heredity, disease conditions, smoking, and drug use (including alcohol) during pregnancy all contribute.[6] Even with optimal nutrition and health during pregnancy, some women give birth to small infants for unknown reasons. But poor nutrition is the major factor in low birthweight—and an avoidable one, as later sections make clear.[7]

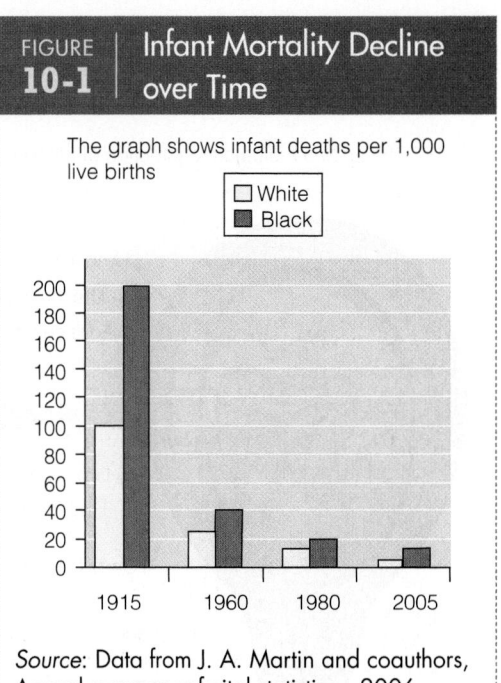

FIGURE 10-1 | Infant Mortality Decline over Time

The graph shows infant deaths per 1,000 live births

☐ White
■ Black

Source: Data from J. A. Martin and coauthors, Annual summary of vital statistics—2006, *Pediatrics* 121 (2008): 788–801

Overweight and Obesity Obese women are also urged to strive for healthy weights before pregnancy. The infant of an obese mother may be larger than normal and may be large even if born prematurely. The large early infant may not be recognized as premature and thus may not receive the special medical care required. Maternal obesity may double the risk for neural tube defects.[8] Folate's role has been examined, but a more likely explanation seems to be poor glycemic control.[9] Obese women are more likely to require drugs to induce labor or require surgical intervention for the birth, and they suffer gestational diabetes, hypertension, and infections after the birth more often than do women of healthy weight.[10] In addition, both overweight and obese women have a greater risk of giving birth to infants with heart defects and other abnormalities.[11] (✚) An appropriate goal for the obese woman who wishes to become pregnant is to strive to attain a healthy prepregnancy body weight so as to minimize her medical risks and those of her future child.

HEALTHY SUPPORT TISSUES

A major reason that the mother's prepregnancy nutrition is so crucial is that it determines whether her **uterus** will be able to support the growth of a healthy **placenta** during the first month of **gestation**. The placenta is both a supply depot and a waste-removal system for the fetus. If the placenta works perfectly, the fetus wants for nothing; if it doesn't, no alternative source of sustenance is available, and the fetus will fail to thrive. Figure 10-2 (p. 274) shows the placenta, a mass of tissue in which maternal and fetal blood vessels intertwine and exchange materials. The two bloods never mix, but the barrier between them is notably thin. To grasp how thin, picture your hands as fetal blood vessels, skintight surgical gloves as the tissue-thin placenta, and finally, your gloved hands immersed in water as the pool of maternal blood. Across this thin barrier, nutrients and oxygen move from the mother's blood into the fetus's blood, and wastes move out of the fetal blood to be excreted by the mother. The **umbilical cord** is the pipeline from the placenta to the fetus. The **amniotic sac** surrounds and cradles the fetus, cushioning it with fluids.

The placenta is an active metabolic organ with many responsibilities of its own. It actively gathers up hormones, nutrients, and protein molecules such as antibodies and transfers them into the fetal bloodstream.[12] The placenta also produces a broad range of hormones that act in many ways to maintain pregnancy and prepare the mother's breasts for **lactation**. A healthy placenta is essential for the developing fetus to attain its full potential.[13]

✚ Neural tube defects and gestational diabetes are discussed in later sections.

uterus (YOO-ter-us): the womb, the muscular organ within which the infant develops before birth.

placenta (pla-SEN-tuh): an organ that develops inside the uterus early in pregnancy, in which maternal and fetal blood circulate in close proximity and exchange materials. The fetus receives nutrients and oxygen across the placenta; the mother's blood picks up carbon dioxide and other waste materials to be excreted via her lungs and kidneys.

gestation: the period of about 40 weeks (three trimesters) from conception to birth; the term of a pregnancy.

umbilical (um-BIL-ih-cul) cord: the ropelike structure through which the fetus's veins and arteries reach the placenta; the route of nourishment and oxygen into the fetus and the route of waste disposal from the fetus.

amniotic (am-nee-OTT-ic) sac: the "bag of waters" in the uterus in which the fetus floats.

lactation: production and secretion of breast milk for the purpose of nourishing an infant.

FIGURE
10-2 | The Placenta

The arrows indicate the direction of blood flow.

Pool of mother's blood

Fetal vein   Fetal artery

Umbilical cord

Uterine wall

Placenta

Fingerlike projections containing fetal blood vessels extend into the pool of mother's blood. No actual mingling of fetal and maternal blood occurs, but substances pass back and forth.

Thus, oxygen and nutrients from the mother's blood enter fetal vessels, and waste products are removed.

Umbilical cord

Umbilical vein

Umbilical arteries

Mother's veins carry fetal wastes away.

Mother's arteries bring fresh blood to the fetus.

Amniotic sac

In the placenta, maternal blood vessels lie side by side with fetal blood vessels that reach the fetus through the umbilical cord.

Fetal portion of placenta

Maternal portion of placenta

Review Notes

- Adequate nutrition before pregnancy establishes physical readiness and nutrient stores to support fetal growth.
- Both underweight and overweight women should strive for appropriate bodyweights before pregnancy.
- Newborns who weigh less than 5½ pounds face greater health risks than normal-weight infants.
- The healthy development of the placenta depends on adequate nutrition before pregnancy.

ovum (OH-vum): the female reproductive cell, capable of developing into a new organism upon fertilization; commonly referred to as an egg.

zygote (ZY-goat): the product of the union of ovum and sperm; a fertilized ovum.

blastocyst (BLASS-toe-sist): the developmental stage of the zygote when it is about five days old and ready for implantation.

implantation: the stage of development in which the blastocyst embeds itself in the wall of the uterus and begins to develop; occurs during the first two weeks after conception.

embryo (EM-bree-oh): the developing infant from two to eight weeks after conception.

fetus (FEET-us): the developing infant from eight weeks after conception until its birth.

THE EVENTS OF PREGNANCY

The newly fertilized **ovum** is called a **zygote**. It begins as a single cell and rapidly divides to become a **blastocyst**. During the first week, the blastocyst floats down into the uterus where it will embed itself in the inner uterine wall—a process known as **implantation**. Minimal growth in size takes place at this time, but it is a crucial period in development. Adverse influences such as smoking, drug abuse, and malnutrition at this time lead to failure to implant or to abnormalities such as neural tube defects that can cause the loss of the developing embryo, possibly before the woman knows she is pregnant.

The Embryo and Fetus During the next six weeks of development, the **embryo** registers astonishing physical changes (see Figure 10-3). At eight weeks, the **fetus** has a complete central nervous system, a beating heart, a fully formed digestive system, well-defined fingers and toes, and the beginnings of facial features.

In the last seven months of pregnancy, the fetal period, the fetus grows 50 times heavier and 20 times longer. Critical periods of cell division and development occur in organ after organ. Most successful pregnancies last 38 to 42 weeks and produce a

FIGURE 10-3 | Stages of Embryonic and Fetal Development

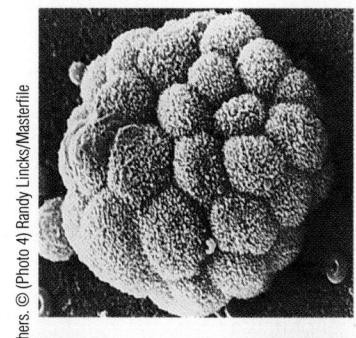

(1) A newly fertilized ovum is called a zygote and is about the size of the period at the end of this sentence. Less than one week after fertilization these cells have rapidly divided multiple times and are ready for implantation.

(3) A fetus after 11 weeks of development is just over an inch long. Notice the umbilical cord and blood vessels connecting the fetus with the placenta.

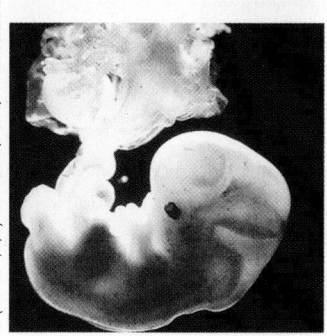

(2) After implantation, the placenta develops and begins to provide nourishment to the developing embryo. An embryo five weeks after fertilization is about ½ inch long.

(4) A newborn infant after nine months of development measures close to 20 inches in length. The average birthweight is about 7½ pounds. From eight weeks to term, this infant grew 20 times longer and 50 times heavier.

© (Photos 1, 2, 3) Petit Format/Nestle/Photo Researchers. © (Photo 4) Randy Lincks/Masterfile

healthy infant weighing between 6.8 and 7.9 pounds.[14] The 40 or so weeks of pregnancy are divided into thirds, each of which is called a **trimester**.

A Note about Critical Periods Each organ and tissue type grows with its own characteristic pattern and timing. The development of each takes place only at a certain time—the **critical period**. Whatever nutrients and other environmental conditions are necessary during this period must be supplied on time if the organ is to reach its full potential. If the development of an organ is limited during a critical period, recovery is impossible. For example, the fetus's heart and brain are well developed at 14 weeks; the lungs, 10 weeks later. Therefore, early malnutrition impairs the heart and brain; later malnutrition impairs the lungs.

The effects of malnutrition during critical periods of pregnancy are seen in defects of the nervous system of the embryo (explained later), in the child's poor dental health, and in the adolescent's and adult's vulnerability to infections and possibly higher risks of diabetes, hypertension, stroke, or heart disease.[15] The effects of malnutrition during critical periods are irreversible: abundant and nourishing food, consumed after the critical time, cannot remedy harm already done.

Table 10-1 (p. 276) identifies characteristics of a **high-risk pregnancy**. A woman with none of these factors is said to have a **low-risk pregnancy**. The more factors that apply, the higher the risk. All pregnant women, especially those in high-risk categories, need prenatal medical care, including dietary advice.

trimester: a period representing one-third of the term of gestation. A trimester is about 13 to 14 weeks.

critical period: a finite period during development in which certain events occur that will have irreversible effects on later developmental stages; usually a period of rapid cell division.

high-risk pregnancy: a pregnancy characterized by risk factors that make it likely the birth will be surrounded by problems such as premature delivery, difficult birth, retarded growth, birth defects, and early infant death.

low-risk pregnancy: a pregnancy characterized by factors that make it likely the birth will be normal and the infant healthy.

Review Notes

- Placental development, implantation, and early critical periods depend on maternal nutrition before and during pregnancy.

TABLE 10-1 | High-Risk Pregnancy Factors

Factor	Condition That Raises Risk
Maternal weight	
• Prior to pregnancy	Prepregnancy BMI either <18.5 or ≥25
• During pregnancy	Insufficient or excessive pregnancy weight gain
Maternal nutrition	Nutrient deficiencies or toxicities; eating disorders
Socioeconomic status	Poverty, lack of family support, low level of education, limited food available
Lifestyle habits	Smoking, alcohol, or other drug use
Age	Teens, especially 15 years or younger; women 35 years or older
Previous pregnancies	
• Number	Many previous pregnancies (three or more to mothers under age 20; four or more to mothers age 20 or older)
• Interval	Short or long intervals between pregnancies (<18 months or >59 months)
• Outcomes	Previous history of problems
• Multiple births	Twins or triplets
• Birthweight	Low- or high-birthweight infants
Maternal health	
• High blood pressure	Development of pregnancy-related hypertension
• Diabetes	Development of gestational diabetes
• Chronic disease	Diabetes; heart, respiratory, and kidney disease; certain genetic disorders; special diets and medications

NUTRIENT NEEDS DURING PREGNANCY

Nutrient needs during pregnancy increase more for certain nutrients than for others. (✚) Figure 10-4 shows the percentage increase in nutrient intakes recommended for pregnant women compared with nonpregnant women. To meet the high nutrient demands of pregnancy, a woman must make careful food choices, but her body will also do its part by maximizing nutrient absorption and minimizing losses.

Energy, Carbohydrate, Protein, and Fat Energy needs vary with the progression of pregnancy. In the first trimester, the pregnant woman needs no additional energy, but as pregnancy progresses, her energy needs rise. She requires an additional 340 kcalories daily during the second trimester and an extra 450 kcalories each day during the third trimester.[16] Well-nourished pregnant women meet these demands for more energy in several ways: some eat more food, some reduce their activity, and some store less of their food energy as fat. A woman can easily meet the need for extra kcalories by selecting more nutrient-dense foods from the five food groups. Table 1-7 (on p. 20) provides suggested eating patterns for several kcalorie levels, and Table 10-2 (p. 278) offers a sample menu for pregnant and lactating women.

If a woman chooses less nutritious options such as sugary soft drinks or fatty snack foods to meet her energy needs, she will undoubtedly come up short on nutrients. The increase in the need for nutrients is even greater than that for energy, so the mother-to-be should choose

✚ Nutrient and energy intake recommendations for pregnant women are listed on the inside front cover.

FIGURE
10-4

Comparison of Nutrient Recommendations for Nonpregnant, Pregnant, and Lactating Women

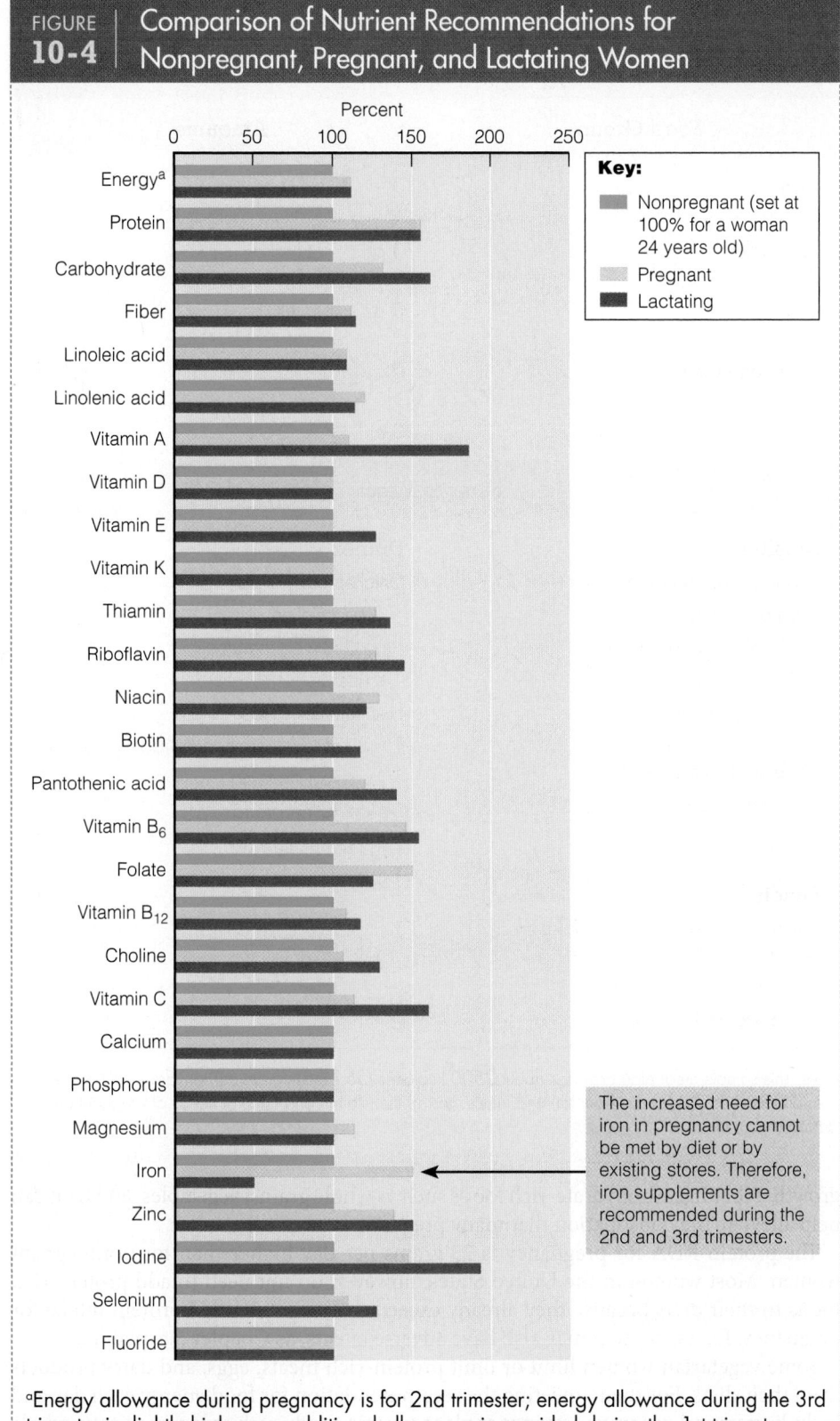

Percent

Key:
- Nonpregnant (set at 100% for a woman 24 years old)
- Pregnant
- Lactating

The increased need for iron in pregnancy cannot be met by diet or by existing stores. Therefore, iron supplements are recommended during the 2nd and 3rd trimesters.

ᵃEnergy allowance during pregnancy is for 2nd trimester; energy allowance during the 3rd trimester is slightly higher; no additional allowance is provided during the 1st trimester. Energy allowance during lactation is for the first 6 months; energy allowance during the second 6 months is slightly higher.

nutrient-dense foods such as whole-grain breads and cereals, legumes, dark green vegetables, citrus fruits, low-fat milk and milk products, and lean meats, fish, poultry, and eggs.

Ample carbohydrate (ideally, 175 grams or more per day and certainly no less than 135 grams) is necessary to fuel the fetal brain and spare the protein needed for fetal

NURSING DIAGNOSIS
Imbalanced nutrition: less than body requirements applies to clients who lack nutrition knowledge or have too little money to purchase food.

TABLE 10-2	Daily Food Choices for Pregnancy (Second and Third Trimesters) and Lactation	

Food Group	Amounts
Fruits	2 c
Vegetables	3 c
Grains	8 oz
Meats and Legumes	6½ oz
Milk	3 c

Sample Menu

Breakfast
1 whole-wheat English muffin
2 tbs peanut butter
1 c low-fat vanilla yogurt
½ c fresh strawberries
1 c orange juice

Midmorning snack
½ c cranberry juice
1 oz pretzels

Lunch
Sandwich (tuna salad on whole-wheat bread)
½ carrot (sticks)
1 c low-fat milk

Dinner
Chicken cacciatore
  3 oz chicken
  ½ c stewed tomatoes
1 c rice
½ c summer squash
1½ c salad (spinach, mushrooms, carrots)
1 tbs salad dressing
1 slice Italian bread
2 tsp soft margarine
1 c low-fat milk

Note: This sample meal plan provides about 2500 kcalories (55 percent from carbohydrate, 20 percent from protein, and 25 percent from fat) and meets most of the vitamin and mineral needs of pregnant and lactating women.

neural tube: the embryonic tissue that later forms the brain and spinal cord.

neural tube defect (NTD): a serious central nervous system birth defect that often results in lifelong disability or death.

anencephaly (AN-en-SEF-a-lee): an uncommon and always fatal type of neural tube defect; characterized by the absence of a brain.
- **an** = not (without)
- **encephalus** = brain

spina (SPY-nah) bifida (BIFF-ih-dah): one of the most common types of neural tube defects; characterized by the incomplete closure of the spinal cord and its bony encasement.
- **spina** = spine
- **bifida** = split

growth. Fiber in carbohydrate-rich foods such as whole grains, vegetables, and fruit can help alleviate the constipation that many pregnant women experience.

The protein RDA for pregnancy is 25 grams per day higher than for nonpregnant women. Most women in the United States, however, do not need to add protein-rich foods to their diets because they already exceed the recommended protein intake for pregnancy. Excess protein may also have adverse effects, as Chapter 5 explained.

Some vegetarian women limit or omit protein-rich meats, eggs, and dairy products from their diets. For them, meeting the recommendation for food energy each day and including several generous servings of plant-protein foods such as legumes, tofu, whole grains, nuts, and seeds are imperative. Protein supplements during pregnancy can be harmful, and their use is discouraged.

The high nutrient requirements of pregnancy leave little room in the diet for excess energy from added purified fats such as oil, margarine, and butter. The essential fatty acids, however, are particularly important to the growth and development of the fetus.[17] The brain contains a substantial amount of lipid material and depends heavily on long-chain omega-3 and omega-6 fatty acids for its growth, function, and structure. (See Table 4-3 on p. 101 for a list of good food sources of the essential fatty acids.)

Review Notes

- Pregnancy brings physiological adjustments that demand increased intakes of energy and nutrients.
- A balanced diet that includes more nutrient-dense foods from each of the five food groups can help to meet these needs.

Of Special Interest: Folate and Vitamin B₁₂

The vitamins famous for their roles in cell reproduction—folate and vitamin B_{12}—are needed in large amounts during pregnancy. New cells are laid down at a tremendous pace as the fetus grows and develops. At the same time, because the mother's blood volume increases, the number of her red blood cells must rise, requiring more cell division and therefore more vitamins. To accommodate these needs, the recommendation for folate during pregnancy (✚) increases from 400 to 600 micrograms a day.

As described in Chapter 8, folate plays an important role in preventing neural tube defects. To review, the early weeks of pregnancy are a critical period for the formation and closure of the **neural tube** that will later develop to form the brain and spinal cord. By the time a woman suspects she is pregnant, usually around the sixth week of pregnancy, the embryo's neural tube normally has closed. A **neural tube defect (NTD)** (✚) occurs when the tube fails to close properly. (✚) In the United States, an estimated 2500 infants with NTD are born each year.[18] When the neural tube fails to close properly and brain development fails, a rare but lethal defect known as **anencephaly** occurs. All infants with anencephaly die shortly after birth.

In a more common NTD, the spinal cord and backbone do not develop normally—and the result is **spina bifida** (see Figure 10-5). The membranes covering the spinal cord often protrude from the spine as a sac, and sometimes a portion of the spinal cord

✚ Folate RDA during pregnancy:
- 600 µg/day

✚ Reminder: Neural tube defects (NTD) are malformations of the brain, spinal cord, or both during embryonic development.

✚ A pregnancy affected by a neural tube defect can occur in any woman, but these factors make it more likely:[19]
- A previous pregnancy affected by a neural tube defect
- Maternal diabetes
- Maternal use of certain antiseizure medications
- Mutations in folate-related enzymes
- Maternal obesity

FIGURE 10-5 | Spina Bifida—A Neural Tube Defect

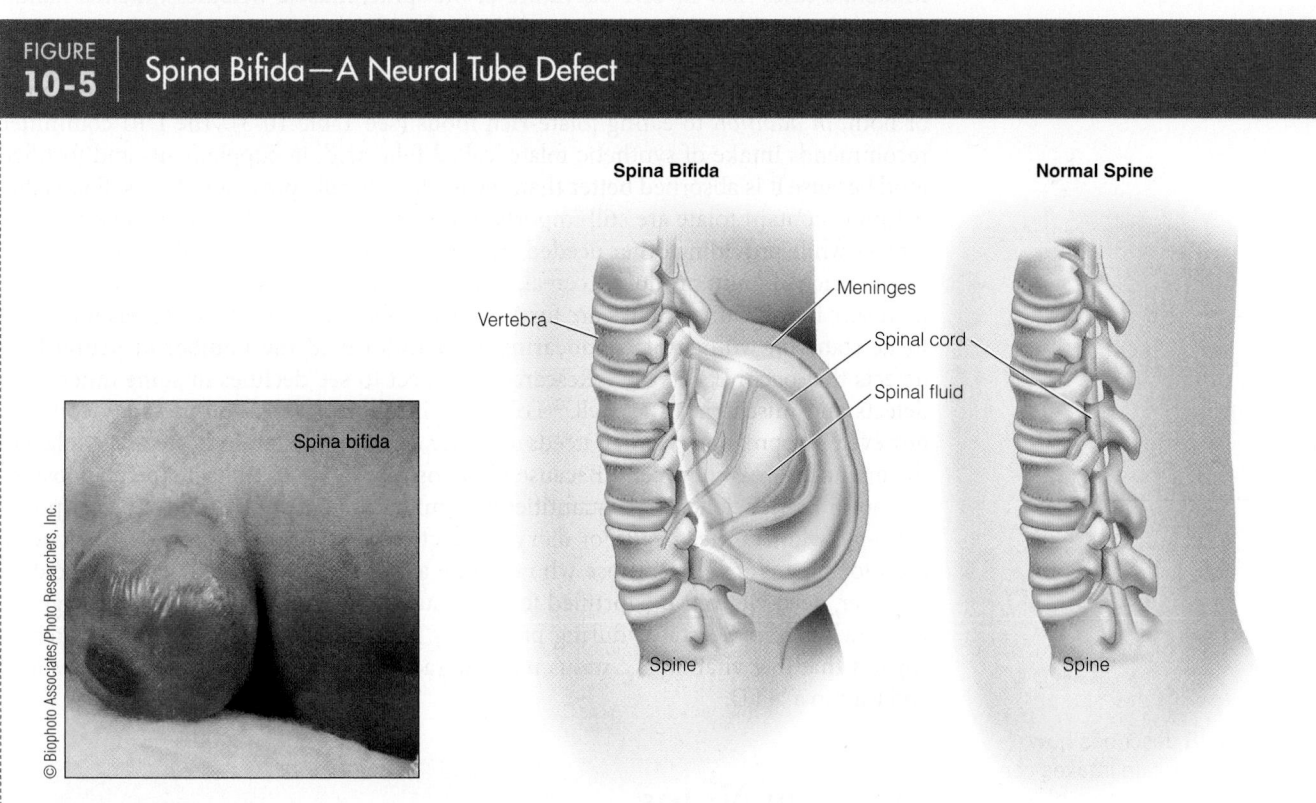

Spina bifida, a common neural tube defect, occurs when the vertebrae of the spine fail to close around the spinal cord, leaving it unprotected. The B vitamin folate helps prevent spina bifida and other neural tube defects.

Source: From the *Journal of the American Medical Association*, June 20, 2001, Vol. 285, No. 23 p. 3050. Reprinted with permission of the American Medical Association.

TABLE 10-3	Rich Folate Sources[a]
Natural Folate Sources	**Fortified Folate Sources**
Liver (3 oz) 221 μg	Multi-Grain Cheerios Plus cereal[b] (1 c) 400 μg
Lentils (½ c) 179 μg	Product 19 cereal[b] (1 c) 400 μg
Chickpeas or pinto beans (½ c) 145 μg	Total cereal[b] (1 c) 400 μg
Asparagus (½ c) 134 μg	Pasta, cooked (1 c) 110 μg
Spinach (1 c raw) 58 μg	Rice, cooked (1 c) 134 μg
Avocado (½ c) 45 μg	Bagel (1 small whole) 75 μg
Orange juice (1 c) 74 μg	Waffles, frozen (2) 36 μg
Beets (½ c) 68 μg	Bread, white (1 slice) 28 μg

[a] Folate amounts for these and 2000 other foods are listed in the Table of Food Composition in Appendix A.
[b] Folate in cereals varies; read the Nutrition Facts panel of the label.

is contained in the sac. Spina bifida is often accompanied by varying degrees of paralysis, depending on the extent of spinal cord damage. Mild cases may not be noticed. Moderate cases may involve curvature of the spine, muscle weakness, mental handicaps, and other ills, while severe cases can lead to death.

To reduce the risk of neural tube defects, women who are capable of becoming pregnant should obtain 400 micrograms of folic acid daily from supplements, fortified foods, or both, *in addition* to eating folate-rich foods (see Table 10-3). The DRI committee recommends intake of synthetic folate, called folic acid, in supplements and fortified food because it is absorbed better than the folate naturally present in foods. Foods that naturally contain folate are still important, however, because they contribute to folate intakes while providing other needed vitamins, minerals, fiber, and phytochemicals.

All enriched grain products (cereal, grits, pasta, rice, bread, and the like) sold commercially in the United States are fortified with folic acid. This measure has improved folate status in women of childbearing age and lowered the number of neural tube defects that occur each year.[20] Researchers expect to see declines in some other birth defects and miscarriages as well.[21] Folate fortification does raise one safety concern, however. The pregnant woman needs a greater amount of vitamin B_{12} to assist folate in the manufacture of new cells. Because high doses of folate complicate the diagnosis of a vitamin B_{12} deficiency, (✚) quantities of 1 milligram or more require a prescription.

People who eat meat, eggs, or dairy products receive all the vitamin B_{12} they need, even for pregnancy. (✚) Those who exclude all animal-derived foods from the diet, however, need vitamin B_{12}-fortified foods or supplements.[22] Limited research suggests that low vitamin B_{12} status during pregnancy is a risk factor for NTD.[23] Researchers suggest that low vitamin B_{12} status may interact synergistically with low folate status and lead to a NTD.

✚ Chapter 8 describes how excessive folate intakes can mask the symptoms of a vitamin B_{12} deficiency.

✚ Vitamin B_{12} RDA during pregnancy:
• 2.6 μg/day

Review Notes
- Due to their key roles in cell reproduction, folate and vitamin B_{12} are needed in large amounts during pregnancy.
- Folate plays an important role in preventing neural tube defects.

Vitamin D and Calcium for Bones

Vitamin D and the minerals involved in building the skeleton—calcium, phosphorus, and magnesium—are in great demand during pregnancy. (✚) Insufficient intakes may produce abnormal fetal bone development. (✚)

Vitamin D plays a vital role in calcium absorption and utilization. Consequently, severe maternal vitamin D deficiency interferes with normal calcium metabolism, which, in rare cases, may cause rickets in the infant.[24] Regular exposure to sunlight and consumption of vitamin D–fortified milk are usually sufficient to provide the recommended amount of vitamin D during pregnancy, although some researchers question whether current recommendations, even with prenatal supplements, are adequate.[25]

Intestinal absorption of calcium doubles early in pregnancy, when the mother's bones store the mineral. Later, as the fetal bones begin to calcify, there is a dramatic shift of calcium across the placenta.[26] Whether the calcium added to the mother's bones early in pregnancy is withdrawn to build the fetus's bones later is unclear. In the final weeks of pregnancy, more than 300 milligrams a day are transferred to the fetus. Recommendations to ensure an adequate calcium intake during pregnancy are aimed at conserving the mother's bone mass while supplying fetal needs.

For women whose prepregnancy calcium intakes are below recommendations, as most are, increased calcium intakes may be especially important. Milk products offer many advantages over supplements, as emphasized in earlier chapters. Because bones are still actively depositing minerals until about age 25, adequate calcium is especially important for young women. Pregnant women under age 25 who consume less than 600 milligrams of calcium a day need to increase their intakes of milk, cheese, yogurt, and other calcium-rich foods. Alternatively, and less preferably, they may need a daily supplement of 600 milligrams of calcium.

Women who exclude milk products need calcium-fortified foods such as soy milk. It is worth noting that not all soy milk is fortified with calcium; products fortified with calcium and vitamin D are recommended. Calcium-fortified orange juice offers folate and vitamin C as well as calcium.

Fluoride

Mineralization of the fetus's teeth begins in the fifth month after conception. For this and for bone development, fluoride may be needed. (✚) Fluoride crosses the placenta, and whether the placenta can defend against excess intakes is questionable. Therefore, fluoride supplements are not recommended for pregnant women who drink fluoridated water. For women who live in communities without fluoridated water, a fluoride supplement may protect fetal teeth.

> ## Review Notes
>
> - All pregnant women, but especially those who are younger than 25 years of age, need to pay special attention to calcium to ensure adequate intakes.
> - Maternal vitamin D deficiency interferes with calcium metabolism in the infant.
> - Fluoride supplements are not recommended for pregnant women who drink fluoridated water, but for those who live in communities where the water is not fluoridated, a fluoride supplement may protect fetal teeth.

Iron

The body conserves iron especially well during pregnancy: menstruation ceases, and absorption of iron increases up to threefold due to a rise in the blood's iron-absorbing and iron-carrying protein transferrin. Still, iron needs are so high that stores dwindle during pregnancy. (✚)

Reminder: Vitamin C–rich foods enhance iron absorption from foods.

The developing fetus draws heavily on the mother's iron stores to create stores of its own to last through the first four to six months of life. Even women with inadequate iron stores transfer significant amounts of iron to the fetus, suggesting that the iron needs of the fetus have priority over those of the mother. Iron losses also occur with the bleeding that is inevitable at birth.

✚ Calcium AI during pregnancy:
- 1300 mg/day (14 to 18 yr)
- 1000 mg/day (19 to 50 yr)

Phosphorus RDA during pregnancy:
- 1250 mg/day (14 to 18 yr)
- 700 mg/day (19 to 50 yr)

Magnesium RDA during pregnancy:
- 400 mg/day (14 to 18 yr)
- 350 mg/day (19 to 30 yr)
- 360 mg/day (31 to 50 yr)

✚ Three cups of milk a day will supply 900 mg of calcium. For other food sources of calcium, see Chapter 9.

✚ Fluoride AI during pregnancy:
- 3 mg/day

✚ Iron RDA during pregnancy:
- 27 mg/day

In pregnancy, hemoglobin values of 12 g are not unusual, and 11 g is where the line defining "too low" is often drawn. Appendix E discusses more sensitive measures of iron status.

Food sources of iron:
- Liver, oysters
- Red meat, fish, other meat
- Dried fruits (raisins, prunes)
- Legumes (dried beans, peas, lima beans)
- Dark green vegetables

Zinc RDA during pregnancy:
- 12 mg/day (≤18 yr)
- 11 mg/day (19 to 50 yr)

Special Supplemental Nutrition Program for Women, Infants, and Children (WIC): a high-quality, cost-effective health care and nutrition services program administered by the U.S. Department of Agriculture for low-income women, infants, and children who are nutritionally at risk. WIC provides supplemental foods, nutrition education, and referrals to health care and other social services.

Few women enter pregnancy with adequate iron stores. Women who enter pregnancy with iron-deficiency anemia have a greater-than-normal risk of delivering low-birthweight or preterm infants.[27] For all women not taking supplements containing iron, a daily iron supplement containing 30 milligrams is recommended during the second and third trimesters of pregnancy. When a low hemoglobin or hematocrit is confirmed by a repeat test, more than 30 milligrams of iron may be prescribed. To enhance iron absorption, the supplement should be taken between meals and with liquids other than milk, coffee, or tea, which inhibit iron absorption.

Zinc Zinc is required for DNA and RNA synthesis and thus for protein synthesis. (✚) Typical zinc intakes for pregnant women are lower than recommendations, but, fortunately, zinc absorption increases when zinc intakes are low.[28] Routine supplementation during pregnancy is not advised.[29] Women taking iron supplements (more than 30 milligrams per day), however, may need zinc supplements because large doses of iron can interfere with the body's absorption and use of zinc. Most supplements for pregnancy provide about 30 to 60 milligrams of iron a day. Zinc is most abundant in protein-rich foods such as shellfish, meat, and nuts.

Review Notes

- A daily iron supplement is recommended for all pregnant women during the second and third trimesters.
- Iron interferes with zinc absorption, so women taking iron supplements (more than 30 milligrams per day) may need zinc supplements as well.

FIGURE 10-6 | Example of a Prenatal Supplement Label

Prenatal Vitamins

Supplement Facts
Serving Size 1 Tablet

Amount Per Tablet	% Daily Value for Pregnant/ Lactating Women
Vitamin A 4000 IU	50%
Vitamin C 100 mg	167%
Vitamin D 400 IU	100%
Vitamin E 11 IU	37%
Thiamin 1.84 mg	108%
Riboflavin 1.7 mg	85%
Niacin 18 mg	90%
Vitamin B6 2.6 mg	104%
Folate 800 mcg	100%
Vitamin B12 4 mcg	50%
Calcium 200 mg	15%
Iron 27 mg	150%
Zinc 25 mg	167%

INGREDIENTS: calcium carbonate, microcrystalline cellulose, dicalcium phosphate, ascorbic acid, ferrous fumarate, zinc oxide, acacia, sucrose ester, niacinamide, modified cellulose gum, di-alpha tocopheryl acetate, hydroxypropyl methylcellulose, hydroxypropyl cellulose, artificial colors (FD&C blue no. 1 lake, FD&C red no. 40 lake, FD&C yellow no. 6 lake, titanium dioxide), polyethylene glycol, starch, pyridoxine hydrochloride, vitamin A acetate, riboflavin, thiamin mononitrate, folic acid, beta carotene, cholecalciferol, maltodextrin, gluten, cyanocobalamin, sodium bisulfite.

Notice that vitamin A is reduced to guard against birth defects, while extra amounts of folate, iron, and other nutrients are provided to meet the specific needs of pregnant women.

Nutrient Supplements Physicians often recommend daily multivitamin-mineral supplements for pregnant women. These prenatal supplements typically provide more folate, iron, and calcium than regular supplements. Prenatal supplements are especially beneficial for women who do not eat adequately and for those in high-risk groups: women carrying twins or triplets, cigarette smokers, and alcohol and drug abusers.[30] For these women, prenatal supplements may be of some help in reducing the risks of preterm delivery, low birthweights, and birth defects (see Figure 10-6). Be aware, however, that supplements cannot prevent the vast majority of fetal harm from tobacco, alcohol, and drugs, which continues unopposed, as later sections explain.

Review Notes

- Women most likely to benefit from multivitamin-mineral supplements during pregnancy include those who do not eat adequately, those carrying twins or triplets, and those who smoke cigarettes or are alcohol or drug abusers.

FOOD ASSISTANCE PROGRAMS

Women of limited financial means may eat diets too low in calcium, iron, vitamins A and C, and protein. Often, they and their children need help in obtaining food and benefit from nutrition counseling. At the federal level, the **Special Supplemental Nutrition Program for Women, Infants, and Children (WIC)** provides vouchers redeemable for nutritious foods, nutrition education, and referrals to health and social services to low-income pregnant and lactating women and their children.[31] The foods offered are milk and cheese, iron-fortified cereals, fruit or vegetable juices, carrots, eggs, dried beans, tuna fish, and peanut butter. Soy-based beverages, tofu, fruits and vegetables, baby foods, whole-wheat bread, and other whole-grain options were recently added. These foods provide nutrients often lacking in diets of low-income women and children. For infants given infant formula, WIC also provides iron-fortified formula. WIC encourages mothers to breastfeed their infants, however, and offers incentives to those who do.[32]

More than 8 million people—most of them infants and young children—receive WIC benefits each month. Participation in the WIC program benefits both the nutrient status and the growth and development of infants and children. WIC participation during pregnancy can effectively reduce infant mortality, low birthweight, and maternal and newborn medical costs.

The Supplemental Nutrition Assistance Program (SNAP) provides a debit card that can also help to stretch the low-income pregnant woman's grocery dollars. Many communities provide educational services and materials, including nutrition, food budgeting, and shopping information through the local agricultural extension service. Organizations such as the American Dietetic Association, the American Diabetes Association, and local hospitals also provide nutrition information.

Review Notes

- Food assistance programs such as WIC can provide nutritious food for pregnant women of limited financial means.

WEIGHT GAIN

Women must gain weight during pregnancy—fetal and maternal well-being depend on it. Ideally, a woman will have begun her pregnancy at a healthy weight, but even more importantly, she will gain within the recommended weight range based on her prepregnancy body mass index (BMI). Table 10-4 presents recommended weight gains for pregnancy. The recommended weight gain for a woman who begins pregnancy at a healthy weight and is carrying a single fetus is 25 to 35 pounds. An underweight woman needs to gain between 28 and 40 pounds, and an overweight woman, between 15 and 25 pounds. Pregnancy weight gains within the recommended ranges are associated with fewer surgical births, a greater number of healthy birthweights, and other positive outcomes for both mothers and infants, but many women do not gain within

TABLE 10-4	Recommended Weight Gains Based on Prepregnancy Weight	
Prepregnancy Weight	**Recommended Weight Gain**	
	For Single Birth	**For Twin Birth**
Underweight (BMI <18.5)	28 to 40 lb (12.5 to 18.0 kg)	Insufficient data to make recommendation
Healthy weight (BMI 18.5 to 24.9)	25 to 35 lb (11.5 to 16.0 kg)	37 to 54 lb (17 to 25 kg)
Overweight (BMI 25.0 to 29.9)	15 to 25 lb (7.0 to 11.5 kg)	31 to 50 lb (14 to 23 kg)
Obese (BMI ≥30)	11 to 20 lb (5 to 9 kg)	25 to 42 lb (11 to 19 kg)

Source: Institute of Medicine, *Weight Gain During Pregnancy: Reexamining the Guidelines.* Reprinted with permission from The National Academies Press, Copyright © 2009, National Academy of Sciences.

these ranges.[33] Among women in the United States, excessive weight gain during pregnancy is more prevalent than inadequate weight gain. To improve pregnancy outcomes, researchers and health care providers are placing greater emphasis on preventing excessive weight gains during pregnancy than in the past.[34]

Weight loss during pregnancy is not recommended.[35] Even obese women are advised to gain between 11 and 20 pounds for the best chance of delivering a healthy infant.[36] Ideally, overweight women will achieve a healthy body weight before becoming pregnant, avoid excessive weight gain during pregnancy, and postpone weight loss until after childbirth.[37]

According to current recommendations, pregnant adolescents who are still growing themselves should strive for gains at the upper end of the target range. Current concerns about obesity raise questions as to whether such recommendations are always appropriate. Compared with older mothers, for example, the risk of lifetime weight retention after pregnancy may be far greater for young adolescents.[38]

The ideal weight gain pattern for a woman who begins pregnancy at a healthy weight is 3½ pounds during the first trimester and 1 pound per week thereafter. (✚) If a woman gains more than is recommended early in pregnancy, she should not restrict her energy intake later on in order to lose weight. A sudden, large weight gain is a danger signal, however, because it may indicate the onset of preeclampsia (discussed later in the chapter).

The weight the pregnant woman gains is nearly all lean tissue: placenta, uterus, blood, milk-producing glands, and the fetus itself (see Figure 10-7). The fat she gains is needed later for lactation. Physical activity can help a pregnant woman cope with the extra weight, as a later section explains.

WEIGHT LOSS AFTER PREGNANCY

The pregnant woman loses some weight at delivery. In the following weeks, she loses more as her blood volume returns to normal and she gets rid of accumulated fluids. The typical woman does not, however, return to her prepregnancy weight. In general, the more weight a woman gains beyond the needs of pregnancy, the more she retains—mostly as body fat.[39] Even with an average weight gain during pregnancy, most women

FIGURE 10-7	Components of Weight Gain during Pregnancy

	Weight gain (lb)
Increase in breast size	2
Increase in mother's fluid volume	4
Placenta	1 1/2
Increase in blood supply to the placenta	4
Amniotic fluid	2
Infant at birth	7 1/2
Increase in size of uterus and supporting muscles	2
Mother's necessary fat stores	7
	30

1st trimester   2nd trimester   3rd trimester

✚ A prenatal weight-gain grid (Appendix E) plots the rate of weight gain during pregnancy.

tend to retain a couple of pounds with each pregnancy. When those couple of pounds become 7 or more and BMI increases by a unit or more, complications such as diabetes and hypertension in future pregnancies as well as chronic diseases later in life can increase—even for women who are not overweight.[40] Those who are successful in losing their pregnancy weight are more likely to limit weight gains through middle adulthood.[41]

Review Notes

- Weight gain is essential for a healthy pregnancy.
- A woman's prepregnancy BMI, her own nutrient needs, and the number of fetuses she is carrying help to determine appropriate weight gain.

PHYSICAL ACTIVITY

Physical activity is important to the pregnant woman, not only to help her carry the extra weight of pregnancy without strain, but also to help ease her upcoming childbirth. Staying active during the course of a normal, healthy pregnancy improves the fitness of the mother-to-be, facilitates labor, helps to prevent or manage gestational diabetes, and reduces psychological stress.[42] Women who remain active during pregnancy report fewer discomforts throughout their pregnancies and retain habits that help in losing excess weight and regaining fitness after the birth.

Pregnant women should take care in choosing their physical activities, however. They should participate in low-impact activities and avoid sports in which they might fall or be hit by other people or objects. Swimming and water aerobics are particularly beneficial because they allow the body to remain cool and move freely with the water's support, thus reducing back pain.[43]

As is true for everyone, the frequency, duration, and intensity of the activity affect the likelihood of the benefits or risks. A pregnant woman should consult her health care provider before taking up additional activity. (✚) A few guidelines are offered in Figure 10-8. Several of the guidelines are aimed at preventing excessively high internal body temperatures and dehydration, both of which can harm fetal development. To this end, a pregnant woman should also stay out of saunas, steam rooms, and hot whirlpools.

Physical Activity Guidelines for Americans, 2008

- Healthy women who are not already highly active or doing vigorous-intensity activity should get at least 150 minutes (2 hours and 30 minutes) of moderate-intensity aerobic activity per week during pregnancy and the postpartum period. Preferably, this activity should be spread throughout the week.
- Pregnant women who habitually engage in vigorous-intensity aerobic activity or are highly active can continue physical activity during pregnancy and the postpartum period, provided that they remain healthy and discuss with their health care provider how and when activity should be adjusted over time.

FIGURE 10-8 | Guidelines for Physical Activity during Pregnancy

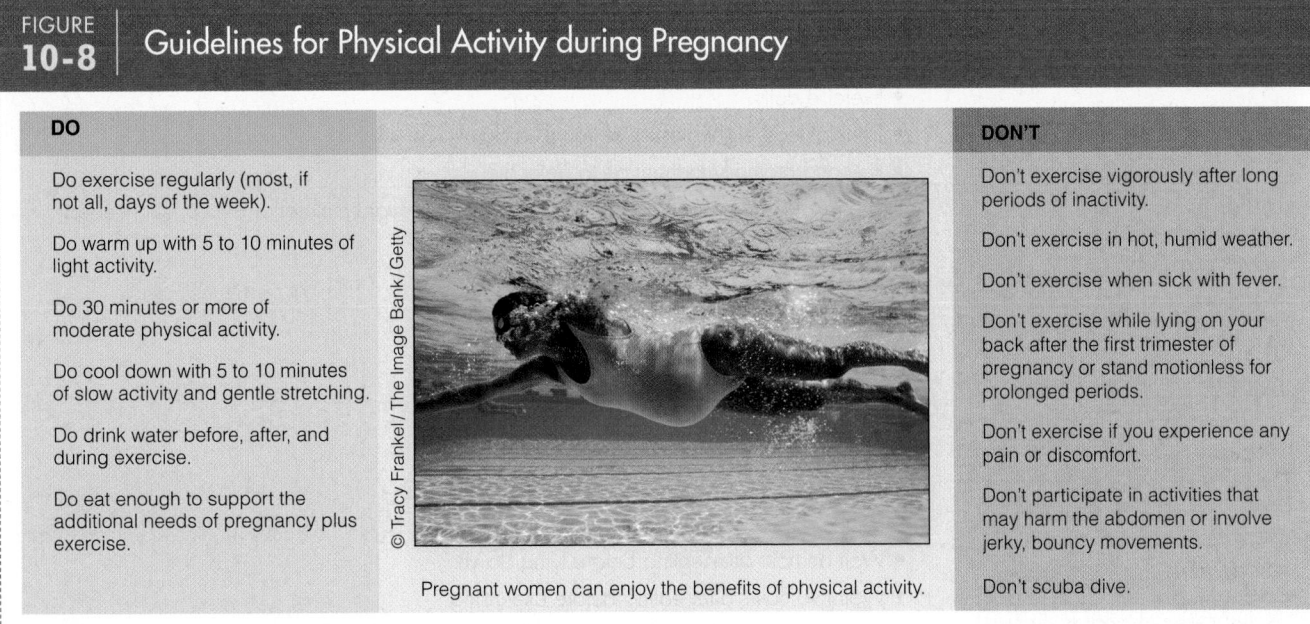

DO

Do exercise regularly (most, if not all, days of the week).

Do warm up with 5 to 10 minutes of light activity.

Do 30 minutes or more of moderate physical activity.

Do cool down with 5 to 10 minutes of slow activity and gentle stretching.

Do drink water before, after, and during exercise.

Do eat enough to support the additional needs of pregnancy plus exercise.

DON'T

Don't exercise vigorously after long periods of inactivity.

Don't exercise in hot, humid weather.

Don't exercise when sick with fever.

Don't exercise while lying on your back after the first trimester of pregnancy or stand motionless for prolonged periods.

Don't exercise if you experience any pain or discomfort.

Don't participate in activities that may harm the abdomen or involve jerky, bouncy movements.

Don't scuba dive.

© Tracy Frankel / The Image Bank/Getty

Pregnant women can enjoy the benefits of physical activity.

Review Notes

- By remaining active throughout pregnancy, a woman can develop the strength she needs to carry the extra weight and maintain habits that will help her lose it after the birth.

COMMON NUTRITION-RELATED CONCERNS OF PREGNANCY

Food sensitivities, nausea, heartburn, and constipation are common during pregnancy. A few simple strategies can help alleviate maternal discomforts (see Table 10-5).

Food Cravings and Aversions Some women develop cravings for, or aversions to, certain foods and beverages during pregnancy. Individual **food cravings** during pregnancy do not seem to reflect real physiological needs. In other words, a woman who craves pickles does not necessarily need salt. Similarly, cravings for ice cream are common during pregnancy but do not signify a calcium deficiency. **Food aversions** and cravings that arise during pregnancy are probably due to hormone-induced changes in taste and sensitivities to smells.

Nonfood Cravings Some pregnant women develop cravings for nonfood items such as laundry starch, clay, soil, or ice—a practice known as pica.[44] Pica may be practiced for cultural reasons that reflect a society's folklore; it is especially common

TABLE 10-5	Strategies to Alleviate Maternal Discomforts

To alleviate the nausea of pregnancy:
- On waking, arise slowly.
- Eat dry toast or crackers.
- Chew gum or suck hard candies.
- Eat small, frequent meals whenever hunger strikes.
- Avoid foods with offensive odors.
- When nauseated, do not drink citrus juice, water, milk, coffee, or tea.

To prevent or alleviate constipation:
- Eat foods high in fiber.
- Exercise daily.
- Drink at least eight glasses of liquids a day.
- Respond promptly to the urge to defecate.
- Use laxatives only as prescribed by a physician; avoid mineral oil—it carries needed fat-soluble vitamins out of the body.

To prevent or relieve heartburn:
- Relax and eat slowly.
- Chew food thoroughly.
- Eat small, frequent meals.
- Drink liquids between meals.
- Avoid spicy or greasy foods.
- Sit up while eating.
- Wait an hour after eating before lying down.
- Wait two hours after eating before exercising.

food cravings: deep longings for particular foods.

food aversions: strong desires to avoid particular foods.

among African American women. Pica is often associated with iron deficiency, but whether iron deficiency leads to pica or pica leads to iron deficiency is unclear.[45] Eating clay or soil may interfere with iron absorption and displace iron-rich foods from the diet. Furthermore, if the soil or clay contains environmental contaminants such as lead or parasites, health and nutrition suffer.

Morning Sickness The nausea of "morning" (actually, anytime) sickness is usually benign, although it is distressing to some women. It arises from the hormonal changes taking place early in pregnancy, ranges from mild queasiness to debilitating nausea, and afflicts more than half of all pregnant women. Many women complain that smells, especially cooking smells, make them sick. Thus, minimizing odors is a key to alleviating morning sickness. Traditional strategies for quelling nausea are listed in Table 10-5, but many women benefit most from simply eating the foods they want when they feel like eating.

Heartburn Heartburn, a burning sensation in the lower esophagus near the heart, is common during pregnancy and is also benign. As the growing fetus puts increasing pressure on the woman's stomach, acid may back up and create a burning sensation in her throat. Tips to relieve heartburn are also listed in Table 10-5.

Constipation As the hormones of pregnancy alter muscle tone and the thriving infant crowds intestinal organs, an expectant mother may complain of constipation, another harmless but annoying condition. A high-fiber diet, physical activity, and plentiful fluids will help relieve this condition. Also, responding promptly to the urge to defecate can help. Laxatives should be used only as prescribed by the physician. Mineral oil should not be used because it interferes with the absorption of fat-soluble vitamins.

Review Notes

- Food cravings typically do not reflect physiological needs.
- The nausea, heartburn, and constipation that sometimes accompany pregnancy can usually be alleviated with a few simple strategies.

PROBLEMS IN PREGNANCY

Just as adequate nutrition and normal weight gain support the health of the mother and growth of the fetus, maternal diseases can have an adverse effect. If discovered early, many diseases can be controlled—another reason why early prenatal care is recommended. Some nutrition measures can help alleviate the most common problems encountered during pregnancy.

Preexisting Diabetes Pregnancy presents special challenges for the management of diabetes.[46] Insulin-induced hypoglycemia has a more rapid onset during pregnancy and is a danger to the mother, especially in those with type 1 diabetes. Women with type 2 diabetes often start pregnancy with insulin resistance and obesity, making optimal glycemic control difficult. The risks of diabetes during pregnancy depend on how well it is managed before, during, and after. Excellent glycemic control in the first trimester and throughout the pregnancy is associated with the lowest frequency of maternal, fetal, and newborn complications.[47] Without proper management, women face high infertility rates, and those who do conceive may experience episodes of severe hypoglycemia or hyperglycemia, preterm labor, and pregnancy-related hypertension. Infants may be large, suffer physical and mental abnormalities, and experience other complications such as severe hypoglycemia or respiratory distress, both of which can be fatal. Signs of fetal health problems are apparent even when maternal glucose is above normal but still below the diagnosis of diabetes.[48] Ideally, a woman will receive the prenatal care needed to achieve glucose

NURSING DIAGNOSIS
Nausea, risk for constipation applies to clients who are pregnant.

gestational diabetes: glucose intolerance with first onset or first recognition during pregnancy.

chronic hypertension: in pregnant women, hypertension that is present and documented before pregnancy; in women whose prepregnancy blood pressure is unknown, the presence of sustained hypertension before 20 weeks of gestation.

gestational hypertension: high blood pressure that develops in the second half of pregnancy and usually resolves after childbirth.

preeclampsia (PRE-ee-KLAMP-see-ah): a condition characterized by hypertension and protein in the urine.

eclampsia (eh-KLAMP-see-ah): a severe complication during pregnancy in which seizures occur.

control before conception and continued glucose control throughout pregnancy. For optimal long-term outcomes, continuation of intensified diabetes management after pregnancy is in the best interest of the mother's health.[49]

Gestational Diabetes

Some women are prone to developing a pregnancy-related form of diabetes, **gestational diabetes**. Gestational diabetes usually resolves after the infant is born, but some women go on to develop diabetes (type 2) later in life, especially if they are overweight.[50] Gestational diabetes can lead to fetal or infant sickness or death. When it is identified early and managed properly, however, the most serious risks fall dramatically.[51] More commonly, gestational diabetes leads to surgical birth and high infant birthweight.[52] To ensure that the problems of gestational diabetes are dealt with promptly, physicians screen for the risk factors listed in the margin (✚) and test high-risk women for glucose intolerance immediately and average-risk women between 24 and 28 weeks gestation.[53] Chapter 20 provides information about medical nutrition therapy for gestational diabetes.

Hypertension

Hypertension (blood pressure ≥140/90 millimeters mercury) complicates pregnancy and affects its outcome in different ways, depending on how severe it becomes. Hypertension during pregnancy is classified as **chronic hypertension** or **gestational hypertension**.[54] Chronic hypertension can be a preexisting condition that develops before a woman becomes pregnant. In women whose prepregnancy blood pressure is unknown, diagnosis of chronic hypertension is based on the presence of sustained hypertension before 20 weeks of gestation.[55] In contrast, gestational hypertension develops after the 20th week of gestation. In women with gestational hypertension, blood pressure usually returns to normal during the first few weeks after childbirth.

Both types of hypertension pose risks to the mother and fetus. In addition to the health risks normally imposed by hypertension (heart attack and stroke), high blood pressure increases the risks of having a low-birthweight infant or of having the placenta separate from the wall of the uterus before the birth, resulting in stillbirth. Both chronic hypertension and gestational hypertension also increase the risk of preeclampsia.

Preeclampsia

Preeclampsia is a condition characterized not only by high blood pressure but also by protein in the urine.[56] (✚) Preeclampsia usually occurs with first pregnancies and almost always appears after 20 weeks' gestation.[57] Symptoms typically regress within 48 hours of delivery.

Preeclampsia affects almost all of the woman's organs—the circulatory system, liver, kidneys, and brain. If it progresses, she may experience seizures; when this occurs, the condition is called **eclampsia**. Maternal mortality during pregnancy is rare in developed countries, but eclampsia is the most common cause. Preeclampsia demands prompt medical attention. Treatment focuses on regulating blood pressure and preventing seizures.

Review Notes

- Conditions such as gestational diabetes, hypertension, and preeclampsia can threaten the health and life of both mother and infant.
- Such conditions require medical and nutrition treatment.

PRACTICES TO AVOID

A general guideline for the pregnant woman is to eat a normal, healthy diet and practice moderation. A woman's daily choices during pregnancy take on enormous importance. Forewarned, pregnant women can choose to abstain from or avoid potentially harmful practices.

Cigarette Smoking

One practice to be avoided during pregnancy is cigarette smoking. A surgeon general's warning states that parental smoke can kill an otherwise healthy fetus or newborn. Unfortunately, an estimated 10 percent of pregnant women in the United States smoke, and rates are even higher for unmarried women and those who have not graduated from high school.[58] Constituents of cigarette smoke, such as nicotine, carbon monoxide, arsenic, and cyanide, are toxic to a fetus.[59] Research shows that smoking during pregnancy can cause damage to fetal chromosomes, which could lead to developmental defects or genetic disorders, including cancer.[60] Smoking also restricts the blood supply to the growing fetus and so limits the delivery of oxygen and nutrients and the removal of wastes. It slows growth, thus retarding physical development of the fetus. Smoking during pregnancy may reduce brain size and impair the intellectual and behavioral development of the child later in life.[61]

A mother who smokes is more likely to have a complicated birth and a low-birthweight infant.[62] The more a mother smokes, the smaller her infant will be. Of all preventable causes of low birthweight in the United States, smoking has the greatest impact. Sudden infant death syndrome (SIDS), the unexplained death that sometimes occurs in an otherwise healthy infant, has been linked to the mother's cigarette smoking during pregnancy.[63] Research suggests that even in women who do not smoke, exposure to **environmental tobacco smoke** (**ETS**, or secondhand smoke) during pregnancy increases the risk of low birthweight and the likelihood of SIDS.[64]

In addition to the harms already described, cigarette (and cigar) smoking adversely affects the pregnant woman's nutrition status and thus impairs fetal nutrition and development. Smokers tend to have lower intakes of dietary fiber, vitamin A, beta-carotene, folate, and vitamin C. The margin (✚) lists complications of smoking during pregnancy.

Medicinal Drugs and Herbal Supplements
Medicinal drugs taken during pregnancy can cause serious birth defects. Pregnant women should not take over-the-counter drugs or any medications not prescribed by a physician. Drug labels warn: "As with any drug, if you are pregnant or nursing a baby, seek the advice of a health professional before using this product." For aspirin and ibuprofen, there is an additional warning: "It is especially important not to use aspirin (or ibuprofen) during the last three months of pregnancy unless specifically directed to do so by a doctor because it may cause problems in the unborn child or complications during delivery." Such warnings should be taken seriously.

Some pregnant women mistakenly consider herbal supplements to be safe alternatives to medicinal drugs and take them to relieve nausea, promote water loss, alleviate depression, help them sleep, or for other reasons. Some herbal products may be safe, but very few have been tested for safety or effectiveness during pregnancy. Pregnant women should stay away from herbal supplements, teas, or other products unless their safety during pregnancy has been ascertained.[65] Nutrition in Practice 14 offers more information about herbal supplements and other alternative therapies.

Drugs of Abuse
Drugs of abuse such as cocaine easily cross the placenta and impair fetal growth and development. Furthermore, such drugs are responsible for preterm births, low-birthweight infants, and sudden infant deaths. If these newborns survive, central nervous system damage is evident: their cries, sleep, and behaviors early in life are abnormal, and their cognitive development later in life is impaired.[66] They may be hypersensitive or underaroused; those who test positive for drugs suffer the greatest effects of toxicity and withdrawal. Their growth throughout childhood continues at a slow rate.[67]

Environmental Contaminants
Infants and young children of pregnant women exposed to environmental contaminants such as lead and mercury show signs of impaired mental and psychomotor development. During pregnancy, lead readily moves across the placenta, inflicting severe damage on the developing fetal nervous system. In addition, infants exposed to even low levels of lead during gestation weigh less at birth and consequently struggle to survive. For these reasons, it is particularly important that pregnant women consume foods and beverages free of contamination. A diet high in calcium will help to defend against lead contamination.

✚ Complications associated with smoking during pregnancy:
- Fetal growth retardation
- Low birthweight
- Complications at birth (prolonged final stage of labor)
- Mislocation of the placenta
- Premature separation of the placenta
- Vaginal bleeding
- Spontaneous abortion
- Fetal death
- Sudden infant death syndrome (SIDS)
- Middle ear diseases
- Cardiac and respiratory diseases

environmental tobacco smoke (ETS): the combination of exhaled smoke (mainstream smoke) and smoke from lighted cigarettes, pipes, or cigars (sidestream smoke) that enters the air and may be inhaled by other people.

Mercury is among the contaminants of concern. As Chapter 4 mentioned, fatty fish are a good source of omega-3 fatty acids, but some fish contain large amounts of the pollutant mercury, which can impair fetal growth and harm the developing brain and nervous system.[68] Because the benefits of seafood consumption seem to outweigh the risks, pregnant (and lactating) women should do the following:[69]

- Avoid shark, swordfish, king mackerel, and tilefish (also called golden snapper or golden bass).
- Limit average weekly consumption to 12 ounces (cooked or canned) of seafood *or* to 6 ounces (cooked or canned) of white (albacore) tuna.

Supplements of fish oil are not recommended because they may contain concentrated toxins and because their effects on pregnancy remain unknown.

Foodborne Illness

The vomiting and diarrhea caused by many foodborne illnesses can leave a pregnant woman exhausted and dangerously dehydrated. Particularly threatening, however, is **listeriosis**, which can cause miscarriage, stillbirth, or severe brain or other infections to fetuses and newborns. Pregnant women are about 20 times more likely than other healthy adults to get listeriosis. A woman with listeriosis may develop symptoms such as fever, vomiting, and diarrhea in about 12 hours after eating a contaminated food, and serious symptoms may develop a week to six weeks later. A blood test can reliably detect listeriosis, and antibiotics given promptly to the pregnant sufferer can often prevent infection of the fetus or newborn. The margin lists preventive measures pregnant women can take to avoid contracting listeriosis. (✚)

Vitamin-Mineral Megadoses

Many vitamins and minerals are toxic when taken in excess. Excessive vitamin A is particularly infamous for its role in fetal malformations of the cranial nervous system. Intakes before the seventh week of pregnancy appear to be the most damaging. For this reason, vitamin A supplements are not given during pregnancy, unless there is specific evidence of deficiency, which is rare.

Dieting

Weight-loss dieting, even for short periods, can be hazardous during pregnancy. Low-carbohydrate diets or fasts that cause ketosis deprive the growing fetal brain of needed glucose and may impair its development. Such diets are also likely to be deficient in other nutrients vital to fetal growth. Regardless of prepregnancy weight, pregnant women need an adequate diet and sufficient weight gain to support healthy fetal development.

Sugar Substitutes

Artificial sweeteners have been studied extensively and found to be acceptable during pregnancy if used within the FDA's guidelines (see Chapter 3).[70] Still, it would be prudent for pregnant women to use sweeteners in moderation and within an otherwise nutritious and well-balanced diet. Women with phenylketonuria should not use aspartame, as Chapter 3 explains.

Caffeine

Caffeine crosses the placenta, and the fetus has only a limited ability to metabolize it. Research studies have not proved that caffeine (even in high doses) causes birth defects in human infants (as it does in animals), but limited evidence suggests that heavy use increases the risk of miscarriage and fetal death.[71] (In these studies, heavy caffeine use is defined as the equivalent of three or more cups of coffee a day.) Depending on the quantities consumed and the mother's metabolism, caffeine may also interfere with fetal growth.[72] In light of this evidence, the most sensible course is to limit caffeine consumption to the equivalent of one cup of coffee or two 12-ounce cola beverages a day. Caffeine amounts in food and beverages are listed in Appendix A.

Alcohol

Drinking alcohol during pregnancy threatens the fetus with irreversible brain damage, growth retardation, mental retardation, facial abnormalities, vision abnormalities, and many more health problems—a spectrum of symptoms known as **fetal alcohol spectrum disorders**, or **FASD**. Children at the most severe end of the spectrum (those with all of the symptoms) are defined as having

✚ To protect their fetuses and newborns from listeriosis, pregnant women should:

- Avoid the following Mexican soft cheeses: queso blanco, queso fresco, queso de hoja, queso de crema, and asadero. Also avoid feta cheese, brie, Camembert, and blue-veined cheeses like Roquefort.
- Use only pasteurized dairy products and juices.
- Eat only thoroughly cooked meat, poultry, and seafood.
- Thoroughly reheat until steaming hot all hot dogs, luncheon meats, and deli meats, including cured meats like salami, before eating them.
- Wash all fruits and vegetables.
- Do not eat refrigerated smoked seafood such as salmon or trout, or any fish labeled "nova-style," "lox," or "kippered," unless it is an ingredient in a cooked dish.
- Do not eat refrigerated pâté or meat spreads. Canned or shelf-stable pâté and meat spreads are safer.

listeriosis: a serious foodborne infection that can cause severe brain infection or death in a fetus or newborn; caused by the bacterium *Listeria monocytogenes*, which is found in soil and water.

fetal alcohol spectrum disorders (FASD): a spectrum of physical, behavioral, and cognitive disabilities caused by prenatal alcohol exposure.

fetal alcohol syndrome (FAS).[73] The fetal brain is extremely vulnerable to a glucose or oxygen deficit, and alcohol causes both by disrupting placental functioning. The lifelong mental retardation and other tragedies of FAS can be prevented by abstaining from drinking alcohol during pregnancy. Once the damage is done, however, the child remains impaired.

The accompanying photo shows the facial abnormalities of FAS, which are easy to depict. A visual picture of the internal harm is impossible, but that damage seals the fate of the child. An estimated 5 to 20 of every 10,000 children are victims of FAS, making it one of the leading known preventable causes of mental retardation in the world.[74]

One out of 8 pregnant women drinks alcohol sometime during her pregnancy; 1 out of 50 pregnant women reports binge drinking (five or more drinks on one occasion).[75] Almost half of all pregnancies are unintended, and many are conceived during a binge-drinking episode.

For women who know they are pregnant and choose to drink alcohol, the question is how much alcohol is too much. Even one drink a day threatens neurological development and behaviors. Low birthweight is reported among infants born to women who drink 1 ounce (two drinks) of alcohol per day during pregnancy, and FAS is also known to occur with as few as two drinks a day. Birth defects have been reliably observed among the children of women who drink 2 ounces (four drinks) of alcohol daily during pregnancy. The most severe impact is likely to occur in the first two months, before the woman may even be aware that she is pregnant.

Research using animals shows that one-fifth of the amount of alcohol needed to produce major visible defects will produce learning impairment or other defects in the offspring. The cluster of mental problems associated with prenatal alcohol exposure and FASD is known as **alcohol-related neurodevelopmental disorder (ARND)**, and the physical malformations are referred to as **alcohol-related birth defects (ARBD)**.

For every child diagnosed with full-blown FAS, many more with FASD go undiagnosed until problems develop in the preschool years. Upon reaching adulthood, such children are ill equipped for employment, relationships, and the other facets of life most adults take for granted. Anyone exposed to alcohol before birth may always respond differently to it, and also to certain drugs, than if no exposure had occurred, making addictions likely.

The American Academy of Pediatrics takes the position that women should stop drinking as soon as they *plan* to become pregnant. Researchers have looked for a "safe" alcohol intake limit during pregnancy and have found none. Their conclusion: abstinence from alcohol is the best policy for pregnant women.

For pregnant women who have already drunk alcohol, the advice is "stop now." A woman who has drunk heavily during the first two-thirds of her pregnancy can still prevent some organ damage by stopping heavy drinking during the third trimester.

These facial traits are typical of fetal alcohol syndrome, caused by drinking alcohol during pregnancy—low nasal bridge, short eyelid opening, underdeveloped groove in the center of the upper lip, small midface, short nose, and small head circumference.

© James W. Hanson, M.D./NICHD

Review Notes

· Abstaining from smoking and other drugs, including alcohol, limiting intake of foods known to contain unsafe levels of contaminants such as mercury, taking precautions against foodborne illness, avoiding large doses of nutrients, refraining from dieting, using artificial sweeteners in moderation, and limiting caffeine use are recommended during pregnancy.

ADOLESCENT PREGNANCY

Many adolescents become sexually active before age 19, and more than 400,000 infants are born to teenage mothers each year in the United States.[76] A pregnant adolescent presents a special case of intense nutrient needs. Young teenage girls have a hard enough time meeting nutrient needs for their own rapid growth and development, let alone those of pregnancy. Many teens enter pregnancy deficient in vitamins B_{12} and D, folate, and iron, which increases the risk of impaired fetal growth.[77] Pregnant

fetal alcohol syndrome (FAS): the cluster of symptoms seen in an infant or child whose mother consumed excessive alcohol during her pregnancy. FAS includes, but is not limited to, brain damage, growth retardation, mental retardation, and facial abnormalities.

alcohol-related neurodevelopmental disorder (ARND): a condition caused by prenatal alcohol exposure. ARND is diagnosed when there is a confirmed history of substantial, regular maternal alcohol intake or heavy episodic drinking and behavioral, cognitive, or central nervous system abnormalities known to be associated with alcohol exposure.

alcohol-related birth defects (ARBD): a condition caused by prenatal alcohol exposure. ARBD is diagnosed when there is a history of substantial, regular maternal alcohol intake or heavy episodic drinking and birth defects known to be associated with alcohol exposure.

+ Energy requirement during lactation:
  - First 6 months: +330 kcal/day
  - Second 6 months: +400 kcal/day

exclusive breastfeeding: an infant's consumption of human milk with no supplementation of any type (no water, no juice, no nonhuman milk, and no foods) except for vitamins, minerals, and medications.

© Ariel Skelley/Corbis

A woman who decides to breastfeed offers her infant a full array of nutrients and protective factors to support optimal health and development.

adolescents are less likely to receive early prenatal care and are more likely to smoke during pregnancy—two factors that predict low birthweight and infant death.[78]

The rates of stillbirths, preterm births, and low-birthweight infants are high for teenagers—both for teen moms and for teen dads.[79] Their greatest risk, though, is death of the infant: mothers under age 16 bear more infants who die within the first year than do women in any other age group. These factors combine to make adolescent pregnancy a major public health problem.

Adequate nutrition is an indispensable component of prenatal care for adolescents and can substantially improve the outlook for both mother and infant. To support the needs of both mother and fetus, a pregnant teenager with a BMI in the normal range is encouraged to gain about 35 pounds to reduce the likelihood of a low-birthweight infant. As mentioned earlier, however, compared with older mothers, the lifetime risk of postpartum weight retention in young adolescents may be far greater. Research shows that women who give birth during adolescence have higher body weights, BMIs, and percent body fat later on than adolescents who do not experience pregnancy.[80] Researchers agree that optimal weight gain recommendations for pregnant adolescents need focused attention. Meanwhile, pregnant and lactating adolescents would do well to follow the eating pattern presented in Table 1-7, making sure to choose a kcalorie level high enough to support adequate, but not excessive, weight gain.

Review Notes

- Proper nutrition and adequate weight gain are especially important in reducing the risk of poor pregnancy outcome in adolescents.

Breastfeeding

The American Academy of Pediatrics (AAP) recommends that infants receive breast milk for at least the first 12 months of life and beyond for as long as mutually desired by mother and child.[81] The American Dietetic Association (ADA) advocates breastfeeding for the nutritional health it confers on the infant as well as for the physiological, social, economic, and other benefits it offers the mother.[82] The AAP and the ADA recognize **exclusive breastfeeding** for 6 months and breastfeeding with complementary foods for at least 12 months as an optimal feeding pattern for infants.[83] Breast milk's unique nutrient composition and protective factors promote optimal infant health and development. The only acceptable alternative to breast milk is iron-fortified formula. Adequate nutrition of the mother supports successful **lactation**, and without it, lactation is likely to falter or fail.

NUTRITION DURING LACTATION

By continuing to eat nutrient-dense foods, not restricting weight gain unduly, and enjoying ample food and fluid at frequent intervals throughout lactation, the mother who chooses to breastfeed her infant will be nutritionally prepared to do so. An inadequate diet does not support the stamina, patience, and self-confidence that nursing an infant demands. Figure 10-4 (on p. 277) shows how a lactating woman's nutrient needs differ from those of a nonpregnant woman, and Table 10-2 (on p. 278) presents a sample menu that meets those needs.

Energy A nursing woman produces about 25 ounces of milk a day, with considerable variation from woman to woman and in the same woman from time to time, depending primarily on the infant's demand for milk. Producing this milk costs a woman almost 500 kcalories per day above her regular need during the first six months of lactation. To meet this energy need, the woman is advised to eat an extra 330 kcalories of food each day. (✚) The other 170 kcalories can be drawn from the fat stores she accumulated during pregnancy. The food energy consumed by the nursing mother should carry with it abundant nutrients. Severe energy restriction hinders milk production and can compromise the mother's health.

Weight Loss After the birth of the infant, many women actively try to lose the extra weight and body fat they accumulated during pregnancy. How much weight a woman retains after pregnancy depends on her gestational weight gain and the duration and intensity of breastfeeding. Many women who follow recommendations for gestational weight gain and breastfeeding can readily return to prepregnancy weight by six months.[84] Neither the quality nor the quantity of breast milk is adversely affected by moderate weight loss, and infants grow normally.

Women often choose to be physically active to lose weight and improve fitness, and this is compatible with breastfeeding and infant growth.[85] A gradual weight loss (1 pound per week) is safe and does not reduce milk output. Too large an energy deficit, however, especially soon after birth, will inhibit lactation.

Vitamins and Minerals A question often raised is whether a mother's milk may lack a nutrient if she fails to get enough in her diet. The answer differs from one nutrient to the next, but, in general, nutritional deprivation of the mother reduces the *quantity*, not the *quality*, of her milk. Women can produce milk with adequate protein, carbohydrate, fat, folate, and most minerals, even when their own supplies are limited. For these nutrients, milk quality is maintained at the expense of maternal stores. This is most evident in the case of calcium: dietary calcium has no effect on the calcium concentration of breast milk, but maternal bones lose some of their density during lactation if calcium intakes are inadequate.[86] Such losses are generally made up quickly when lactation ends, and breastfeeding has no long-term harmful effects on women's bones. The nutrients in breast milk that are most likely to decline in response to prolonged inadequate intakes are the vitamins—especially vitamins B_6, B_{12}, A, and D. Vitamin supplementation of undernourished women appears to help normalize the vitamin concentrations in their milk and may be beneficial.

Water The volume of breast milk produced depends on how much milk the infant demands, not on how much fluid the mother drinks. The nursing mother is nevertheless advised to drink plenty of liquids each day (about 13 cups) to protect herself from dehydration. (✚) To help themselves remember to drink enough liquid, many women make a habit of drinking a glass of milk, juice, or water each time the infant nurses as well as at mealtimes.

Particular Foods Foods with strong or spicy flavors (such as onions or garlic) may alter the flavor of breast milk. A sudden change in the taste of the milk may annoy some infants. Familiar flavors may enhance enjoyment. A mother who is breastfeeding her infant is advised to eat whatever nutritious foods she chooses. Then, if a particular food seems to cause the infant discomfort, she can try eliminating that food from her diet for a few days and see if the problem goes away.

Current evidence does not support a major role for maternal dietary restrictions during lactation to prevent or delay the onset of food allergy in infants.[87] Infants who develop symptoms of food allergy, however, may be more comfortable if the mother's diet excludes the most common offenders—cow's milk, eggs, fish, peanuts, and tree nuts. Generally, infants with a strong family history of food allergies benefit from breastfeeding.[88]

CONTRAINDICATIONS TO BREASTFEEDING

Some substances impair maternal milk production or enter the breast milk and interfere with infant development. Some medical conditions prohibit breastfeeding.

Alcohol Alcohol easily enters breast milk and can adversely affect the production, volume, composition, and ejection of breast milk as well as overwhelm an infant's immature alcohol-degrading system.[89] Alcohol concentration in breast milk peaks

✚ The DRI recommendation for *total* water intake during lactation is 3.8 L/day. This includes 3.1 L or about 13 c as total beverages, including drinking water.

NURSING DIAGNOSIS

Interrupted breastfeeding applies to clients with contraindications to breastfeeding.

within one hour after ingestion of even moderate amounts (equivalent to a can of beer). It may alter the taste of the milk to the disapproval of the nursing infant, who may, in protest, drink less milk than normal.

Caffeine Caffeine can make an infant jittery and wakeful. As during pregnancy, caffeine consumption should be moderate.

Cigarette Smoke Health care professionals should actively discourage smoking by lactating women. Research shows that lactating women who smoke produce less milk, and milk with a lower fat content, than mothers who do not smoke. Consequently, their infants gain less weight than infants of nonsmokers. Furthermore, infants of breastfeeding mothers who smoke sleep less than infants of those who do not smoke.[90]

A lactating woman who smokes not only exposes her infant to nicotine and other chemicals via her breast milk but may also expose the infant to sidestream smoke. Infants who are "smoked over" experience a wide array of health problems—poor growth, hearing impairment, vomiting, breathing difficulties, and even unexplained death.

Medications and Illicit Drugs If a nursing mother must take medication that is secreted in breast milk and is known to affect the infant, then breastfeeding must be put off for the duration of treatment. Meanwhile, the flow of milk can be sustained by pumping the breasts and discarding the milk. Many prescription medications do not reach nursing infants in sufficient quantities to affect them adversely and so have no impact on breastfeeding. Other drugs are not at all compatible with breastfeeding, either because they are secreted into the milk and can harm the infant or because they suppress lactation. A nursing mother should consult with the prescribing physician before taking medicines. Breastfeeding is also contraindicated if the mother uses illicit drugs. Breast milk can deliver such high doses of illicit drugs as to cause irritability, tremors, hallucinations, and even death in infants.

Many women wonder about using oral contraceptives during lactation. One type that combines the hormones estrogen and progestin seems to suppress milk output, lower the nitrogen content of the milk, and shorten the duration of breastfeeding. In contrast, progestin-only pills have no effect on breast milk or breastfeeding and are considered appropriate for lactating women.

Maternal Illness If a woman has an ordinary cold, she can go on nursing without worry. If susceptible, the infant will catch it from her anyway, and, thanks to immunological protection, a breastfed baby may be less susceptible than a formula-fed infant would be. If a woman has active untreated tuberculosis or is receiving therapeutic radioactive isotopes, breastfeeding is contraindicated.[91]

The human immunodeficiency virus (HIV), responsible for causing AIDS, can be passed from an infected mother to her infant during pregnancy, at birth, or through breast milk, especially during the early months of breastfeeding. In developed countries such as the United States, where safe alternatives are available, HIV-positive women should not breastfeed their infants.[92]

Throughout the world, breastfeeding prevents millions of infant deaths each year. In developing countries, where the feeding of inappropriate or contaminated formulas causes 1.5 million infant deaths each year, breastfeeding can be critical to infant survival. Thus, the question of whether HIV-infected women in developing countries should breastfeed comes down to a delicate balance between risks and benefits. For HIV-positive women in developing countries, the most appropriate infant-feeding option depends on individual circumstances, including the health status of the mother and the local situation, as well as the health services, counseling, and support available. The World Health Organization (WHO) recommends exclusive breastfeeding for infants of HIV-infected women for the first six months of life unless replacement feeding is acceptable, feasible, affordable, sustainable, and safe for mothers and their infants before that time.[93]

Nutrition of the Infant

Early nutrition affects later development, and early feeding sets the stage for eating habits that will influence nutrition status for a lifetime. Trends change, and experts argue about the fine points, but properly nourishing an infant is relatively simple, overall. Initially, the infant drinks only breast milk or formula but later begins to eat some foods, as appropriate. Common sense in the selection of infant foods and a nurturing, relaxed environment go far to promote an infant's health and well-being. The remainder of this discussion is devoted to feeding the infant and identifying the nutrients most often deficient in infant diets.

NUTRIENT NEEDS DURING INFANCY

An infant grows faster during the first year than ever again, as Figure 10-9 shows. The growth of infants and children directly reflects their nutritional well-being and is an important parameter in assessing their nutrition status. Health care professionals use growth charts to evaluate the growth and development of children from birth to 20 years of age (see Appendix E).

Nutrients to Support Growth An infant's birthweight doubles by about five months of age and triples by the age of one year, typically reaching 20 to 25 pounds. (Consider that if an adult, starting at 120 pounds, were to do this, the person's weight would increase to 360 pounds in a single year.) The infant's length changes more slowly than weight, increasing about 10 inches from birth to one year. By the end of the first year, the growth rate slows considerably. An infant typically gains less than 10 pounds during the second year and grows about 5 inches in height.

Not only do infants grow rapidly, but, in proportion to body weight, their basal metabolic rate is remarkably high—about twice that of an adult. The rapid growth and metabolism of the infant demand an ample supply of all the nutrients. Of special importance during infancy are the energy nutrients and the vitamins and minerals critical to the growth process, such as vitamin A, vitamin D, and calcium.

Because they are small, infants need smaller *total* amounts of these nutrients than adults do, but as a percentage of body weight, infants need more than twice as much of most nutrients. Infants require about 100 kcalories per kilogram of body weight per day; most adults require fewer than 40 (see Table 10-6 on p. 296). Figure 10-10 (p. 296) compares a five-month-old infant's needs (per unit of body weight) with those of an adult man. You can see that differences in vitamin D and iodine, for instance, are extraordinary. Around six months of age, energy needs begin to increase less rapidly as the growth rate begins to slow, but some of the energy saved by slower growth is spent on increased activity. When their growth slows, infants spontaneously reduce their energy intakes. Parents should expect their infants to adjust their food intakes downward when appropriate and should not force or coax them to eat more.

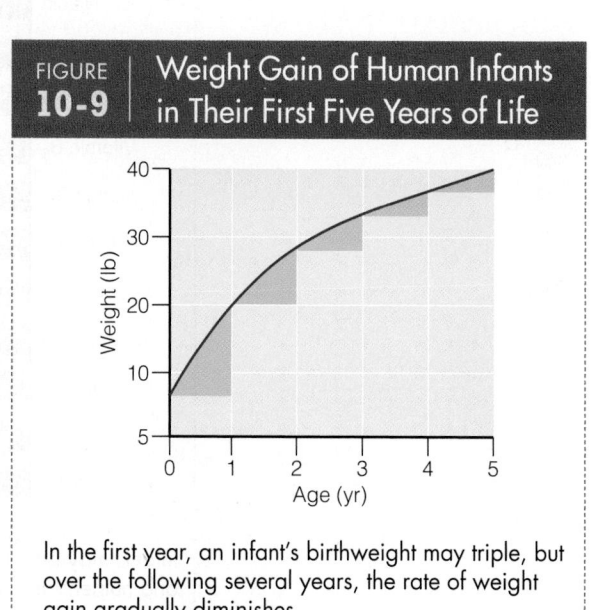

FIGURE 10-9 | Weight Gain of Human Infants in Their First Five Years of Life

In the first year, an infant's birthweight may triple, but over the following several years, the rate of weight gain gradually diminishes.

TABLE 10-6	Infant and Adult Heart Rate, Respiration Rate, and Energy Needs Compared		
		Infants	Adults
Heart rate (beats/minute)		120 to 140	70 to 80
Respiration rate (breaths/minute)		20 to 40	15 to 20
Energy needs (kcal/body weight)		45/lb (100/kg)	<18/lb (<40/kg)

Water One of the most important nutrients for infants, as for everyone, is water. The younger a child is, the more of the child's body weight is water. Breast milk or infant formula normally provides enough water to replace fluid losses in a healthy infant. If the environmental temperature is extremely high, however, infants need supplemental water.[94] Because proportionately more of an infant's body water than an adult's is between the cells and in the vascular space, this water is easy to lose. Consequently, conditions that cause rapid fluid loss, such as vomiting or diarrhea, require an electrolyte solution designed for infants.

FIGURE 10-10	Nutrient Recommendations for a Five-Month-Old Infant and an Adult Male Compared on the Basis of Body Weight

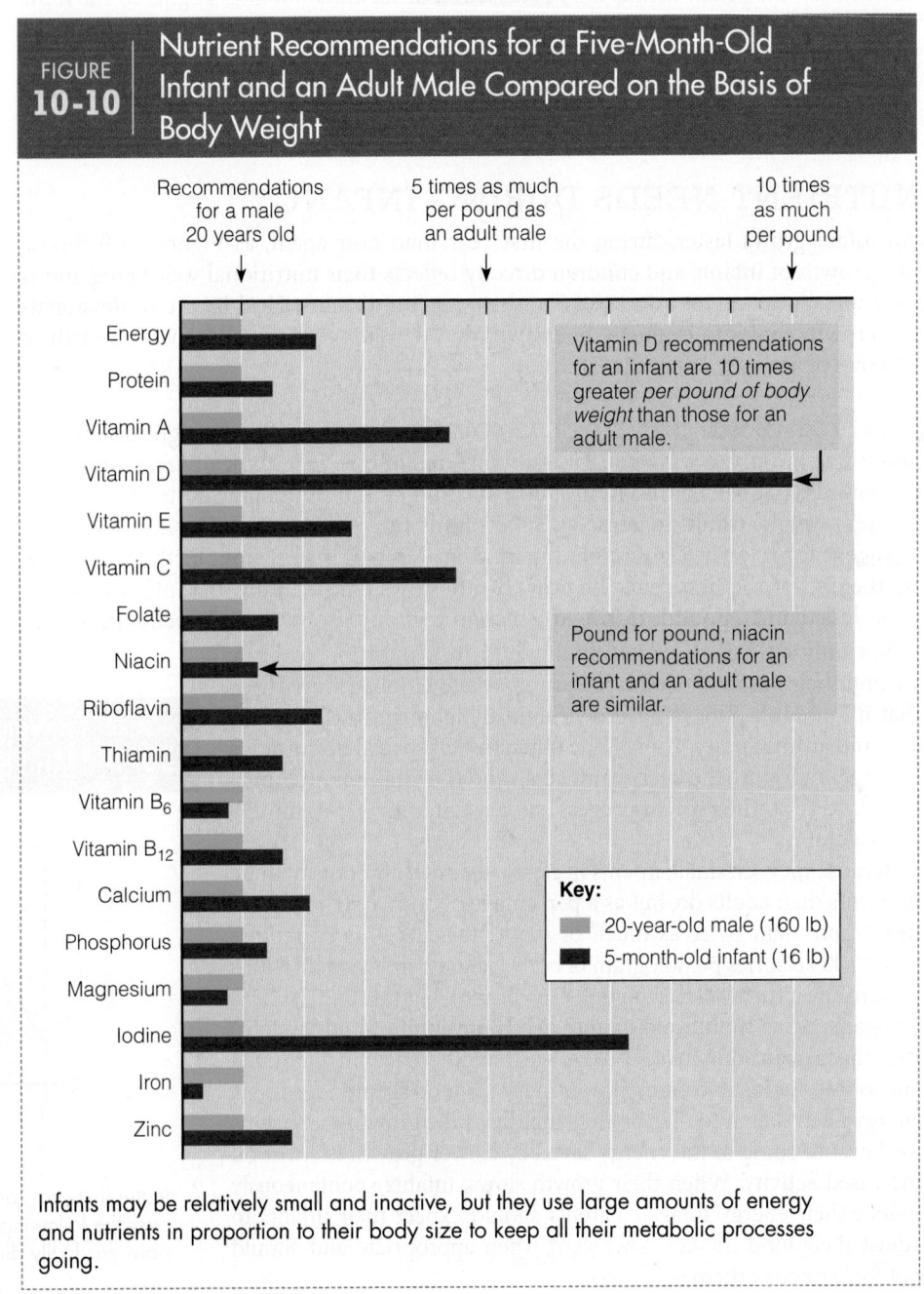

Infants may be relatively small and inactive, but they use large amounts of energy and nutrients in proportion to their body size to keep all their metabolic processes going.

BREAST MILK

Breast milk excels as a source of nutrients for the young infant. With the possible exception of vitamin D (discussed later), breast milk provides all the nutrients a healthy infant needs for the first six months of life.[95] It provides many other health benefits as well.

Frequency and Duration of Breastfeeding Breast milk is more easily and completely digested than formula, so breastfed infants usually need to eat more frequently than formula-fed infants do. During the first few weeks, approximately 8 to 12 feedings a day, on demand, as soon as the infant shows early signs of hunger such as increased alertness, activity, or suckling motions, promote optimal milk production and infant growth.[96] Crying is a late indicator of hunger. An infant who nurses every two to three hours and sleeps contentedly between feedings is adequately nourished. As the infant gets older, stomach capacity enlarges and the mother's milk production increases, allowing for longer intervals between feedings.

Even though the infant obtains about half the milk from the breast during the first two or three minutes of sucking, breastfeeding is encouraged for about 10 to 15 minutes on each breast. The infant's sucking, as well as the complete removal of milk from the breast, stimulates lactation.

Energy Nutrients The balance of energy nutrients in breast milk differs dramatically from the balance recommended for adults (see Figure 10-11). Yet, for infants, breast milk is nature's most nearly perfect food, providing the clear lesson that people at different stages of life have different nutrient needs.

The carbohydrate in breast milk (and standard infant formula) is lactose. In addition to being easily digested, lactose enhances calcium absorption. The carbohydrate component of breast milk also contains abundant oligosaccharides, which are present only in trace amounts in cow's milk and infant formula made from cow's milk.[97] Human milk oligosaccharides help protect the infant from infection by preventing the binding of pathogens to the infant's intestinal cells.[98]

After six months of age, energy saved by slower growth is spent on increased activity.

© Mark Scott/Taxi/Getty Images

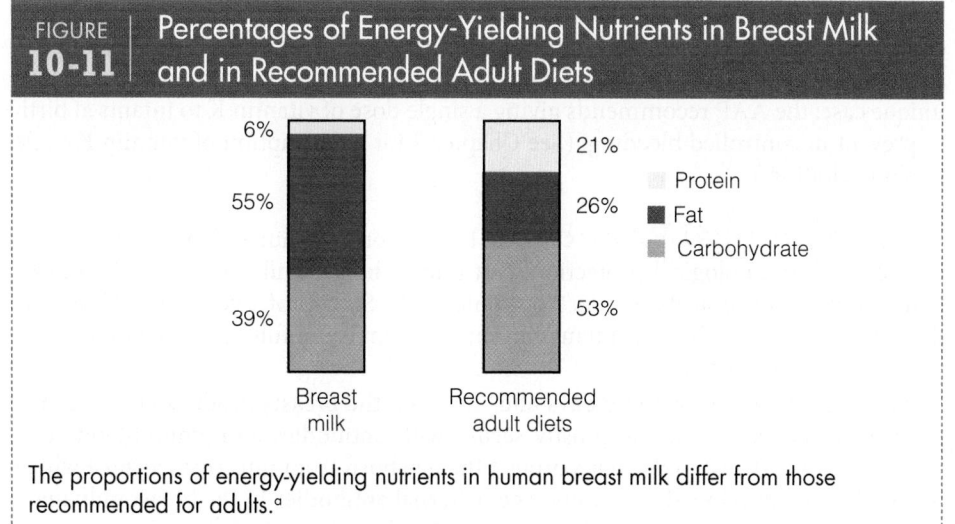

| FIGURE 10-11 | Percentages of Energy-Yielding Nutrients in Breast Milk and in Recommended Adult Diets |

Breast milk: 6% Protein, 55% Fat, 39% Carbohydrate
Recommended adult diets: 21% Protein, 26% Fat, 53% Carbohydrate

The proportions of energy-yielding nutrients in human breast milk differ from those recommended for adults.[a]

[a]The values listed for adults represent approximate midpoints of the acceptable ranges for protein (10 to 35 percent), fat (20 to 35 percent), and carbohydrate (45 to 65 percent).

NURSING DIAGNOSIS

Effective breastfeeding applies to clients with effective mother/infant communication patterns and an infant who is content after feeding.

The amount of protein in breast milk is less than in cow's milk, but this quantity is actually beneficial because it places less stress on the infant's immature kidneys to excrete the major end product of protein metabolism, urea. The protein in breast milk is largely **alpha-lactalbumin**, which is efficiently digested and absorbed.

The lipids in breast milk—and infant formula—provide the main source of energy in the infant's diet. Breast milk contains a generous proportion of the essential fatty acids linoleic acid and linolenic acid, as well as their longer-chain derivatives arachidonic acid and docosahexaenoic acid (DHA). Infant formula used to provide only linoleic and linolenic acid, but now arachidonic acid and DHA are also included. Infants can produce some arachidonic acid and DHA from linoleic and linolenic acid, respectively, but some infants may need more than they can make.

As Chapter 4 mentioned, DHA is the most abundant fatty acid in the brain and is also present in the retina of the eye. DHA accumulation in the brain is greatest during fetal development and early infancy.[99] Research has focused on the mental and visual development of breastfed infants and infants fed standard formula with and without DHA added.[100] One group of researchers found that infants fed formula fortified with DHA had sharper vision at four years of age than those who were fed standard formula.[101] Most studies, however, show no beneficial effect of DHA supplementation of formula for term infants.[102] Adding DHA to standard infant formulas has no adverse effects, however, and most standard formulas are currently fortified with both DHA and arachidonic acid.

Vitamins and Minerals

With the exception of vitamin D, the vitamin content of the breast milk of a well-nourished mother is ample. Even vitamin C, for which cow's milk is a poor source, is supplied generously. The concentration of vitamin D in breast milk is low, however, and vitamin D deficiency impairs bone mineralization. Vitamin D deficiency is most likely in infants who are not exposed to sunlight daily, have darkly pigmented skin, and receive breast milk without vitamin D supplementation.[103] Reports of infants in the United States developing the vitamin D–deficiency disease rickets and recommendations by the AAP to keep infants under six months of age out of direct sunlight have prompted revisions in vitamin D guidelines. The AAP currently recommends a vitamin D supplement for all infants who are breastfed exclusively and for any infants who do not receive at least one liter (1000 milliliters) or one quart (32 ounces) of vitamin D–fortified formula daily.[104]

As for minerals, the calcium content of breast milk is ideal for infant bone growth, and the calcium is well absorbed. Breast milk is also low in sodium. The limited amount of iron in breast milk is highly absorbable, and its zinc, too, is absorbed better than from cow's milk, thanks to the presence of a zinc-binding protein.

Supplements for Infants

Pediatricians may prescribe supplements containing vitamin D, iron, and fluoride (after six months of age). Table 10-7 offers a schedule of supplements during infancy. Vitamin K nutrition for newborns presents a unique case: the AAP recommends giving a single dose of vitamin K to infants at birth to prevent uncontrolled bleeding. (See Chapter 8 for a description of vitamin K's role in blood clotting.)

Immunological Protection

In addition to its nutritional benefits, breast milk offers immunological protection. Not only is breast milk sterile, but it actively fights disease and protects infants from illnesses.[105] Such protection is most valuable during the first year, when the infant's immune system is not fully prepared to mount a response against infections.

During the first two or three days after delivery, the breasts produce **colostrum**, a premilk substance containing mostly serum with antibodies and white blood cells. Colostrum (like breast milk) helps protect the newborn from infections against which the mother has developed immunity. The maternal antibodies in the breast milk inactivate disease-causing bacteria within the infant's digestive tract before they can start infections.[106] This explains, in part, why breastfed infants have fewer intestinal infections than formula-fed infants.

alpha-lactalbumin (lackt-AL-byoo-min): the chief protein in human breast milk, as **casein** (CAY-seen) is the chief protein in cow's milk.

colostrum (co-LAHS-trum): a milk-like secretion from the breasts that is rich in protective factors. Colostrum is present during the first day or so after delivery, before milk appears.

TABLE 10-7	Supplements for Full-Term Infants		
	Vitamin D[a]	Iron[b]	Fluoride[c]
Breastfed infants:			
Birth to six months of age	√		
Six months to one year	√	√	√
Formula-fed infants:			
Birth to six months of age			
Six months to one year		√	√

[a] Vitamin D supplements are recommended for all infants who are exclusively breastfed and for any infants who do not receive at least one liter (1000 milliliters) or one quart (32 ounces) of vitamin D–fortified formula per day.

[b] All infants six months of age need additional iron, preferably in the form of iron-fortified infant cereal and/or infant meats. Formula-fed infants need iron-fortified infant formula.

[c] At six months of age, breastfed infants and formula-fed infants who receive ready-to-use formulas (these are prepared with water low in fluoride) or formula mixed with water that contains little or no fluoride (less than 0.3 ppm) need supplements.

Source: Adapted from Committee on Nutrition, American Academy of Pediatrics, *Pediatric Nutrition Handbook,* 6th ed., ed. R. E. Kleinman (Elk Grove Village, IL: American Academy of Pediatrics, 2009).

In addition to antibodies, colostrum and breast milk provide other powerful agents (✚) that help to fight against bacterial infection. Among them are the oligosaccharides, described earlier, that prevent pathogens from binding to intestinal cells. Also present are **bifidus factors**, which favor the growth of the "friendly" bacterium *Lactobacillus bifidus* in the infant's digestive tract, so that other, harmful bacteria cannot become established. An iron-binding protein in breast milk, **lactoferrin**, keeps bacteria from getting the iron they need to grow, helps absorb iron into the infant's bloodstream, and kills some bacteria directly.[107] The protein **lactadherin** in breast milk binds to, and inhibits replication of, the virus that causes most infant diarrhea.[108] Breastfeeding also protects against other common illnesses of infancy such as middle ear infection and respiratory illness.[109] In addition, a growth factor that is present in breast milk stimulates the development and maintenance of the infant's digestive tract and its protective factors. Several breast milk enzymes such as lipase also help protect the infant against infection. Clearly, breast milk is a very special substance. Nutrition in Practice 10 offers suggestions for successful breastfeeding.

Allergy and Disease Protection In addition to protection against infection, breast milk may offer protection against the development of allergies.[110] Compared with formula-fed infants, breastfed infants have a lower incidence of allergic reactions, such as recurrent wheezing and skin rashes.[111] This protection is especially noticeable among infants with a family history of allergies.[112] Similarly, breast milk may offer protection against the development of cardiovascular disease. Compared with formula-fed infants, breastfed infants have lower blood pressure and lower blood cholesterol as adults.[113]

Other Potential Benefits Breastfeeding may offer some protection against excessive weight gain later, although findings are inconsistent.[114] One extensive review suggests that initial breastfeeding protects against obesity in later life.[115] Another

✚ Protective factors in breast milk:
- Antibodies
- Oligosaccharides
- Bifidus factors
- Lactoferrin
- Lactadherin
- Growth factor
- Lipase enzyme

bifidus (BIFF-id-us, by-FEED-us) factors: factors in colostrum and breast milk that favor the growth of the "friendly" bacterium *Lactobacillus* (lack-toe-ba-SILL-us) *bifidus* in the infant's intestinal tract. These bacteria prevent other, less desirable intestinal inhabitants from flourishing.

lactoferrin (lack-toe-FERR-in): protein in breast milk that binds iron and keeps it from supporting the growth of the infant's intestinal bacteria.

lactadherin (lack-tad-HAIR-in): a protein in breast milk that attacks diarrhea-causing viruses.

The infant thrives on infant formula offered with affection.

study confirms this finding and adds that the longer the duration of breastfeeding, the lower the risk of overweight in childhood.[116] Still another review reports that various studies have shown a protective effect, a protective effect only in certain groups, or no effect.[117] Researchers note that many other factors—socioeconomic status, other infant and child feeding practices, and especially the mother's weight—strongly predict a child's body weight.

Many studies suggest a beneficial effect of breastfeeding on intelligence, but when subjected to strict standards of methodology (for example, large sample size and appropriate intelligence testing), the evidence is less convincing.[118] Nevertheless, the possibility that breastfeeding may positively affect later intelligence is intriguing. It may be that some specific component of breast milk, such as DHA, stimulates brain development or that certain factors associated with the feeding process itself promote intellect.[119] Most likely, a combination of factors is involved. More large, well-controlled studies are needed to confirm the effects, if any, of breastfeeding on later intelligence.

The accompanying Case Study presents a woman who is four months pregnant. Answering the questions offers practice in thinking through some of the issues related to pregnancy and breastfeeding.

INFANT FORMULA

Breastfeeding offers many benefits to both mother and infant, and it should be encouraged whenever possible. The mother who has decided to use formula, however, should be supported in her choice just as the breastfeeding mother should be. She can offer the same closeness, warmth, and stimulation during feedings as the breastfeeding mother can.

Many mothers choose to breastfeed at first but **wean** their children within the first 1 to 12 months. If infants are less than a year of age, mothers must wean them onto *infant formula*, (✚) not onto plain cow's milk of any kind—whole, reduced fat, low fat, or fat free.

Infant Formula Composition
Manufacturers can prepare formulas from cow's milk in such a way that they do not differ significantly from human milk in nutrient content. Figure 10-12 illustrates the energy nutrient balance of breast milk, infant formula, and cow's milk. Notice the higher protein concentration of cow's milk, which stresses the infant's kidneys. The AAP recommends that all formula-fed infants receive iron-fortified infant formulas.[120] Low-iron formulas have no role in infant feeding. Use of iron-fortified formulas has risen in recent decades and is credited with the decline of iron-deficiency anemia in U.S. infants.

Infant Formula Standards
National and international standards have been set for the nutrient contents of infant formulas. U.S. standards are based on AAP recommendations, and the FDA mandates quality control procedures to ensure that

✚Formula preparation:
- Liquid concentrate (moderately expensive, relatively easy)—mix with equal part water.
- Powdered formula (least expensive, lightest for travel)—read label directions.
- Ready-to-feed (easiest, most expensive)—pour directly into clean bottles.

wean: to gradually replace breast milk with infant formula or other foods appropriate to an infant's diet.

CASE STUDY | Woman in Her First Pregnancy

Ellen Cassidy is a 24-year-old woman who is four months pregnant. This is her first pregnancy, and she is eager to learn how to feed herself during pregnancy as well as her infant after birth. She is 5 feet 3 inches tall and currently weighs 150 pounds. Her prepregnancy weight was 148 pounds. Ellen is very concerned about her 2-pound weight gain.

1. Consult the BMI table (inside back cover), and, using the "Healthy Weight" section, find a healthy weight in the middle of the range appropriate for a woman of Ellen's height.

2. Do you think that Ellen's weight at the start of her pregnancy was appropriate for her height? Why or why not? Should

Ellen be concerned about her 2-pound weight gain? Why or why not?

3. What advice should you give Ellen about her weight gain during pregnancy? What other dietary advice would you give her?

4. Discuss methods of infant feeding with Ellen and describe some of the advantages breastfeeding would offer her. What advice will you give Ellen if she decides to breastfeed?

5. What are the advantages of formula feeding? What information should Ellen have about formula feeding?

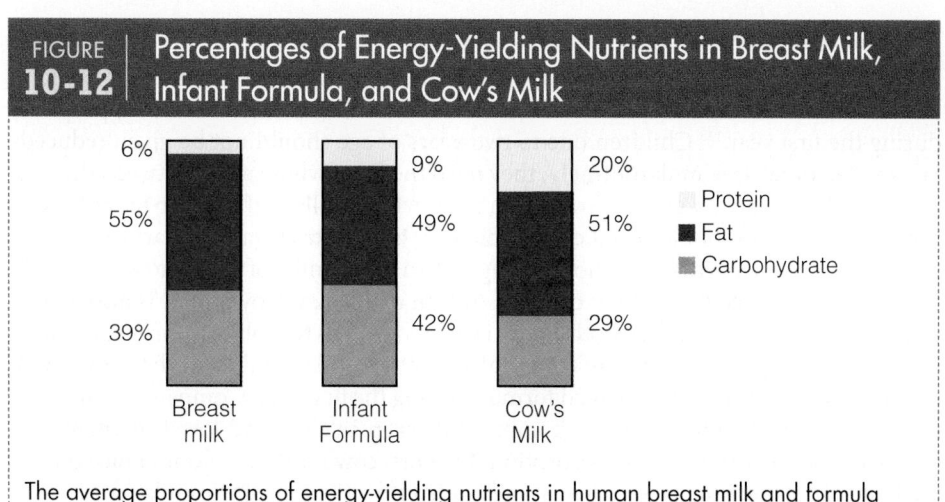

FIGURE 10-12 | Percentages of Energy-Yielding Nutrients in Breast Milk, Infant Formula, and Cow's Milk

Breast milk: 6% Protein, 55% Fat, 39% Carbohydrate

Infant Formula: 9% Protein, 49% Fat, 42% Carbohydrate

Cow's Milk: 20% Protein, 51% Fat, 29% Carbohydrate

- Protein
- Fat
- Carbohydrate

The average proportions of energy-yielding nutrients in human breast milk and formula differ slightly. In contrast, cow's milk provides too much protein and too little carbohydrate.

nursing bottle tooth decay: extensive tooth decay due to prolonged tooth contact with formula, milk, fruit juice, or other carbohydrate-rich liquid offered to an infant in a bottle.

these standards are met. All standard formulas are therefore nutritionally similar. Small differences in nutrient content are sometimes confusing but usually unimportant.

Special Formulas Standard cow's milk–based formulas are inappropriate for some infants. Special formulas have been designed to meet the dietary needs of infants with specific conditions such as prematurity or inherited diseases. Most infants allergic to milk protein can drink formulas based on soy protein.[121] Soy formulas also use cornstarch and sucrose instead of lactose and so are recommended for infants with lactose intolerance as well. They are also useful as an alternative to milk-based formulas for vegan families. Despite these limited uses, soy formulas account for one-fourth of the infant formulas sold today. While soy formulas support the normal growth and development of infants, for infants who don't need them, they offer no advantage over milk formulas.

Some infants who are allergic to cow's milk protein may also be allergic to soy protein.[122] For these infants, special formulas based on hydrolyzed protein are available.

Risks of Formula Feeding Infant formulas contain no protective antibodies for infants, but, in general, vaccinations, purified water, and clean environments in developed countries help protect infants from infections. Formulas can be prepared safely by following the rules of proper food handling and by using water that is free of contamination. Of particular concern is lead-contaminated water, a major source of lead poisoning in infants. Because the first water drawn from the tap each day is highest in lead, a person living in a house with old, lead-soldered plumbing should let the water run a few minutes before drinking or using it to prepare formula or food.

In developing countries and in poor areas of the United States, formula may be unavailable, over diluted in an attempt to save money, or prepared with contaminated water. Over dilution of formula can cause malnutrition and growth failure. Contaminated formula often causes infections leading to diarrhea, dehydration, and malabsorption. Wherever sanitation is poor, breastfeeding should take priority over feeding formula. Breast milk is sterile, and its antibodies enhance an infant's resistance to disease.

Nursing Bottle Tooth Decay Dentists advise against putting an infant to bed with a bottle. Salivary flow, which normally cleanses the mouth, diminishes as the infant falls asleep. Prolonged sucking on a bottle of formula, milk, or juice bathes the upper teeth in a carbohydrate-rich fluid that nourishes decay-producing bacteria. (The tongue covers and protects most of the lower teeth, but they, too, may be affected.) The result is extensive and rapid tooth decay. To prevent **nursing bottle tooth decay**, no child should be put to bed with a bottle as a pacifier.

Nursing bottle tooth decay, an extreme example. The upper teeth have decayed all the way to the gum line.

THE TRANSITION TO COW'S MILK

The age at which whole cow's milk should be introduced to the infant's diet has long been a source of controversy. The AAP advises that whole cow's milk is not appropriate during the first year.[123] Children one to two years of age should not be given reduced-fat, low-fat, or fat-free milk routinely; they need the fat of whole milk. Between the ages of two and five years, a gradual transition from whole milk to the lower-fat milks can take place, but care should be taken to avoid excessive restriction of dietary fat.

In some infants, particularly those younger than six months of age, whole cow's milk causes intestinal bleeding, which can lead to iron deficiency. Cow's milk is also a poor source of iron. Consequently, it both causes iron loss and fails to replace iron. Furthermore, the bioavailability of iron from infant cereal and other foods is reduced when cow's milk replaces breast milk or iron-fortified formula during the first year. Compared with breast milk or iron-fortified formula, cow's milk is higher in calcium and lower in vitamin C, characteristics that reduce iron absorption. In short, cow's milk is a poor choice during the first year of life; infants need breast milk or iron-fortified infant formula.

INTRODUCING FIRST FOODS

Changes in the body organs during the first year affect the infant's readiness to accept solid foods. Until the child is several months old, the immature stomach and intestines can digest milk sugar (lactose) but not starch. This is one of the many reasons why breast milk and formula are such good foods for an infant; they provide simple, easily digested carbohydrate that supplies energy for the infant's growth and activity.

When to Introduce Solid Food The AAP supports exclusive breastfeeding for approximately six months but recognizes that infants are often developmentally ready to accept complementary foods between four and six months of age.[124] The main purpose of introducing solid foods is to provide needed nutrients that are no longer supplied adequately by breast milk or formula alone. The foods chosen must be those that the infant is developmentally capable of handling both physically and metabolically. The exact timing depends on the individual infant's needs and developmental readiness (see Table 10-8), which vary from infant to infant because of differences in growth rates, activities, and environmental conditions. In short, the addition of foods to an infant's diet should be governed by three considerations: the infant's nutrient needs, the infant's physical readiness to handle different forms of foods, and the need to detect and control allergic reactions. With respect to nutrient needs, the nutrient needed earliest is iron and then vitamin C.

Foods to Provide Iron and Vitamin C Rapid growth demands iron. At about four to six months, the infant begins to need more iron than body stores plus breast milk or iron-fortified formula can provide. In addition to breast milk or iron-fortified formula, infants can receive iron from iron-fortified cereals and, once they readily accept solid foods, from meat or meat alternates such as legumes. Iron-fortified cereals contribute a significant amount of iron to an infant's diet, but the iron's bioavailability is poor.[125] Caregivers can enhance iron absorption from iron-fortified cereals by serving vitamin C–rich foods with meals.

The best sources of vitamin C are fruits and vegetables (see p. 223 in Chapter 8). It has been suggested that infants who are introduced to fruits before vegetables may develop a preference for sweets and find the vegetables less palatable, but there is no evidence to support offering these foods in a particular order.[126] Fruit juice is a source of vitamin C, but excessive juice intake can lead to diarrhea in infants and young children.[127] AAP recommendations limit juice consumption for infants and young children (one to six years of age) to between 4 and 6 ounces per day.[128] Too much fruit juice contributes excessive kcalories and displaces other nutrient-rich foods. Fruit juices should be diluted and served in a cup, not a bottle, once the infant is six months of age or older.

Foods such as iron-fortified cereals and formulas, mashed legumes, and strained meats provide iron.

© Polara Studios, Inc.

Physical Readiness for Solid Foods The ability to swallow solid food develops at around four to six months, and food offered by spoon helps to develop

TABLE
10-8 | Infant Development and Recommended Foods

Age (mo)	Feeding Skill	Foods Introduced into the Diet
0–4	Turns head toward any object that brushes cheek. Initially swallows using back of tongue; gradually begins to swallow using front of tongue as well. Strong reflex (extrusion) to push food out during first 2 to 3 months.	Feed breast milk or infant formula.
4–6	Extrusion reflex diminishes, and the ability to swallow nonliquid foods develops. Indicates desire for food by opening mouth and leaning forward. Indicates satiety or disinterest by turning away and leaning back. Sits erect with support at 6 months. Begins chewing action. Brings hand to mouth. Grasps objects with palm of hand.	Begin iron-fortified cereal mixed with breast milk, formula, or water. Begin pureed meats, legumes, vegetables, and fruits.
6–8	Able to self-feed finger foods. Develops pincher (finger to thumb) grasp. Begins to drink from cup.	Begin textured vegetables and fruits. Begin unsweetened, diluted fruit juices from cup.
8–10	Begins to hold own bottle. Reaches for and grabs food and spoon. Sits unsupported.	Begin breads and cereals from table. Begin yogurt. Begin pieces of soft, cooked vegetables and fruit from table. Gradually begin finely cut meats, fish, casseroles, cheese, eggs, and mashed legumes.
10–12	Begins to master spoon but still spills some.	Add variety. Gradually increase portion sizes.[a]

Note: Because each stage of development builds on the previous stage, the foods from an earlier stage continue to be included in all later stages.

[a] Portion sizes for infants and young children are smaller than those for an adult. For example, a grain serving might be ½ slice of bread instead of 1 slice, or ¼ cup rice instead of ½ cup.

Source: Adapted in part from Committee on Nutrition, American Academy of Pediatrics, *Pediatric Nutrition Handbook*, 6th ed., ed. R. E. Kleinman (Elk Grove Village, IL: American Academy of Pediatrics, 2009), pp. 113–142.

swallowing ability. At eight months to a year, an infant can sit up, can handle finger foods, and begins to teethe. At that time, hard crackers and other hard finger foods may be introduced to promote the development of manual dexterity and control of the jaw muscles. These feedings must occur under the watchful eye of an adult because the infant can also choke on such foods.

Some parents want to feed solids at an earlier age, on the theory that "stuffing the baby" at bedtime promotes sleeping through the night. There is no proof for this theory. On average, infants start to sleep through the night at about the same age (three to four months) regardless of when solid foods are introduced.

Allergy-Causing Foods To prevent allergy and to facilitate its prompt identification should it occur, experts recommend introducing single-ingredient foods, one at a time, in small portions, and waiting three to five days before introducing the next new food.[129] For example, rice cereal is usually the first cereal introduced because it is the least allergenic. When it is clear that rice cereal is not causing an allergy, another grain, perhaps barley or oats, is introduced. Wheat cereal is offered last because it is the most common offender. If a cereal causes an allergic reaction such as a skin rash, digestive upset, or respiratory discomfort, it should be discontinued before introducing the next food. Chapter 11 offers more information about food allergies.

Choice of Infant Foods Infant foods should be selected to provide variety, balance, and moderation. Commercial baby foods offer a wide variety of palatable, nutritious foods in a safe and convenient form. Homemade infant foods can be as nutritious as commercially prepared ones, as long as the cook minimizes nutrient losses during preparation. Ingredients for homemade foods should be fresh, whole foods without added salt, sugar, or seasonings. Pureed food can be frozen in ice cube trays, providing convenient-sized blocks of food that can be thawed, warmed, and fed to the infant. To guard against foodborne illnesses, hands and equipment must be kept clean.

Because recommendations to restrict fat do not apply to children under age two, labels on foods for children under two (such as infant meats and cereals) cannot carry information about fat. Fat information is omitted from infant food labels to prevent parents from restricting fat in infants' diets. Fearing that their infant will become overweight, parents may unintentionally malnourish the infant by limiting fat. In fact, infants and young children, because of their rapid growth, need more fat than older children and adults.

Foods to Omit Sweets of any kind (including baby food "desserts") have no place in an infant's diet. The added food energy conveys few, if any, nutrients to support growth and contributes to obesity. Canned vegetables are also inappropriate for infants; they often contain too much sodium. Honey and corn syrup should never be fed to infants because of the risk of botulism. Infants and young children are vulnerable to foodborne illnesses. An infant's caregiver must be on guard against food poisoning and take precautions against it as described in Nutrition in Practice 2.

Infants and even young children cannot safely chew and swallow any of the foods listed in the margin; (+) they can easily choke on these foods, a risk not worth taking. Nonfood items of small size should always be kept out of the infant's reach to prevent choking.

Foods at One Year Whole milk is the best food to supply most of the nutrients the infant needs at one year of age; 2 to 3 cups a day meet those needs sufficiently. More milk than this displaces iron-rich foods and can lead to the iron-deficiency anemia known as milk anemia. (+) Other foods—meat and meat alternates, iron-fortified cereals, whole-grain or enriched bread, fruits, and vegetables—should be supplied in variety and in amounts sufficient to round out total energy needs. Ideally, a one-year-old will sit at the table, eat many of the same foods everyone else eats, and drink liquids from a cup—not a bottle. Table 10-9 shows a sample menu that meets a one-year-old's requirements.

LOOKING AHEAD

Probably the most important single measure to undertake during the first year is to encourage eating habits that will support continued normal weight as the child grows. This means introducing a variety of nutritious foods in an inviting way, not forcing the infant to finish the bottle or the baby food jar, avoiding concentrated sweets and empty-kcalorie foods, and encouraging physical activity. Parents should avoid teaching infants to seek food as a reward, to expect food as comfort for unhappiness, or to associate food deprivation with punishment. Normal dental development is also promoted by supplying nutritious foods, avoiding sweets, and discouraging the association of food with reward or comfort. Oral health is the subject of Nutrition in Practice 17.

MEALTIMES

The nurturing of a young child involves more than nutrition. Those who care for young children are responsible for providing not only nutritious foods, milk, and water but also a safe, loving, secure environment in which the children may grow and develop.

Ideally, a one-year-old eats many of the same healthy foods as the rest of the family.

Jose Luis Pelaez, Inc/Jupiter Images

TABLE 10-9	Sample Meal Plan for a One-Year-Old
	Sample Menu
Breakfast	1 scrambled egg 1 slice whole-wheat toast ½ c whole milk
Morning Snack	½ c yogurt ¼ c fruit[a]
Lunch	½ grilled cheese sandwich: 1 slice whole-wheat bread with 1 slice cheese ½ c vegetables[b] (steamed carrots) ¼ c 100% fruit juice
Afternoon snack	½ c fruit[a] ½ c toasted oat cereal
Dinner	1 oz chopped meat or ¼ c well-cooked mashed legumes ½ c rice or pasta ½ c vegetables[b] (chopped broccoli) ½ c whole milk

Note: This sample menu provides about 1000 kcalories.

[a] Include citrus fruits, melons, and berries.

[b] Include dark green, leafy, and deep yellow vegetables.

The person feeding a one-year-old should be aware that exploring and experimenting are normal and desirable behaviors at this time in a child's life. The child is developing a sense of autonomy that, if allowed to develop, will lay the foundation for later confidence and effectiveness as an individual. In light of the developmental and nutrient needs of one-year-olds, and in the face of their often contrary and willful behavior, a few feeding guidelines may be helpful:

- *Discourage unacceptable behavior (such as standing at the table or throwing food) by removing the child from the table to wait until later to eat.* Be consistent and firm, not punitive. For example, instead of saying "You make me mad when you don't sit down," say "The fruit salad tastes good—please sit down and eat some with me." The child will soon learn to sit and eat.
- *Let young children explore and enjoy food.* This may mean eating with fingers for a while. Learning to use a spoon will come in time. Children who are allowed to touch, mash, and smell their food while exploring it are more likely to accept it.
- *Don't force food on children.* Rejecting new foods is normal, and acceptance is more likely as children become familiar with new foods through repeated opportunities to taste them. Instead of saying "You cannot go outside to play until you taste your carrots," say "You can try the carrots again another time."
- *Provide nutritious foods, and let children choose which ones, and how much, they will eat.* Gradually, they will acquire a taste for different foods.
- *Limit sweets.* Infants and young children have little room for empty-kcalorie foods in their daily energy allowance. Do not use sweets as a reward for eating meals.

These recommendations reflect a spirit of tolerance that serves the best interests of the child emotionally as well as physically. The Nutrition Assessment Checklist helps to identify nutrition-related factors that may help prevent or correct potential problems in pregnant women and infants. Details of nutrition assessment are presented in Chapter 13.

Nutrition Assessment | CHECKLIST FOR PREGNANT WOMEN AND INFANTS

MEDICAL HISTORY

Check the medical record for:

- ○ Alcohol or illicit drug abuse
- ○ Chronic diseases
- ○ Gestational diabetes
- ○ History of previous pregnancies (number, intervals, outcomes, multiple births, and gestational age/birthweights)
- ○ Hypertension
- ○ Neural tube defect in an infant born previously
- ○ Preeclampsia

Note risk factors for complications during pregnancy, including:

- ○ Cigarette smoking
- ○ Food faddism
- ○ Lactose intolerance
- ○ Low socioeconomic status
- ○ Significant or prolonged vomiting
- ○ Very young or old age
- ○ Weight-loss dieting

Note any complaints of:

- ○ Constipation
- ○ Heartburn
- ○ Morning sickness

MEDICATIONS

For pregnant women who are using drug therapy for medical conditions, note:

- ○ Potential for contraindication to breastfeeding
- ○ GI tract side effects that might reduce food intake or change nutrient needs

DIETARY INTAKE

For all pregnant women, especially those considered at risk nutritionally, assess the diet for:

- ○ Total energy
- ○ Protein
- ○ Calcium, phosphorus, magnesium, iron, and zinc

- ○ Folate and vitamin B_{12}
- ○ Vitamin D

For infants, note:

- ○ Method of feeding (breastfeeding, formula, or both)
- ○ Frequency and duration of breastfeeding
- ○ Amount of infant formula
- ○ Practice of putting infant to bed with bottle
- ○ Solid foods the infant is fed, if any
- ○ Amount of food the infant is fed

ANTHROPOMETRIC DATA

Measure baseline height and weight:

- ○ Prepregnancy weight
- ○ Infant birthweight

Reassess weight at each medical checkup and determine whether gains are appropriate. Note:

- ○ Weight gain during pregnancy
- ○ Gestational age
- ○ Weight, length, and head circumference of infants

LABORATORY TESTS

Monitor the following laboratory tests for pregnant women:

- ○ Hemoglobin, hematocrit, or other tests of iron status
- ○ Blood glucose

Monitor the following laboratory tests for infants:

- ○ Blood glucose of infants born to mothers with gestational diabetes
- ○ Results of tests for inborn errors

PHYSICAL SIGNS

Blood pressure measurement is a routine measurement in physical exams but is especially important for pregnant women.

Look for physical signs of:

- ○ Iron deficiency
- ○ Edema
- ○ Protein-energy malnutrition
- ○ Folate deficiency

Self Check

1. The most important single predictor of an infant's future health and survival is:
   a. the infant's birthweight.
   b. the infant's iron status at birth.
   c. the mother's weight at delivery.
   d. the mother's prepregnancy weight.

2. A mother's prepregnancy nutrition is important to a healthy pregnancy because it determines the development of:
   a. the largest baby possible.
   b. adequate maternal iron stores.
   c. an adequate fat supply for the mother.
   d. healthy support tissues—the placenta, amniotic sac, umbilical cord, and uterus.

3. A pregnant woman needs an extra 450 calories above the allowance for nonpregnant women during which trimester(s)?
   a. First
   b. Second
   c. Third
   d. First, second, and third

4. Two nutrients needed in large amounts during pregnancy for rapid cell proliferation are:
   a. vitamin B_{12} and vitamin C.
   b. calcium and vitamin B_6.
   c. folate and vitamin B_{12}.
   d. copper and zinc.

5. For a woman who is at the appropriate weight for height and is carrying a single fetus, the recommended weight gain during pregnancy is:
   a. 40 to 60 pounds.
   b. 25 to 35 pounds.
   c. 10 to 20 pounds.
   d. 20 to 40 pounds.

6. Rewards of physical activity during pregnancy may include:
   a. weight loss.
   b. decreased incidence of pica.
   c. relief from morning sickness.
   d. reduced stress and easier labor.

7. Breast milk is recommended for the first 12 months of life because it offers complete nutrition and ___ to the infant.
   a. fluoride
   b. fructose
   c. immunological protection
   d. pica

8. An acceptable substitute for breast milk during the first year is:
   a. low-fat cow's milk.
   b. apple juice.
   c. water.
   d. iron-fortified infant formula.

9. The addition of solid foods to an infant's diet should be governed by all of the following considerations *except*:
   a. the infant's nutrient needs.
   b. the need to detect and control allergies.
   c. the infant's physical readiness to handle different forms of foods.
   d. the infant's inability to sleep through the night.

10. During the first year of life, the most important step to undertake to encourage healthy eating is to:
    a. give food as a reward or for comfort.
    b. give sweets as a reward for eating vegetables.
    c. introduce a variety of nutritious foods in an inviting way.
    d. restrict fat to less than 30 percent of energy intake.

Answers to these questions can be found in Appendix H.

Clinical Applications

1. Consider the different factors in a pregnant woman's history that can affect her nutrition status and the outcome of her pregnancy. Describe what steps you would take to remedy potential problems for the following clients:
   a. A 15-year-old adolescent of low socioeconomic status is in her first trimester of pregnancy. She began the pregnancy at a normal, healthy weight, but her weight gain during pregnancy so far has been less than expected. Her favorite beverages are soft drinks; her favorite foods are French fries and boxed macaroni and cheese.
   b. A lactose-intolerant, 22-year-old pregnant woman has been eating a vegan diet for the past year or so. She began the pregnancy slightly underweight (BMI = 18.4), but her weight gain has been adequate and consistent during the four months of her pregnancy. She complains of feeling tired all the time.

2 • What information would you give to a pregnant woman who is considering breastfeeding her infant but isn't quite sure why she should?

3 • The parents of a two-month-old infant have been told by the child's grandparents that they should introduce solid foods to help the baby sleep through the night. What advice would you give the parents?

Nutrition on the Net

For further study of the topics in this chapter, access these websites.

- Find updates and quick links to these and other nutrition-related sites at our website: www.cengage.com/nutrition/whitney/nhhc4e
- Visit the pregnancy and child health center of the Mayo Clinic: www.mayohealth.org
- Learn more about having a healthy infant and about birth defects from the March of Dimes: www.modimes.org
- Learn more about neural tube defects from the Spina Bifida Association of America: www.sbaa.org
- Search for "birth defects," "pregnancy," "adolescent pregnancy," "maternal and infant health," and "breastfeeding" at the U.S. government health information site: www.healthfinder.gov

- Search for "pregnancy" at the American Dietetic Association site: www.eatright.org
- Learn more about the WIC program: www.fns.usda.gov/wic/
- Visit the American College of Obstetricians and Gynecologists: www.acog.org
- Learn more about gestational diabetes from the American Diabetes Association: www.diabetes.org
- Learn more about breastfeeding from La Leche League International: www.llli.org/
- Read *A Woman's Guide to Breastfeeding* at the American Academy of Pediatrics site: www.aap.org

Notes

1. Recommendations to improve preconception health and health care—United States, *Morbidity and Mortality Weekly Report* 55 (2006): 1–23.
2. M. Viswanathan and coauthors, Outcomes of maternal weight gain, *Evidence Report/Technology Assessment* 168 (2008): 1–223; R. L. Goldenberg and J. F. Culhane, Low birthweight in the United States, *American Journal of Clinical Nutrition* 85 (2007): 584S–590S.
3. C. Bouchard, Childhood obesity: Are genetic differences involved? *American Journal of Clinical Nutrition* 89 (2009): 1494S–1501S; M. E. Symonds, M. Stephenson, and H. Budge, Early determinants of cardiovascular disease: The role of early diet in later blood pressure control, *American Journal of Clinical Nutrition* 89 (2009): 1518S–1522S; P. D. Gluckman and coauthors, Effect of in utero and early-life conditions on adult health and disease, *New England Journal of Medicine* 359 (2008): 61–73; M. R. Skilton, Intrauterine risk factors for precocious atherosclerosis, *Pediatrics* 121 (2008): 570–574; R. A. Waterland and K. B. Michels, Epigenetic epidemiology of the Developmental Origins Hypothesis, *Annual Review of Nutrition* 27 (2007): 363–388; L. Adair and D. Dahly, Developmental determinants of blood pressure in adults, *Annual Review of Nutrition* 25 (2005): 407–434.
4. D. S. Alam, Prevention of low birthweight, *Nestle Nutrition Workshop Series: Pediatric Program* 63 (2009): 209–225; E. M. Lundgren and T. Tuvemo, Effects of being born small for gestational age on long-term intellectual performance, *Best Practice and Research: Clinical Endocrinology and Metabolism* 22 (2008): 477–488; S. Tong, P. Baghurst, and A. McMichael, Birthweight and cognitive development during childhood, *Journal of Paediatrics and Child Health* 42 (2006): 98–103.
5. J. A. Martin and coauthors, Annual summary of vital statistics: 2006, *Pediatrics* 121 (2008): 788–801.
6. L. M. McCowan and coauthors, Spontaneous preterm birth and small for gestational age infants in women who stop smoking early in pregnancy: Prospective cohort study, *British Medical Journal* 338 (2009): b1081.
7. Position of the American Dietetic Association: Nutrition and lifestyle for a healthy pregnancy outcome, *Journal of the American Dietetic Association* 108 (2008): 553–561; T. O. Scholl, Maternal nutrition before and during pregnancy, *Nestle Nutrition Workshop Series; Pediatrics Program* 61 (2008): 79–89; A. N. Kanade and coauthors, Maternal nutrition and birth size among urban affluent and rural women in India, *Journal of the American College of Nutrition* 27 (2008): 137–145.

8. D. K. Waller and coauthors, Prepregnancy obesity as a risk factor for structural birth defects, *Archives of Pediatrics and Adolescent Medicine* 161 (2007): 745–750.
9. Position of the American Dietetic Association and American Society for Nutrition: Obesity, reproduction, and pregnancy outcomes, *Journal of the American Dietetic Association* 109 (2009): 918–927; J. C. King, Maternal obesity, metabolism, and pregnancy outcomes, *Annual Review of Nutrition* 26 (2006): 271–291.
10. Position of the American Dietetic Association: Nutrition and lifestyle for a healthy pregnancy outcome, *Journal of the American Dietetic Association* 108 (2008): 553–561; E. A. Nohr and coauthors, Combined associations of prepregnancy body mass index and gestational weight gain with the outcome of pregnancy, *American Journal of Clinical Nutrition* 87 (2008): 1750–1759; S. Y. Chu and coauthors, Association between obesity during pregnancy and increased use of health care, *New England Journal of Medicine* 358 (2008): 1444–1453; J. C. King, Maternal obesity, metabolism, and pregnancy outcomes, *Annual Review of Nutrition* 26 (2006): 271–291.
11. K. J. Stothard and coauthors, Maternal overweight and obesity and the risk of congenital anomalies: A systematic review and meta-analysis, *Journal of the American Medical Association* 301 (2009): 636–650; D. K. Waller and coauthors, Prepregnancy obesity as a risk factor for structural birth defects, *Archives of Pediatrics and Adolescent Medicine* 161 (2007): 745–750.
12. V. E. Murphy and coauthors, Endocrine regulation of human fetal growth: The role of the mother, placenta, and fetus, *Endocrine Reviews* 27 (2006): 141–169.
13. J. C. Cross and L. Mickelson, Nutritional influences on implantation and placental development, *Nutrition Reviews* 64 (2006): S12–S18.
14. Position of the American Dietetic Association, 2008.
15. S. H. Zeisel, Epigenetic mechanisms for nutrition determinants of later health outcomes, *American Journal of Clinical Nutrition* 89 (2009): 1488S–1493S; P. D. Gluckman and coauthors, Effect of in utero and early-life conditions on adult health and disease, *New England Journal of Medicine* 359 (2008): 61–73.
16. Standing Committee on the Scientific Evaluation of Dietary Reference Intakes, Food and Nutrition Board, Institute of Medicine, *Dietary Reference Intakes for Energy, Carbohydrate, Fiber, Fat, Fatty Acids, Cholesterol, Protein, and Amino Acids* (Washington, D.C.: National Academies Press, 2005), pp. 185–194.

17. S. M. Innis and R. W. Freisen, Essential n-3 fatty acids in pregnant women and early visual acuity maturation in term infants, *American Journal of Clinical Nutrition* 87 (2008): 548–557; M. von Eijsden and coauthors, Maternal n-3, n-6 and *trans* fatty acid profile early in pregnancy and term birth weight: A prospective cohort study, *American Journal of Clinical Nutrition* 87 (2008): 887–895; E. Oken and coauthors, Associations of maternal fish intake during pregnancy and breastfeeding duration with attainment of developmental milestones in early childhood: A study from the Danish National Birth Cohort, *American Journal of Clinical Nutrition* 88 (2008): 789–796; S. M. Innis, Dietary (n-3) fatty acids and brain development, *Journal of Nutrition* 137 (2007): 855–859; W. C. Heird and A. Lapillonne, The role of essential fatty acids in development, *Annual Review of Nutrition* 25 (2005): 549–571.

18. R. M. Pitkin, Folate and neural tube defects, *American Journal of Clinical Nutrition* 85 (2007): 285S–288S.

19. U.S. Preventive Services Task Force, Folic acid for the prevention of neural tube defects: U.S. Preventive Services Task Force recommendation statement, *Annals of Internal Medicine* 150 (2009): 626–631.

20. P. De Wals and coauthors, Reduction in neural-tube defects after folic acid fortification in Canada, *New England Journal of Medicine* 357 (2007): 135–142; J. I. Rader and B. O. Schneeman, Prevalence of neural tube defects, folate status, and folate fortification of enriched cereal-grain products in the United States, *Pediatrics* 117 (2006): 1394–1399; T. G. Bentley and coauthors, Population-level changes in folate intake by age, gender, and race/ethnicity after folic acid fortification, *American Journal of Public Health* 96 (2006): 2040–2047; M. Eichholzer, O. Tonz, and R. Zimmermann, Folic acid: A public health challenge, *Lancet* 367 (2006): 1352–1361.

21. A. J. Wilcox and coauthors, Folic acid supplements and risk of facial clefts: National population based case-control study, *British Medical Journal* 334 (2007): 464; L. B. Bailey and R. J. Berry, Folic acid supplementation and the occurrence of congenital heart defects, orofacial clefts, multiple births, and miscarriage, *American Journal of Clinical Nutrition* 81 (2005): 1213S–1217S.

22. I. Elmadfa and I. Singer, Vitamin B_{12} and homocysteine status among vegetarians: A global perspective, *American Journal of Clinical Nutrition* 89 (2009): 1693S–1698S.

23. A. M. Molloy and coauthors, Maternal vitamin B_{12} status and risk of neural tube defects in a population with high neural tube defect prevalence and no folic acid fortification, *Pediatrics* 123 (2009): 917–923.

24. C. L. Wagner and F. R. Greer, and the Section on Breastfeeding and Committee on Nutrition, Prevention of rickets and vitamin D deficiency in infants, children, and adolescents, *Pediatrics* 122 (2008): 1142–1152; C. S. Kovacs, Vitamin D in pregnancy and lactation: Maternal, fetal, and neonatal outcomes from human and animal studies, *American Journal of Clinical Nutrition* 88 (2008): 520S–528S.

25. L. M. Bodnar and coauthors, High prevalence of vitamin D insufficiency in black and white pregnant women residing in the northern United States and their neonates, *Journal of Nutrition* 137 (2007): 447–452.

26. K. O'Brien, Maternal and fetal mineral partitioning: Whose needs predominate? *Nutrition Today* 40 (2005): 130–137.

27. S. Mahajan and coauthors, Nutritional anaemia dysregulates endocrine control of fetal growth, *British Journal of Nutrition* 100 (2008): 408–417; F. M. Rioux and C. P. LeBlanc, Iron supplementation during pregnancy: What are the risks and benefits of current practices? *Applied Physiology, Nutrition and Metabolism* 32 (2007): 282–288; T. O. Scholl, Iron status during pregnancy: Setting the stage for mother and infant, *American Journal of Clinical Nutrition* 81 (2005): 1218S–1222S.

28. C. M. Donangelo and coauthors, Zinc absorption and kinetics during pregnancy and lactation in Brazilian women, *American Journal of Clinical Nutrition* 82 (2005): 118–124.

29. D. Shah and H. P. S. Sachdev, Zinc deficiency in pregnancy and fetal outcome, *Nutrition Reviews* 64 (2006):15–30.

30. Position of the American Dietetic Association, 2008.

31. WIC, The Special Supplemental Nutrition Program for Women, Infants, and Children, available at www.fns.usda.gov/fns. Updated April 2009.

32. A. Jacknowitz, D. Novillo, and L. Tiehen, Special supplemental Nutrition Program for Women, Infants, and Children and infant feeding practices, *Pediatrics* 119 (2007): 281–288.

33. Position of the American Dietetic Association and American Society for Nutrition: Obesity, reproduction, and pregnancy outcomes, *Journal of the American Dietetic Association* 109 (2009): 918–927; S. Y. Chu and coauthors, Gestational weight gain by body mass index among U.S. women delivering live births, 2004-2005: Fueling future obesity, *American Journal of Obstetrics and Gynecology* 200 (2009): 271, e1–e7; C. M. Olson, Achieving a healthy weight gain during pregnancy, *Annual Review of Nutrition* 28 (2008): 411–423.

34. Position of the American Dietetic Association and American Society for Nutrition, 2009; E. Oken and coauthors, Gestational weight gain and child adiposity at age 3 years, *American Journal of Obstetrics and Gynecology* 196 (2007): 322, e1–e8.

35. Position of the American Dietetic Association and American Society for Nutrition, 2009.

36. Institute of Medicine, *Weight Gain during Pregnancy: Reexamining the Guidelines* (Washington, D.C.: The National Academies Press, 2009).

37. J. H. Cohen and H. Kim, Sociodemographic and health characteristics associated with attempting weight loss during pregnancy, *Preventing Chronic Disease* 6 (2009): A07.

38. National Research Council, Institute of Medicine, *Influence of Pregnancy Weight on Maternal and Child Health* (Washington, D.C.: National Academies Press, 2007).

39. Position of the American Dietetic Association and American Society for Nutrition, 2009; M. Viswanathan and coauthors, Outcomes of maternal weight gain, *Evidence Report/Technology Assessment* 168 (2008): 1–223; J. L. Baker and coauthors, Breastfeeding reduces postpartum weight retention, *American Journal of Clinical Nutrition* 88 (2008): 1543–1551; N. F. Butte and coauthors, Composition of gestational weight gain impacts maternal fat retention and infant birth weight, *American Journal of Obstetrics and Gynecology* 189 (2003): 1423–1432.

40. D. A. Krummel, Postpartum weight control: A vicious cycle, *Journal of the American Dietetic Association* 107 (2007): 37–40; E. Villamor and S. Cnattingius, Interpregnancy weight change and risk of adverse pregnancy outcomes: A population-based study, *Lancet* 368 (2006): 1164–1170.

41. A. R. Amorium and coauthors, Does excess pregnancy weight gain constitute a major risk for increasing long-term BMI? *Obesity* 15 (2007): 1278–1286.

42. Position of the American Dietetic Association, 2008; R. Artal and M. O'Toole, Guidelines of the American College of Obstetricians and Gynecologists for exercise during pregnancy and the postpartum period, *British Journal of Sports Medicine* 37 (2003): 6–12; American College of Obstetricians and Gynecologists, Exercise during pregnancy and postpartum period, ACOG Committee Opinion no. 267, *Obstetrics and Gynecology* 99 (2002): 171–173.

43. A. B. Granath, M. S. Hellgren, and R. K. Gunnarsson, Water aerobics reduces sick leave due to low back pain during pregnancy, *Journal of Obstetrics, Gynecology, and Neonatal Nursing* 35 (2006): 465-471; S. A. Smith and Y. Michel, A pilot study on the effects of aquatic exercises on discomforts of pregnancy, *Journal of Obstetrics, Gynecology, and Neonatal Nursing* 35 (2006): 315–323.

44. M. E. Mills, Craving more than food: The implications of pica in pregnancy, *Nursing for Women's Health* 11 (2007): 266–273.

45. M. E. Mills, 2007.

46. J. L. Kitzmiller and coauthors, Managing preexisting diabetes for pregnancy: Summary of evidence and consensus recommendations for care, *Diabetes Care* 31 (2008): 1060–1079.

47. J. L. Kitzmiller and coauthors, 2008.

48. The HAPO Study Cooperative Research Group, Hyperglycemia and adverse pregnancy outcomes, *New England Journal of Medicine* 358 (2008): 1991–2002; V. Seshiah and coauthors, "Abnormal" fasting plasma glucose during pregnancy, *Diabetes Care* 31 (2008): e92.

49. J. L. Kitzmiller and coauthors, 2008.

50. Position statement, Standards of medical care in diabetes—2008, *Diabetes Care* 31 (2008): S12-S54; R. J. Kaaja and I. A. Greer, Manifestations of chronic disease during pregnancy, *Journal of the American Medical Association* 294 (2005): 2751–2757; Position statement from the American Diabetes Association: Gestational diabetes mellitus, *Diabetes Care* 26 (2003): S103–S105.

51. C. Mulholland and coauthors, Comparison of guidelines available in the United States for diagnosis and management of diabetes before, during, and after pregnancy, *Journal of Women's Health* 16 (2007): 790–801.

52. The HAPO study Cooperative Research Group, 2008.

53. American Diabetes Association, Diagnosis and classification of diabetes mellitus, *Diabetes Care* 31 (2008): S55–S60.

54. P. E. Marik, Hypertensive disorders of pregnancy, *Postgraduate Medicine* 121 (2009): 69–76.

55. B. M. Sibai, Caring for women with hypertension, *Journal of the American Medical Association* 298 (2007): 1566–1568.

56. Position of the American Dietetic Association, 2008.

57. Position of the American Dietetic Association, 2008.

58. V. T. Tong and coauthors, Trends in smoking before, during, and after pregnancy—Pregnancy Risk Assessment Monitoring System (PRAMS), United States, 31 sites, 2000–2005, *Morbidity and Mortality Weekly Report* 58 (2009): SS-4, pp. 1-31; J. A. Martin and coauthors, Annual summary of vital statistics: 2008, *Pediatrics* 121 (2008): 788–801.

59. J. M. Rogers, Tobacco and pregnancy: Overview of exposures and effects, *Birth Defects Research* (Part C) 84 (2008): 1–15.

60. R. A. de la Chica and coauthors, Chromosomal instability in amniocytes from fetuses of mothers who smoke, *Journal of the American Medical Association* 293 (2005): 1212–1222.

61. M. J. Rivkin and coauthors, Volumetric MRI study of brain in children with intrauterine exposure to cocaine, alcohol, tobacco, and marijuana, *Pediatrics* 121 (2008): 741–750.

62. J. M. Rogers, Tobacco and pregnancy: Overview of exposures and effects, *Birth Defects Research* (Part C) 84 (2008): 1–15.

63. J. M. Rogers, 2008; American Academy of Pediatrics, Task Force on Sudden Infant Death Syndrome, The changing concept of sudden infant death syndrome: Diagnostic coding shifts, controversies regarding the sleeping environment, and new variables to consider in reducing risk, *Pediatrics* 116 (2005): 1245–1255.

64. J. M. Rogers, 2008.

65. Position of the American Dietetic Association, 2008.

66. M. J. Rivkin and coauthors, 2008; H. S. Bada and coauthors, Impact of prenatal cocaine exposure on child behavior problems through school age, *Pediatrics* 119 (2007): e348; B. A. Lewis and coauthors, Prenatal cocaine and tobacco effects on children's language trajectories, *Pediatrics* 120 (2007): e78.

67. G. A. Richardson, L. Goldschmidt, and C. Larkby, Effects of prenatal cocaine exposure on growth: A longitudinal analysis, *Pediatrics* 120 (2007): e1017.

68. T. I. Halldorsson and coauthors, Is high consumption of fatty fish during pregnancy a risk factor for fetal growth retardation? A study of 44,824 Danish pregnant women, *American Journal of Epidemiology* 166 (2007): 687–696.

69. E. Oken and coauthors, Maternal fish intake during pregnancy, blood mercury levels, and child cognition at age 3 years in a U.S. cohort, *American Journal of Epidemiology* 167 (2008): 1171–1181; J. R. Hibbeln and coauthors, Maternal seafood consumption in pregnancy and neuro-developmental outcomes in childhood (ALSPAC study): An observational cohort study, *Lancet* 369 (2007): 578–585; D. Mozaffarian and E. B. Rimm, Fish intake, contaminants, and human health: Evaluating the risks and the benefits, *Journal of the American Medical Association* 296 (2006): 1885–1899; Institute of Medicine report brief, *Seafood Choices: Balancing Benefits and Risks,* October 2006.

70. Position of the American Dietetic Association: Use of nutritive and nonnutritive sweeteners, *Journal of the American Dietetic Association* 104 (2004): 255–275.

71. X. Weng, R. Odouli, and D. Li, Maternal caffeine consumption during pregnancy and the risk of miscarriage: A prospective cohort study, *American Journal of Obstetrics and Gynecology* 198 (2008): 279.e1–279.e8; M. L. Browne, Maternal exposure to caffeine and risk of congenital anomalies: A systematic review, *Epidemiology* 17 (2006): 324–331; A. Matijasevich and coauthors, Maternal caffeine consumption and fetal death: A case-control study in Uruguay, *Paediatric and Perinatal Epidemiology* 20 (2006): 100–109; B. H. Bech and coauthors, Coffee and fetal death: A cohort study with prospective data, *American Journal of Epidemiology* 162 (2005): 983–990.

72. CARE Study Group, Maternal caffeine intake during pregnancy and risk of fetal growth restriction: A large prospective observational study, *British Medical Journal* 337 (2008): a2332.

73. H. E. Hoyme and coauthors, A practical approach to diagnosis of fetal alcohol spectrum disorders: Clarification of the 1996 Institute of Medicine criteria, *Pediatrics* 115 (2005): 39–47.

74. C. H. Denny and coauthors, Alcohol use among pregnant and nonpregnant women of childbearing age—United States, 1991–2005, *Morbidity and Mortality Weekly Report* 58 (2009): 529–532; Centers for Disease Control, Fetal alcohol syndrome, www.cdc.gov/ncbddd/fas/fasask.htm, site visited May 29, 2009.

75. C. H. Denny and coauthors, 2009.

76. J. A. Martin and coauthors, Births: Final data for 2006, *National Vital Statistics Reports* 57 (2009): 1–102.

77. P. N. Baker and coauthors, A prospective study of micronutrient status in adolescent pregnancy, *American Journal of Clinical Nutrition* 89 (2009): 1114–1124; S. Saintonge, H. Bang, and L. M. Gerber, Implications of a new definition of vitamin D deficiency in a multiracial U.S. adolescent population: The National Health and Nutrition examination Survey III, *Pediatrics* 123 (2009): 797–803.

78. Quickstats—Birthrates among females aged 15–19 years, by state—United States, 2004, *Morbidity and Mortality Weekly Report* 55 (2007): 1383.

79. X. Chen and coauthors, Paternal age and adverse birth outcomes: Teenager or 40+, who is at risk? *Human Reproduction* 23 (2008): 1290–1296.

80. E. P. Gunderson and coauthors, Longitudinal study of growth and adiposity in parous compared with nulligravid adolescents, *Archives of Pediatrics and Adolescent Medicine* 163 (2009): 349–356.

81. Breastfeeding, in *Pediatric Nutrition Handbook,* 6th ed., ed. R. E. Kleinman (Elk Grove Village, IL: American Academy of Pediatrics, 2009), pp. 29–59; American Academy of Pediatrics, Policy statement: Breastfeeding and the use of human milk, *Pediatrics* 115 (2005): 496–506.

82. Breastfeeding, in *Pediatric Nutrition Handbook,* 2009; American Academy of Pediatrics, 2005; Position of the American Dietetic Association, 2009.

83. Position of the American Dietetic Association: Promoting and supporting breastfeeding, *Journal of the American Dietetic Association* 109 (2009): 1926–1942.

84. J. Baker and coauthors, Breastfeeding reduces postpartum weight retention, *American Journal of Clinical Nutrition* 88 (2008): 1543–1551.

85. D. Su and coauthors, Breast-feeding mothers can exercise: Results of a cohort study, *Public Health Nutrition* 10 (2007): 1089–1093.

86. K. O. O'Brien and coauthors, Bone calcium turnover during pregnancy and lactation in women with low calcium diets is associated with calcium intake and circulating insulin-like growth factor 1 concentrations, *American Journal of Clinical Nutrition* 83 (2006): 317–323.

87. F. R. Greer, S. H. Sicherer, A. Wesley Burks, and the Committee on Nutrition and Section on Allergy and Immunology, Effects of early nutritional interventions on the development of atopic disease in infants and children: The role of maternal dietary restriction, breastfeeding, timing of introduction of complementary foods, and hydrolyzed formulas, *Pediatrics* 121 (2008): 183–191.

88. F. R. Greer, S. H. Sicherer, A. Wesley Burks, and the Committee on Nutrition and Section on Allergy and Immunology, 2008.

89. American Academy of Pediatrics, 2005.

90. J. A. Mennella, L. M. Yourshaw, and L. K. Morgan, Breastfeeding and smoking: Short-term effects on infant feeding and sleep, *Pediatrics* 120 (2007): 497–502.

91. American Academy of Pediatrics, 2005.

92. P. L. Havens, L. M. Mofenson, and the Committee on Pediatric AIDS, *Pediatrics* 123 (2009): 175–187.

93. World Health Organization, *HIV and Infant Feeding,* available at http://www.who.int/child_adolescent_health/topics/prevention_care/child/nutrition/hivif/en/. Site visited June 1, 2009; M. W. Kline, Early exclusive breastfeeding: Still the cornerstone of child survival, *American Journal of Clinical Nutrition* 89 (2009): 1281–1282.

94. Formula feeding of term infants, in *Pediatric Nutrition Handbook,* 6th ed., ed. R. E. Kleinman (Elk Grove Village, IL: American Academy of Pediatrics, 2009), pp. 61–78.

95. American Academy of Pediatrics, 2005.

96. American Academy of Pediatrics, 2005.

97. L. Bode, Recent advances on structure, metabolism, and function of human milk oligosaccharides, *Journal of Nutrition* 136 (2006): 2127–2130.

98. S. M. Donovan, Human milk oligosaccharides—The plot thickens, *British Journal of Nutrition* 101 (2009): 1267–1269.

99. S. M. Innis, Dietary (n-3) fatty acids and brain development, *Journal of Nutrition* 137 (2007): 855–859.

100. S. E. Carlson, Early determinants of development: A lipid perspective, *American Journal of Clinical Nutrition* 89 (2009): 1523S–1529S; K. Simmer, S. K. Patole, and S. C. Rao, Longchain polyunsaturated fatty acid supplementation in infants born at term, *Cochrane Database of Systematic Reviews* January 23, 2008, CD000376; S. M. Innis, 2007; M. S. Fewtrell, Long-chain polyunsaturated fatty acids in early life: Effects on multiple health outcomes, in *Primary Prevention by Nutrition Intervention in Infancy and Childhood,* eds., A. Lucas and H. A. Sampson, *Nestle Nutrition Workshop Series Pediatric Program* 57 (2006): 203–221; W. C. Heird and A. Lapillonne, The role of essential fatty acids in development, *Annual Review of Nutrition* 25 (2005): 549–571; J. C. McCann and B. N. Ames, Is docosahexaenoic acid, an n-3 long-chain polyunsaturated fatty acid, required for development of normal brain function? An overview of evidence from cognitive and behavioral tests in humans and animals, *American Journal of Clinical Nutrition* 82 (2005): 281–295.

101. E. E. Birch and coauthors, Visual acuity and cognitive outcomes at 4 years of age in a double-blind, randomized trial of long-chain polyunsaturated fatty acid-supplemented infant formula, *Early Human Development* 83 (2007): 279–284.

102. K. Simmer, S. K. Patole, and S. C. Rao, 2008.

103. Fat-soluble vitamins, in *Pediatric Nutrition Handbook,* 6th ed., ed. R. E. Kleinman (Elk Grove Village, IL: American Academy of Pediatrics, 2009), pp. 461–474.

104. C. L. Wagner, and F. R. Greer, and the Section on Breastfeeding and Committee on Nutrition, 2008.

105. Breastfeeding, in *Pediatric Nutrition Handbook*, 2009; American Academy of Pediatrics, 2005; Position of the American Dietetic Association, 2005.

106. K. Sadeharju and coauthors, Maternal antibodies in breast milk protect the child from enterovirus infections, *Pediatrics* 119 (2007): 941–946.

107. L. A. Hanson, Session 1: Feeding and infant development breast-feeding and immune function, *Proceedings of the Nutrition Society* 66 (2007): 384–396.

108. D. S. Newburg, G. M. Ruiz-Palacios, and A. L. Morrow, Human milk glycans protect infants against enteric pathogens, *Annual Review of Nutrition* 25 (2005): 37–58.

109. Breastfeeding, in *Pediatric Nutrition Handbook*, 2009; L. A. Hanson, Session 1: Feeding and infant development breast-feeding and immune function, *Proceedings of the Nutrition Society* 66 (2007): 384–396; C. J. Chantry, C. R. Howard, and P. Auinger, Full breastfeeding duration and associated decrease in respiratory tract infection in U.S. children, *Pediatrics* 117 (2006): 425–432; American Academy of Pediatrics, 2005; Position of the American Dietetic Association, 2005.

110. F. R. Greer, S. H. Sicherer, A. W. Burks, and the Committee on Nutrition and Section on Allergy and Immunology, 2008.

111. F. R. Greer, S. H. Sicherer, A. W. Burks, and the Committee on Nutrition and Section on Allergy and Immunology, 2008; R. S. Zeiger and N. J. Friedman, The relationship of breastfeeding to the development of atopic disorders, *Nestle Nutrition Workshop Series: Pediatric Program* 57 (2006): 93–108.

112. F. R. Greer, S. H. Sicherer, A. W. Burks, and the Committee on Nutrition and Section on Allergy and Immunology, 2008; A. C. Krakowski and coauthors, Management of atopic dermatitis in the pediatric population, *Pediatrics* 122 (2008): 812–824.

113. D. A. Leon and G. Ronalds, Breast-feeding influences on later life—cardiovascular disease, *Advances in Experimental Medicine and Biology* 639 (2009): 153–166; C. G. Owen and coauthors, Does initial breastfeeding lead to lower blood cholesterol in adult life? A quantitative review of the evidence, *American Journal of Clinical Nutrition* 88 (2008): 305–314; L. Schack-Nielsen and K. F. Michaelsen, Advances in our understanding of the biology of human milk and its effects on the offspring, *Journal of Nutrition* 137 (2007): 503S–510S; R. A. Singhal, Early nutrition and long-term cardiovascular health, *Nutrition Reviews* 64 (2006): S44–S49; M. Martin, D. Gunnell, and G. D. Smith, Breastfeeding in infancy and blood pressure in later life: Systematic review and meta-analysis, *American Journal of Epidemiology* 161 (2005): 15–26.

114. A. S. Ryan, Breastfeeding and the risk of childhood obesity, *Collegium Antropologicum* 31 (2007): 19–28; S. Scholtens and coauthors, Breastfeeding, weight gain in infancy, and overweight at seven years of age: The prevention and incidence of asthma and mite allergy birth cohort study, *American Journal of Epidemiology* 165 (2007): 919–926; A. M. Toschke and coauthors, Infant feeding method and obesity: Body mass index and dual-energy X-ray absorptiometry measurements at 9–10 y of age from the Avon Longitudinal Study of Parents and Children (ALSPAC), *American Journal of Clinical Nutrition* 85 (2007): 1578–1585; R. Novotny and coauthors, Breastfeeding is associated with lower body mass index among children of the Commonwealth of the Northern Mariana Islands, *Journal of the American Dietetic Association* 107 (2007): 1743–1746; K. B. Michels and coauthors, A longitudinal study of infant feeding and obesity throughout life course, *International Journal of Obesity* 31 (2007): 1078–1085.

115. C. G. Owen and coauthors, Effect of infant feeding on the risk of obesity across the life course: A quantitative review of published evidence, *Pediatrics* 115 (2005): 1367–1377.

116. T. Harder and coauthors, Duration of breastfeeding and risk of overweight: A meta-analysis, *Journal of Epidemiology* 162 (2005): 397–403.

117. A. S. Ryan, 2007.

118. L. Schack-Nielsen and K. F. Michaelsen, Advances in our understanding of the biology of human milk and its effects on the offspring, *Journal of Nutrition* 137 (2007): 503S–510S; G. Der, G. D. Batty, and I. J. Deary, Effect of breast feeding on intelligence in children; prospective study, sibling pairs analysis, and meta-analysis, *British Medical Journal* 333 (2006): 929–930; M. C. Daniels and L. S. Adair, Breastfeeding influences cognitive development in Filipino children, *Journal of Nutrition* 135 (2005): 2589–2595.

119. L. Schack-Nielsen and K. F. Michaelsen, 2007.

120. Formula feeding of term infants, in *Pediatric Nutrition Handbook*, 2009.

121. Formula feeding of term infants, in *Pediatric Nutrition Handbook*, 2009; L. Seppo and coauthors, A follow-up study of nutrient intake, nutritional status, and growth in infants with cow milk allergy fed either a soy formula or an extensively hydrolyzed whey formula, *American Journal of Clinical Nutrition* 82 (2005): 140–145.

122. Formula feeding of term infants, in *Pediatric Nutrition Handbook*, 2009; L. Seppo and coauthors, 2005.

123. Formula feeding of term infants, in *Pediatric Nutrition Handbook*, 2009.

124. Complementary feeding, in *Pediatric Nutrition Handbook*, 6th ed., ed. R. E. Kleinman (Elk Grove Village, IL: American Academy of Pediatrics, 2009), pp. 113–142.

125. Iron, in *Pediatric Nutrition Handbook*, 6th ed., ed. R. E. Kleinman (Elk Grove Village, IL: American Academy of Pediatrics, 2009), pp. 403–422.

126. Complementary feeding, in *Pediatric Nutrition Handbook*, 2009.

127. Feeding the child, in *Pediatric Nutrition Handbook*, 6th ed., ed. R. E. Kleinman (Elk Grove Village, IL: American Academy of Pediatrics, 2009), pp. 145–174.

128. Feeding the child, in *Pediatric Nutrition Handbook*, 2009.

129. Complementary feeding, in *Pediatric Nutrition Handbook*, 2009; A. Fiocchi, A. Assa'ad, and S. Bahna, Food allergy and the introduction of solid foods to infants: A consensus document, *Annals of Allergy, Asthma and Immunology* 97 (2006): 10–21.

Encouraging Successful Breastfeeding

As discussed in Chapter 10, breastfeeding offers benefits to both mother and infant. The American Academy of Pediatrics (AAP), the American Dietetic Association, and the Canadian Paediatric Society all advocate breastfeeding as the preferred means of infant feeding.[1] Promotion of breastfeeding is an integral part of the WIC program's nutrition education component. National efforts to promote breastfeeding seem to be working, at least to some extent: the percentage of infants who were ever breastfed rose from 60 percent among those born in 1994 to 77 percent among infants born in 2006.[2] Despite this encouraging trend, the rate of breastfeeding at six months of age did not change for infants born between 1993 and 2004.[3] Only about one in three infants is still being breastfed at six months of age. The AAP and many other health organizations recommend exclusive breastfeeding for the first six months of life.[4] Exclusive breastfeeding is defined as an infant's consumption of human milk with no supplementation of any kind (no water, no other type of milk, no juice, and no other foods) except for vitamins, minerals, and medications. The AAP recommends that breastfeeding continue for at least a year and thereafter for as long as mutually desired.[5] In the United States, only about one in five infants is still breastfeeding at one year of age. Increasing the rates of breastfeeding initiation and duration is one of the goals of *Healthy People 2010*:

> Increase the proportion of mothers who breastfeed immediately after birth, for the first six months, and preferably, through the infant's first year of life. Increase the proportion of mothers who breastfeed exclusively.[6]

Despite the trend toward increasing breastfeeding, the percentage of mothers choosing to breastfeed their infants and continuing to do so still falls short of goals.

Why don't more women choose to breastfeed their infants?

Many experts cite two major deterrents: infant formula manufacturers' public advertising and promotion of their products and the medical community's failure to encourage breastfeeding. Infant formula manufacturers spend millions of dollars each year marketing their products, often claiming that formula "is like breast milk." Such advertising efforts seem to be working. According to a recent survey, one out of four people of various ages, races, and socioeconomic backgrounds agree with the statement "infant formula is

as good as breast milk."[7] Infant formula is an appropriate substitute for breast milk when breastfeeding is specifically contraindicated, but for most infants, the benefits of breast milk outweigh those of formula. Despite medical evidence of the benefits of breast milk, medical practice is not always supportive.

As an example of the medical lack of encouragement, some hospitals routinely separate mother and infant soon after birth. The child's first feeding then comes from the bottle rather than the breast. Furthermore, many hospitals send new mothers home with free samples of infant formula.[8] The World Health Organization opposes this practice because it sends a misleading message that medical authorities favor infant formula over breast milk for infants. Even in hospitals where women are encouraged to breastfeed and are supported in doing so, little, if any, assistance is available after hospital discharge when many breastfeeding women still need assistance. Up to half of mothers who initially breastfeed their infants stop within three months—seemingly due to lack of knowledge and support.

Women who receive early and repeated breastfeeding information and support breastfeed their infants longer than other women do.[9] Information and instruction are especially important during the *prenatal* period when most women decide whether to breastfeed or to feed formula. Nurses and other health care professionals can play a crucial role in encouraging successful breastfeeding by offering women adequate, accurate information about breastfeeding that permits them to make informed choices. Table NP10-1 lists ten steps maternity facilities and health care professionals can take to promote successful breastfeeding among new mothers.

If breastfeeding is a natural process, what do mothers need to learn?

Although lactation is an automatic physiological process, breastfeeding requires some learning. This learning is most successful in a supportive environment. It begins with preparatory steps taken before the infant is born.

What are these preparatory steps?

Toward the end of pregnancy and throughout lactation, a woman who intends to breastfeed should stop using soap and lotions on her breasts. The natural secretions of the breasts themselves lubricate the nipple area best. A woman who plans to breastfeed should also acquire at least two nursing bras before her infant is born. The bras should provide good support and have drop-flaps so that either breast can be freed for nursing.

TABLE	
NP10-1	Ten Steps to Successful Breastfeeding

To promote breastfeeding, every maternity facility should:

- Develop a written breastfeeding policy that is routinely communicated to all health care staff.

- Train all health care staff in the skills necessary to implement the breastfeeding policy.

- Inform all pregnant women about the benefits and management of breastfeeding.

- Help mothers initiate breastfeeding within half an hour of birth.

- Show mothers how to breastfeed and how to maintain lactation, even if they need to be separated from their infants.

- Give newborn infants no food or drink other than breast milk, unless medically indicated.

- Practice rooming-in, allowing mothers and infants to remain together 24 hours a day.

- Encourage breastfeeding on demand.

- Give no artificial nipples or pacifiers to breastfeeding infants.

- Foster the establishment of breastfeeding support groups, and refer mothers to them at discharge from the facility.

Sources: U.S. Department of Health and Human Services, Office on Women's Health, Breastfeeding: HHS Blueprint for Action on Breastfeeding (Washington, D.C.: U.S. Department of Health and Human Services, 2000); United Nations Children's Fund and World Health Organization, The UNICEF/Baby-Friendly Hospital Initiative: Ten Steps to Successful Breastfeeding (New York: UNICEF, 1992).

How soon after birth should breastfeeding start?

As soon as possible. Immediately after the delivery, for a short period, the infant is intensely alert and intent on suckling. This is the ideal time for the first breastfeeding and facilitates successful lactation.

What does the new mother need to know to continue breastfeeding her infant successfully?

She needs to learn how to relax and position herself so that she and the infant will be comfortable and the infant can breathe freely while nursing. She also needs to understand that infants have a **rooting reflex** that makes them turn toward any touch on the face. (The glossary on p. 314 defines this and other relevant terms.) Consequently, she should touch the infant's cheek to her nipple so that the infant will turn the right way to nurse. The mother can then place four fingers under the breast and her thumb on top to support the breast and present the nipple to the infant. The mother's fingers and thumb should be behind the areola, the colored ring around the nipple, so as not to interfere with the infant latching onto the breast (see Figure NP10-1 on p. 314).

With the breast supported, the mother tickles the infant's lips with the breast until the infant's mouth opens wide. The mother can then gently bring the infant forward onto the breast. The nipple must rest well back on the infant's tongue so that the infant's gums will squeeze on the glands that release the milk and swallowing will be effortless. To break the suction, if necessary, the mother can slip a finger between the infant's mouth and her breast.

> **NURSING DIAGNOSIS**
>
> *Ineffective breastfeeding* applies to clients whose infants are unable to attach to the maternal breast correctly.

Does it hurt to have the infant sucking so hard on the breast?

Breastfeeding should not be painful if the infant is positioned correctly. The mother has a **letdown reflex** that forces milk to the front of her breast when the infant begins to nurse, virtually propelling the milk into the infant's mouth. Letdown is necessary for the infant to obtain milk easily, and the mother needs to relax for letdown to occur. The mother who assumes a comfortable position in an environment without interruptions will find it easiest to relax.

FIGURE NP10-1 | Infant's Grasp on Mother's Breast

The mother supports the breast with her fingers and thumb behind the areola to present the nipple to the infant. Once the infant latches onto the breast, the infant's lips and gums pump the areola, releasing milk from the mammary glands into the milk ducts that lie beneath the areola.

Glossary

engorgement: overfilling of the breasts with milk.

letdown reflex: the reflex that forces milk to the front of the breast when the infant begins to nurse.

mastitis: infection of a breast.

rooting reflex: a reflex that causes an infant to turn toward whichever cheek is touched, in search of a nipple.

How long should the infant be allowed to nurse at each feeding?

Although the infant sucks half the milk from the breast within the first 2 minutes, and 80 to 90 percent of it within 4 minutes, sucking on each breast for 10 to 15 minutes is encouraged. The sucking itself, as well as the complete removal of milk from the breast, stimulates the mammary glands to produce milk for the next nursing session. Successive sessions should start on alternate breasts to ensure that each breast is emptied regularly. This pattern maintains the same supply and demand for each breast and thus prevents either breast from overfilling.

Infants should be fed "on demand" and not be held to a rigid schedule. The breastfed infant may average 8 to 12 feedings per 24-hour period during the first month or so. Once the mother's milk supply is well established and the infant's capacity has increased, the intervals between feedings will become longer.

What if a mother wants to skip one or two feedings daily—for example, because she works outside the home?

The mother can express breast milk into a bottle ahead of time, freeze the breast milk, and, when needed, substitute the expressed breast milk for a nursing session. Breast milk can be kept refrigerated for 48 hours or frozen. Frozen milk can be kept for one month in a freezer attached to a refrigerator or for three to six months in a zero-degree deep freezer.[10]

The mother can hand express her breast milk or use one of several different breast pumps available. The bicycle-horn type of manual breast pump is difficult to keep clean and is not recommended. Cylinder-type manual pumps or electric breast pumps are safer and are also more efficient. Alternatively, a mother can substitute formula for those missed feedings and continue to breastfeed at other times.

What about problems associated with breastfeeding such as sore nipples or infection of the breast?

Most problems associated with breastfeeding can be resolved. Many mothers experience sore nipples during the initial days of breastfeeding. Sore nipples need to be treated kindly, but nursing can continue. Improper feeding position is a frequent cause of sore nipples: the mother should make sure the infant is taking the entire nipple and part of the areola onto the tongue. She should nurse on the less sore breast first to get letdown going while the infant is sucking hardest; then she can switch to the sore breast. Between times, she should expose her nipples to light and air to heal them.

Before lactation is well established, when the schedule changes, or when a feeding is missed, the breasts may become full and hard—an uncomfortable condition known as **engorgement**. The infant cannot grasp an engorged nipple and so cannot provide relief by nursing. A gentle massage or warming the breasts with a cloth soaked in warm water or in a shower helps to initiate letdown and to release some of the accumulated milk; then the mother can pump out some of her milk and allow the infant to nurse.

Infection of the breast, known as **mastitis**, is best managed by continuing to breastfeed. By drawing off the milk, the infant helps to relieve pressure in the infected area. The infant is safe because the infection is between the milk-producing glands, not inside them.

Even if everything is going smoothly, the nursing mother should ideally have enough help and support so that she can rest in bed a few hours each day for the first week or so. Successful breastfeeding requires the support of all those who care. This, plus adequate nutrition, ample fluids, fresh air, and physical activity, will do much to enhance the well-being of mother and infant.

Notes

1. Breastfeeding, in *Pediatric Nutrition Handbook,* 6th ed., R. E. Kleinman (Elk Grove Village, IL: American Academy of Pediatrics, 2009), pp. 29–59; American Academy of Pediatrics, Policy statement: Breastfeeding and the use of human milk, *Pediatrics* 115 (2005): 496–506; Position of the American Dietetic Association: Promoting and supporting breastfeeding, *Journal of the American Dietetic Association* 105 (2005): 810–818; M. Boland, Exclusive breastfeeding should continue to six months, *Paediatrics and Child Health* 10 (2005): 148–149.

2. Centers for Disease Control and Prevention, National Center for Health Statistics, M. M. McDowell, C. Wang, and J. Kennedy-Stephenson, Breastfeeding in the United States: Findings from the National Health and Nutrition Examination Surveys, 1999-2006, *NCHS Data Brief,* No. 5, April 2008, available at www.cdc.gov/nchs/fastats/Default.htm.

3. Centers for Disease Control and Prevention, National Center for Health Statistics, M. M. McDowell, C. Wang, and J. Kennedy-Stephenson, 2008.

4. Breastfeeding, in *Pediatric Nutrition Handbook,* 2009; American Academy of Pediatrics, 2005.

5. Breastfeeding, in *Pediatric Nutrition Handbook,* 2009; American Academy of Pediatrics, 2005.

6. *Healthy People 2010: National Health Promotion and Disease Prevention Objectives* (Washington, D.C.: U.S. Department of Health and Human Services, 2000).

7. L. Rowell, V. J. Rock, and L. Grummer-Strawn, Changes in public attitudes toward breastfeeding in the United States, *Journal of the American Dietetic Association* 107 (2007): 122–127.

8. Centers for Disease Control and Prevention, Breastfeeding-related maternity practices at hospitals and birth centers—United States, 2007, *Morbidity and Mortality Weekly Report* 57 (2008): 621–625.

9. M. Chung and coauthors, Interventions in primary care to promote breastfeeding: An evidence review for the U.S. Preventive Services Task Force, *Annals of Internal Medicine* 149 (2008): 565–582; I. Mannan and coauthors, Can early postpartum home visits by trained community health workers improve breastfeeding of newborns? *Journal of Perinatology* 28 (2008): 632–640; J. Clifford and E. McIntyre, Who supports breastfeeding? *Breastfeeding Review* 16 (2008): 9–19.

10. Breastfeeding beyond infancy, in *American Academy of Pediatrics, New Mother's Guide to Breastfeeding,* ed. J. Y. Meek and S. Tippins (New York: Bantam Books, 2002), pp. 158–188.

CHAPTER 11

Nutrition Through the Life Span: Childhood and Adolescence

Radius Images/Jupiter Images

CONTENTS

NUTRITION IN PRACTICE

NUTRIENT NEEDS CHANGE THROUGHOUT LIFE, DEPENDING ON RATES of growth, activity, and many other factors. Nutrient needs also vary from individual to individual, but generalizations are possible and useful. Sound nutrition throughout childhood promotes normal growth and development; facilitates academic and physical performance; and helps prevent obesity, diabetes, heart disease, cancer, and other degenerative diseases in adulthood. As children enter the teen years, a foundation built by years of eating nutritious foods best prepares them to meet the upcoming demands of rapid growth.

Nutrition during Childhood

After the age of one, growth rate slows, but the body continues to change dramatically (see Figure 11-1). At one, infants have just learned to stand and toddle; by two, they walk confidently and are learning to run, jump, and climb. Nutrition and physical activity have helped them prepare for these new accomplishments by adding to the mass and density of their bone and muscle tissue. Thereafter, their bones continue to grow longer and their muscles to gain size and strength, though unevenly and more slowly, until adolescence.

ENERGY AND NUTRIENT NEEDS

Children's appetites begin to diminish around the first birthday, consistent with the slowed growth rate. Thereafter, the appetite fluctuates. At times children seem to be insatiable, and at other times they seem to live on air and water. Parents and other caregivers need not worry about this—a child will need and demand more food during periods of rapid growth than during slow periods. The perfect regulation of appetite in children of healthy weight guarantees that their food energy intakes will be right for each stage of growth.

Ideally, children accumulate stores of nutrients before adolescence. Then, when they take off on the adolescent growth spurt and their nutrient intakes cannot keep pace with the demands of rapid growth, they can draw on the nutrient stores accumulated earlier. This is especially true of calcium; the denser the bones are in childhood, the better prepared they will be to support teen growth and still withstand the inevitable bone losses of later life.[1] Consequently, the way children eat influences their nutritional health during childhood, during their teen years, and for the rest of their lives.

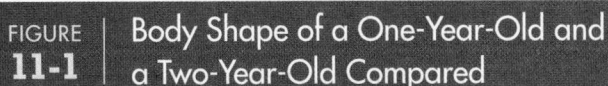

| FIGURE 11-1 | Body Shape of a One-Year-Old and a Two-Year-Old Compared |

© Anthony M. Vanelli (both)

The body shape of a one-year-old (left) changes dramatically by age two (right). The two-year-old has lost much of the baby fat; the muscles (especially in the back, buttocks, and legs) have firmed and strengthened; and the leg bones have lengthened.

Children's Appetites

Many people mistakenly believe that they must "make" their children eat the right amounts of food, and children's erratic appetites often reinforce this belief. Although children's food energy intakes vary widely from meal to meal, total daily energy intake remains remarkably constant.[2] If children eat less at one meal, they typically eat more at the next, and vice versa.

Parents do, however, need to help children choose the right foods, and, with overweight children, they may need to help more, as described later. Overweight children may not adjust their energy intakes appropriately and may disregard appetite-regulation signals and eat in response to external cues, such as television commercials.[3]

Energy

Individual children's energy needs vary widely, depending on their growth and physical activity. A one-year-old child needs approximately 800 kcalories a day; an active six-year-old needs twice as many kcalories a day. By age ten, an active child needs about 2000 kcalories a day. Total energy needs increase gradually with age, but energy needs per kilogram of body weight actually decline. Physically active children of any age need more energy because they expend more, and inactive children can become obese even when they eat less food than the average. Unfortunately, our nation's children are becoming less and less active; schools would serve our children well by offering activities to promote physical fitness.[4]

Some children, notably those adhering to a vegan diet, may have difficulty meeting their energy needs. Grains, vegetables, and fruits provide plenty of fiber, adding bulk, but may provide too few kcalories to support growth. Soy products, other legumes, and nut or seed butters offer more concentrated sources of energy to support optimal growth and development.[5]

Carbohydrate and Fiber

Carbohydrate recommendations are based on glucose use by the brain. After one year of age, brain glucose use remains fairly constant and is within the adult range. Carbohydrate recommendations for children after one year are therefore the same as for adults (see inside front cover).[6]

Fiber recommendations (✚) derive from adult intakes shown to reduce the risk of coronary heart disease and are based on energy intakes. Consequently, fiber recommendations for younger children with low energy intakes are less than those for older ones with high energy intakes.[7]

Fat and Fatty Acids

No RDA for total fat has been established, but the DRI committee recommends a fat intake of 30 to 40 percent of energy for children 1 to 3 years of age and 25 to 35 percent for children 4 to 18 years of age.[8] However, as long as children's energy intakes are adequate, fat intakes below 30 percent of total energy do not impair growth.[9] Children who eat low-fat diets, however, tend to have low intakes of some vitamins and minerals. Recommended intakes of the essential fatty acids are based on average intakes (see inside front cover).

Protein

Like energy needs, total protein needs increase slightly with age but actually decline slightly when the child's body weight is considered (see inside front cover). Protein recommendations must address the requirements for maintaining nitrogen balance, the quality of protein consumed, and the added needs of growth.

Vitamins and Minerals

The vitamin and mineral needs of children increase with age (see inside front cover). A balanced diet of nutritious foods can meet children's needs for these nutrients, with the notable exception of iron, and possibly vitamin D. Iron-deficiency anemia is a major problem worldwide, as well as being prevalent among U.S. and Canadian children, especially toddlers one to three years of age.[10] During the second year of life, toddlers progress from a diet of iron-rich infant foods such as breast milk, iron-fortified formula, and iron-fortified infant cereal to a diet of adult foods and iron-poor cow's milk. In addition, their appetites often fluctuate—some become finicky about the foods they eat, and others prefer milk and juice to solid foods. These situations can interfere with children eating iron-rich foods at a critical time for brain growth and development.

✚Fiber recommendations for children:

Age (yr)	DRI (g/day)
1–3	19
4–8	25
9–13	
Boys	31
Girls	26
14–18	
Boys	38
Girls	26

NURSING DIAGNOSIS

Risk for imbalanced nutrition—more than body requirements applies to clients who eat in response to external cues.

NURSING DIAGNOSIS

Imbalanced nutrition—less than body requirements applies to clients who have a food intake less than the RDA.

To prevent iron deficiency, children's foods must deliver 7 to 10 milligrams of iron per day. To achieve this goal, snacks and meals should include iron-rich foods, and milk intake should be reasonable so that it will not displace lean meats, fish, poultry, eggs, legumes, and whole-grain or enriched products. That means 2 cups of milk per day up to age eight, increasing to 3 cups per day from age nine on. After age two, if reduced-fat or low-fat milk is used instead of whole milk, the saved kcalories can be invested in iron-rich foods such as lean meats, fish, poultry, eggs, and legumes. Whole-grain or enriched breads and cereals also contribute iron. Table 11-1 lists iron-rich foods children like.

The American Academy of Pediatrics recently updated vitamin D guidelines for children. Children who do not obtain 10 micrograms of vitamin D per day by drinking vitamin D–fortified milk (2.5 micrograms per 1-cup serving) and eating fortified foods such as dry cereals (1 microgram per ½-cup serving) should receive a vitamin D supplement of 10 micrograms (400 IU on labels) per day.[11]

Supplements
With the exception of specific recommendations for fluoride, iron, and vitamin D during infancy and childhood, the AAP and other professional groups agree that well-nourished children do not need vitamin and mineral supplements. Despite this, many children and adolescents take supplements.[12] Ironically, children with poor nutrient intakes typically do not receive supplements, while those who do take them usually receive extra nutrients they do not need.[13] Furthermore, researchers are still studying the safety of supplement use by children. The Federal Trade Commission has warned parents about giving children supplements advertised to prevent or cure childhood illnesses such as colds, ear infections, or asthma. Dietary supplements on the market today include many herbal products that have not been tested for safety and effectiveness in children.

Food Patterns for Children
To provide all the needed nutrients, a child's meals and snacks should include a variety of foods from each food group—in amounts suited to the child's appetite and needs. Figure 11-2 presents MyPyramid for Preschoolers, designed for children 2 to 5 years of age, and MyPyramid for Kids, (➕) designed for children 6 to 11 years of age. The figure includes the recommended amounts of food for a 1200-kcalorie intake (appropriate for many preschoolers) and for an 1800-kcalorie intake (appropriate for many older children). Table 11-2 (p. 321) lists recommended amounts from each food group for several kcalorie levels. Estimated daily kcalorie needs for active and sedentary children of various ages are shown in Table 11-3 (p. 321).

Children whose diets follow the pattern presented in Figure 11-2 meet their nutrient needs fully, but few children eat according to these recommendations. One analysis of the quality of children's diets found that most children (up to 88 percent) between two and nine years of age have diets that need substantial improvement.[14] A comprehensive survey, called the Feeding Infants and Toddlers Study (FITS), assessed the food and nutrient intakes of more than 3000 infants and toddlers.[15] The survey found that fruit and vegetable intakes of infants and toddlers are limited, and, in fact, about 25 percent of infants and toddlers older than nine months did not eat a single serving of fruits or vegetables in a day.[16] By 15 to 18 months of age, the most commonly consumed vegetable was French fries, and the most commonly consumed fruit was bananas—neither particularly rich sources of vitamins or minerals. Parents

TABLE 11-1	Iron-Rich Foods Children Like[a]

Breads, cereals, and grains
- Canned macaroni (½ c)
- Canned spaghetti (½ c)
- Cream of wheat (¼ c)
- Fortified dry cereals (1 oz)[b]
- Noodles, rice, or barley (½ c)
- Tortillas (1 flour or whole wheat, 2 corn)
- Whole-wheat, enriched, or fortified bread (1 slice)

Vegetables
- Baked flavored potato skins (½ skin)
- Cooked mung bean sprouts or snow peas (½ c)[c]
- Cooked mushrooms (½ c)
- Green peas (½ c)
- Mixed vegetable juice (1 c)

Fruits
- Canned plums (3 plums)
- Cooked dried apricots (¼ c)
- Dried peaches (4 halves)
- Raisins (1 tbs)

Meats and legumes
- Bean dip (¼ c)
- Canned pork and beans (⅓ c)
- Lean chopped roast beef or cooked ground beef (1 oz)
- Liverwurst on crackers (½ oz)
- Meat casseroles (½ c)
- Mild chili or other bean/meat dishes (¼ c)
- Peanut butter and jelly sandwich (½ sandwich)
- Sloppy joes (½ sandwich)

[a] Each serving provides at least 1 milligram of iron. Vitamin C–rich foods included with these snacks increase iron absorption.

[b] Some fortified breakfast cereals contain more than 10 milligrams of iron per half-cup serving (read the labels).

[c] Raw sprouts may pose a bacterial hazard to young children.

- www.MyPyramid.gov/preschoolers
- www.MyPyramid.gov/kids
- For kcalorie levels over 1800, see Table 1-7 on p. 20.

FIGURE 11-2 | MyPyramid for Preschoolers and for Kids

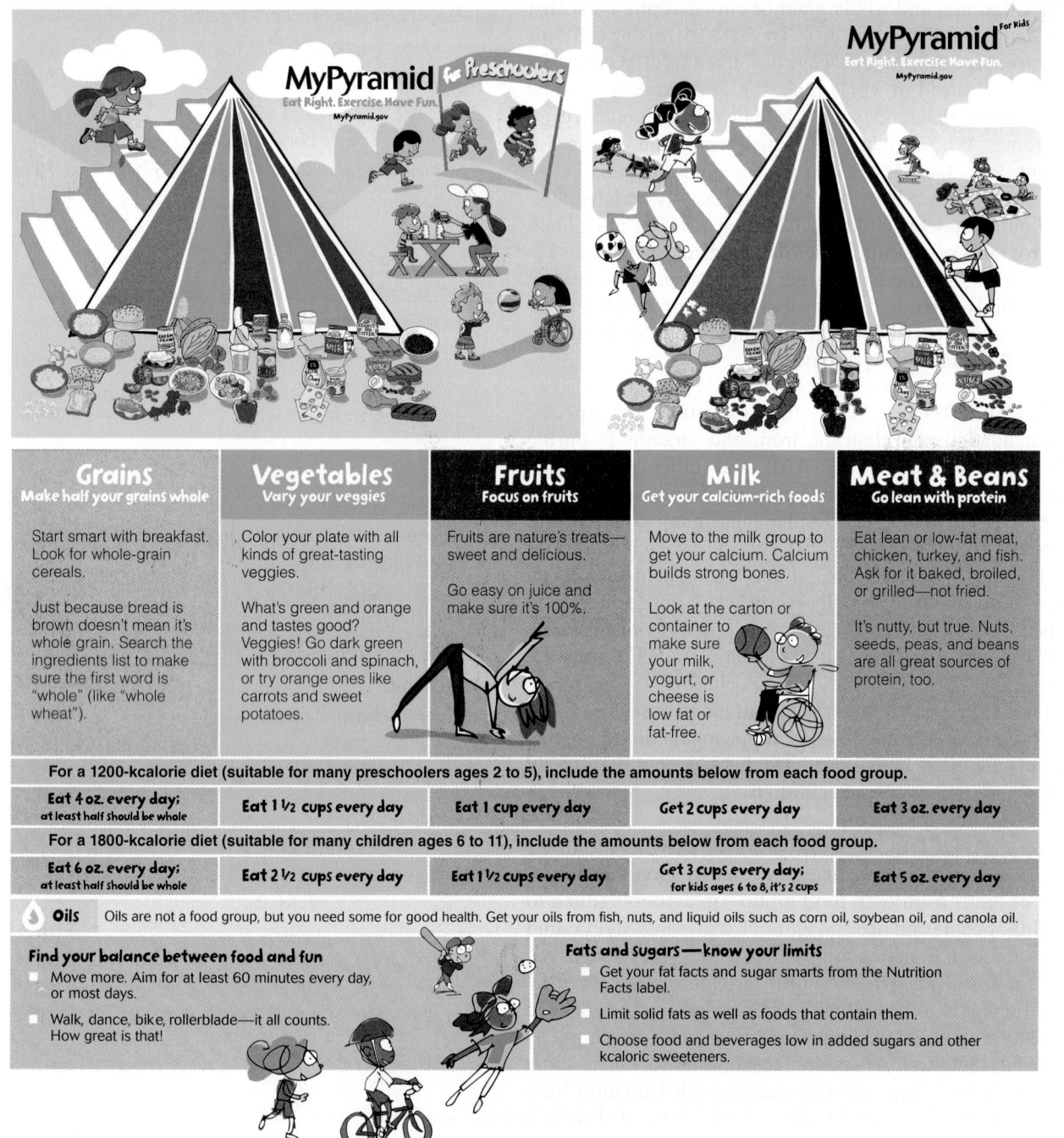

Source: MyPyramid.gov.

and caregivers of infants and toddlers thus need to offer a much greater variety of nutrient-dense vegetables and fruits at meals and snacks to help ensure adequate nutrition. Among other nutrition concerns for U.S. children are inadequate intakes of vitamin E, calcium, magnesium, potassium, and fiber, and excessive intakes of sodium and saturated fat.[17]

TABLE 11-2	Recommended Daily Amounts for Each Food Group (1000 to 1800 kCalories)				
Food Group	1000 kcal	1200 kcal	1400 kcal	1600 kcal	1800 kcal
Fruit	1 c	1 c	1½ c	1½ c	1½ c
Vegetables	1 c	1½ c	1½ c	2 c	2½ c
Grains	3 oz	4 oz	5 oz	5 oz	6 oz
Meat and legumes	2 oz	3 oz	4 oz	5 oz	5 oz
Milk	2 c	2 c	2 c	3 c	3 c
Oils	3 tsp	3 tsp	3 tsp	4 tsp	5 tsp

Note: The discretionary kcalorie allowance for these patterns is about 100 kcalories.

Children's Food Choices Parents and other caregivers can do much to foster the development of healthy eating habits in a child. The challenge is to deliver nutrients in the form of meals and snacks that are both nutritious and appealing so that children will learn to enjoy a variety of nutritious foods.

Candy, cola, and other concentrated sweets must be limited in children's diets. If such foods are permitted in large quantities, the only possible outcomes are nutrient deficiencies, obesity, or both. Children can't be trusted to choose nutritious foods on the basis of taste alone; the preference for sweets is innate, and children naturally gravitate to them. Overweight children, especially, need help in selecting nutrient-dense foods that will meet their nutrient needs within their energy allowances. Underweight children or active, healthy-weight children can enjoy higher-kcalorie foods, but these should still be nutritious. Examples are ice cream and pudding in the milk group and whole-grain or enriched pancakes and crackers in the bread group.

HUNGER AND MALNUTRITION IN CHILDREN

Most children in the United States and Canada have access to regular meals, but hunger and malnutrition do appear in certain circumstances. Children in very low-income families, for example, are more likely to be hungry and malnourished. More than 12 million U.S. children are hungry at least some of the time and are living in poverty.[18] Nutrition in Practice 12 examines the causes and consequences of hunger in the United States.

Hunger and Behavior Both short-term and long-term hunger exert negative effects on behavior and health. Short-term hunger, such as when a child misses a meal, impairs the child's ability to pay attention and to be productive. Hungry children are irritable, apathetic, and uninterested in their environment. Long-term hunger impairs growth and immune defenses. Food assistance programs such as the

TABLE 11-3	Estimated Daily kCalorie Needs for Children	
Children	Sedentary[a]	Active[b]
2 to 3 yr	1000	1400
Females		
4 to 8 yr	1200	1800
9 to 13 yr	1600	2200
Males		
4 to 8 yr	1400	2000
9 to 13 yr	1800	2600

[a] *Sedentary* describes a lifestyle that includes only the activities typical of day-to-day life.

[b] *Active* describes a lifestyle that includes at least 60 minutes per day of moderate physical activity (equivalent to walking more than 3 miles per day at 3 to 4 miles per hour) in addition to the activities of day-to-day life.

Healthy, well-nourished children are alert in the classroom and energetic at play.

WIC program (discussed in Chapter 10) and the School Breakfast and National School Lunch Programs (discussed later in this chapter) are designed to protect against hunger and improve the health of children.

Children who eat nutritious breakfasts improve their school performance and are tardy or absent significantly less often than their peers who do not.[19] A nutritious breakfast is a central feature of a diet that meets the needs of children and supports their healthy growth and development.[20] Children who skip breakfast typically do not make up the deficits at later meals—they simply have lower intakes of energy, vitamins, and minerals than those who eat breakfast. Without breakfast, children perform poorly in tasks requiring concentration, their attention spans are shorter, and they even score lower on intelligence tests than their well-fed peers. Malnourished children are particularly vulnerable. Common sense dictates that it is unreasonable to expect anyone to learn and perform without fuel. For the child who hasn't had breakfast, the morning's lessons may be lost altogether. Even if a child has eaten breakfast, discomfort from hunger may become distracting by late morning. Teachers aware of the late-morning slump in their classrooms wisely request that midmorning snacks be provided; snacks improve classroom performance all the way to lunchtime.

Iron Deficiency and Behavior Iron deficiency has well-known and widespread effects on children's behavior and intellectual performance.[21] In addition to carrying oxygen in the blood, iron transports oxygen within cells, which use it for energy metabolism. Iron is also used to make neurotransmitters—most notably, those that regulate the ability to pay attention, which is crucial to learning. Consequently, iron deficiency not only causes an energy crisis but also directly impairs attention span and learning ability.

Iron deficiency is often diagnosed by a quick, easy, inexpensive hemoglobin or hematocrit test that detects a deficit of iron in the *blood*. A child's *brain,* however, is sensitive to low iron concentrations long before the blood effects appear. Iron deficiency lowers the "motivation to persist in intellectually challenging tasks" and impairs overall intellectual performance. Anemic children perform poorly on tests and are disruptive in the classroom; iron supplementation improves learning and memory. When combined with other nutrient deficiencies, iron-deficiency anemia has synergistic effects that are especially detrimental to learning. Furthermore, children who had iron-deficiency anemia *as infants* continue to perform poorly as they grow older, even if their iron status improves.[22] The long-term damaging effects on mental development make prevention and treatment of iron deficiency during infancy and early childhood a high priority.

Other Nutrient Deficiencies A child with any of several nutrient deficiencies may be irritable, aggressive, and disagreeable, or sad and withdrawn. Such a child may be labeled "hyperactive," "depressed," or "unlikable," when in fact these traits may be due to simple, even marginal, malnutrition. Though parents and medical practitioners often overlook the possibility that malnutrition may account for these abnormalities, any departure from normal, healthy appearance and behavior is a sign of possible poor nutrition (see Table 11-4). In any such case, inspection of the child's diet by a registered dietitian or other qualified health care professional is in order. Any suspicion of dietary inadequacies, *no matter what other causes may be implicated,* should prompt steps to correct those inadequacies immediately.

LEAD POISONING IN CHILDREN

Children who are malnourished are vulnerable to lead poisoning. They absorb more lead if their stomachs are empty; if they have low intakes of calcium, zinc, vitamin C, or vitamin D; and, of greatest concern because it is so common, if they have an iron deficiency. Iron deficiency weakens the body's defenses against lead absorption, and lead poisoning can cause iron deficiency. Common to both iron deficiency and lead poisoning are a low socioeconomic background and a lack of immunizations against infectious diseases. Another common factor is pica—a craving for nonfood

	Well-Nourished	Malnourished	Possible Nutrient Deficiencies
Hair	Shiny, firm in the scalp	Dull, brittle, dry, loose; falls out	Protein-energy malnutrition (PEM)
Eyes	Bright, clear; pink membranes; adjust easily to light	Pale membranes; spots; redness; adjust slowly to darkness	Vitamin A, the B vitamins, zinc, and iron
Teeth and gums	No pain or caries, gums firm, teeth bright	Missing, discolored, decayed teeth; gums bleed easily and are swollen and spongy	Minerals and vitamin C
Face	Clear complexion without dryness or scaliness	Off-color, scaly, flaky, cracked skin	PEM, vitamin A, and iron
Glands	No lumps	Swollen at front of neck, cheeks	PEM and iodine
Tongue	Red, bumpy, rough	Sore, smooth, purplish, swollen	B vitamins
Skin	Smooth, firm, good color	Dry, rough, spotty; "sandpaper" feel or sores; lack of fat under skin	PEM, essential fatty acids, vitamin A, B vitamins, and vitamin C
Nails	Firm, pink	Spoon-shaped, brittle, ridged	Iron
Internal systems	Regular heart rhythm, heart rate, and blood pressure; no impairment of digestive function, reflexes, or mental status	Abnormal heart rate, heart rhythm, or blood pressure; enlarged liver, spleen; abnormal digestion; burning, tingling of hands, feet; loss of balance, coordination; mental confusion, irritability, fatigue	PEM and minerals
Muscles and bones	Muscle tone; posture, long bone development appropriate for age	"Wasted" appearance of muscles; swollen bumps on skull or ends of bones; small bumps on ribs; bowed legs or knock-knees	PEM, minerals, and vitamin D

TABLE 11-4 Physical Signs of Health and Malnutrition in Children

items. Many children with lead poisoning eat dirt or chips of old paint, two common sources of lead.

The anemia brought on by lead poisoning may be mistaken for a simple iron deficiency and therefore may be incorrectly treated. Like iron deficiency, mild lead toxicity has nonspecific symptoms, including diarrhea, irritability, and fatigue. Adding iron to the diet does not reverse the symptoms; exposure to lead must stop and treatment for lead poisoning must begin. With further exposure, the symptoms become more pronounced, and children develop learning disabilities and behavior problems. Still more severe lead toxicity can cause irreversible nerve damage, paralysis, mental retardation, and death.

Recent research suggests that childhood lead exposure disrupts normal brain development—a finding that may partially explain the impaired cognitive and behavioral abilities of lead-exposed children. For six years, researchers measured blood lead levels at intervals in young children who lived in lead-contaminated houses.[23] Years later, brain images revealed that the higher the blood lead concentrations during childhood, the smaller the brain size as a young adult. The brains of boys were more affected than the brains of girls.

NURSING DIAGNOSIS

Risk for poisoning applies to children who have dangerous products placed within their reach.

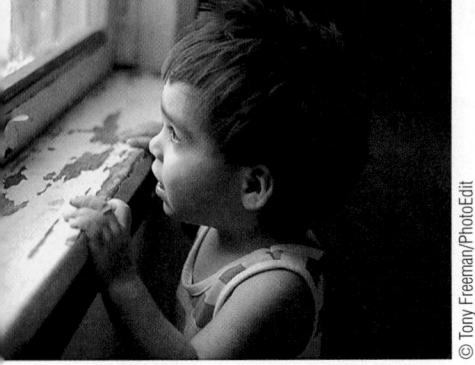
© Tony Freeman/PhotoEdit

Paint is the primary source of lead in children's lives.

More than 300,000 children in the United States—most of them under age six—have blood lead concentrations high enough to cause mental, behavioral, and other health problems.[24] Lead toxicity in young children comes from their own behaviors and activities—putting their hands in their mouths, playing in dirt and dust, and chewing on nonfood items.[25] Unfortunately, the body readily absorbs lead during times of rapid growth and hoards it possessively thereafter. Lead is not easily excreted and accumulates mainly in the bones but also in the brain, teeth, and kidneys. Tragically, a child's neuromuscular system is also maturing during these first few years of life. No wonder children with elevated lead levels experience impairment of balance, motor development, and the relaying of nerve messages to and from the brain. Deficits in intellectual development are only partially reversed when lead levels decline.[26]

Federal laws mandating reductions in leaded gasolines, lead-based solder, and other products over the past four decades have helped to reduce the amounts of lead in food and in the environment in the United States. As a consequence, the prevalence of lead toxicity in children has declined dramatically for most of the United States. Nevertheless, lead exposure is still a threat in certain communities. The accompanying "How to" presents strategies for defending children against lead toxicity.

HOW TO | Protect against Lead Toxicity

Researchers simultaneously made three major discoveries about lead toxicity: lead poisoning has *subtle* effects, the effects are *permanent*, and they occur at *low levels of exposure*. The amount of lead recognized to cause harm is only 10 micrograms per 100 milliliters of blood. Some research shows that blood lead concentration *below* this amount may adversely affect children's physical and mental development.[a] Consequently, consumers should take ultraconservative measures to protect themselves, and especially their infants and young children, from lead poisoning. The American Academy of Pediatrics and the Centers for Disease Control and Prevention recommend screening in communities with a substantial number of houses built before 1950 and in those with a substantial number of children with elevated lead levels. In addition to screening children most likely to be exposed, pediatricians should alert all parents to the possible dangers of lead exposure and explain prevention strategies.
Preventive strategies include:

- In contaminated environments, keep small children from putting dirty or old painted objects in their mouths, and make sure children wash their hands before eating. Similarly, keep small children from eating any nonfood items. Lead poisoning has been reported in young children who have eaten crayons or pool cue chalk.

- Wet-mop floors and damp-sponge walls regularly. Children's blood lead levels decline when the homes they live in are cleaned regularly.

- Be aware that other countries do not have the same regulations protecting consumers against lead. Children have been poisoned by eating crayons made in China, putting toys from China in their mouth, and drinking fruit juice canned in Mexico.

- Do not use lead-contaminated water to make infant formula.

- Once you have opened canned food, store it in a lead-free container to prevent lead migration into the food.

- Do not store acidic foods or beverages (such as vinegar or orange juice) in ceramic dishware or alcoholic beverages in pewter or crystal decanters.

- Many manufacturers are now making lead-safe products. Old, handmade, or imported ceramic cups and bowls may contain lead and should not be used to heat coffee or tea or acidic foods such as tomato soup.

- Feed children nutritious meals regularly.

- Before using your newspaper to wrap food, mulch garden plants, or add to your compost, confirm with the publisher that the paper uses no lead in its ink.

The Environmental Protection Agency (EPA) also publishes a booklet, *Lead and Your Drinking Water*, in which the following cautions appear:

- Have the water in your home tested by a competent laboratory.

- Use only cold water for drinking, cooking, and making formula (cold water absorbs less lead).

- When water has been standing in pipes for more than two hours, flush the cold-water pipes by running water through them for 30 seconds before using it for drinking, cooking, or mixing formulas.

- If lead contamination of your water supply seems probable, obtain additional information and advice from the EPA and your local public health agency.

By taking these steps, parents can protect themselves and their children from this preventable danger.[b]

[a] Centers for Disease Control and Prevention, Interpreting and managing blood lead levels <10 µg/dL in children and reducing childhood exposures to lead: Recommendations of CDC's Advisory Committee on Childhood Lead Poisoning Prevention, *Morbidity and Mortality Weekly Report* 56/RR-8 (2007): 1–16; Policy of Committee on Environmental Health, American Academy of Pediatrics: Lead exposure in children: Prevention, detection, and management, *Pediatrics* 116 (2005): 1036–1046.
[b] Call the National Lead Information Center hotline at (800) 424-LEAD (424-5323) for general information.

FOOD ALLERGY

Food allergy is frequently blamed for physical and behavioral abnormalities in children, but just 6 to 8 percent of children under four years of age are diagnosed with true food allergies.[27] Food allergies diminish with age, until in adulthood they affect less than 4 percent of the population.[28] The prevalence of food allergy, especially peanut allergy, is on the rise, however.[29] Reasons for an increase in peanut allergy are not yet clear, but possible contributing factors include genetics, food preparation methods (roasting peanuts at very high temperatures makes them more allergenic), and exposure to medicinal skin creams containing peanut oil.[30]

A true food allergy occurs when fractions of a food protein or other large molecule are absorbed into the blood and elicit an immunologic response. (Recall that proteins are normally dismantled in the digestive tract to amino acids that are absorbed without such a reaction.) The body's immune system reacts to these large food molecules as it does to other antigens—by producing antibodies or other defensive agents. (✚)(✚)

Asymptomatic and Symptomatic Allergies

Allergies may have one or two components. They always involve antibodies; they may or may not involve symptoms. A person may produce antibodies without having any symptoms (known as *asymptomatic allergy*) or may produce antibodies and have symptoms (known as *symptomatic allergy*). A person who experiences symptoms without producing antibodies, however, does not have an allergy. This means that allergies have to be diagnosed by testing for antibodies. Once a food allergy has been diagnosed, therapy requires strict elimination of the offending food. Children with allergies, like all children, need all their nutrients, so it is important to include other foods that offer the same nutrients as the omitted foods.[31]

Immediate and Delayed Reactions

Allergic reactions to food may be immediate or delayed. In either case, the antigen interacts immediately with the immune system, but symptoms may appear within minutes or after several (up to 24) hours. Identifying the food that causes an immediate allergic reaction is easy because symptoms correlate closely with the time of eating the food. Identifying the food that caused a delayed reaction is more difficult because the symptoms may not appear until a day after the offending food was eaten; by this time, many other foods will have been eaten, too, complicating the picture. Allergic reactions to single foods are common. Reactions to multiple foods are the exception, not the rule.

Anaphylactic Shock

The life-threatening food allergy reaction of **anaphylactic shock** is most often caused by peanuts, tree nuts, milk, eggs, wheat, soybeans, fish, or shellfish. Among these foods, eggs, milk, soy, and peanuts most often cause problems in children.[32] Children are more likely to outgrow allergies to eggs, milk, and soy than allergies to peanuts. Peanuts cause more life-threatening reactions than do all other food allergies combined. Research is currently under way to help those with peanut allergies tolerate small doses, thus saving lives and minimizing reactions.[33] One possible solution depends on finding a natural, hypoallergenic peanut among the 14,000 varieties. Families of children with a life-threatening food allergy and school personnel who supervise them must guard them against any exposure to the allergen. The child must learn to identify which foods pose a problem and then learn and use refusal skills for all foods that may contain the allergen.

✚ Reminder: *Antigens* are substances foreign to the body that elicit the formation of antibodies or an inflammation reaction from immune system cells. Food antigens are usually glycoproteins (large proteins with glucose molecules attached).

✚ Reminder: *Antibodies* are large proteins that are produced in response to antigens and then inactivate the antigens.

food allergy: an adverse reaction to food that involves an immune response; also called *food-hypersensitivity reactions.*

anaphylactic (AN-ah-feh-LAC-tic) shock: a life-threatening whole-body allergic reaction to an offending substance.

These eight normally wholesome foods—milk, shellfish, fish, peanuts, tree nuts, eggs, wheat, and soybeans (and soy products)—may cause life-threatening symptoms in people with allergies.

Parents of allergic children can pack safe foods for lunches and snacks and ask school officials to strictly enforce a "no swapping" policy in the lunchroom. The child must be able to recognize the symptoms of impending anaphylactic shock, (✚) such as a tingling of the tongue, throat, or skin, or difficulty breathing. Any person with food allergies severe enough to cause anaphylactic shock should wear a medical alert bracelet or necklace. Finally, the responsible child and the school staff should be prepared to administer injections of **epinephrine**, which prevents anaphylaxis after exposure to the allergen. Many preventable deaths occur each year when people with food allergies accidentally ingest the allergen but have no epinephrine.

Technology may soon offer new solutions. New drugs are being developed that may interfere with the immune response that causes allergic reactions.[34] Also, through genetic engineering, scientists may one day banish allergens from peanuts, soybeans, and other foods to make them safer.

Food Labeling

Food labels must list the presence of common allergens in plain language, using the names of the eight most common allergy-causing foods.[35] For example, a food containing "textured vegetable protein" must say "soy" on its label. Similarly, "casein" must be identified as "milk," and so forth. Food producers must also prevent cross-contamination during production and clearly label the foods in which it is likely to occur. For example, equipment used for making peanut butter must be scrupulously clean before being used to pulverize cashew nuts for cashew butter to protect unsuspecting cashew butter consumers from peanut allergens.

Other Adverse Reactions to Foods

Not all **adverse reactions** to foods are food allergies, although even physicians may describe them as such. Signs of adverse reactions to foods include stomachaches, headaches, rapid pulse rate, nausea, wheezing, hives, bronchial irritation, coughs, and other such discomforts. Among the causes may be reactions to chemicals in foods, such as the flavor enhancer monosodium glutamate (MSG), the natural laxative in prunes, or the mineral sulfur; digestive diseases, obstructions, or injuries; enzyme deficiencies, such as lactose intolerance; and even psychological aversions. These reactions involve symptoms but no antibody production. Therefore, they are **food intolerances**, not allergies.

Pesticides on produce may also cause adverse reactions. Pesticides that were applied in the fields may linger on the foods. Health risks from pesticide exposure may be low for healthy adults, but children are vulnerable. Therefore, government agencies have set a **tolerance level** for each pesticide by first identifying foods that children commonly eat in large amounts and then considering the effects of pesticide exposure during each developmental stage.

Food Dislikes

Parents are advised to watch for signs of food dislikes and take them seriously. Children's food aversions may be the result of nature's efforts to protect them from allergic or other adverse reactions. Test for allergies, and then apply nutrition knowledge conscientiously in deciding how to alter the diet.

HYPERACTIVITY

Hyperactivity affects behavior and learning in about 5 to 10 percent of young school-aged children.[36] Left untreated, it can interfere with a child's social development and ability to learn. Treatment focuses on relieving the symptoms and controlling the associated problems. Physicians often manage hyperactivity through behavior modification, special educational techniques, and psychological counseling. In many cases, they prescribe medication.[37]

Researchers have debated whether hyperactivity is due to a brain deficit or to a delay in brain development. Recent research supports the view that some areas in the brains of children with hyperactivity develop more slowly than those of other children.[38] Such findings remain controversial, but further support comes from the fact that hyperactivity symptoms tend to improve as children get older.

Parents of hyperactive children often blame sugar as the cause and mistakenly believe that simply eliminating candy and other sweet treats will solve the problem. Despite

✚ Symptoms of impending anaphylactic shock:
- Tingling sensation in mouth
- Swelling of the tongue and throat
- Irritated, reddened eyes
- Difficulty breathing, asthma
- Hives, swelling, rashes
- Vomiting, abdominal cramps, diarrhea
- Drop in blood pressure
- Loss of consciousness

epinephrine: one of the stress hormones secreted whenever emergency action is needed; prescribed therapeutically to relax the bronchioles during allergy or asthma attacks.

adverse reactions: unusual responses to food (including intolerances and allergies).

food intolerances: adverse reactions to foods or food additives that do not involve the immune system.

tolerance level: the maximum amount of residue permitted in a food when a pesticide is used according to the label directions.

hyperactivity: inattentive and impulsive behavior that is more frequent and severe than is typical of others of a similar age; professionally called **attention deficit/hyperactivity disorder (ADHD)**.

Freddie Willis is a six-year-old boy who seldom sits still, often misbehaves, and is frequently sick. Freddie's eating habits are erratic and poor, as is his appetite. He often misses breakfast because he is too tired to get up in time to eat before school. By midmorning, Freddie is irritable and disruptive in the classroom. At lunchtime he trades the peanut butter and banana sandwich his mother packed in his lunchbox for a piece of cake. After school he hurries home to watch television while he eats his favorite snack—cola and potato chips. At dinnertime Freddie picks at his food because he isn't very hungry. Later on, when it's time for bed, Freddie complains that he's hungry. His parents let him stay up to have a bowl of cereal (the kind with marshmallows) before he finally falls asleep.

1. What factors in Freddie's daily routine might be contributing to his restless behavior?

2. Discuss some changes in diet that might improve Freddie's health and disposition.

such speculation, which has been based on personal stories, studies have consistently found no convincing evidence that sugar causes hyperactivity or worsens behavior. Restricting dietary sugar will not cure hyperactivity.

Food additives have also been blamed for hyperactivity and other behavior problems in children, but scientific evidence to substantiate the connection has been elusive—until recently. A well-controlled study of close to 300 children suggests that food additives such as artificial colors or sodium benzoate preservative (or both) exacerbate hyperactive symptoms such as inattention and impulsivity.[39] Additional studies are needed to confirm the findings and to determine which additives studied might be responsible for negative behaviors.

Children can become excitable, rambunctious, and unruly as a result of a desire for attention, lack of sleep, overstimulation, watching too much television or playing too many computer games, too much caffeine from colas or chocolate, or a lack of physical activity. Such behaviors may suggest that more consistent care is needed. It helps to insist on regular hours of sleep, regular mealtimes, and regular outdoor activity. The accompanying Case Study offers an opportunity to think about these issues in relation to a specific child.

Review Notes

- Children's appetites and nutrient needs reflect their stage of growth.
- Long-term hunger and malnutrition impair growth and health.
- Short-term hunger exerts more subtle effects on children's health and behavior—such as poor academic performance.
- Iron deficiency is widespread and has many physical and behavioral consequences.
- Lead toxicity is prevalent among young children and can have irreversible effects on health and behavior.
- True food allergies are somewhat rare in children, and children can outgrow some food allergies.
- Some allergies, however, can cause dangerous, life-threatening reactions in both children and adults.
- "Hyper" behavior is not caused by poor nutrition; misbehavior may reflect inconsistent care.

CHILDHOOD OBESITY

The number of overweight children has increased dramatically over the past three decades (see Figure 11-3 on p. 328). Like their parents, children in the United States are becoming fatter. An estimated 32 percent of U.S. children and adolescents 2 to 19 years of age are overweight, and 17 percent are obese.[40] Based on data from the BMI-for-age

FIGURE
11-3 | Trends in Childhood Obesity

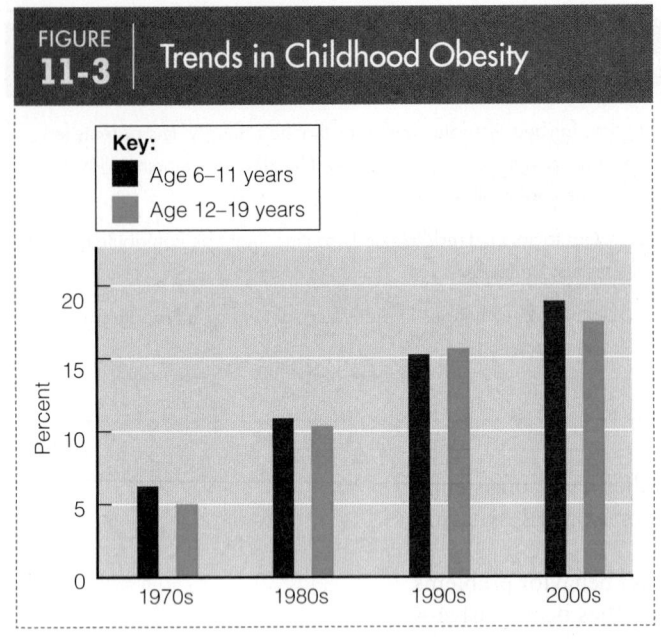

Key:
- ■ Age 6–11 years
- ■ Age 12–19 years

growth charts, children and adolescents are categorized as *overweight* above the 85th percentile and as *obese* at the 95th percentile and above.[41] There are exceptions to the use of the 85th and 95th percentile cutoff points. For older adolescents, BMI at the 95th percentile is higher than 30, the adult obesity cutoff point. Therefore, obesity in young people is defined as BMI at the 95th percentile or BMI of 30 or greater, whichever is lower. For children less than 2 years of age, BMI values are not available. For this age group, weight-for-height values above the 95th percentile are classified as overweight. Figures E-5A and E-5B in Appendix E present the BMI for children and adolescents, indicating cutoff points for obesity and overweight.

The Expert Committee of the American Medical Association recommends a third cutoff point (99th percentile) to define severe obesity in childhood.[42] Unfortunately, severe obesity in children is becoming more prevalent. Many of these children have multiple risk factors for cardiovascular disease and a high risk of severe obesity in adulthood.[43] The special risks and treatment needs of severely obese children need to be recognized.

The problem of obesity in children is especially troubling because overweight children have the potential of becoming obese adults with all the social, economic, and medical ramifications that often accompany obesity. They have additional problems, too, arising from differences in their growth, physical health, and psychological development. In trying to explain the rise in childhood obesity, researchers point to both genetic and environmental factors.

Genetic and Environmental Factors

Parental obesity predicts an early increase in a young child's BMI, and it more than doubles the chances that a young child will become an obese adult. Children with neither parent obese have a less than 10 percent chance of becoming obese in adulthood, whereas overweight teens with at least one obese parent have a greater than 80 percent chance of being obese adults. The chances of an obese child becoming an obese adult grow greater as the child grows older.[44] The link between parental and child obesity reflects both genetic and environmental factors (as described in Chapter 7).

Diet and physical inactivity must also play a role in explaining why children are heavier today than they were 30 or so years ago. As the prevalence of childhood obesity throughout the United States has more than doubled for young children and more than tripled for children 6 to 11 years of age and adolescents, the society our children live in has changed considerably.[45] In many families today, both parents work outside the home and work longer hours; more emphasis is placed on convenience foods and foods eaten away from home; meal choices at school are more diverse and often less nutritious; sedentary activities such as watching television and playing computer games occupy much of children's free time; and opportunities for physical activity and outdoor play both during and after school have declined.[46] All of these factors—and many others—influence children's eating and activity patterns.

Children learn food behaviors from their families, and research confirms the significant roles parents play in teaching their children about healthy food choices, providing nutrient-dense foods, and serving as role models.[47] When parents eat fruits and vegetables frequently, their children do, too.[48] The more fruits and vegetables children eat, the more vitamins, minerals, and fiber, and the less saturated fat, in their diets.[49]

As Chapter 3 discussed, as the prevalence of obesity among both children and adults has surged over the past four decades, so has the consumption of added sugars and, especially, high-fructose corn syrup—the easily consumed, energy-dense liquid sugar added to soft drinks.[50] Each 12-ounce can of soft drink provides the equivalent of about 10 teaspoons of sugar and 150 kcalories. More than half of school-age children consume at least one soft drink each day at school; adolescent males consume the most—four or more cans daily.[51] Research shows that soft drink consumption is associated with increased energy intake and body weight.[52] According to one estimate, the risk of obesity increases by 60 percent with each sugared soft drink consumed daily.

No doubt, the tremendous increase in soft drink consumption plays a role, but much of the obesity epidemic can be explained by lack of physical activity. Children have become more sedentary, and sedentary children are more often overweight.[53] Television watching (✚) may contribute most to physical inactivity. Excessive television time is linked with overweight in children.[54] A child who spends more than an hour or two each day in front of a television, computer monitor, or other media can become overweight even while eating fewer kcalories than a more active child. Playing video games influences children's activity patterns similarly.

Children who have television sets in their bedrooms spend more time watching TV, spend less time being physically active, and are more likely to be overweight than children who do not have televisions in their rooms.[55] Children who watch a great deal of television are most likely to be overweight and least likely to eat family meals or fruits and vegetables.[56] They often snack on the nutrient-poor, energy-dense foods that are advertised.[57] The average child sees an estimated 40,000 TV commercials a year—many peddling foods high in sugar, saturated fat, and salt such as sugar-coated breakfast cereals, candy bars, chips, fast foods, and carbonated beverages.[58] More than half of all food advertisements are aimed specifically at children and market their products as fun and exciting.[59] Not surprisingly, the more time children spend watching television, the more they request these advertised foods and beverages—and they get their requests about half of the time.[60] The most popular foods and beverages are marketed to children and adolescents on the Internet as well, using "advergaming" (advertised product as part of a game), cartoon characters or "spokes-characters," and designated children's areas.[61]

The physically inactive time spent watching television (and playing video and computer games) is second only to time spent sleeping. These activities use no more energy than resting, displace participation in more vigorous activities, and foster snacking on high-fat foods.[62] Simply reducing the amount of time spent watching television (and playing video games) can improve a child's BMI. The American Academy of Pediatrics (AAP) now recommends no television viewing before two years of age and thereafter limiting television and video time to two hours per day as a strategy to help prevent childhood obesity.[63]

Growth Overweight children develop a characteristic set of physical traits. They typically begin puberty earlier and so grow taller than their peers at first, but then they stop growing at a shorter height. They develop greater bone and muscle mass in response to the demand of having to carry more weight—both fat and lean weight. Consequently, they appear "stocky" even when they lose their excess fat.

Physical Health Like overweight adults, overweight children display a blood lipid profile indicating that atherosclerosis is beginning to develop—high levels of total cholesterol, triglycerides, and LDL cholesterol. Overweight children also tend to have high blood pressure; in fact, obesity is a leading cause of pediatric hypertension.[64] Their risks for developing type 2 diabetes and respiratory diseases (such as asthma) are also exceptionally high.[65] These relationships between childhood obesity and chronic diseases are discussed fully in Nutrition in Practice 11.

Psychological Development In addition to the physical consequences, childhood obesity brings a host of emotional and social problems.[66] Because people frequently judge others on appearance more than on character, overweight children are often victims of prejudice. Many suffer discrimination by adults and rejection by their peers. They may have poor self-images, a sense of failure, and a passive approach to life. Television shows, which are a major influence in children's lives, often portray the fat person as the bumbling misfit.[67] Overweight children may come to accept this negative stereotype in themselves and in others, which can lead to additional emotional and social problems. Researchers investigating children's reactions to various body

✚ TV fosters obesity because it:
- Requires no energy beyond basal metabolism.
- Replaces vigorous activities.
- Encourages snacking.
- Promotes a sedentary lifestyle.

types find that both normal-weight and underweight children respond unfavorably to overweight bodies.

Prevention and Treatment of Obesity Medical science has worked wonders in preventing or curing many of even the most serious childhood diseases, but obesity remains a challenge.[68] Once excess fat has been stored, it is challenging to lose. In light of all this, parents are encouraged to make major efforts to prevent childhood obesity, starting at birth, or to begin treatment early—before adolescence.[69] The Expert Committee of the American Medical Association recommends specific eating and physical activity behaviors to prevent obesity for all children (see Table 11-5).

Treatment of obesity must consider the many aspects of the problem and possible solutions. The main goal of obesity treatment is to improve long-term physical health through permanent healthy lifestyle habits.[70] The most successful approach integrates diet, physical activity, psychological support, and behavioral changes.[71] As a first step, the Expert Committee recommends that overweight and obese children and their families adopt the same healthy eating and activity behaviors presented in Table 11-5 for

TABLE 11-5	Recommended Eating and Physical Activity Behaviors to Prevent Obesity

The Expert Committee of the American Medical Association recommends the following healthy habits for children 2 to 18 years of age to help prevent childhood obesity:

- Limit consumption of sugar-sweetened beverages, such as soft drinks and fruit-flavored punches.

- Eat the recommended amounts of fruits and vegetables every day (2 to 4.5 cups per day based on age).

- Learn to eat age-appropriate portions of foods.

- Eat foods low in energy density such as those high in fiber and/or water and modest in fat.

- Eat a nutritious breakfast every day.

- Eat a diet rich in calcium.

- Eat a diet balanced in recommended proportions for carbohydrate, fat, and protein.

- Eat a diet high in fiber.

- Eat together as a family as often as possible.

- Limit the frequency of restaurant meals.

- Limit television watching or other screen time to no more than two hours per day, and do not have televisions or computers in sleeping areas.

- Engage in at least 60 minutes of moderate to vigorous physical activity every day.

Source: S. E. Barlow, Expert Committee recommendations regarding the prevention, assessment, and treatment of child and adolescent overweight and obesity: Summary report, *Pediatrics* 120 (2007): S164–S192.

obesity prevention. The goal for overweight and obese children is to improve BMI. If the child's BMI does not improve after several months, the Expert Committee recommends increasing the intensity of the treatment. The level of intensity depends on treatment response, age, degree of obesity, health risks, and the family's readiness to change. Advanced treatment involves close follow-up monitoring by a health care provider and greater support and structure for the child.[72]

Diet The initial goal for overweight children is to reduce the rate of weight gain, that is, to maintain weight as the child grows taller. Continued growth will then accomplish the desired change in BMI. Weight loss is usually not recommended because diet restriction can interfere with growth and development. Intervention for some overweight children with accompanying medical conditions may warrant weight loss, but this treatment requires an individualized approach based on the degree of overweight and severity of the medical conditions.[73] Dietary strategies begin with those listed in Table 11-5 and progress to more structured family meal plans when necessary. For example, the child or the parent may be instructed to keep detailed logs of dietary intake.

Physical Activity The many benefits of physical activity are well known but often are not enough to motivate overweight people, especially children. Yet regular vigorous activity can improve a child's weight, body composition, and physical fitness.[74] The *Physical Activity Guidelines for Americans 2008* make specific recommendations for children that can be used as a guide for how much activity children need. (✚) Ideally, parents will limit sedentary activities and encourage at least one hour of daily physical activity to promote strong skeletal, muscular, and cardiovascular development and instill in their children the desire to be physically active throughout life. Opportunities to be physically active can include team, individual, and recreational activities (see Figure 11-4). Most importantly, parents need to set a good example. Physical activity is a natural and lifelong behavior of healthy living. It can be as simple as riding a bike, playing tag, jumping rope, or doing chores. The AAP supports the efforts of schools to include more physical activity in the curriculum and encourages parents to support their children's participation.[75]

Psychological Support Weight-loss programs that involve parents and other caregivers in treatment report greater success than those without parental involvement. Because obesity in parents and their children tends to be positively correlated, both benefit when parents participate in a weight-loss program.

✚ *Physical Activity Guidelines for Americans 2008*
- Children and adolescents should engage in 60 minutes (1 hour) or more of physical activity daily.
- Aerobic: Most of the 60 or more minutes a day should be either moderate- or vigorous-intensity aerobic activity and should include vigorous-intensity physical activity at least three days a week.
- Muscle strengthening: As part of their 60 or more minutes of daily physical activity, children and adolescents should include muscle-strengthening physical activity on at least three days of the week.
- Bone strengthening: As part of their 60 or more minutes of daily physical activity, children and adolescents should include bone-strengthening physical activity on at least three days of the week.

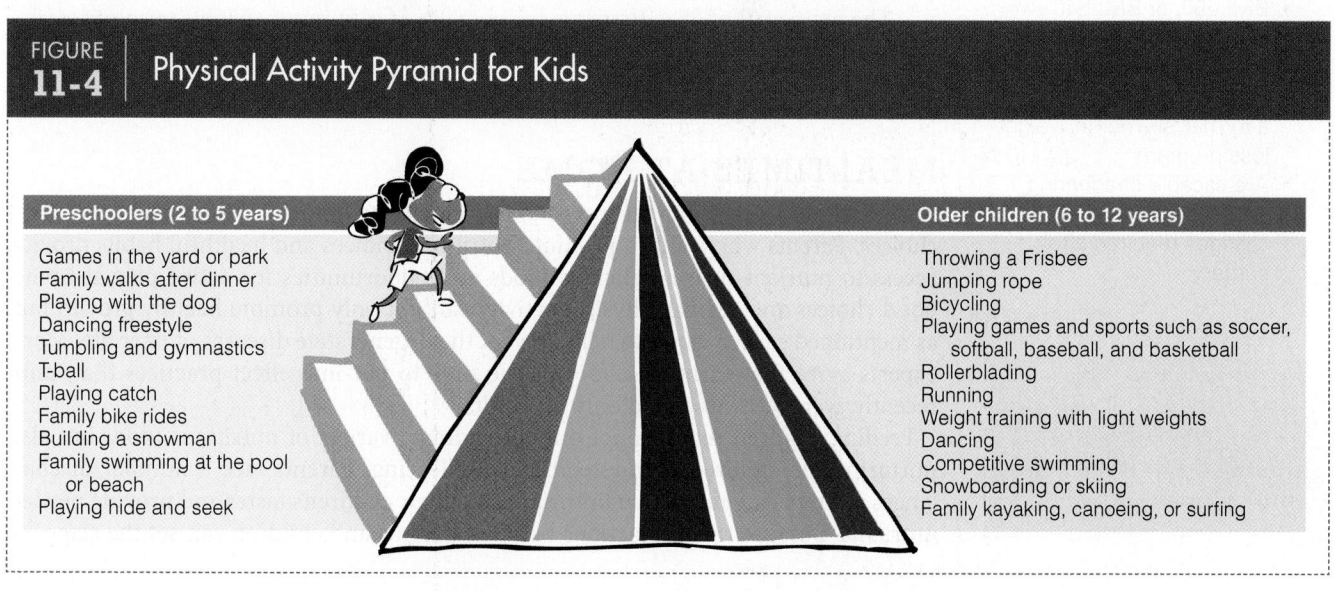

FIGURE 11-4 | Physical Activity Pyramid for Kids

Preschoolers (2 to 5 years)
Games in the yard or park
Family walks after dinner
Playing with the dog
Dancing freestyle
Tumbling and gymnastics
T-ball
Playing catch
Family bike rides
Building a snowman
Family swimming at the pool or beach
Playing hide and seek

Older children (6 to 12 years)
Throwing a Frisbee
Jumping rope
Bicycling
Playing games and sports such as soccer, softball, baseball, and basketball
Rollerblading
Running
Weight training with light weights
Dancing
Competitive swimming
Snowboarding or skiing
Family kayaking, canoeing, or surfing

Parental attitudes about food greatly influence children's eating behavior, so it is important that the influence be positive. Otherwise, eating problems may become exacerbated.

Behavioral Changes In contrast to traditional weight-loss programs that focus on *what* to eat, behavioral programs focus on *how* to eat. These techniques involve changing learned habits that lead a child to eat excessively.

Drugs The use of weight-loss drugs to treat obesity in children merits special concern because the long-term effects of these drugs on growth and development have not been studied.[76] The drugs may be used in addition to structured lifestyle changes for carefully selected children or adolescents who are at high risk for severe obesity in adulthood. Only two obesity drugs, orlistat and sibutramine (see Chapter 7), have been approved for limited use in children and adolescents.

Surgery The use of surgery to treat severe obesity in adults (see Chapter 7) has created interest in its use for adolescents. Limited research shows that, after surgery, extremely obese adolescents lose significant weight and experience improvements in type 2 diabetes and cardiovascular risk factors.[77] The selection criteria for surgery to treat obesity in adolescents (✚) are based on recommendations of a panel of pediatricians and surgeons.[78]

Obesity is prevalent in our society. Because treatment of obesity is frequently unsuccessful, it is most important to prevent its onset. Above all, be sensible in teaching children how to maintain appropriate body weight. Children can easily get the impression that their worth is tied to their body weight. Parents and the media are most influential in shaping self-concept, weight concerns, and dieting practices.[79] Some parents fail to realize that society's ideal of slimness can be perilously close to starvation and that a child encouraged to "diet" cannot obtain the energy and nutrients required for normal growth and development. Even healthy children without diagnosable eating disorders have been observed to limit their growth through "dieting." Weight gain in truly overweight children can be managed without compromising growth, but it should be overseen by a health care professional.

✚ Surgery may be an option for adolescents who meet the following criteria:
- Have reached physical maturity
- BMI ≥50, or BMI ≥40 with significant weight-related health problems
- Have experienced failure in a formal, six-month weight-loss program
- Are capable of adhering to the long-term lifestyle changes required after surgery

Review Notes

- Childhood obesity has become a major health problem.
- Genetics, diet, and physical inactivity play roles in childhood obesity.
- Childhood obesity can impair physical and psychological health.
- The main goal of obesity treatment in children is to improve long-term physical health through permanent healthy lifestyle habits.

MEALTIMES AT HOME

The childhood years are the parents' last chance to influence their children's food choices. Parents who want to promote nutritious choices and healthful habits provide access to nutrient-dense, delicious foods and opportunities for active play at home. Food choices and regular physical activity can not only promote healthy growth but, as mentioned earlier, can also help prevent the degenerative diseases of later life. Many experts agree that early childhood is the time to put into effect practices that, until recently, were recommended only for adults.

Feeding children requires not only providing a variety of nutritious foods but also nurturing the children's self-esteem and well-being. Parents face a number of challenges in preparing meals that both appeal to their children's tastes and provide needed nutrients. Because the interactions between parents and children can set the stage for lifelong attitudes and habits, a child's preferences should be treated with respect, even when nutrient needs must take precedence.

Honoring Children's Preferences Researchers attempting to explain children's food preferences encounter many contradictions. Children say they like colorful foods yet most often reject green and yellow vegetables while favoring brown peanut butter and white potatoes, apple wedges, and bread. They do like raw vegetables better than cooked ones, though, so it is wise to offer vegetables that are raw or slightly undercooked, crunchy, and bright in color. They should be warm, not hot, because a child's mouth is much more sensitive than an adult's. The flavor should be mild (a child has more taste buds), and smooth foods such as mashed potatoes or pea soup should have no lumps (a child wonders, with some disgust, what the lumps might be).

Eating is more fun when friends are there.

Young children like to eat at little tables and to be served little portions of food. They also love to eat with other children and have been observed to stay at the table longer and eat more food when in the company of their peers. Parents who serve food in a relaxed and casual manner, without anxiety, provide an environment in which a child's negative emotions will be minimized.

Avoiding Power Struggles Problems over food often arise during the second or third year, when children begin asserting their independence. Many of these problems stem from the conflict between children's developmental stages and capabilities and parents who, in attempting to do what they think is best for their children, try to control every aspect of eating. Such conflicts can disrupt children's abilities to regulate their own food intakes or to determine their own likes and dislikes. For example, many people share the misconception that children must be persuaded or coerced to try new foods. In fact, the opposite is true. When children are forced to try new foods, especially when offered rewards for eating a particular food (if you eat your vegetables, you can play video games), they are less likely to try those foods again than are children who are left to decide for themselves. Similarly, when children are restricted from eating their favorite foods, they are more likely to want those foods.[80] As dietitian and family therapist Ellyn Satter notes, the parent is responsible for *what* the child is offered to eat, but the child is responsible for *how much* and even *whether* to eat.

When introducing new foods at the table, parents are advised to offer them one at a time and only in small amounts at first. The more often a food is presented to a young child, the more likely the child will accept that food.[81] Between 5 and 10 exposures to a new food are necessary before a toddler shows an enhanced preference for the food. Offer the new food at the beginning of the meal, when the child is hungry, and allow the child to make the decision to accept or reject it. Parents have their own inclinations and dislikes; so do children. Never make an issue of food acceptance.

Choking Prevention Parents must always be alert to the dangers of choking. A choking child is silent, so an adult should be present whenever a child is eating. Make sure the child sits when eating; choking is more likely when a child is running or falling (see p. 304 for a list of foods and nonfood items most likely to cause choking).

Play First Ideally, each meal is preceded, not followed, by the activity the child looks forward to the most. A number of schools have discovered that children eat a much better lunch if it is served after, rather than before, recess. Otherwise, children "hurry up and eat" so that they can go play.

Child Participation Allowing children to help plan and prepare the family's meals provides enjoyable learning experiences and encourages children to eat the

TABLE 11-6	Food Skills of Preschool Children[a]

Age one to two years, when large muscles develop:
- Uses a spoon
- Helps feed self
- Lifts and drinks from a cup
- Helps scrub fruits and vegetables, tear lettuce or greens, snap green beans, or dip foods
- Wipes tables
- Places empty paper and plastic containers in recycle bins

Age three years, when medium hand muscles develop:
- Spears food with a fork
- Feeds self independently
- Adds ingredients to pancake batters, cookie recipes, salads, or other mixed dishes
- Helps wrap, pour, mix, shake, stir, or spread foods
- Helps crack nuts with supervision

Age four years, when small finger muscles develop:
- Uses all utensils and napkin
- Helps roll, juice, or mash foods
- Helps measure dry ingredients
- Cracks egg shells
- Helps make sandwiches and toss salads
- Peels foods such as hard-boiled eggs and bananas

Age five years, when fine coordination of fingers and hands develops:
- Measures liquids
- Helps grind, grate, and cut (soft foods with dull knife)
- Uses hand mixer with supervision

[a] These ages are approximate. Healthy, normal children develop at their own pace.

Source: Adapted from MyPyramid for Preschoolers, Kitchen activities, available at www.mypyramid.gov

foods they have prepared. Vegetables are pretty, especially when fresh, and provide opportunities for children to learn about color, growing things and their seeds, and shapes and textures—all of which are fascinating to young children. Measuring, stirring, decorating, and arranging foods are skills that even a very young child can practice with enjoyment and pride (see Table 11-6).

Snacks Parents may find that their children often snack so much that they aren't hungry at mealtimes. Instead of teaching children *not* to snack, teach them *how* to snack. Provide snacks that are as nutritious as the foods served at mealtime. Snacks can even be mealtime foods that are served individually over time, instead of all at once on one plate. When providing snacks to children, think of the food groups and offer such snacks as pieces of cheese, sliced strawberries, cooked baby carrots, and egg salad on whole-wheat crackers (see Table 11-7). Snacks that are easy to prepare should be readily available to children, especially if the children arrive home after school before their parents.

Preventing Dental Caries Children frequently snack on sticky, sugary foods that stay on the teeth and provide an ideal environment for the growth of bacteria that cause dental caries. Teach children to brush and floss after meals, to

TABLE
11-7

Healthful Snack Ideas—Think Food Groups, Alone and in Combination

Selecting two or more foods from different food groups adds variety and nutrient balance to snacks. The combinations are endless, so be creative.

Grain Products

Grain products are filling snacks, especially when combined with other foods:
- Cereal with fruit and milk
- Crackers and cheese
- Whole-grain toast with peanut butter
- Popcorn with grated cheese
- Oatmeal raisin cookies with milk

Vegetables

Cut-up fresh, raw vegetables make great snacks alone or in combination with foods from other food groups:
- Celery with peanut butter
- Broccoli, cauliflower, and carrot sticks with a flavored cottage cheese dip

Fruits

Fruits are delicious snacks and can be eaten alone—fresh, dried, or juiced—or combined with other foods:
- Apples and cheese
- Bananas and peanut butter
- Peaches with yogurt
- Raisins mixed with sunflower seeds or nuts

Meats and Meat Alternates

Meat and meat alternates add protein to snacks:
- Refried beans with nachos and cheese
- Tuna on crackers
- Luncheon meat on whole-grain bread

Milk and Milk Products

Milk can be used as a beverage with any snack, and many other milk products, such as yogurt and cheese, can be eaten alone or with other foods as listed above.

brush or rinse after eating snacks, to avoid sticky foods, and to select crisp or fibrous foods frequently.

Serving as Role Models In an effort to practice these many tips, parents may overlook perhaps the single most important influence on their children's food habits—themselves.[82] Parents who do not eat oranges should not be surprised when their children refuse to eat oranges. Likewise, parents who dislike the smell of brussels sprouts may not be able to persuade children to try them. Children learn much through imitation. Parents, older siblings, and other caregivers set an irresistible example by sitting with younger children, eating the same foods, and having pleasant conversations during mealtime.

While serving and enjoying food, caregivers can promote both physical and emotional health at every stage of a child's life. They can help their children to develop both a positive self-concept and a positive attitude toward food. If the beginnings are right, children will grow without the conflicts and confusions over foods that lead to nutrition and health problems.

NUTRITION AT SCHOOL

While parents are doing what they can to establish good eating habits in their children at home, others are preparing and serving foods to their children at day-care centers and schools. In addition, children begin learning about food and nutrition in the classroom. Meeting the nutrition and education needs of children is critical to supporting their healthy growth and development.[83]

The U.S. government funds programs to provide nutritious, high-quality meals for children at school. Both the School Breakfast Program and the National School Lunch Program provide meals at a reasonable cost to children from families with the financial means to pay. Meals are available free or at reduced cost to children from low-income families.

School Breakfast The School Breakfast Program (✚) is available in more than 80 percent of the nation's schools that offer school lunch, and 10 million children participate in it.[84] Nevertheless, many children who need the School Breakfast Program either do not have access to the program or do not participate in it.[85] The majority of children who eat school breakfasts are from low-income families. As research results continue to emphasize the positive impact breakfast has on school performance and health, vigorous campaigns to expand school breakfast programs are under way.[86]

School Lunch More than 30 million children receive lunches through the National School Lunch Program—more than half of them free or at a reduced price.[87] School lunches are designed to provide at least a third of the recommendation for energy, protein, vitamin A, vitamin C, iron, and calcium. They must also include specified numbers of servings from each food group. In an effort to help reduce cardiovascular disease risk, all government-funded meals served at schools must follow the Dietary Guidelines for Americans. (✚) Table 11-8 shows school lunch patterns for children of different ages.

Parents often rely on school lunches to meet a significant part of their children's nutrient needs on school days. Indeed, students who regularly eat school lunches have higher intakes of many nutrients and fiber than students who do not.[88] Children don't always like what they are served, however, and school lunch programs must strike a balance between what children want to eat and what will nourish them and guard their health.

Competing Influences at School Serving nutritious lunches is only half the battle; students need to eat them, too. Short lunch periods and long lines prevent some students from eating a school lunch and leave others with too little time to complete their meals.[89] Nutrition efforts at schools are also undermined when students can buy what the USDA labels "competitive foods"—meals from fast-food restaurants or a la carte foods such as pizza or snack foods and carbonated beverages from snack bars, school stores, and vending machines.[90] These foods and beverages compete with nutritious school lunches. Children receive a mixed message when they are left on their own to choose between the health-supporting school lunch and the high-fat, high-salt foods with low nutrient density that their taste buds may prefer. In one study, students who selected competitive foods in addition to, or instead of, school meals consumed more energy and fat and less calcium and vitamin A than those who selected only the school lunch.[91]

Increasingly, school-based nutrition issues are being addressed by legislation. Some states restrict the sale of competitive foods and have higher rates of participation in school meal programs than the national average. Federal legislation mandates that all

---

✚ The school breakfast must contain, at a minimum:
- One serving of fluid milk.
- One serving of fruit or vegetable or full-strength juice.
- Two servings of bread or bread alternatives, or two servings of meat or meat alternatives, or one of each.

✚ The American Dietetic Association has set nutrition standards for child-care programs. Among them, meal plans should:
- Be nutritionally adequate and consistent with the *Dietary Guidelines for Americans*.
- Involve parents in planning.
- Follow recommended meal patterns that balance energy and nutrients with children's ages, appetites, activity levels, and special needs while respecting cultural and ethnic differences.
- Minimize added fat, sugar, and sodium.
- Emphasize fresh fruit, fresh and frozen vegetables, and whole grains.
- Provide furniture and eating utensils that are age appropriate and developmentally suitable to encourage children to accept and enjoy mealtime.

Source: Position of the American Dietetic Association: Benchmarks for nutrition programs in child care settings, *Journal of the American Dietetic Association* 105 (2005): 979–986.

Nutrition Through the Life Span: Childhood and Adolescence

TABLE
11-8 | School Lunch Patterns for Different Ages[a]

Food Group	Preschool (Age)		Grade School through High School (Grade)		
	1 to 2	3 to 4	K to 3	4 to 6	7 to 12
Meat or meat alternative					
One serving:					
Lean meat, poultry, or fish	1 oz	1½ oz	1½ oz	2 oz	3 oz
Cheese	1 oz	1½ oz	1½ oz	2 oz	3 oz
Large egg(s)	½	¾	¾	1	1½
Cooked dry beans or peas	¼ c	⅜ c	⅜ c	½ c	¾ c
Peanut butter	2 tbs	3 tbs	3 tbs	4 tbs	6 tbs
Yogurt	½ c	¾ c	¾ c	1 c	1½ c
Peanuts, soynuts, tree nuts, or seeds[b]	½ oz	¾ oz	¾ oz	1 oz	1½ oz
Vegetable and/or fruit					
Two or more servings, both to total	½ c	½ c	½ c	¾ c	¾ c
Bread or bread alternative[c]					
Servings	5 per week	8 per week	8 per week	8 per week	10 per week
Milk					
One serving of fluid milk	¾ c	¾ c	1 c	1 c	1 c

[a] The quantities listed represent per-lunch minimums for each age and grade except those for the oldest group, which are recommendations. Schools unable to serve the recommended quantities for grades 7 to 12 must provide at least the amount shown for grades 4 to 6.

[b] These meat alternatives may be used to meet no more than half of the meat or meat alternative requirement; therefore, they must be used in a meal with another meat or meat alternative.

[c] Schools must serve daily at least a half serving of bread or bread alternative to the youngest age group and at least one serving to older children.

Source: U.S. Department of Agriculture, National School Lunch Program Regulations, revised January 1, 1998.

school districts that participate in the USDA's National School Lunch Program develop and put in place a local wellness policy.[92] By law, wellness policies must:[93]

- Set goals for nutrition education, physical activity, and other school-based activities.
- Establish nutrition guidelines for all foods available on school campuses during the school day.
- Develop a plan to measure policy implementation.

School districts across the nation have made progress toward meeting these goals, but implementation is inconsistent, and, because wellness policies are established locally, a great deal of variety exists among them. Some are well defined and detailed while others are vague and less detailed.[94] To enhance local wellness policies, standards (see Table 11-9 on p. 338) for competitive foods and beverages served in schools spell out appropriate fat, saturated fat, kcalorie, sugar, and sodium contents.[95] Establishing and implementing these nutrition standards for competitive foods and beverages helps to ensure that all foods served in schools are consistent and comply with the *Dietary Guidelines for Americans*.

Review Notes

- Adults at home and at school need to provide children with nutrient-dense foods and teach them how to make healthful choices.
- Adults also need to provide ample opportunity for children to be physically active.

Preferred Foods for All Students

Foods	Beverages
These foods are fruits, vegetables, whole grains, related combination products,[a] and nonfat and low-fat dairy that are limited to 200 kcalories or less per serving and: • No more than 35 percent of total kcalories from fat. • Less than 10 percent of total kcalories from saturated fats. • *Trans* fat free (≤0.5 g per serving). • 35 percent or less of kcalories from total sugars, except for yogurt with no more than 30 g of total sugars, per 8 oz portion as packaged. • Sodium content of 200 mg or less per portion as packaged.[b]	These beverages are: • Water without flavoring, additives, or carbonation. • Low-fat[c] and nonfat milk: • Lactose-free and soy beverages are included. • Flavored milk with no more than 22 g of total sugars per 8 oz serving. • 100 percent fruit juice in 4 oz portion for elementary/middle school and 8 oz for high school. • Caffeine free, with the exception of trace amounts of naturally occurring caffeine substances.

Snacks for High School Students after School

Foods	Beverages
Snack foods are those that do not exceed 200 kcalories per portion as packaged and: • No more than 35 percent of total kcalories from fat. • Less than 10 percent of total kcalories from saturated fats. • *Trans* fat free (≤0.5 g per serving). • 35 percent or less of kcalories from total sugars. • Sodium content of 200 mg or less per portion as packaged.	These beverages are: • Nonnutritive-sweetened, noncaffeinated, nonfortified beverages with less than 5 kcalories per portion as packaged.

[a] Combination products must contain a total of one or more servings as packaged of fruit, vegetables, or whole-grain products per portion.

[b] Á la carte entrée items meet fat and sugar limits and have a sodium content of 480 mg or less.

[c] 1 percent milk fat

Source: V. A. Stallings and A. L. Yaktine, eds., *Nutrition Standards for Foods in Schools: Leading the Way toward Healthier Youth.* Reprinted with permission from The National Academies Press, Copyright © 2009, National Academy of Sciences.

Nutrition during Adolescence

As children pass through **adolescence** on their way to becoming adults, they change in many ways. Their physical changes make their nutrient needs high, and their emotional, intellectual, and social changes make meeting those needs a challenge.

Teenagers make many more choices for themselves than they did as children. They are not fed; they eat. Food choices made during the teen years profoundly affect health, both now and in the future. At the same time, social pressures thrust choices at them: whether to drink alcoholic beverages and whether to develop their bodies to meet extreme ideals of slimness or athletic prowess. Their interest in nutrition—both valid information and misinformation—derives from personal, immediate experiences. They are concerned with how diet can improve their lives now—they try the latest fad diet to fit into a new bathing suit, avoid greasy foods in an effort to clear acne, or eat a plate of pasta to prepare for a big sporting event. In presenting information on the nutrition and health of adolescents, this chapter includes topics of interest to teens.

adolescence: the period of growth from the beginning of puberty until full maturity. Timing of adolescence varies from person to person.

GROWTH AND DEVELOPMENT DURING ADOLESCENCE

With the onset of adolescence, the steady growth of childhood speeds up abruptly and dramatically, and the growth patterns of females and males become distinct. Hormones direct the intensity and duration of the adolescent growth spurt, profoundly affecting every organ of the body, including the brain. After two to three years of intense growth and a few more at a slower pace, physically mature adults emerge.

In general, the adolescent growth spurt begins at age 10 or 11 for females and at age 12 or 13 for males. It lasts about two and a half years. Before **puberty,** male and female body compositions differ only slightly, but during the adolescent spurt, differences between the genders become apparent in the skeletal system, lean body mass, and fat stores. In females, fat assumes a larger percentage of total body weight, and in males, the lean body mass—principally muscle and bone—increases much more than in females. On average, males grow 8 inches taller, and females, 6 inches taller. Males gain approximately 45 pounds, and females, about 35 pounds.

ENERGY AND NUTRIENT NEEDS

The energy needs of adolescents vary greatly, depending on the current rate of growth, gender, body composition, and physical activity.[96] Boys' energy needs may be especially high; they typically grow faster than girls and, as mentioned, develop a greater proportion of lean body mass. An exceptionally active boy of 15 may need 3500 kcalories or more a day just to maintain his weight. Girls start growing earlier than boys and attain shorter heights and lower weights, so their energy needs peak sooner and decline earlier than those of their male peers. An inactive girl of 15 whose growth is nearly at a standstill may need fewer than 1800 kcalories a day if she is to avoid excessive weight gain. Thus, teenage girls need to pay special attention to being physically active and selecting foods of high nutrient density so that they will meet their nutrient needs without exceeding their energy needs.

Obesity The insidious problem of obesity becomes ever more apparent in adolescence and often continues into adulthood. The problem is most evident in African American females and in Hispanic children of both genders. Without intervention, overweight teens will face numerous physical and socioeconomic consequences for years to come. The consequences of obesity are so dramatic and our society's attitude toward obese people is so negative that even healthy-weight or underweight teens may perceive a need to lose weight. When taken to extremes, restrictive diets bring dramatic physical consequences of their own, as Nutrition in Practice 7 explains.

Vitamin D Recommendations for most vitamins increase during the teen years (see the tables on the inside front cover). Several of the vitamin recommendations for adolescents are similar to those for adults, including the recommendation for vitamin D. Vitamin D is essential for bone growth and development. Recent studies of vitamin D status in adolescents show that as many as half of adolescents are vitamin D deficient.[97] In light of this information, as well as evidence that adequate vitamin D may help prevent diseases such as diabetes and cancer, the American Academy of Pediatrics now recommends doubling the previous intake recommendation from 5 micrograms per day to 10 micrograms per day.[98] Adolescents who do not receive 10 micrograms of vitamin D from vitamin D–fortified foods such as milk (2.5 micrograms per cup) and cereals each day should take a supplement of 10 micrograms (400 IU on supplement labels).[99] Although one quart of vitamin D–fortified milk will provide the recommended amount, the majority of adolescents in the United States drink much less than this.

Iron The need for iron increases during adolescence for both females and males but for different reasons. Iron needs increase for females as they start to menstruate and for males as their lean body mass develops. Hence, the RDA increases at age 14 for both males and females. Because menstruation continues throughout a woman's

puberty: the period in life in which a person becomes physically capable of reproduction.

childbearing years, the RDA for iron remains high for women into late adulthood. For males, the RDA returns to preadolescent values in early adulthood.

In addition, iron needs increase when the adolescent growth spurt begins, whether that occurs before or after age 14. Therefore, boys in a growth spurt need an additional 2.9 milligrams of iron per day above the RDA for their age; girls need an additional 1.1 milligrams per day.

Furthermore, iron recommendations for girls before age 14 do not reflect the iron losses of menstruation, even though the average age of menarche (first menstruation) in the United States is 12.5 years. Therefore, for girls under the age of 14 who have started to menstruate, an additional 2.5 milligrams of iron per day is recommended. Thus, the RDA for iron depends not only on age and gender but also on whether the individual is in a growth spurt or has begun to menstruate, as listed in the margin. (✚)

Iron intakes often fail to keep pace with increasing needs, especially for females, who typically consume fewer iron-rich foods such as meat and fewer total kcalories than males. Not surprisingly, iron deficiency is most prevalent among adolescent girls. Iron-deficient children and teens score lower on standardized tests than those who are not iron deficient.

Calcium Adolescence is a crucial time for bone development, and the requirement for calcium reaches its peak during these years.[100] Unfortunately, low calcium intakes among adolescents have reached crisis proportions: 90 percent of females and 70 percent of males ages 12 to 19 years have calcium intakes below recommendations.[101] Low calcium intakes during times of active growth, especially if paired with physical inactivity, can compromise the development of peak bone mass, which is considered the best protection against adolescent fractures and adult osteoporosis. Increasing milk products in the diet to meet calcium recommendations greatly increases bone density.[102] Once again, however, teenage girls are most vulnerable, for their milk—and therefore their calcium—intakes begin to decline at the time when their calcium needs are greatest. Furthermore, women have much greater bone losses than men in later life. In addition to dietary calcium, physical activity makes bones grow stronger. However, because some high schools do not require students to attend physical activity classes, many adolescents must make a point to be physically active during leisure time.

FOOD CHOICES AND HEALTH HABITS

Teenagers like the freedom to come and go as they choose. They eat what they want if it is convenient and if they have the time. With a multitude of afterschool, social, and job activities, they almost inevitably fall into irregular eating habits. At any given time on any given day, a teenager may be skipping a meal, eating a snack, preparing a meal, or consuming food prepared by a parent or restaurant. Adolescents who frequently eat meals with their families, however, eat more fruits, vegetables, grains, and calcium-rich foods, and drink fewer soft drinks, than those who seldom eat with their families.[103] Some research shows that the more often teenagers eat dinner with their families, the less likely they are to smoke, drink, or use drugs; other research supports these findings only in teenage girls.[104] Many adolescents also begin to skip breakfast on a regular basis, missing out on important nutrients that are not made up at later meals during the day. Compared with those who skip breakfast, teenagers who do eat breakfast have higher intakes of vitamin A, vitamin C, and riboflavin, as well as calcium, iron, and zinc.[105] Teenagers who eat breakfast are therefore more likely to meet their nutrient recommendations.

Breakfast skipping may also lead to weight gain in adolescents. Research shows a dose-response, inverse relationship between breakfast eating and BMI.[106] As adolescents make the transition to adulthood, not only do they skip breakfast more often, they also eat fast food more often. Both skipping breakfast and eating fast foods lead to weight gain.[107]

✚ Iron RDA for males:
- 9-13 yr (8 mg/day)
- 9-13 yr in growth spurt (10.9 mg/day)
- 14-18 yr (11 mg/day)
- 14-18 yr in growth spurt (13.9 mg/day)

Iron RDA for females:
- 9-13 yr (8 mg/day)
- 9-13 yr in menarche (10.5 mg/day)
- 9-13 yr in menarche and growth spurt (11.6 mg/day)
- 14-18 yr (15 mg/day)
- 14-18 yr in growth spurt (16.1 mg/day)

Ideally, in light of adolescents' busy schedules and desire for freedom, the adult becomes a **gatekeeper,** controlling the type and availability of food in the teenager's environment. Teenage sons and daughters and their friends should find plenty of nutritious, easy-to-grab food in the refrigerator (meats for sandwiches; low-fat cheeses; fresh, raw vegetables and fruits; fruit juices; and milk) and more in the cabinets (whole-grain breads, peanut butter, nuts, popcorn, and cereal). In many households today, all the adults work outside the home, and teenagers perform some of the gatekeeper's roles, such as shopping for groceries or choosing fast or prepared foods.

Nutritious snacks contribute valuable nutrients to an active teen's diet.

Snacks On average, about a fourth of an adolescent's total daily energy intake comes from snacks, which, if chosen carefully, can contribute some of the needed nutrients (see Table 11-7 on p. 335). A survey of more than 4000 adolescents found that those who ate snacks more often had higher intakes of fruit compared with those who ate snacks less often.[108] However, adolescents frequently choose foods that are too high in added sugars, saturated fat, and sodium and too low in fiber to support the future health of their arteries.[109]

Beverages Most frequently, adolescents drink soft drinks instead of fruit juice or milk with lunch, supper, and snacks. About the only time they select fruit juices is at breakfast. When teens drink milk, they are more likely to consume it with a meal (especially breakfast) than as a snack. Because of their greater food intakes, boys are more likely than girls to drink enough milk to meet their calcium needs.

Soft drinks, when chosen as the primary beverage, may affect bone density, partly because they displace milk from the diet.[110] Over the past three decades, teens (especially girls) have been drinking more soft drinks and less milk. Adolescents who drink soft drinks regularly have a higher energy intake and a lower calcium intake than those who do not; they are also more likely to be overweight.[111]

Soft drinks containing caffeine present a different problem if caffeine intake becomes excessive. Caffeine seems to be relatively harmless, however, when used in moderate doses (the equivalent of fewer than, say, three 12-ounce cola beverages a day). (✚) In greater amounts, it can cause the symptoms associated with anxiety—sweating, tenseness, and inability to concentrate.

✚ Appendix A provides a table of the caffeine contents of beverages, foods, and medications.

✚ Chapter 13 offers details about nutrition assessment.

gatekeeper: with respect to nutrition, a key person who controls other people's access to foods and thereby exerts a profound impact on their nutrition. Examples are the spouse who buys and cooks the food, the parent who feeds the children, and the caregiver in a day-care center.

Eating Away from Home Adolescents eat about one-third of their meals away from home, and their nutritional welfare is enhanced or hindered by the choices they make. A lunch consisting of a hamburger, a chocolate shake, and french fries supplies substantial quantities of many nutrients at a kcalorie cost of about 800, an energy intake some adolescents can afford. When they eat this sort of lunch, teens can adjust their breakfast and dinner choices to include fruits and vegetables for vitamin A, vitamin C, folate, and fiber, and lean meats and legumes for iron and zinc. Fortunately, many fast-food restaurants are offering more nutritious choices than the standard hamburger meal.

Peer Influence Physical maturity and growing independence present adolescents with new choices. The consequences of those choices will influence their health and nutrition status both today and throughout life. Many of the food and health choices adolescents make reflect the opinions and actions of their peers. When others perceive milk as "babyish," a teen may choose soft drinks instead; when others skip lunch and hang out in the parking lot, a teen may join in for the camaraderie, regardless of hunger. Some teenagers begin using drugs, alcohol, and tobacco; others wisely refrain. Adults can set up the environment so that nutritious foods are available and can stand by with reliable information and advice about health and nutrition, but the rest is up to the adolescents. Ultimately, they make the choices.

Assessment of nutrition status in healthy children and adolescents can confirm that development is normal or can catch potential problems early. (✚) The Nutrition Assessment Checklist (p. 342) highlights problems to look for when working with children and adolescents.

Review Notes

- Nutrient needs rise dramatically as children enter the rapid growth phase of the teen years.
- The busy lifestyles of teenagers add to the challenge of meeting their nutrient needs, especially for iron and calcium.

Nutrition Assessment | CHECKLIST FOR CHILDREN AND ADOLESCENTS

MEDICAL HISTORY

Check the medical record for:

- ❍ Alcohol, tobacco, or illicit drug abuse
- ❍ Attention deficit/hyperactivity disorder (ADHD)
- ❍ Diabetes or other chronic disorders
- ❍ Eating disorders
- ❍ Food allergies
- ❍ Lactose intolerance
- ❍ Obesity
- ❍ Pregnancy

MEDICATIONS

For children or adolescents being treated with drug therapy for medical conditions, note:

- ❍ Side effects that might reduce food intake or change nutrient needs
- ❍ Proper administration of medication with respect to food intake

DIETARY INTAKE

For all children and adolescents, especially those considered at risk nutritionally, assess the diet for:

- ❍ Total energy
- ❍ Protein
- ❍ Calcium and iron
- ❍ Vitamin A, vitamin C, and folate
- ❍ Fiber

Note the following:

- ❍ Number of days each week a nutritious breakfast is eaten
- ❍ Number of hours the child or teen sleeps each day

- ❍ Number of soft drinks the child or teen drinks each day
- ❍ Number of fast-food meals eaten each day
- ❍ Number and type of snacks eaten each day
- ❍ Type and amount of physical activity
- ❍ Amount of caffeine consumed

ANTHROPOMETRIC DATA

Measure baseline height and weight.

- ❍ Reassess height, weight, and growth patterns at each medical checkup.
- ❍ Note significant obesity or underweight and intervention strategies employed.

LABORATORY TESTS

Monitor the following laboratory tests for children and adolescents:

- ❍ Hemoglobin, hematocrit, or other tests of iron status
- ❍ Blood glucose for children or adolescents with diabetes
- ❍ Blood lead concentrations

PHYSICAL SIGNS

Look for physical signs of:

- ❍ Protein-energy malnutrition
- ❍ Iron deficiency
- ❍ Vitamin A deficiency
- ❍ Vitamin C deficiency
- ❍ Folate deficiency

Self-Check

1 • Which of the following is a characteristic of iron deficiency in children?
   a. It rarely develops in those with high intakes of milk.
   b. It affects brain function before anemia sets in.
   c. It is a primary factor in hyperactivity.
   d. Milk deficiency enhances mental performance by lowering physical activity level, thereby leading to increased attention span.

2 • Three symptoms of lead toxicity are:
   a. diarrhea, irritability, and fatigue.
   b. low blood sugar, hair loss, and skin rash.
   c. increased heart rate, hyperactivity, and dry skin.
   d. bleeding gums, brittle fingernails, and swollen glands.

3 • Allergic reactions to foods are more often caused by:
   a. corn, rice, or meats.
   b. eggs, peanuts, or milk.

   c. red meats, milk, or MSG.
   d. seafood, dark greens, or lactose.

4 • When introducing new foods to children:
   a. reward children as they try new foods.
   b. offer many choices to encourage variety.
   c. offer one new food at the end of the meal.
   d. offer one new food at the beginning of the meal.

5 • Which of the following is *not* true? Children who watch a lot of television are likely to:
   a. become obese.
   b. spend less time being physically active.
   c. learn healthy eating tips from programs.
   d. eat the foods most often advertised on television.

6 • Which of the following strategies is *not* effective?
   a. Play first, eat later.
   b. Provide small portions.
   c. Encourage children to help prepare meals.
   d. Use dessert as a reward for eating vegetables.

7 • During the growth spurt of adolescence:
   a. females gain more weight than males.
   b. males gain more fat, proportionately, than females.
   c. differences in body composition between males and females become apparent.
   d. similarities in body composition between males and females become apparent.

8 • Two nutrients that are usually lacking in adolescents' diets are:
   a. zinc and fat.
   b. iron and calcium.
   c. protein and thiamin.
   d. vitamin A and riboflavin.

9 • To help teenagers consume a balanced diet, parents can:
   a. monitor the teens' food intake.
   b. give up—parents can't influence teenagers.
   c. keep the cabinets and refrigerator well stocked.
   d. forbid snacking and insist on regular, well-balanced meals.

10• To balance the day's intake, an adolescent who eats a hamburger, fries, and chocolate shake at lunch might benefit most from a dinner of:
   a. fried chicken, rice, and banana.
   b. ribeye steak, baked potato, and salad.
   c. pork chop, mashed potatoes, and apple juice.
   d. spaghetti with meat sauce, broccoli, and milk.

Answers to these questions are in Appendix H.

Clinical Applications

1 • At two and a half years old, Travis is healthy, though slightly underweight, and headstrong. Travis's mother hovers over him at every meal and insists that he take several bites of every food on his plate, even if he dislikes the food or is not familiar with it. Even though Travis is hungry when he sits down to a meal, his mother's constant urging to get him to eat quickly quells any interest he had in eating. Travis simply folds his arms across his chest, closes his mouth tightly, and refuses to eat any more food. After more begging, pleading, and nagging, Travis's mother becomes angry and sends him away from the table. Travis is not allowed to snack between meals because his mother is concerned that snacks will ruin his appetite.

   • What factors might be contributing to Travis's refusal to eat?
   • Travis's mother is concerned about her son's underweight. What strategies would you suggest to help Travis gain weight?
   • What advice would you offer Travis's mother to help her improve mealtimes with her son?

2 • Loni is a physically inactive, overweight 15-year-old girl who enjoys watching television and playing computer games in her spare time. She typically buys a cola and bag of chips from the vending machine for lunch and then stops by a fast-food restaurant after school for chicken nuggets or a hamburger with french fries. She has noticed that she has gained weight and lacks energy.

   • What nutrients might be excessive or lacking in her current diet plan?
   • What dietary advice would you offer to help Loni look and feel healthier?
   • What would you tell Loni to motivate her to become physically active?

Nutrition on the Net

For further study of the topics in this chapter, access these websites.

• For further study of topics covered in this chapter, log on to **www.cengage.com/nutrition/whitney/nhhc4e**. Go to Chapter 11, and then click on Student Resources.
• Learn how to care for children and adolescents from the American Academy of Pediatrics and the Canadian Paediatric Society: **www.aap.org** and **www.cps.ca**
• Download the current growth charts, and learn about their most recent revision: **www.cdc.gov/growthcharts**
• Get information on MyPyramid for young children from the USDA: **www.mypyramid.gov**
• Get tips for keeping children healthy from the Nemours Foundation: **www.kidshealth.org**
• Visit the National Center for Education in Maternal and Child Health and the National Institute of Child Health and Human Development: **www.ncemch.org** and **www.nichd.nih.gov/**

- Learn about child nutrition programs: www.fns.usda.gov/fns
- Learn how to reduce lead exposure in your home from the U.S. Department of Housing and Urban Development's Office of Lead Hazard Control: www.hud.gov/lead
- Learn more about food allergies from the American Academy of Allergy, Asthma, and Immunology; the Food Allergy and Anaphylaxis Network; and the International Food Information Council: www.aaaai.org, www.foodallergy.org, and www.ific.org
- Learn more about hyperactivity from Children and Adults with Attention Deficit/Hyperactivity Disorder: www.chadd.org

- Learn how to help children develop positive body images and relate to food in a healthy way: www.womenshealth.gov/bodyimage/kids
- Visit the Milk Matters section of the National Institute of Child Health and Human Development (NICHD): www.nichd.nih.gov/milk/milk.cfm
- Get weight-loss tips for children and adolescents: www.shapedown.com
- Read the message for parents and teens on the risks of tobacco use from the American Academy of Pediatrics: www.aap.org/healthtopics/tobacco.cfm
- Visit the Tobacco Information and Prevention Source (TIPS) of the Centers for Disease Control and Prevention: http://cdc.gov/tobacco/

Notes

1. L. L. Moore and coauthors, Effects of average childhood dairy intake on adolescent bone health, *Journal of Pediatrics* 153 (2008): 667–673; K. S. Ondrak and D. W. Morgan, Physical activity, calcium intake and bone health in children and adolescents, *Sports Medicine* 37 (2007): 587–600.
2. M. K. Fox and coauthors, Relationship between portion size and energy intake among infants and toddlers: Evidence of self-regulation, *Journal of the American Dietetic Association* 106 (2006): S77–S83.
3. Position of the American Dietetic Association: Nutrition guidance for healthy children ages 2 to 11 years, *Journal of the American Dietetic Association* 108 (2008): 1038–1047; Position of the American Dietetic Association: Individual-, family-, school-, and community-based interventions for pediatric overweight, *Journal of the American Dietetic Association* 106 (2006): 925–945.
4. American Academy of Pediatrics, Council on Sports Medicine and Fitness and Council on School Health, Active healthy living: Prevention of childhood obesity through increased physical activity, *Pediatrics* 117 (2006): 1834–1842.
5. Nutritional aspects of vegetarian diets, in *Pediatric Nutrition Handbook*, 6th ed., ed. R. E. Kleinman (Elk Grove Village, IL: American Academy of Pediatrics, 2009), pp. 201–224.
6. Committee on the Scientific Evaluation of Dietary Reference Intakes, Food and Nutrition Board, Institute of Medicine, *Dietary Reference Intakes for Energy, Carbohydrate, Fiber, Fat, Fatty Acids, Cholesterol, Protein, and Amino Acids* (Washington, D.C.: National Academies Press, 2005), pp. 265–338.
7. Committee on the Scientific Evaluation of Dietary Reference Intakes, 2005, pp. 339–421.
8. Committee on the Scientific Evaluation of Dietary Reference Intakes, 2005, pp. 769–879.
9. Committee on the Scientific Evaluation of Dietary Reference Intakes, 2005, pp. 422–541.
10. J. M. Brotanek and coauthors, Iron deficiency in early childhood in the United States: Risk factors and racial/ethnic disparities, *Pediatrics* 120 (2007): 568–575; K. C. White, Anemia is a poor predictor of iron deficiency among toddlers in the United States: For heme the bell tolls, *Pediatrics* 115 (2005): 315–320.
11. C. L. Wagner and F. R. Greer, and the Section on Breastfeeding and Committee on Nutrition, Prevention of rickets and vitamin D deficiency in infants, children, and adolescents, *Pediatrics* 122 (2008): 1142–1152.
12. Feeding the child, in *Pediatric Nutrition Handbook*, 6th ed., ed. R. E. Kleinman (Elk Grove Village, IL: American Academy of Pediatrics, 2009), pp. 145–174.
13. U. Shaikh, R. S. Byrd, and P. Auinger, Vitamin and mineral supplement use by children and adolescents in the 1999-2004 National Health and Nutrition Examination Survey: Relationship with nutrition, food security, physical activity, and health care access, *Archives of Pediatrics and Adolescent Medicine* 163 (2009): 150–157; R. Briefel and coauthors, Feeding Infants and Toddlers Study: Do vitamin and mineral supplements contribute to nutrient adequacy or excess among U.S. infants and toddlers? *Journal of the American Dietetic Association* 106 (2006): S52–S65.
14. Position of the American Dietetic Association, 2008.
15. P. Ziegler and coauthors, Feeding Infants and Toddlers Study (FITS): Development of the FITS survey in comparison to other dietary survey methods, *Journal of the American Dietetic Association* 106 (2006): S12–S27.
16. J. Stang, Improving the eating patterns of infants and toddlers, *Journal of the American Dietetic Association* 106 (2006): S7–S9.
17. M. Vadiveloo, L. Zhu, and P. A. Quatromoni, Diet and physical activity patterns of school-aged children, *Journal of the American Dietetic Association* 109 (2009): 145–151; Position of the American Dietetic Association, 2008.
18. Bread for the World, Hunger facts: Domestic, available at www.bread.org/learn/hunger-basics/hunger-facts-domestic.html, updated February, 2008; accessed on January 23, 2009.
19. K. Widenhorn-Muller and coauthors, Influence of having breakfast on cognitive performance and mood in 13- to 20-year-old high school students: Results of a crossover trial, *Pediatrics* 122 (2008): 279–284.
20. W. O. Song and coauthors, Ready-to-eat breakfast cereal consumption enhances milk and calcium intake in the U.S. population, *Journal of the American Dietetic Association* 106 (2006): 1783–1789; G. C. Rampersaud and coauthors, Breakfast habits, nutritional status, body weight, and academic performance in children and adolescents, *Journal of the American Dietetic Association* 105 (2005): 743–760; S. G. Affenito and coauthors, Breakfast consumption by African-American and white adolescent girls correlates positively with calcium and fiber intake and negatively with body mass index, *Journal of the American Dietetic Association* 105 (2005): 938–945.
21. J. C. McCann and B. N. Ames, An overview of evidence for a causal relation between iron deficiency during development and deficits in cognitive or behavioral function, *American Journal of Clinical Nutrition* 85 (2007): 931–945.
22. B. Lozhoff and coauthors, Long-lasting neural and behavioral effects of iron deficiency in infancy, *Nutrition Reviews* 64 (2006): S34–S43.
23. K. M. Cecil and coauthors, Decreased brain volume in adults with childhood lead exposure, *PLos Medicine* 27 (2008): e112.
24. Centers for Disease Control and Prevention, General lead information: Questions and answers, available at www.cdc.gov/nceh/lead/faq/about.htm, accessed January 23, 2009.
25. Centers for Disease Control and Prevention, Interpreting and managing blood lead levels <10µg/dL in children and reducing childhood exposures to lead: Recommendations of CDC's Advisory Committee on Childhood Lead Poisoning Prevention, *Morbidity and Mortality Weekly Report* 56/RR-8 (2007): 1–16; Committee on Environmental Health, American Academy of Pediatrics, Policy statement: Lead exposure in children: Prevention, detection, and management, *Pediatrics* 116 (2005): 1036–1046.
26. Committee on Environmental Health, American Academy of Pediatrics, 2005.
27. National Institutes of Health, National Institute of Allergy and Infectious Diseases, *Food Allergy: Report of the NIH Expert Panel on Food Allergy Research*, March 13-14, 2006, available at www.naid.nih.gov.
28. National Institutes of Health, National Institute of Allergy and Infectious Diseases, 2006.
29. U.S. Food and Drug Administration, Food allergies: Reducing the risks, January 23, 2009, available at www.fda.gov/consumer/updates/foodallergies012209.html.
30. A. Boulay and coauthors, A EuroPrevall review of factors affecting incidence of peanut allergy: Priorities for research and policy, *Allergy* 63 (2008): 797–809; L. A. Lee and A. W. Burks, Food allergies: Prevalence, molecular characterization, and treatment/prevention strategies, *Annual Review of Nutrition* 26 (2006): 539–565.

31. M. Boguniewica, N. Moore, and K. Paranto, Allergic diseases, quality of life, and the role of the dietitian, *Nutrition Today* 43 (2008): 6–10.

32. S. Ramesh, Food allergy overview in children, *Clinical Reviews in Allergy and Immunology* 34 (2008): 217–230.

33. L. A. Lee and A. W. Burks, Food allergies: Prevalence, molecular characterization, and treatment/prevention strategies, *Annual Review of Nutrition* 26 (2006): 539–565.

34. National Institutes of Health, National Institute of Allergy and Infectious Diseases, 2006.

35. Lee and Burks, 2006.

36. P. N. Pastor and C. A. Reuben, Diagnosed attention deficit hyperactivity disorder and learning disability: United States, 2004-2006, *Vital and Health Statistics, Series 10, Data from the National Health Survey* 237 (2008): 1–14; E. Romano and coauthors, Development and prediction of hyperactive symptoms from 2 to 7 years in a population-based sample, *Pediatrics* 117 (2006): 2101–2109.

37. M. L. Wolraich and coauthors, Attention-deficit/hyperactivity disorder among adolescents: A review of the diagnosis, treatment, and clinical implications, *Pediatrics* 115 (2005): 1734–1746.

38. K. Rubia, Neuro-anatomic evidence for the maturational delay hypothesis of ADHD, *Proceedings of the National Academy of Sciences* 104 (2007): 19663–19664.

39. D. McCann and coauthors, Food additives and hyperactive behaviour in 3-year-old and 8/9-year-old children in the community: A randomized, double-blinded, placebo-controlled trial, *Lancet* 370 (2007): 1560–1567.

40. C. L. Ogden and coauthors, Prevalence of high body mass index in U.S. children and adolescents, 2007-2008, *Journal of the American Medical Association* 303 (2010): 242–249.

41. S. E. Barlow and the Expert Committee, Expert Committee recommendations regarding the prevention, assessment, and treatment of child and adolescent overweight and obesity: Summary report, *Pediatrics* 120 (2007): S164–S192.

42. Barlow and the Expert Committee, 2007.

43. D. S. Freedman and coauthors, Cardiovascular risk factors and excess adiposity among overweight children and adolescents: The Bogalusa Heart Study, *Journal of Pediatrics* 150 (2007): 12–17.

44. N. F. Krebs and coauthors, Assessment of child and adolescent overweight and obesity, *Pediatrics* 120 (2007): S193–S228.

45. Barlow and the Expert Committee, 2007.

46. B. A. Spear and coauthors, Recommendations for treatment of child and adolescent overweight and obesity, *Pediatrics* 120 (2007): S254–S287; S. L. Martin, S. M. Lee, and R. Lowry, National prevalence and correlates of walking and bicycling to school, *American Journal of Preventive Medicine* 33 (2007): 98–105; American Academy of Pediatrics, Council on Sports Medicine and Fitness and Council on School Health, 2006; J. P. Koplan, C. T. Liverman, and V. I. Kraak, eds., *Preventing Childhood Obesity: Health in the Balance* (Washington, D.C.: National Academies Press, 2005), pp. 79–123.

47. K. J. Campbell and coauthors, Associations between the home food environment and obesity-promoting eating behaviors in adolescence, *Obesity* 15 (2007): 719–730; Barlow and the Expert Committee, 2007.

48. K. S. Geller and D. A. Dzewaltowski, Longitudinal and cross-sectional influences on youth fruit and vegetable consumption, *Nutrition Reviews* 67 (2009): 65–76; J. Brug and coauthors, Taste preferences, liking and other factors related to fruit and vegetable intakes among schoolchildren: Results from observational studies, *British Journal of Nutrition* 99 (2008): S7–S14; C. A. Forestell and J. A. Mennella, Early determinants of fruit and vegetable acceptance, *Pediatrics* 120 (2007): 1247–1254; C. Arcan and coauthors, Parental eating behaviours, home food environment and adolescent intakes of fruits, vegetables and dairy foods: Longitudinal finding form Project EAT, *Public Health Nutrition* 11 (2007): 1257–1265; M. Wind and coauthors, Correlates of fruit and vegetable consumption among 11-year-old Belgian-Flemish and Dutch schoolchildren, *Journal of Nutrition Education and Behavior* 38 (2006): 211–221.

49. K. E. Leahy, L. L. Birch, and B. Rolls, Reducing the energy density of multiple meals decreases the energy intake of preschool-age children, *American Journal of Clinical Nutrition* 88 (2008): 1459–1468.

50. S. N. Bleich and coauthors, Increasing consumption of sugar-sweetened beverages among U.S. adults: 1988-1994 to 1999-2004, *American Journal of Clinical Nutrition* 89 (2009): 372–381; Spear and coauthors, 2007; L. DuBois and coauthors, Regular sugar-sweetened beverage consumption between meals increases risk of overweight among preschool-aged children, *Journal of the American Dietetic Association* 107 (2007): 924–934; V. S. Malik, M. B. Schultz, and F. B. Hu, Intake of sugar-sweetened beverages and weight gain: A systematic review, *American Journal of Clinical Nutrition* 84 (2006): 274–288.

51. S. Harrington, The role of sugar-sweetened beverage consumption in adolescent obesity: A review of the literature, *Journal of School Nursing* 24 (2008): 3–12; Committee on School Health, American Academy of Pediatrics, Soft drinks in schools, *Pediatrics* 113 (2004): 152–154.

52. L. R. Vartanian, M. B. Schwartz, and K. D. Brownell, Effects of soft drink consumption on nutrition and health: A systematic review and meta-analysis, *American Journal of Public Health* 97 (2007): 667–675.

53. American Academy of Pediatrics, Council on Sports Medicine and Fitness and Council on School Health, 2006.

54. S. Gable, Y. Chang, and J. L. Drull, Television watching and frequency of family meals are predictive of overweight onset and persistence in a national sample of school-aged children, *Journal of the American Dietetic Association* 107 (2007): 53–61; Spear and coauthors, 2007.

55. D. J. Barr-Anderson and coauthors, Characteristics associated with older adolescents who have a television in their bedrooms, *Pediatrics* 121 (2008): 718–724; A. M. Adachi-Mejia and coauthors, Children with a TV in their bedroom at higher risk for being overweight, *International Journal of Obesity* 31 (2007): 644–651.

56. L. Dubois and coauthors, Social factors and television use during meals and snacks is associated with higher BMI among pre-school children, *Public Health Nutrition* 11 (2008): 1267–1279; S. Gable, Y Chang, and J. L. Krull, Television watching and frequency of family meals are predictive of overweight onset and persistence in a national sample of school-aged children, *Journal of the American Dietetic Association* 107 (2007): 53–61.

57. J. L. Wiecha and coauthors, When children eat what they watch: Impact of television viewing on dietary intake in youth, *Archives of Pediatrics & Adolescent Medicine* 160 (2006): 436–442; S. C. Folta and coauthors, Food advertising targeted at school-age children: A content analysis, *Journal of Nutrition Education and Behavior* 38 (2006): 244–248.

58. A. Batada and coauthors, Nine out of 10 food advertisements shown during Saturday morning children's television programming are for foods high in fat, sodium, or added sugars, or low in nutrients, *Journal of the American Dietetic Association* 108 (2008): 673–678; L. M. Powell and coauthors, Nutritional content of television food advertisements seen by children and adolescents in the United States, *Pediatrics* 120 (2007): 576–583; J. L. Wiecha and coauthors, 2006.

59. S. M. Connor, Food-related advertising on preschool television: Building brand recognition in young viewers, *Pediatrics* 118 (2006): 1478–1485; Folta and coauthors, 2006.

60. L. J. Chamberlain, Y. Wang, and T. N. Robinson, Does children's screen time predict requests for advertised products? Cross-sectional and prospective analyses, *Archives of Pediatrics & Adolescent Medicine* 160 (2006): 363–368; Y. Aktas-Arnas, The effects of television food advertisement on children's food purchasing requests, *Pediatrics International* 48 (2006): 138–145; M. O'Dougherty, M. Story, and J. Stang, Observations of parent-child co-shoppers in supermarkets: Children's involvement in food selections, parental yielding, and refusal strategies, *Journal of Nutrition Education and Behavior* 38 (2006): 183–188.

61. K. Weber, M. Story, and L. Harnack, Internet food marketing strategies aimed at children and adolescents: A content analysis of food and beverage brand web sites, *Journal of the American Dietetic Association* 106 (2006): 1463–1466.

62. Spear and coauthors, 2007.

63. Barlow and the Expert Committee, 2007.

64. M. Salvadori and coauthors, Elevated blood pressure in relation to overweight and obesity among children in a rural Canadian community, *Pediatrics* 122 (2008): e821–e827; R. Jago and coauthors, Prevalence of abnormal lipid and blood pressure values among an ethnically diverse population of eighth-grade adolescents and screening implications, *Pediatrics* 117 (2006): 2065–2073.

65. K. L. Jones, Role of obesity in complicating and confusing the diagnosis and treatment of diabetes in children, *Pediatrics* 121 (2008): 361–368; S. Cook and coauthors, Metabolic Syndrome rates in United States adolescents, from the National Health and Nutrition Examination Survey, 1999-2002, *Journal of Pediatrics* 152 (2008): 165–170; C. L. Carroll and coauthors, Childhood overweight increases hospital admission rates for asthma, *Pediatrics* 120 (2007): 734–740; M. L. Cruz and coauthors, Pediatric obesity and insulin resistance: Chronic disease risk and implications for treatment and prevention beyond body weight modification, *Annual Review of Nutrition* 25 (2005): 435–468.

66. D. S. Ludwig, Childhood obesity—The shape of things to come, *New England Journal of Medicine* 357 (2007): 2325–2326; J. Franklin and coauthors, Obesity and risk of low self-esteem: A statewide survey of Australian children, *Pediatrics* 118 (2006): 2481–2487; A. J. Daley and coauthors, Exercise therapy as a treatment for psychopathologic conditions in obese and morbidly obese adolescents: A randomized, controlled trial, *Pediatrics* 118 (2006): 2126–2134.

67. S. M. Himes and J. K. Thompson, Fat stigmatization in television shows and movies: A content analysis, *Obesity* 15 (2007): 712–718.

68. Barlow and the Expert Committee, 2007.

69. M. M. Davis and coauthors, Recommendations for prevention of childhood obesity, *Pediatrics* 120 (2007): S229–S253; Position of the American Dietetic Association: Individual-, family-, school-, and community-based interventions for pediatric overweight, 2006.

70. Barlow and the Expert Committee, 2007.

71. Spear and coauthors, 2007.

72. Barlow and the Expert Committee, 2007.

73. Barlow and the Expert Committee, 2007.

74. American Academy of Pediatrics, Council on Sports Medicine and Fitness and Council on School Health, 2006.

75. American Academy of Pediatrics, Council on Sports Medicine and Fitness and Council on School Health, 2006.

76. Spear and coauthors, 2007.

77. T. H. Inge and coauthors, Reversal of type 2 diabetes mellitus and improvements in cardiovascular risk factors after surgical weight loss in adolescents, *Pediatrics* 123 (2009): 214–222.

78. Spear and coauthors, 2007.

79. Position of the American Dietetic Association, 2008; Position of the American Dietetic Association: Individual-, family-, school-, and community-based interventions for pediatric overweight, 2006.

80. E. Jansen and coauthors, From the Garden of Eden to the land of plenty: Restriction of fruit and sweets intake leads to increased fruit and sweets consumption in children, *Appetite* 51 (2008): 570–575; E. Jansen, S. Mulkens, and A. Jansen, Do not eat the red food: Prohibition of snacks leads to their relatively higher consumption in children, *Appetite* 49 (2007): 572–577.

81. Position of the American Dietetic Association, 2008.

82. Position of the American Dietetic Association, 2008; J. Wardle, S. Carnell, and L. Cooke, Parental control over feeding and children's fruit and vegetable intake: How are they related? *Journal of the American Dietetic Association* 105 (2005): 227–232; A. T. Galloway and coauthors, Parental pressure, dietary patterns, and weight status among girls who are "picky eaters," *Journal of the American Dietetic Association* 105 (2005): 541–548.

83. Position of the American Dietetic Association: Benchmarks for nutrition programs in child care settings, *Journal of the American Dietetic Association* 105 (2005): 979–986.

84. School Breakfast Program: Participation and breakfasts served, USDA, Food and Nutrition Service, www.fns.usda.gov/pd/sbsummar.htm, accessed July 7, 2009; Position of the American Dietetic Association: Local support for nutrition integrity in schools, *Journal of the American Dietetic Association* 106 (2006): 122–133.

85. Position of the American Dietetic Association: Local support for nutrition integrity in schools, 2006.

86. M. K. Crepinsek and coauthors, Meals offered and served in U.S. public schools: Do they meet nutrient standards? *Journal of the American Dietetic Association* 109 (2009): S31–S43; K. Widenhorn-Muller and coauthors, Influence of having breakfast on cognitive performance and mood in 13- to 20-year-old high school students: Results of a crossover trial, *Pediatrics* 122 (2008): 279–284.

87. National School Lunch Program: Participation and lunches served, USDA, Food and Nutrition Service, www.fns.usda.gov/pd/slsummar.htm, site accessed July 7, 2009; Position of the American Dietetic Association: Local support for nutrition integrity in schools, 2006.

88. M. Story, The Third School Nutrition Dietary Assessment Study: Findings and policy implications for improving the health of U.S. children, *Journal of the American Dietetic Association* 109 (2009): S7–S13; Position of the American Dietetic Association, 2008.

89. Position of the American Dietetic Association: Local support for nutrition integrity in schools, 2006.

90. Centers for Disease Control and Prevention, Competitive foods and beverages available for purchase in secondary schools—Selected sites, United States, 2006, *Morbidity and Mortality Weekly Report* 57 (2008): 935–938; Position of the American Dietetic Association: Local support for nutrition integrity in schools, 2006.

91. S. B. Templeton and coauthors, Competitive foods increase the intake of energy and decrease the intake of certain nutrients by adolescents consuming school lunch, *Journal of the American Dietetic Association* 105 (2005): 215–220.

92. Position of the American Dietetic Association: Local support for nutrition integrity in schools, 2006.

93. Institute of Medicine, Food and Nutrition Board, Committee on Nutrition Standards for Foods in Schools, eds. V. A. Stallings and A. L. Yaktine, *Nutrition Standards for Foods in Schools: Leading the Way toward Healthier Youth* (Washington, D.C.: National Academies Press, 2007).

94. Institute of Medicine, Food and Nutrition Board, Committee on Nutrition Standards for Foods in Schools, 2007.

95. Institute of Medicine, Food and Nutrition Board, Committee on Nutrition Standards for Foods in Schools, 2007.

96. Committee on the Scientific Evaluation of Dietary Reference Intakes, 2005, pp. 177–182.

97. Wagner, Greer, and the Section on Breastfeeding and Committee on Nutrition, 2008.

98. C. D. Davis, Vitamin D and cancer: Current dilemmas and future research needs, *American Journal of Clinical Nutrition* 88 (2008): 565S–569S; Wagner, Greer, and the Section on Breastfeeding and Committee on Nutrition, 2008.

99. Wagner, Greer, and the Section on Breastfeeding and Committee on Nutrition, 2008.

100. F. R. Greer, N. F. Krebs, and the Committee on Nutrition, American Academy of Pediatrics, Optimizing bone health and calcium intakes of infants, children, and adolescents, *Pediatrics* 117 (2006): 578–585.

101. Greer, Krebs, and the Committee on Nutrition, 2006.

102. L. Esterie and coauthors, Milk, rather than other foods, is associated with vertebral bone mass and circulating IGF-1 in female adolescents, *Osteoporosis International* 2008 (Epub ahead of print); M. M. Murphy and coauthors, Drinking flavored or plain milk is positively associated with nutrient intake and is not associated with adverse effects on weight status in U.S. children and adolescents, *Journal of the American Dietetic Association* 108 (2008): 631–639; M. L. Savaiano and coauthors, Perceived milk intolerance is related to bone mineral content in 10- to 13-year-old female adolescents, *Pediatrics* 120 (2007):e669–e677.

103. N. I. Larson and coauthors, Family meals during adolescence are associated with higher diet quality and healthful meal patterns during young adulthood, *Journal of the American Dietetic Association* 107 (2007): 1502–1510.

104. M. E. Eisenberg and coauthors, Family meals and substance use: Is there a long-term association? *Journal of Adolescent Health* 43 (2008): 151–156; National Center on Addiction and Substance Abuse (CASA) at Columbia University, *The Importance of Family Dinners,* September 2003.

105. G. C. Rampersaud and coauthors, Breakfast habits, nutritional status, body weight, and academic performance in children and adolescents, *Journal of the American Dietetic Association* 105 (2005): 743–760.

106. M. T. Timlin and coauthors, Breakfast eating and weight change in a 5-year prospective analysis of adolescents: Project EAT (Eating Among Teens), *Pediatrics* 121 (2008): e638–e645.

107. C. M. McDonald and coauthors, Overweight is more prevalent than stunting and is associated with socioeconomic status, maternal obesity, and a snacking dietary pattern in school children from Bogota, Colombia, *Journal of Nutrition* 139 (2009): 370–376; H. M. Niemeier and coauthors, Fast food consumption and breakfast skipping: Predictors of weight gain from adolescence to adulthood in a nationally representative sample, *Journal of Adolescent Health* 39 (2006): 842–849.

108. R. S. Sebastian, L. E. Cleveland, and J. D. Goldman, Effect of snacking frequency on adolescents' dietary intakes and meeting national recommendations, *Journal of Adolescent Health* 42 (2008): 503–511.

109. American Heart Association, S. S. Gidding, and coauthors, Dietary recommendations for children and adolescents: A guide for practitioners, *Pediatrics* 117 (2006): 544–559.

110. L. Libuda and coauthors, Association between long-term consumption of soft drinks and variables of bone modeling and remodeling in a sample of healthy German children and adolescents, *American Journal of Clinical Nutrition* 88 (2008): 1670–1677; Greer, Krebs, and the Committee on Nutrition, 2006; H. Vatanparast and coauthors, Positive effects of vegetable and fruit consumption and calcium intake on bone mineral accrual in boys during growth from childhood to adolescence: The University of Saskatchewan Pediatric Bone Mineral Accrual Study, *American Journal of Clinical Nutrition* 82 (2005): 700–706.

111. L. R. Vartanian, M. B. Schwartz, and K. D. Brownell, Effects of soft drink consumption on nutrition and health: A systematic review and meta-analysis, *American Journal of Public Health* 97 (2007): 667–675; Malik, Schulze, and Hu, 2006.

NUTRITION IN PRACTICE

Childhood Obesity and the Early Development of Chronic Diseases

When people think about the health problems of children and adolescents, they typically think of ear infections, colds, and acne—not heart disease, diabetes, or hypertension. Today, however, unprecedented numbers of U.S. children are being diagnosed with obesity and the serious "adult diseases," such as type 2 diabetes, that accompany overweight.[1] When type 2 diabetes develops before the age of 20, the incidence of diabetic kidney disease and death in middle age increases dramatically, largely because of the long duration of the disease.[2] For children born in the United States in the year 2000, the risk of developing type 2 diabetes sometime in their lives is estimated to be 30 percent for boys and 40 percent for girls.[3] U.S. children are not alone—rapidly rising rates of obesity threaten the health of an alarming number of children around the globe.[4] Without immediate intervention, millions of children are destined to develop type 2 diabetes and hypertension in childhood followed by **cardiovascular disease (CVD)** in early adulthood.[5]

Over the past three decades, researchers have been observing how changes in body weight, blood lipids, blood pressure, and individual behaviors correlate with the development of CVD over time—from infancy to childhood through adolescence and into young adulthood. Some major findings have emerged from this research:

- Changes inside the arteries—changes predictive of CVD—are evident in childhood.
- Obesity in children affects these changes.

- Behaviors that influence the development of obesity and of CVD are learned and begin early in life. These behaviors include overeating, physical inactivity, and cigarette smoking.

This Nutrition in Practice focuses on efforts to prevent childhood obesity, type 2 diabetes, and CVD (see the accompanying glossary for definitions of the relevant terms), but the benefits extend to other obesity-related diseases as well. The years of childhood (ages 2 to 18) are emphasized here, for the earlier in life health-promoting habits become established, the better they will stick.

What about genetics? Do some people inherit the tendency to become obese or develop diabetes or CVD regardless of the lifestyle habits they adopt?

For obesity, as well as for CVD, hypertension, and type 2 diabetes, genetics does not appear to play a *determining* role; that is, a person is not simply destined at birth to develop them. Instead, genetics appears to play a *permissive* role—the potential is inherited and will then develop, if given a push by factors in the environment such as poor diet, sedentary lifestyle, and cigarette smoking.[6] Researchers note that the relationship between genes and the environment is a synergistic one—their combined effects are greater than the sum of their individual effects.

Many experts agree that preventing or treating obesity in childhood will reduce the rate of chronic diseases in adulthood. Without intervention, most overweight children become overweight adolescents who become overweight adults, and being overweight exacerbates every chronic

Glossary

atherosclerosis (ATH-er-oh-scler-OH-sis): a type of artery disease characterized by plaques (accumulations of lipid-containing material) on the inner walls of the arteries (see Chapter 21).
- **athero** = porridge or soft
- **scleros** = hard
- **osis** = condition

cardiovascular disease (CVD): a general term for all diseases of the heart and blood vessels. Atherosclerosis is the main cause of CVD. When the arteries that carry blood to the heart muscle

become blocked, the heart suffers damage known as coronary heart disease (CHD).
- **cardio** = heart
- **vascular** = blood vessels

fatty streaks: accumulation of cholesterol and other lipids along the walls of the arteries.

plaque (PLACK): an accumulation of fatty deposits, smooth muscle cells, and fibrous connective tissue that develops in the artery walls in atherosclerosis. Plaque associated with atherosclerosis is known as **atheromatous (ATH-er-OH-ma-tus) plaque**.

disease that adults face.[7] Fatty liver, a condition that correlates directly with BMI, was not even recognized in pediatric research until recently. Today, fatty liver disease affects about one in three obese children.[8]

What about events that take place during fetal development—malnutrition, for example? Can they affect a person's tendency to develop diseases later in life?

A theory called *fetal programming*, or *fetal origins of disease*, states that maternal malnutrition or other harmful conditions at a critical period of fetal development may have lifelong effects on an individual's pattern of genetic expression and therefore on the tendency to develop obesity and certain diseases.[9] Poor maternal diet or health during pregnancy may alter the infant's bodily functions such as blood pressure, cholesterol metabolism, and immune functions that influence disease development.[10] For example, maternal diet may alter blood vessel growth and program lipid metabolism and lean body mass development in such a way that the infant will develop risk factors for cardiovascular disease as an adult.[11]

Why has type 2 diabetes become so prevalent?

In recent years, type 2 diabetes, a chronic disease closely linked with obesity, has been on the rise among children and adolescents as the prevalence of obesity in U.S. youth has increased.[12] Obesity is the most important risk factor for type 2 diabetes—most of the children diagnosed with type 2 diabetes are obese.[13] Most are diagnosed during puberty, but as children become more obese and less active, the disease is appearing in younger and younger children. Type 2 diabetes is most likely to occur in those who are obese and sedentary and have a family history of diabetes.

> **NURSING DIAGNOSIS**
>
> *Sedentary lifestyle* applies to clients who report a lifestyle that is characterized by a low physical activity level.

How does type 2 diabetes develop?

In type 2 diabetes, the body's cells become insulin resistant—that is, the cells become less sensitive to insulin, reducing the amount of glucose entering the cells from the blood. The combination of obesity and insulin resistance produces a cluster of symptoms, including high blood pressure and high blood lipids, which in turn promotes the development of atherosclerosis and the early development of CVD.[14] Other common problems evident by early adulthood include

kidney disease, blindness, and miscarriages. The complications of diabetes, especially when encountered at a young age, can shorten life expectancy. Chapter 20 offers a detailed discussion of diabetes.

Prevention and treatment of type 2 diabetes depend on weight management, which can be particularly difficult in a young person's world of food advertising, video games, and pocket money for candy bars. The activity and dietary suggestions to help defend against heart disease later in this discussion apply to type 2 diabetes as well.

> **NURSING DIAGNOSIS**
>
> *Risk for unstable blood glucose level* applies to clients who are physically inactive and overweight.

How does CVD develop, and when does its development begin?

Most CVD involves **atherosclerosis**—the accumulation of cholesterol and other blood lipids along the walls of the arteries. Frequently, atherosclerosis and its complications interfere with the flow of blood to the heart and can lead to coronary heart disease (CHD), which, in turn, raises the likelihood of a heart attack. When atherosclerosis interferes with blood flow to the brain, a stroke can result. Infants are born with healthy, smooth, clear arteries, but within the first decade of life, **fatty streaks** may begin to appear. During adolescence, these fatty streaks may begin to turn into **plaques** (Figure 21-2 in Chapter 21 shows the formation of plaques in atherosclerosis).[15] By early adulthood, the fibrous plaques may begin to calcify and become raised lesions, especially in boys and young men. As the lesions grow more numerous and thicken, the heart disease rate begins to rise, and the rise becomes dramatic at about age 45 in men and 55 in women. From this point on, arterial damage and blockage progress rapidly, and heart attacks and strokes threaten life. In short, the consequences of atherosclerosis, which become apparent only in adulthood, have their beginnings in the first decades of life.[16]

Children with the highest risks of developing heart disease are sedentary and obese, with diabetes, high blood pressure, and high blood cholesterol. In contrast, children with the lowest risks of heart disease are physically active and of normal weight, with low blood pressure and favorable lipid profiles.

Parents do not need to worry about their children's blood cholesterol, do they?

Atherosclerotic lesions reflect blood cholesterol: as blood cholesterol increases, lesion coverage increases. Cholesterol values at birth are similar in all populations; differences

TABLE NP11-1	Cholesterol Values for Children and Adolescents	
Disease Risk	Total Cholesterol (mg/dL)	LDL Cholesterol (mg/dL)
Acceptable	<170	<110
Borderline	170–199	110–129
High	≥200	≥130

Note: Adult values appear in Table 21-2 on p. 596.

emerge in early childhood. Standard values for cholesterol screening in children and adolescents are listed in Table NP11-1. Cholesterol concentrations change with age in children and adolescents, however, and are especially variable during puberty.[17] Thus, using a single cut point for all pediatric age groups has limitations.

In general, blood cholesterol tends to rise as dietary saturated fat intakes increase. Blood cholesterol also correlates with childhood obesity, especially abdominal obesity.[18] LDL cholesterol rises with obesity, and HDL declines. These relationships are apparent throughout childhood, and their magnitude increases with age.

Children who are both overweight and have high blood cholesterol are likely to have parents who develop heart disease early. For this reason, selective screening is recommended for children and adolescents who are overweight or obese; those whose parents (or grandparents) have premature (≤55 years of age for men and ≤65 years of age for women) heart disease; those whose parents have elevated blood cholesterol; those who have other risk factors for heart disease such as hypertension, cigarette smoking, or diabetes; and those whose family history is unavailable.[19] Because blood cholesterol in children is a good predictor of adult values, some experts recommend universal screening for all children, and particularly for those who are overweight, smoke, are sedentary, or consume diets high in saturated fat.

Early—but not advanced—atherosclerotic lesions are reversible, making screening and education a high priority. Both those with family histories of heart disease and those with multiple risk factors need intervention.

Is hypertension a concern for children and adolescents?

Pediatricians routinely monitor blood pressure in children and adolescents. High blood pressure may signal an underlying disease or the early onset of hypertension. Hypertension accelerates the development of atherosclerosis.[20] Diagnosing hypertension in children and adolescents requires consideration of age, gender, and height and cannot be assessed using the simple tables applied to adults.[21]

Like atherosclerosis and high blood cholesterol, hypertension may develop in the first decades of life, especially among obese children, and worsen with time. Children can control their hypertension by participating in regular aerobic activity and by losing weight or maintaining their weight as they grow taller. Restricting dietary sodium also causes an immediate drop in most children's and adolescents' blood pressure.[22]

Regular physical activity lowers risks for heart disease and hypertension in adults; does it do so in children as well?

Yes. Research has also confirmed an association between blood lipids and physical activity in children, similar to that seen in adults. Physically active children have a better lipid profile and lower blood pressure than physically inactive children, and these positive findings often persist into adulthood. The *Physical Activity Guidelines for Americans 2008* recommendations for children and adolescents are listed in Chapter 11 on p. 331.

Just as blood cholesterol and obesity track over the years, so does a child's level of physical activity. Those who are inactive now are likely to still be inactive years later. Similarly, those who are physically active now tend to remain so. Compared with inactive teens, those who are physically active weigh less, smoke less, eat a diet lower in saturated fats, and have better blood lipid profiles. Both obesity and blood cholesterol correlate with the inactive pastime of watching television. The message is clear: physical activity offers numerous health benefits, and children who are active today are most likely to be active for years to come.

Are adult dietary recommendations appropriate for children?

Regardless of family history, all children over age two should eat a variety of foods and maintain desirable weight (see Table NP11-2 on p. 350). Children (4 to 18 years of age) should receive at least 25 percent and no more than 35 percent of total energy from fat, less than 10 percent from saturated fat, and less than 300 milligrams of cholesterol per day.[23]

Recommendations limiting fat and cholesterol are not intended for infants or children under two years old. Infants and toddlers need a higher percentage of fat to support their rapid growth. For children between one year of age and two years of age who are overweight or obese, or have a family history of heart disease, obesity, or abnormal blood lipids, however, the use of reduced-fat milk is appropriate.[24]

<table>
<tr><td>TABLE
NP11-2</td><td>American Heart Association Dietary Guidelines and Strategies for Children[a]</td></tr>
</table>

- Balance dietary kcalories with physical activity to maintain normal growth.

- Every day, engage in 60 minutes of moderate to vigorous play or physical activity.

- Eat vegetables and fruits daily. Use fresh, frozen, and canned vegetables and fruits and serve at every meal; limit those with added fats, salt, and sugar.

- Limit juice intake (4 to 6 ounces per day for children 1 to 6 years of age, 8 to 12 ounces for children 7 to 18 years of age).

- Use vegetable oils (canola, soybean, olive, safflower, or other unsaturated oils) and soft margarines low in saturated fat and *trans* fatty acids instead of butter or most other animal fats in the diet.

- Choose whole-grain breads and cereals rather than refined products; read labels and make sure that "whole grain" is the first ingredient.

- Reduce the intake of sugar-sweetened beverages and foods.

- Consume low-fat and nonfat milk and milk products daily.

- Include two servings of fish per week, especially fatty fish such as broiled or baked salmon.

- Choose legumes and tofu in place of meat for some meals.

- Choose only lean cuts of meat and reduced-fat meat products; remove the skin from poultry.

- Use less salt, including salt from processed foods. Breads, breakfast cereals, and soups may be high in salt and/or sugar so read food labels and choose high-fiber, low-salt, low-sugar alternatives.

- Limit the intake of high-kcalorie add-ons such as gravy, Alfredo sauce, cream sauce, cheese sauce, and hollandaise sauce.

- Serve age-appropriate portion sizes on appropriately sized plates and bowls.

[a] These guidelines are for children three years of age and older.

SOURCE: Adapted from American Heart Association, S. S. Gidding, and coauthors, Dietary recommendations for children and adolescents: A guide for practitioners, *Pediatrics* 117 (2006): 544–559.

Healthy children over age two can begin the transition to eating according to recommendations by eating fewer foods high in saturated fat and selecting more fruits and vegetables. Healthy meals can occasionally include moderate amounts of a child's favorite foods, even those that are high in saturated fat such as french fries and ice cream. A steady diet of some restaurants' "children's menu" items, such as chicken nuggets, hot dogs, and french fries, easily exceeds a prudent intake of saturated fat, *trans* fat, and kcalories, however, and invites both nutrient shortages and weight gains.[25] Fortunately, most restaurant chains are changing children's menus to include steamed vegetables, fruit cups, and broiled or grilled chicken—additions welcomed by busy parents who often dine out or purchase take-out foods.

Other fatty foods, such as nuts, vegetable oils, and some varieties of fish such as tuna or salmon, contribute essential fatty acids. Low-fat milk and milk products also deserve special attention in a child's diet for the needed calcium and other nutrients they supply.[26]

Parents and caregivers play a key role in helping children establish healthy eating habits. Balanced meals need to provide lean meat, poultry, fish, and legumes; fruits and vegetables; whole grains; and low-fat milk products. Such meals can provide enough energy and nutrients to support growth and maintain blood cholesterol within a healthy range.

Pediatricians warn parents to avoid extremes. Although intentions may be good, excessive food restriction may create nutrient deficiencies and impair growth. Furthermore, parental control over eating may instigate battles and foster attitudes about foods that can lead to inappropriate eating behaviors.

Do pediatricians ever prescribe drugs to lower blood cholesterol in children?

Experts agree that children with high blood cholesterol should first be treated with diet. If high blood cholesterol persists despite dietary intervention in children eight years of age and older, then drugs may be necessary to lower blood cholesterol. Drugs can effectively lower blood cholesterol without interfering with adolescent growth or development.[27]

Can parents or caregivers do anything else to help children reduce their risks of CVD?

Even though the focus of this text is nutrition, another risk factor for heart disease that starts in childhood and carries over into adulthood must also be addressed—cigarette smoking. Each day 3000 children light up for the first time—typically in grade school. Among high school students, almost two out of three have tried smoking, and one in five smokes regularly.[28] Approximately 80 percent of all adult smokers began smoking before the age of 18.

Of those teenagers who continue smoking, half will eventually die of smoking-related causes. Efforts to teach children about the dangers of smoking need to be aggressive. Children are not likely to consider the long-term health consequences of tobacco use. They are more likely to be struck by the immediate health consequences, such as shortness of breath when playing sports, or social consequences, such as having bad breath. Whatever the context, the message to all children and teens should be clear: Don't start smoking. If you've already started, quit.

In conclusion, *adult* heart disease is a major *pediatric* problem. Without intervention, some 60 million children are destined to suffer its consequences within the next 30 years. Optimal prevention efforts focus on children, especially on those who are overweight.[29] Just as young children receive vaccinations against infectious diseases, they need screening for, and education about, chronic diseases. Many health education programs have been implemented in schools around the country. These programs are most effective when they include education in the classroom, heart-healthy meals in the lunchroom, fitness activities on the playground, and parental involvement at home.

Notes

1. C. J. Lavie, R. V. Milani, and H. O. Ventura, Obesity and cardiovascular disease, *Journal of the American College of Cardiology* 53 (2009): 1925–1933; D. S. Freedman and coauthors, Risk factors and adult body mass index among overweight children: The Bogalusa Heart Study, *Pediatrics* 123 (2009): 750–757; C. L. Ogden, M. D. Carroll, and K. M. Flegal, High body mass index for age among U.S. children and adolescents, 2003-2006, *Journal of the American Medical Association* 299 (2008): 2401–2405; K. L. Jones, Role of obesity in complicating and confusing the diagnosis and treatment of diabetes in children, *Pediatrics* 121 (2008): 361–368; M. Gardner, D. W. Gardner, and J. R. Sowers, The cardiometabolic syndrome in the adolescent, *Pediatric Endocrinology Reviews* Suppl. 4 (2008): 964–968; S. Cook and coauthors, Metabolic Syndrome rates in United States adolescents, from the National Health and Nutrition Examination survey, 1999-2002, *Journal of Pediatrics* 152 (2008): 165–170; D. S. Ludwig, Childhood obesity—The shape of things to come, *New England Journal of Medicine* 357 (2007): 2325–2327; J. P. Kaplan, C. T. Liverman, and V. I. Kraak, eds., *Preventing Childhood Obesity: Health in the Balance* (Washington, D.C.: National Academies Press, 2005), pp. 1–20; M. L. Cruz and coauthors, Pediatric obesity and insulin resistance: Chronic disease risk and implications for treatment and prevention beyond body weight modification, *Annual Review of Nutrition* 25 (2005): 435–468.
2. M. E. Pavkov and coauthors, Effect of youth-onset type 2 diabetes mellitus on incidence of end-stage renal disease and mortality in young and middle-aged Pima Indians, *Journal of the American Medical Association* 296 (2006): 421–426.
3. Kaplan, Liverman, and Kraak, 2005.
4. C. Bouchard, Childhood obesity: Are genetic differences involved? *American Journal of Clinical Nutrition* 89 (2009): 1494S–1501S; W. Maziak, K. D. Ward, and M. B. Stockton, Childhood obesity: Are we missing the big picture? *Obesity Reviews* 9 (2008): 35–42; Y. Wang and T. Lobstein, Worldwide trends in childhood overweight and obesity, *International Journal of Pediatric Obesity* 1 (2006): 11–25; Cruz and coauthors, 2005.
5. Freedman and coauthors, 2009; H. Zhu and coauthors, Relationships of cardiovascular phenotypes with healthy weight, at risk of overweight, and overweight in US youths, *Pediatrics* 121 (2008): 115–122; D. S. Freedman and coauthors, Cardiovascular risk factors and excess adiposity among overweight children and adolescents: The Bogalusa Heart Study, *Journal of Pediatrics* 150 (2007): 12–17.
6. E. C. Brito and coauthors, Previously associated type 2 diabetes variants may interact with physical activity to modify the risk of impaired glucose regulation and type 2 diabetes, *Diabetes* 58 (2009): 1411–1418; C. Bouchard, Childhood obesity: Are genetics differences involved? *American Journal of Clinical Nutrition* 89 (2009): 1494S–1501S; J. M. Ordovas, Genetic influences on blood lipids and cardiovascular disease risk: Tools for primary prevention, *American Journal of Clinical Nutrition* 89 (2009): 1509S–1517S.
7. S. E. Barlow and the Expert Committee, Expert Committee recommendations regarding the prevention, assessment, and treatment of child and adolescent overweight and obesity: Summary report, *Pediatrics* 120 (2007): S164–S192; Ludwig, 2007.
8. Ludwig, 2007.
9. M. E. Symonds, T. Stephenson, and H. Budge, Early determinants of cardiovascular disease: The role of early diet in later blood pressure control, *American Journal of Clinical Nutrition* 89 (2009): 1518S–1522S; S. H. Zeisel, Epigenetic mechanisms for nutrition determinants of later health outcomes, *American Journal of Clinical Nutrition* 89 (2009): 1488S–1493S; P. D. Gluckman and coauthors, Effect of in utero and early-life conditions on adult health and disease, *New England Journal of Medicine* 359 (2008): 61; L. Adair and D. Dahly, Developmental determinants of blood pressure in adults, *Annual Review of Nutrition* 25 (2005): 407–434.
10. W. Palinski and coauthors, Developmental programming: Maternal hypercholesterolemia and immunity influence susceptibility to atherosclerosis, *Nutrition Reviews* 65 (2007): S182–S187.
11. R. C. Painter and coauthors, Early onset of coronary artery disease after prenatal exposure to the Dutch famine, *American Journal of Clinical Nutrition* 84 (2006): 322–327; O. A. Kensara and coauthors, Fetal programming of body composition: Relation between birth weight and body composition measured with dual-energy X-ray absorptiometry and anthropometric methods in older Englishmen, *American Journal of Clinical Nutrition* 82 (2005): 980–987.
12. Jones, 2008; T. S. Hannon, F. Rao, and S. A. Arslanian, Childhood obesity and type 2 diabetes mellitus, *Pediatrics* 116 (2005): 473–480; Cruz and coauthors, 2005.
13. Jones, 2008; Hannon, Rao, and Arslanian, 2005; Cruz and coauthors, 2005.
14. E. M. Urbina and coauthors, Youth with obesity and obesity-related type 2 diabetes mellitus demonstrate abnormalities in carotid structure and function, *Circulation* 119 (2009): 2913–2919; Cook and coauthors, 2008; G. S. Boyd and coauthors, Effect of obesity and high blood pressure on plasma lipid levels in children and adolescents, *Pediatrics* 116 (2005): 442–446.
15. W. Insull, The pathology of atherosclerosis: Plaque development and plaque responses to medical treatment, *The American Journal of Medicine* 122 (2009): S3–S14.
16. Zhu and coauthors, 2008; Freedman and coauthors, 2007; D. R. Thompson and coauthors, Childhood overweight and cardiovascular disease risk factors: The National Heart, Lung, and Blood Institute Growth and Health Study, *Journal of Pediatrics* 150 (2007): 18–25; J. Botton and coauthors, Cardiovascular risk factor levels and their relationships with overweight and fat distribution in children: The Fleurbaix Laventie Ville Sante II Study, *Metabolism* 56 (2007): 614–622; J. C. Eisenmann and coauthors, Fatness, fitness, and cardiovascular disease risk factors in children and adolescents, *Medicine & Science in Sports & Exercise* 39 (2007): 1251–1256.
17. S. R. Daniels, F. R. Greer, and the Committee on Nutrition, Lipid screening and cardiovascular health in childhood, *Pediatrics* 122 (2008): 198–208.
18. Freedman and coauthors, 2009; Cook and coauthors, 2008; Botton and coauthors, 2007; Thompson and coauthors, 2007.
19. Daniels, Greer, and the Committee on Nutrition, 2008.

CHAPTER 12 | **Nutrition Through the Life Span: Later Adulthood**

Ulrich Kerth/Getty Images

CONTENTS

Commonly used age groups:
- Young old (65–74 years)
- Old (75–84 years)
- Oldest old (≥85 years)

life expectancy: the average number of years lived by people in a given society.

life span: the maximum number of years of life attainable by a member of a species.

longevity: long duration of life.

quality of life: a person's perceived physical and mental well-being.

THE LAST TWO CHAPTERS WERE DEVOTED TO STAGES OF THE LIFE cycle that require special nutrition attention: pregnancy, lactation, infancy, childhood, and adolescence. Much of the text before that focused on nutrition to support wellness during adulthood. This chapter describes the special nutrition needs of the later adult years.

The most urgent nutrition need of older people, however, is to have made good food choices in the past! All of life's nutrition choices incur health consequences for the better or for the worse. A single day's intakes of nutrients may exert only a minute effect on body organs and their functions, but, over years and decades, the repeated effects accumulate to have major impacts. This being the case, it is of great importance for everyone, of every age, to pay close attention today to nutrition.

The "graying" of America is a continuing trend.[1] The majority of citizens are now middle aged, and the ratio of old people to young is increasing, as Figure 12-1 shows. Our society uses the arbitrary age of 65 to define the transition point between middle age and old age, but growing "old" happens day by day, with changes occurring gradually over time.(✚) Since 1950 the population aged 65 and over has almost tripled. Remarkably, the fastest-growing age group has been people over 85 years; since 1950 their numbers have increased sevenfold. The number of people in the United States age 100 or older doubled in the past decade. Similar trends are occurring in populations worldwide. The U.S. Bureau of the Census projects that by the year 2040 more than a million Americans will be 100 years old or older.

Life expectancy in the United States is 78 years, up from about 47 years in 1900.[2] Advances in medical science—antibiotics and other treatments—are largely responsible for almost doubling the life expectancy in the 20th century. Improved nutrition and an abundant food supply have also contributed to lengthening life expectancy. Ironically, this abundant food supply has also jeopardized the chances of further lengthening life expectancy as obesity rates increase.[3]

The human **life span**, currently estimated at 130 years, is the upper limit of human **longevity**, even given optimal nutrition. With work progressing in medical and genetic technologies, however, the human life span may be extended significantly.

Research in the field of aging is active—and difficult. Researchers are challenged by the diversity of older adults. When older adults experience health problems, it is hard to know whether to attribute these problems to genetics, aging, or other environmental factors such as nutrition. The idea that nutrition can influence the way the human body ages is particularly appealing because diet is a factor that people can control and change.

Nutrition and Longevity

What has been learned so far about the effects of nutrition and environment on longevity provides incentive for researchers to keep asking questions about how and why human beings age. Among their questions are:

- To what extent is aging inevitable, and can it be slowed through changes in lifestyle and environment?
- What role does nutrition play in aging, and what role can it play in slowing aging?

With respect to the first question, it seems that aging is an inevitable, natural process, programmed into the genes at conception. People can, however, slow the process within the natural limits set by heredity by adopting healthy lifestyle habits such as eating nutritious food and engaging in physical activity. In fact, an estimated 70 to 80 percent of the average person's life expectancy may depend on individual health-related behaviors; genes determine the remaining 20 to 30 percent.

With respect to the second question, good nutrition helps to maintain a healthy body and can therefore ease the aging process in many significant ways.[4] Clearly, nutrition can improve the **quality of life** in the later years.

| FIGURE 12-1 | The Aging of the U.S. Population |

Percentage of population 65 years or older

Percentage of total population

In 1940, 6.8 percent of the population was 65 or older. In 1990, 12.7 percent of us had reached age 65; by 2040, 21.7 percent will have reached age 65; and by 2090, nearly one out of four Americans will be 65 or older.

SLOWING THE AGING PROCESS

One approach researchers use to search out the secret of long life is to study older people. Some people are young for their ages, whereas others are old for their ages. What makes the difference?

Healthy Habits Six lifestyle habits seem to have a profound influence on people's health and therefore on their **physiological age**:[5]

- Sleeping regularly and adequately
- Eating well-balanced meals rich in fruits and vegetables regularly
- Maintaining a healthy body weight
- Engaging in regular physical activity
- Not smoking
- Not using alcohol, or using it in moderation

Over the years, the effects of these lifestyle choices accumulate—that is, those who follow all of these practices live longer and have fewer disabilities as they age. They are in better health, even if older in **chronological age**, than people who do not adopt these behaviors.[6] Even though people cannot alter their birth dates, they may be able to add years to, and enhance the quality of, their lives.[7] Physical activity seems to be most influential in preventing or slowing the many changes that many people seem to accept as an inevitable consequence of old age. In other words, physical activity and long life seem to go together.[8]

Physical Activity The many and remarkable benefits of regular physical activity are not limited to the young. Compared with those who are inactive, older adults who are active weigh less; have greater flexibility, more endurance, better balance, and better health; and live longer.[9] They reap additional benefits from various types of activities as well: aerobic activities improve cardiorespiratory endurance, blood pressure, and blood lipid concentrations; moderate endurance activities improve the quality of sleep; and strength training significantly improves posture and mobility. In fact, regular physical activity is a powerful predictor of a person's mobility in the later years. Physical activity also increases blood flow to the brain, thereby preserving mental ability, alleviating depression, and supporting independence.[10]

Muscle mass and muscle strength tend to decline with aging, making older people vulnerable to falls and immobility.[11] Falls are a major cause of fear, injury, disability, dependence, and even death among older adults. Regular physical activity tones, firms, and strengthens muscles, helping to improve confidence, reduce the risk of falling, and minimize the risk of injury should a fall occur. Strength training, even in frail, elderly people over 85 years of age, has been shown not only to improve balance, muscle strength, and mobility but also to increase energy expenditure and energy intake. This finding highlights another reason to be physically active: a person spending energy on physical activity can afford to eat more food and, with it, more nutrients. People who are committed to an ongoing fitness program have higher energy and nutrient intakes than more sedentary people.

Activities of all kinds are recommended to maintain and promote health.[12] Strength training improves muscle strength, which enhances a person's ability to perform many of life's daily tasks such as climbing stairs and carrying packages.[13] Muscle strength during midlife (between the ages of 45 and 65) predicts health and disability 25 years later. Greater muscle strength during midlife may act as a strength *reserve* later on, protecting older adults from disability even when chronic conditions develop. In short, improving overall strength during early and middle adulthood could potentially lower the risk of later physical disability.

Ideally, physical activity should be part of each day's schedule and should be intense enough to prevent muscle atrophy and to speed up the heartbeat and respiration rate. Although aging affects both speed and endurance to some degree, older adults can still train and achieve exceptional performances. Healthy older adults who have not been active can ease into a suitable routine. They can start by walking short distances until they are walking at least 10 minutes continuously and then gradually increase

physiological age: a person's age as estimated from her or his body's health and probable life expectancy.

chronological age: a person's age in years from his or her date of birth.

NURSING DIAGNOSIS

Impaired physical mobility applies to clients with slowed movement, decreased muscle mass, and decreased muscle strength.

NURSING DIAGNOSIS

Risk for falls applies to clients who are 65 years of age or older, those who have a history of falls, those who live alone, and those who use assistive devices such as a walker or a cane.

Regular physical activity promotes a healthy, independent lifestyle.

© Warren Morgan/CORBIS

TABLE
12-1 | Exercise Guidelines for Older Adults

	Aerobic	Strength	Balance	Flexibility
Examples				
Start easy and progress gradually	Be active five minutes on most or all days	Using 0- to 2-pound weights, do one set of 8–12 repetitions twice a week	Hold onto table or chair with one hand, then with one finger	Hold stretch for 10 seconds; do each stretch three times
Frequency	At least five days per week of moderate activity or at least three days per week of vigorous activity	At least two (nonconsecutive) days per week	Three days each week	At least two days per week, preferably on all days that aerobic or strength activities are performed
Intensity[a]	Moderate, vigorous, or combination	Moderate to high; 10 to 15 repetitions per exercise		At least 10 minutes per day
Duration	At least 30 minutes of moderate activity in bouts of at least 10 minutes each or at least 20 minutes of continuous vigorous activity	8 to 10 exercises involving the major muscle groups		Stretch major muscle groups for 10–30 seconds, repeating each stretch three to four times
Cautions and comments	Stop if you are breathing so hard you can't talk or if you feel dizziness or chest pain	Breathe out as you contract and in as you relax (do not hold breath); use smooth, steady movements	Incorporate balance techniques with strength exercises as you progress	Stretch after strength and endurance exercises for 20 minutes, three times a week; use slow, steady movements; bend joints slightly

Note: Activity recommendations are in addition to routine activities of daily living (such as getting dressed, cooking, and grocery shopping) and moderate activities lasting less than 10 minutes.

Source: M. E. Nelson and coauthors, Physical activity and public health in older adults: Recommendation from the American College of Sports Medicine and the American Heart Association, *Medicine and Science in Sports and Exercise* 39 (2007): 1435–1445.

[a]On a 10-point scale, where sitting = 0 and maximum effort = 10, moderate intensity = 5 to 6 and vigorous intensity = 7 to 8.

their distance to a 30-minute walk at least five days a week.[14] With persistence, people can achieve great improvements at any age. Table 12-1 provides exercise guidelines for seniors; people with medical conditions should check with a physician before beginning an exercise routine, as should sedentary men over 40 and women over 50 who want to participate in a vigorous program.

Restriction of kCalories In their efforts to understand longevity, researchers have not only observed people but have also manipulated influencing factors, such as diet, in animals. This research has produced some interesting and suggestive findings. For example, animals live longer and have fewer age-related diseases when their energy intakes are restricted. These life-prolonging benefits become evident when the diet provides enough food to prevent malnutrition and energy intake of about 70 percent of normal; benefits decline as the age of starting the energy restriction is delayed.[15]

Exactly how energy restriction prolongs life remains unexplained, although gene activity appears to play a key role. Energy restriction in animals prevents alterations in gene expression that are associated with aging.[16] Food restriction may also extend the life span by preventing damaging lipid oxidation, thereby delaying the onset of age-related diseases, such as atherosclerosis.[17] Other research suggests that energy restriction beneficially alters several aspects of fat cell metabolism, which may play a role in reducing chronic disease risk and extending life.[18] Experiments with food restriction and longevity in animals have *not* suggested any direct applications to human nutrition.

Moderate energy restriction (80 percent of usual intake) in human beings may be valuable. When people restrict energy intake moderately, body weight, body fat, and blood pressure drop, and HDL cholesterol rises—favorable changes for preventing chronic diseases.[19] The reduction in oxidative damage that occurs with energy restriction in animals also occurs in people whose diets include antioxidant nutrients and phytochemicals. Diets such as the Mediterranean diet that include an abundance of fruits, vegetables, olive oil, whole grains, and legumes—with their array of antioxidants and phytochemicals—support good health and long life.

NUTRITION AND DISEASE PREVENTION

Nutrition alone, even if ideal, cannot ensure a long and robust life. Nevertheless, nutrition clearly affects aging and longevity in human beings by way of its role in disease prevention. Among the better-known relationships between nutrition and disease are the following:

- Appropriate energy intake helps prevent *obesity*, *diabetes*, and related *cardiovascular diseases* such as atherosclerosis and hypertension (Chapters 7, 20, and 21) and may influence the development of some forms of *cancer* (Chapter 23).
- Adequate intakes of essential nutrients prevent *deficiency diseases* such as scurvy, goiter, anemia, and the like (Chapters 8 and 9).
- Variety in food intake, as well as ample intakes of certain fruits and vegetables, may be protective against certain types of *cancer* (Chapter 23).
- Moderation in sugar intake helps prevent *dental caries* (Nutrition in Practice 17).
- Appropriate fiber intakes help prevent disorders of the digestive tract such as *constipation*, *diverticulosis*, and possibly *colon cancer* (Chapters 3, 18, and 23).
- Moderate sodium intake and adequate intakes of potassium, calcium, and other minerals help prevent *hypertension* (Chapters 9 and 21).
- An adequate calcium intake throughout life helps protect against *osteoporosis* (Chapter 9).

Other, less well-established links between nutrition and disease are being discovered each day. Research that focuses on how life factors affect aging and disease processes is vital to ensuring that more and more people can look forward to long, healthy lives.

Review Notes

- Life expectancy in the United States increased dramatically in the twentieth century.
- Factors that enhance longevity include limited or no alcohol use, regular balanced meals rich in fruits and vegetables, weight control, adequate sleep, abstinence from smoking, and regular physical activity.
- Nutrition alone, even if ideal, cannot guarantee a long and robust life. At the very least, however, nutrition—especially when combined with regular physical activity—can influence aging and longevity in human beings by supporting good health and preventing disease.

Nutrition-Related Concerns during Late Adulthood

Nutrition through the prime years may play a greater role than has been realized in preventing many changes once thought to be inevitable consequences of growing older. The following discussions of cataracts and macular degeneration, arthritis, and the aging brain show that nutrition may provide at least some protection against some of the conditions commonly associated with aging.

CATARACTS AND MACULAR DEGENERATION

Cataracts are age-related thickenings in the lenses of the eye that impair vision. If not surgically removed, they ultimately lead to blindness. Oxidative stress appears to play a significant role in the development of cataracts, and the antioxidant nutrients and phytochemicals in fruits and vegetables may help minimize the damage. Some studies suggest that a diet providing ample carotenoids, vitamin C, and vitamin E may be especially important for preventing early onset of cataracts.[20] Also, people who follow the *Dietary Guidelines for Americans* are reported to have fewer cataracts, though cataracts can occur even in well-nourished individuals due to exposure to ultraviolet light, oxidative damage, viral infections, toxic substances, genetic disorders, injury, or other trauma. Most cataracts are vaguely called "senile" cataracts, meaning "caused by aging." In the United States, more than half of all adults age 65 and older have a cataract.

One other diet-related factor may play a role in cataract development: obesity. How obesity may influence the development of cataracts is not known, but researchers speculate that conditions that typically accompany obesity such as glucose intolerance and insulin resistance may provide clues.

The leading cause of visual loss among older people is **macular degeneration**, a deterioration of the macular region of the eye.[21] As with cataracts, risk factors for age-related macular degeneration include oxidative stress from sunlight. Preventive factors for macular degeneration may include supplements of the omega-3 fatty acid DHA and the carotenoids lutein and zeaxanthin.[22]

ARTHRITIS

More than 46 million people in the United States have some form of **arthritis**.[23] As the population ages, it is expected that the prevalence will increase to 60 million by 2020. The most common type of arthritis that disables older people is **osteoarthritis**, a painful swelling of the joints. During movement, the ends of bones are normally protected from wear by cartilage and by small sacs of fluid that lubricate the joint. With age, the cartilage sometimes disintegrates, and the joints become malformed and painful to move.

One known connection between osteoarthritis and nutrition is overweight. Weight loss can help overweight people with osteoarthritis, partly because the joints affected are often weight-bearing joints that are stressed and irritated by having to carry excess poundage. Interestingly, though, weight loss often relieves the worst pain of osteoarthritis in the hands as well, even though they are not weight-bearing joints. Jogging and other weight-bearing activities do not worsen osteoarthritis. In fact, both aerobic activity and weight training offer modest improvements in physical performance and pain relief, especially when accompanied by even modest weight loss.[24]

Nutrition quackery to treat arthritis is abundant, but no one universally effective diet for arthritis relief is known. Table 12-2 presents some of the many ineffective dietary treatments for osteoarthritis. Traditional medical intervention for arthritis includes medication and surgery. Two popular supplements for treating osteoarthritis—glucosamine and chondroitin—may alleviate pain and improve mobility, but mixed reports from studies emphasize the need for additional research.[25] Drugs and supplements used to relieve arthritis can impose nutrition risks; some affect appetite and alter the body's use of nutrients, as Chapter 14 explains.

cataracts: thickenings of the eye lenses that impair vision and can lead to blindness.

macular (MACK-you-lar) degeneration: deterioration of the macular area of the eye that can lead to loss of central vision and eventual blindness. The **macula** is a small, oval, yellowish region in the center of the retina that provides the sharp, straight-ahead vision so critical to reading and driving.

arthritis: inflammation of a joint, usually accompanied by pain, swelling, and structural changes.

osteoarthritis: a painful, chronic disease of the joints that occurs when the cushioning cartilage in a joint breaks down; joint structure is usually altered, with loss of function; also called *degenerative arthritis*.

Another type of arthritis, known as **rheumatoid arthritis**, has a possible link to diet through the immune system. In rheumatoid arthritis, the immune system mistakenly attacks the bone coverings as if they were made of foreign tissue. In some individuals, certain foods, notably a Mediterranean-type diet of fish, vegetables, and olive oil, may moderate the inflammatory responses and provide some relief.[26]

The omega-3 fatty acids commonly found in fish oil reduce joint tenderness and improve mobility in some people with rheumatoid arthritis. The same diet recommended for heart health—one low in saturated fat from meats and milk products and high in omega-3 fats from fish—helps prevent or reduce the inflammation in the joints that makes arthritis so painful. Fish, not fish oil supplements, is the preferred source of omega-3 fatty acids, except for persons with cardiovascular disease who cannot obtain enough EPA and DHA from fish, and then only under a physician's supervision.[27]

TABLE 12-2	Ineffective Dietary Strategies for Arthritis
• Alfalfa tea	• Garlic
• Aloe vera liquid	• Honey
• Amino acid supplements	• Inositol
• Blackstrap molasses	• Kelp
• Burdock root	• Lecithin
• Calcium	• Para-amino benzoic acid (PABA)
• Celery juice	• Raw liver
• Cod liver oil	• Superoxide dismutase (SOD)
• Copper supplements	• Vitamin D
• Dimethyl sulfoxide (DMSO)	• Vitamin megadoses
• Fasting	• Watercress
• Fresh fruit	• Yeast

THE AGING BRAIN

The brain, like all of the body's organs, responds to both inherited and environmental factors that can enhance or diminish its amazing capacities. (✚) One of the challenges researchers face when studying the aging of the human brain is to distinguish among changes caused by normal, age-related, physiological processes; changes caused by diseases; and changes caused by cumulative, extrinsic factors such as diet.

The brain normally changes in some characteristic ways as it ages. For one thing, its blood supply decreases. For another, the number of **neurons**, the brain cells that specialize in transmitting information, diminishes as people age. When the number of nerve cells in one part of the **cerebral cortex** diminishes, hearing and speech are affected. Losses of neurons in other parts of the cortex can impair memory and cognitive function. When the number of neurons in the hindbrain diminishes, balance and posture are affected. Losses of neurons in other parts of the brain affect still other functions.

Nutrient Deficiencies and Brain Function Clinicians now recognize that much of the cognitive loss and forgetfulness generally attributed to aging is due in part to extrinsic, and therefore controllable, factors such as nutrient deficiencies. The ability of neurons to synthesize specific neurotransmitters depends in part on the availability of precursor nutrients that are obtained from the diet. The neurotransmitter serotonin, for example, derives from the amino acid tryptophan. In addition, the enzymes involved in neurotransmitter synthesis require vitamins and minerals to function properly. Thus, nutrient deficiencies may contribute to the loss of memory and cognition that some older adults experience.[28] Such losses may be preventable or at least diminished or delayed through diet. Table 12-3 (p. 360) summarizes some of the better-known connections between brain function and nutrients.

In some instances, the degree of cognitive loss is extensive. Such **senile dementia** may be attributable to a specific disorder such as a brain tumor or Alzheimer's disease. Table 12-4 (p. 360) lists common signs of dementia.

Alzheimer's Disease In **Alzheimer's disease**, the most prevalent form of senile dementia, brain cell death occurs in the areas of the brain that coordinate memory and cognition (see the margin on p. 361). (✚) Alzheimer's disease afflicts an estimated 5 million people in the United States, and that number is expected to almost triple by the year 2050.[29] Diagnosis of Alzheimer's depends on its characteristic

✚ Factors that protect brain function:
- Physical activities
- Intellectual challenges
- Social interactions
- Balanced diet rich in antioxidants

rheumatoid arthritis: a disease of the immune system involving painful inflammation of the joints and related structures.

neurons: nerve cells; the structural and functional units of the nervous system. Neurons initiate and conduct nerve transmissions.

cerebral cortex: the outer surface of the cerebrum, which is the largest part of the brain.

senile dementia: the loss of brain function beyond the normal loss of physical adeptness and memory that occurs with aging.

Alzheimer's disease: a progressive, degenerative disease that attacks the brain and impairs thinking, behavior, and memory.

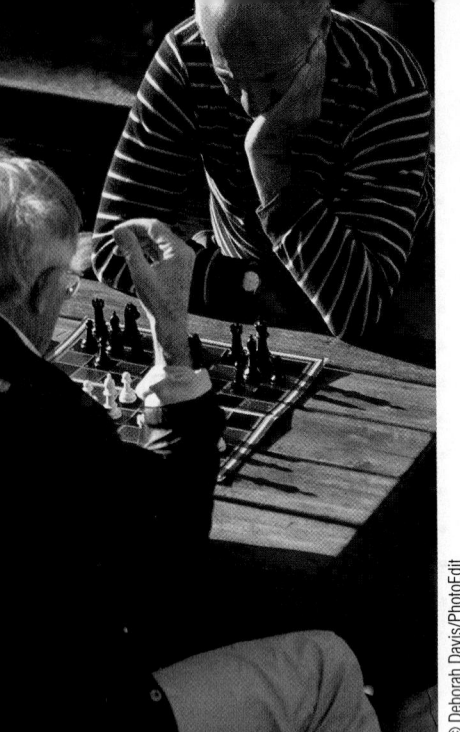

Both foods and mental challenges nourish the brain.

© Deborah Davis/PhotoEdit

TABLE 12-3	Summary of Nutrient-Brain Relationships
Brain Function	**Depends on an Adequate Intake of:**
Short-term memory	Vitamin B_{12}, vitamin C, vitamin E
Performance in problem-solving tests	Riboflavin, folate, vitamin B_{12}, vitamin C
Mental health	Thiamin, niacin, zinc, folate
Cognition	Folate, vitamin B_6, vitamin B_{12}, iron, vitamin E
Vision	Essential fatty acids, vitamin A
Neurotransmitter synthesis	Tyrosine, tryptophan, choline

symptoms: the victim gradually loses memory and reasoning ability, the ability to communicate, physical capabilities, and eventually life itself.

Researchers are closing in on the cause of Alzheimer's disease.* Clearly, genetic factors are involved.[30] Free radicals and oxidative stress also seem to be involved.[31] Nerve cells in the brains of people with Alzheimer's disease show evidence of free-radical attack—damage to DNA, cell membranes, and proteins[32]—and of the minerals that trigger these attacks—iron, copper, zinc, and aluminum. Some research suggests that the antioxidant nutrients can limit free-radical damage and delay or prevent Alzheimer's disease.[33]

Increasing evidence also suggests that overweight and obesity in middle age are associated with dementia, in general, and with Alzheimer's disease, in particular.[34] The possible relationship between obesity and Alzheimer's disease is disturbing given the current obesity epidemic. Efforts to prevent and treat obesity, however, may also help prevent Alzheimer's disease.

In Alzheimer's disease, the brain develops **senile plaques** and **neurofibrillary tangles**. Senile plaques are clumps of a protein fragment called beta-amyloid, whereas neurofibrillary tangles are snarls of the fibers that extend from the nerve cells. Both seem to occur in response to oxidative stress.[35] Researchers question whether these characteristics are the cause or the result of Alzheimer's disease.[36] In fact, scientists are unsure whether these plaques and tangles are causing the damage, serving as markers, or even protecting the brain by sequestering the proteins that begin the dementia process.[37] In any case, treatment research focuses on lowering beta-amyloid levels.[38]

Research suggests that cardiovascular disease risk factors such as high blood pressure, diabetes, and elevated levels of homocysteine may be related to the development of Alzheimer's disease.[39] Diets designed to support a healthy heart, which include the omega-3 fatty acids of oily fish, may benefit brain health as well.[40] Similarly, physical activity supports heart health and slows the cognitive decline of Alzheimer's disease.[41]

Treatment for Alzheimer's disease involves providing care to clients and support to their families. Drugs are used to improve or at least to slow the loss of short-term memory and cognition, but they do not cure the disease. Other drugs may be used to control depression, anxiety, and behavior problems.

TABLE 12-4	Common Signs of Dementia

- Agitated behavior
- Becoming lost in familiar surroundings or circumstances
- Confusion
- Delusions
- Loss of interest in daily activities
- Loss of memory
- Loss of problem-solving skills
- Unclear thinking

---

*A report on the genetic and other aspects of Alzheimer's is available from Alzheimer's Disease Education and Referral Center, P.O. Box 8250, Silver Springs, MD 20907-8250.

Maintaining appropriate body weight may be the most important nutrition concern for the person with Alzheimer's disease. Depression and forgetfulness can lead to changes in eating behaviors and poor food intake. Furthermore, changes in the body's weight-regulation system may contribute to weight loss. Perhaps the best that a caregiver can do nutritionally for a person with Alzheimer's disease is to supervise food planning and mealtimes. Providing well-liked and well-balanced meals and snacks in a cheerful atmosphere encourages food consumption. To minimize confusion, offer a few ready-to-eat foods, in bite-size pieces, with seasonings and sauces. To avoid mealtime disruptions, control distractions such as music, television, children, and the telephone.

Review Notes

- Cataracts, age-related macular degeneration, and arthritis afflict millions of older adults, while others face senile dementia and other losses of brain function.
- Some of these problems may be inevitable, but others are preventable, and good nutrition may play a key preventive role.

Energy and Nutrient Needs during Late Adulthood

Knowledge about the nutrient needs and nutrition status of older adults has grown considerably in recent years. The Dietary Reference Intakes (DRI) cluster people over the age of 50 into two age categories—51 to 70 years old, and 71 years and older. Research is showing that the nutrition needs of people 50 to 70 years old may be very different from those of people over 70—a pattern that makes sense considering the wide age span involved.

Setting standards for older people is difficult, though, because individual differences become more pronounced as people grow older. People start out with different genetic predispositions and ways of handling nutrients, and the effects of these differences become magnified with years of unique dietary habits. For example, one person may tend to omit fruits and vegetables from his diet, and by the time he is old, he may have a set of nutrition problems associated with a lack of fiber and antioxidants. Another person who omitted milk and milk products all her life may have nutrition problems related to a lack of calcium. Also, as people age, they may suffer different chronic diseases and take different medications—both have impacts on nutrient needs. Table 12-5 (p. 362) lists some changes of aging that can affect nutrition. For all these reasons, researchers have difficulty even defining "healthy aging," a prerequisite to developing recommendations that are designed to meet the "needs of practically all healthy persons." Still, some generalizations are valid. The next sections give special attention to a few nutrients of concern.

ENERGY AND ENERGY NUTRIENTS

Energy needs decline with advancing age. As a general rule, adult energy needs decline an estimated 5 percent per decade. One reason is that people usually reduce their physical activity as they age, although they need not do so. Another reason is that basal metabolic rate declines 1 to 2 percent per decade, in part because lean body mass and thyroid hormones diminish. Loss of muscle mass, known as **sarcopenia**, can be significant in the later years (its prevalence is more than 50 percent among those older than 80), and its consequences, dramatic (see Figure 12-2 on p. 362). As skeletal muscle mass diminishes, people lose their ability to move and to maintain balance, making falls likely. The limitations that accompany the loss of muscle mass and strength play a key role in the diminishing health that often accompanies aging.[42] To some extent, however,

A person with typical benign memory loss of aging may:
- Forget names or places temporarily.
- Need more time to remember a task the person set out to do.
- Misplace items in typical places, such as leaving reading glasses in the car.
- Joke about apparent forgetfulness.
- Experience little interference in living a full and productive life.

A person in the early stages of Alzheimer's disease may:
- Ask the same questions repeatedly.
- Have difficulty remembering common words—saying "that thing for my mouth" instead of "toothbrush," for example.
- Mix words up—saying "bed" instead of "table," for example.
- Be unable to complete familiar tasks, such as cooking a meal or making a phone call.
- Misplace items in uncommon places, such as putting the phone in the refrigerator.
- Get lost while driving on familiar streets.
- Have sudden, unexplained mood or behavior changes.
- Become less able to follow directions.
- Be unaware of memory loss or forgetfulness.
- Experience worsening memory loss that progressively diminishes the quality of life.

senile plaques: clumps of the protein fragment beta-amyloid on the nerve cells, commonly found in the brains of people with Alzheimer's dementia.

neurofibrillary tangles: snarls of the threadlike strands that extend from the nerve cells, commonly found in the brains of people with Alzheimer's dementia.

sarcopenia (SAR-koh-PEE-nee-ah): loss of skeletal muscle mass, strength, and quality.

TABLE 12-5	Examples of Physical Changes of Aging That Affect Nutrition
Mouth	Tooth loss, gum disease, and reduced salivary output impede chewing and swallowing. Swallowing disorders and choking may become likely. Discomfort and pain associated with eating may reduce food intake.
Digestive tract	Intestines lose muscle strength, resulting in sluggish motility that leads to constipation (see Chapter 18). Stomach inflammation, abnormal bacterial growth, and greatly reduced acid output impair digestion and absorption. Pain may cause food avoidance or reduced intake.
Hormones	For example, the pancreas secretes less insulin and cells become less responsive, causing abnormal glucose metabolism.
Sensory organs	Diminished senses of smell and taste can reduce appetite; diminished sight can make food shopping and preparation difficult.
Body composition	Weight loss and decline in lean body mass lead to lowered energy requirements. May be preventable or reversible through physical activity.
Urinary tract	Increased frequency of urination may limit fluid intake.

declines in lean body mass and energy needs may not be entirely inevitable. Optimal nutrition with sufficient protein and regular physical activity can help maintain muscle mass and strength and minimize the changes in body composition associated with aging.[43] Physical activity not only increases energy expenditure but, along with sound nutrition, enhances bone density and supports many body functions as well.[44]

The lower energy expenditures of many older adults require that they eat less food energy to maintain their weights. Accordingly, the estimated energy requirements for adults decrease steadily after age 19. Energy intakes typically decline in parallel with needs. Still, many older adults are overweight, indicating that their food intakes do not

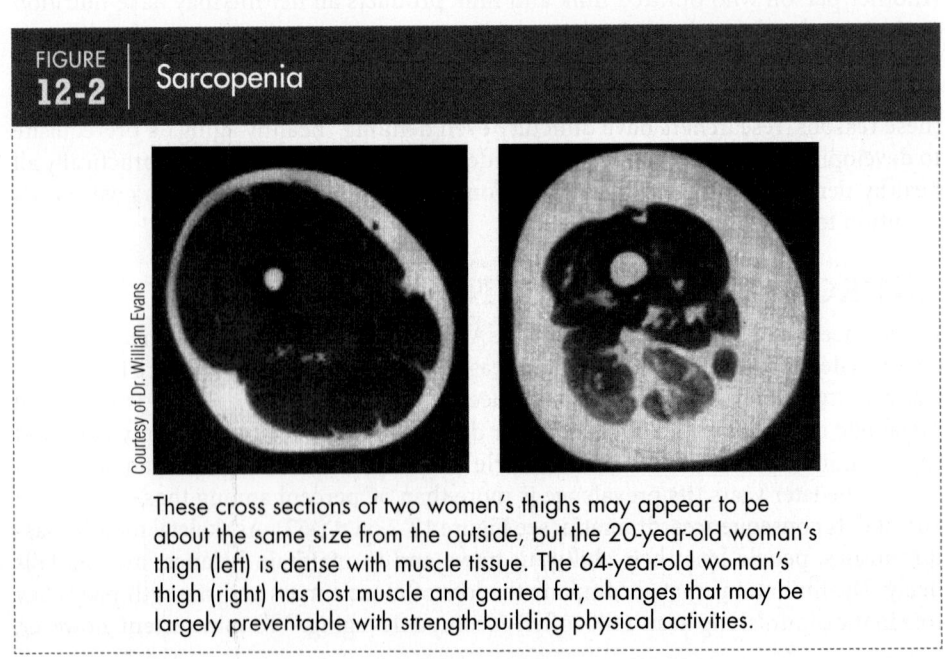

FIGURE 12-2 | Sarcopenia

Courtesy of Dr. William Evans

These cross sections of two women's thighs may appear to be about the same size from the outside, but the 20-year-old woman's thigh (left) is dense with muscle tissue. The 64-year-old woman's thigh (right) has lost muscle and gained fat, changes that may be largely preventable with strength-building physical activities.

decline enough to compensate for their reduced energy expenditures. Overweight and obesity in older adults increase the risk for many diseases and for disabilities as well.[45]

On limited energy allowances, people must select mostly nutrient-dense foods. There is little leeway for added sugars, solid fats, or alcohol. Older adults can follow the USDA Food Guide (see pp. 18–19), making sure to choose the recommended daily amounts of food from each food group that are appropriate to their energy needs (see Table 1-8 on p. 21).

Protein The protein needs of older adults appear to be about the same as those of younger people. Protein is especially important for older adults to support a healthy immune system and to prevent muscle wasting. Because energy needs decrease, however, the protein has to be obtained from low-kcalorie sources of high-quality protein, such as lean meats, poultry, fish, and eggs; fat-free and low-fat milk products; and legumes.

Underweight or malnourished older adults need protein- and energy-dense snacks such as hard-boiled eggs, tuna fish and crackers, peanut butter on wheat toast, and hearty soups. Drinking liquid nutritional formulas between meals can also boost energy and nutrient intakes.

Carbohydrate and Fiber As always, abundant carbohydrate is needed to protect protein from being used as an energy source. The recommendation to obtain ample amounts of mostly whole-grain breads, cereals, rice, and pasta holds true for older people. As for younger people, a steady supply of carbohydrate is essential for optimal brain functioning. With age, fiber takes on extra importance for its role in alleviating constipation, a common complaint among older adults and among nursing home residents in particular. Fruits and vegetables supply viscous (soluble) fibers thought to help ward off diseases of aging, but factors such as transportation problems, limited cooking facilities, and chewing problems limit some elderly people's intakes of fresh fruits and vegetables.[46] Most older adults do not obtain the recommended daily 25 or more grams of fiber (14 grams per 1000 kcalories).[47] When low fiber intakes are combined with low fluid intakes, inadequate physical activity, and constipating medications, constipation becomes inevitable.

Fat As is true for people of all ages, fat intake needs to be moderate in the diets of most older adults—enough to enhance flavors and provide valuable essential fatty acids and other nutrients, but not so much as to raise risks of cancer, atherosclerosis, and other degenerative diseases. The recommendation should not be taken too far; limiting fat too severely may lead to nutrient deficiencies and weight loss—two problems that carry greater health risks in the elderly than overweight.

WATER

Dehydration is a risk for older adults, who may not notice or pay attention to their thirst or who find it difficult and bothersome to get a drink or to get to a bathroom.[48] Older adults who have lost bladder control may be afraid to drink too much water. Despite real fluid needs, older people do not seem to feel as thirsty or notice mouth dryness as readily as younger people. Many nursing home employees say it is hard to persuade their elderly clients to drink enough water and fruit juices.

Total body water decreases as people age, so even mild stresses such as fever or hot weather can precipitate rapid dehydration in older adults. Dehydrated older adults seem to be more susceptible to urinary tract infections, pneumonia, pressure ulcers, confusion, and disorientation.[49] An intake of 9 cups a day of total beverages, including water, is recommended for women; for men, the recommendation is 13 cups a day of total beverages, including water.[50]

VITAMINS AND MINERALS

As research reveals more about how specific vitamins and minerals influence disease prevention and how age-related physiological changes affect nutrient metabolism, optimal intakes of vitamins and minerals for different groups of older adults are being defined. This section highlights the vitamins and minerals of greatest concern to older adults.

> **NURSING DIAGNOSIS**
> *Risk for deficient fluid volume* applies to clients who have deviations affecting fluid intake and access.

Vitamin D Older adults face a greater risk of vitamin D deficiency than younger people do. Vitamin D–fortified milk is the most reliable source of vitamin D, but many older adults drink little or no milk. Consequently, the vitamin D intakes of many older adults are less than half of recommendations. Further compromising the vitamin D status of many older people, especially those in nursing homes, is their limited exposure to sunlight. Finally, aging reduces the skin's capacity to make vitamin D and the kidneys' ability to convert it to its active form. Not only are older adults not getting enough vitamin D, but they may actually need more to improve both muscle and bone strength.[51] The margin lists vitamin D recommendations to prevent bone loss and to maintain vitamin D status in older people, especially those who engage in minimal outdoor activity.(✚)

Vitamin B$_{12}$ The DRI committee recommends that adults aged 51 years and older obtain 2.4 micrograms of vitamin B$_{12}$ daily *and* that vitamin B$_{12}$–fortified foods (such as fortified cereals) or supplements be used to meet much of the DRI recommended intake.[52] (✚) The committee's recommendation reflects the finding that an estimated 10 to 30 percent of adults older than 50 years lose the ability to produce enough stomach acid to make the protein-bound form of vitamin B$_{12}$ available for absorption. Synthetic vitamin B$_{12}$ is reliably absorbed, however. Given the poor cognition, anemia, and devastating neurological effects associated with a vitamin B$_{12}$ deficiency, an adequate intake is imperative.[53]

One cause of the malabsorption of protein-bound vitamin B$_{12}$ is a condition known as **atrophic gastritis**. The prevalence of atrophic gastritis among those 60 years of age and older is high.

Folate As is true of vitamin B$_{12}$, folate intakes of older adults typically fall short of recommendations. (✚) The elderly are also more likely to have medical conditions or to take medications that can compromise folate status.

Iron Among the minerals, iron deserves first mention. (✚) Iron-deficiency anemia is less common in older adults than in younger people, but it still occurs in some, especially in those with low food energy intakes. Aside from diet, other factors in many older people's lives make iron deficiency likely: chronic blood loss from disease conditions and medicines, and poor iron absorption due to reduced secretion of stomach acid and antacid use. Anyone concerned with older people's nutrition should keep these possibilities in mind.

Zinc Zinc intake is commonly low in older people. Zinc deficiency can depress the appetite and blunt the sense of taste, thereby leading to low food intakes and worsening of zinc status. Zinc deficiency may also increase the likelihood of infection.[54] Many medications that older adults commonly use can impair zinc absorption or enhance its excretion and thus lead to deficiency. (✚)

Calcium The importance of abundant dietary calcium throughout life to protect against osteoporosis has been emphasized throughout this book. The calcium intakes of many people, especially women, in the United States are well below the recommended amount. (✚) If milk causes stomach discomfort, as many older adults report, then lactose-modified milk or other calcium-rich foods should take its place.

NUTRIENT SUPPLEMENTS FOR OLDER ADULTS

People judge for themselves how to manage their nutrition, and more than half of older adults turn to dietary supplements. When recommended by a physician or registered dietitian, vitamin D and calcium supplements for osteoporosis or vitamin B$_{12}$ for pernicious anemia may be beneficial. Advertisers target older people with appeals to take

✚ Vitamin D AI during late adulthood:
- 10 µg/day (51–70 yr)
- 15 µg/day (>70 yr)

✚ Vitamin B$_{12}$ RDA during late adulthood:
- 2.4 µg/day

✚ Folate RDA during late adulthood:
- 400 µg/day

✚ Iron RDA during late adulthood:
- 8 mg/day

✚ Zinc RDA during late adulthood:
- 11 mg/day (men)
- 8 mg/day (women)

✚ Calcium AI during late adulthood:
- 1200 mg/day

atrophic gastritis (a-TRO-fik gas-TRI-tis): a condition characterized by chronic inflammation of the stomach accompanied by a diminished size and functioning of the mucosa and glands.

supplements and eat "health" foods, claiming that these products prevent disease and promote longevity. Quite often those who take supplements are not deficient in the nutrients being supplemented.

Elderly people often benefit from a balanced low-dose vitamin and mineral supplement, however.[55] Such supplements supply many of the needed minerals along with the vitamins often lacking in older people's diets without providing too much of any one nutrient.

Food is still the best source of nutrients for everybody, however. Supplements are just that—supplements to foods, not substitutes for them. For anyone who is motivated to obtain the best possible health, it is never too late to learn to eat well, become physically active, and adopt other lifestyle changes such as quitting smoking, moderating alcohol use, and the like. Table 12-6 summarizes the nutrient concerns of aging. Table 12-7 (p. 366) offers strategies for growing old healthfully.

THE EFFECTS OF DRUGS ON NUTRIENTS

As people grow older, the use of medicines—from over-the-counter types such as aspirin and laxatives to prescription medications of all kinds—becomes commonplace. Most drugs interact with one or more nutrients in several ways, usually resulting in greater-than-normal needs for these nutrients. Chapter 14 offers a discussion of diet-drug interactions and describes the many reasons why elderly people are vulnerable to such interactions.

The most common drug that can affect nutrition in older people is alcohol. The effects of alcohol on people of all ages are explained in Nutrition in Practice 19.

TABLE 12-6	Summary of Nutrient Concerns of Aging	
Nutrient	**Effect of Aging**	**Comments**
Water	Lack of thirst and decreased total body water make dehydration likely.	Mild dehydration is a common cause of confusion. Difficulty obtaining water or getting to the bathroom may compound the problem.
Energy	Need decreases as muscle mass decreases (sarcopenia).	Physical activity moderates the decline.
Fiber	Likelihood of constipation increases with low intakes and changes in the GI tract.	Inadequate water intakes and lack of physical activity, along with some medications, compound the problem.
Protein	Needs may stay the same or increase slightly.	Low-fat, high-fiber legumes and grains meet both protein and other nutrient needs.
Vitamin B$_{12}$	Atrophic gastritis is common.	Deficiency causes neurological damage; supplements may be needed.
Vitamin D	Increased likelihood of inadequate intake; skin synthesis declines.	Daily sunlight exposure in moderation or supplements may be beneficial.
Calcium	Intakes may be low; osteoporosis is common.	Stomach discomfort commonly limits milk intake; calcium substitutes or supplements may be needed.
Iron	In women, status improves after menopause; deficiencies are linked to chronic blood losses and low stomach acid output.	Adequate stomach acid is required for absorption; antacid or other medicine use may aggravate iron deficiency; vitamin C and meat increase absorption.

TABLE
12-7 | Strategies for Growing Old Healthfully

- Choose nutrient-dense foods.
- Be physically active. Walk, run, dance, swim, bike, or row for aerobic activity. Lift weights, do calisthenics, or pursue some other activity to tone, firm, and strengthen muscles. Practice balancing on one foot or doing simple movements with your eyes closed. Modify activities to suit changing abilities and tastes.
- Maintain appropriate body weight.
- Reduce stress (cultivate self-esteem, maintain a positive attitude, manage time wisely, know your limits, practice assertiveness, release tension, and take action).
- For women, discuss with a physician the risks and benefits of estrogen replacement therapy.
- For people who smoke, discuss with a physician strategies and programs to help you quit.
- Expect to enjoy sex, and learn new ways of enhancing it.
- Use alcohol only moderately, if at all; use drugs only as prescribed.
- Take care to prevent accidents.
- Expect good vision and hearing throughout life; obtain glasses and hearing aids if necessary.
- Take care of your teeth; obtain dentures if necessary.
- Be alert to confusion as a disease symptom, and seek diagnosis.

- Take medications as prescribed; see a physician before selfprescribing medicines or herbal remedies and a registered dietitian before self-prescribing supplements.
- Control depression through activities and friendships; seek professional help if necessary.
- Drink plenty of water every day.
- Practice mental skills. Keep on solving math problems and crossword puzzles, playing cards or other games, reading, writing, imagining, and creating.
- Make financial plans early to ensure security.
- Accept change. Work at recovering from losses; make new friends.
- Cultivate spiritual health. Cherish personal values. Make life meaningful.
- Go outside for sunshine and fresh air as often as possible.
- Be socially active—play bridge, join an exercise or dance group, take a class, teach a class, eat with friends, volunteer time to help others.
- Stay interested in life—pursue a hobby, spend time with grandchildren, take a trip, read, grow a garden, or go to the movies.
- Enjoy life.

Review Notes

- Table 12-6 summarizes the nutrient concerns of aging.
- The ever-growing number of older people creates an urgent need to know more about how their nutrient requirements differ from those of others and how such knowledge can enhance their health.

Food Choices and Eating Habits of Older Adults

To provide any benefit, strategies and interventions to improve a person's nutrition status must be based on knowledge of food preferences and eating patterns. Menus and feeding programs for older adults must take into consideration not only the food likes and dislikes but also the living conditions, economic status, and medical conditions of this diverse group of people. If nutrition intervention is to be successful, it is essential to know what foods people will eat, in what settings they like to eat these foods, and whether they can buy and prepare meals.

Older people are, for the most part, independent, socially sophisticated, mentally lucid, fully participating members of society who report themselves to be happy and healthy. In fact, chronic disabilities among the elderly have declined dramatically in recent years. Older people spend more money per person on foods to eat at home than other age groups and less money on foods away from home. Manufacturers would be wise to cater to the preferences of older adults by providing good-tasting, nutritious foods in easy-to-open, single-serving packages with labels that are easy to read. Such products enable older adults to maintain their independence; most of them want to take care of themselves and need to feel a sense of control and involvement in their own lives. As discussed earlier, another way older adults can take care of themselves is by remaining or becoming physically active. Physical activity helps preserve one's ability to perform daily tasks and so promotes independence.[56]

Shared meals can brighten the day and enhance the appetite

INDIVIDUAL PREFERENCES

Familiarity, taste, and health beliefs are most influential on older people's food choices. Eating foods that are familiar, especially ethnic foods that recall family meals and pleasant times, can be comforting. Older adults are choosing poultry and fish, low-fat milk and milk products, and high-fiber breads and grains, indicating that they recognize the importance of diet in supporting good health. Few older adults, however, consume the recommended amounts of milk products.

MEAL SETTING

The food choices and eating habits of older adults are also affected by the changes in lifestyle that often accompany aging in this society. Whether people live alone, with others, or in institutions affects the way they eat. For example, men living alone are most likely to be poorly nourished. Older adults who live alone do not make poorer food choices than those who live with companions; rather, they consume too little food: loneliness is directly related to inadequacies, especially of energy intakes.

DEPRESSION

Another factor affecting food intake and appetite in older people is depression. Loss of appetite and motivation to cook or even to eat frequently accompanies depression. An overwhelming feeling of grief and sadness at the death of a spouse, friend, or family member may leave many people, particularly elderly people, with a feeling of powerlessness to overcome the depression. The support and companionship of family and friends, especially at mealtimes, can help overcome depression and enhance appetite. The accompanying Case Study presents a man who has several of these problems. Use the suggestions here, and in the last section of this chapter, to help develop solutions. The Nutrition Assessment Checklist for Older Adults at the end of this chapter helps to pinpoint nutrition-related factors to look for when working with older adults. To *determine* the risk of malnutrition in older clients, health care providers can keep in mind the characteristics listed in the margin. (✚)

Risk factors for malnutrition in older adults:
- **D**isease
- **E**ating poorly
- **T**ooth loss or oral pain
- **E**conomic hardship
- **R**educed social contact
- **M**ultiple medications
- **I**nvoluntary weight loss or gain
- **N**eeds assistance with self-care
- **E**lderly person older than 80 years

FOOD ASSISTANCE PROGRAMS

Federally funded programs can provide food and nutrition services for older adults.[57] The Older Americans Act (OAA) provides many different services and support to help older adults remain independent. An integral component of the OAA is the OAA

CASE STUDY | Elderly Man with a Poor Diet

Mr. Brezenoff is 75 years old and lives alone. He has slowly been losing weight since his wife died a year ago. At 5 feet 8 inches tall, he currently weighs 124 pounds. His previous weight was 150 pounds. In talking with Mr. Brezenoff, you realize that he doesn't even like to talk about food, let alone eat it. "My wife always did the cooking before, and I ate well. Now I just don't feel like eating." You manage to find out that he skips breakfast, has soup and bread for lunch, and sometimes eats a cold-cut sandwich or a frozen dinner for supper. He seldom sees friends or relatives. Mr. Brezenoff has also lost several teeth and doesn't eat any raw fruits or vegetables because he finds them hard to chew. He lives on a meager but adequate income.

1. Consult the BMI table (inside back cover), and judge whether Mr. Brezenoff is at a healthy weight. What other assessments might you use to back up your judgment? Is his weight loss significant?

2. What factors are contributing to Mr. Brezenoff's poor food intake? What nutrients are probably deficient in his diet?

3. Look at Mr. Brezenoff as an individual and suggest ways he can improve his diet and his lifestyle.

4. What other aspects of Mr. Brezenoff's physical and mental health should you consider in helping him to improve his food intake?

TABLE 12-8	Food Assistance Programs for Older Adults

OAA Nutrition Program

Services: Provides congregate and home-delivered meals to improve older people's nutrition status. Includes transportation to congregate meal sites; shopping assistance; information and referral; and, to some extent, nutrition counseling and education.

Impact: Improves the nutrient content of high-risk older adults' diets and offers socialization and recreation. Many of the nutrition programs around the country go above and beyond federal requirements of congregate and home meals by offering lunch clubs, ethnic meals, and meals for older homeless people.

Supplemental Nutrition Assistance Program (SNAP)

Services: Supplements income for low-income households by means of a card similar to a debit card that can be used to purchase food.

Impact: Serves more as an income supplement for some elderly participants than as a device to improve nutrition status. For other elderly participants, nutrient intakes are higher than those of nonparticipants with similar incomes.

Meals on Wheels

Services: Delivers meals directly to the homebound elderly; integrated into the meal delivery services provided by the OAA Program.

Impact: Focuses on filling the need for weekend and holiday meals for the homebound elderly people, a service that is limited in the OAA Nutrition Program.

Senior Farmers Market Nutrition Program

Services: Provides low-income older adults with coupons that can be exchanged for fresh fruits, vegetables, and herbs at community-supported farmers' markets and roadside stands; administered by the USDA. State agencies may limit sales to specific foods that are locally grown to encourage recipients to support farmers in their own states.

Impact: Increases fresh fruit and vegetable consumption, provides nutrition information, and even reaches the homebound elderly, a group of people who normally do not have access to farmers' markets.

Nutrition Program, formerly known as the Elderly Nutrition Program, which offers services that promote health to older adults. Table 12-8 summarizes food assistance programs available to the elderly.

MEALS FOR SINGLES

Many older adults live alone, and singles of all ages face challenges in purchasing, storing, and preparing food. Large packages of meat and vegetables are often intended for families of four or more, and even a head of lettuce can spoil before one person can use it all. Many singles live in small dwellings and have little storage space for foods. A limited income presents additional obstacles. This section offers suggestions that can help to solve some of the problems singles face, beginning with a note about the dangers of foodborne illness.

Foodborne Illness The risk of older adults getting a foodborne illness is greater than for other adults. The consequences of an upset stomach, diarrhea, fever, vomiting, abdominal cramps, and dehydration are oftentimes more severe, sometimes leading to paralysis, meningitis, or even death. For these reasons, older adults need to carefully follow the food safety suggestions presented in Nutrition in Practice 2.

Spend Wisely People who have the means to shop and cook for themselves can cut their food bills just by being wise shoppers. Large supermarkets are usually less expensive than convenience stores. A grocery list helps reduce impulse buying, and specials and coupons can save money when the items featured are those that the shopper needs and uses.

Buying the right amount so as not to waste any food is a challenge for people eating alone. They can buy fresh milk in the size best suited for personal needs. Pint-size and even cup-size boxes (✚) of milk are available and can be stored unopened on a shelf for up to three months without refrigeration.

Many foods that offer a variety of nutrients for practically pennies have a long shelf life; staples such as rice, pastas, dry powdered milk, and dried legumes can be purchased in bulk and stored for months at room temperature. Other foods that are usually a good buy include whole pieces of cheese rather than sliced or shredded cheese, fresh produce in season, variety meats such as chicken livers, and cereals that require cooking instead of ready-to-serve cereals.

A person who has ample freezing space can buy large packages of meat, such as pork chops, ground beef, or chicken, when they are on sale. Then the meat can be immediately wrapped in individual servings for the freezer. All the individual servings can be put in a bag marked appropriately with the contents and the date.

Frozen vegetables are more economical in large bags than in small boxes. The amount needed can be taken out, and the bag closed tightly with a twist tie or rubber band. If the package is returned quickly to the freezer each time, the vegetables will stay fresh for a long time.

Finally, breads and cereals usually must be purchased in larger quantities. Again the amount needed for a few days can be taken out and the rest stored in the freezer.

People who do not have freezers can ask the grocer to break open a package of wrapped meat and rewrap the portion needed. Similarly, eggs can be purchased by the half-dozen. Eggs do keep for long periods, though, if stored properly in the refrigerator.

Fresh fruits and vegetables can be purchased individually. A person can buy fresh fruit at various stages of ripeness: a ripe one to eat right away, a semiripe one to eat soon after, and a green one to ripen on the windowsill. If vegetables are packaged in large quantities, the grocer can break open the package so that a smaller amount can be purchased. Small cans of fruits and vegetables, even though they are more expensive per unit, are a reasonable alternative, considering that it is expensive to buy a regular-size can and let the unused portion spoil.

Be Creative Creative chefs think of various ways to use foods when only large amounts are available. For example, a head of cauliflower can be divided into thirds. Then one-third is cooked and eaten hot, another third is put into a vinegar and oil marinade for use in a salad, and the last third can be used in a casserole or stew.

A variety of vegetables and meats can be enjoyed stir-fried; inexpensive vegetables such as cabbage, celery, and onion are delicious when crisp cooked in a little oil with herbs or lemon added. Interesting frozen vegetable mixtures are available in larger grocery stores. Cooked, leftover vegetables can be dropped in at the last minute. A bonus of a stir-fried meal is that there is only one pan to wash. Similarly, a microwave oven allows a home chef to use fewer pots and pans. Meals and leftovers can also be frozen or refrigerated in microwavable containers to reheat as needed.

Many frozen dinners or grocery store take-out foods offer nutritious options. Adding a fresh salad, a whole-wheat roll, and a glass of milk can make a nutritionally balanced meal. The "How to" (p. 370) offers time-saving tips to turn convenience foods into nutritious meals.

Also, single people shouldn't hesitate to invite someone to share meals with them whenever there is enough food. It's likely that the person will return the invitation, and both parties will get to enjoy companionship and a meal prepared by others.

✚ Boxes of milk that can be stored at room temperature have been exposed to temperatures above those of pasteurization just long enough to sterilize the milk—a process called *ultrahigh temperature (UHT)*.

These time-saving tips can turn convenience foods into nutritious meals:

- Add extra nutrients and a fresh flavor to canned stews and soups by tossing in some frozen ready-to-use mixed vegetables. Choose vegetables frozen without salty, fatty sauces—prepared foods generally contain enough salt to season the whole dish, including added vegetables.

- Buy frozen vegetables in a bag, toss in a variety of herbs, and use as needed.

- When grilling burgers or chicken, wrap a mixture of frozen broccoli, onion, and carrots in a foil packet with a tablespoon of Italian dressing and grill alongside the meat for seasoned grilled vegetables.

- Use canned fruits in their own juices as desserts. Toss in some frozen berries or peach slices and top with flavored yogurt for an instant fruit salad.

- Prepared rice or noodle dishes are convenient, but those claiming to contain broccoli, spinach, or other vegetables seldom contain enough to qualify as a serving of vegetables. Pump up the nutrient value by adding a half-cup of frozen vegetables per serving of pasta or rice just before cooking.

- Purchase frozen onion, mushroom, and pepper mixtures to embellish jarred spaghetti sauce or small frozen pizzas. Top with parmesan cheese.

- Use frozen shredded potatoes, sold for hash browns, in soups or stews or mix with a handful of shredded reduced-fat cheese or a can of fat-free "cream of anything" soup and bake for a quick and hearty casserole.

- Purchase a bag of triple-washed, ready-to-eat salad and add any or all of the following to make a hearty, healthy salad: a small can of garbanzo beans or a package of frozen edamame (soy beans); a handful of shredded reduced-fat cheese; a hardboiled egg; a handful of toasted almonds or other nuts.

- Open a can of pinto beans or black beans, heat a tablespoon of olive oil, and sauté a little bit of frozen onion and pepper mixture. Add the beans and mash them in the oil and vegetables. Serve the bean mixture in a soft taco shell with shredded reduced-fat cheese, lettuce, and salsa for a tasty, nutritious bean taco.

Review Notes

- Food choices of older adults are affected by health status and changed life circumstances.
- Older people can benefit from both the nutrients provided and the social interaction available at congregate meals. Other government programs deliver meals to those who are homebound.
- With creativity and careful shopping, those living alone can prepare nutritious, inexpensive meals.

Nutrition Assessment | CHECKLIST FOR OLDER ADULTS

MEDICAL HISTORY

Check the medical record for:

- ○ Alcohol abuse
- ○ Alzheimer's disease or other dementia or confusion
- ○ Arthritis
- ○ Cataracts
- ○ Chronic diseases (cancer, heart disease, hypertension, diabetes)
- ○ Cigarette, cigar, or pipe smoking; use of other tobacco products
- ○ Constipation
- ○ Dehydration
- ○ Dental disease or tooth loss
- ○ Depression
- ○ Inflammation of the stomach (gastritis)
- ○ Swallowing disorders

MEDICATIONS

For older adults being treated with drug therapy for medical conditions, note:

- ○ Use of multiple medications—prescription and/or over-the-counter medications such as laxatives and pain relievers
- ○ Side effects that might reduce food intake or change nutrient needs

- Proper administration of medication with respect to food intake
- Malnutrition—is the person's nutrition status questionable even before considering side effects of medications that worsen nutrition status?
- Diminished mental capacity that might interfere with taking correct medications and doses
- Dehydration (can alter effects of medications)

DIETARY INTAKE

For all older adults, especially those at risk nutritionally, assess the diet for:

- Total energy
- Protein
- Calcium, iron, and zinc
- Vitamin B_6, vitamin B_{12}, folate, and vitamin D

Note the following:

- Number of meals eaten each day
- Number and ages of people in household
- Amount of milk consumed each day
- Type and frequency of outdoor activity
- Type and frequency of physical activity
- Financial resources
- Transportation resources
- Physical disabilities
- Mental alertness

ANTHROPOMETRIC DATA

Measure baseline height and weight.

- Reassess height and weight at each medical checkup.
- Note significant overweight or underweight, which warrants intervention.
- Use skinfold measures to reveal altered body composition that may indicate malnutrition and loss of lean tissue.

LABORATORY TESTS

- Hemoglobin, hematocrit, or other tests of iron status
- Serum albumin or other measures of protein status
- Serum folate
- Serum B_{12}

PHYSICAL SIGNS

Look for physical signs of:

- Protein-energy malnutrition
- Iron and zinc deficiency
- Folate deficiency

Self Check

1. The fastest-growing age group in the United States is:
   a. under 21 years of age.
   b. 30 to 45 years of age.
   c. 50 to 70 years of age.
   d. over 85 years of age.

2. Which of the following lifestyle habits can enhance the length and quality of people's lives?
   a. Moderate smoking
   b. Six hours of sleep daily
   c. Regular physical activity
   d. Skipping breakfast

3. Which of the following is among the better-known relationships between nutrition and disease prevention?
   a. Appropriate fiber intake helps prevent goiter.
   b. Moderate sodium intake helps prevent obesity.
   c. Moderate sugar intake helps prevent hypertension.
   d. Appropriate energy intake helps prevent diabetes and cardiovascular disease.

4. A disease of the immune system that involves painful inflammation of the joints is:
   a. sarcopenia.
   b. osteoarthritis.
   c. senile dementia.
   d. rheumatoid arthritis.

5. Examples of low-kcalorie, high-quality protein foods include:
   a. cottage cheese, sour cream, and eggs.
   b. green and yellow vegetables and citrus fruits.
   c. potatoes, rice, pasta, and whole-grain breads.
   d. lean meats, poultry, fish, legumes, fat-free milk, and eggs.

6. For malnourished and underweight people, protein- and energy-dense snacks include:
   a. fresh fruits and vegetables.
   b. yogurt and cottage cheese.
   c. whole grains and high-fiber legumes.
   d. hard-boiled eggs and peanut butter and graham crackers.

7. Which of the following does not explain why dehydration is a risk for older adults?
   a. They do not seem to feel thirsty.
   b. Total body water increases with age.
   c. They may find it difficult to get a drink.
   d. They may have difficulty swallowing liquids.

8. Inadequate milk intake and limited exposure to sunlight contribute to older adults' risk of:
   a. vitamin A deficiency.
   b. vitamin D deficiency.
   c. riboflavin deficiency.
   d. vitamin B_{12} deficiency.

9. Two risk factors for malnutrition in older adults are:
   a. loneliness and multiple medication use.
   b. increased energy needs and lack of fiber.
   c. decreased mineral absorption and antioxidant intake.
   d. high carbohydrate intake and lack of physical activity.

10. Two strategies to improve nutrition status when growing old include:
    a. increase vitamin A intake and exercise 30 minutes daily.

b. choose nutrient-dense foods and maintain appropriate weight.
c. avoid high-fiber foods and take a daily vitamin-mineral supplement.
d. eat at least one big meal per day and drink at least 10 glasses of water daily.

Answers to these questions appear in Appendix H.

Clinical Applications

1. Ms. Hamilton is an 80-year-old woman in excellent health who lives alone, eats a well-balanced diet, enjoys an active social life, and walks every day. Consider the way Ms. Hamilton's health and nutrition status might be affected by the following situations:

   - Many of Ms. Hamilton's friends pass away or move into extended care facilities.
   - Ms. Hamilton falls and breaks her hip.
   - Ms. Hamilton begins to feel isolated and depressed.

   Describe interventions the health care professional can take to help Ms. Hamilton deal with each situation to prevent her from falling into a downward spiral.

Nutrition on the Net

For further study of the topics in this chapter, access these websites.

- Find updates and quick links to these and other nutrition-related sites at our website: www.cengage.com/nutrition/whitney/nhhc4e
- Search for "aging," "arthritis," and "Alzheimer's" on the U.S. government health information site: www.healthfinder.gov
- Visit the National Aging Information Center of the Administration on Aging: www.aoa.gov
- Visit the American Geriatrics Society Foundation for Health in Aging: www.healthinaging.org
- Visit the National Institution on Aging: www.nia.nih.gov
- Visit the American Association of Retired Persons: www.aarp.org
- Get nutrition tips for growing older in good health from the American Dietetic Association: www.eatright.org
- Learn more about cataracts and macular degeneration from the National Eye Institute, the Macular Degeneration Partnership, and the American Society of Cataract and

Refractive Surgery: www.nei.nih.gov, www.amd.org, and www.ascrs.org
- Learn more about arthritis from the Arthritis Society, the Arthritis Foundation, and the National Institute of Arthritis and Musculoskeletal and Skin Diseases: www.arthritis.ca, www.arthritis.org, and www.niams.nih.gov
- Learn more about Alzheimer's disease from the NIA Alzheimer's Disease Education and Referral Center and the Alzheimer's Association: www.nia.nih.gov/alzheimers and www.alz.org
- Learn more about malnutrition in older adults and the Nutrition Screening Initiative from the American Academy of Family Physicians: www.aafp.org
- Find out about federal government programs designed to help senior citizens maintain good health: www.seniors.gov
- Visit the National Council on Aging: www.ncoa.org

Notes

1. National Center for Health Statistics, Life expectancy at age 65 years, by sex and race—United States, 2000-2006, *Morbidity and Mortality Weekly Report* 58 (2009): 473.
2. H. Kung and coauthors, Deaths: Final data for 2005, *National Vital Statistics Reports* 56 (2008): 1–120; S. Harper and coauthors, Trends in the black-white life expectancy gap in the United States, 1983–2003, *Journal of the American Medical Association* 297 (2007): 1224–1232.
3. C. J. Lavie and coauthors, Obesity and cardiovascular disease, *Journal of the American College of Cardiology* 53 (2009): 1925–1932; R. S. Blacklow, Actuarially speaking: An overview of life expectancy. What can we expect? *American Journal of Clinical Nutrition* 86 (2007): 1560S–1562S.
4. Position of the American Dietetic Association: Nutrition across the spectrum of aging, *Journal of the American Dietetic Association* 105 (2005): 616–633.

5. L. B. Yates and coauthors, Exceptional longevity in men: Modifiable factors associated with survival and function to age 90 years, *Archives of Internal Medicine* 168 (2008): 284–290; R. S. Rivlin, Keeping the young-elderly healthy: Is it too late to improve our health through nutrition? *American Journal of Clinical Nutrition* 86 (2007): 1572S–1576S; N. M. Peel, R. J. McClure, and H. P. Bartlett, Behavioral determinants of health aging, *American Journal of Preventive Medicine* 28 (2005): 298–304.

6. Yates and coauthors, 2008; K. Khaw and coauthors, Combined impact of health behaviours and mortality in men and women: The EPIC-Norfolk Prospective Population Study, *PLoS Medicine* 5 (2008): e12.

7. Yates and coauthors, 2008.

8. Yates and coauthors, 2008; X. Sui and coauthors, Cardiorespiratory fitness and adiposity as mortality predictors in older adults, *Journal of the American Medical Association* 298 (2007): 2507–2516.

9. American College of Sports Medicine, Position stand: Exercise and physical activity for older adults, *Medicine and Science in Sports and Exercise* 41 (2009): 1510–1530; P. Kokkinos and coauthors, Exercise capacity and mortality in black and white men, *Circulation* 117 (2008): 614–622; Position of the American Dietetic Association, 2005.

10. R. C. Cassilhas and coauthors, The impact of resistance exercise on the cognitive function of the elderly, *Medicine and Science in Sports and Exercise* 39 (2007): 1401–1407; W. R. Bixby and coauthors, The unique relation of physical activity to executive function in older men and women, *Medicine and Science in Sports and Exercise* 39 (2007): 1408–1416.

11. Rivlin, 2007.

12. M. E. Nelson and coauthors, Physical activity and public health in older adults: Recommendation for the American College of Sports Medicine and the American Heart Association, *Medicine and Science in Sports and Exercise* 39 (2007): 1435–1445.

13. R. Koopman and L. J. van Loon, Aging, exercise, and muscle protein metabolism, *Journal of Applied Physiology*, 106 (2009): 2040–2048; K. A. Martin Ginis and coauthors, Weight training to activities of daily living: Helping older adults make a connection, *Medicine and Science in Sports and Exercise* 38 (2006): 116–121.

14. Nelson and coauthors, 2007.

15. J. R. Speakman and C. Hambly, Starving for life: What animal studies can and cannot tell us about the use of caloric restriction to prolong human lifespan, *Journal of Nutrition* 137 (2007): 1078–1086.

16. L. Fontana and S. Klein, Aging, adiposity, and calorie restriction, *Journal of the American Medical Association* 297 (2007): 986–994; Position of the American Dietetic Association, 2005.

17. Fontana and Klein, 2007.

18. K. A. Varady and M. K. Hellerstein, Do calorie restriction or alternate-day fasting regimens modulate adipose tissue physiology in a way that reduces chronic disease risk? *Nutrition Reviews* 66 (2008): 333–342.

19. Fontana and Klein, 2007.

20. W. G. Christen and coauthors, Dietary carotenoids, vitamins C and E, and risk of cataract in women. A prospective study, *Archives of Ophthalmology* 126 (2008): 102–109; A. G. Tan and coauthors, Antioxidant nutrient intake and the long-term incidence of age-related cataract: The Blue Mountains Eye Study, *American Journal of Clinical Nutrition* 87 (2008): 1899–1905; W. G. Christen and coauthors, Fruit and vegetable intake and the risk of cataract in women, *American Journal of Clinical Nutrition* 81 (2005): 1417–1422.

21. R. D. Jager, W. F. Mieler, and J. W. Miller, Age-related macular degeneration, *New England Journal of Medicine* 358 (2008): 2606–2617.

22. C. Augood and coauthors, Oily fish consumption, dietary docosahexaenoic acid and eicosapentaenoic acid intakes, and associations with neovascular age-related macular degeneration, *American Journal of Clinical Nutrition* 88 (2008): 398–406; E. J. Johnson and coauthors, The influence of supplemental lutein and docosahexaenoic acid on serum, lipoproteins, and macular pigmentation, *American Journal of Clinical Nutrition* 87 (2008): 1521–1529; E. D. O'Connell and coauthors, Diet and risk factors for age-related maculopathy, *American Journal of Clinical Nutrition* 87 (2008): 712–722; H. Coleman and E. Chew, Nutritional supplementation in age-related macular degeneration, *Current Opinion in Ophthalmology* 18 (2007): 220–223; P. R. Trumbo and K. C. Ellwood, Lutein and zeaxanthin intakes and risk of age-related macular degeneration and cataracts: An evaluation using the Food and Drug Administration's evidence-based review system for health claims, *American Journal of Clinical Nutrition* 84 (2006): 971–974.

23. Prevalence of doctor-diagnosed arthritis and arthritis-attributable activity limitation—United States, 2003–2005, *Morbidity and Mortality Weekly* 55 (2006): 1089–1092.

24. L. E. Hart and coauthors, The relationship between exercise and osteoarthritis in the elderly, *Clinical Journal of Sport Medicine* 18 (2008): 508–521; L. Devos-Comby, T. Cronan, and S. C. Roesch, Do exercise and

self-management interventions benefit patients with osteoarthritis of knee? A metaanalytic review, *Journal of Rheumatology* 33 (2006): 744–756.

25. C. T. Vangsness, W. Spiker, and J. Erickson, A review of evidence-based medicine for glucosamine and chondroitin sulfate use in knee osteoarthritis, *Arthroscopy* 25 (2009): 86–94; National Center for Complimentary and Alternative Medicine, The NIH Glucosamine/Chondroitin Arthritis Intervention Trial (GAIT), *Journal of Pain and Palliative Care Pharmacotherapy* 22 (2008): 39–43; S. Dahmer and R. M. Schiller, Glucosamine, *American Family Physician* 78 (2008): 471–476; O. Bruyere and J. Y. Reginster, Glucosamine and chondroitin sulfate as therapeutic agents for knee and hip osteoarthritis, *Drugs and Aging* 24 (2007): 573–580; D. O. Clegg and coauthors, Glucosamine, chondroitin sulfate, and two in combination for painful knee osteoarthritis, *New England Journal of Medicine* 354 (2006): 795–808.

26. G. McKellar and coauthors, A pilot study of a Mediterranean-type diet intervention in female patients with rheumatoid arthritis living in areas of social deprivation in Glasgow, *Annals of the Rheumatic Diseases* 66 (2007): 1239–1243.

27. P. M. Kris-Etherton and A. M. Hill, n-3 Fatty acids: Foods or supplements? *Journal of the American Dietetic Association* 108 (2008): 1125–1130.

28. A. D. Smith and H. Refsum, Vitamin B-12 and cognition in the elderly, *American Journal of Clinical Nutrition* 89 (2009): 707S–711S; D. M. Lee and coauthors, Association between 25-hydroxyvitamin D levels and cognitive performance in middle-aged and older European men, *Journal of Neurology, Neurosurgery, and Psychiatry* 80 (2009): 722–729; W. J. Lukiw and N. G. Bazan, Docosahexaenoic acid and the aging brain, *Journal of Nutrition* 138 (2008): 2510–2514; B. M. van Gelder and coauthors, Fish consumption, n-3 fatty acids, and subsequent 5-y cognitive decline in elderly men: The Zutphen Elderly Study, *American Journal of Clinical Nutrition* 85 (2007): 1142–1147; L. M. L. de Lau and coauthors, Plasma folate concentration and cognitive performance: Rotterdam Scan Study, *American Journal of Clinical Nutrition* 86 (2007): 728–734; M. N Haan and coauthors, Homocysteine, B vitamins, and the incidence of dementia and cognitive impairment: Results from the Sacramento Area Latino Study on Aging, *American Journal of Clinical Nutrition* 85 (2007): 511–517.

29. Centers for Disease Control and Prevention, Alzheimer's Disease, available at www.cdc.gov/Features/Alzheimer's. Site accessed August 17, 2009.

30. A. Burns and S. Lliffe, Clinical review—Alzheimer's disease, *British Medical Journal* 338 (2009): b158; T. D. Bird, Genetic factors in Alzheimer's Disease, *New England Journal of Medicine* 352 (2005): 862–864.

31. D. Praticò, Evidence of oxidative stress in Alzheimer's disease brain and antioxidant therapy: Lights and shadows, *Annals of the New York Academy of Sciences* 1147 (2008): 70–78; I. G. Onyango and S. M. Khan, Oxidative stress, mitochondrial dysfunction, and stress signaling in Alzheimer's disease, *Current Alzheimer Research* 3 (2006): 339–349; P. I. Moreira and coauthors, Oxidative stress: The old enemy in Alzheimer's disease pathophysiology, *Current Alzheimer Research* 2 (2005): 403–408.

32. Praticò, 2008; P. I. Moreira and coauthors, Alzheimer disease and the role of free radicals in the pathogenesis of the disease, *CNS and Neurological Disorders Drug Targets* 7 (2008): 3–10; A. Nunomura and coauthors, Involvement of oxidative stress in Alzheimer disease, *Journal of Neuropathology and Experimental Neurology* 65 (2006): 631–641.

33. W. Wang and coauthors, Nutritional biomarkers in Alzheimer's disease: The association between carotenoids, n-3 fatty acids, and dementia severity, *Journal of Alzheimer's Disease* 13 (2008): 31–38; H. J. Wengreen and coauthors, Antioxidant intake and cognitive function of elderly men and women: The Cache County Study, *Journal of Nutrition, Health, and Aging*, 11 (2007): 230–237; F. C. Lau, B. Shukitt-Hale, and J. A. Joseph, Nutritional intervention in brain aging: Reducing the effects of inflammation and oxidative stress, *Sub-cellular Biochemistry* 42 (2007): 299–318; L. Letenneur and coauthors, Flavonoid intake and cognitive decline over a 10-year period, *American Journal of Epidemiology* 165 (2007): 1364–1371.

34. J. A. Luchsinger and D. R. Gustafson, Adiposity and Alzheimer's disease, *Current Opinion in Clinical Nutrition and Metabolic Care* 12 (2009): 15–21; D. B. Miller and J. P. O'Callaghan, Do early-life insults contribute to the late-life development of Parkinson and Alzheimer diseases? *Metabolism* 57 (2008): S44–S49; R. A. Whitmer, The epidemiology of adiposity and dementia, *Current Alzheimer Research* 4 (2007): 117–122.

35. Moreira and coauthors, 2008; R. J. Castellani and coauthors, Antioxidant protection and neurodegenerative disease: The role of amyloid-beta and tau, *American Journal of Alzheimer's Disease and Other Dementias* 21 (2006): 126–130; P. Zafrilla and coauthors, Oxidative stress in Alzheimer

patients in different stages of the disease, *Current Medicinal Chemistry* 13 (2006): 1075–1083.

36. R. A. Armstrong, Plaques and tangles and the pathogenesis of Alzheimer's disease, *Folia Neuropathologica* 44 (2006): 1–11; G. L. Wenk, Neuropathologic changes in Alzheimer's disease: Potential targets for treatment, *Journal of Clinical Psychiatry* 67 (2006): 3–7.

37. R. J. Castellani and coauthors, Reexamining Alzheimer's disease; Evidence for a protective role for amyloid-beta protein precursor and amyloid-beta, *Journal of Alzheimer's Disease* 18 (2009): 447–452; A. Nunomura and coauthors, Neuropathology in Alzheimer's disease: Awaking from a hundred-year-old dream, *Science of Aging Knowledge Environment* (2006): pe10; R. E. Tanzi, Tangles and neurodegenerative disease—A surprising twist, *New England Journal of Medicine* 353 (2005): 1853–1855.

38. D. J. Selkoe, Developing preventive therapies for chronic diseases: Lessons learned from Alzheimer's disease, *Nutrition Reviews* 65 (2007): S239–S243.

39. J. A. Luchsinger and D. R. Gustafson, Adiposity, type 2 diabetes, and Alzheimer's disease, *Journal of Alzheimer's Disease* 16 (2009): 693–704; M. N. Haan and coauthors, Homocysteine, B vitamins, and the incidence of dementia and cognitive impairment: Results from the Sacramento Area Latino Study on Aging, *American Journal of Clinical Nutrition* 85 (2007): 511–517; G. Ravaglia and coauthors, Homocysteine and folate as risk factors for dementia and Alzheimer disease, *American Journal of Clinical Nutrition* 82 (2005): 636–643; K. L. Tucker and coauthors, High homocysteine and low B vitamins predict cognitive decline in aging men: The Veterans Affairs Normative Aging Study, *American Journal of Clinical Nutrition* 82 (2005): 627–635.

40. L. J. Whalley and coauthors, n-3 Fatty acid erythrocyte membrane content, APOE ε4, and cognitive variation: An observational follow-up study in late adulthood, *American Journal of Clinical Nutrition* 87 (2008): 449–454; M. A. Beydoun and coauthors, Plasma n-3 fatty acids and the risk of cognitive decline in older adults: The Atherosclerosis Risk in Communities study, *American Journal of Clinical Nutrition* 85 (2007): 1103–1111; W. E. Connor and S. L. Connor, The importance of fish and docosahexaenoic acid in Alzheimer disease, *American Journal of Clinical Nutrition* 85 (2007): 929–930; C. Dullemeijer and coauthors, n-3 Fatty acid proportions in plasma and cognitive performance in older adults, *American Journal of Clinical Nutrition* 86 (2007): 1479–1485; B. M. V. Gelder and coauthors, Fish consumption, n-3 fatty acids, and subsequent 5-y cognitive decline in elderly men: The Zutphen Elderly study, *American Journal of Clinical Nutrition* 85 (2007): 1142–1147; E. Nurk and coauthors, Cognitive performance among the elderly and dietary fish intake: The Hordaland Health study, *American Journal of Clinical Nutrition* 86 (2007): 1470–1478; E. J. Schaefer and coauthors, Plasma phosphatidylcholin docosahexaenoic acid content and risk of dementia and Alzheimer disease, *Archives of Neurology* 63 (2006): 1545–1550; R. Uauy and A. D. Dangour, Nutrition in brain development and aging: Role of essential fatty acids, *Nutrition Reviews* 64 (2006): S24–S33.

41. N. Scarmeas and coauthors, Physical activity, diet, and risk of Alzheimer disease, *Journal of the American Medical Association* 302 (2009): 627–637; T. Liu-Ambrose and M. G. Donaldson, Exercise and cognition in older adults: Is there a role for resistance training programmes? *British Journal of Sports Medicine* 43 (2009): 25–27; E. B. Larson, Physical activity for older adults at risk for Alzheimer disease, *Journal of the American Medical Association* 300 (2008): 1077–1079; N. T. Lautenschlager and coauthors, Effect of physical activity on cognitive function in older adults at risk for Alzheimer disease, *Journal of the American Medical Association* 300 (2008): 1027–1037.

42. Koopman and van Loon, 2009; M. Cesari and coauthors, Frailty syndrome and skeletal muscle: Results from the Invecchiare in Chianti Study, *American Journal of Clinical Nutrition* 83 (2006): 1142–1148.

43. Koopman and van Loon, 2009; D. K. Houston and coauthors, Dietary protein intake is associated with lean mass change in older, community-dwelling adults: The Health, Aging, and Body Composition (Health ABC) Study, *American Journal of Clinical Nutrition* 87 (2008): 150–155;

D. Paddon-Jones and coauthors, Role of dietary protein in the sarcopenia of aging, *American Journal of Clinical Nutrition* 87 (2008): 1562S–1566S; H. B. Iglay and coauthors, Resistance training and dietary protein: Effects on glucose tolerance and contents of skeletal muscle insulin signaling proteins in older persons, *American Journal of Clinical Nutrition* 85 (2007): 1005–1013; W. W. Campbell, Synergistic use of higher-protein diets or nutritional supplements with resistance training to counter sarcopenia, *Nutrition Reviews* 65 (2007): 416–422.

44. S. Karinkanta and coauthors, A multi-component exercise regimen to prevent functional decline and bone fragility in home-dwelling elderly women: Randomized, controlled trial, *Osteoporosis International* 18 (2007): 453–462; Rivlin, 2007.

45. Rivlin, 2007; Position of the American Dietetic Association, 2005.

46. R. B. Ervin and B. A. Dye, The effect of functional dentition on Healthy Eating Index scores and nutrient intakes in a nationally representative sample of older adults, *Journal of Public Health Dentistry* 69 (2009): 207–216; R. B. Ervin, Healthy Eating Index scores among adults 60 years of age and over by sociodemographic and health characteristics: United States, 1999–2002, *Advance Data* 20 (2008): 1–16; Position of the American Dietetic Association, 2005.

47. Standing Committee on the Scientific Evaluation of Dietary Reference Intakes, Food and Nutrition Board, Institute of Medicine, *Dietary Reference Intakes for Energy, Carbohydrate, Fiber, Fat, Fatty Acids, Cholesterol, Protein, and Amino Acids* (Washington D.C.: National Academies Press, 2005), pp. 387–389.

48. Effect of aging on regional cerebral blood flow responses associated with osmotic thirst and its satiation by water drinking: A PET study, *Proceedings of the National Academy of Sciences of the United States of America* 105 (2008): 382–387; Position of the American Dietetic Association, 2005.

49. Standing Committee on the Scientific Evaluation of Dietary Reference Intakes, Food and Nutrition Board, Institute of Medicine, *Dietary Reference Intakes for Water, Potassium, Sodium, Chloride, and Sulfate* (Washington, D.C.: National Academies Press, 2005), pp. 118–127; Position of the American Dietetic Association: Liberalization of the diet prescription improves quality of life for older adults in long-term care, *Journal of the American Dietetic Association* 105 (2005): 1955–1965.

50. Standing Committee on the Scientific Evaluation of Dietary Reference Intakes, *Dietary Reference Intakes for Water, Potassium, Sodium, Chloride, and Sulfate,* 2005, pp. 149–150.

51. B. Dawson-Hughes, Serum 25-hydroxyvitamin D and functional outcomes in the elderly, *American Journal of Clinical Nutrition* 88 (2008): 537S–540S.

52. R. Chernoff, Micronutrient requirements in older women, *American Journal of Clinical Nutrition* 81 (2005): 1240S–1245S.

53. A. D. Smith and H. Refsum, Vitamin B-12 and cognition in the elderly, *American Journal of Clinical Nutrition* 89 (2009): 707S–711S; R. Clarke and coauthors, Low vitamin B-12 status and risk of cognitive decline in older adults, *American Journal of Clinical Nutrition* 86 (2007): 1384–1391.

54. A. S. Prasad and coauthors, Zinc supplementation decreases incidence of infections in the elderly: Effect of zinc on generation of cytokines and oxidative stress, *American Journal of Clinical Nutrition* 85 (2007): 837–844.

55. R. S. Sebastian and coauthors, Older adults who use vitamin/mineral supplements differ from nonusers in nutrient intake adequacy and dietary attitudes, *Journal of the American Dietetic Association* 107 (2007): 1322–1332; Position of the American Dietetic Association: Nutrition across the spectrum of aging, *Journal of the American Dietetic Association* 105 (2005): 616–633.

56. Karinkanta and coauthors, 2007.

57. Position of the American Dietetic Association, American Society for Nutrition, and Society for Nutrition Education: Food and nutrition programs for community-residing older adults, *Journal of the American Dietetic Association* 110 (2010): 463–472; Position of the American Dietetic Association: Nutrition across the spectrum of aging, *Journal of the American Dietetic Association* 105 (2005): 616–633.

Hunger and Community Nutrition

Worldwide, one person in every seven experiences persistent hunger—not the healthy appetite triggered by anticipation of a hearty meal, but the painful sensation caused by a lack of food.[1] Hunger deprives a person of the physical and mental energy needed to enjoy a full life and often leads to severe malnutrition and death. Tens of thousands die of starvation each day—one child every five seconds.

In the United States, where most people enjoy a life of relative abundance, about one in every nine households has one or more members who experience pain from hunger caused by lack of food. In these households, almost 13 million children do not know where their next meal is coming from or when it will come.[2] Given the agricultural bounty and enormous wealth in this country, do these numbers surprise you? The limited or uncertain availability of nutritionally adequate and safe foods is known as **food insecurity** and is a major social problem in our nation today.[3] Table NP12-1 (p. 376) presents the questions used in national surveys to identify food insecurity in the United States, and Figure NP12-1 presents the most recent findings. Surveys like these provide crude, but necessary, data to estimate the degree of hunger in this country. The glossary (p. 377) defines related terms.

Why is hunger a problem in developed countries such as the United States where food is abundant?

Hunger has many causes, but in developed countries, the primary cause is **food poverty**. People are hungry not because there is no food nearby to purchase, but because they lack sufficient money with which to buy nutritious food and pay for other necessities, such as housing, clothing, medicines, and utilities. More than 12 percent of the population of the United States lives in poverty. Even those above the poverty line may not have **food security**. Physical and mental illnesses and disabilities, sudden job losses, and high living expenses threaten their financial stability. Further contributing to food poverty are other problems such as abuse of alcohol and other drugs; lack of awareness of available food assistance programs; and the reluctance of people, particularly the elderly, to accept what they perceive as "welfare" or "charity." Lack of resources remains the major cause of food poverty in developed countries, and solving this problem would do a lot to relieve hunger.

In the United States, food poverty and hunger reach into many segments of society, affecting not only the chronic poor (migrant workers, the unskilled and unemployed, the homeless, and some elderly) but also the so-called working poor. Some are displaced farm families. Some are former blue-collar and white-collar workers forced out of their trades and professions into minimum-wage jobs. These people outnumber the chronic poor, and they are not on welfare—they have jobs, but the pay is too low to meet their needs. Families with incomes below a certain level are simply unable to buy sufficient amounts of nourishing foods, even if they are skilled in food shopping. Consequently, their diets tend to be inadequate.[4] For many of the children in these families, school lunch (and breakfast, where available) may be the only nourishment for the day. Otherwise, they go hungry, waiting for an adult to find money for food. Not surprisingly, these children are more likely to have health problems than those who eat regularly.[5] They also tend to perform poorly in school and in social situations.[6]

| FIGURE NP12-1 | Prevalence of Food Security, Food Insecurity, and Hunger in U.S. Households, 2007 |

Food secure (89%)
Very low food security (4%)
Low food security (7%)

Source: USDA Economic Research Service; available at www.ers.usda.gov/publication/, update November 2008.

To determine the extent of food insecurity in a household, surveys ask questions about behaviors and conditions known to characterize households having difficulty meeting basic food needs during the past 12 months. Most often, adults tend to protect their children from hunger. In the most severe cases, children also suffer from hunger and eat less.

1. Did you worry whether your food would run out before you got money to buy more?

2. Did you find that the food you bought just didn't last, and you didn't have money to buy more?

3. Were you unable to afford to eat balanced meals?

4. Did you or other adults in your household ever cut the size of your meals or skip meals because there wasn't enough money for food?

5. Did this happen in three or more months during the previous year?

6. Did you ever eat less than you felt you should because there wasn't enough money for food?

7. Were you ever hungry but didn't eat because you couldn't afford enough food?

8. Did you lose weight because you didn't have enough money for food?

9. Did you or other adults in your household ever not eat for a whole day because there wasn't enough money for food?

10. Did this happen in three or more months during the previous year?

11. Did you rely on only a few kinds of low-cost food to feed your children because you were running out of money to buy food?

12. Were you unable to feed your children a balanced meal because you couldn't afford it?

13. Were your children not eating enough because you just couldn't afford enough food?

14. Did you ever cut the size of your children's meals because there wasn't enough money for food?

15. Were your children ever hungry but you just couldn't afford more food?

16. Did your children ever skip a meal because there wasn't enough money for food?

17. Did this happen in three or more months during the previous year?

18. Did your children ever not eat for a whole day because there wasn't enough money for food?

The more positive responses, the greater the food insecurity. Households with children answer all of the questions and are categorized as follows:

≤2 positive responses = food secure

3–7 positive responses = low food security

≥8 positive responses = very low food security

Households without children answer the first 10 questions and are categorized as follows:

≤2 positive responses = food secure

3–5 positive responses = low food security

≥6 positive responses = very low food security

Source: United States Department of Agriculture, *Household Food Security in the United States, 2008*, available at www.ers.usda.gov

Glossary

emergency shelters: facilities that are used to provide temporary housing.

food bank: a facility that collects and distributes food donations to authorized organizations feeding the hungry.

food insecurity: limited or uncertain access to foods of sufficient quality or quantity to sustain a healthy and active life. Food insecurity categories:

Low food security: reduced quality of diet with little or no indication of reduced food intake.

Very low food security: multiple indications of disrupted eating patterns and reduced food intake.

food pantries: programs that provide groceries to be prepared and eaten at home.

food poverty: hunger resulting from inadequate access to available food for various reasons, including inadequate resources, political obstacles, social disruptions, poor weather conditions, and lack of transportation.

food recovery: collecting wholesome food for distribution to low-income people who are hungry. Four common methods of food recovery are:

Field gleaning: collecting crops from fields that either have already been harvested or are not profitable to harvest.

Perishable food rescue or salvage: collecting perishable produce from wholesalers and markets.

Prepared food rescue: collecting prepared foods from commercial kitchens.

Nonperishable food collection: collecting processed foods from wholesalers and markets.

food security: access to enough food to sustain a healthy and active life.

High food security: no indications of food-access problems or limitations.

Marginal food security: one or two indications of food-access problems but with little or no change in food intake.

soup kitchens: programs that provide prepared meals to be eaten on-site.

These people and many others like them in the United States face food insecurity daily.

What U.S. food programs are directed at relieving hunger in the United States?

The American Dietetic Association (ADA) calls for aggressive action to bring an end to domestic hunger and to achieve food and nutrition security for all residents of the United States.[7] Many federal and local programs aim to prevent or relieve malnutrition and hunger in the United States.

An extensive network of federal assistance programs provides life-giving food daily to millions of U.S. citizens. One out of every five Americans receives food assistance of some kind, at a total cost of almost $60 billion per year. Even so, the programs are not fully successful in preventing hunger, but they do seem to improve the nutrient intakes of those who participate. Programs described in the life cycle chapters include the WIC program for low-income pregnant women, breastfeeding mothers, and their young children (Chapter 10); the school lunch and breakfast programs for children (Chapter 11); and the food assistance programs for older adults such as congregate meals and Meals on Wheels (Chapter 12).

The centerpiece of food programs for low-income people in the United States is the Supplemental Nutrition Assistance Program (SNAP), administered by the U.S. Department of Agriculture (USDA). The USDA issues debit cards through state agencies to households—people who buy and prepare food together. The amount a household receives depends on its size, resources, and income. Recipients may use the cards to purchase food and food-bearing plants and seeds but not to buy tobacco, cleaning items, alcohol, or other nonfood items. The "How to" (p. 378) offers shopping tips for those on a limited budget.

SNAP is the largest of the federal food assistance programs, both in amount of money spent and in number of people participating. It provides assistance to more than 28 million people at a cost of more than $34 billion per year; about half of the recipients are children.[8]

Although food assistance programs improve nutrient intakes significantly, hunger continues to plague the United States. Of the estimated 2 million homeless people in the United States who are eligible for food assistance, only 15 percent of single adults and 50 percent of families receive SNAP benefits. For some, reading, understanding, and

Chapter 1 introduces the USDA MyPyramid Food Guide and principles for planning a healthy diet. Meeting that goal on a limited budget adds to the challenge. To save money and spend wisely, plan and shop for healthy meals with the following tips in mind:

Planning

- Make a grocery list before going to the store to avoid expensive "impulse" items.
- Do not shop when hungry.
- Use leftovers.
- Center meals on rice, noodles, and other grains.
- Use small quantities of meat, poultry, fish, or eggs.
- Use legumes instead of meat, poultry, fish, or eggs several times a week.
- Use cooked cereals such as oatmeal instead of ready-to-eat breakfast cereals.
- Cook large quantities when time and money allow.
- Check for sales and clip coupons for products you need; plan meals to take advantage of sale items.

Shopping

- Buy day-old bread and other products from a bakery outlet.
- Select whole foods instead of convenience foods (potatoes instead of instant mashed potatoes, for example).
- Try store brands.
- Buy fresh produce that is in season; buy canned or frozen items at other times.
- Buy only the amount of fresh foods that you will eat before it spoils. Buy large bags of frozen items or dry goods; when cooking, take out the amount needed and store the remainder.
- Buy fat-free dry milk; mix and refrigerate quantities needed for a day or two. Buy fresh milk by the gallon or half-gallon.
- Buy less expensive cuts of meat. Chuck and bottom round roast are usually inexpensive; cover during cooking and cook long enough to make meat tender. Buy whole chickens instead of pieces.
- Compare the unit price (cost per ounce, for example) of similar foods so that you can select the least expensive brand or size.
- Buy nonfood items such as toilet paper and laundry detergent at discount stores instead of grocery stores.

For daily menus and recipes for healthy, thrifty meals, visit the USDA Center for Nutrition Policy and Promotion: **www.usda.gov/cnpp.**

---

completing the application can be difficult. For others, having to show identification and proof of homelessness can be frustrating. For many, accepting hunger is simply easier than meeting these challenges.

Why do health care professionals need to know about food assistance programs?

Health care professionals who work in public health are generally well acquainted with food assistance programs, and often many of their clients receive such assistance. Regardless of the setting in which health care professionals see clients, however, it is important to encourage those who may be having financial problems to talk with a social worker who can assess their eligibility for food assistance programs. The subject of food assistance must be approached in a nonjudgmental and tactful manner—the client may feel uncomfortable about seeking assistance.

Are there other programs aimed at reducing hunger in the United States?

Efforts to resolve the problem of hunger in the United States do not depend solely on federal assistance programs.

National **food recovery** programs have made a dramatic difference; the largest program, Feeding America, coordinates the efforts of more than 40,000 **food pantries, emergency shelters**, and **soup kitchens** that feed an estimated 24 to 27 million people a year. Table NP12-2 lists addresses, phone numbers, and websites for Feeding America and other hunger relief organizations.

Each year, an estimated one-fifth of our food supply is wasted in fields, commercial kitchens, grocery stores, and restaurants—that's enough food to feed 49 million people. Food recovery programs collect and distribute good food that would otherwise go to waste. Volunteers might

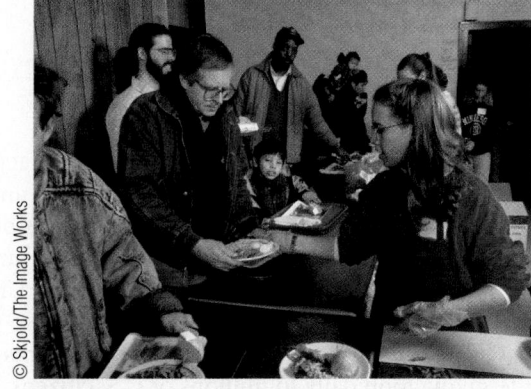

Feeding the hungry in the United States.

TABLE NP12-2 | Hunger-Relief Organizations

Organization	Mission Statement
Action without Borders www.idealist.org	International organization seeking to connect people, organizations, and resources to help build a world where all people can live free and dignified lives.
Bread for the World www.bread.org	Nonpartisan, Christian citizens' movement seeking to influence reform in policies, programs, and conditions that allow hunger and poverty to persist globally.
Catholic Relief Services www.crs.org	Humanitarian service agency assisting the impoverished and disadvantaged through community-based, sustainable development initiatives.
Community Food Security Coalition www.foodsecurity.org	North American coalition of diverse people and organizations working from the local to the international levels to build community food security.
Congressional Hunger Center www.hungercenter.org	Bipartisan organization training and inspiring leaders with the intent to end hunger and advocating public policies to create a food-secure world.
Feeding America www.feedingamerica.org	Domestic charity organization providing food assistance through a nationwide network of member food banks and facilitating education to end hunger nationally.
Food and Agriculture Organization (FAO) of the United Nations www.fao.org	International organization leading efforts to defeat hunger by helping to develop and modernize countries' agriculture, forestry, and fishery practices.
Oxfam America www.oxfamamerica.org	International relief and development organization aiming to create lasting solutions to poverty, hunger, and injustice.
Pan American Health Organization www.paho.org	International public health agency aiming to strengthen national and local health systems with the purpose of improving the quality of, and lengthening, the lives of the peoples in the Americas.
Society of St. Andrew www.endhunger.org	Ecumenical Christian ministry salvaging and redirecting large amounts of fresh produce to hunger agencies for distribution to the poor.
The Hunger Project www.thp.org	International relief organization emphasizing sustainable solutions such as rural development and self-reliance to facilitate food security.
United Nations Children's Fund (UNICEF) www.unicef.org	International organization advocating for the protection of children's rights, to help meet their basic needs and to expand their opportunities to reach their full potentials.
World Food Programme www.wfp.org	Food aid branch of the United Nations aiming to prepare for, protect during, and provide assistance after emergencies, as well as reduce hunger and undernutrition.
World Health Organization (WHO) www.who.int	United Nations agency acting as the authority on international public health by influencing policy, setting research agendas, establishing standards, and providing technical support to monitor and assess health trends.
World Hunger Year (WHY) www.whyhunger.org	Domestic organization supporting and funding community-based organizations intent on empowering individuals and building self-reliance to provide long-term solutions to hunger and poverty.

pick corn left in an already harvested field, a grocer might deliver ripe bananas to a local **food bank**, and a caterer might take leftover chicken salad to a community shelter, for example. All of these efforts help to feed the hungry in the United States.

What about local efforts and community nutrition programs?

Food recovery programs depend on volunteers. Concerned citizens work through local agencies and churches to feed the hungry. Community-based food pantries provide groceries, and soup kitchens serve prepared meals. Meals often deliver adequate nourishment, but most homeless people receive fewer than one and a half meals a day, so many are still inadequately nourished. Health care professionals can serve as valuable members of community groups seeking to provide food assistance.

Community-based efforts to feed citizens include food pantries that provide groceries.

Notes

1. *State of Food Insecurity in the World, 2008*, Food Security Statistics, available from Food and Agriculture Organization, www.fao.org.
2. United States Department of Agriculture, *Household Food Security in the United States, 2007*, ERS Report Summary, November 2008, available at www.ers.usda.gov/Publications/ERR66.
3. Position of the American Dietetic Association: Food insecurity and hunger in the United States, *Journal of the American Dietetic Association* 106 (2006): 446–458.
4. C. M. Champagne and coauthors, Poverty and food intake in rural America: Diet quality is lower in food insecure adults in the Mississippi Delta, *Journal of the American Dietetic Association* 107 (2007): 1886–1894; M. L. Kropf and coauthors, Food security status and produce intake and behaviors of Special Supplemental Nutrition Program for Women, Infants, and Children and

Farmer's Market Nutrition Program participants, *Journal of the American Dietetic Association* 107 (2007): 1903–1908.
5. R. Rose-Jacobs and coauthors, Household food insecurity: Associations with at-risk infant and toddler development, *Pediatrics* 121 (2008): 65–72.
6. D. F. Jyoti, E. A. Frongillo, and S. J. Jones, Food insecurity affects school children's academic performance, weight gain, and social skills, *Journal of Nutrition* 135 (2005): 2831–2839.
7. Position of the American Dietetic Association, 2006.
8. *Leading the Fight against Hunger—Federal Nutrition Assistance*, June 2008, www.fns.usda.gov/fns.hunger.pdf; P. S. Landers, The Food Stamp Program: History, nutrition education, and impact, *Journal of the American Dietetic Association* 107 (2007): 1945–1951.

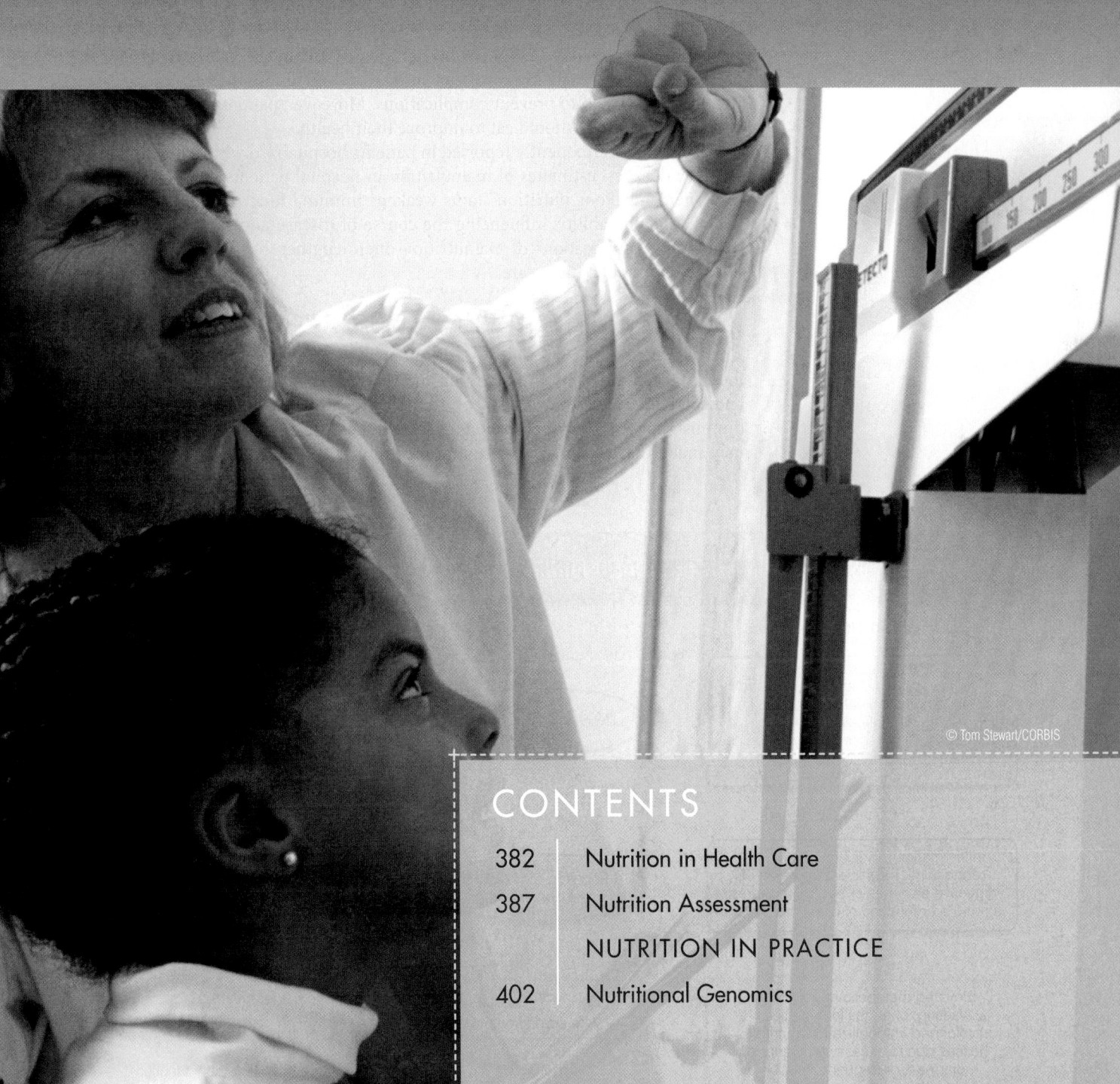

CHAPTER 13 | **Nutrition Care and Assessment**

CONTENTS

EARLIER CHAPTERS OF THIS BOOK INTRODUCED THE NUTRIENTS AND described how the appropriate dietary choices can support good health. Turning now to clinical nutrition, the remaining chapters describe how illnesses and their treatments can influence nutrition status and nutrient needs. Nurses and other health care providers who consider nutrition care in their treatment decisions are best prepared to help patients (✚) recover from disease and maintain an optimal quality of life. This chapter introduces the process used for providing nutrition care and strategies used for evaluating nutrition status.

Nutrition in Health Care

The busy nurse with many responsibilities may be tempted to put a patient's nutrition needs on the back burner. After all, the benefits of nutrition therapy are not always as obvious or immediate as those of other medical treatments. Correcting nutritional problems, however, may improve both short-term and long-term outcomes of medical treatments and help to prevent complications. Moreover, patients are often concerned about the foods they should eat to improve their health.

Malnutrition is frequently reported in patients hospitalized with acute illness. In the past few decades, estimates of malnutrition in hospital patients have ranged from 38 to 62 percent.[1] Poor nutrition status weakens immune function and compromises a person's healing ability, influencing the course of disease and the body's response to treatment. Complications of malnutrition often lengthen hospital stays and increase the overall cost of patient care.

HOW ILLNESS AFFECTS NUTRITION STATUS

An illness, its symptoms, and its treatments may lead to malnutrition by reducing food intake, interfering with digestion and absorption, or altering nutrient metabolism and excretion (see Figure 13-1). For example, the nausea caused by some illnesses can diminish appetite and thereby reduce food intake. An inflamed mouth or esophagus may make the physical act of eating uncomfortable. Certain medications can cause

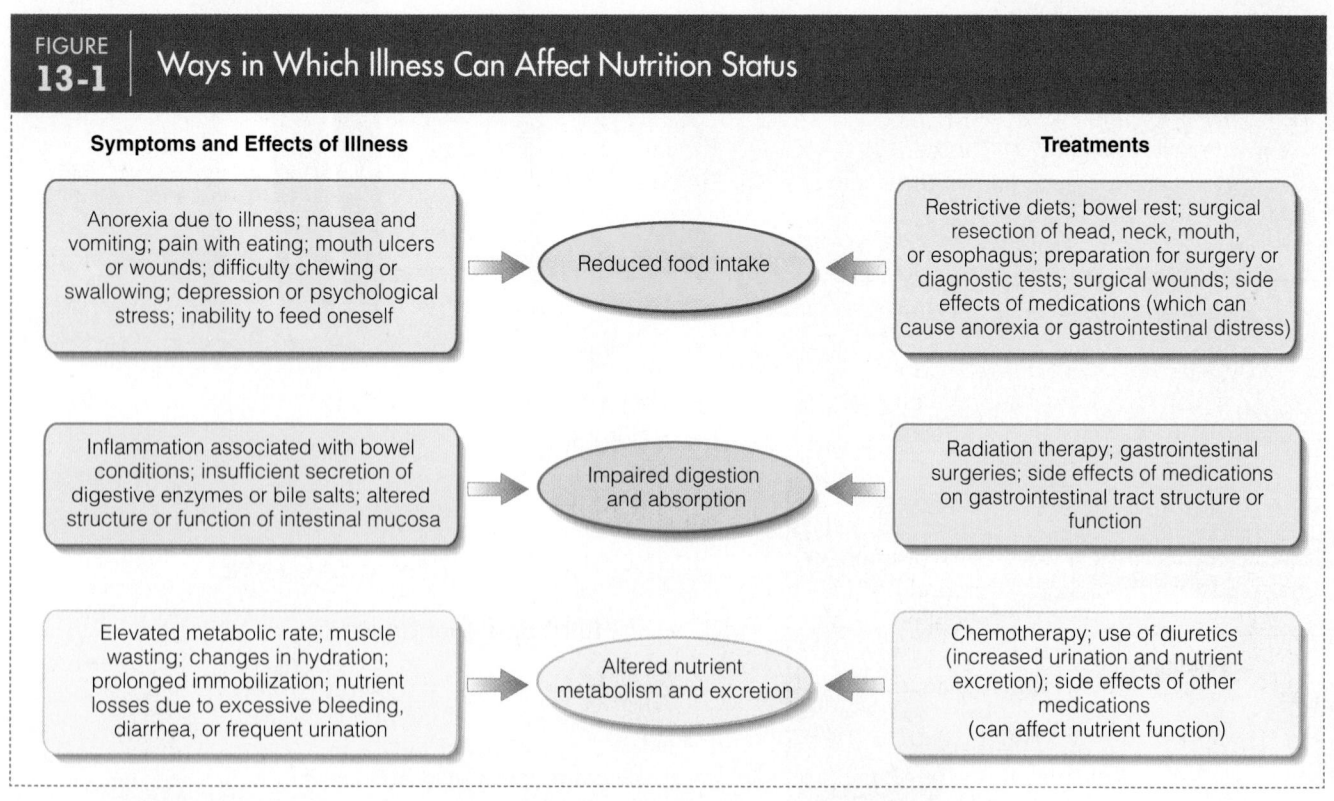

FIGURE 13-1 | Ways in Which Illness Can Affect Nutrition Status

Symptoms and Effects of Illness

Anorexia due to illness; nausea and vomiting; pain with eating; mouth ulcers or wounds; difficulty chewing or swallowing; depression or psychological stress; inability to feed oneself

→ **Reduced food intake** ←

Treatments

Restrictive diets; bowel rest; surgical resection of head, neck, mouth, or esophagus; preparation for surgery or diagnostic tests; surgical wounds; side effects of medications (which can cause anorexia or gastrointestinal distress)

Inflammation associated with bowel conditions; insufficient secretion of digestive enzymes or bile salts; altered structure or function of intestinal mucosa

→ **Impaired digestion and absorption** ←

Radiation therapy; gastrointestinal surgeries; side effects of medications on gastrointestinal tract structure or function

Elevated metabolic rate; muscle wasting; changes in hydration; prolonged immobilization; nutrient losses due to excessive bleeding, diarrhea, or frequent urination

→ **Altered nutrient metabolism and excretion** ←

Chemotherapy; use of diuretics (increased urination and nutrient excretion); side effects of other medications (can affect nutrient function)

anorexia or gastrointestinal discomfort or interfere with nutrient function and metabolism. Prolonged bed rest often results in **pressure sores**, which increase metabolic stress and raise protein and energy needs.

The dietary changes required during acute illness are usually temporary and can be tailored to accommodate an individual's preferences and lifestyle. Chronic illnesses, however, may require long-term dietary modifications. For example, diabetes treatment requires lifelong changes in diet and lifestyle that some people may find difficult to adhere to. The challenge for nurses and other health professionals is to help their patients appreciate the potential benefits of nutrition therapy and accept the dietary changes that can improve their health.

In addition to the direct effects of an illness on nutrition status, the cost of health care can drain financial resources and limit the ability to obtain high-quality foods. Some individuals may lack the space and equipment necessary to store and prepare special meals. Many persons lack the strength and energy required for meal preparation while recovering from illness. Emotional health may also suffer as a result of chronic disease or terminal illness, causing a lack of appetite and disinterest in food preparation.

RESPONSIBILITY FOR NUTRITION CARE

The members of the health care team work together to ensure that the nutritional needs of patients are met. The roles of health professionals may vary among different institutions, and their responsibilities may sometimes overlap. Sometimes the nutrition care of a patient is incorporated into the medical care plan developed by the entire health care team. Such plans, called **critical pathways**, outline coordinated plans of care for specific medical diagnoses, treatments, or procedures.

Physicians Physicians are responsible for meeting all of a patient's medical needs, including nutrition. They prescribe **diet orders** and other orders related to nutrition care, including those for nutrition assessment and dietary counseling. Physicians rely on nurses, registered dietitians, and other health professionals to alert them to nutrition problems, suggest strategies for handling nutrition care, and provide nutrition services.

Nurses Nurses interact closely with patients and thus are in an ideal position to identify people who would benefit from nutrition services. Nurses often screen patients for nutrition problems and may participate in nutrition and dietary assessments. Nurses also provide direct nutrition care, such as encouraging patients to eat, finding practical solutions to food-related problems, recording a patient's food intake, and answering questions about special diets. As members of **nutrition support teams**, nurses are responsible for administering tube and intravenous feedings. In facilities that do not employ registered dietitians, nurses often assume responsibility for much of the nutrition care.

Registered Dietitians Registered dietitians (**+**) are food and nutrition experts who are qualified to provide **medical nutrition therapy**. They conduct nutrition and dietary assessments; diagnose nutritional problems; develop, implement, and evaluate **nutrition care plans** (described in a later section); plan and approve menus; and provide dietary counseling and nutrition education services. Registered dietitians may also work as managers of food and cafeteria services in health care institutions.

Registered Dietetic Technicians Registered dietetic technicians work in partnership with registered dietitians and assist in the implementation and monitoring of nutrition services. Depending on their background and experience, they may screen patients for nutrition problems, provide patient education and counseling, develop menus and recipes, ensure appropriate meal delivery, and monitor patients' food choices and intakes. Dietetic technicians sometimes supervise foodservice operations and may have roles in purchasing, inventory, quality control, sanitation, or safety.

Other Health Care Professionals Other heath care professionals may also assist with nutrition care. Pharmacists, physical therapists, occupational

+Reminder: A registered dietitian has met the academic and professional requirements to qualify for the RD credential conferred by the American Dietetic Association (or Dietitians of Canada), including a bachelor's degree in nutrition or dietetics, a supervised internship, and the successful completion of a national examination.

pressure sores: regions of damaged skin and tissue due to prolonged pressure on the affected area by an external object, such as a bed, wheelchair, or cast; vulnerable areas of the body include buttocks, hips, and heels. Also called *decubitus* (deh-KYU-bih-tus) *ulcers*.

critical pathways: coordinated programs of treatment that merge the care plans of different health practitioners; also called *clinical pathways*.

diet orders: specific instructions concerning dietary management including the type, amount, and frequency of feedings; also called *diet prescriptions* or *nutrition prescriptions*.

nutrition support teams: health care professionals responsible for the provision of nutrients by tube feeding or intravenous infusion.

medical nutrition therapy: nutrition care provided by a registered dietitian; includes assessment of nutrition status, diagnosis of nutrition problems, development of nutrition care plans, and provision of dietary counseling and nutrition education.

nutrition care plans: strategies for meeting an individual's nutritional needs.

nutrition screening: a brief assessment of health-related variables to identify patients who are malnourished or at risk for malnutrition.

Joint Commission: a nonprofit organization that sets standards for health care performance and safety and confers accreditation to health care organizations and programs that meet those standards.

nursing diagnoses: clinical judgments about actual or potential health problems that provide the basis for selecting appropriate nursing interventions.

therapists, speech therapists, social workers, nursing assistants, and home health care aides can be instrumental in alerting dietitians or nurses to nutrition problems or may share relevant information about a patient's health status or personal needs.

IDENTIFYING RISK FOR MALNUTRITION

To identify patients who are malnourished or at risk for malnutrition, a **nutrition screening** is conducted when a patient is admitted to a hospital or other extended-care facility. The screening may also be included in certain types of outpatient services and community health programs. A nutrition screening involves collecting health-related data that can indicate the presence of protein-energy malnutrition (PEM) (✚) or other nutrition problems. The screening should be sensitive enough to identify patients who require nutrition care but simple enough to be completed within 10 to 15 minutes. Usually a nurse, nursing assistant, registered dietitian, or dietetic technician performs and documents the screening. The **Joint Commission**, a nonprofit organization that provides accreditation for health care organizations and programs, recommends that nutrition screening be conducted within 24 hours of a patient's admission to a health care institution.

The information collected in a nutrition screening varies according to the patient population, the type of care offered by the health care facility, and the patient's medical problems. Often included are the admitting diagnosis, information from the medical record, physical measurements and laboratory test results obtained during the admission process, and responses given by the patient or caregiver in an interview or questionnaire. Table 13-1 lists examples of information that can help to identify individuals at risk of developing malnutrition. A number of screening tools that use different combinations of these variables have become popular in recent years; one such example is the Subjective Global Assessment, which combines elements of the medical history and physical examination to determine malnutrition risk (see Table 13-2). More rapid screening methods may use just two or three variables; for example, several tools screen for malnutrition risk by evaluating unintentional weight changes and reduced appetite or food intake.[2]

Nursing care plans often include **nursing diagnoses** that suggest the need for nutrition interventions (see Table 13-3). For example, a nursing diagnosis of "impaired swallowing" alerts the nurse to potential problems with food consumption and suggests the need for a modified diet. Such a diagnosis can accompany various medical disorders, including developmental disabilities, diseases involving the esophagus, and neurological conditions. Examples of relevant nursing diagnoses are provided throughout the clinical nutrition chapters.

A nutrition screening may lead to a referral for nutrition care. The following section describes the next stage of the process: the method used by dietitians to address nutritional concerns.

TABLE 13-1	Criteria for Identifying Malnutrition Risk

- Age, medical diagnosis, severity of illness
- Height and weight, body mass index (BMI), unintentional weight changes
- Tissue wasting, loss of subcutaneous fat
- Changes in appetite or food intake
- Problems that interfere with food intake (such as chewing or swallowing difficulty, or nausea and vomiting)
- Food allergies or intolerances, extensive dietary restrictions
- Laboratory test results that indicate poor health status
- History of diabetes, renal disease, or other chronic illness
- Presence of anemia or pressure sores
- Use of medications that can impair nutrition status
- Depression, social isolation, dementia

	Subjective Global Assessment
TABLE 13-2	

The Subjective Global Assessment evaluates a person's risk of malnutrition by ranking key variables of the medical history and physical examination. These variables are each given an A, B, or C rating: A for well nourished, B for potential or mild malnutrition, and C for severe malnutrition. Patients are classified according to the final numbers of A, B, and C ratings.

Medical History	• Body weight changes: percentage change in past six months; weight change in past two weeks • Dietary changes: suboptimal, low kcalorie, liquid diet, or starvation • GI symptoms: nausea, diarrhea, vomiting, or anorexia for more than two weeks • Functional ability: full capacity versus suboptimal, walking versus bedridden • Degree of disease-related metabolic stress: low, medium, or high
Physical Examination	• Subcutaneous fat loss (triceps or chest) • Muscle loss (quadriceps or deltoids) • Ankle edema • Sacral (lower spine) edema • Ascites (abdominal edema)
Classification:	**A: Well nourished:** if no significant loss of weight, fat, or muscle tissue and no dietary difficulties, functional impairments, or GI symptoms; also applies to patients with recent weight gain and improved appetite, functioning, or medical prognosis **B: Moderate malnutrition:** if 5 to 10 percent weight loss, mild loss of muscle or fat tissue, decreased food intake, and digestive or functional difficulties that impair food intake; the B classification usually applies to patients with an even mix of A, B, and C ratings **C: Severe malnutrition:** if more than 10 percent weight loss, severe loss of muscle or fat tissue, edema, multiple GI symptoms, and functional impairments

Sources: R. S. Gibson, *Principles of Nutritional Assessment* (New York: Oxford University Press, 2005), pp. 809–826; A. S. Detsky and coauthors, What is subjective global assessment of nutritional status? *Journal of Parenteral and Enteral Nutrition* 11 (1987): 8–13.

THE NUTRITION CARE PROCESS

Registered dietitians use a systematic approach to medical nutrition therapy called the **nutrition care process**. The steps of this process include nutrition assessment, nutrition diagnosis, nutrition intervention, and nutrition monitoring and evaluation, as shown in Figure 13-2.[3] (✚) Although the process is easiest to visualize as a series of steps, previous steps are often revisited to reassess and revise diagnoses and intervention strategies. Each step of the nutrition care process must be documented in the medical record, providing a record for future reference and facilitating communication among members of the health care team.

Nutrition Assessment Nutrition assessment involves the collection and analysis of health-related information in order to identify specific nutrition problems and their underlying causes. The information may be obtained from the medical record, physical examination, laboratory analyses, medical procedures, interview with the patient or caregiver, and consultation with other health professionals. The assessment data are used to develop a plan of action to prevent or correct energy or nutrient imbalances, or to determine whether a care plan is working. The second half of this chapter describes the components of nutrition assessment in detail.

Nutrition Diagnosis Each nutrition problem identified by the nutrition assessment receives a separate diagnosis.[4] Nutrition diagnoses, similar to nursing diagnoses, are formatted to include the specific nutrition problem, the etiology or cause, and signs and symptoms that provide evidence of the problem. For example, a

✚ As a comparision, the *nursing process* consists of five steps:
1. Assessment
2. Nursing diagnosis
3. Planning
4. Implementation
5. Evaluation

nutrition care process: a problem-solving method that dietetics professionals use to evaluate and treat nutrition-related problems.

TABLE 13-3	Nursing Diagnoses with Nutritional Implications

- Chronic confusion
- Chronic pain
- Constipation
- Diarrhea
- Disturbed body image
- Feeding self-care deficit
- Imbalanced nutrition: less than body requirements
- Imbalanced nutrition: more than body requirements
- Impaired dentition
- Impaired oral mucous membrane
- Impaired physical mobility
- Impaired swallowing
- Ineffective breastfeeding
- Nausea
- Readiness for enhanced nutrition
- Risk for aspiration
- Risk for deficient fluid volume
- Risk for unstable blood glucose

Source: NANDA International, *Nursing Diagnoses: Definitions and Classification 2009–2011* (Oxford: Wiley-Blackwell, 2009).

nutrition diagnosis might state, "Unintentional weight loss *(the problem)* related to insufficient kcaloric intake *(the etiology or cause)* as evidenced by a 10-pound weight loss (8 percent of body weight) in the past few months *(the sign or symptom).*" Like nursing diagnoses, a nutrition diagnosis can change during the course of an illness.

Nutrition Intervention After nutrition problems are identified, the appropriate nutrition care can be planned and implemented. An intervention may include counseling or education about appropriate dietary and lifestyle practices, changes in a medication or other treatment, or modifications in the meals offered to a hospital patient. To be successful, the intervention must consider an individual's food habits, lifestyle, and other personal factors. Goals are stated in terms of measurable outcomes; for example, goals for an overweight person with diabetes might include changes in blood glucose levels and body weight. Desirable outcomes may also include changes in dietary behaviors and lifestyle; for example, a diabetes patient may need to learn how to control carbohydrate intake and may benefit from regular exercise. Chapter 14 gives additional information about nutrition intervention.

Nutrition Monitoring and Evaluation

The effectiveness of the nutrition care plan must be evaluated periodically: the patient's progress should be monitored closely, and updated assessment data or diagnoses may require adjustments in goals or outcome measures. Sometimes a new situation alters nutritional needs; for example, a change in the medical treatment or a new medication may alter a person's tolerance to certain foods. The nutrition care plan must be flexible enough to adapt to the new situation.

If progress is slow or a patient is unwilling or unable to make the suggested changes, the care plan should be redesigned and take into account the reasons why the earlier plan was not successful. The new plan may need to include motivational techniques or additional patient education. If the patient remains unwilling to modify behaviors despite the expected benefits, the health care provider can try again at a later time when the patient may be more receptive.

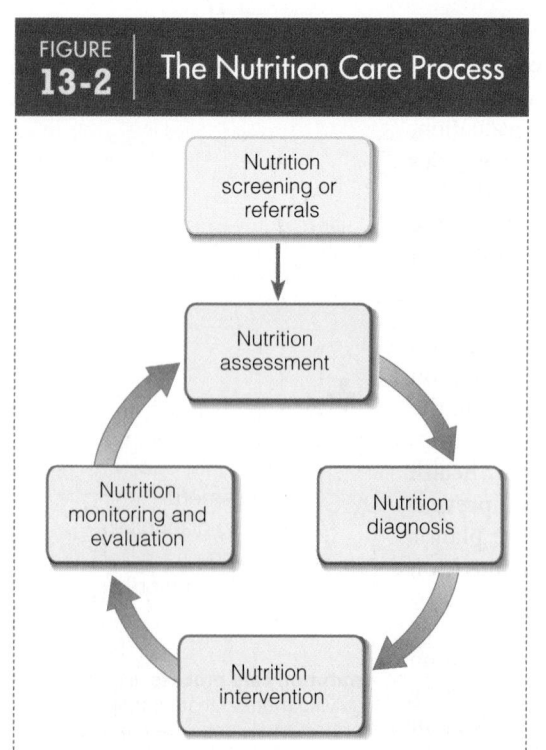

FIGURE 13-2	The Nutrition Care Process

Review Notes

- Illnesses and their treatments can affect food intake and nutrient needs, leading to malnutrition. In turn, poor nutrition status can influence the course of illness and the effectiveness of medical treatment.

- The combined efforts of each member of the health care team ensure that patients receive optimal nutrition care.

- Nutrition screening identifies individuals who can benefit from nutrition assessment and follow-up care. Nursing diagnoses can also identify potential nutrition problems.

- The nutrition care process includes four interrelated steps: nutrition assessment, nutrition diagnosis, nutrition intervention, and nutrition monitoring and evaluation.

Nutrition Assessment

As described earlier in this chapter, a nutrition assessment provides the information needed for diagnosing nutrition problems and designing a nutrition care plan; follow-up assessments help to determine whether the care plan has been effective. Ideally, the assessment should be sensitive enough to detect subtle nutrition problems and specific enough to identify problem nutrients. The remainder of this chapter describes the types of information and measures that are most often obtained in a nutrition assessment.

HISTORICAL INFORMATION

Historical information provides valuable clues about nutrition status and nutrient requirements; it also reveals personal preferences that need consideration when developing a nutrition care plan. Table 13-4 summarizes the various types of historical data that contribute to a nutrition assessment. This information can be obtained from the medical record or by interviewing the patient or caregiver.

Medical History A substantial number of medical problems and their treatments can interfere with food intake or require dietary changes; Table 13-5 lists examples. The medical history generally includes the family medical history as well; this information may reveal a person's genetic susceptibilities for diseases that can potentially be prevented with dietary and lifestyle changes.

Medication and Supplement History Medications can sometimes have detrimental effects on nutrition status, and some dietary components can alter the absorption and metabolism of drugs. Ingredients in dietary and herbal supplements can also interact with medications. Chapter 14 describes examples of notable diet-drug interactions that may need consideration when planning nutrition care.

Personal and Social History Personal and social factors influence food choices as well as a person's ability to manage health and nutrition problems. For example, financial concerns may restrict access to health care and nutritious foods. Cultural background or religious beliefs can affect food preferences. Some individuals may depend on others to prepare or procure food. An individual who lives alone or is depressed may eat poorly or be unable to follow complex dietary instructions. Use of tobacco or illegal drugs may alter food intake and have disruptive effects on health and nutrition status.

> **NURSING DIAGNOSIS**
>
> *Readiness for enhanced nutrition* is appropriate for a person who is willing to improve dietary practices.

TABLE 13-4	Historical Information Used in Nutrition Assessment[a]		
Medical History	**Medication and Supplement History**	**Personal and Social History**	**Food and Nutrition History**
Age	Prescription drugs	Employment status	Food intake
Current complaint(s)	Over-the-counter drugs	Educational level	Alcohol consumption
Past medical conditions	Dietary and herbal supplements	Socioeconomic status	Dietary restrictions
Surgical history		Cultural/ethnic identity	Food allergies and intolerances
Family medical history		Religious beliefs	Nutrition and health knowledge
Chronic disease risk		Home/family situation	Food availability
Allergies		Cognitive abilities	Physical activity and exercise habits
Mental/emotional health status		Use of tobacco or illegal drugs	

[a] Historical information is classified in different ways among medical institutions.

Source: American Dietetic Association, *Nutrition Diagnosis and Intervention: Standardized Language for the Nutrition Care Process* (Chicago: American Dietetic Association, 2007).

TABLE 13-5	Medical Problems Often Associated with Malnutrition

- Acquired immune deficiency syndrome (AIDS)
- Alcoholism
- Anorexia nervosa
- Bulimia
- Burns (extensive or severe)
- Cancer and cancer treatments
- Cardiovascular diseases
- Celiac disease
- Chewing or swallowing difficulties
- Chronic kidney disease
- Dementia
- Diabetes mellitus
- Feeding disabilities
- Infections
- Inflammatory bowel diseases
- Liver disease
- Malabsorption
- Mental illness
- Pressure sores
- Surgery (major)
- Vomiting (prolonged or severe)

Food and Nutrition History A food and nutrition history (often called a *diet history*) is a detailed account of a person's dietary practices. It includes data about food intake, lifestyle habits, and other factors that may influence food choices, such as food allergies or beliefs about nutrition and health. The procedure often includes an interview about recent food intake (for example, a *24-hour recall*) and a survey about usual food choices (such as a *food frequency questionnaire*). In the hospital setting, direct observation of patients' food intakes is possible. The following section describes the most common methods of gathering food intake information.

DIETARY ASSESSMENT METHODS

Obtaining accurate food intake data is challenging, and results may vary depending on both the individual's memory and honesty and the assessor's skill and training. In addition, each method has its own strengths and weaknesses, so best results are obtained from using a combination of methods. Table 13-6 summarizes the methods most commonly used and each method's advantages and disadvantages.

The 24-Hour Recall The **24-hour recall** is a guided interview in which an individual recounts all of the foods and beverages consumed in the past 24 hours or during the previous day. The interviewer includes questions about the times when meals or snacks were eaten, amounts consumed, and ways in which foods were prepared. Accuracy can be improved by prompting the respondent to recall items that are often forgotten, such as condiments, snacks, and beverages.[5]

In a typical interview, the assessor may begin by asking, "What is the first thing you ate or drank yesterday morning?" After the respondent describes the first food items, follow-up questions might be, "What time was that?" and "How much did you eat?" Questioning continues until the intake record for the day is complete. Food models or measuring cups and spoons can be used to help the individual visualize and describe the amounts consumed. After the day's intake is recounted, the interviewer asks whether the intake that day is fairly typical and, if not, how it varies from the person's usual intake. A recall interview may be conducted on several nonconsecutive days to get a better representation of a person's usual diet.

A recall interview can yield useful data for developing an acceptable nutrition care plan and identifying food items that may need to be restricted due to illness. It is a poor technique, however, for determining the adequacy of a diet because it does not take into account fluctuations in food intake or seasonal variations. Moreover, food intakes are often underestimated because the process relies on an individual's memory and reporting accuracy. People often forget to mention alcohol, soft drinks, snack foods, and desserts unless specifically prompted to do so, and some individuals find it embarrassing to report consumption of foods such as chocolate, butter, and red meat.[6]

Food Frequency Questionnaire A **food frequency questionnaire** surveys the foods and beverages regularly consumed during a specific time period. Some questionnaires are qualitative only: food lists contain common foods, organized by food group, with check boxes to indicate frequency of consumption. Other types of questionnaires provide semiquantitative information by including portion sizes as well. Figure 13-3 shows a sample section of a semiquantitative questionnaire that surveys fruit intake over the previous year. Because the respondent is often asked to estimate food intakes over a one-year period, the results should not be affected by seasonal

24-hour recall: a record of foods consumed in the previous 24 hours; sometimes modified to include foods consumed in a typical day.

food frequency questionnaire: a survey of foods routinely consumed. Some questionnaires ask about the types of food eaten and yield only qualitative information, whereas others include questions about portions consumed and yield semiquantitative data as well.

TABLE 13-6	Methods for Obtaining Food Intake Data		
Method	**Description**	**Advantages**	**Disadvantages**
24-hour recall	Guided interview in which the foods and beverages consumed in a 24-hour period are described in detail.	• Results are not dependent on literacy or educational level of respondent. • Interview occurs after food is consumed, so method does not influence dietary choices. • Results are obtained quickly; method is relatively easy to conduct.	• Process is reliant on memory. • Underestimation and overestimation of food intakes are common. • Food items that cause embarrassment (alcohol, desserts) may be omitted. • Data from a single day cannot accurately represent the respondent's usual intake. • Seasonal variations may not be addressed. • Skill of interviewer affects outcome.
Food frequency questionnaire	Written survey of food consumption during a specific period of time, often a one-year period.	• Process examines long-term food intake, so day-to-day and seasonal variability should not affect results. • Questionnaire is completed after food is consumed, so method does not influence food choices. • Method is inexpensive to administer.	• Process is reliant on memory. • Food lists often include common foods only. • Serving sizes are often difficult for respondents to evaluate without assistance. • Calculated nutrient intakes may not be accurate. • Food lists for the general population are of limited value in special populations. • Method is not effective for monitoring short-term changes in food intake.
Food record	Written account of food consumed during a specified period, usually several consecutive days. Accuracy is improved by including weights or measures of foods.	• Process does not rely on memory. • Recording foods as they are consumed may improve accuracy of food intake data. • Process is useful for controlling intake because keeping records increases awareness of food choices.	• Recording process itself influences food intake. • Underreporting and portion size errors are common. • Process is time-consuming and burdensome for respondent; requires high degree of motivation. • Method requires literacy and the physical ability to write. • Seasonal changes in diet are not taken into account.
Direct observation	Observation of meal trays or shelf inventories before and after eating; possible only in residential facilities.	• Process does not rely on memory. • Method does not influence food intake. • Method can be used to evaluate the acceptability of a prescribed diet.	• Process is possible only in residential situations. • Method is labor-intensive.

changes in diet. Conversely, a disadvantage of this method is its inability to determine recent changes in food intake. Another limitation is that the questionnaires typically include only common food items, so the accuracy of food intake data is reduced if an individual consumes atypical foods.

Food models and measuring utensils can help an individual visualize portion sizes.

Simple versions of food frequency questionnaires focus on food categories relevant to a person's medical condition. For example, a questionnaire designed to evaluate calcium intake may include only milk products, fortified foods, certain fruits and vegetables, and dietary supplements that contain calcium. A computer analysis can then quickly estimate the individual's calcium intake and compare it to recommendations.

Food Record A **food record** is a written account of foods and beverages consumed during a specified time period, usually several consecutive days. Foods are recorded as they are consumed in order to obtain the most complete and accurate record possible; thus, the process does not rely on memory. A detailed food record includes the types and amounts of foods and beverages consumed, times of consumption, and methods of preparation. It may also include information about medication use, disease symptoms, and daily physical activity.

The food record provides valuable information about food intake and can also be used to evaluate a person's compliance with nutrition therapy. Unfortunately, food records require a great deal of time to complete, and people need to be highly motivated to keep accurate records. Another drawback is that the recording process itself may influence food intake. Furthermore, it is difficult to obtain accurate estimates of nutrient intakes in just a few days or even a week due to day-to-day and seasonal variations in food intake.

Direct Observation In facilities that serve meals, food intakes can be directly observed and analyzed. This method can also reveal a person's food preferences, changes in appetite, and any problems with a prescribed diet. Although a useful means of discerning patients' intakes, direct observation requires regular and careful documentation and can be labor-intensive and costly.

Nurses use direct observation to conduct patients' **kcalorie counts**, which are estimates of the food energy (and often protein) consumed by patients during a single day

food record: a detailed log of food eaten during a specified time period, usually several days; also called a *food diary*. A food record may also include information regarding medications, disease symptoms, and physical activity.

kcalorie counts: estimates of food energy (and often protein) consumed by patients for one or more days.

FIGURE 13-3 | Sample Section of a Food Frequency Questionnaire

FRUIT	Never or less than once per month	1 per mon.	2–3 per mon.	1 per week	2 per week	3–4 per week	5–6 per week	Every day	MEDIUM SERVING	YOUR SERVING SIZE S	M	L
EXAMPLE: Bananas	○	○	○	●	○	○	○	○	1 medium	○ 1/2	● 1	○ 2
Bananas	○	○	○	○	○	○	○	○	1 medium	○ 1/2	○ 1	○ 2
Apples, applesauce	○	○	○	○	○	○	○	○	1 medium or 1/2 cup	○ 1/2	○ 1	○ 2
Oranges (not including juice)	○	○	○	○	○	○	○	○	1 medium	○ 1/2	○ 1	○ 2
Grapefruit (not including juice)	○	○	○	○	○	○	○	○	1/2 medium	○ 1/4	○ 1/2	○ 1
Cantaloupe	○	○	○	○	○	○	○	○	1/4 medium	○ 1/8	○ 1/4	○ 1/2
Peaches, apricots (fresh, in season)	○	○	○	○	○	○	○	○	1 medium	○ 1/2	○ 1	○ 2
Peaches, apricots (canned or dried)	○	○	○	○	○	○	○	○	1 medium or 1/2 cup	○ 1/2	○ 1	○ 2
Prunes, or prune juice	○	○	○	○	○	○	○	○	1/2 cup	○ 1/4	○ 1/2	○ 1
Watermelon (in season)	○	○	○	○	○	○	○	○	1 slice	○ 1/2	○ 1	○ 2
Strawberries, other berries (in season)	○	○	○	○	○	○	○	○	1/2 cup	○ 1/4	○ 1/2	○ 1
Any other fruit, including kiwi, fruit cocktail, grapes, raisins, mangoes	○	○	○	○	○	○	○	○	1/2 cup	○ 1/4	○ 1/2	○ 1

Nutrition Care and Assessment

or several consecutive days. To perform a kcalorie count, the nurse records the dietary items that a patient is given at meals and subtracts the amounts remaining after meals are completed; this procedure allows an analysis of the caloric value of foods and beverages that are actually consumed.

ANTHROPOMETRIC DATA

Measures of body size, known as **anthropometric** measurements, can reveal problems related to both overnutrition and PEM. Height (or length) and weight are the most common anthropometric measures and are used to evaluate growth in children and nutrition status in adults. Other helpful values include skinfold measurements (described in Appendix E) and circumferences of the head, waist, and limbs.

Height (or Length)

Poor growth in children can be a sign of malnutrition. In adults, height measurements alone do not reflect current nutrition status but can be used for estimating a person's energy needs or appropriate body weight. Length is measured in infants and children younger than 24 months of age, and height is usually measured in older children and adults. (✚) Length can also be measured in adults and children who cannot stand unassisted due to physical or medical reasons. The "How to" below describes some standard techniques for measuring length and height.

✚ *Length* is measured while a person is recumbent (lying down), whereas *height* is measured while a person is standing upright.

anthropometric (AN-throw-poe-MEH-trik): related to physical measurements of the human body, such as height, weight, body circumferences, and percentage of body fat.

HOW TO | Measure Length and Height

To improve the accuracy of length and height measurements, keep the following in mind:

- Always measure—never ask! Self-reported heights are less accurate than measured heights. If height is not measured, document that the height is self-reported.

- Measure the length of infants and young children by using a measuring board with a fixed headboard and a movable footboard. It generally takes two people to measure length: one person gently holds the infant's head against the headboard; the other straightens the infant's legs and moves the footboard to the bottom of the infant's feet. The measurement is taken while the infant is lying flat on its back, with chin and toes pointing upward and heels flat against the footboard.

- Measure height next to a wall on which a nonstretchable measuring tape or board has been fixed. Ask the person to stand erect without shoes and with heels together. The person's eyes and head should be facing forward, with heels, buttocks, and shoulder blades touching the wall. Place a ruler or other flat, stiff object on the top of the head at a right angle to the wall and carefully note the height measurement.

- Immediately record length and height measurements to the nearest ⅛ inch or 0.1 centimeter.

- For evaluating growth rate in young children, use the appropriate growth chart (Appendix E) when plotting results. If length is measured, use the growth chart for children between 0 and 36 months; if height is measured, use the chart for individuals between 2 and 20 years.

- Higher values are obtained from supine measurements than from vertical height measurements due to gravity.

Janine Wiedel Photolibrary/Alamy

It generally takes two people to measure the length of an infant.

© Tony Freeman/PhotoEdit

Standing erect allows for an accurate height measurement.

In adults who are unable to stand, height can be estimated from equations that include either the knee height or the full arm span, both of which correlate well with height.[7] Knee height, which extends from the heel to the top of the knee when the leg is bent at a 90-degree angle, can be measured in either a sitting or recumbent position with a knee-height caliper; specific formulas are available for different age, gender, and ethnic groups. The full arm span is the distance from the tip of one middle finger to the other while the arms are extended horizontally. In children with disabilities that affect stature, alternative measures of linear growth include the full arm span, lower-leg lengths (knee to heel, similar to the knee height measure), and upper-arm lengths (shoulder to elbow), all of which can be compared with reference percentiles.

Body Weight During clinical care, health care providers monitor body weights closely: weight changes may reflect changes in hydration status, and involuntary weight loss can be a sign of PEM. Body weights can be compared with healthy ranges on height-weight tables and growth charts or used to calculate the body mass index (BMI). (✚) A healthy body weight typically falls within a BMI range of 18.5 to 25; thus, an appropriate body weight can usually be estimated by using a BMI table or graph (see the inside back cover of this book).[8] The "How to" below includes suggestions for improving the accuracy of weight measurements.

HOW TO | Measure Weight

Tips for measuring weight include:

- Always measure—never ask! Self-reported weights are often inaccurate. If weight is not measured, document that the weight is self-reported.

- Valid weight measurements require scales that have been carefully maintained, calibrated, and checked for accuracy at regular intervals. Beam balance and electronic scales are the most accurate. Bathroom scales are inaccurate and inappropriate in the clinical setting.

- Measure an infant's weight with a scale that allows the infant to sit or lie down. The tray should be large enough to support an infant or young child up to 40 pounds, and weight graduations should be in ½-ounce or 10-gram increments. For accurate results, weigh infants without clothes or diapers. Excessive movement by the infant can reduce accuracy.

- Children who can stand are weighed in the same way as adults, using beam balance or electronic scales with platforms large enough for standing comfortably. If repeated weight measurements are needed, each weighing should take place at the same time of day (preferably before breakfast), in the same amount of clothing, after the person has voided, and using the same scale. Record weights to the nearest ¼ pound or 0.1 kilogram.

- Special scales and hospital beds with built-in scales are available for weighing people who are bedridden.

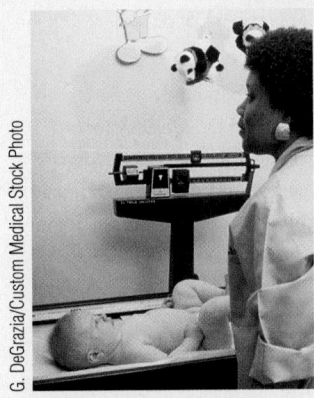

Infants are weighed on scales that allow them to sit or lie down.

Beam balance scales allow accurate weight measurements for older children and adults.

Nutrition Care and Assessment

Head circumference measurements can help to assess brain growth.

Head Circumference A head circumference measure helps to assess brain growth and malnutrition in children up to three years of age, although this measure is not necessarily reduced in a malnourished child. Head circumference values can also track brain development in premature and small-for-gestational-age infants. To measure head circumference, the assessor encircles the largest circumference measure of a child's head with a nonstretchable measuring tape: the tape is placed just above the eyebrows and ears, and around the occipital prominence at the back of the head. The measurement is read to the nearest 1/8th inch or 0.1 centimeter.

Circumferences of Waist and Limbs Circumferences of the waist and limbs are useful for evaluating body fat and muscle mass, respectively. Waist circumference correlates with intra-abdominal fat and can help in assessing overnutrition (see Chapter 6, p. 153). Circumferences of the mid-upper arm, mid-thigh, and mid-calf regions can help in evaluating the effects of illness, aging, and PEM on skeletal muscle tissue. For improved accuracy, circumference measurements are often used together with skinfold measurements to correct for the subcutaneous fat in limbs. In individuals with edema, upper body measurements may be more useful than those in the lower body, where excess body water tends to accumulate.[9]

Anthropometric Assessment in Infants and Children To evaluate growth patterns, the nurse takes periodic measurements of height (or length), weight, and head circumference and plots them on growth charts, such as those provided in Appendix E. The most commonly used growth charts compare height (or length) to age, weight to age, head circumference to age, weight to length, and BMI to age. A number of specialized growth charts are available for children with medical conditions that influence height and weight, such as Down syndrome and Prader-Willi syndrome. (✚) Although individual growth patterns vary, a child's growth will generally stay at about the same percentile throughout childhood; a sharp drop in a previously steady growth pattern suggests malnutrition. Growth patterns that fall below the 5th percentile may also be cause for concern, although genetic influences must be considered when interpreting low values. Growth charts with BMI-for-age percentiles can be used to assess risk of underweight and overweight in children over two years of age: the 5th and 85th percentiles are used as cutoffs to identify children who may be malnourished or overweight, respectively.[10]

Anthropometric Assessment in Adults To evaluate the nutritional risks associated with illness, clinicians monitor both the total reduction in weight and the rate of weight loss over time.[11] Weight changes need to be evaluated carefully, however: although unintentional weight *loss* can indicate malnutrition, weight *gain* may result from fluid retention rather than recovery of muscle tissue or overnutrition. Fluid retention often accompanies worsening disease in patients with heart failure, liver cirrhosis, and kidney failure, and it can mask the weight loss associated with PEM. Some medications can also contribute to weight changes.

Weight data are frequently expressed as percent of ideal body weight (%IBW) or percent of usual body weight (%UBW). The %UBW is more effective than %IBW for interpreting weight changes that occur in underweight, overweight, or obese individuals. In overweight persons, the %IBW may fail to identify significant weight loss. Conversely, in underweight individuals, the %IBW can overstate the degree of weight loss due to illness. The "How to" on p. 394 describes how to estimate %IBW and %UBW, and Table 13-7 shows how to interpret these values. As noted previously, the rate of weight loss should be considered as well as the amount; for example, an involuntary weight loss of more than 10 percent within a six-month period suggests risk of PEM.[12] Table 13-8 provides additional information about the rates of weight loss that indicate nutritional risk.

✚ *Down syndrome* is a genetic abnormality that causes mental disability, short stature, and flattened facial features. *Prader-Willi syndrome* is a genetic disorder characterized by excessive appetite, obesity, and short stature.

%IBW: To estimate %IBW, compare an individual's current weight with a reasonable (ideal) weight from a BMI table or other appropriate reference:

$$\%IBW = \frac{current\ weight}{ideal\ weight} \times 100$$

For example, suppose you wish to calculate the %IBW for a woman who is 5 feet 8 inches tall and weighs 116 pounds. The midpoint of the healthy BMI range is approximately 22, so using a BMI table (as shown on the inside back cover of this book), you estimate that a reasonable weight for this woman would be about 144 pounds:

$$\%IBW = \frac{116}{144} \times 100 = 80.6\%$$

The woman in this example weighs about 80.6 percent of her ideal body weight. A look at Table 13-7 suggests that, at 80.6 percent of IBW, she may be mildly malnourished. Keep in mind that the calculation of "ideal body weight" is somewhat arbitrary, because the BMI table and various other references provide a range of weights for individuals of a given height.

%UBW: To estimate %UBW, compare a person's current weight with the weight that the person generally maintains:

$$\%UBW = \frac{current\ weight}{usual\ weight} \times 100$$

For example, if a man loses 32 pounds during illness and his usual weight is 180 pounds, his current weight would be 148 pounds. These values can be incorporated into the above equation:

$$\%UBW = \frac{148}{180} \times 100 = 82.2\%$$

The man in this example weighs 82.2 percent of his usual weight. A look at Table 13-7 shows that a person at 82 percent of UBW may be moderately malnourished.

Many of the illnesses discussed in later chapters are associated with losses in muscle tissue that resist nutrition intervention. In addition, losses of both muscle tissue and height are common with aging even though body weights may remain stable. Thus, health care providers may utilize skinfold and limb circumference measurements to evaluate body composition changes that need to be addressed in the treatment plan.

BIOCHEMICAL ANALYSES

Biochemical data provide information about protein-energy nutrition, vitamin and mineral status, fluid and electrolyte balance, and organ function. Most tests are based on analyses of blood and urine samples, which contain proteins, nutrients, and metabolites that reflect nutrition and health status. Repeated measures are more helpful than single values, as serial data can indicate whether a condition is improving or worsening. Table 13-9 lists and describes common blood tests (✚) that have nutritional implications. Laboratory tests relevant to specific diseases will be discussed in the chapters that follow.

Interpreting laboratory values can be challenging because a number of factors influence the test results. For example, serum protein values can be affected by fluid imbalances, (✚) pregnancy, infections, and some medications. Similarly, serum levels of vitamins and minerals are often poor indicators of nutrient deficiency because their values are affected by multiple variables; therefore, a variety of tests are generally needed to diagnose a nutrition problem. Taken together with other assessment data, however, laboratory test results help to present a clearer picture than is possible to obtain otherwise.

✚ Blood test results are reported in terms of either *plasma* or *serum* levels. *Plasma* is the yellow fluid that remains after cells are removed, and it still contains clotting factors. *Serum* is the fluid remaining after both cells and clotting factors are removed.

✚ Fluid retention can cause lab results to be deceptively low. Dehydration may cause lab results to be deceptively high.

TABLE 13-7	Body Weight and Nutritional Risk		
%IBW	**%UBW**		**Nutritional Risk**
80–90	85–95		Risk of mild malnutrition
70–79	75–84		Risk of moderate malnutrition
<70	<75		Risk of severe malnutrition

Plasma Proteins Plasma protein levels can help in the assessment of protein-energy status, but the levels may fluctuate for other reasons as well.[13] For example, plasma proteins are synthesized in the liver, so plasma levels of these proteins can reflect liver function. Metabolic stress alters plasma protein levels, because the liver responds by increasing its synthesis of some proteins and reducing synthesis of others. Values are also influenced by pregnancy, kidney function, zinc status, and some medications. Because plasma proteins are affected by so many factors, their values must be considered along with other data to evaluate nutrition status. The following paragraphs describe several of the plasma proteins commonly measured during illness.

Albumin Albumin is the most abundant plasma protein, and its levels are routinely monitored during illness. Although many medical conditions influence albumin, it is slow to reflect changes in nutrition

TABLE 13-8	Rate of Involuntary Weight Loss and Nutritional Risk	
% Weight Loss*	**Time Period**
>2%	1 week
>5%	1 month
>7.5%	3 months
>10%	6 months

* % weight loss $= \dfrac{\text{usual weight} - \text{current weight}}{\text{usual weight}} \times 100$

TABLE 13-9	Routine Laboratory Tests with Nutritional Implications

This table presents a partial listing of some uses of commonly performed lab tests that have implications for nutritional problems.

Laboratory Test	Acceptable Range	Description
Hematology		
Red blood cell (RBC) count	Male: 4.3–5.7 million/µL Female: 3.8–5.1 million/µL	Number of RBC; aids anemia diagnosis.
Hemoglobin (Hb)	Male: 13.5–17.5 g/dL Female: 12.0–16.0 g/dL	Hemoglobin content of RBC; aids anemia diagnosis.
Hematocrit (Hct)	Male: 39–49% Female: 35–45%	Percentage RBC in total blood volume; aids anemia diagnosis.
Mean corpuscular volume (MCV)	80–100 fL	RBC size; helps to distinguish between microcytic and macrocytic anemia.
Mean corpuscular hemoglobin concentration (MCHC)	31–37% Hb/cell	Hb concentration within RBC; helps to distinguish iron-deficiency anemia.
White blood cell (WBC) count	4500–11,000 cells/µL	Number of WBC; general assessment of immunity.
Serum Proteins		
Total protein	6.4–8.3 g/dL	Protein levels are not specific to disease or highly sensitive; they can reflect body protein, illness or infections, changes in hydration or metabolism, pregnancy, or use of certain medications.
Albumin	3.4–4.8 g/dL	May reflect illness or PEM; slow to respond to improvement or worsening of disease.
Transferrin	200–400 mg/dL >60 yr: 180–380 mg/dL	May reflect illness, PEM, or iron deficiency; slightly more sensitive to health status changes than albumin.

(Continued)

Prealbumin (transthyretin)	10–40 mg/dL	May reflect illness or PEM; more responsive to health status changes than albumin or transferrin.
C-reactive protein	68–8200 ng/mL	Indicator of inflammation or disease.
Serum Enzymes		
Creatine kinase (CK)	Male: 38–174 U/L Female: 26–140 U/L	Different forms of CK are found in muscle, brain, and heart. High levels in blood may indicate heart attack, brain tissue damage, or skeletal muscle injury.
Lactate dehydrogenase (LDH)	208–378 U/L	LDH is found in many tissues. Specific types may be elevated after heart attack, lung damage, or liver disease.
Alkaline phosphatase	25–100 U/L	Found in many tissues; often measured to evaluate liver function.
Aspartate aminotransferase (AST, formerly SGOT)	10–30 U/L	Usually monitored to assess liver damage; elevated in most liver diseases. Levels are somewhat increased after muscle injury.
Alanine aminotransferase (ALT, formerly SGPT)	Male: 10–40 U/L Female: 7–35 U/L	Usually monitored to assess liver damage; elevated in most liver diseases. Levels are somewhat increased after muscle injury.
Serum Electrolytes		
Sodium	136–146 mEq/L	Helps to evaluate hydration status or neuromuscular, kidney, and adrenal functions.
Potassium	3.5–5.1 mEq/L	Helps to evaluate acid-base balance and kidney function; can detect potassium imbalances.
Chloride	98–106 mEq/L	Helps to evaluate hydration status and detect acid-base and electrolyte imbalances.
Other		
Glucose (fasting)[a]	74–106 mg/dL >60 yr: 80–115 mg/dL	Detects risk of glucose intolerance, diabetes mellitus, and hypoglycemia; helps to monitor diabetes treatment.
Glycated hemoglobin (Hb A$_{1c}$)	5.0–7.5% of total Hb	Used to monitor long-term blood glucose control (approximately 1 to 3 months prior).
Blood urea nitrogen (BUN)	6–20 mg/dL	Primarily used to monitor kidney function; value is altered by liver failure, dehydration, or shock.
Uric acid	Male: 3.5–7.2 mg/dL Female: 2.6–6.0 mg/dL	Used for detecting gout or changes in kidney function; levels affected by age and diet; varies among different ethnic groups.
Creatinine (serum or plasma)	Male: 0.7–1.3 mg/dL Female: 0.6–1.1 mg/dL	Used to monitor renal function.

[a] Fasting glucose levels that repeatedly exceed 100 mg/dL suggest prediabetes.

Note: μL = microliter; dL = deciliter; fL = femtoliter; ng = nanogram; U/L = units per liter; mEq = milliequivalents.

Source: L. Goldman and D. Ausiello, coeditors, *Cecil Medicine* (Philadelphia: Saunders, 2008).

status because of its large body pool and slow rate of degradation. (✚) In people with chronic PEM, albumin levels remain normal for long periods of time despite depletion of body proteins; levels fall only after prolonged malnutrition. Likewise, albumin levels increase slowly when malnutrition is treated, so albumin is not a sensitive indicator of effective treatment.

Transferrin Transferrin is an iron-transport protein, and its concentrations can respond to both iron status and PEM. Transferrin levels rise as iron status worsens and fall as iron status improves, so using transferrin values to evaluate protein-energy status is difficult if an iron deficiency is also present. Transferrin is degraded more rapidly than albumin, (✚) but its levels change relatively slowly in response to nutrition therapy.

Prealbumin and Retinol-Binding Protein Levels of prealbumin (also called transthyretin) and retinol-binding protein decrease rapidly during PEM and respond quickly to improvements in protein intake. Thus, these proteins are more sensitive than albumin to changes in protein status. (✚) Like other plasma proteins, their usefulness in nutrition assessment is limited because they are affected by a number of different factors, including metabolic stress, zinc deficiency, and various medical conditions. Prealbumin and retinol-binding protein are more expensive to measure than albumin, so they are not routinely included during nutrition assessment.

PHYSICAL EXAMINATIONS

As with other assessment methods, interpreting physical signs of malnutrition requires skill and clinical judgment. Most physical signs are nonspecific; they can reflect any of several nutrient deficiencies, as well as conditions unrelated to nutrition. For example, cracked lips may be caused by several B vitamin deficiencies, but they can also result from sunburn, windburn, or dehydration. Dietary and laboratory data are usually needed as additional evidence to confirm suspected nutrient deficiencies.

Clinical Signs of Malnutrition Signs of malnutrition tend to appear most often in parts of the body where cell replacement occurs at a rapid rate, such as the hair, skin, and digestive tract (including the mouth and tongue). Table 13-10 lists some clinical signs of nutrient deficiencies. Many of the symptoms listed occur only in advanced stages of deficiency. Chapters 8 and 9 provide additional examples of clinical signs that develop during nutrient imbalances.

Hydration State As mentioned previously, fluid imbalances may accompany some illnesses and can also result from the use of certain medications. Recognizing the physical signs of fluid retention or dehydration is necessary for the correct interpretation of blood test results and the body weight measurement.

Fluid retention (also called *edema*) can accompany malnutrition, infection, or injury. It can be caused by impaired blood circulation and frequently accompanies disorders of the heart and blood vessels, kidneys, liver, and lungs. Physical signs of fluid retention include weight gain, facial puffiness, swelling of limbs, abdominal distention, and tight-fitting shoes.

Dehydration can result from vomiting, diarrhea, fever, sweating, excessive urination, and skin injury or burns (due to fluid loss through skin lesions). Dehydration risk is greatest in elderly individuals, who have a reduced thirst response and various other impairments in fluid regulation.[14] Symptoms of dehydration include thirst, dry skin or mouth, reduced skin tension, dark yellow or amber urine, and low urine volume.

Functional Assessment Nutrient deficiencies sometimes impair physiological functions, so health care providers may conduct tests or procedures to help them evaluate the changes that develop in malnutrition. For example, both PEM and zinc deficiency can depress immunity, which can be evaluated by testing the skin's

✚ In blood tests, the term *half-life* describes the length of time that a substance remains in plasma. The albumin in plasma has a half-life of 14 to 20 days, meaning that half of the amount circulating in plasma is degraded in this time period.

✚ Transferrin's half-life in plasma is approximately 8 to 10 days.

✚ Half-lives of prealbumin and retinol-binding protein are 2 to 3 days and 12 hours, respectively.

TABLE
13-10 | Clinical Signs of Nutrient Deficiencies

Body System	Acceptable Appearance	Signs of Malnutrition	Other Possible Causes
Hair	Shiny, firm in scalp	Dull, brittle, dry, loose; falls out (PEM); corkscrew hair (vitamin C)	Excessive hair bleaching, hair loss from aging, chemotherapy, or radiation therapy
Eyes	Bright; clear; shiny; pink, moist membranes; adjust easily to light	Pale membranes (iron); spots, dryness, night blindness (vitamin A); redness at corners of eyes (B vitamins)	Anemia that is unrelated to nutrition; eye disorders; allergies
Lips	Smooth	Dry, cracked, or with sores in the corners of the lips (B vitamins)	Sunburn, windburn, excessive salivation from ill-fitting dentures or various disorders
Mouth and gums	Oral tissues without lesions, swelling, or bleeding; red tongue; normal sense of taste; teeth without caries; ability to chew and swallow	Bleeding gums (vitamin C); smooth or magenta tongue (B vitamins), poor taste sensation (zinc)	Medications, periodontal disease (poor oral hygiene)
Skin	Smooth, firm, good color	Poor wound healing (PEM, vitamin C, zinc); dry, rough, lack of fat under skin (essential fatty acids, PEM, vitamin A, B vitamins); bruising or bleeding under skin (vitamins C and K); pale (iron)	Poor skin care, diabetes mellitus, aging, medications
Nails	Smooth, firm, pink	Ridged (PEM); spoon shaped, pale (iron)	
Other	—	Dementia, peripheral neuropathy (B vitamins); swollen glands at front of neck (PEM, iodine); bowed legs (vitamin D)	Disorders of aging (dementia), diabetes mellitus (peripheral neuropathy)

wasting: the gradual atrophy (loss) of body tissues; associated with protein-energy malnutrition or chronic illness.

response to antigens that ordinarily cause redness and swelling when immune function is adequate. Muscle weakness due to **wasting,** or loss of muscle tissue, can be assessed by testing hand-grip strength. Exercise tolerance, which is reduced in heart and lung disorders, can be assessed using a treadmill or cycle ergometer. The chapters that follow include additional examples of functional assessment. The accompanying Case Study can help you review the different components of a nutrition assessment.

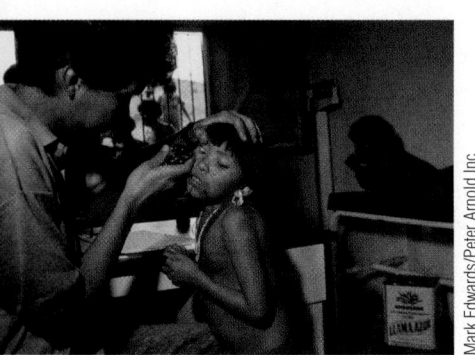

Mark Edwards/Peter Arnold Inc.

Physical signs of malnutrition are often evident in parts of the body where cells are replaced at a rapid rate.

Review Notes

- Nutrition assessments include historical information, anthropometric data, biochemical analyses, and physical examinations. Health care providers assess food intake using 24-hour recall interviews, food frequency questionnaires, food records, and direct observation.
- Anthropometric measurements help clinicians evaluate growth patterns, overnutrition and undernutrition, and body composition.
- Biochemical analyses help in the assessment of nutrient imbalances but are also influenced by various other medical problems.
- Physical examinations allow the detection of nutrient deficiencies, fluid imbalances, and functional impairments that are related to nutritional problems.

Elise Walden is an 85-year-old retired businesswoman who has been a widow for 10 years. She uses a walker and has poorly fitting dentures. She was recently admitted to the hospital with pneumonia and also has congestive heart failure and diabetes. She routinely takes several medications to control her blood glucose levels, hypertension, and heart function. In addition to these medications, the physician has recently ordered antibiotics to treat the pneumonia. During an initial nutrition screening, Mrs. Walden stated that she had been eating very poorly over the past two weeks. She said that she usually weighs about 125 pounds—a fact that was documented in her medical chart from a previous visit. Although she felt she was losing weight, she didn't know how much weight she may have lost or when she started losing weight. Upon admission to the hospital, Mrs. Walden weighed 110 pounds and was 5 feet 3 inches tall. Her serum albumin level was 3.0 grams per deciliter. A physical exam revealed edema, and several other laboratory tests confirmed that she was retaining fluid. As a result of the nutrition screening, Mrs. Walden was referred to a nurse for a nutrition assessment.

1. From the brief description provided, which items in Mrs. Walden's medical history, personal and social history, and food and nutrition history might alert the nurse that this patient is at risk of malnutrition?

2. Identify a healthy body weight for Mrs. Walden, and calculate her %IBW and %UBW. What do the results reveal? What effect does fluid retention have on Mrs. Walden's weight?

3. How can fluid retention alter Mrs. Walden's serum protein levels? What physical symptoms may have suggested that she was retaining excess fluid?

4. What tools can be used to estimate Mrs. Walden's usual food intake? What medical, physical, and personal factors are likely to influence her dietary intake?

5. Describe other types of assessment information that may help the nurse determine whether Mrs. Walden should be referred to a registered dietitian.

Self Check

1 • Mr. Hom experiences loss of appetite, difficulty swallowing, and mouth pain as a consequence of illness. Mr. Hom is at risk of malnutrition due to:
   a. altered metabolism.
   b. reduced food intake.
   c. altered excretion of nutrients.
   d. altered digestion and absorption.

2 • The central role of nurses in health care makes them well positioned for:
   a. calculating patients' nutrient needs.
   b. providing medical nutrition therapy.
   c. conducting complete nutrition assessments.
   d. identifying patients at risk for malnutrition.

3 • Of the following data collected during a nutrition screening, which item does *not* place the person at risk for malnutrition?
   a. Having a health problem that is frequently associated with PEM
   b. The use of prescription medications that affect nutrient needs
   c. Residing with a spouse in a middle-income neighborhood

   d. A significant reduction in food intake over the past five or more days

4 • The nutrition care process is a systematic approach for:
   a. identifying the nutrient content of foods.
   b. ordering special diets.
   c. conducting nutrition screening.
   d. identifying and meeting the nutrition needs of patients.

5 • To conduct complete nutrition assessments, clinicians rely on several sources of information, which include all of the following *except*:
   a. nutrition care plans.
   b. body measurements.
   c. medical, medication, and social histories.
   d. biochemical analyses.

6 • Which dietary assessment method does a nurse use to conduct a kcalorie count?
   a. 24-hour recall interview
   b. Food frequency questionnaire
   c. Food record
   d. Direct observation

7 • The %UBW of a person who weighs 135 pounds and has a usual body weight of 150 pounds is:
   a. 111 percent.
   b. 90 percent.
   c. 86 percent.
   d. 74 percent.

8 • A malnourished, acutely ill patient has just begun to eat after days without significant amounts of food. Which of the following blood test results would change most quickly as the patient's nutrition and health status improves?
   a. Albumin
   b. Transferrin
   c. Serum electrolytes
   d. Retinol-binding protein

9 • Which sign of PEM would be unlikely to show up in a physical examination?
   a. Low plasma protein levels
   b. Dull, brittle hair
   c. Poor wound healing
   d. Wasting

10• Fluid retention can cause all of the following effects *except*:
   a. lab results that are deceptively high.
   b. facial puffiness.
   c. lab results that are deceptively low.
   d. tight-fitting shoes.

Answers: Answers to these questions appear in Appendix H.

Clinical Applications

1 • Describe the potential nutritional implications of these findings from a patient's medical, personal, and social histories: age 78, lives alone, recently lost spouse, uses a walker, has no natural teeth or dentures, has a history of hypertension and diabetes, uses medications that cause frequent urination.

2 • Calculate the %IBW and %UBW for a man who is 5 feet 11 inches tall with a current weight of 150 pounds and a usual body weight of 180 pounds. What additional information do you need to interpret the implications of his weight loss?

3 • Nurses and nurses' aides frequently shoulder much of the responsibility for collecting food intake data for kcalorie counts because they typically deliver food trays and snacks and later retrieve them. Why is it important to verify and record both what the patient receives (foods and amounts) and the foods that remain uneaten? When might patients be enlisted in the collection of food intake data, and when might such a course be unwise?

Nutrition on the Net

For further study of topics covered in this chapter, access these websites.

- Find updates and quick links to these and other nutrition-related sites at our website: www.cengage.com/nutrition/whitney/nhhc4e
- Learn more about nursing diagnoses at the website of NANDA International: www.nanda.org
- Visit the website of the Joint Commission to learn about accreditation of health care institutions: www.jointcommission.org

- Learn about the Mini Nutritional Assessment, a nutrition screening and assessment tool developed by Nestle Nutrition Institute, at this website: www.mna-elderly.com
- Analyze your diet by following the process described at this website: www.mypyramid.gov

Notes

1. D. C. Heimburger, Adulthood, in M. E. Shils and coeditors, *Modern Nutrition in Health and Disease* (Baltimore: Lippincott Williams & Wilkins, 2006), pp. 830–842.
2. P. Charney and M. Marian, Nutrition screening and nutrition assessment, in P. Charney and A. M. Malone, eds., *ADA Pocket Guide to Nutrition Assessment* (Chicago: American Dietetic Association, 2009), pp. 1–19.
3. Writing Group of the Nutrition Care Process/Standardized Language Committee, Nutrition care process and model part I: The 2008 update, *Journal of the American Dietetic Association* 108 (2008): 1113–1117; K. Lacey and E. Pritchett, Nutrition care process and model: ADA adopts road map to quality care and outcomes management, *Journal of the American Dietetic Association* 103 (2003): 1061–1072.
4. Writing Group of the Nutrition Care Process/Standardized Language Committee, 2008.
5. F. E. Thompson and A. F. Subar, Dietary assessment methodology, in A. M. Coulston and C. J. Boushey, eds., *Nutrition in the Prevention and Treatment of Disease* (Burlington, MA: Elsevier Academic Press, 2008), pp. 3–39.
6. L. C. Tapsell, V. Brenninger, and J. Barnard, Applying conversation analysis to foster accurate reporting in the diet history interview, *Journal of the American Dietetic Association* 100 (2000): 818–824.
7. E. Saltzman and M. A. McCrory, Physical assessment of nutritional status, in A. M. Coulston and C. J. Boushey, eds., *Nutrition in the Prevention and Treatment of Disease* (Burlington, MA: Elsevier Academic Press, 2008), pp. 57–73.
8. B. Shah, K. Sucher, and C. B. Hollenbeck, Comparison of ideal body weight equations and published height-weight tables with body mass index tables for healthy adults in the United States, *Nutrition in Clinical Practice* 21 (2006): 312–319.
9. Saltzman and McCrory, 2008.
10. S. E. Barlow and the Expert Committee, Expert Committee recommendations regarding the prevention, assessment, and treatment of child and adolescent overweight and obesity: Summary report, *Pediatrics* 120 (2007): S164–S192.
11. S. B. Heymsfield and R. N. Baumgartner, Body composition and anthropometry, in M. E. Shils and coeditors, *Modern Nutrition in Health and Disease* (Baltimore: Lippincott Williams & Wilkins, 2006), pp. 751–770.
12. American Dietetic Association, *Nutrition Care Manual* (Chicago: American Dietetic Association, 2009).
13. C. W. Thompson, Laboratory assessment, in P. Charney and A. M. Malone, eds., *ADA Pocket Guide to Nutrition Assessment* (Chicago: American Dietetic Association, 2009), pp. 62–153.
14. Standing Committee on the Scientific Evaluation of Dietary Reference Intakes, Food and Nutrition Board, Institute of Medicine, *Dietary Reference Intakes for Water, Potassium, Sodium, Chloride, and Sulfate* (Washington, D.C.:National Academies Press, 2005, pp. 147–150.

NUTRITION IN PRACTICE

Nutritional Genomics

Imagine this scenario: A physician scrapes a sample of cells from inside your cheek and submits it to a **genomics** lab. In a short time, you receive a report that reveals your disease susceptibilities and recommends dietary and lifestyle changes that can maintain your health. You may even be given a prescription for a dietary supplement that will best meet your personal nutrient requirements. Unlikely? Perhaps, but these possibilities are being explored by scientists working in the field of **nutritional genomics**, the study of dietary effects on **gene expression**. Recent research suggests that some dietary factors may be more helpful (or more harmful) in people who have particular genetic variations. The promise of nutritional genomics is a custom-designed dietary prescription that fits each person's specific needs. The Glossary on p. 403 defines genomics and related terms.

What is a genome?

Genetic information is encoded in DNA molecules within the nuclei of almost all of the cells in our bodies. Figure NP13-1 shows how the genetic material is organized within the **genome**, the complete set of genetic information within our cells. The DNA molecules are tightly packed along with associated proteins within the 46 **chromosomes**. Segments of a DNA strand that can eventually be translated into proteins are called **genes**. The sequence of **nucleotides** within each gene encodes the amino acid sequence of a particular protein. Scientists estimate that there are between 20,000 and 24,000 genes in the human genome.[1] However, only a

---

FIGURE **NP13-1** | The Human Genome

1. The human genome is a complete set of genetic material organized into 46 chromosomes, located within the nucleus of a cell.

2. A chromosome is made of DNA and associated proteins.

3. The double helical structure of a DNA molecule is made up of two long chains of nucleotides. Each nucleotide is composed of a phosphate group, a 5-carbon sugar, and a base.

4. The sequence of nucleotide bases (C, G, A, T) determines the amino acid sequence of proteins. These bases are connected by hydrogen bonding to form base pairs: adenine (A) with thymine (T) and guanine (G) with cytosine (C).

5. A gene is a segment of DNA that includes the information needed to synthesize one or more proteins.

Source: Adapted from "A Primer: From DNA to Life," Human Genome Project, U.S. Department of Energy Office of Science, www.ornl.gov/sci/techresources/Human_Genome/primer_pic.shtml.

Glossary

chromosomes: structures within the nucleus of a cell that contain the cell's DNA and associated proteins.

epigenetics: the study of heritable changes in DNA structure that do not change the DNA nucleotide sequence.

gene expression: the process by which a cell converts the genetic code into RNA and protein.

genes: segments of DNA that contain the information needed to make proteins.

genome (JEE-nome): the full complement of genetic material in the chromosomes of a cell.

genomics (jee-NO-miks): the study of genomes.

inherited disorders: medical conditions resulting from genetic defects.

methylation: the addition of methyl ($-CH_3$) groups.

microarray technology: research technology that monitors the expression of thousands of genes simultaneously.

multigene or polygenic: involving a number of genes, rather than a single gene.

noncoding sequences: regions of DNA that do not code for proteins. Some noncoding sequences may have regulatory or structural properties, but most have no known function.

nucleotides: the subunits of DNA and RNA molecules. These compounds—cytosine (C), thymine (T), uracil (U), guanine (G), and adenine (A)—are each composed of a phosphate group, a 5-carbon sugar (ribose), and a nitrogen-containing base. A DNA molecule is made up of two long chains of nucleotides held together by hydrogen bonding between nucleotide bases on opposing strands; each hydrogen-bonded nucleotide couple is called a *base pair*.

nutritional genomics: the study of dietary effects on genetic expression; also known as **nutrigenomics**.

polymorphisms: differences in the DNA sequences among individuals. **A single-nucleotide polymorphism** involves a single nucleotide at a particular area in the DNA strand.

- *poly* = many
- *morph* = form
- *ism* = condition

promoter: a region of DNA involved with gene activation.

transcription factors: proteins that bind DNA at specific sequences to regulate gene expression.

---

small percentage of the genome codes for proteins: most DNA consists of **noncoding sequences**, which may help to regulate gene expression or have other functions.

When proteins are made, the information in the DNA sequence is first transcribed (copied) to messenger RNA molecules, which carry the genetic information out of the nucleus. Gene expression can be measured by determining the amounts of messenger RNA in a tissue sample. The expression of thousands of genes can be measured simultaneously using **microarray technology** (see photo).

A DNA microarray allows researchers to monitor the expression of thousands of genes simultaneously.

© Science VU/Visuals Unlimited

How did research in nutritional genomics begin?

The Human Genome Project, an international effort by industry and government scientists to sequence the human genome, was completed in April 2003. The project led to enormous advances in the research technologies needed to study genes and genetic variation. Knowing the DNA sequences within human chromosomes allows researchers to study how alterations in diet and lifestyle can alter the expression of a multitude of genes. Scientists are working to identify the individual genes in the genome and the roles of their protein products, the genes and proteins associated with diseases, and the dietary and lifestyle choices that influence the expression of genes involved in disease. Furthermore, researchers are studying how variations in the noncoding regions of DNA molecules—which regulate gene expression—influence disease risks.[2]

Genetic differences among individuals have been studied for years, as have the specialized dietary therapies used to treat various **inherited disorders**. For example, an individual may inherit a genetic defect that inhibits the normal metabolism of an essential nutrient and may therefore need to consume a diet that contains either more or less of this nutrient. An example of this type of condition is phenylketonuria (PKU), discussed in Nutrition in Practice 15. Genomic research takes this concept further: instead of focusing on alterations in one or two genes, researchers are studying the expression of *multiple* genes.

How do nutrients alter gene expression?

Some nutrients can switch gene expression on or off.[3] The **promoter** region of a gene (a DNA region involved with gene activation) acts as the master switch. A large variety of proteins known as **transcription factors** can bind to areas on the promoter and either enhance or inhibit gene expression. A combination of dietary factors and hormones influences the types of transcription factors that reach the nucleus and their tendency to bind to DNA. Specific examples of how nutrients can influence transcription factors include:

- The transcription factor that enhances the gene expression of enzymes required for cholesterol synthesis enters the nucleus only when the cellular cholesterol content is low.
- The transcription factor that inhibits the expression of ferritin, an iron-storage protein, changes its affinity for DNA based on the iron content of the cell.

Gene expression is also influenced by modifications in the structure of DNA and its packaging in chromosomes. For example, **methylation** of DNA molecules (the addition of methyl groups) alters the expression of numerous genes and depends on both inherited factors and the availability of various nutrients. In individuals who are susceptible for a disease that is influenced by DNA methylation, nutrient supplementation may reduce the risk of disease.[4] The study of heritable changes in DNA structure that are separate from the underlying DNA nucleotide sequence is called **epigenetics**.

How much genetic variation is there among people?

Except for identical twins, no two individuals are genetically identical. However, the variation in the genomes of any two persons is only about 0.1 percent, a difference of only one base in every 1000.[5] The most common genetic differences, known as **polymorphisms**, are changes in single nucleotides. A **single-nucleotide polymorphism** is due to a nucleotide insertion, deletion, or substitution within the DNA molecule. Such variations are significant only if they affect a protein's amino acid sequence in a way that alters the protein's function, or if the change in the DNA molecule changes how a particular gene is regulated.

Genetic variation gives rise to the diversity among human beings—it explains most of the differences in our physical appearances and metabolic characteristics. Along with environmental factors, it also determines our susceptibilities to disease. Diseases affected by a single gene tend to be relatively rare and usually exert their effects early in life. In contrast, common diseases such as heart disease and cancer are influenced by many genes and typically develop over several decades or even longer. In these more complex **multigene**, or **polygenic**, disorders, many genes can contribute to disease risk, but no single gene may be sufficient to cause the disease on its own.

What are some examples of single-gene disorders?

Examples of single-gene disorders include PKU, sickle-cell anemia, and the iron-overload disease hemochromatosis. Single-gene disorders may seriously disrupt metabolism and often require significant dietary or medical intervention. However, not all single-gene disorders have life-threatening ramifications. For example, lactose intolerance can result from an alteration in the promoter of the lactase gene; it may cause gastrointestinal discomfort but is readily managed by simple dietary changes.

How are multigene disorders different from single-gene disorders?

Multigene disorders are usually sensitive to a number of environmental influences, including diet and lifestyle. These environmental factors can directly influence the expression of the genes involved. Multigene disorders tend to develop over many years, so determining genetic susceptibility may allow a person to modify diet and lifestyle appropriately and reduce the risk of developing a disease.

Heart disease is an example of a disease with multiple gene influences. Its many risk factors represent the involvement of an assortment of genes, which affect disparate aspects of physiology and metabolism. Consider that the major risk factors for heart disease include elevated blood cholesterol levels, obesity, diabetes, and hypertension. The underlying cause of any of these risk factors is rarely known; currently, clinicians screen for the presence of risk factors but not the reasons why they occur. Should genomic research prove successful, a future assessment approach might be to identify specific genetic alterations and changes in metabolism that lead to the development of individual risk factors. For example, tests may determine whether blood cholesterol levels are high due to excessive cholesterol absorption, excessive cholesterol production in the liver, or reduced cholesterol degradation.[6] This information could then guide health care providers to the most appropriate intervention, allowing a better match between treatment recommendations and a person's genetic profile.

Can genomic research be used to explore the differences in nutrient needs among people?

Even though most people apparently can meet their nutrient needs by consuming nutrients at recommended levels, it would be useful to learn more about genetic variations within healthy populations. The techniques that have emerged from genomic research may provide a means for fine-tuning nutrient recommendations for different individuals.[7] Moreover, ideal indicators of nutrient status are still lacking for several of the minerals, such as zinc, magnesium, and chromium. Scientists hope to eventually produce genomic maps that will indicate how various nutrient deficiencies and combinations of deficiencies affect gene expression. These maps may eventually provide data that can help diagnose nutrient deficiencies.

Will knowledge about the human genome substantially change the manner in which health care is provided?

The enthusiasm surrounding genomic research must be put into perspective in terms of both the status of clinical medicine at present and people's willingness to make difficult lifestyle choices. Critics have questioned whether genetic markers for disease would be more useful than simple and inexpensive clinical measurements, which reflect both genetic *and* environmental influences. In other words, knowing that a person is genetically predisposed toward high cholesterol levels is not necessarily more useful than knowing the person's actual blood cholesterol level.[8] Furthermore, a person's family history is already a simple "genomic tool" that indicates a higher genetic risk for certain illnesses. Understanding the family's medical history prompts the clinician to use risk-reduction strategies that are appropriate to the culture and literacy of the patient, rather than focusing on genetic risk alone.[9]

Obtaining additional knowledge about disease risk is not necessarily useful unless people are motivated to make serious lifestyle changes. For example, despite the present abundance of disease prevention recommendations, many people seem unwilling to make the changes known to improve health. Researchers have estimated that heart disease and type 2 diabetes are 80 percent and 90 percent preventable, respectively, by changing one's lifestyle to include an appropriate diet, a healthy body weight, and regular exercise, among other factors.[10] Given the difficulty that people have with current recommendations, it is unlikely that they will enthusiastically adopt an even more detailed list of dietary and lifestyle modifications.

What ethical concerns are raised by having extensive knowledge about an individual's genome?

The ability to obtain detailed genetic information raises a number of concerns. A primary consideration is confidentiality: should information about a person's susceptibility to disease be released to others (including other family members at risk) without that person's consent? Because environmental factors play such an important role in disease risk, genetic predisposition alone usually cannot predict whether a person will develop a particular disease. Concern about privacy issues has led to federal and state legislation that prevents discrimination by group health plans, health insurers, and employers on the basis of an individual's genetic predisposition to disease.[11]

Genetic information can potentially reveal information that has been kept hidden from a person's spouse or children, such as the true paternity of a couple's child or an undisclosed adoption. Such findings may pose difficulty for health practitioners, who may be unable to answer family members' questions honestly yet cannot legally provide false information. The best practice may be to encourage honesty among family members before individuals undergo genetic testing.

Although genomic research has the potential to improve our ability to diagnose and treat disease, it is still unclear how knowledge of the genome will be translated into useful medical treatments. Still, health care professionals will need to keep informed of the ethical, legal, and social implications of nutritional and medical genomics as this remarkable research continues.

Notes

1. S. Barnes, Nutritional genomics, polyphenols, diets, and their impact on dietetics, *Journal of the American Dietetic Association* 108 (2008): 1888–1895; International Human Genome Sequencing Consortium, Finishing the euchromatic sequence of the human genome, *Nature* 431 (2004): 931–945.
2. J. Hardy and A. Singleton, Genomewide association studies and human disease, *New England Journal of Medicine* 360 (2009): 1759–1768.
3. R. J. Cousins, Nutritional regulation of gene expression and nutritional genomics, in M. E. Shils and coeditors, *Modern Nutrition in Health and Disease* (Baltimore: Lippincott Williams & Wilkins, 2006), pp. 615–626.
4. P. J. Stover and M. A. Caudill, Genetic and epigenetic contributions to human nutrition and health: Managing genome–diet interactions, *Journal of the American Dietetic Association* 108 (2008): 1480–1487.
5. P. J. Stover and C. Garza, Polymorphisms: Effect on nutrient utilization and metabolism, in M. E. Shils and coeditors, *Modern Nutrition in Health and Disease* (Baltimore: Lippincott Williams & Wilkins, 2006), pp. 627–635.
6. J. B. German, M.-A. Roberts, and S. M. Watkins, Personal metabolomics as a next generation nutritional assessment, *Journal of Nutrition* 133 (2003): 4260–4266.
7. Stover and Caudill, 2008.
8. W. C. Willett, Balancing life-style and genomics research for disease prevention, *Science* 296 (2002): 695–698.
9. M. J. Khoury and coauthors, Do we need genomic research for the prevention of common diseases with environmental causes? *American Journal of Epidemiology* 161 (2005): 799–805.
10. Khoury and coauthors, 2005; Willett, 2002.
11. P. R. Reilly and R. M. DeBusk, Ethical and legal issues in nutritional genomics, *Journal of the American Dietetic Association* 108 (2008): 36–40.

CHAPTER 14

Nutrition Intervention and Diet-Drug Interactions

© Brooke Fasani/Corbis

CONTENTS

NUTRITION IN PRACTICE

THIS CHAPTER DESCRIBES THE IMPLEMENTATION OF NUTRITION CARE in clinical practice. A key part of this process is ensuring that dietary needs are met, so the chapter also introduces common dietary modifications and describes some of the procedures and challenges involved in foodservice delivery. The final section discusses diet-drug interactions that need consideration when health practitioners administer nutrition care.

Implementing Nutrition Care

As explained in Chapter 13, nurses are well positioned to identify patients with nutritional problems. In addition, nursing care plans may include nursing diagnoses that suggest the need for nutritional intervention. This section provides examples of typical nutrition interventions and describes how the nurse can incorporate nutrition care into a care plan.

CARE PLANNING

Once the dietitian or nurse has collected and analyzed assessment information, the next steps of nutrition care can be carried out. Table 14-1 lists examples of nutrition interventions that may be appropriate in either the hospital or outpatient setting; note that some interventions may fall within the scope of nursing practice whereas others require the assistance of other health professionals. Many interventions include a diet order (prescribed by the patient's physician), which provides specific dietary recommendations regarding food, nutrient, or energy intake or feeding method. The care plan may also involve nutrition education or counseling (typically provided by a registered dietitian) to provide the knowledge, skills, and motivation that enable the patient to make dietary and lifestyle changes.

Table 14-2 shows an example of how nutrition care might be incorporated into a nursing care plan. The example describes a patient at risk for protein-energy malnutrition

TABLE 14-1	Examples of Nutrition Interventions
Intervention	**Examples**
Food and/or nutrient delivery	Providing appropriate meals, snacks, and dietary supplements
	Providing specialized nutrition support (tube and intravenous feedings)
	Determining need for feeding assistance or adjustment in feeding environment
	Managing nutrition-related medication problems
Nutrition education	Providing basic nutrition-related instruction
	Providing in-depth training to increase dietary knowledge or skills
Nutrition counseling	Helping individuals set priorities and establish goals
	Motivating individuals to change behaviors
	Solving problems that interfere with the nutrition care plan
Coordination of nutrition care	Providing referrals or consulting other health professionals or agencies that can assist with treatment
	Organizing treatments that involve other health professionals or health care facilities
	Arranging transfer of nutrition care to another professional or location

Source: American Dietetic Association, *Nutrition Diagnosis and Intervention: Standardized Language for the Nutrition Care Process* (Chicago: American Dietetic Association, 2007).

TABLE
14-2 | Incorporating Nutrition Care into the Nursing Care Plan

The following example illustrates how the nurse can address nutrition problems while working through the different phases of the nursing process.

Nursing Process	Nutrition-Related Features
Assessment. The nurse includes nutrition assessment data in the overall assessment database.	The assessment data related to nutrition care are categorized and documented. *Subjective data:* • 74-year-old man with emphysema and dysphagia (difficulty swallowing); lives with wife. • Uses oxygen therapy at home but mostly while sleeping; frequently feels "out of breath" during the day. • Reports coughing while eating; senses that food gets "stuck" in his throat. • Believes he has lost weight recently because his clothes seem looser than usual. Says usual weight is 160 pounds, which is documented in the medical record. • Physically inactive; mostly watches TV during the day. *Objective data:* Height: 5' 9"; weight: 145 lb; BMI: 21.5; %UBW: 90.6%; albumin: 3.6 g/dL; continually needs to clear throat; exhibits dyspnea (labored breathing) with walking.
Nursing diagnosis. The nurse develops diagnoses that indicate the need for nutrition intervention.	Nursing diagnoses with nutritional implications include: • *Impaired swallowing:* related to neuromuscular impairment. • *Risk for aspiration:* related to ineffective swallowing reflex. • *Imbalanced nutrition: less than body requirements* related to inability to ingest foods. • *Activity intolerance:* related to imbalance between oxygen supply and demand.
Planning: outcome identification. The nurse identifies outcomes associated with improved nutrition status.	Appropriate outcomes include the patient's ability to: • Identify foods and beverages that can be consumed without difficulty. • Consume meals without coughing or aspiration. • Consume adequate amounts of food and beverages to meet nutritional needs. • Show no further evidence of weight loss. • Use oxygen therapy as needed to permit a steady increase in activity.
Planning: interventions. The nurse develops strategies to help the patient achieve the expected outcomes.	To achieve the expected outcomes, the nurse plans to: • Educate the patient about body positioning and feeding techniques that can improve his ability to eat without coughing or discomfort. • Provide the patient with information about high-kcalorie and high-protein foods to minimize further weight and lean tissue loss. • Explain the need for daily physical activity, including suggestions that may improve the patient's ability to tolerate additional activity. • Teach the patient to conserve energy while performing activities of daily living. • Provide information about lightweight, portable, supplemental oxygen that can assist the patient during the day. Examples of interventions that would require the involvement of other health professionals include: • The attending physician may need to prescribe dysphagia testing to help determine the most appropriate dysphagia diet. • A dysphagia specialist may need to provide specific feeding recommendations related to the patient's type of dysphagia. • A registered dietitian may need to review and modify the patient's diet so that he can improve his energy intake and make more appropriate food and beverage selections.

Implementation. The nurse performs the appropriate interventions and refers patient to other health practitioners, as necessary.

Evaluation: The nurse continually monitors and evaluates the patient's progress in achieving each outcome. The nursing care plan is revised as needed.

and wasting due to his swallowing difficulty and intolerance to physical activity. After diagnosing his nutrition-related problems, the nurse identifies **expected outcomes** and plans strategies that can correct the problems. This example includes interventions that require referrals to other health practitioners.

expected outcomes: patient-oriented goals that are derived from nursing diagnoses.

APPROACHES TO NUTRITION CARE

A nutrition care plan often involves significant dietary modifications. To ensure better compliance, the plan must be compatible with the desires and abilities of the person it is designed to help. The challenge is greater if dietary changes are required for extended periods.

Long-Term Dietary Intervention When long-term changes are necessary, a care plan must take into account the person's current food practices, lifestyle, and degree of motivation. Behavior change is a process that occurs in stages; therefore, more than one consultation is usually necessary. The following approaches may be helpful in implementing long-term dietary changes:[1]

- *Determine the individual's readiness for change.* Some people have little desire to change their dietary behaviors, and even those who are willing may not be fully prepared to take the necessary steps. The health practitioner needs to consider a patient's readiness to adopt new dietary behaviors before attempting to implement an ambitious care plan.
- *Emphasize what to eat, rather than what not to eat.* Emphasizing foods to include in the diet, rather than those to restrict, can make dietary changes more appealing. For example, encouraging additional fruits and vegetables is a more attractive message than telling the patient to restrict butter, cream sauces, and ice cream.
- *Suggest only one or two changes at a time.* People are more likely to adopt a dietary plan that does not deviate too much from their usual diet. If they succeed in adopting one or two changes, they are more likely to stick to the plan and be open to additional suggestions. Stricter plans may yield quicker results but are useful only for highly motivated people.

Nutrition Education Nutrition education allows patients to learn about the dietary factors that affect their particular medical condition. Ideally, this knowledge can motivate them to change their diet and lifestyle to improve their health status.

A nutrition education program should be tailored to a person's age, level of literacy, and cultural background. Learning style should also be considered: some people learn best by discussion supplemented with written materials, whereas others prefer visual examples, such as food models and measuring devices.[2] Information can be provided in one-on-one sessions or group discussions. The meeting should include an assessment of the person's understanding of the material and commitment to making changes. Follow-up sessions can reveal whether the person has successfully adopted a dietary plan. For example, a nurse who counsels a woman who is lactose intolerant and hesitant to use milk products might proceed as follows:

- The nurse provides sample menus of a nutritionally adequate diet that limits milk and milk products. Together, the nurse and the woman design menus that consider her food preferences.
- The nurse describes the types and amounts of milk products that are unlikely to cause symptoms and explains how to gradually incorporate these foods into the diet.
- Using diet analysis software, the nurse demonstrates how altering intakes of calcium-containing foods changes a meal's calcium content.
- The nurse explains how to use the Daily Values information on food labels to estimate the calcium content of packaged foods.
- The nurse provides information about the advantages and disadvantages of different calcium supplements.
- The nurse assesses the woman's understanding by having her identify nonmilk products that are high in calcium.

Ideally, the nurse would be able to monitor the woman's progress in a subsequent session.

© ACE STOCK LIMITED/Alamy

Dietary counseling requires sensitivity to cultural orientation, educational background, and motivation for change.

CASE STUDY | Implementing Nutrition Care

Max is an 11-year-old boy who was admitted to the hospital after he passed out while playing with friends. Tests confirm a diagnosis of type 1 diabetes mellitus. Max remains in the hospital for several days until his blood glucose and ketone levels are under control. During this time, he and his family learn about diabetes, the diet Max needs to follow, the use of insulin, the monitoring of blood glucose levels, and the required coordination of diet, insulin, and physical activity. The details of diabetes mellitus are reserved for Chapter 20, but for now you can consider the steps that are necessary for implementing Max's nutrition care.

1. The nurse handling Max's case must identify expected outcomes when she writes her care plan. What expected outcomes are appropriate for Max's situation?

2. Given the chronic nature of Max's illness and his age, what approaches should the nurse use when discussing the required dietary and medical treatments with Max and his family?

3. What factors need consideration when designing a nutrition education program for Max and his parents?

4. Max will need additional care to learn more about diabetes and to make the adjustments that will allow him to cope with his condition. Why is it important to address follow-up care before Max leaves the hospital?

Follow-up Care For optimal success, health practitioners should periodically evaluate the effectiveness of nutrition care plans. Doing so usually involves comparing relevant outcome measures (such as the results of blood tests) with initial values and meeting with the patient to learn whether the plan has been satisfactory from the patient's point of view. Such follow-up efforts can reveal whether the care plan needs to be revised or updated, as is often the case when a person's medical condition changes. The accompanying Case Study provides an opportunity for you to review the implementation of nutrition care.

Review Notes

- Nutrition interventions are designed to correct the nutrition problems associated with illness. Using the steps of the nursing process, a nurse can incorporate nutrition care into a nursing care plan.

- A nutrition intervention should take into account a person's food practices, lifestyle, and degree of motivation. Nutrition education should be individualized to accommodate a patient's needs and learning style.

- Nutrition care can be evaluated by reviewing relevant outcome measures of health status and determining the patient's understanding and acceptance of the intervention.

Dietary Modifications

During many illnesses, a person can meet energy and nutrient needs by following a **standard diet**. In other cases, adjustments in energy or nutrient intakes or a **modified diet** may be necessary. Modified diets contain foods with altered texture, consistency, or nutrient content, or they may include or omit specific foods. This section introduces several types of dietary modifications and explains their uses during illness.

DETERMINING ENERGY REQUIREMENTS

To determine energy requirements for hospital patients, clinicians typically measure or estimate the resting metabolic rate (RMR) and then adjust the RMR value with "stress factors" that account for medical problems or, in some cases, medical treatments. In ambulatory patients, a factor for activity level may also be applied. Table 14N3 presents examples of RMR equations in common use, and the "How to" on p. 411 presents an example of this method. Note that in individuals who are overweight or obese, the Mifflin–St. Jeor equation has been found to yield the most accurate results.[3]

standard diet: a diet that includes all foods and meets the nutrient needs of healthy people; also called a *regular diet*.

modified diet: a diet that contains foods altered in texture, consistency, or nutrient content or that includes or omits specific foods; also called a *therapeutic diet*.

TABLE
14-3

Selected Equations for Estimating Resting Metabolic Rate

Harris–Benedict[a]

Women: RMR = 655.1 + [9.563 × weight (kg)] + [1.85 × height (cm)] − [4.676 × age (years)].

Men: RMR = 66.5 + [13.75 × weight (kg)] + [5.003 × height (cm)] − [6.755 × age (years)].

Mifflin–St. Jeor

Women: RMR = [9.99 × weight (kg)] + [6.25 × height (cm)] − [4.92 × age (years)] − 161

Men: RMR = [9.99 × weight (kg)] + [6.25 × height (cm)] − [4.92 × age (years)] + 5

[a] Although these equations are sometimes used for estimating basal metabolic rate (BMR), they were derived from data measured during resting conditions in most cases.

In critical-care patients, energy needs may be considerably higher than normal due to fever, mechanical ventilation, restlessness, or the presence of open wounds. Patients who are critically ill are usually bedridden and inactive, however, so the energy needed for physical activity is minimal. Energy requirements for critical-care patients are described in Chapter 16.

MODIFIED DIETS

Diets with altered texture and consistency may be necessary for individuals with chewing or swallowing impairments. Diets with modified nutrient or food content may be prescribed to correct malnutrition, relieve disease symptoms, or reduce the risk of developing complications. If a patient has a number of medical problems, several aspects of the diet may need to be modified. Keep in mind that modified diets should be adjusted to satisfy individual preferences and tolerances and may also need to be altered as a patient's condition changes. Table 14-4 lists examples of modified diets that are often prescribed during illness.[4] Later chapters discuss other types of modified diets and additional dietary strategies for treating nutritional problems.

HOW TO | Estimate the Energy Requirements of a Hospital Patient

To determine the energy requirements of a hospital patient, the health practitioner calculates the patient's resting metabolic rate (RMR) and then applies a "stress factor" to accommodate the additional energy needs imposed by illness. The stress factor 1.25 has been shown to be reasonably accurate for many hospitalized patients; other examples are listed in Table 16-2 on p. 473.

The following example uses the Mifflin–St. Jeor equation (shown in Table 14-3) and the stress factor 1.25 to determine the energy needs of a 57-year-old female patient who is 5 feet 3 inches tall, weighs 115 pounds, and is confined to bed.

Step 1: The patient's weight and height are converted to the units used in the equation:

Weight in kilograms = 115 lb ÷ 2.2 lb/kg = 52.3 kg
Height in centimeters = 63 in × 2.54 cm/in = 160 cm

Step 2: Using the Mifflin–St. Jeor equation for estimating RMR in women:

RMR = [9.99 × weight (kg)] + [6.25 × height (cm)] − [4.92 × age (years)] − 161

= (9.99 × 52.3) + (6.25 × 160) − (4.92 × 57) − 161
= 522 + 1000 − 280 − 161 = 1081 kcal

Step 3: The RMR value is multiplied by the appropriate stress factor:

RMR × stress factor = 1081 × 1.25 = 1351 kcal

Thus, an appropriate energy intake for this patient would be approximately 1351 kcal. Her weight should be monitored to determine if her actual needs are higher or lower.

For a patient who is not confined to bed, an additional activity factor can be applied to accommodate the extra energy needs. For example, if the patient in the example begins limited activity while in the hospital, an activity factor of 1.2 can be multiplied by the results obtained in Step 3:

1351 × activity factor = 1351 × 1.2 = 1621 kcal

The activity factor for a hospitalized patient often falls between 1.1 and 1.4, and it is likely to change as the patient's condition improves.

| TABLE 14-4 | Examples of Modified Diets |

Type of Diet	Description of Diet	Appropriate Uses
Modified Texture and Consistency		
Mechanically altered diets	Contain foods that are modified in texture. Pureed diets include only pureed foods; mechanical soft diets may include solid foods that are mashed, minced, ground, or soft.	Pureed diets are used for people with swallowing difficulty, poor lip and tongue control, or oral hypersensitivity. Mechanical soft diets are appropriate for people with limited chewing ability or certain swallowing impairments.
Blenderized liquid diet	Contains fluids and foods that are blenderized to liquid form.	For people who cannot chew, swallow easily, or tolerate solid foods.
Clear liquid diet	Contains clear fluids or foods that are liquid at room temperature and leave minimal residue in the colon.	For preparation for bowel surgery or colonoscopy, for acute GI disturbances (such as after GI surgeries), or as a transition diet after intravenous feeding. For short-term use only.
Modified Nutrient or Food Content		
Fat-controlled diet	Limits dietary fat to low (<50 g/day) or very low (<25 g/day) intakes.	For people who have certain malabsorptive disorders or symptoms of diarrhea, flatulence, or steatorrhea (fecal fat) resulting from dietary fat intolerance.
Fiber-restricted diet	Limits dietary fiber; degree of restriction depends on the patient's condition and reason for restriction.	For acute phases of intestinal disorders or to reduce fecal output before surgery. Not recommended for long-term use.
Sodium-controlled diet	Limits dietary sodium; degree of restriction depends on symptoms and disease severity.	To help lower blood pressure or prevent fluid retention; used in hypertension, congestive heart failure, renal disease, and liver disease.
High-kcalorie, high-protein diet	Contains foods that are kcalorie and protein dense.	Used for patients with high kcalorie and protein requirements (due to cancer, AIDS, burns, trauma, and other conditions); also used to reverse malnutrition, improve nutritional status, or promote weight gain.

Source: American Dietetic Association, *Nutrition Care Manual* (Chicago: American Dietetic Association, 2009).

Mechanically Altered Diets Individuals who have difficulty chewing or swallowing may benefit from mechanically altered diets. Chewing difficulties usually result from dental problems. Impaired swallowing, or **dysphagia,** may accompany neurological disorders, surgical procedures involving the head and neck, and physiological or anatomical abnormalities that restrict the movement of food within the throat or esophagus. Dysphagia diets are highly individualized because swallowing problems vary in severity and swallowing ability can fluctuate over time. Chapter 17 provides details about the specific diets used for treating dysphagia.

Table 14-5 provides examples of foods included in mechanically altered diets. Although the names for these diets vary, a more restrictive diet may contain mostly pureed foods (*pureed diet*), whereas a less restrictive diet may include moist, soft-textured foods that easily form a bolus (*mechanical soft diet*, or simply *soft diet*). Diets for people with chewing problems typically include foods that are ground or minced (*ground/minced diet*). Note that the foods used in these diets can overlap, and individual tolerances ultimately determine whether foods are included or excluded.

dysphagia: difficulty swallowing.

TABLE
14-5 | Foods Included in Mechanically Altered Diets

Depending on the feeding problem, a mechanically altered diet may include foods that are pureed, mashed, ground, minced, or soft textured. Foods vary according to tolerance.

Pureed Diets	Mechanical Soft Diets
Milk products: Milk, smooth yogurt, pudding, custard	**Milk products:** Milk, yogurt with soft fruit, pudding, cottage cheese
Fruits: Pureed fruits and juices without pulp, seeds, skins, or chunks; well-mashed fresh bananas; applesauce	**Fruits:** Canned or cooked fruits without seeds or skin, fruit juices with small amounts of pulp, ripe bananas
Vegetables: Pureed cooked vegetables without seeds, skins, or chunks; mashed potatoes, pureed potatoes with gravy	**Vegetables:** Soft, well-cooked vegetables that are not rubbery or fibrous; well-cooked, moist potatoes
Meats and meat substitutes: Pureed meats; smooth, homogenous souffles; hummus or other pureed legume spreads	**Meats and meat substitutes:** Ground, minced, or tender meat, poultry, or fish with gravy or sauce; tofu; well-cooked, moist legumes; scrambled or soft-cooked eggs
Breads and cereals: Smooth cooked cereals such as Cream of Wheat, slurried breads and pancakes,ª pureed rice and pasta	**Breads and cereals:** Cooked cereals or moistened dry cereals with minimal texture, soft pancakes or breads, well-cooked noodles or dumplings in sauce or gravy

ª Slurried foods are mixed with liquid until the consistency is appropriate; they may be gelled and shaped to improve their appearance.

Source: American Dietetic Association, *Nutrition Care Manual* (Chicago: American Dietetic Association, 2009).

Blenderized Liquid Diet

Blenderized diets are most often recommended following oral or facial surgeries (for example, jaw wiring). Soft or tender foods that can be blenderized (often with added liquid) are available from all food groups; they include cereals and breads; cooked vegetables; fresh or cooked fruits without skins or seeds; cooked, tender meats and fish; and potatoes, rice, and pasta. Foods that do not blend well should be excluded; these include hard or rubbery foods such as nuts and seeds, dried fruits, coconut, hard cheeses, sausages and frankfurters, and some raw vegetables.

Clear Liquid Diet

Clear liquids, which require minimal digestion and are easily tolerated by the gastrointestinal (GI) tract, are often the foods recommended before some GI procedures (including GI examinations, X-rays, or surgeries), after GI surgery, or after fasting or intravenous feeding. The **clear liquid diet** consists of clear fluids and foods that are liquid at room temperature and leave little undigested material (called **residue**) in the colon. Permitted foods include clear or pulp-free fruit juices, carbonated beverages, clear meat and vegetable broths (such as consommé and bouillon), fruit-flavored gelatin, fruit ices made from clear juices, frozen juice bars, and plain hard candy. Although the clear liquid diet provides fluid and electrolytes, its nutrient and energy contents are extremely limited. If used for longer than a day or two, the diet should be supplemented with commercially prepared low-residue formulas that provide required nutrients. Figure 14-1 gives an example of a one-day clear liquid menu.

Fat-Controlled Diet

Fat restriction may be necessary for reducing the symptoms of fat malabsorption, which often accompanies diseases of the liver, gallbladder, pancreas, and intestines. Fat restriction may also alleviate the symptoms of heartburn. Although the fat intake is occasionally limited to as little as 25 grams daily, it should not be restricted more than necessary because fat is an important source of kcalories. Chapter 18 gives additional information about fat-controlled diets.

Most foods included in a fat-controlled diet provide less than 1 gram of fat per serving. The diet includes fat-free milk products, most breads and cooked grains, fat-free broths and soups, vegetables prepared without fats, most fruits, and fat-free candies

clear liquid diet: a diet that consists of foods that are liquid at room temperature, require minimal digestion, and leave little residue (undigested material) in the colon.

residue: material left in the intestine after digestion; includes mostly dietary fiber and undigested starches and proteins.

FIGURE
14-1

Menu—Clear Liquid Diet

Sample Menu

Breakfast	Strained orange juice
	Flavored gelatin
	Ginger ale
	Coffee or tea, sugar
Lunch	Bouillion or consommé
	Flavored gelatin
	Frozen juice bars
	Apple or grape juice
	Coffee or tea, sugar
Supper	Bouillion or consommé
	Flavored gelatin
	Fruit ice
	Cranberry juice
	Coffee or tea, sugar
Snacks	Soft drinks
	Fruit ices
	Hard candy

and sweets (see Table 18-5 on p. 520). Restricted foods include low-fat and whole-milk products, baked products with added fat (like muffins), and most prepared desserts. Lean meat and meat substitutes are permitted but may be restricted to 4 to 6 ounces per day, depending on the degree of restriction. Some patients with malabsorptive disorders cannot tolerate large amounts of lactose or dietary fiber, so foods that include these substances may also be excluded from the diet.

Fiber-Restricted Diet Fiber restriction is recommended during acute phases of intestinal disorders, when the presence of fiber may exacerbate intestinal discomfort or cause diarrhea or blockages. Fiber-restricted diets are sometimes used before surgery to minimize fecal volume and after surgery during transition to a regular diet. Long-term fiber restriction is discouraged, however, because it is associated with constipation, diverticulosis, and other problems.

Fiber-restricted diets often eliminate whole-grain breads and cereals, nuts and nut butters, most fresh fruits (except peeled apples, ripe bananas, and melons), dried fruits, dried beans and peas, and many vegetables (including broccoli, cabbage, corn, onions, peppers, spinach, and winter squash). If required, even greater reductions in colonic residue can be achieved by excluding foods high in resistant starch (see p. 67), milk products, and foods that contain fructose or sugar alcohols (such as sorbitol); these foods contribute to colonic residue because some of their nutrients may be poorly digested or absorbed. Information about the fiber content of specific foods can be found in Chapter 3 (p. 81) and Appendix A.

Sodium-Controlled Diet A sodium-controlled diet can help to prevent or correct fluid retention and may be recommended for treatment of hypertension, congestive heart failure, kidney disease, and liver disease. The degree of sodium restriction depends on the illness, the severity of symptoms, and the drug treatment prescribed. In most cases, sodium is restricted to 2000 or 3000 milligrams daily, although more severe restrictions may be used in the hospital setting. Many patients find it difficult to significantly reduce their sodium intake, so while the sodium-controlled diet is an attempt to improve the patient's medical problem, the sodium recommendation may sometimes exceed the Tolerable Upper Intake Level (UL) for sodium of 2300 milligrams.(✚)

A sodium-controlled diet limits the use of salt when cooking and at the table, eliminates most prepared foods and condiments, and limits consumption of milk and milk products (if excessive). Because so many processed foods are high in sodium, people following a sodium-controlled diet should check food labels and consume only low-sodium products. Sodium restrictions are difficult to implement on a long-term basis because many people find the diet unpalatable. Additional information about controlling dietary sodium is provided in Chapters 21 and 22.

High-kCalorie, High-Protein Diet The high-kcalorie, high-protein diet is used to increase kcalorie and protein intakes in patients who have unusually high requirements or in those who are eating poorly. High-fat foods are added to increase energy intakes; consequently, the diet may exceed 35 percent kcalories from fat.(✚) Consuming small, frequent meals and commercial liquid supplements (such as Ensure or Boost) can also help a patient meet increased energy, protein, and other nutrient needs.

Examples of foods included in high-kcalorie, high-protein diets are listed in Table 14-6. Some of these foods are high in saturated fat, which is limited in heart-healthy diets. These foods are used liberally in diets for malnourished patients to help correct their immediate nutrition problems—weight loss and muscle wasting. Chapter 23 offers additional suggestions for increasing the kcalorie and protein contents of meals.

✚ The average sodium intake in the United States is approximately 3400 mg per day. The sodium UL was set at 2300 mg to help prevent hypertension.

✚ Reminder: Current guidelines recommend a total fat intake between 20 and 35 percent of kcalories, with most fats coming from polyunsaturated and monounsaturated fats.

TABLE 14-6	Foods Included in High-kCalorie, High-Protein Diets
Milk products	Whole milk, half-and-half, cream
	Milk shakes, eggnog
	Cheese
	Ice cream, whipped cream
Fruits	Dried fruits
	Canned fruits in heavy syrup
	Avocado
Vegetables	High-kcalorie vegetables such as potatoes, corn, and peas
	Vegetables prepared with butter, margarine, sour cream, cheese sauces, mayonnaise, or salad dressing
	Cream of vegetable soups
Meats and high-protein foods	All meats, fish, and poultry, including bacon, frankfurters, and luncheon meats; eggs; beans; tofu
	All meats, prepared fried or covered in cream sauces or gravies
	Protein bars
	Nuts and seeds, peanut and other nut butters, coconut
Breads and cereals	Granola and dry cereals prepared with whole milk or cream and dried fruit
	Hot cereals with whole milk or cream, or added fat
	Pasta, rice, and biscuits with added fat
	Pancakes, waffles, French toast
Beverages	Fruit juices, sweetened beverages
	Meal replacement drinks
	Beverages with added protein powders

VARIATIONS IN THE DIET ORDER

As mentioned previously, the physician usually has the primary responsibility for prescribing an appropriate diet for a patient in a medical facility. Diet orders must be precise to avoid confusion; for example, a "sodium-controlled diet" should specify the amount of sodium permitted, as "sodium control" could be interpreted to mean any amount between 500 and 3000 milligrams. The physician often relies on the dietitian or nurse to recommend changes in the diet order when warranted. If a diet order seems inappropriate or outdated, the nurse should alert the physician that a mistake may have been made.

Diet Progression A change in diet as a patient's food tolerance improves is called **diet progression.** For example, the diet order may read, "progress diet from clear liquids to a regular diet as tolerated." In practice, this means that the patient would be given clear beverages initially and then gradually be provided with other beverages or solid foods that are unlikely to cause discomfort. As another example, the diet may progress from small, frequent feedings to larger meals as tolerance improves. The nurse is often responsible for monitoring a patient's tolerance to a diet; symptoms such as nausea, vomiting, diarrhea, and gastrointestinal pain suggest intolerance.

Nothing by Mouth (NPO) An order to not give a patient anything at all—food, beverages, or medications—is indicated by NPO, an abbreviation for *non per os,*

diet progression: a change in diet as a patient's tolerances permit.

meaning "nothing by mouth." For example, an order may read "NPO for 24 hours" or "NPO until after X-ray." The NPO order is commonly used during certain acute illnesses or diagnostic tests involving the GI tract.

Alternative Feeding Routes In most cases, patients can meet their nutrient needs by consuming regular foods. Sometimes, however, a person's medical condition makes it difficult to meet nutrient needs orally. In such cases, the physician may order **tube feedings** or **intravenous feedings**, which are described in detail in Chapter 15.

- *Tube feedings.* Nutritionally complete formulas can be delivered through a tube placed directly into the stomach or intestine. Tube feedings are preferred to intravenous feedings if the GI tract is functioning normally.
- *Intravenous feedings.* A person's medical condition sometimes prohibits the use of the GI tract to deliver nutrients. If the person is malnourished and the GI tract cannot be used for a significant period of time, intravenous feedings (also called *parenteral nutrition*) can meet nutritional needs.

IMPROVING FOOD INTAKE

People in hospitals and other medical facilities often lose their appetites as a result of their medical condition, treatment, or emotional distress. Moreover, some medications and other treatments can dramatically alter taste perceptions. Patients usually receive meals at specified times, whether they are hungry or not, and often must eat in bed without companionship. Under these types of conditions, eating can become more of a chore than a pleasurable experience. Meals may also be unwelcome if the person is in pain or has been sedated.

Nurses often play a central role in helping patients to eat. Whenever possible, the patient's room should remain calm and quiet during mealtime. Excessive activity, like room maintenance or ward rounds, can distract patients and reduce appetite. If the patient's appetite or sense of taste is affected by illness, the nurse should work with the patient to identify foods that are the most enjoyable. When meals are served, the nurse can help the patient wash up before eating and check to see that foods and utensils are arranged attractively. Placing an occasional "surprise" on the tray—a decoration or funny card, for example—may help patients look forward to meals or perk up sagging spirits. The "How to" below includes additional suggestions that may help to improve food intake at mealtimes.

HOW TO | Help Hospital Patients Improve Their Food Intakes

1. Empathize with the patient. Show that you understand how difficult eating may be. Imagine feeling too sick to move or too tired to sit up.

2. Motivate. Be sure the patient understands how important nutrition is to recovery.

3. Help patients select the foods they like and mark menus appropriately. When appropriate and permissible, let friends or family members bring favorite foods from outside the hospital.

4. For patients who are weak, suggest foods that require little effort to eat. Eating a roast beef sandwich, for example, requires less effort than cutting and eating a steak. Drinking soup from a cup may be easier than eating it with a spoon.

5. During mealtimes, make sure the patient's room is quiet and has sufficient lighting for viewing the food. See that the room is free of odors that may interfere with the appetite.

6. Help patients prepare for meals. Help them get comfortable, either in bed or in a chair. Adjust the extension table to a comfortable distance and height, and make sure it is clean. Take these steps before the tray arrives, so the meal can be served promptly and at the right temperature.

7. When the food cart arrives, check the patient's tray. Confirm that the patient is receiving the right diet, the foods on the tray are those selected from the menu, appropriate condiments are available, and the foods look appealing. Order a new tray if the foods are not appropriate.

8. Help with eating, if necessary. Help patients to open containers or cut foods, and assist with feeding if patients cannot feed themselves. Have somebody sit with the patient during meals if the patient is uninterested in eating while alone.

9. Try to solve eating problems. Encourage patients with little appetite to eat the most nutritious foods first and to drink liquids between meals.

10. Take a positive attitude toward the hospital's food. Never say something like "I couldn't eat this either." Instead, say, "The food-service department really tries to make foods appetizing. I'm sure we can find a solution."

Review Notes

- Dietary modifications prescribed during illness include changes in food texture or consistency, modified energy or nutrient content, or the inclusion or exclusion of certain foods.
- Energy requirements for hospital patients are typically estimated by multiplying a person's resting metabolic rate (RMR) by factors that account for the medical condition, medical treatments, and activity level.
- Mechanically altered diets may be prescribed for people with swallowing and chewing difficulties.
- Clear liquid diets may be recommended before various diagnostic tests or after acute gastrointestinal disturbances, intravenous feedings, or fasts.
- Some medical conditions require the restriction of specific nutrients, such as fat, fiber, or sodium.
- A high-kcalorie, high-protein diet may help to prevent or reverse malnutrition, improve nutrition status, or promote weight gain.
- The diet order must include specific instructions about dietary modifications to avoid confusion. The diet prescribed may change during the course of illness.
- Hospital patients may need assistance at mealtime and encouragement to consume adequate amounts of food.

diet manual: a resource that specifies the exact foods or preparation methods to include or exclude in modified diets and provides sample menus.

selective menus: menus that provide choices in some or all menu categories.

Foodservice

The work of a foodservice department may appear deceptively simple: appropriate foods are delivered to patients who need specific types of diets. Behind the scenes, however, a complex system is at work. A foodservice department faces a daily challenge in planning, producing, and delivering hundreds of nutritious meals and accommodating dozens of special diets and food preferences.

When designing menus for modified diets, the dietary and foodservice personnel refer to a **diet manual,** which details the exact foods or preparation methods to include or exclude in a modified diet. The diet manual may also outline the rationale and indications for use of the diets and include sample menus. The manual may be compiled by the dietetics staff or adopted from another health care facility or a dietetics organization.

FOOD SELECTION

Most hospitals provide **selective menus** from which patients can select their meals. The patient who must follow a modified diet receives menus that include only the foods specified in the hospital's diet manual for that particular diet (examples of menus are shown in Figure 14-2). Often, patients need to make menu selections a day or two in advance so that the foodservice department can estimate the amounts and types of food they need to purchase and prepare. A member of the foodservice staff may later check the menus to make sure that the selections are appropriate.

If a menu is not marked correctly or is misplaced, the patient may receive a meal selected by the foodservice department. Other potential problems that may arise when selective menus are used include the following:

- Patients may have difficulty reading, understanding, or physically marking menus.
- Patients may not understand that their selections will be for the next (or another) day.
- Patients may be out of their rooms (for tests, procedures, or physical activity) or asleep when the menus arrive and may miss the menu pickup time.
- Patients may be too ill or too uninterested in food to make menu selections.

Problems with menu procedures can often be corrected by explaining the system or by taking the time to help patients mark menus.

Foodservice departments strive to prepare appetizing and nutritious meals and may accommodate dozens of special diets.

FIGURE 14-2 | Sample Lunch Menus

LOW FAT/LOW CHOLESTEROL/CARDIAC SUNDAY

✤〜 *Lunch* 〜✤

LF = Low Fat   LSLF = Low Sodium, Low Fat

Meats

LSLF Baked chicken   LSLF Baked fish (cod)

Starchy Vegetables

LSLF Rice   LSLF Boiled potatoes

Vegetables

LSLF Baby carrots   LSLF Green beans

Soup/Salad/Juice	Dressings
LSLF Coleslaw	Diet French
Gelatin	Diet Thousand Island
Tomato soup	Diet Italian
Tossed salad	

Desserts

Pears	Fresh fruit

Breads

LF Dinner roll	Bran bread
White bread	LS Crackers
Whole wheat bread	

Beverages & Condiments

Coffee	Creamer
Decaf. coffee	Sugar
Hot tea	Sugar substitute
Decaf. hot tea	Herb seasoning
Iced tea	Lemon
Buttermilk	Margarine
Fat-free milk	Mustard
	Diet mayonnaise
	Catsup

Name _____   Room _____

SODIUM-CONTROLLED   SUNDAY

✤〜 *Lunch* 〜✤

LF = Low Fat   LSLF = Low Sodium, Low Fat

Meats

LSLF Baked chicken   LSLF Baked fish (cod)

Starchy Vegetables

LSLF Rice   LSLF Boiled potatoes

Vegetables

LSLF Baby carrots   LSLF Green beans

Soup/Salad/Juice	Dressings
LSLF Coleslaw	Diet French
LS Chicken broth	Diet Thousand Island
Apple juice	Diet Italian
Tossed salad	

Desserts

Pears	Fresh fruit

Breads

Dinner roll	Bran bread
White bread	LS Crackers
Whole wheat bread	

Beverages & Condiments

Coffee	Sugar
Decaf. coffee	Sugar substitute
Hot tea	Creamer
Decaf. hot tea	Lemon
Iced tea	Herb seasoning
Whole milk	Margarine
2% milk	Diet mustard
Fat-free milk	Diet mayonnaise
No salt	Diet catsup

Name _____   Room _____

RENAL   SUNDAY

✤〜 *Lunch* 〜✤

LF = Low Fat   LSLF = Low Sodium, Low Fat

Meats

LSLF Baked chicken   LSLF Baked fish

Starchy Vegetables

LSLF Rice   LSLF Dialyzed potatoes

Vegetables

LSLF Baby carrots   LSLF Green beans

Soup/Salad/Juice	Dressings
Lemonade	Diet French
LSLF Coleslaw	Diet Thousand Island
Tossed salad	Diet Italian
(no tomato)	

Desserts

Pears	Apple pie

Breads

Dinner roll	Bran bread
White bread	LS Crackers
Whole wheat bread	

Beverages & Condiments

Coffee	Sugar
Decaf. coffee	Sugar substitute
Hot tea	Creamer
Decaf. hot tea	Lemon
Iced tea	Margarine
	Diet mustard
	Mayonnaise
No salt	

Name _____   Room _____

Some hospitals do not offer selective menus. Instead, they may provide **nonselective menus** (menus with preselected food items) or menus that include some elements of both systems (**semiselective menus**). Nonselective menus have been gaining popularity in hospital foodservice because they simplify operations and may help to cut costs.

FOOD SAFETY

Each institution has protocols for handling food products based on the identification of potential hazards and critical control points in food preparation, usually referred to as **Hazard Analysis and Critical Control Points (HACCP).** Generally, a HACCP program addresses food handling, cooking, and storage procedures; cleaning and disinfecting of utensils, surfaces, and equipment; and staff sanitation issues. Personnel involved with preparing or delivering meals need to be aware of the specific HACCP systems at their facility.

nonselective menus: menus that do not allow choices and list only preselected food items.

semiselective menus: menus that combine aspects of both selective and nonselective menus.

Hazard Analysis and Critical Control Points (HACCP): systems of food or formula preparation that identify food safety hazards and critical control points during foodservice procedures; pronounced *hassip*.

Review Notes

- Hospital foodservice departments may accommodate the special needs of hundreds of patients daily. Diet manuals specify the foods to include or exclude in modified diets.
- Many hospitals provide selective menus from which patients can choose meals that are appropriate for their medical conditions.
- Foodservice departments must follow the specific HACCP protocols adopted by their institutions to ensure food safety.

Diet-Drug Interactions

When working with patients, nurses should be alert to possible interactions between drugs and dietary substances. These interactions can raise health care costs and result in serious, and sometimes fatal, complications. With hundreds of diet-drug interactions known and more to be identified in the future, nurses and other health professionals must learn to take steps to prevent or lessen their adverse consequences. Diet-drug interactions generally fall into the following categories:

- Drugs may alter food intake by reducing the appetite or by causing complications that make food consumption difficult or unpleasant. Other drugs may increase appetite and cause weight gain.
- Drugs may alter the absorption, metabolism, or excretion of nutrients. Conversely, nutrients and other food components may alter the absorption, metabolism, and excretion of drugs.
- Some interactions between dietary components and drugs can be toxic.

Examples of these types of diet-drug interactions are shown in Table 14-7. The remaining sections of this chapter describe some specific diet-drug interactions and their clinical significance.[5]

DRUG EFFECTS ON FOOD INTAKE

Some drugs can make food intake difficult or unpleasant: they may suppress the appetite, alter the sense of taste, induce nausea or vomiting, cause mouth dryness, or lead to inflammation or lesions in the mouth or GI tract. Certain side effects of drugs, including abdominal discomfort, constipation, and diarrhea, may be aggravated by food consumption. Medications that cause drowsiness, such as sedatives and some painkillers, can make a person too tired to eat.

Drug complications that reduce food intake are significant only when they continue for a long period. Although many drugs can cause nausea in some individuals, the nausea often subsides after the first few doses of the medication and therefore has little effect on nutrition status. If side effects persist, other medications may be prescribed to treat them; for example, antinauseants and antiemetics can help to reduce nausea and vomiting and thereby improve food intake.

Some medications stimulate food intake and encourage weight gain. Unintentional weight gain may result from the use of some antipsychotics, antidepressants, and corticosteroids (such as prednisone). People using these drugs may be unable to feel satiated and may gain 40 to 60 pounds in just a few months. For some conditions, however, weight gain is desirable. Patients with diseases that cause wasting, such as cancer or AIDS, are sometimes prescribed appetite enhancers such as megestrol acetate, a progesterone analog, or dronabinol, which is derived from the active ingredient in marijuana.

DRUG EFFECTS ON NUTRIENT ABSORPTION

The medications that most often cause widespread nutrient malabsorption are those that damage the intestinal mucosa. Antineoplastic and antiretroviral drugs (✚)are especially detrimental, although nonsteroidal anti-inflammatory drugs (NSAIDs) and some antibiotics can have similar, though milder, effects. This section describes additional ways in which medications may alter nutrient absorption.

Drug-Nutrient Binding Some medications bind to nutrients in the GI tract, preventing their absorption. For example, bile acid binders, which reduce blood cholesterol levels, may bind to fat-soluble vitamins. Some antibiotics, notably tetracycline and ciprofloxacin, bind to the calcium in foods and supplements, reducing the absorption of both the calcium and the antibiotic. Certain antibiotics can bind to other minerals, including iron, magnesium, and zinc. Consumers are advised to use dairy products and all mineral supplements at least two hours apart from these medications.

✚ *Antineoplastic drugs* combat tumor growth. *Antiretroviral drugs* treat HIV infection.

TABLE 14-7 | Examples of Diet-Drug Interactions

Drugs may alter food intake by:

- Altering the appetite (amphetamines suppress appetite; corticosteroids increase appetite).
- Interfering with taste or smell (amphetamines change taste perceptions).
- Inducing nausea or vomiting (digitalis may do both).
- Interfering with oral function (some antidepressants may cause dry mouth).
- Causing sores or inflammation in the mouth (methotrexate may cause painful mouth ulcers).

Drugs may alter nutrient absorption by:

- Changing the acidity of the digestive tract (antacids may interfere with iron and folate absorption).
- Damaging mucosal cells (cancer chemotherapy may damage mucosal cells).
- Binding to nutrients (bile acid binders bind to fat-soluble vitamins).

Foods and nutrients may alter drug absorption by:

- Stimulating the secretion of gastric acid (the antifungal agent ketoconazole is absorbed better with meals due to increased acid secretion).
- Altering the rate of gastric emptying (intestinal absorption of drugs may be delayed when they are taken with food).
- Binding to drugs (calcium binds to tetracycline, reducing the absorption of both substances).
- Competing for absorption sites in the intestine (dietary amino acids interfere with levodopa absorption).

Drugs and nutrients may interact and alter metabolism by:

- Acting as structural analogs (as do warfarin and vitamin K).
- Using similar enzyme systems (phenobarbital induces liver enzymes that increase the metabolism of folate, vitamin D, and vitamin K).
- Competing for transport on plasma proteins (fatty acids and drugs may compete for the same sites on the plasma protein albumin).

Drugs may alter nutrient excretion by:

- Altering nutrient reabsorption in the kidneys (some diuretics increase the excretion of sodium and potassium).
- Causing diarrhea or vomiting (diarrhea and vomiting may cause electrolyte losses).

Food substances may alter drug excretion by:

- Inducing the activities of liver enzymes that metabolize drugs, increasing drug excretion (components of charcoal-broiled meats increase the metabolism of warfarin, theophylline, and acetaminophen).

Food substances and drugs may interact and cause toxicity by:

- Increasing side effects of the drug (the caffeine in beverages can increase the adverse effects of stimulants).
- Increasing drug action to excessive levels (grapefruit components inhibit the enzymes that degrade certain drugs, increasing drug concentrations in the body).

Altered Stomach Acidity Medications that reduce stomach acidity can impair the absorption of vitamin B_{12}, folate, and iron. Examples include antacids, which neutralize stomach acid by acting as weak bases, and antiulcer drugs (such as proton pump inhibitors and H2 blockers), which interfere with acid secretion.

Direct Inhibition Several drugs impede nutrient absorption by interfering with their intestinal metabolism or transport into mucosal cells. For example, the antibiotics trimethoprim and pyrimethamine compete with folate for absorption into intestinal cells.

DIETARY EFFECTS ON DRUG ABSORPTION

Most drugs are absorbed in the upper small intestine. Major influences on drug absorption include the stomach-emptying rate, the level of acidity in the stomach, and direct interactions with dietary components. The drug's formulation may also influence its absorption. The instructions included with medications typically advise whether food should be included or avoided with use.

Stomach-Emptying Rate Drugs reach the small intestine more quickly when the stomach is empty. Therefore, taking a medication with meals may delay its absorption, although the total amount absorbed may not be lower. As an example, aspirin works faster when taken on an empty stomach, but taking it with food is often encouraged to reduce stomach irritation.

Slow stomach emptying can enhance drug absorption because the drug's absorption sites in the small intestine do not become saturated. However, a slower absorption rate (due to slow stomach emptying) can be a problem if high drug concentrations are needed for effectiveness, as when a hypnotic is taken to induce sleep.

Stomach Acidity Some drugs are better absorbed in an acidic environment, so conditions that are too alkaline may reduce their absorption. Hence, antacid medications may reduce the absorption of these drugs. Other drugs can be damaged by acid and are often available in coated forms that resist the stomach's acidity.

Binding between Food Components and Drugs Some dietary substances can bind to drugs and inhibit their absorption. For example, the phytates in foods can bind to digoxin, a drug prescribed for heart disease.(✚) High-fiber diets may decrease the absorption of some tricyclic antidepressants due to binding between the fiber and the drugs. As mentioned earlier, calcium can bind to some antibiotics, reducing absorption of both the calcium and the drug.

DRUG EFFECTS ON NUTRIENT METABOLISM

Drugs and nutrients use similar enzyme systems in the small intestine and liver. Consequently, some drugs may enhance or inhibit the activities of enzymes needed for nutrient metabolism. For example, the anticonvulsants phenobarbital and phenytoin increase levels of the liver enzymes that metabolize folate, vitamin D, and vitamin K; therefore, persons using these drugs may require supplements of these vitamins.

The drug methotrexate, used to treat cancer and inflammatory conditions, acts by interfering with folate metabolism and thus depriving rapidly dividing cancer cells of the folate they need to multiply. Methotrexate resembles folate in structure (see Figure 14-3) and competes with folate for the enzyme that converts folate to its active form. The adverse effects of using methotrexate therefore include symptoms of folate deficiency. These adverse effects can be reduced by using a preactivated form of folate (called leucovorin), which is often prescribed along with methotrexate to ensure that the body's rapidly dividing cells (such as cells of the digestive tract, skin cells, and red blood cells) receive adequate folate.

Isoniazid (INH) is an antituberculosis drug similar in structure to vitamin B_6. The drug can interfere with both the vitamin's activation and its normal functioning.[6] Because INH must be taken for at least six months to treat infection, vitamin B_6 supplements are often given simultaneously to prevent deficiency.

Corticosteroids, used as anti-inflammatory agents and immunosuppressants, have actions that mimic those of the hormone cortisol. Long-term(✚) corticosteroid use can have broad effects on nutritional health and may cause weight gain, muscle wasting, bone loss, and hyperglycemia, with eventual development of osteoporosis and diabetes.

Tetra Images/Jupiter Images

Because nurses interact closely with patients, they are often responsible for educating patients about potential diet-drug interactions.

✚ Reminder: *Phytates* are compounds found in many plant foods, including whole grains and legumes. Phytates can bind to minerals and other substances and reduce their absorption.

✚ Cortisol is a steroid hormone secreted by the adrenal cortex as part of the body's stress response.

FIGURE 14-3 Folate and Methotrexate

By competing for the enzyme that activates folate, methotrexate prevents cancer cells from obtaining the folate they need to multiply. In the process, normal cells are also deprived of the folate they need.

DIETARY EFFECTS ON DRUG METABOLISM

Some food components alter the activities of enzymes that metabolize drugs or may counteract drug effects in other ways. Compounds in grapefruit juice (and whole grapefruit) have been found to inhibit or inactivate enzymes that metabolize a number of different drugs. As a result of the reduced enzyme action, blood concentrations of the drugs increase, leading to stronger physiological effects. The effect of the grapefruit juice lasts for a substantial period after the juice is consumed; for example, in experiments with a drug prescribed for heart disease, the juice's effect had an estimated half-life of 12 hours.[7](✚) Table 14-8 provides examples of drugs that interact with grapefruit juice, as well as some common drugs that are unaffected.

A number of dietary substances can alter the activity of the anticoagulant drug warfarin. The most important interaction is with vitamin K, which is structurally similar to warfarin. Warfarin acts by blocking the enzyme that activates vitamin K, thereby preventing the synthesis of blood-clotting factors.(✚) The amount of warfarin prescribed is dependent, in part, on how much vitamin K is in the diet. If vitamin K consumption from foods or supplements increases substantially, it can weaken the effect of the drug. Individuals using warfarin are advised to consume similar amounts of vitamin K daily to keep warfarin activity stable. The dietary sources highest in vitamin K are green leafy vegetables.

Several popular herbs contain natural compounds that may enhance the activity of warfarin and therefore should be avoided during warfarin treatment. These herbs include St. John's wort, garlic, ginseng, dong quai, danshen, and others.[8]

DRUG EFFECTS ON NUTRIENT EXCRETION

Drugs that enhance urinary excretion may reduce nutrient reabsorption in the kidneys and consequently cause greater urinary losses of the nutrients.(✚) For example, some diuretics can increase the excretion of calcium, potassium, magnesium, and thiamin, and dietary supplements may be necessary to avoid deficiency. Risk of nutrient depletion is higher if multiple drugs with the same effect are used, if kidney function is impaired, or if the medications are used for a long time. Note that some diuretics can cause certain minerals to be retained, rather than excreted.[9]

DIETARY EFFECTS ON DRUG EXCRETION

Inadequate excretion of medications can cause toxicity, whereas excessive losses may reduce the amount available for therapeutic effect. Some food components affect drug excretion by altering the amount reabsorbed in the kidneys. For example, the amount of the medication lithium(✚) reabsorbed in the kidneys is similar to the amount of

✚ Reminder: The term *half-life* can be used to define the time period of a chemical effect. If the grapefruit effect has a 12-hour half-life, this means that, after 12 hours, its biological effect is half of the maximum effect measured.

✚ Reminder: Vitamin K is required for the synthesis of prothrombin and several other blood-clotting proteins.

✚ When the kidneys reabsorb a substance, they retain it in the blood. Substances that are not reabsorbed are excreted in urine.

✚ Lithium is used to prevent mood swings in patients with bipolar disorder.

TABLE 14-8 | Examples of Grapefruit Juice–Drug Interactions

Drug Category	Drugs Affected by Grapefruit Juice	Drugs Unaffected by Grapefruit Juice
Cardiovascular drugs	Amiodarone Felodipine Nicardipine	Amlodipine Digoxin Diltiazem
Cholesterol-lowering drugs	Atorvastatin Lovastatin Simvastatin	Fluvastatin Pravastatin Rosuvastatin
Central nervous system drugs	Buspirone Carbamazepine Diazepam	Alprazolam Haloperidol Lorazepam
Anti-infective drugs	Erythromycin Saquinavir	Clarithromycin Quinine
Estrogens	Ethinylestradiol	17-β-estradiol
Anticoagulants	—	Acenocoumarol Warfarin
Immunosuppressants	Cyclosporine Tacrolimus	Prednisone

sodium that is reabsorbed. Thus, both sodium depletion and dehydration, which increase sodium reabsorption, can result in lithium retention. Similarly, a person with a high sodium intake will excrete more sodium in the urine and, therefore, more lithium. Individuals using lithium are advised to maintain a consistent sodium intake from day to day to maintain a stable blood level of lithium.[10]

Urine acidity can affect drug excretion due to the effects of pH on a compound's ionic (chemical) form. The medication quinidine, used to treat arrhythmias, is excreted more readily in acidic urine. Foods or drugs that cause urine to become more alkaline may reduce quinidine excretion and raise blood levels of the medication.

DIET-DRUG INTERACTIONS AND TOXICITY

Interactions between food components and drugs can cause toxicity or exacerbate a drug's side effects. The combination of tyramine, a food component, and monoamine oxidase (MAO) inhibitors, which include some antidepressants and a medication that treats Parkinson's disease, can be fatal. MAO inhibitors block an enzyme that normally inactivates tyramine, as well as the hormones epinephrine and norepinephrine. When people who take MAO inhibitors consume excessive tyramine, the increased tyramine in the blood can induce a sudden release of stored norepinephrine. This surge in norepinephrine results in severe headaches, rapid heartbeat, and a dangerous rise in blood pressure. For this reason, people taking MAO inhibitors are advised to restrict their intakes of foods rich in tyramine.

Tyramine occurs naturally in foods and is also formed when bacteria degrade the protein in foods. Thus, the tyramine content of a food usually increases when a food ages or spoils. Individuals at risk of tyramine toxicity are advised to buy mainly fresh foods and consume them promptly.[11] Foods that often contain substantial amounts of tyramine are listed in Table 14-9.

| TABLE 14-9 | Examples of Foods with a High Tyramine Content[a] |

- Aged cheeses (cheddar, Gruyère)
- Aged or cured meats (sausage, salami)
- Beer
- Fermented vegetables (sauerkraut, kim chee)
- Fish, smoked or pickled
- Mushrooms
- Prepared soy foods (miso, tempeh, tofu)
- Soy sauce
- Wine (red)
- Yeast extract (Marmite, Vegemite)

[a] The tyramine content of foods depends on storage conditions and processing; thus, the amounts in similar products can vary substantially.

Considering the number of medications available and the many ways in which drugs and dietary substances can interact, it is not surprising that serious side effects are increasingly being recognized. Nurses and other health professionals should attempt to understand the mechanisms of diet-drug interactions, identify them when they occur, and prevent them whenever possible. The accompanying "How to" offers some practical advice about preventing diet-drug interactions.

Review Notes

- Medications can alter food intake and affect the absorption, metabolism, and excretion of nutrients. Components of foods can similarly affect the absorption, metabolism, and excretion of medications.
- Drugs can alter food intake by reducing appetite, altering the sense of taste, causing GI discomfort, or damaging the lining of the GI tract.
- Drugs can affect nutrient absorption by binding to nutrients, changing stomach acidity, or interfering with nutrient transport into intestinal cells. Dietary substances can influence drug absorption by altering the stomach emptying rate, changing stomach acidity, or directly binding to drugs.
- Drugs and nutrients may interfere with each other's metabolism because they use similar enzymes in the small intestine and liver.
- Diet-drug interactions may cause nutrient losses in urine and alter the urinary excretion of drugs. Some interactions between food components and drugs may result in toxicity.

HOW TO | Prevent Diet-Drug Interactions

The Joint Commission, an accreditation agency for health care organizations, has recommended that all patients be educated about potential diet-drug interactions. Nurses can help by informing patients of precautions related to medications and watching for signs of problems that may arise.

To prevent diet-drug interactions, first list the types and amounts of over-the-counter drugs, prescription medications, and dietary supplements that the patient uses on a regular basis. Look up each medication in a drug reference and make a note of:

- The appropriate method of administration (twice daily or at bedtime, for example).
- How the medication should be administered with respect to foods, beverages, and specific nutrients (for example, take on an empty stomach, take with food, do not take with milk, or do not drink alcoholic beverages while using the medication).
- How the medication should be used with respect to other medications.
- The side effects that may influence food intake (nausea and vomiting, diarrhea, constipation, or sedation, for example) or nutrient needs (interference with nutrient absorption or metabolism, for example).

A similar process can be used to review the dietary supplements that a person is taking. A reliable reference may list their appropriate uses, possible side effects, and potential interactions with food and medications.

Patients who take multiple medications may need to time their medications carefully to avoid drug-drug or diet-drug interactions. The nurse can use information from a patient's food and nutrition history (see Chapter 13) to help the patient coordinate meals and drugs so as to avoid interactions.

Some medications have well-known effects on nutritional status. The nurse should remain alert for signs of problems, especially when:

- Nutritional problems are a frequent result of using the medication.
- A patient uses multiple medications.
- The patient is in a high-risk group; for example, a child, a pregnant or lactating woman, an older adult, or a person who is malnourished, abuses alcohol, or has impaired liver or kidney function.
- The patient needs to use the medication for a long period of time.

Check with the pharmacist for additional information about medications and potential interactions.

Self Check

1 • A successful nutrition intervention would include a long list of:
   a. dietary changes that the patient should consider making.
   b. foods that the patient should avoid.
   c. appetizing meals and foods that the patient can include in the diet.
   d. reasons why the patient should make dietary changes.

2 • The most important factor(s) that affect(s) how nutrition education is presented is (are):
   a. the person's nutrient needs and nutrition status.
   b. the person's abilities and motivation.
   c. the person's medical history.
   d. the entries in the medical record.

3 • Mechanically altered diets are often prescribed for individuals with:
   a. disorders of the liver, gallbladder, and pancreas.
   b. unusually high kcalorie and protein requirements.
   c. chewing and swallowing difficulties.
   d. malabsorptive disorders.

4 • The modified diet *least* likely to provide adequate nutrients and kcalories is the:
   a. blenderized diet.
   b. clear liquid diet.
   c. ground/minced diet.
   d. high-kcalorie, high-protein diet.

5 • Fiber restriction may be recommended:
   a. for patients with dysphagia.
   b. for patients who are unable to absorb fat normally.
   c. for patients with heartburn.
   d. during the acute phases of some intestinal disorders.

6 • A nurse notices a food on a patient's tray and is not sure if the food is allowed on the patient's particular type of diet. An appropriate action for the nurse to take would be to check the:
   a. diet manual.
   b. nutrition care plan.
   c. nutrition prescription.
   d. medical record.

7 • Factors that typically interfere with drug absorption include:
   a. binding between drugs and food components.
   b. use of antacid therapies.
   c. a rapid stomach-emptying rate.
   d. all of the above.

8 • Compounds in grapefruit juice:
   a. bind to antibiotics, reducing absorption.
   b. cause excessive drug excretion.
   c. strengthen the effects of certain drugs.
   d. alter acidity in the stomach, impairing drug absorption.

9 • Vitamin K consumption should be consistent in patients using:
   a. tetracycline.
   b. isoniazid.
   c. lithium.
   d. warfarin.

10 • People who use MAO inhibiters must limit consumption of:
   a. aged cheeses.
   b. whole milk and yogurt.
   c. dark green leafy vegetables.
   d. grapefruit juice.

Answers to these questions appear in Appendix H.

Clinical Applications

1 • David is a 49-year-old male who is 6 feet 2 inches tall and has a usual body weight of 180 pounds. He was admitted to the hospital following an automobile accident and was treated for minor injuries. Using the method described in the "How to" on p. 411, estimate his energy requirement using the Mifflin–St. Jeor equation and the stress factor 1.25.

2 • A hospital patient with a dysphagia problem has been receiving a mechanical soft diet. You notice that she coughs repeatedly while eating meals and eats only small portions of the foods on her plate. You suspect that the diet is inappropriate and that she may need a more restrictive dysphagia diet, but her medical chart doesn't specify the severity of the dysphagia.
   • To address these problems in your nursing care plan, which health professionals would you need to consult, and what information would you require from each of them?

- The next meal is due within the hour, and you suspect the woman will be intolerant to the foods she is scheduled to receive. You haven't yet heard from the health practitioners you consulted while developing your care plan. What options might you consider in handling this immediate problem?

3 • An elderly man in a residential home has been losing weight since his arrival there. He has been taking several medications to treat both a heart problem and a mild case of bronchitis. You notice that he eats only a few bites at mealtimes and seems uninterested in food. Describe several steps you can take to learn whether the medications are interfering with his food intake in some way.

Nutrition on the Net

For further study of topics covered in this chapter, access these websites.

- Find updates and quick links to these and other nutrition-related sites at our website: www.cengage.com/nutrition/whitney/nhhc4e
- Visit the website of the American Dietetic Association to learn more about nutrition services in clinical care: www.eatright.org
- Design patient education materials with information from the Medline Plus website: www.nlm.nih.gov/medlineplus/

- This Food and Drug Administration website discusses issues of clinical interest and is targeted to health professionals: www.fda.gov/ForHealthProfessionals/default.htm
- Visit the home page of the U.S. Food and Drug Administration (FDA), the agency that regulates all drugs in the United States: www.fda.gov
- The FDA provides safety information about drugs and other medical products on the MedWatch website: www.fda.gov/medwatch

Notes

1. K. Glanz, Current theoretical bases for nutrition intervention and their uses, in A. M. Coulston and C. J. Boushey, eds., *Nutrition in the Prevention and Treatment of Disease* (Burlington, MA: Elsevier Academic Press, 2008), pp. 127–138.
2. L. M. Delahanty and J. M. Heins, Tools and techniques to facilitate nutrition intervention, in A. M. Coulston and C. J. Boushey, eds., *Nutrition in the Prevention and Treatment of Disease* (Burlington, MA: Elsevier Academic Press, 2008), pp. 149–167.
3. J. Boullata and coauthors, Accurate determination of energy needs in hospitalized patients, *Journal of the American Dietetic Association* 107 (2007): 393–401.
4. American Dietetic Association, *Nutrition Care Manual* (Chicago: American Dietetic Association, 2009).
5. L.-N. Chan, Drug-nutrient interactions, in M. E. Shils and coeditors, *Modern Nutrition in Health and Disease* (Baltimore: Lippincott Williams & Wilkins, 2006), pp. 1539–1553.
6. P. Preziosi, Isoniazid: Metabolic aspects and toxicological correlates, *Current Drug Metabolism* 8 (2007): 839–851.
7. D. G. Bailey, Grapefruit juice–drug interaction issues, in J. I. Boullata and V. T. Armenti, eds., *Handbook of Drug-Nutrient Interactions* (Totowa, NJ: Humana Press, 2004), pp. 175–194.
8. M. L. Chavez, M. A. Jordan, and P. I. Chavez, Evidence-based drug–herbal interactions, *Life Sciences* 78 (2006): 2146–2157.
9. S. A. Shapses, Y. R. Schlussel, and M. Cifuentes, Drug-nutrient interactions that impact mineral status, in J. I. Boullata and V. T. Armenti, eds., *Handbook of Drug-Nutrient Interactions* (Totowa, NJ: Humana Press, 2004), pp. 301–328; B. J. McCabe, E. H. Frankel, and J. J. Wolfe, Monitoring nutritional status in drug regimens, in B. J. McCabe, E. H. Frankel, and J. J. Wolfe, eds., *Handbook of Food-Drug Interactions* (Boca Raton, FL: CRC Press, 2003), pp. 73–108.
10. McCabe, Frankel, and Wolfe, 2003.
11. W. Marcason, What is the bottom line for dietary guidelines when taking monoamine oxidase inhibitors? *Journal of the American Dietetic Association* 105 (2005): 163.

Complementary and Alternative Therapies

The medical treatments described in the clinical chapters are based on current scientific understanding of human physiology and biochemistry and are generally supported by well-conducted clinical research. This Nutrition in Practice examines therapies that have *not* been scientifically validated and are therefore not currently accepted by conventional medical professionals; these therapies fall into a category called *complementary and alternative medicine (CAM)*. When the therapies are used together with conventional medicine, they are called *complementary*; when used in place of conventional medicine, they are called *alternative*.[1] Note that the term "alternative" may be misleading because it inappropriately implies that unproven methods of treatment are valid alternatives to conventional treatments.

How popular is CAM in the United States?

An estimated 38 percent of adults in the United States use some form of CAM (excluding the use of prayer).[2] CAM is most prevalent among people with chronic, debilitating diseases; for example, 84 percent of AIDS patients reportedly use CAM.[3] Many patients use CAM as an adjunct to conventional medicine—often for symptoms or illnesses that are not sufficiently helped by conventional treatments. CAM therapies remain popular despite the dearth of evidence demonstrating their effectiveness. Reasons for their popularity include consumers' growing interest in self-help measures, the noninvasive nature of many CAM therapies, and the positive interactions consumers have with CAM practitioners.[4]

In response to the enormous popularity of CAM in the United States, in 1998 Congress established the National Center for Complementary and Alternative Medicine (NCCAM), which is now one of the 27 institutes that make up the National Institutes of Health (NIH). The missions of NCCAM are to investigate complementary and alternative therapies by funding well-designed scientific studies and to provide authoritative information for consumers and health professionals. If enough evidence is found to support the use of a complementary or alternative therapy, it will likely become a treatment regularly offered by conventional health practitioners.[5]

Why should mainstream health professionals learn more about CAM?

Due to the enormous consumer interest in trying novel treatments, health professionals need to be familiar with CAM therapies so that they can better communicate with patients regarding their medical care and advise them when an alternative approach conflicts with standard therapy or presents a danger to health. To provide medical students with objective information about CAM, about half of the medical schools in the United States offer elective courses about alternative forms of treatment.[6] Physicians who practice *integrative medicine* may refer patients for complementary therapies while continuing to provide standard treatments.

What kinds of practices are considered CAM therapies?

CAM encompasses any and all therapies that are not normally part of conventional medicine. Consequently, the list of CAM approaches includes hundreds of advertised therapies purchased and used by consumers. Unfortunately, CAM has become a marketing buzzword and is used by unscrupulous sellers of worthless treatments. The NCCAM has classified CAM therapies as shown in Table NP14-1 and defined in the Glossary of Alternative Therapies on p. 433. Several popular examples are described in this highlight. Other examples are discussed on the NCCAM website (**http://nccam.nih.gov/health**).

In what ways do alternative medical systems differ from conventional medicine?

Alternative medical systems are based on beliefs that lack the scientific basis of the theories underlying conventional medicine. Virtually all of these alternative systems were developed well over 100 years ago, before our bodies' biochemical and physiological processes were well understood. The alternative forms of diagnoses and treatments may appeal to consumers because the interventions are nontechnical and seem nonthreatening. In general, however, the alternative theories and practices remain rooted in the past and have not been updated to include our current knowledge. Examples of alternative medical systems include the following:

- **Naturopathic medicine** proposes that a person's natural "life force" can foster self-healing. This life force is allegedly stimulated by certain health-promoting factors and

TABLE NP14-1	Examples of Complementary and Alternative Medicine

Alternative Medical Systems

- Naturopathic medicine
- Homeopathic medicine
- Traditional Chinese medicine
- Ayurveda

Mind-Body Interventions

- Meditation
- Faith healing (prayer)
- Mental healing (including hypnotherapy)
- Music, art, and dance therapy

Biologically Based Therapies

- Dietary supplements
- Foods and special diets
- Herbal products
- Hormones
- Aromatherapy

Manipulative and Body-Based Methods

- Chiropractic
- Massage therapy
- Osteopathic manipulation
- Reflexology

Energy Therapies

- Biofield therapies (including therapeutic touch, acupuncture, and qi gong)
- Bioelectrical therapies (including electrical and magnetic fields)

suppressed by excesses and deficiencies. Naturopaths believe that ill health results from an internal disruption rather than from external disease-causing agents. Naturopathic therapies aim to enhance the natural healing powers of the body and may include special diets or fasting, herbal remedies and other dietary supplements, acupuncture, homeopathy, massage, and various other interventions.

- **Homeopathic medicine** is based on the dubious theory that "like cures like." Homeopaths believe that a substance that causes a particular set of symptoms can be used to cure a disease that has similar symptoms. Homeopathic medicines are usually natural substances that are substantially diluted in the belief that dilution increases potency, and most remedies are so extremely diluted that the original substance is no longer present. Homeopaths theorize that even though their remedies no longer

contain a diluted substance, they still have powerful healing effects because the water structure is somehow altered during the dilution process used to prepare homeopathic medicines. This theory, however, conflicts with scientific understanding of water structure and properties.

- **Traditional Chinese medicine (TCM)** includes a large number of folk practices that originated in China. TCM is based on the theory that the body has pathways (called *meridians*) that conduct energy (called *qi*; pronounced "chee"). The interrupted flow of qi is believed to cause illness. TCM practices allegedly improve the flow of qi and include acupuncture, qi gong, herbal remedies, dietary practices, and massage. Ironically, TCM is used by relatively few in the Chinese population, as Chinese physicians have largely adopted the Western approach to managing illness.[7]

What is the theory underlying mind-body interventions?

Mind-body interventions attempt to improve a person's sense of psychological or spiritual well-being despite the presence of illness. The treatments are also used in the hope of reducing stress, dealing with pain, or lowering blood pressure. Some of these therapies have been incorporated into mainstream medicine for stress reduction or relaxation. For example, **biofeedback** training, in which individuals learn to monitor skin temperature, muscle tension, or brain wave activity while practicing relaxation techniques, is frequently taught by behavioral medicine specialists to help patients reduce stress or anxiety. Other techniques to reduce stress and promote relaxation include **meditation,** art and music therapy, and prayer.

The clinical applications of other mind-body therapies are far more questionable. An example is guided **imagery,** in which a person tries to reverse the disease process (for example, shrink a tumor) by using mental pictures. Another

© Cindy Charles/PhotoEdit

Biofeedback training is a stress reduction and relaxation technique.

Nutrition Intervention and Diet-Drug Interactions

example is the use of **faith healing** in place of proven conventional treatments to cure disease.

What are some examples of biologically based therapies?

Biological therapies involve the use of natural products, such as dietary supplements, herbal and plant extracts, and special foods. The most common of these treatments include the use of vitamin and mineral supplements (discussed in Nutrition in Practice 9) and herbal products. Table NP14-2 lists examples of popular herbs, their common uses, and potential adverse effects associated with their use.

How effective are herbal remedies in the treatment of disease?

Herbs contain naturally occurring compounds that can exert physiological effects, and they have been used for centuries to treat a variety of medical conditions. Despite their popularity, however, the benefits of their use are uncertain. Few herbal products have been rigorously tested, many make unfounded claims, and some contain contaminants or produce toxic effects.[8] Only a limited number of clinical studies support the traditional uses, and the results of studies that suggest little or no benefit are rarely publicized by the supplement industry. The NCCAM is currently funding large, controlled trials of several popular herbal treatments in an effort to obtain reliable efficacy and safety data.

Determining the effectiveness of herbal remedies can be complicated. Herbs contain numerous compounds, and it is often unclear which of these ingredients, if any, might produce the implied beneficial effects. Because the compounds in herbs vary among species and are affected by a plant's growing conditions, different samples of an herb can have different chemical compositions. Even when the active ingredients in an herbal product have been shown to be effective, the dosage suggested on the label may not provide the quantity of active ingredients found to be effective. For example, a consumer group (ConsumerLab. com) tested seven *Ginkgo biloba* products and found that four of the products, when consumed at the recommended dosage, lacked the amounts of the compounds indicated on their labels.[9] In a university study of echinacea preparations, 10 percent of the 59 products tested contained no measurable echinacea, and only 52 percent of the samples contained the variety of echinacea listed on the label.[10]

How safe are the herbal products that are available in the marketplace?

Consumers of herbal supplements often assume that because plants are "natural," herbal products must be harmless. Many herbal remedies have toxic effects, however. The most common adverse effects of herbs include diarrhea, nausea, and vomiting.[11] The popular herbs kava, chaparral, and comfrey have caused liver damage. The use of yohimbe (promoted for bodybuilding) has been linked to renal failure, seizures, and heart palpitations. Note that the adverse effects of herbs are seldom listed on supplement labels.

Unlike drugs, herbal products do not need FDA approval before they are marketed. According to the Dietary Supplement Health and Education Act (DSHEA) of 1994, the companies that produce or distribute dietary (including herbal) supplements are responsible for determining their safety, yet these companies are not required to provide any evidence or conduct safety studies. If a company receives reports of illness or injury related to the use of its products, it is not required to submit this information to the FDA. In addition, the FDA must show that a supplement is unsafe before it can take action to remove the product from the marketplace.

Contamination of herbal products is another safety concern. Some products have been found to contain lead and other toxic metals in excessive amounts.[12] Other contaminants frequently found in herbal products include molds, bacteria, and pesticides that have been banned for use on food crops.[13] Adulteration of imported products has been a serious concern: several studies found that some herbal products imported from China and India contained synthetic drugs that were not declared on the label.[14] There have also been reports of serious illnesses and fatalities occurring from the intentional or accidental substitutions of one plant species for another.[15]

Is there any risk that herbs may interact with medications like other dietary substances do?

Yes. Like drugs, herbs may either intensify or interfere with the effects of other herbs and drugs, or they may raise the risk of toxicity. For example, garlic, ginkgo, and ginseng may increase the risk of bleeding when used with anticoagulant drugs.[16] St. John's wort has been found to inhibit the actions of oral contraceptives, anticoagulants, and other drugs. Ginseng contains compounds that raise blood pressure and may increase the toxicity of drugs that have the same side effect. Unfortunately, information about herb-drug interactions is limited, and much of what is known has been obtained from case studies rather than from controlled clinical trials. Table NP14-3 provides examples of herb-drug interactions.

Aside from herbal products, have other types of dietary supplements been found to be effective therapies?

As with herbal products, the efficacy and safety of other types of dietary supplements are uncertain. Remember that

TABLE NP14-2 | Popular Herbs, Their Common Uses, and Adverse Effects

Herb	Scientific Name	Common Uses	Adverse Effects
Black cohosh	*Cimicifuga racemosa*	Relief of menopausal symptoms	Rare; occasional stomach upset, headache, weight gain
Chaparral	*Larrea tridentata*	General tonic, treatment of infection, cancer, and arthritis	Hepatitis, liver failure
Comfrey	*Symphytum officinale*	Wound healing (topical use), treatment of lung and GI disorders	Liver damage
Echinacea	*Echinacea augustifolia, E. pallida, E. purpurea*	Prevention and treatment of upper respiratory infections	Rare; occasional allergic reactions
Feverfew	*Tanacetum parthenium*	Prevention of migraine headache	Mouth and tongue sores, swelling of lips, GI upset
Garlic	*Allium sativum*	Reduction of blood clotting, atherosclerosis, blood pressure, and blood cholesterol	Bad breath, body odor; occasional dyspepsia, flatulence, excessive bleeding, anorexia, allergic reactions
Ginger	*Zingiber officinale*	Prevention and treatment of nausea and motion sickness	Rare; occasional heartburn
Ginkgo	*Ginkgo biloba*	Treatment of dementia, memory defects, and circulatory impairment	Rare; occasional stomach upset, headache, skin hypersensitivity, excessive bleeding
Ginseng	*Panax ginseng, P. quinquefolius*	General tonic, reduction of blood glucose levels	Rare
Kava kava	*Piper methysticum*	Treatment of anxiety, stress, and insomnia	Dyspepsia, restlessness, drowsiness, tremor, headache, dermatitis (with heavy use), occasional hepatitis and liver failure
St. John's wort	*Hypericum perforatum*	Treatment of mild to moderate depression	Rare; occasional stomach upset, fatigue, dizziness, headache, dry mouth, dermatitis, skin photosensitivity
Saw palmetto	*Serenoa repens*	Reduction of symptoms associated with enlarged prostate	Rare
Valerian	*Valeriana officinalis*	Sedation, treatment of insomnia	Rare
Yohimbe	*Pausinystalia yohimbe*	Treatment of erectile dysfunction	Anxiety, headache, dizziness, nausea, rapid heartbeat, hypertension, increased urinary frequency; isolated reports of renal failure, blood disorders, and airway constriction

TABLE NP14-3	Examples of Herb-Drug Interactions	
Herb	**Drugs**	**Interaction**
Echinacea	Immunosuppressant drugs	Suppresses drug effects
Feverfew	Anticoagulants, aspirin	Enhances drug effects
Garlic, ginkgo, ginseng	Anticoagulants, antiplatelet drugs	Increases risk of hemorrhaging
Kava kava	Acetaminophen, antifungal drugs, methotrexate, steroids	Increases risk of liver damage
St. John's wort	Various	Suppresses drug effects
Valerian	Antidepressants, antiepileptics, anesthetics, analgesics, barbiturates	May enhance drug effects, increase sedation

Source: J. A. Rindfleisch and B. Barrett, Herbs and other dietary supplements, in R. E. Rakel, ed., *Textbook of Family Medicine* (Philadelphia: Saunders, 2007), pp. 243–266.

manufacturers are free to market the supplements even if studies fail to show measurable health benefits, and the products are not regulated or tested for safety. Dietary supplements that are currently popular include the following:

- **Hormones.** Some hormones or hormone-like products derived from foods are considered dietary supplements and can be sold over the counter. One example is melatonin, a hormone made by the pineal gland and alleged to correct sleep disorders and prevent jet lag. Another example is the adrenal hormone dehydroepiandrosterone (DHEA), which is promoted to enhance immunity, increase muscle mass, improve memory, and defend against aging.
- **Glucosamine-chondroitin supplements.** The use of glucosamine and chondroitin supplements is an example of a CAM therapy that is being considered for adoption by mainstream medicine, depending on the outcome of studies of their safety and effectiveness. Glucosamine and chondroitin are produced in the body and help to maintain joint cartilage. Early studies suggested that glucosamine and chondroitin supplements reduced moderate to severe symptoms of osteoarthritis better than a placebo, prompting some physicians to suggest

using these supplements for pain relief.[17] Recent studies have cast doubt on the earlier findings, however, and several trials are still in progress.[18]

Is there any evidence supporting the use of various foods or supplements to cleanse or detoxify the body?

No; these practices are useless for the intended purpose. "Cleansing" practices are promoted based on the incorrect idea that the organs, blood, and intestines are "clogged" by toxins and undigested foods and that some types of dietary substances can rid the body of these accumulated toxins and wastes. Consumers who have little or no knowledge about physiology perceive this idea as plausible and are vulnerable to deceptive claims. A common scam is the sale of supplements or recipes for liver and gallbladder "flushes," which are said to cleanse the liver, remove gallstones, or improve medical conditions ranging from allergies to cancer.[19] In many instances, the ingested substances are partially or wholly indigestible and the individual using them passes semisolid materials that resemble gallstones to the untrained eye. Similarly, "colon cleanse" products are combinations of dietary substances such as clay and gelling fibers that cause the users to pass large fecal casts claimed to represent years of accumulated wastes; such wastes are alleged to cause an array of health problems. Note that there is no scientific support for the alleged benefits of products said to "flush" the liver, gallbladder, or colon.

Which alternative practices involve physical manipulation, and how do they work?

Manipulative interventions include physical touch, forceful movement of different parts of the body, and the application of pressure. Some practitioners maintain that special energy fields are also manipulated during the physical treatment and that proper energy flow induces healing. The most popular practices include the following:

- **Chiropractic** theory proposes that keeping the nervous system free from obstruction allows the body to heal itself, because the healing process stems from the brain and is conducted via the spinal cord and nerves to all parts of the body. Chiropractors claim to diagnose illnesses by detecting subluxations in the spine, which are variously described as misaligned vertebrae or pinched nerves that allegedly cause subtle interferences within the nervous system. The main treatment is the adjustment, a manual manipulation that is said to correct a subluxation and restore the body's natural healing ability. Although spinal manipulation has mainly been found to be helpful for improving back pain, many chiropractors still assert that chiropractic can cure disease rather than simply relieve symptoms.[20] For example, many chiropractors promote spinal manipulation to treat infectious diseases, prevent cancer, and regulate menstrual periods, even though the nervous system and spinal alignment do not play roles in the pathology of these conditions.

- **Massage therapy** is the manipulation of muscle and connective tissue to improve muscle function, reduce pain, or promote relaxation. Massage therapists may also apply heat or cold and give advice about exercises that may improve muscle tone and range of motion. Massage is often integrated into conventional physical therapy, although some massage therapists may incorrectly suggest that massage is a valid treatment for a wide range of medical conditions.

Acupuncture involves the shallow insertion of stainless steel needles into the skin, sometimes accompanied by a low-frequency current.

What are the alleged effects of "energy" therapies?

Two categories of therapies involve the alleged curative power of "energy":

- **Biofield therapies** are said to influence the energy that surrounds or pervades the human body, and their proponents claim that an energy therapy can strengthen or restore a person's "energy flow" and induce healing. Acupuncture, qi gong, and therapeutic touch are among the therapies that subscribe to these theories. Note that CAM adherents often use the term "energy" unscientifically and that there is no objective evidence of this sort of energy flow.
- **Bioelectrical** or **bioelectromagnetic therapies** use electric or magnetic fields to allegedly promote healing; for example, magnets have been marketed with claims that they can improve circulation, reduce inflammation, and speed recovery from injuries.

Acupuncture, a component of traditional Chinese medicine, is the most well known of the therapies involving "energy flow." Acupuncture is based on the theory that disease is caused by the disrupted flow of qi through the body, and the treatment allegedly corrects such disruptions and restores health. The practice involves the shallow insertion of stainless steel needles into the skin at designated points on the body, sometimes accompanied by a low-frequency current to produce greater stimulation.

Qi gong is another therapy originating in China that is said to improve the flow of qi within the body. Qi gong masters allegedly cure disease by releasing energy from their body and passing it to the person being treated. Self-help practices include deep breathing, certain types of physical exercise, and concentration and relaxation techniques.

Therapeutic touch is based on the premise that the "healing force" of a practitioner can be used to cure disease. Practitioners claim to identify and correct energy imbalances by passing their hands above a patient's body and transferring "excess energy" to the patient.

Do conventional health practitioners consider CAM treatments to be safe and effective?

As mentioned earlier, CAM treatments are generally excluded from mainstream medical practice because there is no evidence proving that they are effective for treating the diseases and medical conditions for which they are used. Many consumers think otherwise and seem satisfied that these treatments work. How is this dichotomy to be explained?

Surveys suggest that consumers perceive their visits to CAM therapists as far more pleasant than their visits to conventional health practitioners. As explained earlier, CAM therapists spend more time with patients, are more attentive, and use less invasive interventions.[21] Self-help measures are encouraged, so the consumer has more control over the treatment. The therapies appear to be more "natural" and to have fewer side effects. Possible explanations for "cures" include the following:

- A person may seem cured because of misdiagnosis; that is, the condition diagnosed by the CAM practitioner may not have actually existed.
- The condition may have been self-limiting, or it may have gone into temporary remission after the treatment.
- Undue credit may be inappropriately assigned to the CAM therapy when the improvement was actually due to a previous or concurrent conventional treatment.
- The placebo effect may have had an influence on the course of disease.

The central question remains: Do the CAM therapies merely make people *feel* better, or do they really *get* better? This question can be answered only by well-controlled research studies.

Nutrition Intervention and Diet-Drug Interactions

Are any potential dangers associated with the use of CAM?

One of the attractions of alternative therapies is the assumption that they are safe. Recall, however, the concerns associated with the use of herbal products, which include the potential toxicity of herbal ingredients, product contamination or adulteration, and interactions with conventional medications. Between 1990 and 1999, the FDA recalled more than 100 dietary supplements due to hazards associated with their use.[22]

Another concern is that use of CAM therapies may delay the use of reliable treatments that have demonstrable benefits.[23] Various reports have described people with treatable medical conditions who suffered permanent disability or death when they were misdiagnosed or improperly treated by CAM practitioners. For example, a rare but well-known risk of spinal cord injury or stroke is associated with a type of cervical manipulation performed by chiropractors.[24] Unfortunately, because most CAM therapies are not regulated or monitored, there are no accurate estimates of their adverse effects.

What should nurses do if they think their patients are using CAM?

Nurses should be aware when their patients are using CAM therapies that may have consequences influencing the course of a disease and its treatment. Accordingly, it is important to routinely inquire about the use of CAM therapies in a respectful, nonjudgmental manner and to educate patients about the hazards of postponing or stopping conventional treatment. Patients should also be told about potential interactions between conventional treatments and

Glossary of Alternative Therapies

acupuncture (AK-you-PUNK-chur): a therapy that involves inserting thin needles into the skin at specific anatomical points, allegedly to correct disruptions in the flow of energy within the body.

aromatherapy: inhalation of oil extracts from plants to cure illness or enhance health.

ayurveda: a traditional medical system from India that promotes the use of diet, herbs, meditation, massage, and yoga for preventing and treating illness.

bioelectrical or bioelectromagnetic therapies: therapies that involve the unconventional use of electric or magnetic fields to cure illness.

biofeedback: a technique in which individuals are trained to gain voluntary control of certain physiological processes, such as skin temperature or brain wave activity, to help reduce stress and anxiety.

biofield therapies: healing methods based on the belief that illnesses can be cured by manipulating energy fields that purportedly surround and penetrate the body. Examples include *acupuncture, qi gong,* and *therapeutic touch.*

chiropractic (KYE-roh-PRAK-tic): an alternative medical system based on the unproven theory that spinal manipulation can restore health.
- A *subluxation* is a misaligned vertebra or other spinal alteration that may cause illness.
- *Adjustment* is the manipulative therapy practiced by chiropractors.

faith healing: the use of prayer or belief in divine intervention to promote healing.

homeopathic (HO-mee-oh-PATH-ic) medicine: a practice based on the theory that "like cures like"; that is, substances believed to cause certain symptoms are prescribed for curing the same symptoms but are given in extremely diluted amounts.
- **homeo** = like
- **pathos** = suffering

hypnotherapy: a technique that uses hypnosis and the power of suggestion to improve health behaviors, relieve pain, and promote healing.

imagery: the use of mental images of things or events to aid relaxation or promote self-healing.

massage therapy: manual manipulation of muscles to reduce tension, increase blood circulation, improve joint mobility, and promote healing of injuries.

meditation: a self-directed technique of calming the mind and relaxing the body.

naturopathic (NAY-chur-oh-PATH-ic) medicine: an approach to medical care using practices alleged to enhance the body's natural healing abilities. Treatments may include a variety of alternative therapies including dietary supplements, herbal remedies, exercise, and homeopathy.

osteopathic (OS-tee-oh-PATH-ic) manipulation: a CAM technique performed by a doctor of osteopathy (D.O., or osteopath) that includes deep tissue massage and manipulation of the joints, spine, and soft tissues. A D.O. is a fully trained and licensed medical physician, although osteopathic manipulation has not been proved to be an effective treatment.

qi gong (chee-GUNG): a traditional Chinese practice that combines movement, meditation, and breathing techniques and allegedly cures illness by enhancing the flow of qi (energy) within the body.

reflexology: a technique that applies pressure or massage on areas of the hands or feet to allegedly cure disease or relieve pain in other areas of the body; sometimes called *zone therapy.*

therapeutic touch: a technique of passing hands over a patient to purportedly identify energy imbalances and transfer healing power from therapist to patient; also called *laying on of hands.*

traditional Chinese medicine (TCM): an approach to medical care based on the concept that illness can be cured by enhancing the flow of qi (energy) within a person's body. Treatments may include herbal therapies, physical exercises, meditation, acupuncture, and remedial massage.

CAM therapies. Some patients may want to learn about differences between evidence-based medical practices and untested CAM theories and may be interested in the integrative medicine options available.

All alternative therapies have one characteristic in common: their effectiveness is, for the most part, unproven.[25] As mentioned previously, patients often choose alternative therapies because of positive interactions with CAM practitioners. Thus, all health practitioners should realize that empathizing with patients may go a long way toward winning their trust and improving their compliance with therapy. In addition, health practitioners need to regularly use reliable, objective resources to update their knowledge about unconventional practices so that they can knowledgeably discuss these options with patients.

Notes

1. S. E. Straus, Complementary and alternative medicine, in L. Goldman and D. Ausiello, eds., *Cecil Medicine* (Philadelphia: Saunders, 2008), pp. 206–209.

2. P. M. Barnes, B. Bloom, and R. Nahin, Complementary and alternative medicine use among adults and children: United States, 2007, *CDC National Health Statistics Report* 12 (December 10, 2008): 1–24.

3. J. D. Berman and S. E. Straus, Implementing a research agenda for complementary and alternative medicine, *Annual Review of Medicine* 55 (2004): 239–254.

4. A. M. McCaffrey, G. F. Pugh, B. B. O'Connor, Understanding patient preference for integrative medical care: Results from patient focus groups, *Journal of General Internal Medicine* 22 (2007): 1500–1505; E. Ernst, The role of complementary and alternative medicine, *British Medical Journal* 321 (2000): 1133–1135.

5. Straus, 2008.

6. B. Barzansky, H. S. Jonas, and S. I. Etzel, Educational programs in U.S. medical schools, 1999–2000, *Journal of the American Medical Association* 284 (2000): 1114–1120.

7. D. Normile, The new face of Chinese medicine, *Science* 299 (2003): 188–190.

8. R. B. van Breemen, H. H. S. Fong, and N. R. Farnsworth, Ensuring the safety of botanical dietary supplements, *American Journal of Clinical Nutrition* 87 (2008): 509S–513S; J. J. Mucksavage and L.-N. Chan, Dietary supplement interactions with medication, in J. I. Boullata and V. T. Armenti, eds., *Handbook of Drug-Nutrient Interactions* (Totowa, NJ: Humana Press, 2004), pp. 217–233.

9. ConsumerLab.com, Product review: Supplements for memory and cognition enhancement (ginkgo, huperzine A, and acetyl-L-carnitine), available at **www.consumerlab.com**, posted April 27, 2009; site visited May 26, 2009.

10. C. M. Gilroy and coauthors, Echinacea and truth in labeling, *Archives of Internal Medicine* 163 (2003): 699–704.

11. C. H. Halsted, Dietary supplements and functional foods: 2 sides of a coin? *American Journal of Clinical Nutrition* 77 (2003): 1001S–1007S.

12. ConsumerLab.com, 2009.

13. V. H. Tournas, E. Katsoudas, and E. J. Miracco, Moulds, yeasts, and aerobic plate counts in ginseng supplements, *International Journal of Food Microbiology* 108 (2006): 178–181; K. S. Leung and coauthors, Systematic evaluation of organochlorine pesticide residues in Chinese materia medica, *Phytotherapy Research* 19 (2005): 514–518.

14. R. J. Ko, A U.S. perspective on the adverse reactions from traditional Chinese medicines, *Journal of the Chinese Medical Association* 67 (2004): 109–116; E. Ernst, Toxic heavy metals and undeclared drugs in Asian herbal medicines, *Trends in Pharmacological Sciences* 23 (2002): 136–139.

15. Breemen, Fong, and Farnsworth, 2008.

16. C. E. Dennehy and C. Tsourounis, Botanicals ("herbal medications") and nutritional supplements, in B. G. Katzung, ed., *Basic and Clinical Pharmacology* (New York: The McGraw-Hill Companies, Inc., 2007), pp. 1050–1062; J. A. Rindfleisch and B. Barrett, Herbs and other dietary supplements, in R. E. Rakel, ed., *Textbook of Family Medicine* (Philadelphia: Saunders, 2007), pp. 243–266.

17. O. Bruyere and J. Y. Reginster, Glucosamine and chondroitin sulfate as therapeutic agents for knee and hip osteoarthritis, *Drugs and Aging* 24 (2007): 573–580.

18. A. D. Sawitzke and coauthors, The effect of glucosamine and/or chondroitin sulfate on the progression of knee osteoarthritis: A report from the glucosamine/chondroitin arthritis intervention trial, *Arthritis and Rheumatism* 58 (2008): 3183–3191; R. M. Rozendaal and coauthors, Effect of glucosamine sulfate on hip osteoarthritis, *Annals of Internal Medicine* 148 (2008): 268–277; S. Reichenbach and coauthors, Meta-analysis: Chondroitin for osteoarthritis of the knee or hip, *Annals of Internal Medicine* 146 (2007): 580–590.

19. P. Moran, The truth about liver and gallbladder "flushes," available at **http://quackwatch.com/01QuackeryRelatedTopics/flushes.html,** posted March 9, 2007, site visited May 27, 2009; C. W. Sies and J. Brooker, Could these be gallstones? *Lancet* 365 (2005): 1388–1389.

20. J. C. Keating and coauthors, Subluxation: Dogma or science? *Chiropractic and Osteopathy* epub 10 August 2005 (DOI 10.1186/1746-1340-13-17).

21. McCaffrey, Pugh, and O'Connor, 2007.

22. Berman and Straus, 2004.

23. Straus, 2008.

24. W.-L. Chen and coauthors, Vertebral artery dissection and cerebellar infarction following chiropractic manipulation, *Emergency Medical Journal* 23 (2006): e1.doi:10.1136/emj.2004.015636; W. S. Smith and coauthors, Spinal manipulative therapy is an independent risk factor for vertebral artery dissection, *Neurology* 13 (2003):1424–1428; R. Dziewas and coauthors, Cervical artery dissection—Clinical features, risk factors, therapy and outcome in 126 patients, *Journal of Neurology* 250 (2003): 1179–1184.

25. Barnes, Bloom, and Nahin, 2008.

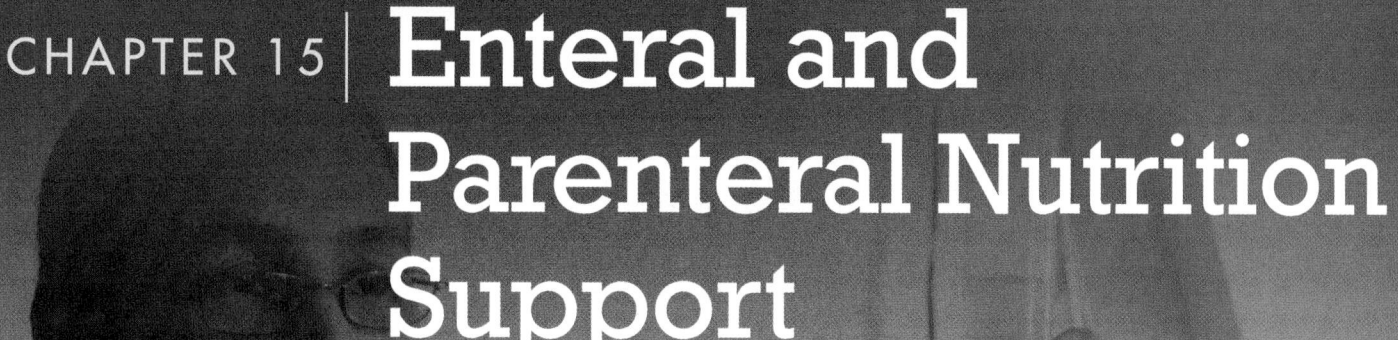

CHAPTER 15

Enteral and Parenteral Nutrition Support

© David Gee/ Alamy

CONTENTS

FIGURE
15-1 | Selecting a Feeding Route

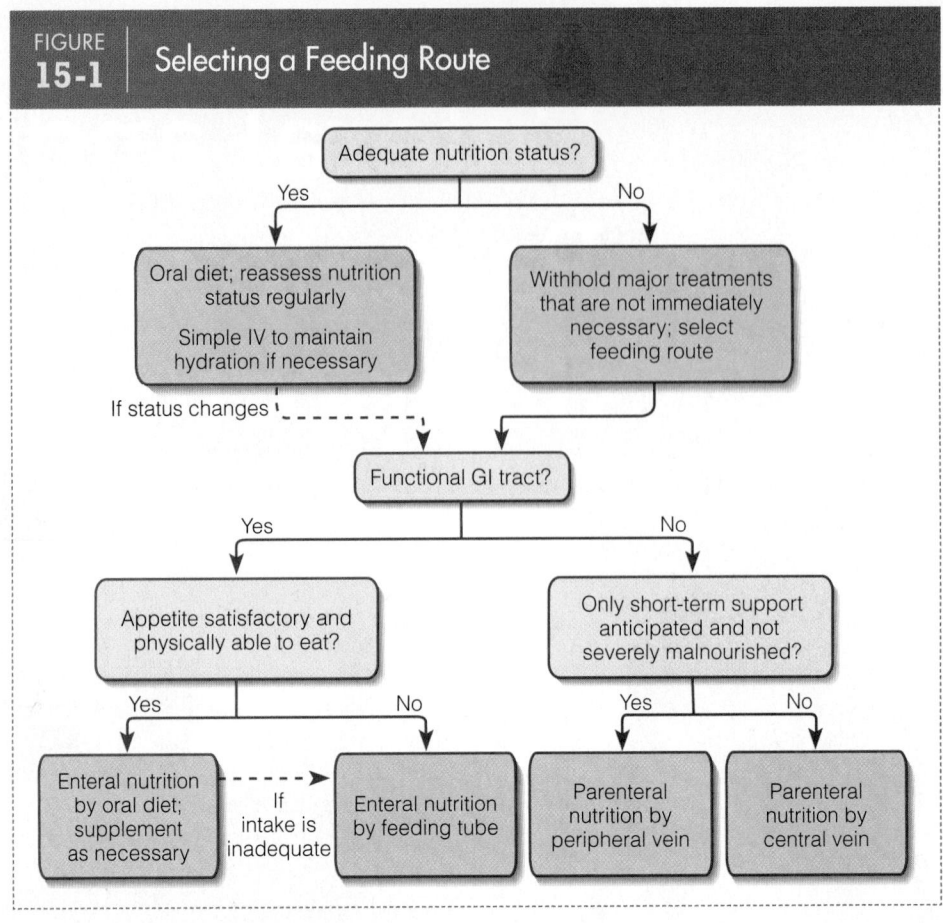

PATIENTS ARE OFTEN TOO SICK TO OBTAIN THE ENERGY AND NUTRIENTS they need by consuming foods. Moreover, some illnesses may interfere with eating, digestion, or absorption to such a degree that conventional foods cannot supply the necessary nutrients. In such cases, **nutrition support**—the delivery of nutrients using a feeding tube or intravenous infusions—can meet a patient's nutritional needs. **Enteral nutrition** provides nutrients using the gastrointestinal (GI) tract. Enteral nutrition includes oral diets or supplements but most often refers to the use of tube feedings, which supply nutrients directly to the stomach or intestine via a thin, flexible tube. **Parenteral nutrition** provides nutrients intravenously to patients who do not have adequate gastrointestinal function to handle enteral feedings. If the GI tract remains functional, enteral nutrition support is preferred, partly to avoid the expense and complications associated with intravenous infusions and partly to preserve healthy GI function. Figure 15-1 summarizes the decision-making process for selecting the most appropriate feeding method.

Enteral Nutrition Support

If gastrointestinal function is normal and a poor appetite is the primary nutrition problem, patients can drink enteral formulas to supplement their usual diet. If patients cannot consume enough food or drink enough formula to meet nutrient needs, tube feedings can be used to deliver the required nutrients.

ENTERAL FORMULAS

Most enteral formulas can supply all of an individual's nutrient requirements when consumed in sufficient volume, a necessity for the patient who is using a tube feeding or oral liquid diet for more than a few days. The formulas can be used alone or provided along with other foods.

nutrition support: the delivery of nutrients using a feeding tube or intravenous infusions.

enteral (EN-ter-al) nutrition: the provision of nutrients using the GI tract, including the use of tube feedings and oral diets.

parenteral (par-EN-ter-al) nutrition: the intravenous provision of nutrients that bypasses the GI tract.
- **par** = beside
- **entero** = intestine

Types of Enteral Formulas

More than 100 enteral formulas are currently marketed;[1] Appendix G lists examples. The main types of formulas include the following:

- **Standard formulas**, also called *polymeric formulas*, are provided to individuals who can digest and absorb nutrients without difficulty. They contain intact proteins extracted from milk or soybeans or a combination of **protein isolates** (proteins isolated from foods). The carbohydrate sources include modified starches, glucose polymers (such as maltodextrin), and sugars. A few formulas, called **blenderized formulas**, are made from whole foods and derive their protein primarily from pureed meat or poultry.
- **Elemental formulas**, also called *hydrolyzed*, *chemically defined*, or *monomeric formulas*, are prescribed for patients who have compromised digestive or absorptive functions. Elemental formulas contain proteins and carbohydrates that have been partially or fully broken down to fragments that require little (if any) digestion. The formulas are often low in fat or may provide fat from **medium-chain triglycerides (MCT)** to ease digestion and absorption.
- **Specialized formulas**, also called *disease-specific formulas*, are designed to meet the specific nutrient needs of patients with particular illnesses. Enteral products have been developed for individuals with liver, kidney, and lung diseases; glucose intolerance; and metabolic stress. Specialized formulas are generally expensive, and their effectiveness is controversial.
- **Modular formulas**, created from individual macronutrient (✚) preparations called *modules*, are prepared for patients who require specific nutrient combinations to treat their illnesses. Vitamin and mineral preparations are also included in these formulas so that they can meet all of a person's nutrient needs. In some cases, one or more modules may be added to other enteral formulas to adjust their nutrient composition.

Macronutrient Composition

The percentages of protein, carbohydrate, and fat vary substantially among enteral formulas. The protein content of most formulas ranges from 12 to 20 percent of total kcalories;[2] note that protein needs are high in patients with severe metabolic stress, whereas protein restrictions are necessary for patients with chronic kidney disease. Carbohydrate and fat provide most of the energy in enteral formulas; standard formulas generally provide 40 to 60 percent of kcalories from carbohydrate and 30 to 40 percent of kcalories from fat.

Energy Density

The energy density of enteral formulas ranges from 0.5 to 2.0 kcalories per milliliter of fluid. Standard formulas typically provide 1.0 to 1.2 kcalories per milliliter and are appropriate for patients with average fluid requirements. Formulas that have higher energy densities can meet energy and nutrient needs in a smaller volume of fluid and therefore benefit patients who have high nutrient needs or fluid restrictions. Individuals with high fluid needs can be given a formula with low energy density or be supplied with additional water via the feeding tube or intravenously.

Fiber Content

The fiber content may strongly influence the selection of an enteral formula. Fiber-containing formulas can be helpful for normalizing intestinal function, treating diarrhea or constipation, and maintaining blood glucose control. Conversely, fiber-containing formulas may be avoided in patients with acute intestinal conditions, pancreatitis, or procedures involving the intestines.

Osmolality

Osmolality refers to the moles of osmotically active solutes (or *osmoles*) per kilogram of solvent. (✚) An enteral formula with an osmolality similar to that of blood serum (about 300 milliosmoles per kilogram) is an **isotonic formula**, whereas a **hypertonic formula** has an osmolality greater than that of blood serum.

Most enteral formulas have osmolalities between 300 and 700 milliosmoles per kilogram; generally, hydrolyzed formulas and nutrient-dense formulas have higher osmolalities than standard formulas. Most people are able to tolerate both isotonic and hypertonic feedings without difficulty. When medications are infused along with enteral feedings, however, the osmotic load increases substantially and may contribute to the diarrhea experienced by many tube-fed patients.

✚ Reminder: The *macronutrients* are proteins, carbohydrates, and fats.

✚ Osmotically active solutes affect *osmosis*, the movement of water across semipermeable membranes.

standard formulas: enteral formulas that contain mostly intact proteins and polysaccharides; also called *polymeric formulas*.

protein isolates: proteins that have been isolated from foods.

blenderized formulas: enteral formulas that are prepared by using a food blender to mix and puree whole foods.

elemental formulas: enteral formulas that contain carbohydrates and proteins that are partially or fully hydrolyzed; also called *hydrolyzed, chemically defined,* or *monomeric formulas.*

medium-chain triglycerides (MCT): triglycerides that contain fatty acids that are 8 to 10 carbons in length. MCT do not require digestion and can be absorbed in the absence of lipase or bile.

specialized formulas: enteral formulas designed to meet the nutrient needs of patients with specific illnesses; also called *disease-specific formulas.*

modular formulas: enteral formulas prepared in the hospital from *modules* that contain single macronutrients; used for people with unique nutrient needs.

osmolality (OZ-moe-LAL-ih-tee): the concentration of osmotically active solutes in a solution, expressed as milliosmoles (mOsm) per kilogram of solvent.

isotonic formula: a formula with an osmolality similar to that of blood serum (about 300 milliosmoles per kilogram).

- **iso** = equal
- **tono** = pressure

hypertonic formula: a formula with an osmolality greater than that of blood serum.

FIGURE
15-2 | Selecting a Formula

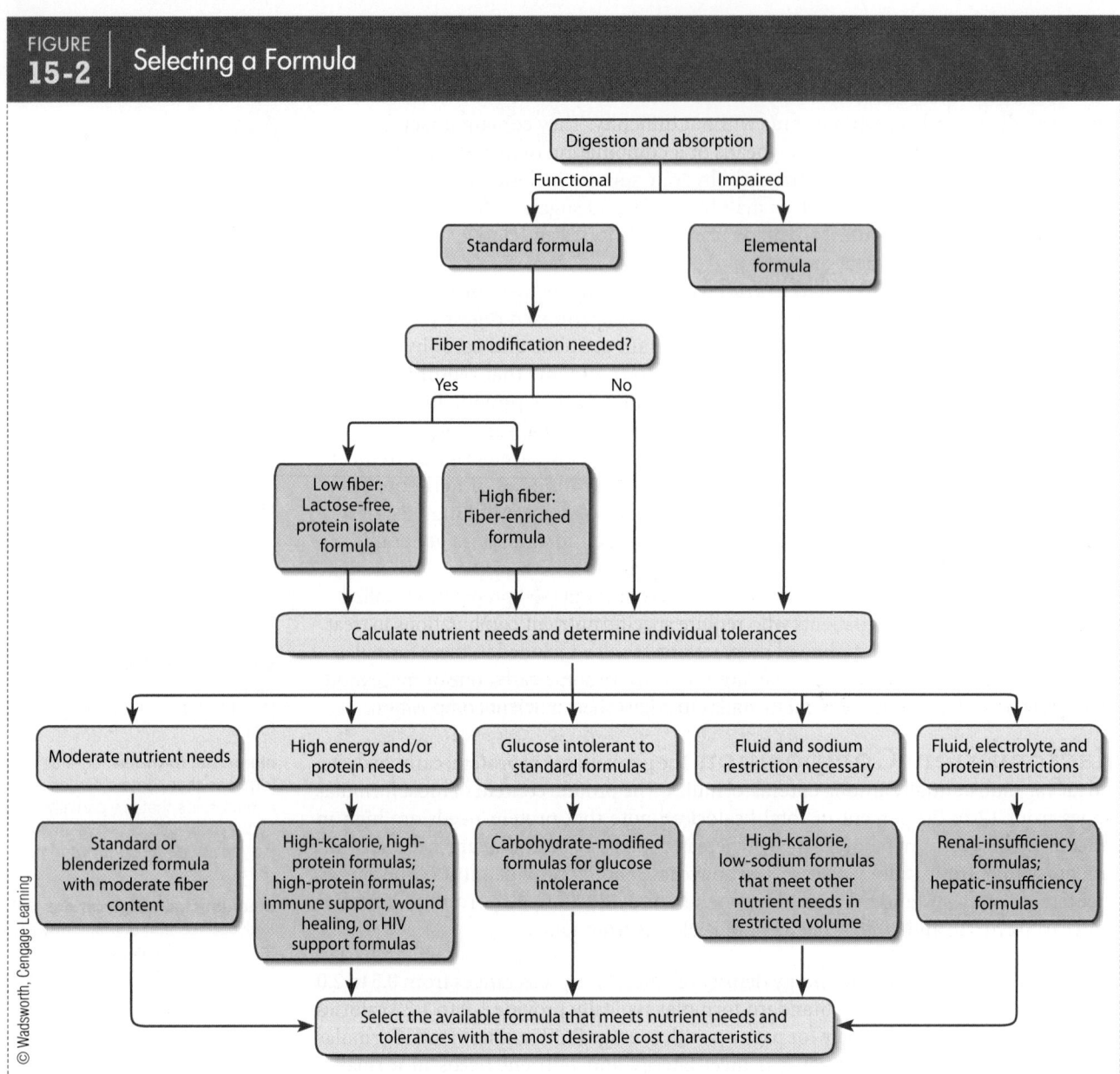

Formula Selection The formula is selected after careful assessment of the patient's medical problems, fluid and nutrition status, and ability to digest and absorb nutrients; some of the factors considered are shown in Figure 15-2. Generally, the best formula is one that meets the patient's medical and nutrient needs with the lowest risk of complications and the lowest cost. The vast majority of patients can use standard formulas. A person with a functional, but impaired, GI tract may require an elemental formula. Factors that influence formula selection include:

- *Nutrient and energy needs.* As with patients consuming regular diets, an adjustment in macronutrient and energy intakes may be necessary for tube-fed patients. For example, critical-care patients may have high protein and energy requirements, individuals with diabetes may need to control carbohydrate intake, and patients with chronic kidney disease may need to limit intakes of protein and several minerals.

- *Fluid requirements.* High nutrient needs must be met using the volume of formula a patient can tolerate. If fluids are restricted, the formula should have adequate nutrient content and energy density to deliver the required nutrients in the volume prescribed.

- *The need for fiber modifications.* The choice of formulas is narrower if fiber intake needs to be low or high.
- *Individual tolerances (food allergies and sensitivities).* Most formulas are lactose-free because many patients who need enteral formulas have some degree of lactose intolerance. Many formulas are also gluten-free and can accommodate the needs of individuals with celiac disease (gluten sensitivity).

Health care facilities stock a limited number of formulas, so formula selection is influenced by availability. Initially, the medical staff may choose a formula based on the criteria previously mentioned and then reevaluate the decision according to the patient's response to the formula. Note that few research studies have assessed the effectiveness of the various specialized formulas,[3] so their additional expense may be difficult to justify.

ENTERAL NUTRITION IN CLINICAL CARE

A person with a functioning GI tract who cannot meet nutrient needs with conventional foods alone may be a candidate for enteral nutrition support. Enteral feedings are preferred over parenteral nutrition because they help to stimulate or maintain gut function, cause fewer complications, and are less costly.[4] Similarly, oral feedings are preferred to tube feedings when the person is able to drink enteral formulas, because drinking the formulas prevents the stress, complications, and expense associated with tube feedings.

Oral Use of Enteral Formulas
As mentioned previously, enteral formulas can fully meet a person's nutritional needs. In most cases, however, patients drink enteral formulas to supplement their diets when they are unable to consume enough food to meet their needs. Enteral formulas provide a reliable source of nutrients and add energy and protein to the diets of malnourished patients. Moreover, those who are weak or debilitated may find it easier to manage formulas than meals.

When a patient drinks a formula, taste becomes an important consideration. Allowing patients to sample different products and flavors and to select the ones they prefer helps to promote acceptance. The "How to" offers additional suggestions for helping patients accept and enjoy oral formulas.

Several enteral products are sold in pharmacies and grocery stores for home use; examples include Ensure, Boost, and Carnation Instant Breakfast. These products are sometimes used as convenient meal replacements or supplements by healthy individuals. The products are available in ready-to-drink liquid form or in powdered forms that need to be reconstituted with water or milk.

© Caro/Alamy

Patients can drink enteral formulas when they are unable to consume enough food from a conventional diet.

HOW TO | Help Patients Accept Oral Formulas

People using enteral formulas are often quite ill and have poor appetites. Even when a person enjoys a formula, the taste can become monotonous in time. Elemental formulas are usually less palatable than standard formulas, and patients may find them difficult to drink. Nurses can motivate patients to drink formulas by trying these suggestions:

- Let the patient sample different formulas that are appropriate for his or her needs, and use only those that the patient enjoys.
- Serve formulas attractively, and remind patients to drink them. Formulas offered in a glass on an attractive plate may be more appealing than those served from a can with an unfamiliar name.
- If a patient finds the smell of a formula unappealing, it may help to cover the top of the glass with plastic wrap or a lid, leaving just enough room for a straw.

- Provide easy access. Keep the formula close to the patient's bed where it can be reached with little effort and within sight so that the patient is reminded to drink it. Patients who are very ill may lack the motivation to reach for the formula, let alone drink it.
- Try keeping the formula in an ice bath so that it will be cool and refreshing when the patient drinks it. Check with the patient to make sure the colder temperature is suitable.
- For patients with little appetite, offer the formula in small amounts that are easy to tolerate, and serve it more frequently during the day.
- If the patient stops enjoying the formula, recommend different flavors or try other formulas. Check with the pharmacy to see if alternative enteral products are available, such as milkshakes, puddings, or snack bars.

Candidates for Tube Feedings

Tube feedings are typically recommended for patients at risk of developing protein-energy malnutrition who are unable to consume adequate food or formula for at least seven days.[5] The following medical conditions or treatments may indicate the need for tube feedings:

- Severe swallowing disorders
- Impaired motility in the upper GI tract
- Gastrointestinal obstructions and **fistulas** that can be bypassed with a feeding tube
- Certain types of intestinal surgeries
- Mechanical ventilation
- Extremely high nutrient requirements
- Little or no appetite for extended periods, especially if the patient is malnourished
- Mental incapacitation due to confusion, neurological disorders, or coma

Contraindications for tube feedings include severe GI bleeding, high-output fistulas, **intractable** vomiting or diarrhea, complete intestinal obstruction, and severe malabsorption.[6] In addition, some clinical studies suggest that tube feedings are not always effective in some of the patient populations in which they are routinely used; thus, the decision to use tube feedings should be considered in light of the most recent research evidence.[7]

Feeding Routes

The feeding route chosen depends on the patient's medical condition, the expected duration of tube feeding, and the potential complications of a particular route. Figure 15-3 illustrates the main feeding routes, and the Glossary of Tube Feeding Routes on p. 441 describes each route.

When a patient is expected to be tube fed for less than four weeks, a **nasogastric** or **nasoenteric** route is generally chosen; for these routes, the feeding tube is passed into

---

FIGURE 15-3 | Tube Feeding Routes

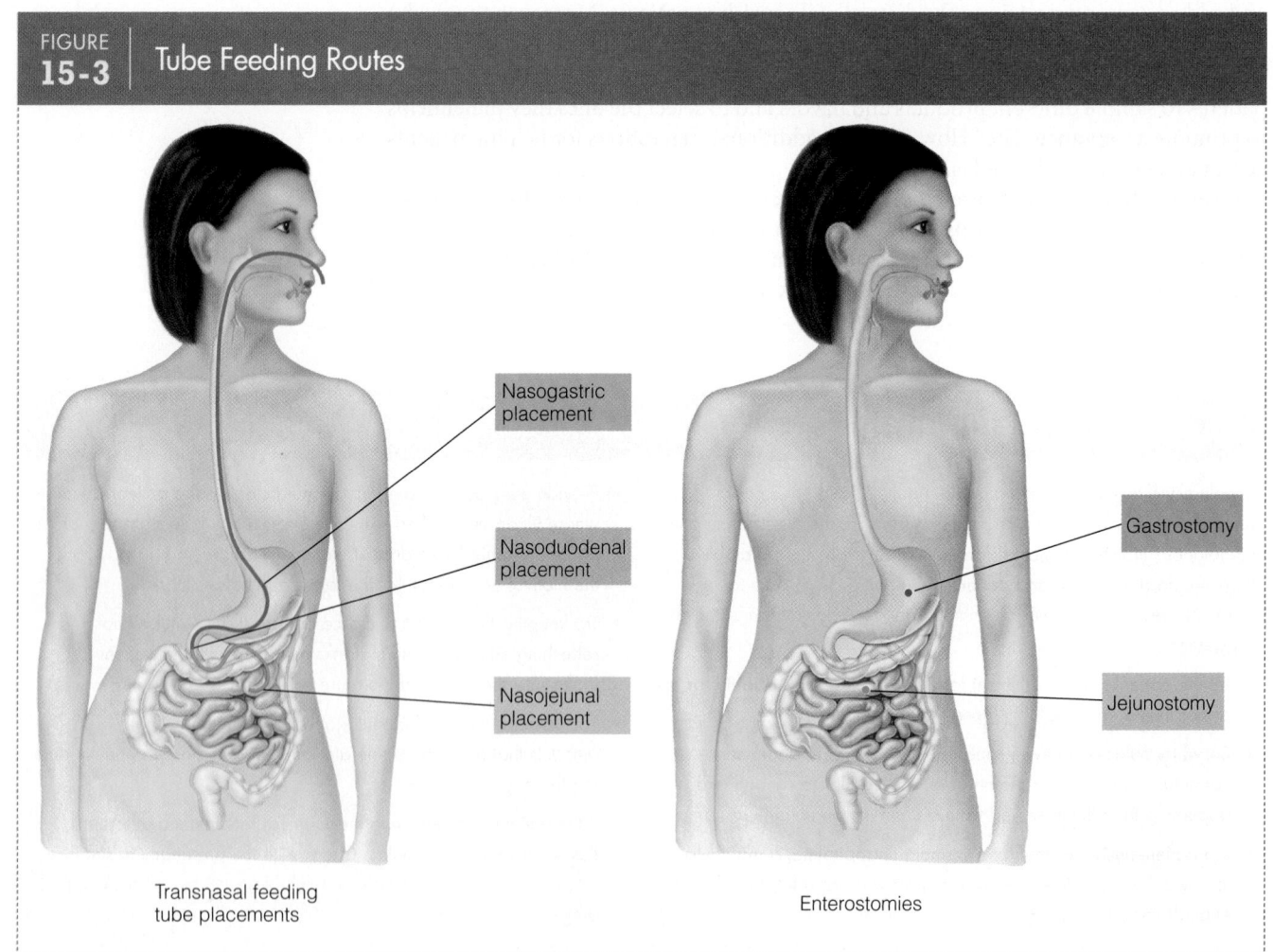

Nasogastric placement

Nasoduodenal placement

Nasojejunal placement

Gastrostomy

Jejunostomy

Transnasal feeding tube placements

Enterostomies

Enteral and Parenteral Nutrition Support

Glossary of Tube Feeding Routes

For each type of tube placement, the terms are listed in order from the upper to lower organs of the digestive system.

transnasal: a *transnasal feeding tube* is one that is inserted through the nose.

- **nasogastric (NG):** tube is placed into the stomach via the nose.
- **nasoenteric:** tube is placed into the GI tract via the nose. (*Nasoenteric feedings* usually refer to *nasoduodenal* and *nasojejunal* feedings.)
- **nasoduodenal (ND):** tube is placed into the duodenum via the nose.
- **nasojejunal (NJ):** tube is placed into the jejunum via the nose.

orogastric: tube is inserted into the stomach through the mouth. This method is often used to feed infants because a nasogastric tube may hinder the infant's breathing.

enterostomy (EN-ter-AH-stoe-mee): an opening into the GI tract through the abdominal wall.

- **gastrostomy (gah-STRAH-stoe-mee):** an opening into the stomach through which a feeding tube can be passed. A nonsurgical technique for creating a gastrostomy under local anesthesia is called *percutaneous endoscopic gastrostomy (PEG)*.
- **jejunostomy (JEH-ju-NAH-stoe-mee):** an opening in the jejunum through which a feeding tube can be passed. A nonsurgical technique for creating a jejunostomy is called *percutaneous endoscopic jejunostomy (PEJ)*. The tube can either be guided into the jejunum via a gastrostomy or passed directly into the jejunum (*direct PEJ*).

---

the GI tract via the nose. The patient is frequently awake during **transnasal** (through-the-nose) placement of a feeding tube. While the patient is in a slightly upright position with head tilted, the tube is inserted into a nostril and passed into the stomach (naso-gastric placement), duodenum (**nasoduodenal** placement), or jejunum (**nasojejunal** placement). If the patient is awake and alert, he or she can swallow water to ease the tube's passage. The final position of the feeding tube tip is verified by abdominal X-ray or other means. In infants, **orogastric** placement, in which the feeding tube is passed into the stomach via the mouth, is sometimes preferred over transnasal routes; this placement allows the infant to breathe more normally during feedings.

When a patient will be tube fed for longer than four weeks or if the nasoenteric route is inaccessible due to an obstruction or other medical reasons, a direct route to the stomach or intestine may be created by passing the tube through an **enterostomy**, an opening in the abdominal wall that leads to the stomach (**gastrostomy**) or jejunum (**jejunostomy**). An enterostomy can be made by either surgical incision or needle puncture.

© Wadsworth, Cengage Learning

A transnasal feeding tube accesses the GI tract via the nose.

© Wadsworth, Cengage Learning

In a gastrostomy, the feeding tube accesses the GI tract through the abdominal wall.

Aspiration risk is high in patients with esophageal disorders, neuromuscular diseases, and conditions that reduce consciousness or cause dementia.

aspiration: drawing in by suction or breathing; a common complication of enteral feedings in which foreign material enters the lungs, often from GI secretions or the reflux of stomach contents.

aspiration pneumonia: a lung disease resulting from the abnormal entry of foreign material; caused by either bacterial infection or irritation of the lower airways.

NURSING DIAGNOSIS

The nursing diagnosis *risk for aspiration* may apply to certain patients using tube feedings.

Selecting a Feeding Route

As mentioned, transnasal access is usually preferred when the tube feeding duration is expected to be less than four weeks, and enterostomies are often appropriate when tube feedings are planned for longer periods. Gastric feedings, such as the nasogastric and gastrostomy routes, are preferred whenever possible. These feedings are more easily tolerated and less complicated to deliver than intestinal feedings because the stomach controls the rate at which nutrients enter the intestine. Gastric feedings are not possible, however, if patients have gastric obstructions or motility disorders that interfere with the stomach's ability to empty. Gastric feedings are also avoided in patients at high risk of **aspiration**, (✚) a common complication in which formula or GI secretions enter the lungs, possibly from the backflow of stomach contents. **Aspiration pneumonia**, a lung disease that is sometimes fatal, may result. Although health practitioners frequently administer nasoenteric feedings to minimize the possibility of aspiration, studies have not consistently shown that gastric feedings are associated with increased aspiration risk.[8] Table 15-1 summarizes the advantages and disadvantages of the various tube feeding routes.

Feeding Tubes

Feeding tubes are made from soft, flexible materials (usually silicone, polyurethane, or polyvinyl chloride) and come in a variety of lengths and diameters. The tube selected largely depends on the patient's age and size, the feeding route, and the formula viscosity. In many cases, the tube selected is the smallest-diameter tube through which the formula will flow without clogging.

TABLE 15-1	Comparison of Tube Feeding Routes[a]	
Insertion Method or Feeding Site	**Advantages**	**Disadvantages**
Transnasal	Does not require surgery or incisions for placement; tubes can be placed by a nurse or trained dietitian.	Easy to remove by disoriented patients; long-term use may irritate the nasal passages, throat, and esophagus.
Nasogastric	Easiest to insert and confirm placement; least expensive method; feedings can often be given intermittently and without an infusion pump.	Highest risk of aspiration in compromised patients;[b] risk of tube migration to small intestine.
Nasoduodenal and nasojejunal	Lower risk of aspiration in compromised patients;[b] allows for earlier tube feedings than gastric feedings during severe stress; may allow enteral feedings even when obstructions, fistulas, or other medical conditions prevent gastric feedings.	More difficult to insert and confirm placement; risk of tube migration to stomach; tube feedings require an infusion pump for administration; may take longer to reach nutrition goals.
Tube enterostomies	Allow the lower esophageal sphincter to remain closed, reducing the risk of aspiration;[b] more comfortable than transnasal insertion for long-term use; site is not visible under clothing.	Tubes must be placed by physician or surgeon; general anesthesia may be required for surgically placed tubes; risk of complications from the insertion procedure; risk of infection at insertion site.
Gastrostomy	Feedings can often be given intermittently and without a pump; easier insertion procedure than a jejunostomy.	Moderate risk of aspiration in high-risk patients.[b]
Jejunostomy	Lowest risk of aspiration;[b] allows for earlier tube feedings than gastrostomy during severe stress; may allow enteral feedings even when obstructions, fistulas, or medical conditions prevent gastric feedings.	Most difficult insertion procedure; most costly method; feedings require an infusion pump for administration; may take longer to reach nutrition goals.

[a] Relative to other tube feeding routes. The actual advantages and disadvantages of different insertion procedures depend on the person's medical condition.

[b] The risk of aspiration associated with the different feeding routes is controversial and still under investigation.

The outer diameter of a feeding tube is measured in **French units**, in which each unit equals ⅓ millimeter; thus, a "12 French" feeding tube has a 4-millimeter diameter. (✚)The inner diameter depends on the thickness of the tubing material. Double-lumen tubes are also available; these allow a single tube to be used for both intestinal feedings and **gastric decompression**, a procedure in which the stomach contents of patients with motility disorders are removed by suction.

The thin wires protruding from the ends of these feeding tubes are stylets, which stiffen the tubes to ease insertion and are discarded thereafter. The Y-connector (shown here in orange) provides a port for administering water or medications without disrupting the feeding.

ADMINISTRATION OF TUBE FEEDINGS

After the feeding route and formula have been selected, the formula must be safely delivered. The methods of tube feeding administration vary somewhat from one health care facility to the next. The procedures presented in the following sections are suggested guidelines.

Safe Handling Individuals who are ill or malnourished often have suppressed immune systems, making them vulnerable to infection from foodborne illness. Thus, the personnel involved with preparing or delivering formula—usually individuals in the foodservice department or pharmacy—should be aware of the specific protocols at their facility that prevent formula contamination. (✚)

Formulas are available in open feeding systems and closed feeding systems. With an **open feeding system**, the formula needs to be transferred from its original packaging to a feeding container. Examples include formulas that are packaged in cans or bottles, concentrates that need to be diluted, and powders that require reconstitution. In a **closed feeding system**, the formula is prepackaged in a container that can be connected directly to a feeding tube. Closed systems are less likely to become contaminated, require less nursing time, and can hang for longer periods of time than open systems. Although closed systems cost more initially, they may be less expensive in the long run because they prevent bacterial contamination and thus avoid the costs of treating infections.

✚ 1 French = 1/3 mm
12 French = 12 × 1/3 mm
= 4 mm

✚ Reminder: Health care facilities have protocols for handling food products and formulas based on the potential hazards and critical control points in food preparation, referred to as *Hazard Analysis and Critical Control Points* (*HACCP*).

Safety Guidelines After the formula reaches the nursing station, the nursing staff assumes responsibility for its safe handling. Hands should be carefully washed

In an open feeding system, the formula is transferred from its original packaging to a feeding container.

In a closed feeding system, the formula is prepackaged in a container that can be attached directly to a feeding tube, such as the bottle shown on the left. The formula in the can at right can be used in an open feeding system.

before handling formulas and feeding containers. Some facilities require that nonsterile gloves be worn whenever formulas are handled. The following steps can reduce the risk of formula contamination when using open feeding systems:

- Before opening a can of formula, clean the lid with a disposable alcohol wipe and wash the can opener with detergent and hot water. (Check HACCP protocols for details.) If you do not use the entire can at one feeding, label the can with the date and time it was opened.
- Store opened cans or mixed formulas in clean, closed containers. Refrigerate the unused portion of formula promptly.
- Discard unlabeled or improperly labeled containers and all opened containers of formula that are not used within 24 hours.
- Hang no more than an 8-hour supply of formula when using an open feeding system. Discard any formula that remains, rinse out the feeding bag and tubing, and add fresh formula to the feeding bag. Use a new feeding container and tubing (except for the feeding tube itself) every 24 hours.

For closed feeding systems, the hang time should be no longer than 24 to 48 hours. Contamination is more likely with the longer time periods.

Preparing for Tube Feedings

Before starting a tube feeding, nurses can ease fears by fully discussing the procedure with the patient and family members, who may feel anxious about the use of a feeding tube. The discussion should address the reasons why tube feeding is appropriate as well as the benefits and risks of the procedure. The "How to" offers suggestions that may help ease the concerns of patients who may benefit from tube feeding.

HOW TO | Help Patients Cope with Tube Feedings

The thought of being "force-fed" is frightening to many people. Some may envision thick feeding tubes or fear that the procedure will be painful. Others may associate tube feedings with disabling injury or irreversible illness. Patients may be less apprehensive once they understand the insertion procedure, the expected duration of the tube feeding, and the strategic role that nutrition plays in recovery from disease. The pointers that follow can help nurses prepare patients for transnasal tube feedings:

- Allow the patient to see and touch the feeding tube. Seeing first-hand that the tube is soft and narrow (only about half the diameter of a pencil) often alleviates anxiety.

- Show the patient how the feeding apparatus is attached to the feeding tube, and explain how the feeding will work. For young children, use dolls or stuffed toys to demonstrate tube insertion and feeding procedures.

- Explain that the patient remains fully alert during the procedure and helps pass the tube by swallowing. A numbing solution sprayed on the back of the throat minimizes discomfort and prevents gagging during the procedure.

- Tell the patient that once the tube has been inserted, most people become accustomed to its presence within a few hours. In most cases, the patient can easily swallow foods and liquids with the tube in place. If permitted, favorite foods or beverages can still be enjoyed.

- Assure the patient that the tube feeding will be temporary, if such assurance is appropriate.

A tube feeding may be frightening for some patients, but others may be relieved to know that they can receive sound nutrition without any effort. As they feel better and begin to eat again, the volume of the feeding can be reduced and then discontinued when oral intake is adequate.

Tube feedings may cause some patients to feel that they have lost control over an important aspect of their lives. They may also feel self-conscious about how the feeding tube looks or feel awkward when moving around with the equipment. A few measures can help:

- Involve patients in the decision-making and care process whenever possible. Patients can help to arrange their daily feeding schedules and can perform some of the feeding procedures themselves.

- Show patients how to manipulate the feeding equipment so that they can get out of bed and move around.

- Encourage patients to maintain contact with friends and keep busy with the hobbies and activities they enjoy. This measure is especially important for children, teens, and those on long-term feedings.

When caring for infants and children, keep the developmental age of the child in mind and work with parents to ensure that appropriate feeding skills are mastered. Infants can be provided with a pacifier during feedings to help maintain the associations between sucking, swallowing, and fullness. When possible, the formula can be provided by bottle to an infant, or by spoon to a child, to further develop skills.

The more complex the procedure, the easier it becomes for health care professionals to focus on the procedure and disregard a patient's emotional response. No matter how many technicalities you have to keep in mind, remember to stay focused on the person receiving your care.

Enteral and Parenteral Nutrition Support

Serious complications can develop if a transnasal tube is accidentally inserted into the respiratory tract or if formula or GI secretions are aspirated into the lungs. To minimize the risk of incorrect tube placement, clinicians use X-rays to verify the position of the feeding tube before a feeding is initiated. After the tube's placement has been confirmed, the nurse secures the tube to the patient's nose and cheek with tape and monitors the position of the tubing throughout the day. Tube placement can also be monitored by testing the pH of a sample of bodily fluid drawn into the feeding tube; recall that the pH of stomach fluid is much lower than the pH of fluid obtained from the intestine or respiratory tract. (✛)

To reduce the risk of aspiration, the patient's upper body is elevated to at least a 30- to 45-degree angle during the feeding and for 30 minutes after the feeding whenever possible. The addition of blue food coloring to formula was formerly suggested as a means of identifying aspirated formula in lung secretions; however, this practice is now discouraged due to its lack of reliability and because several deaths have been attributed to its use.[9]

Formula Delivery Methods

A day's nutrient needs can be met by delivering relatively large amounts of formula several times per day (**intermittent feedings**) or smaller amounts continuously during the day (**continuous feedings**). A patient may also start with continuous feedings and gradually transition to intermittent feedings. Each method has specific uses, advantages, and disadvantages.

Intermittent feedings are best tolerated when they are delivered into the stomach (not the intestine). Generally, a total of about 250 to 400 milliliters of formula is delivered over 20 to 40 minutes using a gravity drip method or an infusion pump. The exact amount is determined by dividing the required volume of formula into several daily feedings, as shown in the "How to" below. Due to the relatively high volume of formula delivered at one time, intermittent feedings may be difficult for some patients to tolerate, and the risk of aspiration may be higher than with continuous feedings. An advantage of intermittent feedings is that they are similar to the usual pattern of eating and allow the patient freedom of movement between meals.

Rapid delivery of a large volume of formula into the stomach (250 to 500 milliliters in less than 20 minutes) is called a **bolus feeding**. This type of feeding may be given every 3 to 4 hours using a syringe. Bolus feedings can cause abdominal discomfort, nausea, and cramping in some patients, and the risk of aspiration is greater than with other methods of feeding. For these reasons, bolus feedings are used only in patients who are not critically ill.

Continuous feedings are delivered slowly and at a constant rate over a period of 8 to 24 hours. Continuous feedings are used to deliver intestinal feedings and are generally recommended for critically ill patients because the slower delivery rate is easier to tolerate. An infusion pump is required to ensure accurate and steady flow rates; consequently, the feedings can limit the patient's freedom of movement and are also more costly.

✛ A gastric sample usually has a pH between 1 and 4. An intestinal sample should have a pH between 6 and 8.

intermittent feedings: delivery of about 250 to 400 milliliters of formula over 20 to 40 minutes.

continuous feedings: slow delivery of formula at a constant rate over an 8- to 24-hour period.

bolus (BOH-lus) feeding: delivery of about 250 to 500 milliliters of formula in less than 20 minutes.

HOW TO | Plan a Tube Feeding Schedule

After selecting a suitable formula, the clinician must determine the volume of formula that meets the patient's nutritional needs. Consider a patient who needs 2000 kcalories daily and is using a standard formula that provides 1.0 kcalorie per milliliter. The total volume of formula required would be 2000 milliliters per day:

$$\chi \text{ mL} \times 1.0 \text{ kcal/mL} = 2000 \text{ kcal}$$

$$\chi \text{ mL} = \frac{2000 \text{ kcal}}{1.0 \text{ kcal/mL}} = 2000 \text{ mL}$$

If the patient is to receive intermittent feedings six times a day, he will need about 333 milliliters of formula at each feeding:

$$2000 \text{ mL} \div 6 \text{ feedings} = 333 \text{ mL/feeding}$$

Alternatively, if he is to receive intermittent feedings eight times a day, he will need 250 milliliters (or about one can of ready-to-feed formula) at each feeding:

$$2000 \text{ mL} \div 8 \text{ feedings} = 250 \text{ mL/feeding}$$

He will probably tolerate this volume of formula best if it is delivered over a 20- to 40-minute period at each feeding. If the patient is to receive the formula continuously over 24 hours, he will need about 83 milliliters of formula each hour:

$$2000 \text{ mL} \div 24 \text{ hours} = 83 \text{ mL/hr}$$

The delivery of intermittent and continuous feedings can be controlled with an infusion pump.

© Wadsworth, Cengage Learning

Initiating and Advancing Tube Feedings Formula administration techniques vary widely among institutions, so protocols should be reviewed carefully before working with patients. In addition, patient tolerance must be considered when adjusting formula delivery rates. Keep in mind that few studies have evaluated the various methods for initiating and advancing enteral feedings.

Formulas are typically provided full-strength, although they may occasionally be diluted if the patient's fluid requirements are high and water needs cannot be met by other means.[10] Intermittent feedings may start with 60 to 120 milliliters at the initial feeding and be increased by 30 to 60 milliliters at each feeding until the goal volume is reached. Continuous feedings may start at about 20 to 50 milliliters per hour and be raised by 10 to 25 milliliters per hour every 4 to 8 hours.[11] Concentrated formulas are often started at the slower rates. If the patient cannot tolerate an increased rate of delivery, the feeding rate is slowed until the person adapts. In some patients, formula delivery can be started at the goal rate immediately, which significantly improves the patient's overall caloric intake.[12]

Checking the Gastric Residual Volume When a patient receives a gastric feeding, the nurse regularly measures the **gastric residual volume** (the volume of formula remaining in the stomach after feeding) to ensure that the stomach is emptying properly. The gastric residual volume is measured by gently withdrawing the gastric contents through the feeding tube using a syringe, usually before each intermittent feeding and every 4 to 6 hours during continuous feedings.[13] Although opinions vary, some experts recommend that an evaluation be conducted if the gastric residual volume exceeds 200 milliliters and that feedings be withheld if it exceeds 500 milliliters.[14] If the tendency to accumulate fluids persists, the physician may recommend intestinal feedings or begin drug therapy to improve gastric emptying.

Meeting Water Needs Attention must also be paid to the patient's fluid requirements. Although water needs vary (✚), many adults require about 2000 milliliters (about 2 quarts) of water daily. Fluids may be restricted in persons with kidney, liver, or heart disease. Additional water is required in patients with fever, high urine output, diarrhea, excessive sweating, severe vomiting, fistula drainage, high-output ostomies, blood loss, or open wounds.

The water in formulas meets a substantial portion of water needs. Standard formulas contain about 85 percent water, or about 850 milliliters of water per liter of formula. Nutrient-dense formulas contain about 70 to 75 percent water; exact amounts can be obtained from the product label or manufacturer's information sheet.

In addition to the water in formulas, water can be provided by flushing water separately through the feeding tube. To prevent clogging, feeding tubes are routinely flushed with 20 to 30 milliliters of warm water before and after each intermittent feeding and about every 4 hours during continuous feedings.[15] The water used for routine flushes should be included when estimating fluid intakes.

MEDICATION DELIVERY THROUGH FEEDING TUBES

Patients receiving tube feedings sometimes require one or more medications that need to be delivered through feeding tubes. Because medications can interact with substances in enteral formulas in the same ways that they interact with food substances, potential diet-drug interactions must be considered. In addition, some medications may need to be exposed to the acidic stomach environment and thus cannot be administered via an intestinal feeding tube. Medications can also cause feeding tubes to clog. The "How to" provides some guidelines that may help to prevent complications.

Diarrhea Medications are a major cause of the diarrhea that frequently accompanies tube feedings. Diarrhea is especially associated with the administration of sorbitol-containing medications, laxatives, and some types of antibiotics.[16] The high osmolality of many liquid medications can also cause diarrhea, so dilution of hypertonic medications may be helpful.

✚ To estimate fluid requirements in adults and children:
- Adults: allow 30 to 40 mL/kg; 25 to 30 mL/kg in adults ≥65 years old
- Children: allow 50 to 60 mL/kg
- Infants: allow 100 to 150 mL/kg

gastric residual volume: the volume of formula remaining in the stomach from a previous feeding.

NURSING DIAGNOSIS

The nursing diagnoses *deficient fluid volume* and *excess fluid volume* may apply to patients who are receiving too little or too much water relative to needs.

NURSING DIAGNOSIS

The nursing diagnosis *diarrhea* often applies to patients using tube feedings.

The pharmacist is your best resource for learning how and when medications can be administered via feeding tubes, especially when you are dealing with an unfamiliar drug. Check with the pharmacist to learn the following:

- Whether a particular medication is known to be incompatible with formulas.

- The proper timing of medication administration to avoid drug-nutrient interactions.

- For patients using intestinal feedings, whether a medication can be absorbed without exposure to stomach acid.

- Whether a liquid form of a medication is available and, if so, the appropriate dosage of the liquid form.

- If only tablets are available, whether the tablets can be crushed and mixed with water. Enteric-coated and sustained-release medications should not be crushed due to the potential for adverse effects.

In general, it is best to give medications by mouth instead of by tube whenever possible. In some cases, the injectable form of a medication may be the best option. For medications that must be given by feeding tube:

- Do not mix medications with enteral formulas. Do not mix medications together.

- Before administering medications, ensure that the feeding tube is placed correctly, that it is not clogged, and that the gastric residual volume is not excessive.

- Position the patient in a semi-upright position (30 degrees or higher) to prevent aspiration.

- Flush the feeding tube with 20 to 30 milliliters of warm water before and after administering a medication. When more than one medication is administered, flush the feeding tube with water after each medication is given.

- Use liquid forms of medications whenever possible. Dilute very viscous or hypertonic liquid medications with 10 to 30 milliliters of water before administering them through the feeding tube.

- If tablets are used, crush tablets to a fine powder and mix with 10 milliliters of warm water before administering.

Medications and Continuous Feeding A continuous feeding is ordinarily stopped for 15 minutes before and after the administration of a medication so that the components of enteral formulas do not interfere with the medication's absorption. Some medications may require a longer formula-free interval; for example, feedings need to be stopped for one to two hours before and after administering phenytoin, a medication that controls seizures.[17] In such cases, the formula's delivery rate needs to be increased so that the correct amount of formula can be delivered.

TUBE FEEDING COMPLICATIONS

Complications are a frequent occurrence during tube feedings. Possible complications include gastrointestinal problems, such as constipation and diarrhea; mechanical problems related to the tube feeding process; and metabolic problems, such as biochemical alterations and nutrient deficiencies. Examples of the most common complications, along with some preventive and corrective measures, are summarized in Table 15-2.

Many complications of tube feeding can be prevented by choosing the most appropriate feeding route, formula, and delivery method. Attention to a patient's primary medical condition and medication use is important as well. Nurses responsible for day-to-day care of the patient routinely monitor body weight, hydration status, and results of laboratory tests to detect problems before complications develop.

TRANSITION TO TABLE FOODS

After the patient's condition improves, the volume of formula can be tapered off as the patient gradually shifts to an oral diet. The steps in the transition depend on the patient's medical condition and the type of feeding the patient has been receiving. Individuals using continuous feedings are often switched to intermittent feedings initially. In some patients, swallowing function may need to be evaluated before oral feedings begin. Patients receiving elemental formulas may begin the transition by using a standard formula, either orally or via tube feeding. If the patient has not consumed lactose for several weeks, a diet with minimal lactose may be better tolerated. Oral intake should supply about two-thirds of estimated nutrient needs before the tube feeding is discontinued completely.[18] The Case Study allows you to consider the many factors involved in tube feedings.

TABLE
15-2

Causes and Management of Tube Feeding Complications

Complications	Possible Causes	Preventive/Corrective Measures
Aspiration of formula	Inappropriate tube placement	Ensure correct placement of feeding tube.
	Delayed gastric emptying	Ensure that head of bed is properly elevated during and after feeding; evaluate gastric residual volume and decrease formula delivery rate or halt feeding if necessary; consider using intestinal feedings in high-risk patients.
	Excessive sedation	Minimize use of medications that cause sedation.
Clogged feeding tube	Excessive formula viscosity	Ensure that tube size is appropriate; flush tubing with water before and after giving formula. Remedies to unclog feeding tubes include flushes with warm water or solutions that contain pancreatic enzymes and sodium bicarbonate; consult pharmacist for more options.
	Improper administration of medications	Use oral, liquid, or injectable medications whenever possible; flush tubing with water before and after medications are given; avoid mixing medications with formula; dilute thick or sticky liquid medications with water before administering; crush tablets to a fine powder and mix with water (except enteric-coated or sustained-release medications).
Constipation	Inadequate dietary fiber	Use a formula with appropriate fiber content.
	Dehydration	Provide additional fluids.
	Lack of exercise	Encourage walking and other activities, if appropriate.
	Medication side effect	Consult physician about minimizing or replacing medications that cause constipation.
Diarrhea	Medication intolerance	Dilute hypertonic medications before administering; replace poorly tolerated medications with injectable or more easily tolerated oral medications.
	Infection in GI tract	Consult physician about specific diagnosis and appropriate treatment.
	Formula contamination	Review safety guidelines for formula preparation and delivery.
	Excessively rapid formula administration	Decrease formula delivery rate or use continuous feedings.
	Lactose or gluten intolerance	Use lactose-free or gluten-free formula in patients with intolerances.
	Unknown cause	Review medical record for conditions that predispose to diarrhea; try an alternative formula that contains adequate fiber; consult physician about appropriateness of antidiarrheal or antimotility medications.
Fluid and electrolyte imbalances	Diarrhea	See items under *Diarrhea*.
	Inappropriate fluid intake or excessive losses	Monitor daily weights, intake and output records, serum electrolyte levels, and clinical signs that indicate dehydration or overhydration; ensure that water intake and formula delivery rates are appropriate.
	Inappropriate nutrient intake	Use a formula with appropriate nutrient content; ensure that nutrient intakes of malnourished patients are not excessive.[a]
	Inappropriate insulin, diuretic, or other therapy	Ensure that medication doses are appropriate.
Irritation or inflammation of skin or mucous membranes	Inappropriate feeding tube	Use small-bore tubes made from soft materials.
	Friction from feeding tube movement	Tape feeding tube securely to prevent excessive movement.
	Infection at insertion site	Keep site clean; inspect area for redness, tenderness, and drainage; use protective dressing or ointment; treat with antibiotics, if necessary.

Nausea and vomiting, cramps	Delayed stomach emptying	Decrease formula delivery rate or use continuous feedings; halt feeding if gastric residual volume is excessive (>500 mL); evaluate for obstruction; consider use of medications to improve emptying rate.
	Formula intolerance	Ensure that formula is at room temperature, delivery rate is appropriate, and formula odor is not objectionable; consider using formula that is low in fat, low in fiber, or elemental.
	Medication intolerance	Consult physician about replacing medications that are poorly tolerated.
	Response to disease or disease treatment	Consider use of medications that control nausea and vomiting.

ª See section on refeeding syndrome (p. 456) for details.

Review Notes

- Enteral formulas are liquid diets that can supplement conventional diets or be used for tube feedings. They differ in their macronutrient composition, energy density, fiber content, and osmolality.

- A nasoenteric feeding route is preferred for short-term tube feedings, whereas enterostomies are used for longer-term feedings. Gastric feedings are preferred but are avoided in patients at risk of aspiration.

- Depending on the feeding route and the patient's medical condition, the formula can be delivered in bolus feedings, intermittently, or continuously. Medications should be given separately and accompanied by water flushes to prevent tube clogging.

- Formulas can meet a substantial portion of the patient's water requirements, and additional water can be provided by flushing water through the feeding tube.

- Complications of tube feedings can be gastrointestinal, mechanical, or metabolic in nature.

CASE STUDY | Injured Hiker Requiring Enteral Nutrition Support

Sharyn Eschler is a 24-year-old graphics designer who suffered multiple fractures when she fell from a cliff while hiking. She has been in the hospital for two weeks and has no appetite. Sharyn weighed 140 pounds upon her arrival in the hospital, but she has lost 8 pounds over the course of her hospitalization. Due to the nature of her injuries, she is in traction and is immobile, although the head of her bed can be elevated 45 degrees. From the food and nutrition history, it appears that Sharyn's nutrition status was adequate prior to hospitalization. The health care team agrees that nasoduodenal tube feeding should be instituted before her nutrition status deteriorates further. The standard formula selected for the feeding is lactose-free, and Sharyn's nutrient requirements can be met with 2200 milliliters of the formula per day.

1. What steps can be taken to prepare Sharyn for tube feeding? What are some general reasons why nasoduodenal placement of the feeding tube might be preferred over nasogastric placement?

2. The physician's orders specify that the feeding should be given continuously over 18 hours. Using the method shown in the "How to" on p. 445, determine an appropriate tube feeding schedule.

3. Estimate Sharyn's fluid needs using her current weight and the fluid intake range suggested in the margin on p. 446. Will Sharyn receive enough water from the formula she is given daily? If not, estimate the amount of additional fluid she would need, and explain how this fluid could be provided.

4. Describe precautions that should be taken if Sharyn is to receive medications through the feeding tube.

5. After three days of feeding, Sharyn develops diarrhea. Check Table 15-2 to determine the possible causes. What measures can be taken to correct the diarrhea?

Parenteral Nutrition Support

The first half of this chapter described how enteral formulas can supplement or replace a conventional diet. Enteral formulas cannot be used when intestinal function is inadequate, however, and therefore the ability to meet nutrient needs intravenously is a lifesaving option for critically ill persons. The procedure is costly, however, and is associated with a number of potentially dangerous complications. As previous sections suggested, enteral nutrition support is preferred if the GI tract is functional.

CANDIDATES FOR PARENTERAL NUTRITION

Parenteral nutrition may be recommended for patients who do not have functioning GI tracts and who are either malnourished or likely to become so (review Figure 15-1). Parenteral support is also beneficial if using the GI tract would cause harm to the patient, as when severe tissue damage in the small intestine requires bowel rest for an extended period. Thus, patients with the following conditions are often considered candidates for parenteral nutrition:

- Intestinal obstructions or fistulas
- Paralytic ileus (intestinal paralysis)
- Short bowel syndrome (a substantial portion of the small intestine has been removed)
- Intractable vomiting or diarrhea
- Severe pancreatitis
- Bone marrow transplants
- Severe malnutrition and intolerance to enteral nutrition

VENOUS ACCESS

Once the decision to use parenteral nutrition has been made, the access site must be selected. The access sites for parenteral nutrition fall into two main categories: nutrients may be delivered into the **peripheral veins** located in the arms and legs or into the large-diameter **central veins** located near the heart.

Peripheral Parenteral Nutrition

In **peripheral parenteral nutrition (PPN)**, nutrient needs are met using only the peripheral veins. Peripheral veins can be damaged by overly concentrated solutions, however—**phlebitis** may develop, characterized by redness, swelling, and tenderness at the infusion site. To prevent phlebitis, the **osmolarity** of parenteral solutions used for PPN is generally kept below 900 milliosmoles per liter,[19] a concentration that also limits the amounts of energy and protein the solution can provide. The "How to" below compares the terms *osmolarity* and *osmolality*, both of which can be used to express the osmolar concentration of a solution.

HOW TO | Express the Osmolar Concentration of a Solution

The movement of water across biological membranes (called *osmosis*) is influenced by a solution's concentration of *milliosmoles*, the ions and molecules that contribute to water's osmotic pressure. The terms *osmolarity* and *osmolality* are both used to express the concentration of these types of solutes:

- *Osmolarity* refers to the milliosmoles per liter of solution (mOsm/L).
- *Osmolality* refers to the milliosmoles per kilogram of solvent (mOsm/kg).

The main difference between the terms is that osmolarity refers to a volume of solution that includes the solutes of interest (milliosmoles contained in a liter of the solution), whereas osmolality refers to the solutes separately from the solvent in which they are dissolved (milliosmoles per kilogram of solvent). Osmolarity and osmolality are roughly equivalent when describing dilute aqueous solutions at room or body temperature; this is because 1 liter of water weighs 1 kilogram, and the solutes contribute little to the volume of the solution.

Osmolarity and osmolality are both used in clinical practice, but they are derived in different ways. Osmolarity is typically calculated using equations that account for the nutrients and electrolytes in biological solutions. Osmolality is usually a measured value obtained using an *osmometer,* a common instrument in hospital laboratories.

PPN is used most often in patients who require short-term nutrition support (about 7 to 10 days) and who do not have high nutrient needs or fluid restrictions. The use of PPN is not possible if the peripheral veins are too weak to tolerate the procedure. In many cases, clinicians must rotate venous access sites to avoid damaging veins.

Total Parenteral Nutrition Most patients meet their nutrient needs using the larger, central veins, where blood volume is greater and nutrient concentrations do not need to be limited. Because this method can reliably meet a person's complete nutrient requirements, it is called **total parenteral nutrition (TPN).** Central veins lie close to the heart, where the large volume of blood rapidly dilutes parenteral solutions. Therefore, patients with very high nutrient needs or fluid restrictions are able to receive the nutrient-dense solutions they require. TPN is also preferred for patients who require long-term parenteral nutrition.

There are several ways to access central veins. The tip of a central venous **catheter** can be placed directly into a large-diameter central vein or threaded into a central vein through a peripheral vein (see Figure 15-4). Peripheral insertion of central catheters is less invasive and lower in cost than the direct insertion of catheters into central veins; this method is usually preferred for short-term venous access (about two months or less in duration).[20]

The peripheral veins can provide access to the blood for delivery of parenteral solutions.

PARENTERAL SOLUTIONS

The pharmacies located within health care institutions are often responsible for preparing parenteral solutions. This arrangement is convenient because the pharmacist can customize formulations to meet patients' nutrient needs and because the solutions have a limited shelf life. The physician typically submits an order form to the pharmacy such as the one shown in Figure 15-5. Prescriptions for parenteral solutions are highly individualized and may need to be recalculated daily until the patient's condition is stable. Because the nutrients are provided intravenously, they must be given in forms that are safe to inject directly into the bloodstream.

total parenteral nutrition (TPN): the infusion of nutrient solutions into a central vein.

catheter: a thin tube placed within a narrow lumen (such as a blood vessel) or body cavity; can be used to infuse or withdraw fluids or keep a passage open.

FIGURE 15-4 | Accessing Central Veins for Total Parenteral Nutrition

- IV solution
- Right subclavian vein
- Catheter
- Hub of catheter
- Filter
- IV tubing
- Internal jugular vein
- External jugular vein
- Left subclavian vein
- Left cephalic vein
- Left basilic vein
- Right superior vena cava
- Catheter

1 Traditionally, central catheters enter the circulation at the right subclavian vein and are threaded into the superior vena cava with the tip of the catheter lying close to the heart. Sometimes catheters are threaded into the superior vena cava from the left subclavian vein, the internal jugular vein, or the external jugular vein.

2 Peripherally inserted central catheters usually enter the circulation at the basilic or cephalic vein and are guided up toward the heart so that the catheter tip rests in the superior vena cava.

FIGURE
15-5 | Sample Parenteral Nutrition Order Form

Physician Orders
PARENTERAL NUTRITION (PN) – ADULT

Primary Diagnosis: _____ Ht: _____ cm Dosing Wt: _____ kg

PN Indication: _____ Allergies _____

Instructions: This form must be completed for a new order or continuation of PN and faxed to the Pharmacy by [Insert Time] to receive same day preparation. PN administration begins at [Insert Time]. Contact the Nutrition Support Service at (XXX) XXX-XXXX for additional information.

Administration Route: CVC or PICC   Note: Proper tip placement of the CVC or PICC must be confirmed prior to PN infusion

Peripheral IV (PIV) (Final PN Osmolarity ≤ _____ mOsm/L)

Monitoring: Daily weights, Strict input & output, Bedside glucose monitoring every _____ hours

Na, K, Cl, CO_2, Glucose, BUN, Scr, Mg, PO_4 every _____

T, Bili, Alk Phos, AST, ALT, Albumin, Triglycerides, Calcium every _____

Base Solution:	Parenteral nutrition MUST be administered through a dedicated infusion port and filtered with a 1.2-micron in-line
Select one	filter at all times. Discard any unused volume after 24 hours.

PERIPHERAL 2-in-1
Dextrose _____ g
Amino Acids (Brand _____) ____ g

For patients with PIV and established glucose tolerance; Provides _____ kcal; Maximum Rate not to exceed _____ mL/hour

CENTRAL 2-in-1
Dextrose _____ g
Amino Acids (Brand _____) ____ g

For patients with CVC or PICC and established glucose tolerance; Provides _____ kcal; Maximum Rate not to exceed _____ mL/hour

CENTRAL 3-in-1
Dextrose _____ g
Amino Acids (Brand _____) ____ g
Fat Emulsion (Brand _____) ____ g

For patients with CVC or PICC and established glucose/fat emulsion tolerance; Provides _____ kcal; Maximum Rate not to exceed _____ mL/hour

Use of additional fat emulsion not required with 3-in-1 base solution

RATE & VOLUME: _____ mL/hour for _____ hours = _____ mL/day
Must specify

or **CYCLIC INFUSION:** _____ mL/hour for _____ hours, then _____ mL/hour for _____ hours = _____ mL/day

Fat Emulsion (Brand _____) – via PIV or CVC with 2-in-1 base solutions (Select caloric density & volume)

| 10% | 250 mL | Infuse at _____ mL/hour over _____ hours | Frequency _____ |
| 20% | 500 mL | (Note: infusions < 4 or > 12 hours not recommended) | Discard any unused volume after 12 hours. |

Additives: (per day)
Sodium Chloride _____ mEq
   as Acetate _____ mEq
   as Phosphate _____ mmol of PO_4
Potassium Chloride _____ mEq
   as Acetate _____ mEq
   as Phosphate _____ mmol of PO_4
Calcium **Gluconate** _____ mEq

Magnesium **Sulfate** _____ mEq
Adult **Multivitamins** _____ mL/day
Adult **Trace Elements** _____ mL/day
H_2 **Antagonist** _____ _____ mg
Other:

Normal Dosages
1-2 mEq Sodium/kg/day
pH or CO_2 dependent
Consider if hyperkalemic
1-2 mEq Potassium/kg/day
pH or CO_2 dependent
20-40 mmol/day (1 mmol Phos = 1.5 mEq K)
5-15 mEq/day

8-24 mEq/day
Contains Vitamin K 150 mcg
Zn ___ mg, Cu ___ mg, Mn ___ mg, Cr ___ mcg, Se ___ mcg (with normal hepatic function)
____ mg/day with normal renal function

Additives: (per day)
Regular Insulin _____ units
Recommend if hyperglycemic, start with 1 unit for every 10 g of dextrose

Pharmacy Use Only: Ca/PO_4
Limit Checked _____
(Note: Some brands of amino acids contain phosphate)

Physician's Signature: _____ Pager Number: _____ Date/time: _____
Orders transcribed by: _____ Date/time: _____ Orders verified by: _____ Date/time: _____
SEND COMPLETED ORDERS TO PHARMACY

© Wadsworth, Cengage Learning

Amino Acids

Parenteral solutions contain all of the essential amino acids and various combinations of the nonessential amino acids. Amino acid concentrations range from 3.5 to 15 percent; (✚) the more concentrated solutions are used only for TPN. Just as in regular foods, the amino acids provide 4 kcalories per gram. Disease-specific amino acid solutions are available for patients with liver disease, kidney disease, and metabolic stress.

Carbohydrate

Glucose is the main source of energy in parenteral solutions. It is provided in the form dextrose monohydrate, in which each glucose molecule is associated with a single water molecule. Dextrose monohydrate provides 3.4 kcalories per gram, slightly less than pure glucose, which provides 4 kcalories per gram. Commercial dextrose solutions are available in concentrations between 2.5 and 70 percent. (✚) Concentrations greater than 12.5 percent are used only in TPN solutions.[21]

In parenteral solutions, the dextrose concentration is indicated by a "D" followed by its concentration in water (W) or normal saline (NS). For example, D5 or D5W indicates that a solution contains 5 percent dextrose in water. Similarly, D5NS means that a solution contains 5 percent dextrose in normal saline.

Lipids

Lipid emulsions supply essential fatty acids and are a significant source of energy. The emulsions usually contain triglycerides from soybean oil and safflower

✚ A 10 percent amino acid solution supplies 10 g of amino acids per 100 mL of solution.

✚ A 10 percent dextrose solution provides 10 g of dextrose monohydrate per 100 mL of solution.

✚ 500 mL of a 10% lipid emulsion: 500 mL × 1.1 kcal/mL= 550 kcal
500 mL of a 20% lipid emulsion: 500 mL × 2 kcal/mL = 1000 kcal

oil, phospholipids to serve as emulsifying agents, and glycerol to make the solutions isotonic. Lipid emulsions are available in 10, 20, and 30 percent solutions, containing 1.1, 2.0, and 3.0 kcalories per milliliter, respectively. Therefore, a 500-milliliter container of 10 percent lipid emulsion would provide 550 kcalories; the same volume of a 20 percent lipid emulsion would provide 1000 kcalories. (✚) In the United States, the 30 percent lipid emulsion can be used for preparing mixed parenteral solutions but cannot be directly infused into patients.[22]

Lipid emulsions are often provided daily and may supply 20 to 30 percent of total kcalories. Including lipids as an energy source reduces the need for energy from dextrose and lowers the risk of hyperglycemia in glucose-intolerant patients. Lipid infusions must be restricted in patients with hypertriglyceridemia, however. There is also some concern that lipid emulsions that contain excessive linoleic acid can suppress some aspects of the immune response.

Fluids and Electrolytes

Daily fluid needs usually range from 30 to 40 milliliters per kilogram of body weight in young adults and 25 to 30 milliliters per kilogram of body weight in adults who are 65 years and older, averaging between 1500 and 2500 milliliters for most people. The amounts are adjusted according to daily fluid losses and the results of hydration assessment.

The electrolytes added to parenteral solutions include sodium, potassium, chloride, calcium, magnesium, and phosphorus. The amounts in parenteral solutions differ from DRI values because the nutrients are infused directly into the blood and are not influenced by absorption, as they are when consumed orally. Because electrolyte imbalances can be lethal, electrolyte management by experienced professionals is necessary whenever intravenous therapies are used. Blood tests are administered daily to monitor electrolyte levels until patients have stabilized.

The electrolyte content of parenteral solutions is expressed in *milliequivalents (mEq)*, which are units indicating the number of ionic charges provided by electrolytes. (✚) The body's fluids and parenteral solutions are neutral solutions that contain equal numbers of positive and negative charges.

Vitamins and Trace Minerals

Commercial multivitamin and trace mineral preparations are routinely added to parenteral solutions. All of the vitamins are usually included, although a preparation without vitamin K is available for patients using warfarin therapy.[23] (✚) The trace minerals usually added to parenteral solutions include zinc, copper, chromium, selenium, and manganese. Iron is excluded because it alters the stability of other ingredients in parenteral mixtures; therefore, special forms of iron need to be injected separately.

Osmolarity

Recall that the osmolarity of PPN solutions is limited to 900 milliosmoles per liter because peripheral veins are sensitive to high nutrient concentrations, whereas TPN solutions may be as nutrient dense as necessary. The components of a solution that contribute most to its osmolarity are amino acids, dextrose, and electrolytes: as concentrations of these nutrients increase, the osmolarity of a solution increases. Because lipids contribute little to osmolarity, lipid emulsions are used to increase the energy provided in PPN solutions.

Medications

To avoid the need for a separate infusion site, medications are occasionally added directly to parenteral solutions or infused through a separate port (attached via a Y-connector). The administration of a second solution using a separate port in a catheter is called a **piggyback**. Insulin, for example, is sometimes added by piggyback to improve glucose tolerance. In practice, few medications are added to parenteral solutions so that potential drug-nutrient interactions can be avoided.

Parenteral Formulations

When a parenteral solution contains dextrose, amino acids, and lipids, it is called a **total nutrient admixture (TNA)**, a **3-in-1 solution**, or an **all-in-one solution**. A **2-in-1 solution** excludes lipids, and the lipid emulsion is administered separately, often by piggyback administration. The administration of

A lipid emulsion gives the parenteral solution a milky white color.

© Wadsworth, Cengage Learning

✚ Milliequivalents are determined by dividing an ion's molecular weight (MW) by its number of charges. For example:
- For calcium, MW = 40, and the ion has 2 positive charges: 40 ÷ 2 = 20. Thus, 1 mEq of Ca^{++} is equivalent to 20 mg of calcium.
- For sodium, MW = 23, and the ion has 1 positive charge: 23 ÷ 1 = 23. Thus, 1 mEq of Na^+ is equivalent to 23 mg of sodium.
- *1 mEq of Ca^{++} has the same number of charges as 1 mEq of Na^+.*

✚ Reminder: The anticoagulant warfarin works by interfering with vitamin K's blood-clotting function (see Chapter 14).

piggyback: the administration of a second solution using a separate port in an intravenous catheter.

total nutrient admixture (TNA): a parenteral solution that contains dextrose, amino acids, and lipids; also called a **3-in-1 solution** or an **all-in-one solution**.

2-in-1 solution: a parenteral solution that contains dextrose and amino acids, but excludes lipids.

Suppose a patient is receiving 1.25 liters (1250 milliliters) of a parenteral solution that contains 5 percent amino acids and 30 percent dextrose, supplemented by 250 milliliters of a 20 percent lipid emulsion daily. How many grams of protein and carbohydrate is the person receiving, and what is the total energy intake for the day?

Amino acids:

$$5\% \text{ amino acids} = \frac{5 \text{ g amino acids}}{100 \text{ mL}}$$

$$\frac{5 \text{ g amino acids}}{100 \text{ mL}} \times 1250 \text{ mL} = 62.5 \text{ g of amino acids}$$

$$62.5 \text{ g amino acids} \times 4.0 \text{ kcal/g} = 250 \text{ kcal}$$

Carbohydrate:

$$30\% \text{ dextrose} = \frac{30 \text{ g dextrose}}{100 \text{ mL}}$$

$$\frac{30 \text{ g dextrose}}{100 \text{ mL}} \times 1250 \text{ mL} = 375 \text{ g of dextrose}$$

$$375 \text{ g dextrose} \times 3.4 \text{ kcal/g} = 1275 \text{ kcal}$$

Lipids:

Recall that a 20 percent lipid emulsion provides 2.0 kcalories per milliliter. If the patient is given 250 milliliters of the emulsion:

$$250 \text{ mL} \times 2.0 \text{ kcal/mL} = 500 \text{ kcal}$$

Total energy intake:

$$250 \text{ kcal} + 1275 \text{ kcal} + 500 \text{ kcal} = 2025 \text{ kcal}$$

TNA solutions is simpler because only one infusion pump is required; however, the addition of lipid emulsion to solutions reduces their stability, a major concern when TNA solutions are compounded. Thus, lipids are usually provided separately when they are not a major energy source and are used only to provide essential fatty acids. The "How to" above describes a method for calculating the macronutrient and energy content of a parenteral solution.

ADMINISTERING PARENTERAL NUTRITION

Parenteral nutrition is a complex treatment that requires skills from a variety of disciplines. Many hospitals organize nutrition support teams, (✚) consisting of physicians, nurses, dietitians, and pharmacists, that specialize in the provision of both intravenous and tube feedings. The nurse, who performs direct patient care, plays a central role in administering and monitoring parenteral infusions.

Insertion and Care of Intravenous Catheters
Although a skilled nurse can place catheters into peripheral veins, only qualified physicians can insert catheters directly into central veins. Patients may be awake for the procedure and given local anesthesia. Unnecessary apprehension can be avoided by explaining the procedure to the patient beforehand.

Catheter-related problems frequently cause complications (see Table 15-3). Catheters may be improperly positioned or may dislodge after placement. Air can leak into catheters and escape into the bloodstream, obstructing blood flow. Catheters in peripheral veins may cause phlebitis, necessitating reinsertion at an alternate site. A catheter may become clogged from blood clotting or from a buildup of scar tissue around the catheter tip. Catheters are also a leading cause of infection: contamination may be introduced during insertion or may develop at the placement site.

To reduce the risk of complications, nurses use aseptic techniques when inserting catheters, changing tubing, or changing a dressing that covers the catheter site. Unusual bleeding or a wet dressing suggests a problem with catheter placement. A change in infusion rate may indicate a clogged catheter. Infection may be indicated by redness or swelling around the catheter site or by an unexplained fever. Routine inspections of equipment and frequent monitoring of patients' symptoms help to minimize the problems associated with catheter use.

Administration of Parenteral Solutions
The method used to initiate and advance a parenteral solution depends on the patient's condition and the potential for complications.[24] One approach is to start the infusion at a slow rate and

✚ Reminder: A *nutrition support team* is a multidisciplinary team of health care professionals who are responsible for the provision of nutrients by tube feeding or intravenous infusion.

TABLE 15-3	Potential Complications of Parenteral Nutrition	
Catheter-Related	**Metabolic**
Air embolism	Abnormal liver function
Blood clotting at catheter tip	Electrolyte imbalances
Clogging of catheter	Gallbladder disease
Dislodgment of catheter	Hyperglycemia, hypoglycemia
Improper placement	Hypertriglyceridemia
Infection, sepsis	Metabolic bone disease
Phlebitis	Nutrient deficiencies
Tissue injury	Refeeding syndrome

increase the rate gradually over a two- to three-day period. For example, 40 milliliters per hour can be infused during the first 24 hours of administration (supplying 960 milliliters) and the volume increased to the goal rate on the second day. Another method is to give the full volume of a nutrient-dilute solution on the first day and advance nutrient concentrations as tolerated. Solutions can often be started at full strength unless there is a risk of hyperglycemia or other complications.

Parenteral solutions may be infused continuously over 24 hours (**continuous parenteral nutrition**) or during 10- to 16-hour periods only (**cyclic parenteral nutrition**). Continuous infusions are given to critically ill and malnourished patients who cannot receive adequate nutrients in the shorter time periods. Cyclic infusions are sometimes provided at night so that patients can participate in routine activities during the day. This method is especially suited to patients who require long-term parenteral support or who will be infusing parenteral solutions at home. Patients may begin with continuous parenteral nutrition and transition to cyclic parenteral nutrition as their condition improves.

Regular monitoring can help to prevent complications. The parenteral solution and tubing are checked frequently for signs of contamination. Routine testing of glucose, lipid, and electrolyte levels helps to determine tolerance to solutions. Frequent reassessment of nutrition status may be necessary until a patient has stabilized. Rapid changes in infusion rate are discouraged in some patients due to a risk of developing hyperglycemia or hypoglycemia.[25]

Discontinuing Intravenous Infusions
The patient must have adequate GI function before parenteral nutrition can be tapered off and enteral feedings begun. During the transition to oral feedings, a combination of methods is often necessary. Parenteral infusions are usually tapered off at the same time that tube feedings or oral feedings are begun, such that the two methods can together supply the needed nutrients. Clear liquids are generally the first foods offered and include pulp-free fruit juices, soft drinks, and clear broths; small amounts are given initially to determine tolerance. (✚) Later feedings include beverages and solid foods that are unlikely to cause discomfort. If gastrointestinal symptoms (such as nausea, vomiting, bloating, or diarrhea) develop, oral feedings are limited in size or frequency until the intestines adapt. Once about two-thirds to three-fourths of nutrient needs can be provided enterally, the intravenous infusions may be discontinued.

✚ Chapter 14 provides more information about the clear liquid diet.

continuous parenteral nutrition: continuous administration of parenteral solutions over a 24-hour period.

cyclic parenteral nutrition: administration of parenteral solutions over a 10- to 16-hour period each day.

Transitioning to an oral diet is sometimes difficult because a person's appetite remains suppressed for several weeks after parenteral nutrition is terminated. Patients receiving continuous parenteral nutrition may have better appetites during the day if they are switched to nocturnal cyclic infusions before beginning oral intakes.

MANAGING METABOLIC COMPLICATIONS

As discussed previously, the catheters used for intravenous infusions may cause a number of serious complications. This section describes some metabolic complications that may result from parenteral nutrition (review Table 15-3) and some suggestions for managing them.[26]

Hyperglycemia

Hyperglycemia (✚) most often occurs in patients who are glucose intolerant or undergoing severe metabolic stress. It can be prevented by providing insulin along with parenteral solutions or by restricting the amount of dextrose in a solution. Dextrose infusions are generally limited to less than 5 milligrams per kilogram of body weight per minute in critically ill adult patients so that the carbohydrate intake does not exceed the maximum glucose oxidation rate.

Hypoglycemia

Although uncommon, hypoglycemia sometimes occurs when parenteral nutrition is interrupted or discontinued or if excessive insulin is given. In patients at risk, such as young infants, infusions may be tapered off over several hours before discontinuation. Another option is to infuse a 10 percent dextrose solution at the same time that parenteral nutrition is interrupted or stopped.[27]

Hypertriglyceridemia

Hypertriglyceridemia may develop in critically ill patients who cannot tolerate the amount of lipid emulsion supplied. Patients at risk include those with severe infection, liver disease, kidney failure, hyperglycemia, and use of immunosuppressant or corticosteroid medications. If blood triglyceride levels exceed 500 milligrams per deciliter, lipid infusions should be reduced or stopped.[28]

Refeeding Syndrome

Severely malnourished patients who are fed aggressively (parenterally or otherwise) may develop **refeeding syndrome,** characterized by electrolyte and fluid imbalances and hyperglycemia. These effects occur because dextrose infusions raise circulating insulin levels, which promote anabolic processes that quickly remove phosphate, potassium, and magnesium from the blood. The altered electrolyte levels can lead to fluid retention and life-threatening changes in organ systems.

Refeeding syndrome generally develops within two weeks of beginning parenteral infusions.[29] The patients at highest risk are those who have experienced chronic malnutrition or substantial weight loss. To prevent refeeding syndrome, health practitioners start parenteral infusions slowly and carefully monitor electrolyte and glucose levels when malnourished patients begin receiving nutrition support.

Abnormal Liver Function

Fatty liver often results from parenteral nutrition, but it is usually corrected when the parenteral infusions are discontinued. Long-term parenteral nutrition, however, may result in chronic, irreversible liver disease that can eventually lead to liver failure. To minimize the risk, practitioners are careful to avoid giving the patient excess energy, dextrose, or lipids, which create additional work for the liver. If appropriate, some oral feedings may be encouraged to reduce the amount of parenteral support necessary.[30]

Gallbladder Disease

When parenteral nutrition continues for more than four weeks, sludge (thickened bile) often builds up in the gallbladder and may eventually lead to gallstone formation. Prevention is sometimes possible by initiating oral feedings before problems develop. Patients requiring long-term parenteral nutrition may be given cholecystokinin injections to induce gallbladder contraction and bile release or may have their gallbladders removed surgically.

NURSING DIAGNOSIS

The nursing diagnoses *risk for unstable blood glucose level* and *risk for electrolyte imbalance* often apply to critically ill patients who begin parenteral nutrition.

NURSING DIAGNOSIS

The nursing diagnosis *risk for impaired liver function* may apply to patients who undergo parenteral nutrition.

✚ For most patients receiving parenteral nutrition, blood glucose levels should not exceed 200 mg/dL.

refeeding syndrome: a condition that sometimes develops when a severely malnourished person is aggressively fed; characterized by electrolyte and fluid imbalances and hyperglycemia.

Jerry Huang, a 27-year-old geologist with an inflammatory intestinal disease, underwent a surgical procedure in which a substantial portion of his small intestine was removed. He had received TPN prior to surgery and continued to receive it afterward. After 10 days, tube feeding, which initially delivered very small feedings, was begun.

1. How would you explain the need for parenteral nutrition to Jerry? List some reasons why the nutrition support team initially chose TPN to provide nutrition support to this patient.

2. Describe the components of a typical TPN solution. Calculate the energy content of 1 liter of a solution that provides 140 grams of dextrose monohydrate, 45 grams of amino acids, and 90 milliliters of 20 percent lipid emulsion. If Jerry's energy requirement is 2100 kcalories per day, how many liters of solution will he need each day?

3. Why is it important that Jerry begin enteral feedings as soon as possible? Assuming that Jerry eventually tolerates a tube feeding, in what ways can the health care team help Jerry make the transition from parenteral nutrition to tube feedings? Consider some of the physiological problems that Jerry might face when he begins eating an oral diet.

4. If Jerry is unable to meet his nutrient needs orally, he may need to continue tube feeding or TPN at home. As you read through the section on nutrition support at home, consider the factors that would make Jerry a good candidate for a home nutrition support program. Consider both the benefits of a proposed program and the problems he could encounter.

Metabolic Bone Disease Long-term parenteral nutrition is associated with lower bone density, which may be related to altered calcium, phosphorus, magnesium, and sodium metabolism. Imbalanced intakes of vitamin D, vitamin K, and phosphorus have also been implicated. The ideal intervention for metabolic bone disease varies among patients; it may include dietary adjustments, nutrient supplements, medications, and physical activity.[31]

Review Notes

- Peripheral parenteral nutrition is provided to patients who need short-term parenteral support and do not have high nutrient needs or fluid restrictions. Total parenteral nutrition supplies nutrient-dense solutions for long-term parenteral support.

- Parenteral solutions include amino acids, dextrose, electrolytes, vitamins, and minerals. Lipid emulsions may be included in the mixture or may be administered separately.

- Catheters are frequently the cause of complications, which include improper placement or dislodgment, infection, clotting, embolism, and phlebitis.

- Critically ill patients may require continuous parenteral nutrition, whereas stable patients and long-term users may prefer cyclic parenteral nutrition.

- Metabolic complications include hyperglycemia, hypoglycemia, hypertriglyceridemia, refeeding syndrome, and diseases affecting the liver, gallbladder, and bone. The Case Study checks your understanding of the concepts introduced in this section.

Nutrition Support at Home

Some individuals may require nutrition support—either tube feedings or parenteral nutrition—after a medical condition has stabilized and they no longer require hospital services. For such a person, home nutrition support may be a suitable option.

The use of home nutrition support is rapidly expanding. Current medical technology allows for the safe administration of nutrition support in home settings, and insurance

Portable pumps and convenient carrying cases allow freedom of movement for individuals using home nutrition support.

coverage often pays a substantial portion of the costs. Medical equipment providers and home infusion companies can provide the supplies, enteral formulas or parenteral solutions, and services necessary for home nutrition care. Most important, patients using these services can continue to receive specialized nutrition care while leading normal lives.

CANDIDATES FOR HOME NUTRITION SUPPORT

Individuals referred for home nutrition support usually need long-term nutrition care for chronic medical conditions. Users of home nutrition services (or their families and other caregivers) must be intellectually capable of learning the necessary procedures, monitoring the treatment, and managing complications as necessary. The home should be clean and have adequate storage for formulas or solutions and equipment. The costs should be clearly explained to families who cannot get insurance reimbursement. Candidates for home nutrition support include the following:[32]

- For home enteral nutrition, individuals who have disorders that prevent food from reaching the intestines or interfere with nutrient absorption. Examples include people with head and neck cancers, severe dysphagia, gastric outlet obstructions, and pancreatic or intestinal conditions that cause malabsorption.
- For home parenteral nutrition, individuals who have disorders that severely impede nutrient absorption or interfere with intestinal motility. Examples include people with short bowel syndrome, inflammatory bowel diseases, and intestinal obstructions.

PLANNING HOME NUTRITION CARE

As with the nutrition support provided in health care facilities, planning for home nutrition care involves decisions about access sites, formulas, and nutrient delivery methods. Users of home services should be involved in the decision making to ensure long-term compliance and satisfaction.

Home Enteral Nutrition Access to the GI tract is possible using either nasal tubes or enterostomies. People sometimes learn to place nasogastric tubes themselves, which may improve acceptance of the treatment. Active children and adults often prefer low-profile gastrostomy tubes, which allow them to lead a more normal lifestyle. Jejunostomy tubes may be required for some individuals but are less convenient because the frequent feedings required can interfere with daytime activities.

The choice of formula for home use is influenced by its cost and availability. Insurance reimbursements do not always include the cost of enteral formulas, which are considered to be "food" products. For this reason, some people choose to prepare simple formulas at home. Blenderizing home-cooked foods is possible, but the foods need to be strained to remove particles and clumps that may obstruct the tube. Closed (ready-to-hang) feeding systems are useful for avoiding contamination risk but are not appropriate for intermittent feedings that require smaller amounts of formula.

The advantages and disadvantages associated with the different administration methods should be fully discussed with patients. For gastric feedings, bolus infusions are simplest and can be quickly delivered. Gravity drip infusions eliminate the need for an infusion pump, but the delivery rates are less reliable. If intermittent feedings are appropriate, they need to be tailored to daily routines. Portable pumps can free individuals from the need to infuse formula at home and can also be used when traveling.

Home Parenteral Nutrition Although both peripheral parenteral nutrition and total parenteral nutrition (TPN) can be provided at home, long-term therapy requires access to the larger, central veins that are appropriate for TPN. The catheter can be inserted so that the exit site is in a region that is accessible to the patient.

Parenteral solutions need to be sterile and aseptically prepared, and individuals who mix their own solutions must be carefully trained. Ready-made parenteral solutions require refrigeration and are stable for limited periods; for example, TNA (total nutrient admixture) solutions may be stable for only a week when refrigerated.

Most people prefer cyclic infusions over continuous infusions and transition to cyclic infusions before discharge from the hospital. Because an infusion pump is required for home TPN, sufficient battery backup should be on hand in case electrical service is interrupted. Portable pumps are helpful for individuals who lead an active lifestyle or prefer to infuse during the day.

QUALITY-OF-LIFE ISSUES

Although home nutrition programs can help to improve health and extend life, consumers of home services and their families may struggle with the lifestyle adjustments required. In addition to the economic impact of nutrition support, home feedings are often time consuming and inconvenient. Activities and work schedules must be planned around feedings. Extra planning is needed and precautions must be taken when a person wants to travel or participate in sports activities. Explaining one's medical needs to friends and acquaintances may be embarrassing.

Among physical difficulties, people receiving nocturnal feedings often cite disturbed sleep as a major problem. Disruptions may be due to multiple nighttime bathroom visits, noisy infusion pumps, or difficulty finding a comfortable sleeping position when "hooked up." People using parenteral support sometimes prefer infusing solutions during the day to improve their sleeping patterns.

Among social issues, the inability to consume meals with family and friends is often a great concern. Some individuals may be able to eat small amounts of food or may decide to sit at the table to participate in the conversation. Joining friends at restaurants and attending certain types of social events, however, can be problematic.

People who depend on nutrition support face a number of stressful issues that can affect quality of life. Although parenteral and enteral nutrition are life-sustaining treatments, both are associated with serious complications. Many people find that their lifestyles need to be greatly altered to accommodate nutrition therapy and may experience fear, anxiety, and depression. Support groups or counseling resources may help patients cope with ongoing stresses. (✚)

Review Notes

- Candidates for home enteral nutrition services have disorders that interfere with swallowing ability, GI motility, or nutrient absorption. Candidates for home parenteral nutrition have disorders that severely impair nutrient absorption or cause intestinal motility problems.
- Patients and caregivers should participate in decisions about access sites, formulas, and nutrient delivery methods. Enteral formulas and parenteral solutions can be purchased or prepared in the home.
- The use of portable pumps may help individuals lead a normal lifestyle. Nevertheless, lifestyle adjustments to nutrition support may be difficult and stressful.

✚ The Oley Foundation is an excellent source of outreach services, emotional support, and current information for people who require home nutrition support **(www.oley.org)**.

Nutrition Assessment | CHECKLIST FOR PEOPLE RECEIVING ENTERAL NUTRITION SUPPORT

MEDICAL HISTORY

Check the medical record for medical conditions that:

○ Alter nutrient needs and influence the formula selection
○ Influence the selection of tube placement sites and feeding routes
○ Suggest the length of time that the tube feeding will be needed

Monitor the medical record for complications or risks that may influence the formula selection or delivery technique, including:

○ Aspiration
○ Constipation
○ Fluid and electrolyte imbalances
○ Diarrhea
○ Hyperglycemia
○ Nausea and vomiting
○ Skin irritation

MEDICATIONS

Check medications for those that can cause side effects similar to the complications of tube feeding, such as:

○ Nausea and vomiting
○ Diarrhea
○ Constipation
○ GI discomfort

For medications delivered through the feeding tube, check:

○ Form of medication and possible alternatives
○ Viscosity of liquid medications
○ Potential for diet-drug interactions

DIETARY INTAKE

To assess nutritional adequacy, check to see whether:

○ The formula is appropriate for patient's needs
○ Supplemental water is provided to meet needs
○ The formula is administered as prescribed

ANTHROPOMETRIC DATA

Measure baseline height and weight, and monitor body weight regularly. If weight is not appropriate:

○ Determine whether energy needs have been correctly assessed
○ Check to see if the formula is being delivered as prescribed
○ Check for signs of dehydration or overhydration

LABORATORY TESTS

Check serum and urine tests for signs of:

○ Fluid and electrolyte imbalances
○ Glucose intolerance
○ Inadequate protein status (serum protein levels)
○ Improvement or deterioration of the medical condition

PHYSICAL SIGNS

Look for physical signs of:

○ Dehydration or overhydration
○ Delayed gastric emptying
○ Malnutrition

Nutrition Assessment | CHECKLIST FOR PEOPLE RECEIVING PARENTERAL NUTRITION SUPPORT

MEDICAL HISTORY

Check the medical record for medical conditions that:

○ Prevent the use of enteral nutrition
○ Suggest the time period that parenteral nutrition will be required

Monitor the medical record for complications or risks that may influence the parenteral solution formulation or delivery technique, including:

○ Acid-base imbalances
○ Fluid and electrolyte imbalances
○ Hyperglycemia or hypoglycemia
○ Hypertriglyceridemia
○ Preexisting liver disease
○ Refeeding syndrome

MEDICATIONS

For medications added to the parenteral solution, determine the:

○ Medication's compatibility with the parenteral solution
○ Length of time that the medication can remain stable in solution

For medications infused separately, determine:

○ Length of time that the infusion may need to be stopped
○ Necessary adjustments in parenteral infusions to compensate for medication delivery

DIETARY INTAKE

To assess nutritional adequacy, check to see whether:

○ Patient's nutrient needs were correctly determined
○ Solution is administered as prescribed
○ Infusion pump is operating correctly

ANTHROPOMETRIC DATA

Measure baseline height and weight, and monitor daily weights. If weight is not appropriate:

○ Determine whether energy needs have been correctly assessed
○ Check to see if the parenteral solution is being delivered as prescribed
○ Check for signs of dehydration or overhydration

LABORATORY TESTS

Check serum and urine tests for signs of:

○ Fluid, electrolyte, and acid-base imbalances
○ Hyperglycemia or hypoglycemia
○ Hypertriglyceridemia

○ Abnormal liver function
○ Inadequate protein status (serum protein levels)
○ Improvement or deterioration of medical condition

PHYSICAL SIGNS

Routinely monitor the following:

○ Catheter insertion site for signs of infection or inflammation
○ Blood pressure, temperature, pulse, and respiration for signs of fluid, electrolyte, and acid-base imbalances

Look for physical signs of:

○ Dehydration or overhydration
○ Protein-energy malnutrition
○ Malnutrition

Self Check

1. ● An important measure that may prevent bacterial contamination in tube feeding formulas is:
   a. nonstop feeding of formula.
   b. using the same feeding bag and tubing each day.
   c. discarding opened containers of formula not used within 24 hours.
   d. adding formula to the feeding container before it empties completely.

2. ● Compared with intermittent tube feedings, continuous feedings:
   a. require an infusion pump.
   b. allow greater freedom of movement.
   c. are more similar to normal patterns of eating.
   d. are associated with more GI side effects.

3. ● A patient needs 1800 milliliters of formula a day. If the patient is to receive formula intermittently every four hours, how many milliliters of formula will she need at each feeding?
   a. 225
   b. 300
   c. 400
   d. 425

4. ● The term that describes the amount of enteral formula remaining in the stomach from a previous feeding is:
   a. residue.
   b. osmolar load.
   c. gastric residual volume.
   d. intermittent feeding.

5. ● The nurse using a feeding tube to deliver medications recognizes that:
   a. medications given by feeding tube generally do not cause GI complaints.

   b. medications can usually be added directly to the feeding container.
   c. enteral formulas do not interact with medications in the same way that foods do.
   d. thick or sticky liquid medications and crushed tablets can clog feeding tubes.

6. ● TPN is preferred over PPN for a patient who:
   a. does not have high nutrient requirements.
   b. needs long-term parenteral nutrition support.
   c. has strong peripheral veins and moderate nutrient needs.
   d. needs parenteral infusions as a supplement to tube feedings.

7. ● For a patient receiving central TPN who also receives intravenous lipid emulsions two or three times a week, the lipid emulsions serve primarily as a source of:
   a. essential fatty acids.
   b. cholesterol.
   c. fat-soluble vitamins.
   d. concentrated energy.

8. ● Which nutrient is often omitted from parenteral solutions because it may destabilize other ingredients in the solution?
   a. Calcium
   b. Vitamin K
   c. Iron
   d. Chromium

9. ● Refeeding syndrome causes dangerous fluctuations in:
   a. electrolytes.
   b. liver enzymes.
   c. triglycerides.
   d. ketone bodies.

10. Patients using home parenteral nutrition:
    a. are unable to use TNA solutions.
    b. are usually given continuous rather than cyclic infusions.
    c. are generally unable to work out of the home or travel.
    d. require infusion pumps for use at home.

    Answers to these questions can be found in Appendix H.

Clinical Applications

1. Appendix G provides examples of enteral formulas on the market and lists their energy and macronutrient contents. Select one standard formula and one elemental formula from Tables G-1 and G-2, respectively. For the two formulas you selected, calculate the volume of formula that would meet the energy needs of a patient who requires about 1750 kcalories daily. Use these results in answering the following questions:
    a. What is the amount of protein, carbohydrate, and fat that the patient would obtain in a typical day? Determine the percentages of kcalories that come from carbohydrate and fat. Do these percentages fall within the Acceptable Macronutrient Distribution Ranges described in Chapter 1 (pp. 9–10)?
    b. Tables G-1 and G-2 show the formula volumes that would meet the Reference Daily Intakes (RDI). Would the volumes you obtained meet typical vitamin and mineral needs?

2. A liter of a TPN solution contains 500 milliliters of 50 percent dextrose solution and 500 milliliters of 5 percent amino acid solution. Determine the daily energy and protein intakes of a person who receives 2 liters per day of such a solution. Calculate the average daily energy intake if the person also receives 500 milliliters of a 20 percent fat emulsion three times a week.

3. Consider the social, psychological, clinical, and financial ramifications of using home parenteral nutrition, with no foods allowed by mouth, in answering the following questions:
    a. What would be the advantages of living at home instead of in a hospital or other residential facility? Can you think of some disadvantages?
    b. Think about how you, as the patient, might manage daily feedings: consider the time, cost, and commitment required to maintain the therapy.
    c. If not allowed to consume foods, what possible difficulties might you encounter? How would you handle holidays and special occasions that center around food?

Nutrition on the Net

For further study of topics covered in this chapter, access these websites.

- Find updates and quick links to these and other nutrition-related sites at our website: www.cengage.com/nutrition/whitney/nhhc4e
- To learn more about the appropriate uses of enteral and parenteral nutrition, visit the websites of these organizations:
  - American Society for Parenteral and Enteral Nutrition: www.nutritioncare.org
- British Association for Parenteral and Enteral Nutrition: www.bapen.org.uk
- To learn about home nutrition support, visit the website of the Oley Foundation, a national nonprofit organization that provides information, outreach services, and emotional support for consumers of home enteral and parenteral services: www.oley.org

Notes

1. A. M. Malone, Enteral formula selection, in P. Charney and A. Malone, eds., *ADA Pocket Guide to Enteral Nutrition* (Chicago: American Dietetic Association, 2006), pp. 63–122.
2. M. Shike, Enteral feeding, in M. E. Shils and coeditors, *Modern Nutrition in Health and Disease* (Baltimore: Lippincott Williams & Wilkins, 2006), pp. 1554–1566.
3. J. L. Rombeau, Enteral nutrition, in L. Goldman and D. Ausiello, eds., *Cecil Medicine* (Philadelphia: Saunders, 2008), pp. 1617–1621; Shike, 2006.
4. N. Gupta and R. G. Martindale, Parenteral vs. enteral nutrition, in G. Cresci, ed., *Nutrition Support for the Critically Ill Patient: A Guide to Practice* (Boca Raton, FL: Taylor & Francis Group, 2005), pp. 193–208.
5. Rombeau, 2008.

Enteral and Parenteral Nutrition Support

6. M. Marian and P. Charney, Patient selection and indications for enteral feedings, in P. Charney and A. Malone, eds., *ADA Pocket Guide to Enteral Nutrition* (Chicago: American Dietetic Association, 2006), pp. 1–25; Shike, 2006.

7. R. L. Koretz, Do data support nutrition support? Part II. Enteral artificial nutrition, *Journal of the American Dietetic Association* 107 (2007): 1374–1380.

8. K. K. Kattelmann and coauthors, Preliminary evidence for a medical nutrition therapy protocol: Enteral feedings for critically ill patients, *Journal of the American Dietetic Association* 106 (2006): 1226–1241; B. Taylor and J. E. Mazuski, Enteral feeding access in the critically ill, in G. Cresci, ed., *Nutrition Support for the Critically Ill Patient: A Guide to Practice* (Boca Raton, FL: Taylor & Francis Group, 2005), pp. 235–252.

9. Kattelmann, 2006.

10. C. Thompson, Initiation, advancement, and transition of enteral feedings, in P. Charney and A. Malone, eds., *ADA Pocket Guide to Enteral Nutrition* (Chicago: American Dietetic Association, 2006), pp. 123–154.

11. Thompson, 2006; C. R. Parrish, J. Krenitsky, and C. Kusenda, Enteral feeding challenges, in G. Cresci, ed., *Nutrition Support for the Critically Ill Patient: A Guide to Practice* (Boca Raton, FL: Taylor & Francis Group, 2005), pp. 321–340.

12. A. Desachy and coauthors, Initial efficacy and tolerability of early enteral nutrition with immediate or gradual introduction in intubated patients, *Intensive Care Medicine* 34 (2008): 1054–1059.

13. M. K. Russell, Monitoring complications of enteral feedings, in P. Charney and A. Malone, eds., *ADA Pocket Guide to Enteral Nutrition* (Chicago: American Dietetic Association, 2006), pp. 155–192.

14. S. A. McClave and coauthors, Guidelines for the provision and assessment of nutrition support therapy in the adult critically ill patient: Society of Critical Care Medicine (SCCM) and American Society for Parenteral and Enteral Nutrition (A.S.P.E.N.), *Journal of Parenteral and Enteral Nutrition* 33 (2009): 277–316; Russell, 2006.

15. Russell, 2006.

16. Russell, 2006.

17. Russell, 2006.

18. Thompson, 2006.

19. C. Hamilton, Vascular access, in P. Charney and A. Malone, eds., *ADA Pocket Guide to Parenteral Nutrition* (Chicago: American Dietetic Association, 2007), pp. 33–51.

20. Hamilton, 2007.

21. M. L. Christensen, Parenteral formulations, in G. Cresci, ed., *Nutrition Support for the Critically Ill Patient: A Guide to Practice* (Boca Raton, FL: Taylor & Francis Group, 2005), pp. 279–302.

22. R. O. Brown and G. Minard, Parenteral nutrition, in M. E. Shils and coeditors, *Modern Nutrition in Health and Disease* (Baltimore: Lippincott Williams & Wilkins, 2006), pp. 1567–1597.

23. A. M. Malone, Parenteral nutrients and formulations, in P. Charney and A. Malone, eds., *ADA Pocket Guide to Parenteral Nutrition* (Chicago: American Dietetic Association, 2007), pp. 52–63.

24. S. Roberts, Initiation, advancement, and acute complications, in P. Charney and A. Malone, eds., *ADA Pocket Guide to Parenteral Nutrition* (Chicago: American Dietetic Association, 2007), pp. 76–102.

25. E. E. Szeszycki and S. Benjamin, Complications of parenteral feeding, in G. Cresci, ed., *Nutrition Support for the Critically Ill Patient: A Guide to Practice* (Boca Raton, FL: Taylor & Francis Group, 2005), pp. 303–319.

26. M. P. Fuhrman, Complications of long-term parenteral nutrition, in P. Charney and A. Malone, eds., *ADA Pocket Guide to Parenteral Nutrition* (Chicago: American Dietetic Association, 2007), pp. 103–117; Roberts, 2007; Szeszycki and Benjamin, 2005.

27. A. Wilmer and G. Van den Berghe, Parenteral nutrition, in L. Goldman and D. Ausiello, eds., *Cecil Medicine* (Philadelphia: Saunders, 2008), pp. 1621–1626; Szeszycki and Benjamin, 2005.

28. Roberts, 2007.

29. Wilmer and Van den Berghe, 2008.

30. Roberts, 2007.

31. Fuhrman, 2007.

32. C. Hamilton and T. Austin, Home parenteral nutrition, in P. Charney and A. Malone, eds., *ADA Pocket Guide to Parenteral Nutrition* (Chicago: American Dietetic Association, 2007), pp. 118–146; A. Pattinson and J. Buchholtz, Home enteral nutrition, in P. Charney and A. Malone, eds., *ADA Pocket Guide to Enteral Nutrition* (Chicago: American Dietetic Association, 2006), pp. 193–227.

Inborn Errors of Metabolism

An **inborn error of metabolism** is an inherited trait, caused by a genetic **mutation,** that results in the absence, deficiency, or malfunction of a protein that has a critical metabolic role.[1] The severity of the inborn error's effects are ultimately related to the degree of impairment caused by the altered or missing protein. This Nutrition in Practice describes some inborn errors of metabolism and discusses the role of diet in two of these disorders: phenylketonuria and galactosemia. The accompanying glossary defines the relevant terms.

What problems can result from inborn errors of metabolism?

The protein affected by an inborn error may function as an enzyme, receptor, transport protein, or structural protein. When the body fails to make a protein, the functions that depend on that protein are impaired. For example, when an enzyme is missing or malfunctioning in a metabolic pathway that typically converts compound A to compound B, compound A will accumulate and compound B will not be made. The excess of compound A and the lack of compound B may have harmful effects. Furthermore, the imbalances in one pathway may affect other pathways and ultimately cause a number of metabolic and physiologic disturbances.

What role can diet play in treating inborn errors of metabolism?

Medical nutrition therapy is the primary treatment for many inborn errors that involve nutrient metabolism. Once the biochemical pathway affected by a mutation is identified, a health practitioner may be able to manipulate elements of the diet to compensate for deficiencies and excesses. Dietary intervention generally involves restricting substances that cannot be properly metabolized and supplying substances that cannot be produced. Thus, dietary changes may be able to improve outcomes of some inborn errors by:

- Preventing the accumulation of toxic metabolites
- Replacing nutrients that are deficient as a result of a defective metabolic pathway
- Providing a diet that supports normal growth and development and maintains health

Successful treatment for an inborn error of metabolism depends on the ability to screen newborns and diagnose metabolic diseases before irreversible damage can occur. After a genetic defect is identified, family members undergo **genetic counseling** to evaluate the likelihood that they may pass on the disorder to future offspring. During counseling, couples may learn about reproductive options such as artificial insemination, *in vitro* fertilization, or prenatal monitoring after conception.

Are there treatments for inborn errors that don't involve dietary changes?

Nondietary therapies can treat some inborn errors of metabolism, although the options are somewhat limited. In some cases, the missing protein is infused; this is the primary means of treating **hemophilia,** caused by deficiency of one of the plasma proteins needed for clotting blood. Drug therapy is the main treatment for some inborn errors, including **cystic fibrosis** (discussed in Chapter 18), which is characterized by a defect that prevents normal chloride transport across cell membranes. Future approaches may include **gene therapy,** a treatment that introduces DNA sequences into the chromosomes of affected cells, prompting the cells to express the protein needed to correct the abnormality.

What is an example of an inborn error that benefits from dietary treatment?

A classic example is **phenylketonuria (PKU),** a metabolic disorder that affects amino acid metabolism. PKU occurs in approximately 1 out of every 10,000 births in the United States each year.[2] In PKU, the missing or defective protein is a liver enzyme that converts the essential amino acid phenylalanine to the amino acid tyrosine (see Figure NP15-1). Without this enzyme, phenylalanine and its **metabolites** (metabolic products) accumulate and damage the developing nervous system. The impairment in the metabolic pathway also prevents liver synthesis of tyrosine and tyrosine-derived compounds (such as the neurotransmitter epinephrine). Under these conditions, tyrosine becomes essential: the body cannot produce tyrosine, and therefore the diet must supply it.

Although PKU's most debilitating effect is on brain development, other symptoms may manifest if the condition is untreated. Infants with PKU may have poor appetites and grow slowly. They may be irritable or have tremors or seizures. Their bodies and urine may have a musty odor. Their skin may be unusually pale, and they may develop skin rashes. In older children and adults who discontinue treatment, neurological and psychological problems are common.

FIGURE NP15-1 | Biochemical Alterations in PKU

Normal:

Normally, the amino acid phenylalanine follows two pathways, one in the liver and the other in the kidneys. In the liver, the enzyme phenylalanine hydroxylase adds a hydroxyl group (OH) to produce the amino acid tyrosine. Tyrosine, in turn, produces melanin, the pigmented compound found in skin and brain cells; the neurotransmitters epinephrine and norepinephrine; and the hormone thyroxin. In the kidneys, enzymes convert phenylalanine to by-products that are excreted.

In the liver:

Phenylalanine →(Phenylalanine hydroxylase)→ Tyrosine → Melanin / Epinephrine / Norepinephrine / Thyroxin

In the kidneys:

Phenylalanine → Phenylpyruvic acid (a ketone body) → Other phenyl acids (excreted)

In PKU:

Individuals with PKU lack the liver enzyme phenylalanine hydroxylase, impairing conversion of phenylalanine to tyrosine. Phenylalanine accumulates in the liver and blood, reaching the kidneys in abnormally high concentrations. In the kidneys, an aminotransferase enzyme converts phenylalanine to the ketone body phenylpyruvic acid, which spills into the urine—thus the name phenylketonuria.

In the liver:

Phenylalanine (accumulates) →(Phenylalanine hydroxylase (deficient))→ Tyrosine (deficient)

In the kidneys:

Phenylalanine (accumulates) → Phenylpyruvic acid (accumulates) → Other phenyl acids (accumulate)

How is PKU diagnosed?

Although PKU is not evident at birth, it must be diagnosed in the first few days of life so that early treatment can prevent its devastating effects. For this reason, newborns are screened for PKU in all 50 states.[3] A standard blood test for phenylalanine is typically conducted by heel puncture after the infant has consumed several meals containing protein (usually after 24 hours). Abnormal results require further testing.

The screening of newborns for PKU is one of the most common genetic tests in the United States and many other countries. Before widespread newborn screening, infants with PKU demonstrated developmental delays (for example, inability to crawl) by six to nine months of age. By the time parents recognized the problem, the damage was irreversible. Most of the damaging consequences of this disorder are now prevented due to the early detection and treatment of PKU.

What is the treatment for PKU?

The only current treatment for PKU is a diet that restricts phenylalanine and supplies tyrosine so that the blood levels of these amino acids are maintained within safe ranges. Because phenylalanine is an essential amino acid, the diet cannot exclude it completely. Children with PKU need phenylalanine to grow, but they cannot handle excesses without detrimental effects. Therefore, their diets must provide enough phenylalanine to support growth and health but not so much as to cause harm. The diets must also provide tyrosine, which is an essential nutrient for individuals with PKU. To ensure that blood concentrations of phenylalanine and tyrosine are close to normal, blood tests are performed periodically, and diets are adjusted when necessary. If the dietary treatment is conscientiously followed, it can prevent the symptoms described earlier. Adults with PKU must continue to follow the PKU diet as well to prevent deterioration in brain function.

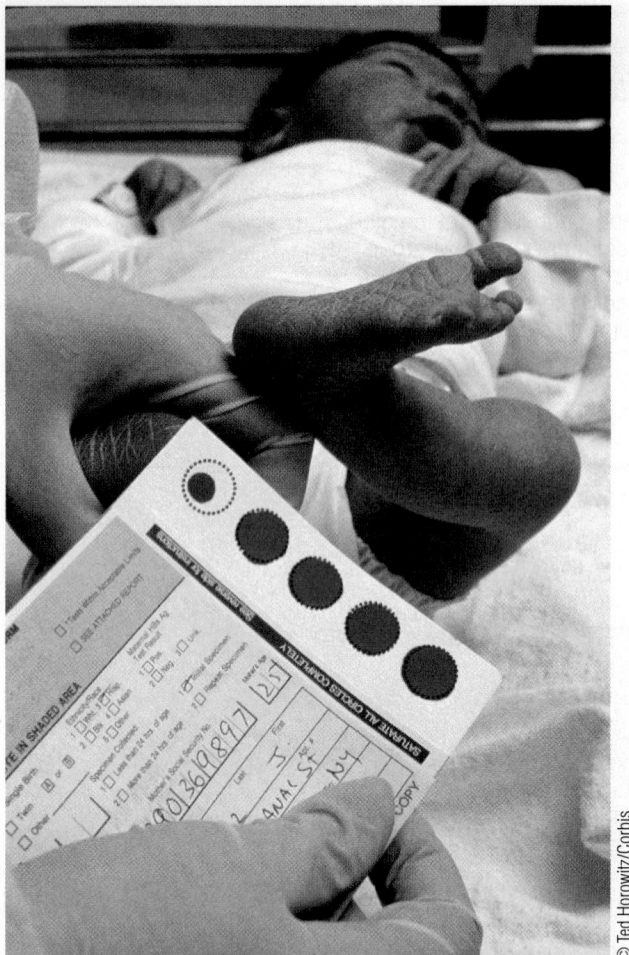

A simple blood test screens newborns for PKU—a common inborn error of metabolism.

What are the main features of the PKU diet?

Central to the PKU diet is the use of an enteral formula that is phenylalanine-free yet supplies energy, amino acids, vitamins, and minerals. For infants, the phenylalanine-free formula can be supplemented with measured amounts of breast milk or regular infant formula to provide the phenylalanine needed for growth. Low-phenylalanine formulas are available for infants who must meet all of their nutrient needs with formula. Formula requirements need to be recalculated periodically to accommodate the growing infant's shifting needs for protein, phenylalanine, tyrosine, and energy.

Once food consumption begins, a phenylalanine-free formula supplies the needed amino acids, and foods that contain phenylalanine are carefully monitored. All proteins contain some phenylalanine; therefore, high-protein foods such as meat, fish, poultry, milk, cheese, legumes, and nuts (including peanut butter) are omitted. Fruits, vegetables, and cereals also contain phenylalanine, so

only limited amounts are allowed. Low-protein flours and mixes are available for making low-phenylalanine breads, pasta, cakes, and cookies. Foods that do not contain phenylalanine, such as jams, jellies, and most sweeteners, can be used freely. Growth rates and nutrition status are monitored to ensure that the diet is adequate. Note that older children, teens, and adults with PKU should continue to use the phenylalanine-free formulas to help meet their protein and energy needs.

Parents and children should be encouraged to develop creative ways to make these diets enjoyable. The formula can be flavored or combined with fruits or juices to make smoothies or frozen juice bars. Sandwiches can include low-phenylalanine breads and fillings such as mashed bananas or avocados, shredded carrots and olives, or tomato slices with mayonnaise. Children often enjoy creating special recipes with permitted foods to make their choices more varied and to share meals with friends.

How long should a person with PKU continue the dietary treatment?

Lifelong adherence to a phenylalanine-restricted diet is currently recommended for all individuals with PKU. Elevated phenylalanine levels can adversely affect cognitive function at any age. Case studies have suggested that individuals with PKU who discontinue dietary management may have problems with attention span, concentration, and memory. It is especially important that women with PKU maintain safe phenylalanine concentrations during pregnancy. Elevated phenylalanine levels, especially during the first trimester, have been associated with mental retardation and organ malformations in the offspring of PKU mothers who have discontinued dietary treatment.[4]

What is another example of an inborn error that requires dietary changes?

Galactosemia is an example of an inborn error of carbohydrate metabolism. Individuals with galactosemia are deficient in one of the enzymes needed to metabolize galactose, a sugar that is primarily found in milk products (recall that each lactose molecule contains galactose). An accumulation of galactose can cause damage in multiple tissues. Infants with galactosemia who are given milk react with severe vomiting and liver jaundice within days of the initial feeding. Serious liver damage can develop and progress to symptomatic cirrhosis. Other complications may include kidney failure, cataracts, and brain damage. Treatment in the first weeks of life can prevent the most detrimental effects of galactose accumulation, but if treatment is delayed, the damage to the brain is irreversible.[5]

Enteral and Parenteral Nutrition Support

What is the dietary treatment for galactosemia?

The diet for galactosemia is much simpler than the diet for PKU. For one thing, galactose is not an essential nutrient. The galactosemia diet essentially eliminates galactose from the diet and does not need to provide a carefully determined amount of any nutrient, as the PKU diet does. In addition, dietary galactose is primarily obtained from lactose (the milk sugar), so the main focus of dietary treatment is the exclusion of milk and milk products. A number of other foods that contain galactose in substantial amounts, such as organ meats and some legumes, fruits, and vegetables, must also be avoided or restricted. Patients receive food lists that identify the galactose content of common foods.

Infants diagnosed with galactosemia are given lactose-free formulas to meet their nutrient needs. Once a child can consume adequate amounts of regular foods, special formulas are unnecessary. However, care must be taken to ensure that the diet supplies adequate calcium.

How effective is the dietary treatment for galactosemia?

Although the early introduction of a galactose-restricted diet can eliminate the acute toxic effects of galactosemia, complications of the disease may develop despite an individual's compliance with diet therapy. For example, most patients experience delays in speech and language development. Ovarian failure occurs in up to 85 percent of women who have galactosemia.[6] In addition, some evidence suggests that IQ declines as a person with galactosemia ages. The reasons for these long-term complications are not fully understood.

As our scientific understanding of human genetics and biochemistry increases, more inborn errors of metabolism are being recognized. Mainstays of management for these diseases include effective diagnosis, early treatment, and control of environmental factors that cause toxicity. In some cases, dietary changes are central to treatment and can prevent serious complications. Not all inborn errors are easily treated, however. Future developments in biotechnology may someday allow medical practitioners to correct genetic errors using gene therapy.

Glossary

cystic fibrosis: an inherited disorder that affects the transport of chloride across epithelial cell membranes; primarily affects the gastrointestinal and respiratory systems.

galactosemia (ga-LAK-toe-SEE-me-ah): an inherited disorder that affects galactose metabolism. Accumulated galactose causes damage to the liver, kidneys, and brain in untreated patients.

gene therapy: treatment for inherited disorders, in which DNA sequences are introduced into the chromosomes of affected cells, prompting the cells to express the protein needed to correct the disease.

genetic counseling: support for families at risk of genetic disorders; involves diagnosis of disease, identification of inheritance patterns within the family, and review of reproductive options.

hemophilia (HE-moh-FEEL-ee-ah): an inherited bleeding disorder characterized by deficiency or malfunction of a plasma protein needed for clotting blood.

inborn error of metabolism: an inherited trait (one that is present at birth) that causes the absence, deficiency, or malfunction of a protein that has a critical metabolic role.

metabolites: products of metabolism; compounds produced by a biochemical pathway.

mutation: an inheritable alteration in the DNA sequence of a gene.

phenylketonuria (FEN-il-KEY-toe-NU-ree-ah) or PKU: an inherited disorder that affects the conversion of the essential amino acid phenylalanine to the amino acid tyrosine.

Notes

1. L. J. Elsas II, Approach to inborn errors of metabolism, in L. Goldman and D. Ausiello, eds., *Cecil Medicine* (Philadelphia: Saunders, 2008), pp. 1539–1546.
2. S. D. Cederbaum, Disorders of phenylalanine and tyrosine metabolism, in L. Goldman and D. Ausiello, eds., *Cecil Medicine* (Philadelphia: Saunders, 2008), pp. 1573–1576.
3. L. J. Elsas II and P. B. Acosta, Inherited metabolic disease: Amino acids, organic acids, and galactose, in M. E. Shils and coeditors, *Modern Nutrition in Health and Disease* (Baltimore: Lippincott Williams & Wilkins, 2006), pp. 909–959.
4. Cederbaum, 2008.
5. L. J. Elsas II, Galactosemia, in L. Goldman and D. Ausiello, eds., *Cecil Medicine* (Philadelphia: Saunders, 2008), pp. 1555–1558.
6. Elsas, Galactosemia, 2008.

CHAPTER 16 | # Nutrition in Metabolic and Respiratory Stress

David Hanover/Getty Images

CONTENTS

THE BODY'S DRAMATIC RESPONSE TO SEVERE STRESS CAN alter metabolism enough to threaten survival. Many patients with severe stress require life support measures and intensive monitoring. Stress also raises nutritional needs considerably—increasing the risk of malnutrition even in previously healthy individuals. **Metabolic stress**, a disruption in the body's internal chemical environment, can result from uncontrolled infections or extensive tissue damage, such as deep, penetrating wounds or multiple broken bones. As the first part of this chapter explains, the body's stress response is an attempt to restore balance, but it can have both helpful and harmful effects. The final sections of this chapter describe **respiratory stress**, which is characterized by inadequate oxygen and excessive carbon dioxide in the blood and tissues. Both metabolic and respiratory stress can lead to **hypermetabolism** (above-normal metabolic rate), **wasting** (breakdown of muscle mass and loss of strength), and, in severe circumstances, life-threatening complications. The accompanying glossary defines some terms related to metabolic stress.

Although severe metabolic stress can have damaging consequences, the healthy body handles minor stresses quickly and efficiently.

The Body's Responses to Stress and Injury

The **stress response** is the body's *nonspecific* response to a variety of stressors, such as infection, fractures, surgery, and burns. During stress, the metabolic processes that support immediate survival are given priority, while those of lesser consequence are delayed. Energy is of primary importance, and therefore the energy nutrients are mobilized from storage and made available in the blood. Heart rate and respiration (breathing rate) increase to deliver oxygen and nutrients to cells more quickly, and blood pressure rises. Meanwhile, energy is diverted from processes that are not life sustaining, such as growth, reproduction, and long-term immunity. If stress continues

Glossary of Terms Related to Metabolic Stress

acute-phase response: changes in body chemistry resulting from infection, inflammation, or injury; characterized by alterations in plasma proteins.

complement: a group of plasma proteins that assist the activities of antibodies.

C-reactive protein: an acute-phase protein released from the liver during acute inflammation or stress.

cytokines (SIGH-toe-kines): signaling proteins produced by the body's cells; those produced by white blood cells regulate various aspects of immune function.

eicosanoids (eye-KO-sa-noids): 20-carbon molecules derived from dietary fatty acids that help to regulate blood pressure, blood clotting, and other body functions.
- **eicosa** = twenty

hypermetabolism: a higher-than-normal metabolic rate.

inflammatory response: a group of nonspecific immune responses to infection or injury.

mast cells: cells within connective tissue that produce and release histamine.

metabolic stress: a disruption in the body's chemical environment due to the effects of disease or injury. Metabolic stress is characterized by changes in metabolic rate, heart rate, blood pressure, hormonal status, and nutrient metabolism.

phagocytes (FAG-oh-sites): white blood cells (neutrophils and macrophages) that have the ability to engulf and destroy antigens.
- **phagein** = to eat

respiratory stress: abnormal gas exchange between the air and blood, resulting in lower-than-normal oxygen levels and higher-than-normal carbon dioxide levels.

sepsis: a whole-body inflammatory response caused by infection; characterized by symptoms similar to those of *systemic inflammatory response syndrome* (see definition below).

shock: a severe reduction in blood flow that deprives the body's tissues of oxygen and nutrients; characterized by reduced blood pressure, raised heart and respiratory rates, and muscle weakness.

stress response: the chemical and physical changes that occur within the body during stress.

systemic (sih-STEM-ic): relating to the entire body.

systemic inflammatory response syndrome (SIRS): a whole-body inflammatory response caused by severe illness or trauma; characterized by raised heart and respiratory rates, increased white blood cell counts, and elevated body temperature.

wasting: the breakdown of muscle tissue that results from disease or malnutrition.

TABLE 16-1	Metabolic Effects of Hormones Released during the Stress Response

Hormone	Metabolic Effects
Catecholamines	• Increase in metabolic rate • Glycogen breakdown in liver and muscle • Glucose production from amino acids • Release of fatty acids from adipose tissue • Glucagon secretion from pancreas
Glucagon	• Glycogen breakdown in liver • Glucose production from amino acids • Release of fatty acids from adipose tissue
Cortisol	• Protein degradation • Enhancement of glucagon's action on liver glycogen • Glucose production from amino acids • Release of fatty acids from adipose tissue
Aldosterone	• Sodium reabsorption in kidneys
Antidiuretic hormone	• Water reabsorption in kidneys

for a long period, interference with these processes begins to cause damage, possibly resulting in growth retardation and illness.

HORMONAL RESPONSES TO STRESS

The stress response is mediated by several hormones, which are released into the blood soon after the onset of injury (see Table 16-1).[1] The catecholamines (epinephrine and norepinephrine), often called the *fight-or-flight hormones*, stimulate heart muscle, raise blood pressure, and increase metabolic rate. Epinephrine also promotes glucagon secretion from the pancreas, prompting the release of nutrients from storage. The steroid hormone cortisol enhances protein degradation, raising amino acid levels in the blood and making amino acids available for conversion to glucose. All of these hormones have similar effects on glucose and fat metabolism, causing the breakdown of glycogen, the production of glucose from amino acids, and the breakdown of triglycerides in adipose tissue. (✚) Thus, the combined effects of these hormones contribute to hyperglycemia, which often accompanies critical illness. Two other hormones induced by stress, aldosterone and antidiuretic hormone, help to maintain blood volume by stimulating the kidneys to reabsorb more sodium and water, respectively.

Cortisol's effects can be detrimental when stress is prolonged. In excess, cortisol causes the depletion of protein in muscle, bone, connective tissue, and skin. It impairs wound healing, so high cortisol levels are especially dangerous for a patient with severe injuries. Because cortisol inhibits protein synthesis, consuming more protein cannot easily reverse tissue losses. Excess cortisol also leads to insulin resistance, contributing to hyperglycemia. In addition, cortisol suppresses immune responses, increasing susceptibility to infection. Note that the pharmaceutical forms of cortisol are common anti-inflammatory medications (such as *cortisone* and *prednisone*); their long-term use may cause undesirable side effects such as muscle wasting, thinning of the skin, diabetes, and early osteoporosis.

✚ The catecholamines, glucagon, and cortisol have actions that oppose those of insulin and are therefore referred to as *counterregulatory hormones*.

NURSING DIAGNOSIS

Impaired tissue integrity and *risk for infection* may apply to a person who undergoes prolonged stress.

Nutrition in Metabolic and Respiratory Stress

THE INFLAMMATORY RESPONSE

Cells of the immune system mount a quick, nonspecific response to infection or tissue injury. This so-called **inflammatory response** serves to contain and destroy infectious agents (and their products) and prevent further tissue damage. As in the stress response, however, there is a delicate balance between a response that protects tissues from further injury and an excessive response that can cause additional damage to tissue.

The Inflammatory Process The inflammatory response begins with the dilation of blood vessels that deliver blood to the site of an injury (arterioles) and the constriction of small blood vessels that carry blood away from an infected area (venules). The capillaries within the damaged tissue become more permeable, allowing some blood plasma to escape into the tissue and cause local edema (see Figure 16-1). These changes in blood vessels (✚) limit or prevent the spread of infection and encourage the entry of immune cells that can destroy foreign agents. Among the first cells to arrive are the **phagocytes**, which slip through gaps between the endothelial cells that form the vessel walls. The phagocytes engulf microorganisms and destroy them with hydrolytic enzymes and reactive forms of oxygen. When inflammation becomes chronic, these normally useful products of phagocytes can damage healthy tissue.

Mediators of Inflammation Numerous chemical substances control the inflammatory process. These *mediators* are released from damaged tissue, blood vessel cells, and activated immune cells. Many of them help to regulate more than one step in the process. Histamine, a small molecule similar to an amino acid in structure, is released from granules within **mast cells**, causing vasodilation and capillary permeability. (✚) Other compounds that participate in the inflammatory process include **cytokines**, produced by white blood cells (and several other types of cells), and **eicosanoids**, which are derived from dietary fatty acids. Note that most anti-inflammatory medications, including steroidal drugs (such as cortisone and prednisone) and nonsteroidal anti-inflammatory drugs (such as aspirin and ibuprofen), act by blocking eicosanoid synthesis.

Changing dietary fat sources can have subtle effects on the inflammatory process.[2] The major precursor for the eicosanoids is arachidonic acid, which derives from the omega-6 fatty acids in vegetable oils. Some omega-3 fatty acids compete with

✚ The classic signs of inflammation that accompany altered blood flow are:
- *Swelling*—from the accumulation of fluid at the site of injury
- *Redness*—from the dilation of small blood vessels in the injured area
- *Heat*—from the influx of warm arterial blood
- *Pain*—from the pressure of edema within the damaged tissue and the actions of certain chemical mediators on pain receptors

✚ *Antihistamines* are medications taken to reduce the effects of histamine.

FIGURE 16-1 | The Inflammatory Process

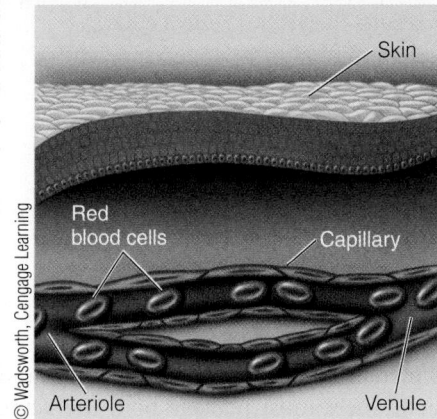

Cells lining the blood vessels lie close together and normally do not allow the contents to cross into tissue.

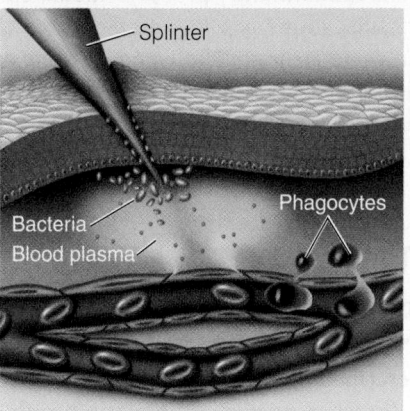

When tissues are damaged, immune cells release histamine, which dilates some blood vessels, increasing blood flow to the damaged area. Fluid leaks out of capillaries (causing swelling), and phagocytes escape between the small gaps in the blood vessel walls.

Phagocytes engulf bacteria and disable them with hydrolytic enzymes and reactive forms of oxygen.

arachidonic acid and inhibit the production of the most powerful inflammatory mediators. Partially replacing vegetable oils rich in omega-6 fatty acids with food sources high in omega-3 fatty acids (such as fish oil) helps to suppress inflammation, but it is not a reliable treatment.

Systemic Effects of Inflammation Cytokines released during the inflammatory process induce **systemic** effects as well as the localized effects described earlier. Within hours (or, in some cases, days) after inflammation, infection, or severe injury, the liver steps up its production of certain proteins in an effort known as the **acute-phase response.**[3] These acute-phase proteins include **C-reactive protein, (✚) complement**, blood-clotting proteins such as fibrinogen and prothrombin, and others. At the same time, plasma concentrations of albumin, iron, and zinc fall (recall from Chapter 13 that albumin levels are often measured to assess health and nutrition status). The acute-phase response is accompanied by muscle catabolism to make amino acids available for glucose production, tissue repair, and immune protein synthesis; consequently, negative nitrogen balance (and wasting) frequently results. Other clinical features include an elevated metabolic rate, increased neutrophil levels in the blood, lethargy, anorexia, and, often, fever.

If inflammation does not resolve, the continued production of pro-inflammatory cytokines may lead to the **systemic inflammatory response syndrome (SIRS)**, which is diagnosed when the patient's symptoms include substantial increases in heart rate, respiratory rate, white blood cell counts, and/or body temperature. If these symptoms result from a severe infection, the condition is called **sepsis.** Complications associated with severe cases of SIRS or sepsis include fluid retention and tissue edema, low blood pressure, and impaired blood flow. If the reduction in blood flow is severe enough to deprive the body's tissues of oxygen and nutrients (a condition known as **shock**), multiple organs may fail simultaneously, as discussed in Nutrition in Practice 16.

✚ C-reactive protein, the best clinical indicator of the acute-phase response, becomes elevated during many chronic diseases.

abscesses (AB-sess-es): accumulations of pus.

debridement: the surgical removal of dead, damaged, or contaminated tissue resulting from burns or wounds; helps to prevent infection and hasten healing.

Review Notes

- The stress and inflammatory responses are nonspecific responses to stressors that cause infection and injury.
- The stress response is mediated by the catecholamine hormones, cortisol, and glucagon, which together raise nutrient levels in blood, stimulate heart rate, raise blood pressure, and increase metabolic rate. Aldosterone and antidiuretic hormone help to maintain adequate blood volume.
- The inflammatory process—mediated by compounds released from damaged tissues, immune cells, and blood vessels—results in systemic effects that alter nutrient metabolism, heart rate, blood pressure, body temperature, and immune cell functions. Persistent, severe inflammation may lead to shock and increases the risk of multiple organ dysfunction.

Nutrition Treatment of Acute Stress

As described earlier, an excessive response to metabolic stress can worsen illness and even threaten survival. Therefore, health practitioners must manage both the acute medical condition that initiated stress and the complications that arise as a result of the stress and inflammatory responses. Immediate concerns during severe stress are to restore lost fluids and electrolytes and to remove underlying stressors. Thus, initial treatments include administering intravenous solutions to correct fluid and electrolyte imbalances, treating infections, repairing wounds, draining **abscesses** (accumulated pus), and removing dead tissue (**debridement**). After stabilization, nutrient needs can be assessed and medical nutrition therapy provided.

DETERMINING NUTRITIONAL REQUIREMENTS

The most notable metabolic changes in patients undergoing metabolic stress include hypermetabolism, negative nitrogen balance, insulin resistance, and hyperglycemia. Hypermetabolism and negative nitrogen balance can result in wasting, which may impair organ function and delay recovery. Hyperglycemia increases the risk of infection, a dangerous problem during critical illness. Therefore, the principal goals of medical nutrition therapy are to preserve lean tissue, maintain immune defenses, and promote healing.

Feeding an acutely stressed patient is often challenging. Overfeeding increases the risks of refeeding syndrome (✚) and its associated hyperglycemia. Underfeeding can worsen negative nitrogen balance and increase lean tissue losses. Assessing nutritional needs can be complicated, however, because fluid imbalances prevent accurate weight measurements, and laboratory data may reflect the metabolic alterations of illness rather than the person's nutrition status.

The amounts of protein and energy to provide during acute illness are controversial and still under investigation. Research results have been mixed, in part because a wide assortment of conditions can lead to metabolic stress and each patient's situation is somewhat different. Moreover, protein and energy needs can vary substantially over the course of illness. The guidelines presented here are subject to change as new findings help to resolve the complex issues related to nutrient intakes and delivery methods. In all cases, clinicians need to closely observe patients' responses to feedings and readjust nutrient intakes as necessary.

Estimating Energy Needs in Acute Stress A common method for determining the energy needs of acutely stressed individuals is to estimate or measure the resting metabolic rate (RMR) and then multiply the result by a stress factor to account for the increased energy requirements of stress and healing. This method was introduced in Chapter 14 (see p. 410 and the "How to" on p. 411); Table 16-2 reviews

✚ Reminder: *Refeeding syndrome* can develop when a severely malnourished person is aggressively fed; it is associated with fluid and electrolyte imbalances and hyperglycemia.

TABLE 16-2	Using Disease-Specific Stress Factors to Estimate Energy Needs in Hospital Patients

Method:

Step 1. Estimate the energy needed to support resting metabolic rate (RMR) using indirect calorimetry or a predictive equation (see Table 14-3, p. 411).

Step 2. Multiply the estimated RMR by an appropriate stress factor for acute illness (see the "How to" box on p. 411).

Examples of disease-specific stress factors:
- Advanced liver disease: 1.0 to 1.16
- Inflammatory bowel disease (active): 1.05 to 1.10
- Pancreatitis: 1.13 to 1.21
- Surgery: 1.2 to 1.4
- Leukemia: 1.25 to 1.35
- Mechanical ventilation: 1.32 to 1.34
- Burns (20 to 30 percent of body surface): 1.6 to 1.7
- Burns (30 to 40 percent of body surface): 1.8 to 1.9
- Burns (40 to 45 percent of body surface): 2.0

Adjustment for obesity:

In some individuals with BMI >30, using an adjusted body weight in RMR equations may provide more accurate results.[a] One popular method is to use a weight that falls between the person's actual body weight and an ideal body weight (IBW):

$$\text{Adjusted weight} = \text{IBW} + [0.5 \times (\text{actual body weight} - \text{IBW})]$$

[a] The use of adjusted body weights for determining energy requirements in obese individuals is controversial and under investigation.

Sources: American Dietetic Association, *Nutrition Care Manual* (Chicago: American Dietetic Association, 2009); N. Barak, E. Wall-Alonso, and M.D. Sitrin, Evaluation of stress factors and body weight adjustments currently used to estimate energy expenditure in hospitalized patients, *Journal of Parenteral and Enteral Nutrition* 26 (2002): 231–238.

+ 72.7 kg×25 kcal/kg=1818 kcal
72.7 kg×30 kcal/kg=2181 kcal

+ Reminder: The protein RDA for adults is 0.8 grams per kilogram body weight.

the use of stress factors for determining energy requirements and provides examples. Generally, energy needs are increased by fever, mechanical ventilation, restlessness, and the presence of open wounds; patients with burns and infections typically have the highest energy requirements. Note that hospital patients undergoing acute stress are usually bedridden, so the energy needed for physical activity is minimal.

Predictive equations used for determining energy needs sometimes include "built-in" stress factors to account for stress, injury, or intensive treatment. Table 16-3 lists examples of equations used for critical care patients and describes the use of the Ireton–Jones equation, which includes multipliers for the presence of trauma and burn injuries.

A quick method for estimating energy needs is to multiply a person's body weight by a factor appropriate for the medical condition. For example, daily energy needs for critical care patients often fall within the range of 25 to 30 kcalories per kilogram of body weight;[4] a patient weighing 160 pounds (72.7 kilograms) may therefore require between 1818 and 2181 kcalories per day. (+) The energy intake can be started within this range and then adjusted as the patient's body weight and other determinants of nutrition status change.

Protein Requirements in Acute Stress

To maintain lean tissue, the protein intakes recommended during acute stress are higher than DRI values. (+) In many critically ill patients, protein needs may range between 1.2 and 2 grams per kilogram body weight per day;[5] burn patients may require between 2 and 3 grams per kilogram body weight each day due to the substantial losses of protein associated with burn wounds.[6] Even with adequate protein, however, negative nitrogen balance cannot be prevented during acute stress because hormonal changes encourage the degradation of body protein. The bed rest required during critical illness also contributes substantially to muscle breakdown.

The amino acids glutamine and arginine are sometimes added to the diets of acutely stressed and immune-compromised patients. Studies have suggested that glutamine supplementation may improve immune function, preserve muscle mass, and

TABLE 16-3	Selected Equations for Estimating Energy Needs in Critical Care Patients[a]

Ireton–Jones

Energy needs (kcal/day) = 1925 + [5 × wt (kg)] − [10 × age (yr)] + (281 × sex) + (292 × trauma) + (851 × burn)

where sex is male (×1) or female (×0), trauma is the presence of physical injury (×1) or not (×0), and burn is the presence of a burn injury (×1) or not (×0).

Penn State

Energy needs (kcal/day) = [RMR × 0.85] + [V_E × 33] + [T_{max} × 175] − 6433

where RMR is calculated using the Harris–Benedict equation (see Table 14-3, p. 411), V_E is minute ventilation in liters per minute (reading taken from the ventilator), and T_{max} is the patient's maximum body temperature (in degrees Celsius) in the preceding 24 hours.

Example (Ireton–Jones equation): Erin is a 27-year-old female patient who weighs 140 pounds (63.6 kilograms). Two days ago, she was severely injured in an automobile accident and is currently being cared for in a critical care unit where she is receiving mechanical ventilation. She did not suffer a burn injury. Using the Ireton–Jones equation shown above, her daily energy needs can be estimated as follows:

Energy needs (kcal/day)

= 1925 + [5 × wt (kg)] − [10 × age (yr)] + (281 × sex) + (292 × trauma) + (851 × burn)

= 1925 + (5 × 63.6 kg) − (10 × 27 yr) + (281 × 0) + (292 × 1) + (851 × 0)

= 1925 + 318 − 270 + 0 + 292 + 0 = 2265 kcal

[a] The equations shown here were developed for ventilator-dependent patients.

reduce mortality rates in critically ill patients.[7] Arginine supplementation may have beneficial effects on the immune responses and nitrogen balance of critically ill and postoperative patients.[8] Although glutamine and arginine are often added to enteral formulas promoted for wound healing and enhanced immunity, their use remains controversial.

Carbohydrate and Fat Intakes in Acute Stress

The bulk of energy needs are supplied from carbohydrate and fat. Carbohydrate is usually the main source of energy, providing 50 to 60 percent of total energy requirements.[9] (✚) In patients who have severe hyperglycemia, fat may supply up to 50 percent of kcalories, although high fat intakes may suppress immune function and increase the risks of developing infections and hypertriglyceridemia. Patients with blood triglyceride levels above 300 to 400 milligrams per deciliter may require fat restriction.[10]

Micronutrient Needs in Acute Stress

Acutely stressed patients are believed to have increased micronutrient needs, but specific requirements remain unknown.[11] In hypermetabolic patients, the need for B vitamins may be higher to support the increase in energy metabolism. A number of micronutrients, such as vitamin A, vitamin C, and zinc, have critical roles in immunity and wound healing, and their supplementation may speed recovery under certain circumstances. Patients with burns and tissue injuries may have increased requirements for trace minerals due to tissue losses; in several studies, supplementation of zinc, copper, and selenium improved immune responses in severely burned patients.[12]

Plasma levels of micronutrients are often altered during critical illness. The acute-phase response causes a redistribution in the tissue content of some micronutrients that either raises or lowers their blood levels; therefore, micronutrient status is sometimes difficult to interpret. (✚) Blood concentrations of trace minerals are monitored in patients receiving parenteral nutrition support to ensure that excessive amounts are not given intravenously.

APPROACHES TO NUTRITION CARE IN ACUTE STRESS

As mentioned earlier, the initial care following acute stress focuses on maintaining fluid and electrolyte balances. Simple intravenous solutions often contain dextrose, providing minimal kcalories. Once patients are stable, nutrition support may be necessary if poor appetite, the medical condition, or a medical procedure (such as mechanical ventilation) interferes with food intake. For patients with a functional GI tract, early enteral feedings—started in the first 24 to 48 hours after hospitalization—are associated with fewer complications and shorter hospital stays compared with delayed feedings. If enteral nutrition is not possible, malnourished patients may receive parenteral nutrition support soon after admission to the hospital. In previously healthy patients, however, parenteral nutrition support may be withheld during the first seven days of hospitalization to avoid the risk of infectious complications.[13]

Once patients can tolerate oral feedings, a high-kcalorie, high-protein diet is often prescribed, although care must be taken not to overfeed patients who are at risk of developing refeeding syndrome or hyperglycemia. Because meeting protein and energy needs may be difficult, enteral formulas are often provided to supplement the diet. Many such formulas have high nutrient density, and some contain extra amounts of nutrients believed to promote healing or benefit immune function, such as the amino acids arginine and glutamine, omega-3 fatty acids, and the antioxidant nutrients. Nutrient needs should be reassessed frequently until the patient's condition improves. The accompanying Case Study reviews the nutrition care of a patient undergoing acute metabolic stress.

✚ Reminder: When parenteral infusions are necessary, dextrose is usually limited to 5 milligrams per kilogram body weight per minute.

✚ During the acute-phase response, plasma levels of iron and zinc fall, whereas plasma copper levels rise.

NURSING DIAGNOSIS
Imbalanced nutrition: less than body requirements may apply to a patient recovering from acute stress.

David Bray, a 42-year-old mortgage broker, has been admitted to intensive care. He suffered a severe burn covering 35 percent of his body when he was trapped inside a burning building. His wife told the nurse that Mr. Bray's height is 6 feet and that he usually weighs about 175 pounds. The physician ordered lab tests, including serum protein concentrations, but the results have not yet been received.

1. Identify Mr. Bray's immediate needs after the injury. Describe the initial concerns of the health care team and the measures they might take soon after Mr. Bray's arrival at the hospital.

2. Considering Mr. Bray's condition, what problems might the health care team encounter when they attempt to obtain information that can help them assess his nutrition status? What additional concerns might they have if Mr. Bray was malnourished before he experienced the burn?

3. Estimate Mr. Bray's energy and protein needs (use a protein factor of 2.5 grams per kilogram). What problems may interfere with Mr. Bray's ability to meet his nutrient needs?

4. After Mr. Bray transitions to oral feedings, he is able to obtain only 65 percent of his energy requirements. What other feeding options may be considered?

Review Notes

- In patients who are hospitalized with acute stress, initial treatments include restoring fluid and electrolyte balances and treating infections and wounds.
- Metabolic stress can cause hypermetabolism and negative nitrogen balance, and may result in wasting. The objective of nutrition care is to provide a diet that can preserve muscle tissue, maintain immune defenses, and promote healing.
- To determine energy needs during acute stress, RMR values are modified with stress factors that account for the increased demands of the medical condition or treatment. Protein recommendations are higher than DRI levels to help prevent tissue losses and allow healing of damaged tissue.
- Micronutrient needs may be increased during acute stress, but specific requirements remain unknown.
- Enteral and parenteral nutrition support or oral enteral formulas may be used to meet the nutritional needs of acutely stressed patients.

chronic obstructive pulmonary disease (COPD): a group of lung diseases characterized by persistent obstructed airflow through the lungs and airways; includes chronic bronchitis and emphysema.

bronchi (BRON-key), bronchioles (BRON-key-oles): the main airways of the lungs. The singular form of bronchi is *bronchus*.

alveoli (al-VEE-oh-lie): air sacs in the lungs. One air sac is an *alveolus*.

chronic bronchitis (bron-KYE-tis): a lung disorder characterized by persistent inflammation and excessive secretions of mucus in the main airways of the lungs; diagnosis is based on the presence of a chronic, productive cough for at least three months of the year for two successive years.

emphysema (EM-fih-ZEE-mah): a progressive lung condition characterized by the breakdown of the lungs' elastic structure and destruction of the walls of the bronchioles and alveoli, reducing the surface area involved in respiration.

Nutrition and Respiratory Stress

Some medical problems upset the process of gas exchange between the air and blood and result in respiratory stress, which is characterized by a reduction in the blood's oxygen supply and an increase in carbon dioxide levels. Excessive carbon dioxide in the blood may disturb the breathing pattern enough to interfere with food intake. Moreover, the labored breathing caused by many respiratory disorders entails a higher energy cost than normal breathing does, raising energy needs and increasing carbon dioxide production further. Lung diseases make physical activity difficult and can lead to muscle wasting. Weight loss and malnutrition therefore become dangerous outcomes of some types of respiratory illnesses.

CHRONIC OBSTRUCTIVE PULMONARY DISEASE

Chronic obstructive pulmonary disease (COPD) refers to a group of conditions characterized by the persistent obstruction of airflow through the lungs. Figure 16-2 illustrates the main airways (**bronchi** and **bronchioles**) and air sacs (**alveoli**) of the normal respiratory system, and Figure 16-3 shows how they are altered in COPD. The two main types of COPD are **chronic bronchitis** and **emphysema**, and many patients display features of both conditions:[14]

FIGURE
16-2 | The Respiratory System

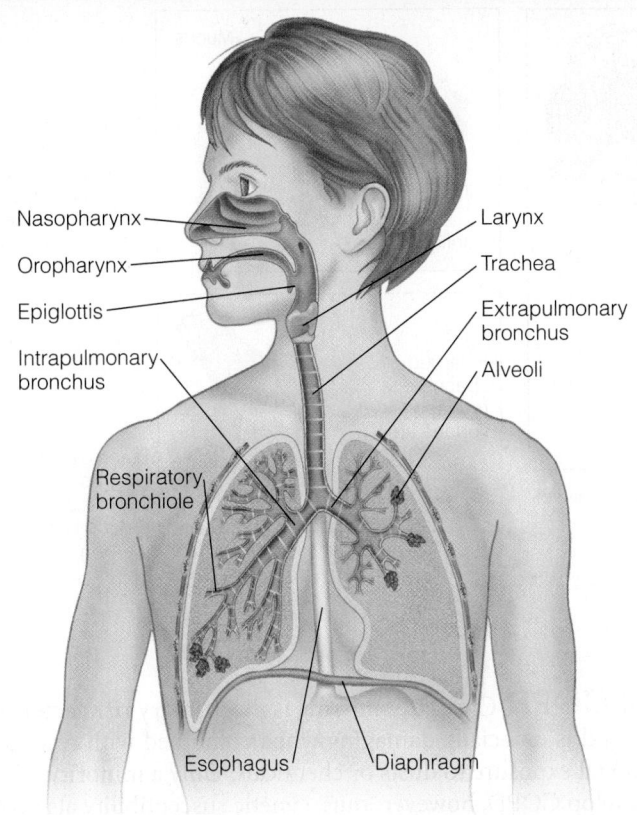

Nasopharynx
Oropharynx
Epiglottis
Intrapulmonary bronchus
Respiratory bronchiole
Larynx
Trachea
Extrapulmonary bronchus
Alveoli
Esophagus
Diaphragm

Based on a drawing in Carol Mattson Porth, Pathophysiology, 5th ed. (Lippincott Williams and Wilkins, 1998).

Inhaled air travels via the trachea to the bronchi and bronchioles, the major airways of the lungs. Oxygen and carbon dioxide are exchanged across the thin-walled alveoli, which are surrounded by capillaries.

- *Chronic bronchitis* is characterized by persistent inflammation and excessive secretions of mucus in the main airways of the lungs, which may ultimately thicken and become too narrow for adequate mucus clearance. Chronic bronchitis is diagnosed when a chronic, productive cough persists for at least three months of the year for two consecutive years.
- *Emphysema* is characterized by the breakdown of the lungs' elastic structure and destruction of the walls of the bronchioles and alveoli, changes that significantly reduce the surface area needed for respiration. Emphysema is diagnosed on the basis of clinical signs and the results of lung function tests.

Both chronic bronchitis and emphysema are associated with abnormal levels of oxygen and carbon dioxide in the blood and shortness of breath (**dyspnea**). COPD may eventually lead to respiratory or heart failure and ranks as the fourth leading cause of death in the United States.[15]

COPD is a debilitating condition. Generally, dyspnea worsens as the disease progresses, resulting in dramatic reductions in physical activity and quality of life. Activities of daily living such as bathing or dressing may cause exhaustion or breathlessness. Weight loss and wasting are common in the advanced stages of disease and may result from hypermetabolism, poor food intake, and the actions of various inflammatory proteins. As with other chronic illnesses, anxiety and depression are a concern, and psychological distress may reduce a COPD patient's ability to cope with the demands of treatment.

dyspnea (DISP-nee-ah): shortness of breath.

FIGURE
16-3 | Chronic Obstructive Pulmonary Disease

Bronchus (plural: bronchi)

Alveolus (plural: alveoli)

Bronchiole

© Wadsworth, Cengage Learning

Healthy bronchi provide an open passageway for air. Healthy alveoli permit gas exhange between the air and blood.

Mucus

Chronic bronchitis is characterized by inflammation, excessive secretion of mucus, and narrowing of the bronchi—factors that reduce normal airflow.

Inflammation

Enlarged air spaces with reduced surface area

Emphysema is characterized by gradual destruction of the walls separating alveoli and reduced lung elasticity.

NURSING DIAGNOSIS

Nursing diagnoses that may apply to people with COPD include *impaired gas exchange*, *ineffective breathing pattern*, *ineffective airway clearance*, and *activity intolerance*.

Patients who need supplemental oxygen can use lightweight, portable equipment that allows them to move around freely.

© Courtesy of AirSep Corporation

Causes of COPD Cigarette smoking is the primary risk factor in 90 percent of COPD cases[16] and is especially damaging when combined with respiratory infections or an occupational exposure to dusts or chemicals. Only a minority of smokers (about 15 percent) develop COPD, however; thus, genetic susceptibility also contributes to its development. Genetic factors are especially likely in patients with early-onset COPD. Alpha-1-antitrypsin deficiency, an inherited disorder, accounts for 1 to 2 percent of COPD cases.[17] Individuals with this defect have inadequate blood levels of a plasma protein (alpha-1 antitrypsin) that normally inhibits enzymatic breakdown of the lungs' connective tissue.

Treatment of COPD The primary objectives of COPD treatment are to prevent the disease from progressing and relieve major symptoms (dyspnea and coughing). Individuals with COPD are encouraged to quit smoking to prevent disease progression and to get vaccinated against influenza and pneumonia to avoid complications. The most frequently prescribed medications are bronchodilators, which improve airflow, and corticosteroids (anti-inflammatory medications), which help to prevent symptom recurrence; note that corticosteroids promote catabolic processes and can exacerbate the muscle loss that often accompanies COPD. For people with severe COPD, supplemental oxygen therapy (12 hours daily) can maintain normal oxygen levels in the blood and reduce mortality risk. The Diet-Drug Interactions feature lists nutrition-related effects of the medications used to treat COPD.

Medical Nutrition Therapy for COPD The main goals of nutrition therapy for COPD are to correct malnutrition (which affects up to 60 percent of patients with COPD),[18] promote the maintenance of a healthy body weight, and prevent muscle wasting. Research studies have found that underweight COPD patients have higher mortality rates;[19] thus, encouraging adequate food intake is generally the main focus of the nutrition care plan. Energy needs of COPD patients are usually raised due to hypermetabolism (about 20 percent above normal), which results from chronic inflammation and the increased workload of respiratory muscles.[20] Because excess body weight places an

DIET-DRUG INTERACTIONS

Check this table for notable nutrition-related effects of the medications discussed in this chapter.

	GASTROINTESTINAL EFFECTS	INTERACTIONS WITH DIETARY SUBSTANCES	METABOLIC EFFECTS
Bronchodilators (theophylline, dyphylline)	Increased gastric acid secretion, acid reflux	Caffeine enhances drug effects (daily caffeine intake should be consistent); excessive alcohol intake can reduce drug clearance.	—
Corticosteroids (prednisone)	—	—	Glucose intolerance, sodium retention, negative nitrogen balance, decreased bone mineral density, appetite stimulation, weight gain, growth suppression in children

additional strain on the respiratory system, COPD patients who are overweight or obese may benefit from energy restriction and gradual weight reduction.

Food intake often declines as COPD progresses, although the causes of poor intake vary among patients. Dyspnea may interfere with chewing or swallowing. Physical changes in the diaphragm and lungs may reduce abdominal volume, leading to early satiety. Appetite may be reduced by medications, depression or anxiety, or altered taste perception. (✚) Some patients may become too disabled to shop or prepare food or may lack adequate support at home. The dietitian or nurse must assess the unique needs of a COPD patient before proposing a nutrition care plan.

Some patients may benefit from eating frequent, small meals spaced throughout the day rather than two or three large ones. The lower energy content of small meals reduces the carbon dioxide load, and abdominal discomfort and dyspnea may be reduced when less food is consumed at one time. Some individuals may eat better if they receive supplemental oxygen at mealtimes. Consuming adequate fluids should be encouraged to help prevent the secretion of overly thick mucus; however, some patients should consume liquids between meals so as not to interfere with food intake. For undernourished persons, a high-kcalorie, high-protein diet may be helpful, but high energy intakes increase the amount of carbon dioxide produced and can increase respiratory stress. Patients are sometimes encouraged to drink liquid supplements between meals to improve weight gain or exercise endurance, but they should be cautioned not to reduce energy intake at mealtime as a result of between-meal snacks.

Pulmonary Formulas Enteral formulas designed for use in COPD provide more kcalories from fat and fewer from carbohydrate than standard formulas. The ratio of carbon dioxide production to oxygen consumption is lower when fat is consumed, so theoretically these formulas should lower respiratory requirements. However, research studies have not confirmed that the reduced-carbohydrate formulas improve clinical outcomes more than moderate energy intakes, so the benefits of using these pulmonary formulas are uncertain.[21]

Incorporating an Exercise Program Loss of muscle can be more readily prevented or reversed if the treatment plan includes an effective exercise program. With exercise, patients are likely to see improvements in their endurance and become less fearful of their physical limitations. For some patients, the combination of an exercise plan and oral supplements may be better for maintaining weight and improving muscle mass than either component of treatment alone.[22] The accompanying Case Study allows you to review the nutrition care for a patient with COPD.

✚ The altered sense of taste in patients with COPD may be due to chronic mouth breathing, which dries the mouth. Taste is also affected by the use of certain medications, including some bronchodilators.

acute respiratory distress syndrome (ARDS): respiratory failure triggered by severe lung injury; a medical emergency that is characterized by dyspnea and pulmonary edema and usually requires mechanical ventilation.

hypoxemia (high-pock-SEE-me-ah): a low level of oxygen in the blood.

hypercapnia (high-per-CAP-nee-ah): excessive carbon dioxide in the blood.

hypoxia (high-POCK-see-ah): a low amount of oxygen in body tissues.

acidosis: acid accumulation in body tissues; depresses the central nervous system and may lead to disorientation and, eventually, coma.

cyanosis (sigh-ah-NOH-sis): a bluish cast in the skin due to the color of deoxygenated hemoglobin. Cyanosis is most evident in individuals with lighter, thinner skin; it is mostly seen on lips, cheeks, and ears and under the nails.

Mechanical ventilation controls the rate and amount of oxygen supplied to a person's airways.

RESPIRATORY FAILURE

In respiratory failure, the gas exchange between the air and circulating blood is severely impaired, causing abnormal levels of tissue gases that can be life threatening. Any of a large number of conditions that cause lung injury or impair lung function can be the underlying cause of failure. Possible causes of respiratory failure include infection (such as pneumonia or sepsis), aspiration of stomach contents, physical trauma, neuromuscular disorders, smoke inhalation, and airway obstruction.[23]

Severe lung damage can lead to **acute respiratory distress syndrome** (**ARDS**), a life-threatening condition that requires the use of mechanical ventilation to restore normal oxygen and carbon dioxide levels. In ARDS, the lungs exhibit extensive inflammation and fluid buildup (called *pulmonary edema*) that interfere with lung ventilation and gas exchange in the alveoli. Later stages are associated with a proliferation of lung cells, which causes fibrosis and disrupts lung structure. A dangerous complication of ARDS is the progression to multiple organ dysfunction syndrome, described in the Nutrition in Practice following this chapter.

Consequences of Respiratory Failure
Respiratory failure is characterized by severe **hypoxemia** (low oxygen levels in the blood) and **hypercapnia** (excessive carbon dioxide in the blood). The low oxygen content of tissues (**hypoxia**) impedes cellular function and may lead to cell death. Severe hypercapnia can cause **acidosis**, which interferes with normal functioning of the central nervous system. To compensate for respiratory failure, a person breathes more rapidly, and the heart rate increases. The skin may become sweaty and develop a bluish cast (**cyanosis**). Headache, confusion, and drowsiness may occur. Severe cases of respiratory failure can cause heart arrhythmias and, ultimately, coma.

Treatment of Respiratory Failure
The treatment of respiratory failure focuses on supporting lung function and correcting the underlying disorder. Because respiratory failure can be caused by a number of different conditions, treatment plans vary considerably. Individuals with chronic lung disorders may be provided with oxygen therapy via a face mask or nasal tubing to relieve symptoms, whereas patients with ARDS receive mechanical ventilation until they are able to breathe independently. Diuretics may be prescribed to mobilize the fluid that has accumulated in lung tissue. Medications are given to treat infections, keep airways open, or relieve inflammation. Complications are common in ARDS and must be forestalled to prevent multiple organ dysfunction.

Medical Nutrition Therapy for Respiratory Failure
Patients with lung injuries or ARDS are frequently hypermetabolic and/or catabolic and at high risk of muscle wasting. The primary concerns are therefore to provide enough energy and protein to sustain muscle mass and lung function without overtaxing the respiratory system. Fluid restrictions may be necessary to help correct pulmonary edema.

When nutrition support is necessary, enteral nutrition is preferred over parenteral nutrition. Specific recommendations for respiratory failure include the following:

- *Energy.* Energy needs typically range from 25 to 35 kilocalories per kilgram.[24] The body weight used to determine energy needs may need to be corrected for pulmonary edema. Energy needs can also be estimated using predictive equations such as those described in Tables 16-2 and 16-3. Overfeeding should be avoided because it can cause excessive carbon dioxide production and worsen respiratory function.
- *Protein.* Protein needs are increased in patients with lung inflammation or ARDS. For mild or moderate lung injury, protein recommendations range from 1.0 to 1.5 grams of protein per kilogram body weight per day. Patients with ARDS may require 1.5 to 2 grams of protein per kilogram body weight daily.
- *Fluids.* Although most patients have normal fluid requirements, fluid status should be monitored daily to prevent fluid imbalance. Some patients may require fluid restriction to prevent edema in lung tissue, whereas others may become dehydrated due to diuretic therapy.

Nutrition Support in Respiratory Failure

Patients with severe cases of respiratory failure may be unable to eat meals and may require nutrition support. Tube feedings are used if the intestine is functional, and intestinal feedings may be preferred over gastric feedings because they reduce the risk of aspiration. Patients with acute lung injuries or ARDS may benefit from enteral formulas designed to reduce inflammation and promote healing, which are typically fortified with omega-3 fatty acids and antioxidant nutrients.[25] Nutrient-dense formulas (1.5 to 2.0 kcalories per milliliter) are prescribed for patients with fluid restrictions. If the risk of aspiration is too high to continue enteral feedings, parenteral nutrition support may be considered.

Review Notes

- Chronic obstructive pulmonary disease (COPD) is a debilitating, progressive illness that can lead to malnutrition, muscle wasting, and activity intolerance. The main types of COPD are chronic bronchitis and emphysema.
- The goals of nutrition therapy for COPD are to improve food intake, maintain proper weight, preserve muscle tissue, and improve exercise endurance.
- Respiratory failure, which is characterized by severe hypoxemia and hypercapnia, can be caused by conditions that cause lung injury or impair lung function. Acute respiratory distress syndrome (ARDS) is a severe form of respiratory failure that requires mechanical ventilation.
- The main goals of nutrition therapy for respiratory failure are to supply enough energy and protein to support lung function without burdening the respiratory system. Fluid restrictions are sometimes necessary to reverse pulmonary edema.

Nutrition Assessment | CHECKLIST FOR PEOPLE UNDERGOING METABOLIC OR RESPIRATORY STRESS

MEDICAL HISTORY

Check the medical record to determine:

- ❍ Cause of stress
- ❍ Severity of stress
- ❍ Whether any organ system is compromised
- ❍ Whether nutrition support is required

For patients with COPD, check to determine:

- ❍ Degree of breathing difficulty
- ❍ Use of oxygen therapy
- ❍ Activity tolerance

Review the medical record for complications related to underfeeding or overfeeding, such as:

○ Dehydration or fluid overload
○ Electrolyte imbalances
○ Fatty liver
○ Hyperglycemia
○ Hypertriglyceridemia

MEDICATIONS

Record all medications and note:

○ Side effects that may alter food intake or nutrition status
○ Use of theophylline, in patients who may need to monitor caffeine intake

DIETARY INTAKE

If the patient is not meeting nutrition goals:

○ Monitor intakes to ensure that the patient is receiving the diet prescribed.
○ Investigate appetite problems or difficulties with eating.
○ Consider interventions to improve food intake.
○ Consider the need for supplementation.
○ In patients with COPD, consider problems that may hamper the patient's ability to prepare or consume foods.

ANTHROPOMETRIC DATA

Measure baseline height and weight, and monitor daily weights. Remember that body weight can fluctuate in acutely ill patients who undergo fluid resuscitation. After the patient's weight has stabilized:

○ Reevaluate protein and energy needs.
○ Consider the need to alter the energy prescription to meet weight goals.

LABORATORY TESTS

Laboratory tests that may be affected by stress and therefore require careful interpretation include:

○ Albumin
○ C-reactive protein
○ Prealbumin
○ Serum iron and zinc
○ Transferrin
○ White blood cell count

Monitor laboratory tests for signs of:

○ Dehydration or fluid overload
○ Electrolyte and acid-base imbalances
○ Hyperglycemia
○ Hypertriglyceridemia
○ Nutrient deficiencies
○ Negative nitrogen balance
○ Organ dysfunction or organ function that has normalized

PHYSICAL SIGNS

Regularly assess vital signs, including:

○ Blood pressure
○ Body temperature
○ Pulse
○ Respiratory rate

Look for physical signs of:

○ Protein-energy malnutrition
○ Dehydration or fluid overload
○ Nutrient deficiencies and excesses

Self Check

1 • Which of the following metabolic changes accompanies acute stress?
  a. Reduced plasma concentrations of glucose and fatty acids
  b. Reduced blood volume and blood pressure
  c. Increased insulin action
  d. Catabolism of protein in muscle and connective tissue

2 • Tissue injury is followed by:
  a. fluid accumulation in damaged tissue.
  b. reduced blood flow to injured tissue.
  c. reduced capillary permeability.
  d. decreased body temperature.

3 • What is a possible effect of replacing vegetable oils rich in omega-6 fatty acids with oils rich in omega-3 fatty acids?
  a. Improvement in blood circulation
  b. Suppression of inflammation
  c. Protection against sepsis
  d. Hypertriglyceridemia

4 • The acute-phase response results in an increased plasma concentration of:
  a. albumin.
  b. iron.
  c. C-reactive protein.
  d. zinc.

5 • Which of the following statements concerning protein and energy recommendations during acute metabolic stress is true?
  a. Protein and energy recommendations are similar to those for healthy people.
  b. Protein and energy recommendations are reduced because a stressed individual cannot metabolize nutrients normally.
  c. Acutely stressed individuals can benefit from as much protein and energy as can be provided.
  d. Protein and energy recommendations are increased to minimize muscle tissue losses.

6 • The amount of protein recommended for an acutely stressed patient who weighs 150 pounds usually ranges from about _____ grams of protein per day.
   a. 55 to 68
   b. 82 to 136
   c. 102 to 170
   d. 136 to 205

7 • The primary risk factor for COPD is:
   a. alpha-1 antitrypsin deficiency.
   b. occupational exposure to dusts or chemicals.
   c. cigarette smoking.
   d. respiratory infections.

8 • A primary feature of emphysema is:
   a. obstruction within the bronchi.
   b. obstruction within the bronchioles.
   c. destruction of the walls separating the alveoli.
   d. excessive lung elasticity.

9 • The weight loss and wasting that often occur in COPD can be caused by:
   a. reduced food intake.
   b. increased metabolic rate.
   c. reduced exercise tolerance.
   d. all of the above.

10 • Medical nutrition therapy for a person with respiratory failure includes:
   a. careful attention to providing enough, but not too much, energy.
   b. a generous fluid intake to facilitate mucus clearance.
   c. a high fat intake to prevent weight loss.
   d. a high carbohydrate intake to increase carbon dioxide production.

Answers to these questions appear in Appendix H.

Clinical Applications

1 • Adam is a 49-year-old male who is 6 feet 2 inches tall and has a usual body weight of 180 pounds. He was physically injured by an explosion in the chemistry lab where he works and is now in the intensive care unit. Using the Ireton–Jones equation shown in Table 16-3 on p. 474, estimate Adam's energy requirement. Estimate his protein requirement, using the factor 1.5 grams per kilogram of body weight.

2 • Ayla is a 23-year-old law student who was admitted to the hospital following an automobile accident in which she broke several bones and ruptured part of her small intestine. She has been in the hospital for several weeks and has just begun eating table foods. Her brother, who was driving the vehicle, was also seriously injured and nearly lost his life. Aside from the increased nutritional needs imposed by the stress of the accident, discuss how the following factors might interfere with Ayla's ability to improve her nutrition status:

   • Ayla's injuries are painful.
   • Ayla's medications cause drowsiness.
   • Ayla is depressed.
   • Ayla is often out of her room for X-rays and other diagnostic tests when the menus and food trays arrive.
   • Ayla's food intake is sometimes restricted due to the procedures she is undergoing.

   How might these problems be resolved to improve Ayla's food intake?

Nutrition on the Net

For further study of topics covered in this chapter, access these websites.

• Find updates and quick links to these and other nutrition-related sites at our website: www.cengage.com/nutrition/whitney/nhhc4e
• To uncover additional information relevant to critical care, visit these sites:
   • American Association of Critical-Care Nurses: www.aacn.org
   • American Society for Parenteral and Enteral Nutrition: www.nutritioncare.org

• This nonprofit group provides comprehensive, up-to-date information for burn care professionals: www.burnsurgery.org
• To learn more about lung diseases, visit these sites:
   • American Lung Association: www.lungusa.org
   • The Lung Association (Canada): www.lung.ca
   • National Heart, Lung, and Blood Institute: www.nhlbi.nih.gov

Notes

1. S. F. Lowry and J. M. Perez, The hypercatabolic state, in M. E. Shils and coeditors, *Modern Nutrition in Health and Disease* (Baltimore: Lippincott Williams & Wilkins, 2006), pp. 1381–1400; M. I. T. D. Correia and C. T. de Almeida, Metabolic response to stress, in G. Cresci, ed., *Nutrition Support for the Critically Ill Patient: A Guide to Practice* (Boca Raton, FL: Taylor & Francis Group, 2005), pp. 3–13.

2. N. D. Riediger and coauthors, A systemic review of the roles of n-3 fatty acids in health and disease, *Journal of the American Dietetic Association* 109 (2009): 668–679; P. C. Calder, Polyunsaturated fatty acids, inflammatory processes and inflammatory bowel diseases, *Molecular Nutrition and Food Research* 8 (2008): 885–897.

3. V. Kumar and coauthors, Acute and chronic inflammation, in V. Kumar and coeditors, *Robbins and Cotran Pathologic Basis of Disease* (Philadelphia: Saunders, 2010), pp. 43–77; D. S. Pisetsky, Laboratory testing in the rheumatic diseases, in L. Goldman and D. Ausiello, eds., *Cecil Medicine* (Philadelphia: Saunders, 2008), pp. 1966–1970.

4. K. A. Kudsk and G. S. Sacks, Nutrition in the care of the patient with surgery, trauma, and sepsis, in M. E. Shils and coeditors, *Modern Nutrition in Health and Disease* (Baltimore: Lippincott Williams & Wilkins, 2006), pp. 1414–1435.

5. S. A. McClave and coauthors, Guidelines for the provision and assessment of nutrition support therapy in the adult critically ill patient: Society of Critical Care Medicine (SCCM) and American Society for Parenteral and Enteral Nutrition (A.S.P.E.N.), *Journal of Parenteral and Enteral Nutrition* 33 (2009): 277–316.

6. American Dietetic Association, *Nutrition Care Manual* (Chicago: American Dietetic Association, 2009).

7. McClave and coauthors, 2009; Lowry and Perez, 2006.

8. M. Zhou and R. G. Martindale, Arginine in the critical care setting, *Journal of Nutrition* 137 (2007): 1687S–1692S; P. Furst, Protein and amino acid metabolism: Comparison of stressed and nonstressed states, in G. Cresci, ed., *Nutrition Support for the Critically Ill Patient: A Guide to Practice* (Boca Raton, FL: Taylor & Francis Group, 2005), pp. 27–47.

9. Kudsk and Sacks, 2006.

10. J. Lefton and P. P. Lopez, Macronutrient requirements: Carbohydrate, protein, and lipid, in G. Cresci, ed., *Nutrition Support for the Critically Ill Patient: A Guide to Practice* (Boca Raton, FL: Taylor & Francis Group, 2005), pp. 99–108.

11. K. Sriram and J. I. Cué, Micronutrient and antioxidant therapy in critically ill patients, in G. Cresci, ed., *Nutrition Support for the Critically Ill Patient: A Guide to Practice* (Boca Raton, FL: Taylor & Francis Group, 2005), pp. 109–123.

12. Kudsk and Sacks, 2006.

13. McClave and coauthors, 2009.

14. A. N. Husain, The lung, in V. Kumar and coeditors, *Robbins and Cotran Pathologic Basis of Disease* (Philadelphia: Saunders, 2010), pp. 677–737; N. Anthonisen, Chronic obstructive pulmonary disease, in L. Goldman and D. Ausiello, eds., *Cecil Medicine* (Philadelphia: Saunders, 2008), pp. 619–627.

15. Husain, 2010.

16. T. J. Prendergast and S. J. Ruoss, Pulmonary disease, in S. J. McPhee and W. F. Ganong, eds., *Pathophysiology of Disease: An Introduction to Clinical Medicine* (New York: McGraw-Hill/Lange, 2006), pp. 218–258.

17. M. H. Beers and coeditors, *The Merck Manual of Diagnosis and Therapy* Whitehouse Station, NJ: Merck Research Laboratories, 2006), pp. 400–422.

18. B. Suckling, M. M. Johnson, and R. Chin, Jr., Nutrition, respiratory function, and disease, in M. E. Shils and coeditors, *Modern Nutrition in Health and Disease* (Baltimore: Lippincott Williams & Wilkins, 2006), pp. 1462–1474.

19. D. A. King, F. Cordova, and S. M. Scharf, Nutritional aspects of chronic obstructive pulmonary disease, *Proceedings of the American Thoracic Society* 5 (2008): 519–523.

20. King, Cordova, and Scharf, 2008.

21. McClave and coauthors, 2009; A. Malone, Enteral formula selection, in P. Charney and A. Malone, eds., *ADA Pocket Guide to Enteral Nutrition* (Chicago: American Dietetic Association, 2006), pp. 63–122.

22. M. C. Steiner and coauthors, Nutritional enhancement of exercise performance in chronic obstructive pulmonary disease: A randomised controlled trial, *Thorax* 58 (2003): 745–751.

23. L. D. Hudson and A. S. Slutsky, Acute respiratory failure, in L. Goldman and D. Ausiello, eds., *Cecil Medicine* (Philadelphia: Saunders, 2008), pp. 723–734.

24. American Dietetic Association, 2009.

25. McClave and coauthors, 2009.

Multiple Organ Dysfunction Syndrome

Multiple organ dysfunction syndrome (MODS), also called *multiple organ failure,* is a frequent cause of death in intensive care patients. Described as the progressive dysfunction of two or more of the body's organ systems, MODS most often involves the lungs, liver, kidneys, and gastrointestinal (GI) tract. MODS is not a disease, per se, but rather a late stage of severe illness or injury that results from a severe inflammatory response (discussed in Chapter 16).[1] MODS can be initiated by a number of very different critical illnesses and conditions, including respiratory failure, sepsis, burn injuries, extensive surgery, and pancreatitis. This Nutrition in Practice discusses how MODS develops, the manner in which it is treated, and the importance of its prevention.

How long has MODS been a major clinical problem?

MODS was recognized as a clinical entity only after World War II. Prior to the mid-20th century, patients with severe illnesses or multiple injuries frequently died of shock or circulatory failure. After fluid replacement and blood transfusions became standard treatments, the kidneys became the organs at highest risk, and kidney failure became the most common cause of death. Eventually, physicians learned to better support kidney function by providing appropriate electrolyte solutions and improving urine output. With improved kidney care, the lungs became the most vulnerable organ after severe injury. Improved treatment of respiratory failure eventually led to the current situation: advances in critical care allow patients to survive severe illnesses and injuries, but the body's defenses often overburden organs that were not originally injured.

Why does critical illness sometimes lead to MODS?

As discussed earlier in Chapter 16, injury and infection cause the release of chemical mediators that have systemic (whole-body) effects. A severe, persistent inflammatory response can lead to systemic inflammatory response syndrome (SIRS), which is associated with a constellation of symptoms including fever, raised heart and respiratory rates, and abnormal white blood cell counts. SIRS is a normal adaptive response to a severe insult, but if not reversed quickly enough it can progress to shock, which is characterized by extremely low blood pressure and an inadequate blood supply for the tissues and organs of the body.[2]

As might be expected from a systemic reduction in blood availability, shock can impair numerous organ systems. The abnormal delivery of oxygen and nutrients to tissues and insufficient removal of wastes result in irreversible injury to cells and tissues. Although each organ system is affected differently, ultimately one or more organs may begin to fail. The failure of one organ may place excessive demands on another, causing the second to fail as well. The progression of SIRS to MODS reflects the inability of the body's defenses and medical treatments to counter the detrimental effects of a sustained and potent inflammatory response.

The specific pathophysiology of MODS is poorly understood. Although early reports attempted to link the development of MODS directly to sepsis, sepsis is not present in all cases. Infection often results from impaired immune function and therefore is a frequent consequence of MODS, but it is not necessarily the underlying trigger of organ dysfunction. Recall from this chapter that sepsis gives rise to symptoms identical to those seen in SIRS. Figure NP16-1

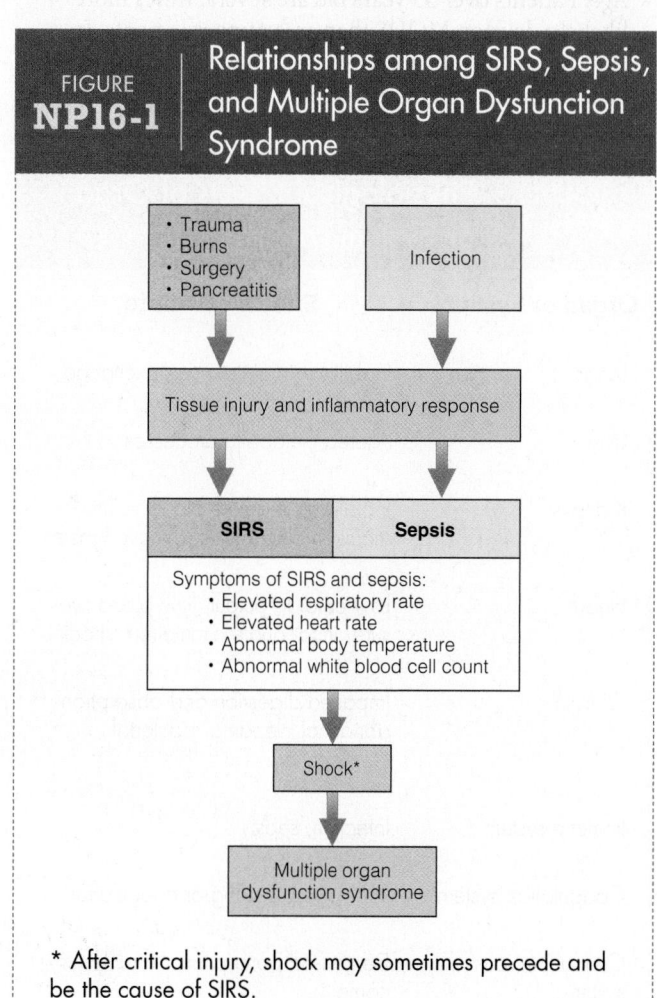

FIGURE NP16-1 Relationships among SIRS, Sepsis, and Multiple Organ Dysfunction Syndrome

* Trauma
* Burns
* Surgery
* Pancreatitis

Infection

Tissue injury and inflammatory response

| SIRS | Sepsis |

Symptoms of SIRS and sepsis:
* Elevated respiratory rate
* Elevated heart rate
* Abnormal body temperature
* Abnormal white blood cell count

Shock*

Multiple organ dysfunction syndrome

* After critical injury, shock may sometimes precede and be the cause of SIRS.

illustrates the relationships among SIRS, infection, sepsis, and MODS.

Do organs fail in a specific pattern?

Although the clinical course differs substantially among patients, the sequence of organ dysfunction often follows a similar pattern: first the lungs fail, then the liver, and finally the kidneys, GI tract, or heart.[3] Other organs or systems may also become involved, and each additional failure reduces the likelihood of survival. Table NP16-1 lists the organs and systems most often involved in MODS and the potential consequences of their failure.

Are there any risk factors for MODS?

Epidemiological studies have identified a number of factors that increase risk. For example, people who develop MODS are often older, have multiple or severe injuries, and develop severe infections. Table NP16-2 lists the major risk factors associated with MODS, some of which are discussed below:

- *Age.* Patients over 55 years old are several times more likely to develop MODS than are younger patients. In elderly patients, the increased risk may be due to the presence of chronic illnesses that directly affect organ function,

TABLE NP16-1	Physiological Effects of Organ or System Failure
Organ or System	**Effects of Failure**
Lungs	Inability to maintain gas exchange
Liver	Altered metabolic processes
Kidneys	Inability to regulate blood volume, maintain electrolytes, remove wastes
Heart	Low cardiac output, low blood pressure, inadequate circulation, shock
GI tract	Impaired digestion and absorption, abnormal bleeding, bacterial translocation
Immune system	Infection, sepsis
Coagulation system	Excessive bleeding or coagulation
Central nervous system	Decreased perceptions, brain injury, coma

TABLE NP16-2	Factors That Influence Risk of Multiple Organ Dysfunction Syndrome
Age over 55 years	
Prior chronic disease	
Persistent SIRS	
Major infection	
Blood transfusions	
Severity of tissue injury	
Length of time between injury and arrival at hospital	
Malnutrition	

such as heart disease, lung disease, diabetes, or liver damage. Aging also decreases the functional reserve of organs, thereby reducing an older patient's ability to deal with the additional stress that arises during critical illness.

- *Severity of SIRS.* The length of time that SIRS persists is related to the development of MODS. In one study, patients who had SIRS that persisted for more than three days were more likely to develop MODS than patients who had SIRS for less than two days.[4]
- *Infection.* Prolonged SIRS can suppress immune function and increase the risk of developing an infection. During hospital stays, critically ill patients often contract pneumonia—the principal infection associated with MODS. The risks of infection and sepsis greatly increase with the use of invasive catheters, which are frequently needed during intensive care to provide oxygen support, intravenous fluid resuscitation, nutrition support, and urine clearance.
- *Blood transfusions.* Blood transfusions are immunosuppressive and may increase a patient's risks of developing infection or sepsis. Blood transfusions frequently have adverse effects that can add further stress; they may cause acute lung injury, allergic reactions, red blood cell hemolysis (breakdown), and other complications.

What is the treatment for MODS?

Once MODS has developed, extensive medical support is needed until the inflammatory response has abated. Unfortunately, aggressive treatments can have damaging effects of their own and may cause further injury to organs that are already weakened by illness. Health practitioners should be aware of the adverse effects of aggressive thera-pies and remain alert to a patient's responses to treatments. Therapies that are often used to manage MODS include:

- *Lung support.* Mechanical ventilation is used to assist injured lungs and sustain gas exchange.
- *Fluid resuscitation.* Fluids and electrolytes are supplied to restore blood volume and maintain electrolyte balance.
- *Support of heart and blood vessel function.* Medications help to sustain or increase cardiac output and maintain adequate blood pressure.
- *Kidney support.* Hemofiltration or dialysis helps to prevent the buildup of toxic metabolites in blood.
- *Protection against infection.* Antibiotic therapy may reverse or prevent infections.
- *Nutrition support.* Enteral and parenteral nutrition support provide nutrients, help to prevent excessive wasting, and promote recovery.

What can be done to reduce the incidence of MODS?

Because mortality rates for MODS are so high, prevention must be considered at the earliest stages of injury and treat-ment, before an excessive inflammatory response can cause further damage. Health practitioners have learned to iden-tify the conditions that can increase organ stress whether they are due to a disease process, an inflammatory response, or an aggressive treatment that is intended to provide organ support. Although improvements in care over the past few decades have reduced some of the complications that arise during intensive care, rates of mortality from MODS have not changed. Thus, a focus on prevention is criti-cal until a better understanding of the pathophysiology of MODS, which may lead to additional therapeutic options, is achieved.

Notes

1. J. Parrillo, Approach to the patient with shock, in L. Goldman and D. Ausiello, eds., *Cecil Medicine* (Philadelphia: Saunders, 2008), pp. 742–750; D. Johnson and I. Mayers, Multiple organ dysfunction syndrome: A narrative review, *Canadian Journal of Anesthesia* 48 (2001): 502–509.
2. J. A. Russell, Shock syndromes related to sepsis, in L. Goldman and D.Ausiello, eds., *Cecil Medicine* (Philadelphia: Saunders, 2008), pp. 755–763.
3. P. J. Offner and E. E. Moore, Risk factors for MOF and pattern of organ failure following severe trauma, in A. E. Baue, E. Faist, and D. E. Fry, eds., *Multiple Organ Failure: Pathophysiology, Prevention, and Therapy* (New York: Springer-Verlag, 2000), pp. 30–43.
4. Offner and Moore, 2000.

CHAPTER 17

Nutrition and Upper Gastrointestinal Disorders

Ryan McVay/Getty Images

CONTENTS

GASTROINTESTINAL (GI) ILLNESSES ACCOUNT FOR A SIGNIFICANT fraction of hospital admissions and visits to health practitioners each year. Diagnosis is not always straightforward, however, because many patients with GI complaints exhibit no physical abnormalities. Evaluation therefore requires a detailed review of a patient's symptoms and responses to dietary adjustments. Because GI complications frequently accompany other illnesses, the medical history can sometimes uncover the underlying source of distress. This chapter describes upper GI symptoms and disorders; the next chapter discusses conditions that involve the lower GI tract.

Conditions Affecting the Mouth and Esophagus

Chapter 14 described several types of mechanically altered diets that can be used by individuals who have difficulty chewing and swallowing (see pp. 412–413). This section describes how people with dry mouth can relieve discomfort, and it examines the causes and treatments of the two most common disorders involving the esophagus: dysphagia (difficulty swallowing) and gastroesophageal reflux disease.

DRY MOUTH

Dry mouth (**xerostomia**), caused by reduced salivary flow, is a side effect of many medications and is associated with a number of diseases and disease treatments. Antihistamines, antihypertensive drugs, antidepressants, decongestants, and other medications can cause dry mouth. Poorly controlled diabetes mellitus is often associated with dry mouth, as are conditions that directly affect salivary gland function, such as **Sjögren's syndrome**. Radiation therapy that treats head and neck cancers often damages salivary glands, sometimes permanently. Mouth breathing is also a common cause of dry mouth.[1]

A reduction in salivary flow can impair health in a variety of ways. Dry mouth can interfere with speech and cause bad breath. Mouth infections and dental diseases are more common. Chewing and swallowing are more difficult, and taste sensation is diminished. Dentures may be uncomfortable to wear, and ulcerations may develop where they contact the mouth. Dry mouth may cause a person to reduce food intake and may thereby increase malnutrition risk. Table 17-1 (p. 490) offers suggestions that can help to manage dry mouth.

DYSPHAGIA

The act of swallowing involves multiple processes. In the initial, or **oropharyngeal**, phase of swallowing, muscles in the mouth and tongue propel the bolus of food through the pharynx and into the esophagus. At the same time, tissues of the soft palate prevent food from entering the nasal cavity, and the epiglottis blocks the opening to the trachea to prevent aspiration of food substances or saliva into the lungs. In the second, or **esophageal**, phase of swallowing, peristalsis forces the bolus through the esophagus, and the lower esophageal sphincter relaxes to allow passage of the bolus into the stomach. Due to the many tasks involved in swallowing, dysphagia can result from a number of different physical or neurological conditions. Prevalence increases with age, affecting as many as 35 percent of individuals over 50 years of age at least weekly.[2] Table 17-2 lists some potential causes of dysphagia, which are categorized according to the phase of swallowing that is impaired.

Oropharyngeal Dysphagia A person with **oropharyngeal dysphagia** typically has a neuromuscular condition that upsets the swallowing reflex or impairs the necessary movements of the tongue and other oral tissues. Symptoms include an inability to initiate swallowing, coughing during or after swallowing (due to aspiration), and nasal regurgitation. Other signs include bad breath, a gurgling noise after swallowing, a hoarse or "wet" voice, or a speech disorder. Oropharyngeal dysphagia is common in elderly persons and frequently follows a stroke.[3]

Esophageal Dysphagia A person with **esophageal dysphagia** usually has an obstruction in the esophagus or a motility disorder. The main symptom is the

xerostomia (ZEE-roh-STOE-me-ah): dry mouth caused by reduced salivary flow.
- *xero* = dry
- *stomia* = mouth

Sjögren's (SHOW-grenz) syndrome: an autoimmune disease characterized by the destruction of secretory glands, resulting in dry mouth and dry eyes.

oropharyngeal (OR-oh-fah-ren-JEE-al): involving the mouth and pharynx.

esophageal (eh-SOF-ah-JEE-al): involving the esophagus.

oropharyngeal dysphagia: an inability to transfer food from the mouth and pharynx to the esophagus; usually caused by a neurological or muscular disorder.

esophageal dysphagia: an inability to move food through the esophagus; usually caused by an obstruction or a motility disorder.

stricture: abnormal narrowing of a passageway; often due to inflammation, scarring, or a congenital abnormality.

achalasia (ack-ah-LAY-zhah): an esophageal disorder characterized by weakened peristalsis and impaired relaxation of the lower esophageal sphincter.
- *a* = without
- *chalasia* = relaxation

> NURSING DIAGNOSIS
>
> *Impaired oral mucous membrane* is appropriate for a person with dry mouth.

> NURSING DIAGNOSIS
>
> *Impaired swallowing* is appropriate for a person with dysphagia.

> NURSING DIAGNOSIS
>
> *Imbalanced nutrition: less than body requirements* and *risk for aspiration* often apply to a patient with dysphagia.

TABLE 17-1 | Suggestions for Managing Dry Mouth

Take frequent sips of water or another sugarless beverage.

Chew sugarless gum to help stimulate salivary flow.

Suck on ice cubes or frozen fruit juice bars (unless their coldness causes discomfort).

Avoid citrus juices and spicy or salty foods if they cause mouth irritation.

Avoid dry foods like toast, chips, and crackers.

Avoid caffeine, alcohol, and smoking, which may dry the mouth.

Consume foods that have a high fluid content such as soups, stews, sauces and gravies, yogurt, and pureed fruits.

Try over-the-counter saliva substitutes (available as gels, sprays, and tablets), especially just before meals and at bedtime.

Try rinsing the mouth with small amounts of vegetable oil or softened margarine.

Use a humidifier during the night.

Pay strict attention to oral hygiene, brushing and flossing at least twice daily. Try to brush immediately after each meal.

Avoid alcohol- and detergent-containing mouthwashes that may dry and irritate the mouth.

If dry mouth is caused by a medication, ask your physician about possible alternatives.

Ask your physician if using a medication to stimulate saliva secretion may be of benefit; examples include nicotinic acid tablets and pilocarpine.

TABLE 17-2 | Selected Causes of Dysphagia

Oropharyngeal Dysphagia

- Alzheimer's disease (advanced stages)
- Developmental disabilities
- Lou Gehrig's disease (amyotrophic lateral sclerosis)
- Multiple sclerosis
- Muscular dystrophy
- Myasthenia gravis
- Parkinson's disease
- Poliomyelitis
- Stroke

Esophageal Dysphagia

- Achalasia
- Enlarged right atrium (upper right chamber of heart)
- Esophageal cancer
- Esophageal spasm
- Scleroderma
- Strictures (from inflammation, scarring, or a congenital abnormality)

sensation of food "sticking" in the esophagus after it is swallowed. An obstruction can be caused by a **stricture** (abnormal narrowing), tumor, or compression of the esophagus by surrounding tissues. Whereas an obstruction can prevent the passage of solid foods but may not affect liquids, a motility disorder hinders the passage of both solids and liquids. **Achalasia**, the most common motility disorder, is a degenerative nerve condition affecting the esophagus; it is characterized by impaired peristalsis and incomplete relaxation of the lower esophageal sphincter when swallowing.[4]

Complications of Dysphagia Nurses should be alert to the various complications that may accompany dysphagia. If food consumption is reduced due to dysphagia, malnutrition and weight loss may occur. Individuals who cannot swallow liquids are at increased risk of dehydration. A potentially life-threatening complication associated with dysphagia is aspiration, which can cause airway obstruction, choking, or respiratory infections, including pneumonia. If the cough reflex is absent, aspiration is more difficult to diagnose and may go unnoticed.

Nutrition Intervention for Dysphagia To compensate for swallowing difficulties, people with dysphagia can consume foods and beverages that have been physically modified so that they are easier to swallow. Because a wide variety of defects can cause dysphagia, finding the best diet is often a challenge. Even after careful assessment of a person's swallowing abilities, the most appropriate foods may be determined only by trial and error. Furthermore, a person's swallowing ability can fluctuate over time, so the dietary plan needs frequent reassessment.

The National Dysphagia Diet, developed in 2002 by a panel of dietitians, speech and language therapists, and a food scientist, has helped to standardize the nutrition care of dysphagia patients.[5] Table 17-3 presents brief descriptions of the different levels of the diet and some sample meals.[6] After the appropriate dietary level is selected, it must be adjusted to suit the person's swallowing abilities and tolerances. A consultation with a swallowing expert, such as a speech and language therapist, is often necessary.

Diamond Crystal Specialty Foods

Can you tell that the foods in this photo are pureed foods shaped with food molds?

Food Properties and Preparation
Foods included in dysphagia diets should have easy-to-manage textures and consistencies. Soft, cohesive foods are easier to swallow than hard or crumbly foods. Moist foods are better tolerated than dry foods. Some foods within a category may be acceptable and others may not; for example, some cookies are soft and tender, whereas others are hard and brittle. Sticky or gummy foods, such as peanut butter and cream cheese, may be difficult to clear from the mouth and throat.

The textures of foods are typically altered to make them easier to swallow. Foods are often pureed, mashed, ground, or minced (review Table 14-5 on p. 413). Foods that have more than one texture, such as vegetable soup or cereal with milk, are harder to manage, so ingredients may be blended to a single consistency with items such as nuts and seeds omitted.

Consuming foods that have a similar consistency can quickly become monotonous. By using commercial thickeners and food molds, pureed foods can be formed into attractive shapes. Including a variety of flavors and colors can also make a meal more appealing. The "How to" offers additional suggestions for improving the acceptance of pureed and other mechanically altered foods.

Properties of Liquids
Thickened liquids are easier to swallow than thin liquids such as water or juice. Table 17-3 describes the four levels of liquid consistencies prescribed for dysphagia patients, referred to as thin, nectarlike, honeylike, and spoon-thick. To increase viscosity, commercial starch thickeners are stirred into beverages and soup broths. Some beverages can lose their appeal when thickened; for example, individuals may find thickened coffee and tea unacceptable. Moreover, hydration is more difficult to maintain when a patient has access to only thickened beverages, which are often less acceptable for quenching thirst.

Alternative Feeding Strategies for Dysphagia
Some patients may be able to learn alternative feeding methods that help them compensate

---

HOW TO | Improve Acceptance of Mechanically Altered Foods

Take a moment to think about a meal of pureed or ground foods. A typical dinner of baked chicken, potatoes, carrots, and green beans can look like mounds of differently colored mush. The foods may taste great, but a person may have little appetite before trying a first bite. To improve appetite, be creative when preparing and serving meals:

- Help to stimulate the appetite by preparing favorite foods and foods with pleasant smells. Enliven food flavors with seasonings and spices.

- Use attractive plates and silverware to improve the visual appeal of a meal. Consider colors and shapes when arranging foods on a plate; colorful garnishes can add color and eye appeal. Substitute

brightly colored vegetables for white vegetables; for example, replace mashed potatoes with mashed sweet potatoes.

- Try layering ingredients so that the entrée looks like a fancy casserole. For example, recipes can resemble such popular entrées as lasagna, shepherd's pie, and moussaka.

- Shape pureed and ground foods to resemble traditional dishes. Flatten a spoonful of pureed meat to make a patty, or use small scoops so that meat resembles meatballs. Use food molds to restore slurried breads and pureed meats to their traditional shapes.

Efforts to improve the visual appearance of foods can go a long way toward helping people eat nourishing meals and maintain a healthy weight.

TABLE
17-3 | National Dysphagia Diet

Level 1: Dysphagia Pureed

Foods should be pureed or well mashed, homogeneous, and cohesive. This diet is for patients with moderate to severe dysphagia and poor oral or chewing ability.

Sample menus:

- *Breakfast:* Cream of wheat, slurried muffins or pancakes,ᵃ pureed scrambled eggs, plain or vanilla yogurt, well-mashed bananas, fruit juice without pulp (thickened as needed), coffee or tea (if thin liquids are acceptable).
- *Lunch or dinner:* Pureed tomato soup, slurried crackers, pureed meat or poultry, zucchini soufflé, mashed potatoes with gravy, pureed carrots or green beans, smooth applesauce, pureed peaches, chocolate pudding.

Foods to avoid: Dry breads and cereals, oatmeal, rice, fruit yogurt, cheese (including cottage cheese), peanut butter, nuts and seeds, raw fruits and vegetables, chunky applesauce, fruit preserves with chunks or seeds, tomato sauce with seeds, beverages with pulp, coarsely ground pepper, herbs.

Level 2: Dysphagia Mechanically Altered

Foods should be moist, cohesive, and soft textured and should easily form a bolus. This diet is for patients with mild to moderate dysphagia; some chewing ability is required.

Sample menus:

- *Breakfast:* Moist oatmeal, cornflakes or puffed rice cereal with milk (thickened as needed), moist pancakes or muffins (with butter, margarine, or jam; without nuts or seeds), soft scrambled eggs, cottage cheese, ripe bananas or cooked fruit without skin or seeds, fruit juice (thickened as needed), coffee or tea (if thin liquids are allowed).
- *Lunch or dinner:* Soup with easy-to-chew meat and vegetables; slurried bread or crackers; minced, tender-cooked meat; well-cooked pasta with moist meatballs and meat sauce; baked potato with gravy; soft, tender-cooked vegetables (not fibrous or rubbery); canned peach slices; soft fruit pie (with bottom crust only); soft, smooth chocolate bar.

Foods to avoid: Dry or coarse foods; breads and cereals with nuts, seeds, or dried fruit; frankfurters and sausages; hard-cooked eggs; corn and clam chowders; sandwiches; pizza; sliced cheese; rice; potato skins; french fries; raw vegetables; fibrous, rubbery, or nontender cooked vegetables such as asparagus, broccoli, brussels sprouts, cabbage, celery, corn, and peas; peanut butter; coconut; nuts and seeds; raw fruit (except banana); cooked fruits with skin or seeds; pineapple; mango; uncooked dried fruit; popcorn; chewy candies (such as caramel or licorice).

Level 3: Dysphagia Advanced

Foods should be moist and be in bite-sized pieces when swallowed; foods with mixed textures are included. This diet is for patients with mild dysphagia and adequate chewing ability.

Sample menus:

- *Breakfast:* Cereal with milk, moist pancakes or muffins (with butter, margarine, or jam; without nuts or seeds), poached or scrambled eggs, fruit yogurt, soft fresh fruit (peeled) or berries, coffee or tea (if thin liquids are tolerated).
- *Lunch or dinner:* Chicken noodle soup; moistened crackers or moist bread; thin-sliced tender meat; cheese; moist, soft-cooked potatoes or rice; tender-cooked vegetables; shredded lettuce with dressing; fresh, peeled peach or melon; canned fruit salad; moist chocolate chip cookie (without nuts).

Foods to avoid: Dry or coarse foods; breads and cereals with nuts, seeds, or dried fruit; corn and clam chowders; potato skins; raw vegetables (except shredded lettuce); corn; chunky peanut butter; coconut; nuts and seeds; hard fruit (such as apples or pears); fruit with skin, seeds, or stringy textures (such as mango or pineapple); uncooked dried fruit; fruit leathers; popcorn; chewy candies (such as caramel or licorice).

Liquid Consistencies (only those tolerated are allowed in the diet)

- *Thin:* Watery fluids; may include milk, coffee, tea, juices, carbonated beverages.
- *Nectarlike:* Fluids thicker than water that can be sipped through a straw; may include buttermilk, eggnog, tomato juice.
- *Honeylike:* Fluids that can be eaten with a spoon but do not hold their shape; may include honey, tomato sauce, yogurt.
- *Spoon-thick:* Thick fluids that must be eaten with a spoon and can hold their shape; may include milk pudding, thickened applesauce.

ᵃ Slurried foods are mixed with liquid until the consistency is appropriate; they may be gelled and shaped to improve appearance.

for their swallowing problem. For example, changing the position of the head and neck while eating and drinking can minimize some swallowing difficulties. (As an example, cups designed for dysphagia patients allow drinking without tilting the head back.) Individuals with oropharyngeal dysphagia can be taught exercises that strengthen the jaws, tongue, or larynx, or they can learn new methods of swallowing that allow them to consume a normal diet. Speech and language therapists are often responsible for teaching patients these techniques.

GASTROESOPHAGEAL REFLUX DISEASE

Gastroesophageal reflux disease (GERD) is a condition in which the stomach's acidic contents back up into the esophagus, causing discomfort and, sometimes, tissue damage. People who suffer from GERD often refer to these symptoms as *heartburn* or *acid indigestion*. Reflux does not necessarily cause symptoms or injury—it occurs occasionally in healthy people and is a problem only if it creates complications and requires lifestyle changes or medical treatment.

Causes of GERD The lower esophageal sphincter is the main barrier to gastric reflux, so GERD can result if the sphincter muscle is weak or relaxes inappropriately. Medical conditions that either interfere with the sphincter's function or prevent rapid clearance of acid from the esophagus can predispose a person to GERD.

Conditions associated with high rates of GERD include pregnancy, obesity, asthma, and **hiatal hernia**, a condition in which a portion of the stomach protrudes above the diaphragm (see Figure 17-1). Pregnancy is the most common predisposing condition—as many as two-thirds of pregnant women report heartburn, which usually worsens during the third trimester.[7] Some medications can increase the risk of reflux, as does

---

FIGURE 17-1 | The Upper GI Tract, Acid Reflux, and Hiatal Hernia

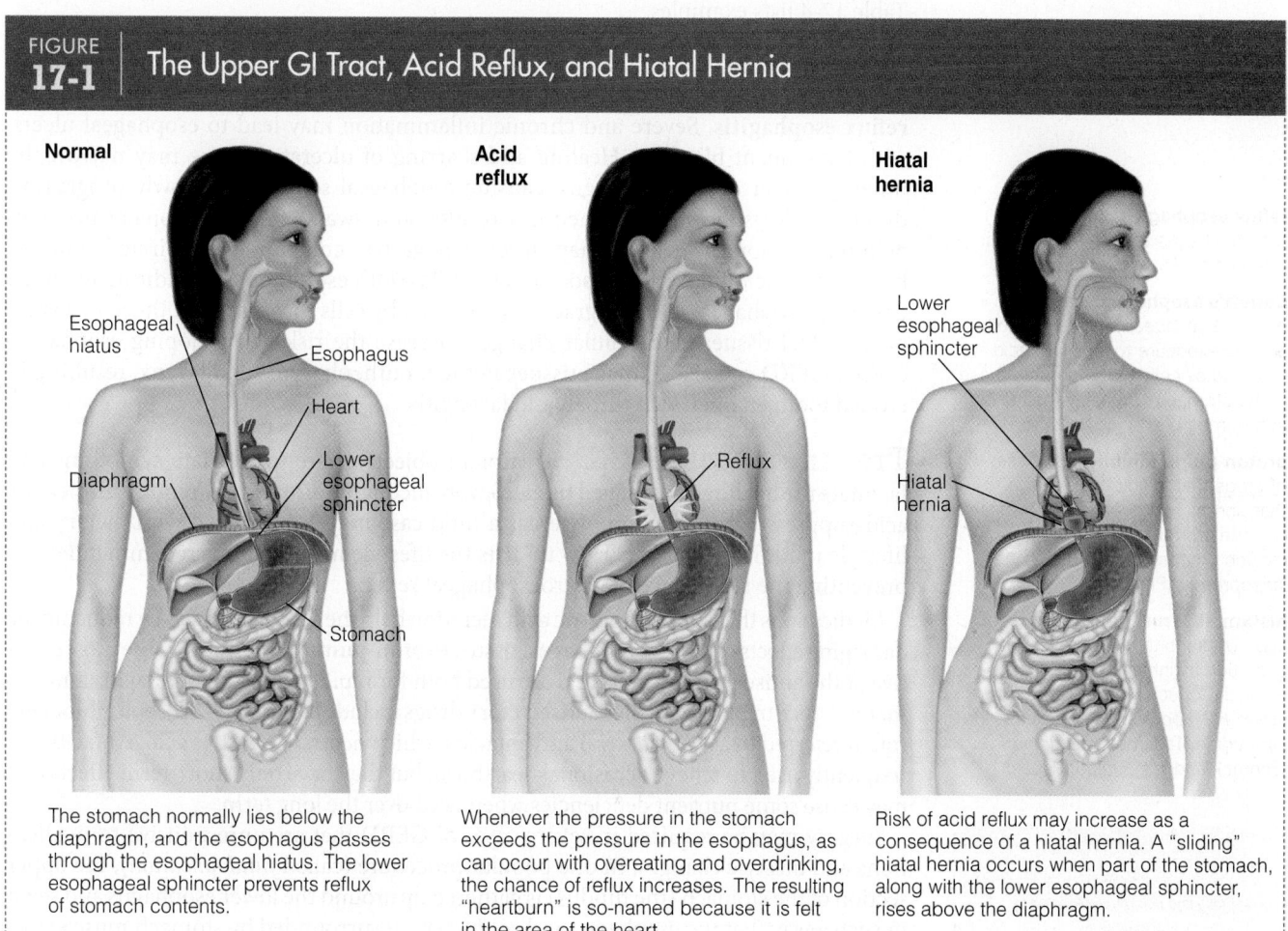

Normal

Esophageal hiatus
Esophagus
Heart
Diaphragm
Lower esophageal sphincter
Stomach

The stomach normally lies below the diaphragm, and the esophagus passes through the esophageal hiatus. The lower esophageal sphincter prevents reflux of stomach contents.

Acid reflux

Reflux

Whenever the pressure in the stomach exceeds the pressure in the esophagus, as can occur with overeating and overdrinking, the chance of reflux increases. The resulting "heartburn" is so-named because it is felt in the area of the heart.

Hiatal hernia

Lower esophageal sphincter
Hiatal hernia

Risk of acid reflux may increase as a consequence of a hiatal hernia. A "sliding" hiatal hernia occurs when part of the stomach, along with the lower esophageal sphincter, rises above the diaphragm.

TABLE 17-4	Conditions and Substances Associated with Esophageal Reflux	
Conditions That Increase Pressure within the Stomach	**Substances That Weaken the Lower Esophageal Sphincter**	
Ascites (abdominal fluid accumulation)	Alcohol	
Delayed gastric emptying	Anticholinergic drugs	
Eating large meals	Antihistamines	
Lying down after eating	Caffeinated beverages	
Obesity	Calcium channel blockers	
Pregnancy	Chocolate	
Wearing tight clothing around the waist or abdomen	Cigarette smoking	
	Diazepam	
	Fatty foods	
	Peppermint and spearmint	
	Progesterone	
	Theophylline	
	Tricyclic antidepressants	

the use of nasogastric tubes in tube feedings. Various other conditions can exacerbate GERD by increasing stomach distention or weakening the lower esophageal sphincter; Table 17-4 lists examples.

reflux esophagitis: inflammation in the esophagus that is related to the reflux of acidic stomach contents.

Barrett's esophagus: a condition in which esophageal cells damaged by chronic exposure to stomach acid are replaced by cells that resemble those in the stomach or small intestine, sometimes becoming cancerous.

proton-pump inhibitors: a class of drugs that inhibit the enzyme that pumps hydrogen ions (protons) into the stomach. Examples include omeprazole (Prilosec) and lansoprazole (Prevacid).

histamine-2 receptor blockers: a class of drugs that suppress acid secretion by inhibiting receptors on acid-producing cells; commonly called *H2 blockers*. Examples include cimetidine (Tagamet), ranitidine (Zantac), and famotidine (Pepcid).

Consequences of GERD If gastric acid remains in the esophagus long enough to damage the esophageal lining, the resulting inflammation is called **reflux esophagitis**. Severe and chronic inflammation may lead to esophageal ulcers, with consequent bleeding. Healing and scarring of ulcerated tissue may narrow the inner diameter of the esophagus, causing esophageal stricture. A slowly progressive dysphagia for solid foods sometimes results, and swallowing occasionally becomes painful. Pulmonary disease may develop if gastric contents are aspirated into the lungs. Chronic reflux is also associated with **Barrett's esophagus**, a condition in which damaged esophageal cells are gradually replaced by cells that resemble those in gastric or intestinal tissue; such cellular changes increase the risk of developing esophageal cancer. GERD can also damage tissues in the mouth, pharynx, and larynx, resulting in eroded tooth enamel, sore throat, and laryngitis.[8]

Treatment of GERD Treatment objectives are to alleviate symptoms and facilitate the healing of damaged tissue. Severe ulcerative disease may require immediate acid-suppressing medication, whereas a mild case may be managed with dietary and lifestyle modifications. The "How to" lists the lifestyle modifications recommended for preventing the recurrence of gastroesophageal reflux.

Medications that suppress gastric acid secretion help the healing process by reducing the damaging effects of acid on esophageal tissue. **Proton-pump inhibitors** are the most effective of the antisecretory agents and are used both for rapid healing of esophagitis and as a maintenance treatment. Other antisecretory drugs include **histamine-2 receptor blockers** (often referred to as *H2 blockers*) and antacids, which neutralize gastric acid. Antacids are frequently used to relieve occasional heartburn, but they have only short-term effects and may cause some nutrient deficiencies when used over the long term.

Surgery may be required in severe cases of GERD that are unresponsive to medications and lifestyle changes. In one popular procedure (called *fundoplication*), the upper section of the stomach (the fundus) is gathered up around the lower esophagus and sewn in such a way that the esophagus and sphincter are surrounded by stomach muscle; this technique increases pressure within the esophagus and fortifies the sphincter muscle.

NURSING DIAGNOSIS

Acute pain and *risk for aspiration* may apply to a person with GERD.

Management of GERD may require modifications in diet and lifestyle to minimize discomfort and reduce the recurrence of acid reflux. Recommendations typically include the following:

- Avoid eating bedtime snacks or lying down after meals. Meals should be consumed at least three hours before bedtime.

- Reduce nighttime reflux by elevating the head of the bed on 6-inch blocks, inserting a foam wedge under the mattress, or propping pillows under the head and upper torso.

- Consume only small meals, and drink liquids between meals so that the stomach does not become overly distended, which can exert pressure on the lower esophageal sphincter.

- Limit foods that weaken lower esophageal sphincter pressure or increase gastric acid secretion; these include chocolate, fried and fatty foods, spearmint and peppermint, coffee (both caffeinated and decaffeinated), and tea.

- Avoid cigarettes and alcohol; both relax the lower esophageal sphincter.

- Avoid bending over and wearing tight-fitting garments; both can cause pressure in the stomach to increase, heightening the risk of reflux.

- During periods of esophagitis, avoid foods and beverages that may irritate the esophagus, such as citrus fruits and juices, tomato products, garlic, onions, pepper, spicy foods, carbonated beverages, and very hot or very cold foods (depending on individual tolerances).

- Avoid using nonsteroidal anti-inflammatory drugs (NSAIDs) such as aspirin, naproxen, and ibuprofen, which can damage the esophageal mucosa.

Food tolerances among people with GERD can vary markedly. Nurses can help patients pinpoint food intolerances by advising them to keep a record of the foods and beverages consumed, as well as any resulting symptoms.

Esophageal strictures are often treated by dilating the esophagus with an inflatable balloon-like device or a fixed-size dilator, or by using surgical approaches. The Case Study will help you to review the treatments available for a patient with GERD.

Review Notes

- Dry mouth can increase the risk of developing oral infections, diminish taste sensation, and lead to reduced food intake. It can be managed with oral hygiene, dietary changes, and saliva substitutes.

- Dysphagia may interfere with food intake and increase the risk of aspiration. Treatment may include dietary adjustments, strengthening exercises, and use of different swallowing techniques.

- Gastroesophageal reflux disease (GERD) may lead to esophageal ulcers, inflammation, bleeding, and stricture. Treatment includes the use of acid-suppressing drugs and lifestyle changes.

CASE STUDY | Woman with GERD

Gina Rinaldi is a 39-year-old accountant who is 5 feet 4 inches tall and weighs 165 pounds. During a recent physical examination, she mentioned to her physician that she had been feeling fairly well until she began experiencing heartburn, which has progressively become more frequent and painful. The heartburn often occurs after she eats a large meal and is particularly bad after she goes to bed at night. By directly examining the esophageal lumen using an endoscope (a thin, flexible tube equipped with an optical device), the physician found evidence of reflux esophagitis and a slight narrowing throughout the length of the esophagus.

Ms. Rinaldi's medical history does not indicate any significant health problems. During her last physical exam, her physician advised her to stop smoking cigarettes and to lose 20 pounds, but she has not attempted to do either. The nutrition assessment reveals that Ms. Rinaldi is feeling stressed because it is the middle of the tax season. She usually has little time for breakfast, eats a lunch of fast foods while continuing to work at her desk, and eats a large dinner at around 8 P.M. She generally has wine with dinner and another alcoholic beverage later in the evening.

1. Explain to Ms. Rinaldi the meaning of the medical diagnoses *reflux esophagitis* and *esophageal stricture*.

2. From the brief history provided, list the factors and behaviors that increase Ms. Rinaldi's risks of experiencing reflux. What recommendations can you make to help her change these behaviors?

3. What medications might the physician prescribe, and why?

Conditions Affecting the Stomach

Stomach disorders range from occasional bouts of discomfort to severe conditions that require surgery. This section begins with a discussion of *dyspepsia* (often called "indigestion"), the sensation of pain or discomfort in the upper abdomen that occurs after food consumption. More serious stomach conditions that may benefit from medical treatment and dietary adjustments include *gastritis* and *peptic ulcers,* which most often result from bacterial infection or the use of medications that damage the stomach lining.

DYSPEPSIA

Dyspepsia refers to the general symptoms of indigestion in the upper abdominal region, which may include stomach pain, gnawing sensations, early satiety, nausea, vomiting, and bloating. These symptoms sometimes indicate the presence of more serious illnesses, such as GERD or peptic ulcer disease. Although about 25 percent of the population experiences dyspepsia, only one person in four seeks medical attention.[9]

Causes of Dyspepsia
Abdominal symptoms don't always lead to a clear diagnosis, as the cause of the symptoms may be difficult to identify. Various medical problems can cause abdominal discomfort, including peptic ulcers, GERD, gastric motility disorders, gallbladder and pancreatic diseases, and tumors in the upper GI tract. Chronic diseases such as diabetes mellitus, heart disease, and hypothyroidism can sometimes be accompanied by gastric symptoms. Some medications, including aspirin (and other NSAIDs), antibiotics, digitalis, and theophylline, can cause gastrointestinal distress. Some dietary supplements, such as iron and potassium supplements and some herbal products, may cause gastrointestinal problems. Intestinal conditions such as irritable bowel syndrome or lactose intolerance can mimic dyspepsia. Although pinpointing the cause of the symptoms can be difficult, a complete examination is in order if the individual experiences unintentional weight loss, persistent vomiting, dysphagia, anemia, or GI bleeding, which suggest the presence of serious illness.[10]

Potential Food Intolerances
Some people report that their symptoms worsen after eating certain foods or spices. Coffee can induce symptoms in about 50 percent of dyspepsia patients, and it also increases gastric acid production and acid reflux.[11] Spicy foods may cause some injury to the mucosal lining and exacerbate the pain from a preexisting ulcer. High-fat meals can slow gastric emptying and thereby exacerbate dyspepsia. To minimize symptoms, people with dyspepsia are typically advised to avoid consuming excessively large meals, fatty or highly spiced foods, and specific foods believed to trigger symptoms.[12]

Bloating and Stomach Gas
The feeling of bloating may be caused by excessive gas in the stomach, which accumulates when air is swallowed. Air swallowing often accompanies gum chewing, smoking, rapid eating, drinking carbonated beverages, and using a straw. Omitting these practices generally helps to correct the problem.

NAUSEA AND VOMITING

Nausea and vomiting accompany many illnesses and are common side effects of medications. Although occasional vomiting is not dangerous, prolonged vomiting can cause fluid and electrolyte imbalances and may require medical care. Chronic vomiting can reduce food intake and lead to malnutrition and nutrient deficiencies.

The timing of vomiting gives clues about its cause. Vomiting that occurs within an hour after a meal suggests a peptic ulcer or a psychological cause. If it occurs more than one hour after a meal, possible causes include food poisoning, an obstruction that prevents stomach emptying, or a stomach motility disorder.

dyspepsia: a feeling of pain, bloating, or discomfort in the upper abdominal area, often called *indigestion;* a symptom of illness rather than a disease itself.
- *dys* = bad; impaired
- *pepsis* = digestion

NURSING DIAGNOSIS

Acute pain and *nausea* may be appropriate for a person with dyspepsia.

Treatment of Nausea and Vomiting

Most cases are short lived and require no treatment. When treatment is necessary, the main goal is to find and correct the underlying disorder. Restoring hydration may also be necessary in some individuals. If a medication is the cause, taking it with food may help. If the cause is unknown or the underlying disorder cannot be corrected, medications that suppress nausea and vomiting may be prescribed. People with **intractable vomiting**—vomiting that is not easily controlled—may require intravenous nutrition support.

Dietary Interventions

Sometimes nausea can be prevented or improved with dietary measures.[13] Patients should consume small meals to minimize stomach distention and avoid lying down after meals. Beverages should be consumed between meals rather than during a meal. Dry, starchy foods such as toast, crackers, and pretzels may help to reduce nausea, whereas fatty or spicy foods and foods with strong odors may worsen symptoms. Foods that are cold or at room temperature may be better tolerated than hot foods. Individuals often have strong food aversions when nauseated, and tolerances vary greatly.

GASTRITIS

Gastritis is a general term that refers to inflammation of the stomach mucosa. (✚) Acute cases of gastritis typically result from irritating substances or treatments that damage the gastric mucosa, resulting in tissue erosions, ulcers, or hemorrhaging (severe bleeding). Chronic cases may be caused by long-term infections or autoimmune disease and can progress to widespread gastric inflammation and tissue atrophy. Most often, gastritis results from *Helicobacter pylori* infection or the use of NSAIDs, both primary causes of peptic ulcer disease as well. Table 17-5 lists some potential causes of gastritis.

Complications of Gastritis

The extensive tissue damage that sometimes develops in chronic gastritis can disrupt gastric secretory functions. If hydrochloric acid secretions become abnormally low (**hypochlorhydria**) or absent (**achlorhydria**), absorption of nonheme iron and vitamin B_{12} can be impaired, and the risk of deficiency increases. Pernicious anemia, a condition characterized by the destruction of stomach cells that produce intrinsic factor, is a late complication of chronic gastritis and a primary cause of vitamin B_{12} deficiency (see p. 220).

Dietary Interventions for Gastritis

Dietary recommendations depend on an individual's symptoms. In asymptomatic cases, no dietary adjustments are needed. If pain or discomfort is present, the patient should avoid irritating foods and beverages; these often include alcohol, coffee (including decaffeinated), tea, cola beverages, spicy foods, and fried or fatty foods. If food consumption causes intense pain or nausea and vomiting, food intake should be avoided for 24 to 48 hours to rest the stomach. If hypochlorhydria or achlorhydria is present, supplementation of iron and vitamin B_{12} may be warranted.

PEPTIC ULCER DISEASE

A **peptic ulcer** is an open sore that develops in the gastrointestinal mucosa when gastric acid and pepsin overwhelm mucosal defenses and destroy mucosal tissue. A primary factor in peptic ulcer development is *Helicobacter pylori* infection, which is present in about 60 percent of patients with gastric ulcers and 80 percent of those with duodenal ulcers.[14] (✚) Another major factor is the use of NSAIDs, which have both topical and systemic effects that can damage

---

✚ The suffix *-itis* refers to the presence of inflammation in an organ or tissue.

✚ The specific reasons why ulcers develop are not known; only 10 to 15 percent of individuals with chronic *Helicobacter pylori* infection actually develop a peptic ulcer.

intractable vomiting: vomiting that is not easily managed or controlled.

gastritis: inflammation of stomach tissue.

Helicobacter pylori: a species of bacterium that colonizes gastric mucosa; a primary cause of gastritis and peptic ulcer disease.

hypochlorhydria (HIGH-poe-clor-HIGH-dree-ah): abnormally low gastric acid secretions.

achlorhydria (AY-clor-HIGH-dree-ah): an absence of gastric acid secretions.

peptic ulcer: an open sore in the gastrointestinal mucosa resulting from the destructive effects of gastric acid and pepsin; may develop in the esophagus, stomach, or duodenum.
• *peptic* = related to digestion

TABLE 17-5	Potential Causes of Gastritis

Infection
- Bacterial: *Helicobacter pylori, Actinomyces israelii*
- Fungal: *Candida albicans*
- Parasitic: Cryptosporidiosis, nematode infection
- Viral: Cytomegalovirus, herpes simplex virus

Chemical Substances
- Alcohol
- Cancer chemotherapy
- Drugs (especially aspirin and other NSAIDs)
- Ingestion of toxins or corrosive materials

Internal (Bodily) Causes
- Autoimmune disease
- Bile reflux
- Severe stress
- Systemic illness or sepsis

Miscellaneous
- Food allergy
- Foreign bodies
- High salt intake
- Radiation therapy

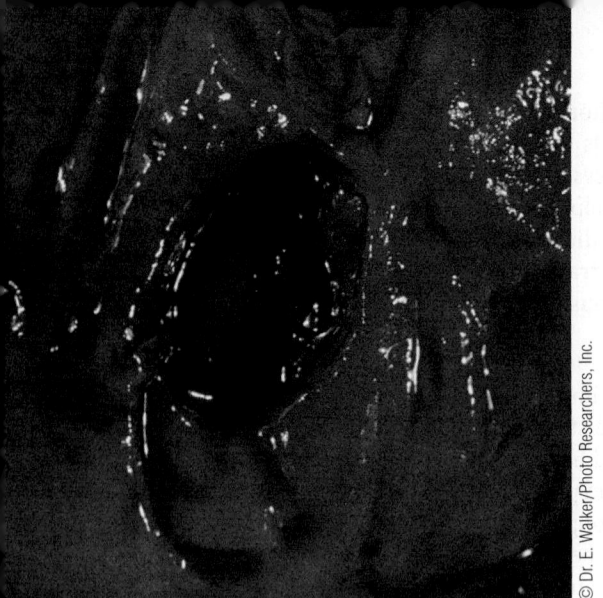

A peptic ulcer, such as the gastric ulcer shown here, damages mucosal tissue and may cause pain and bleeding.

mucosal tissue. In rare cases, ulcers may develop from disorders that cause excessive acid secretion. Ulcer risk can be increased by cigarette smoking and psychological stress.

Effects of Psychological Stress Although most ulcers are associated with *H. pylori* infection or NSAID use, about a quarter of ulcers develop in people for other reasons.[15] Psychological stress is not believed to cause ulcers per se, but it has effects on physiological processes and behaviors that may increase a person's vulnerability. The physiological effects of stress vary among individuals but may include hormonal changes that impair immune responses and wound healing, increased secretions of hydrochloric acid and pepsin, and rapid stomach emptying (which increases the acid load in the duodenum). Stress may also lead to behavioral changes, including the increased use of cigarettes, alcohol, and NSAIDs—all potential risk factors for ulcers. Thus, stress may play a contributory role in ulcer development, although its precise effects are not fully understood.

Symptoms of Peptic Ulcers Peptic ulcer symptoms vary. Some people are asymptomatic or experience only mild discomfort. Ulcer "pain" may be experienced as a hunger pain, a sensation of gnawing, or a burning pain in the stomach region. The pain or discomfort of ulcers may be relieved by food and recur several hours after a meal, especially if the ulcer is duodenal. (✚) Gastric ulcers may be aggravated by food and can cause loss of appetite and eventual weight loss. Ulcer symptoms tend to go into remission regularly and recur every few weeks or months.

Complications of Peptic Ulcers Peptic ulcers are a major cause of gastrointestinal bleeding, which occurs in up to 15 percent of ulcer cases.[16] Bleeding is a potential cause of death and, if severe, may indicate the need for surgical intervention. Severe bleeding is evidenced by black, tarry stool samples or, occasionally, vomit that resembles coffee grounds. Other serious complications of ulcers include perforations of the stomach or duodenum (sometimes leading directly into the peritoneal cavity) and **gastric outlet obstruction** due to scarring or inflammation.

Drug Therapy for Peptic Ulcers The goals of ulcer treatment are to relieve pain, promote healing, and prevent recurrence. In most cases, treatment requires using a combination of antibiotics to eradicate *H. pylori* infection and/or discontinuing the use of aspirin and other NSAIDs, which can irritate the gastric mucosa and delay healing. The antibiotics used to treat *H. pylori* infection most often include amoxicillin, clarithromycin, metronidazole, and tetracycline. Antisecretory drugs are prescribed to relieve pain and allow healing; these include proton-pump inhibitors, H2 blockers, and antacids (as used in GERD; see the earlier discussion on p. 494). The most frequently prescribed drug regimen is a "triple therapy" that includes two antibiotics and an antisecretory drug. Bismuth preparations (such as Pepto-Bismol) and sucralfate may also help to heal ulcers by coating the gastrointestinal lining and preventing further tissue erosion. See the Diet-Drug Interactions feature on p. 499 for nutrition-related effects of the medications used in ulcer treatment.

Nutrition Care for Peptic Ulcers The goals of nutrition care are to correct nutrient deficiencies, if necessary, and encourage dietary and lifestyle practices that minimize symptoms.[17] Patients should avoid dietary items that increase acid secretion or irritate the gastrointestinal lining; examples include alcohol, coffee and other caffeine-containing beverages, chocolate, and pepper, although individual tolerances vary. Small meals may be better tolerated than large ones. Patients should avoid food consumption for at least two hours before bedtime. Cigarette smoking is discouraged, as it can delay healing and increase the risk of ulcer recurrence. There is no evidence that dietary adjustments alter the rate of healing.[18]

✚ In the United States, most ulcers are duodenal ulcers. In Asian countries, gastric ulcers are more common.

gastric outlet obstruction: an obstruction that prevents the normal emptying of stomach contents into the duodenum.

NURSING DIAGNOSIS

For people with peptic ulcers may include *acute pain* and *nausea*. For patients with bleeding ulcers, appropriate diagnoses may include *risk for deficient fluid volume, imbalanced nutrition: less than body requirements,* and *fatigue.*

Nutrition and Upper Gastrointestinal Disorders

Check this table for notable nutrition-related effects of the medications discussed in this chapter.

	GASTROINTESTINAL EFFECTS	INTERACTIONS WITH DIETARY SUBSTANCES	METABOLIC EFFECTS
Antacids (aluminum hydroxide, magnesium hydroxide, calcium carbonate)	Constipation (aluminum- or calcium-containing antacids), diarrhea (magnesium-containing antacids)	May decrease iron, folate, or vitamin B_{12} absorption.	Hypophosphatemia (from excess aluminum, magnesium, or calcium)
Antibiotics (for *Helicobacter pylori* infection; include amoxicillin, metronidazole, tetracycline)	Diarrhea (amoxicillin, tetracycline), nausea and vomiting (tetracycline), altered taste sensation (metronidazole)	Avoid alcohol with metronidazole; tetracycline decreases iron absorption and binds calcium in the GI tract, reducing absorption of both the tetracycline and the calcium.	–
Antisecretory drugs (proton-pump inhibitors, H2 blockers)	Constipation, nausea and vomiting, abdominal pain (proton-pump inhibitors)	May decrease iron, folate, and vitamin B_{12} absorption.	–
Coating agents (bismuth preparations, sucralfate)	Constipation, diarrhea	–	Hypophosphatemia, calcium retention (sucralfate)

Review Notes

- Dyspepsia refers to general symptoms of indigestion such as abdominal pain, nausea, and vomiting, which can be caused by a variety of medical conditions. Dietary measures may include avoiding large meals, fatty or spicy foods, and foods that trigger symptoms.
- Gastritis and peptic ulcer disease are most often associated with *Helicobacter pylori* infection, which can be eradicated by antibiotic therapy. NSAID use can promote gastritis and peptic ulcer disease by damaging the mucosal lining.
- Extensive damage to the mucosa may reduce gastric secretions and increase the risks of developing iron and vitamin B_{12} deficiencies.
- The nutrition care for gastritis and peptic ulcer disease includes correcting any nutritional deficiencies that develop and eliminating dietary substances that cause pain or discomfort.

Gastric Surgery

Gastric surgery is sometimes necessary for treating stomach cancer, some ulcer complications, and ulcers that are resistant to drug therapy. In recent years, gastric surgeries have also become popular treatments for severe obesity. This section describes **gastrectomy**, the surgery that removes diseased areas of the stomach, and **bariatric surgery**, the type of surgery that treats severe obesity.

gastrectomy (gah-STREK-ta-mee): the surgical removal of part of the stomach (partial gastrectomy) or the entire stomach (total gastrectomy).

bariatric (BAH-ree-AH-trik) surgery: surgery that treats severe obesity.
- *baros* = weight

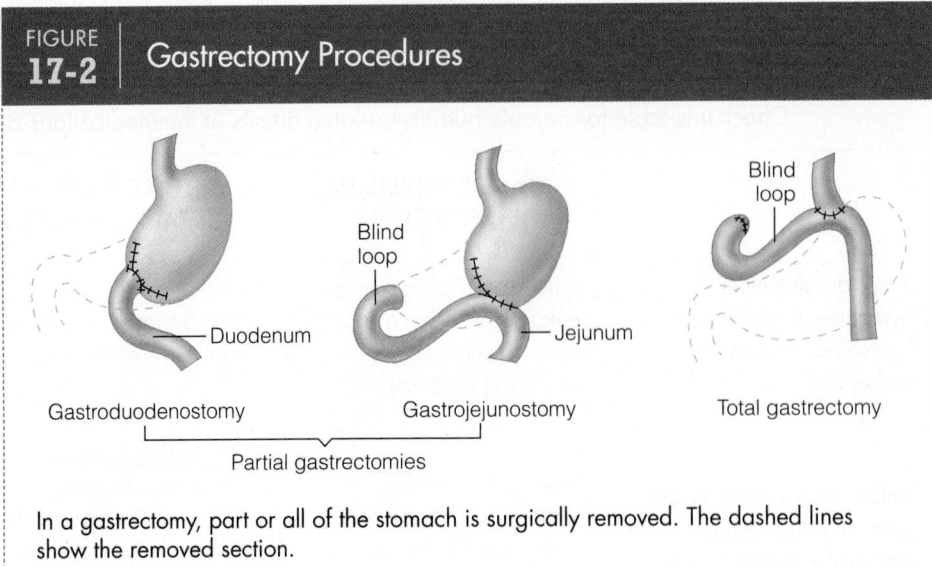

GASTRECTOMY

Figure 17-2 illustrates some typical gastrectomy procedures. In a partial gastrectomy, only part of the stomach is removed, and the remaining portion is connected to the duodenum or jejunum. In a total gastrectomy, the surgeon removes the entire stomach and connects the esophagus directly to the small intestine.

Nutrition Care after Gastrectomy The primary objectives of nutrition care after a gastrectomy are to meet the nutrient needs of the postsurgical patient and promote the healing of stomach tissue. Another goal is to prevent discomfort or nutrient deficiencies that may arise due to altered stomach function. As the next section will describe, some gastric surgeries increase the risk of **dumping syndrome**, a group of symptoms that result when a large amount of food passes rapidly into the small intestine.

Following a gastrectomy, oral intake of fluids and foods is suspended until some healing has occurred, and fluids are supplied intravenously. Ice chips (melted in the mouth), small sips of water, and broth are usually the first fluids given orally. Once fluids are tolerated, patients are offered liquid meals (with no sugars) at first, and they usually progress to a soft food diet by the fourth or fifth day after surgery. Tube feedings may be necessary if complications prevent a normal progression to solid foods.[19]

Dietary measures after gastrectomy are influenced by the size of the remaining stomach, which influences meal size, and the stomach emptying rate, which affects food tolerances. Initially, the patient is offered small meals and snacks that include only one or two food items; these foods may contain protein (fish, lean meats, and eggs), fat, and complex carbohydrates (bread, potatoes, and vegetables). Depending on the amount of food tolerated, the patient may require as many as six to eight small meals and snacks per day. The patient should avoid sweets and sugars because they increase osmolarity in the small intestine and potentiate the dumping syndrome (discussed below). Some patients may need to avoid milk products due to lactose intolerance. Soluble fibers may be added to meals to help delay stomach emptying and reduce diarrhea. Although tolerances vary, patients may have difficulty with fatty foods, highly spiced foods, carbonated drinks, caffeine-containing beverages, alcohol, extremely hot or cold foods, peppermint, and chocolate. Liquids are restricted during meals due to the limited stomach capacity and because liquids can increase the stomach emptying rate. Table 17-6 lists foods that are often permitted and those that are limited in postgastrectomy diets.[20]

Dumping Syndrome The dumping syndrome, a common complication of gastrectomy, is characterized by a group of symptoms resulting from rapid gastric emptying. Ordinarily, the pyloric sphincter controls the rate of flow from the stomach

dumping syndrome: symptoms that result from the rapid emptying of an osmotic load from the stomach into the small intestine. Early symptoms include nausea, abdominal cramping, and diarrhea; later symptoms are those of hypoglycemia and include confusion, headache, and hunger.

TABLE 17-6	Postgastrectomy Diet	
Food Category	Foods Recommended (as tolerated)	Foods to Limit (unless tolerated)
Meat and meat alternates	Lean tender meats, fish, poultry, shellfish, eggs, smooth nut butters	Fried, tough, or chewy meats; frankfurters and sausages; bacon; luncheon meats; dried peas and beans
Milk and milk products	Milk, plain yogurt, mild cheeses	Milk shakes, chocolate milk, fruit yogurt
Breads and cereals	Breads, crackers, bagels, pasta, and breakfast cereals made from enriched white flour (cereals should contain no added sugars)	Breads and cereals with more than 2 grams of fiber per serving; baked goods with dried fruits, nuts, or seeds; granola; frosted cereals; pastries; doughnuts
Vegetables	Tender-cooked vegetables without peels, skins, or seeds; raw lettuce	Raw vegetables (except lettuce), beets, broccoli, brussels sprouts, cabbage, cauliflower, collard and mustard greens, corn, potato skins
Fruit	Canned fruit without added sugars, bananas, melon	Canned fruits in syrup, raw fruits (except bananas and melons), dried fruits, fruit juices
Beverages	Decaffeinated coffee and tea, beverages sweetened with artificial sweeteners	Caffeinated beverages; alcoholic beverages; beverages sweetened with sugars, corn syrup, or honey

into the duodenum. After some types of stomach surgery, the hypertonic gastric contents are no longer regulated and can rush into the small intestine more quickly after meals, causing a number of unpleasant effects. Early symptoms can occur within 30 minutes and may include nausea, vomiting, abdominal cramping, diarrhea, lightheadedness, rapid heartbeat, and others (see Table 17-7). These symptoms may be due to intestinal distention (which triggers the release of GI hormones that affect digestive processes), a shift of fluid from blood vessels to the intestine that lowers blood volume, and an increase in peristaltic activity. Several hours later, symptoms of hypoglycemia may occur (see Table 17-7) because the unusually large spike in blood glucose following the meal (due to rapid nutrient influx and absorption) can result in an excessive insulin response.

Dietary adjustments can greatly minimize or prevent dumping syndrome. The goals are to limit the amount of food material that reaches the intestine, slow the rate of gastric emptying, and reduce foods that increase hypertonicity. Therefore, meal size is limited, fluids are restricted during meals, and sugars (including milk sugar) are restricted. In some cases, drugs that inhibit gastrointestinal motility may help. The "How to" on p. 502 lists practical suggestions for reducing the occurrence of dumping syndrome. The Case Study on p. 502 provides the opportunity to design a menu for a postgastrectomy patient who is at risk for dumping syndrome.

Nutrition Problems following Gastrectomy
After a gastrectomy, it may take time for the patient to learn the amount of food that can be consumed without discomfort. The symptoms associated with meals may lead to food avoidance, substantial weight loss, and eventually malnutrition. Other nutrition problems that may occur after gastrectomy include the following:[21]

TABLE 17-7	Symptoms of Dumping Syndrome	
Early Dumping Syndrome		**Late Dumping Syndrome**
Symptoms may begin within 30 minutes after eating.		Symptoms may begin one to three hours after eating.
• Abdominal pain, cramping		• Anxiety
• Diarrhea		• Confusion
• Dizziness		• Headache
• Flushing, sweating		• Hunger
• Nausea and vomiting		• Palpitations
• Rapid heartbeat		• Sweating
• Weakness, feeling faint		• Weakness, feeling faint

Dietary adjustments can minimize or prevent symptoms of dumping syndrome. The following suggestions may help:

- Eat smaller meals that suit the reduced capacity of the stomach. Increase the number of meals consumed daily so that energy intake is adequate.
- Eat in a relaxed setting. Eat slowly, and chew food thoroughly.
- Limit the amount of fluid included in meals. Avoid drinking beverages within 45 minutes before and after meals, but be sure to consume adequate fluid during the day to avoid dehydration.
- Avoid juices and sweetened beverages and foods that contain high amounts of sugar. Avoid carbonated beverages if they cause bloating.
- Use artificial sweeteners to sweeten beverages and desserts.

- Avoid foods and beverages that are very hot or very cold, unless tolerated.
- Include fiber-rich foods in each meal. Sometimes adding soluble fibers like pectin or guar gum to meals can help to control symptoms.
- Avoid milk and most milk products, which are high in lactose. Enzyme-treated milk should also be avoided because the breakdown products of lactose (glucose and galactose) can also cause symptoms. Cheese may be better tolerated because its lactose content is low. Make an effort to consume nonmilk calcium sources such as green leafy vegetables, tofu, and fish with bones.
- If symptoms of hypoglycemia continue, try including a protein-rich food in each meal.
- Lie down for 20 to 30 minutes (or longer) after eating to help slow the transit of food to the small intestine. While eating a meal, sit upright.

+ Bacterial overgrowth may be a consequence of reduced gastric acid secretions, altered motility of intestinal contents, or changes in intestinal anatomy due to surgical reconstruction. Chapter 18 describes bacterial overgrowth in detail.

+ Fat malabsorption reduces calcium absorption because the negatively charged fatty acids combine with calcium (which is positively charged) and prevent its absorption.

- *Fat malabsorption.* Fat digestion and absorption may become impaired for a number of reasons after gastrectomy. The accelerated transit of food material may prevent the normal mixing of fat with lipase and bile. If the duodenum has been removed or bypassed, less lipase is available for fat digestion. Bacterial overgrowth, a common consequence of gastrectomy, (+) leads to changes in bile acids that interfere with normal bile function. The fat malabsorption that results from these changes may lead to deficiencies of fat-soluble vitamins and some minerals. Supplemental pancreatic enzymes are sometimes provided to improve fat digestion. Medium-chain triglycerides, which are more easily digested and absorbed, can be used to supply additional fat kcalories.
- *Bone disease.* Osteoporosis and osteomalacia are common outcomes following a gastrectomy. The fat malabsorption described earlier can cause malabsorption of both vitamin D and calcium; (+) furthermore, patients at risk of dumping syndrome may need to avoid milk products, which are among the best sources of these nutrients. Bone density should be monitored during the years following surgery, and supplementation of calcium and vitamin D is often recommended.
- *Anemia.* After gastrectomy, iron and vitamin B_{12} deficiencies may develop and eventually lead to anemia. The reduction in gastric secretions impairs the absorption of both iron and vitamin B_{12}. If the duodenum has been removed or is bypassed, the risk of iron deficiency increases because the duodenum is a major site of iron absorption. Supplementation of both iron and vitamin B_{12} is usually warranted after surgery.

CASE STUDY | Nutrition Care for Patient after Gastric Surgery

Dirk Hanson, a 58-year-old biology teacher, was admitted to the hospital for gastric surgery after numerous medical treatments failed to manage his severe peptic ulcer disease. A gastrojejunostomy was performed, and after about 24 hours, Mr. Hanson was able to take small sips of warm water. The health care team anticipates multiple nutrition-related problems and is taking measures to prevent them.

1. Review Figure 17-2 to better understand Mr. Hanson's surgical procedure. Consider the possibilities that he might experience the following symptoms: early satiety, nausea and vomiting, weight

loss, dumping syndrome, fat malabsorption, anemia, and bone disease. Explain why each of these conditions may occur.

2. What type of diet will the physician prescribe for Mr. Hanson after he begins eating solid foods? Create a day's worth of menus, using foods from Table 17-6.

3. What advice can you give Mr. Hanson that will help to prevent dumping syndrome? List several foods from each major food group that may cause symptoms of dumping syndrome.

BARIATRIC SURGERY

Bariatric surgery is currently considered the most effective and durable treatment for morbid obesity.[22] (✚) Candidates for bariatric surgery are obese individuals who have a body mass index (BMI) greater than 40, or a BMI between 35 and 40 accompanied by severe weight-related problems such as diabetes, hypertension, or debilitating osteo-arthritis (recall that a healthy BMI usually falls between 20 and 25). In addition, the individual who seeks bariatric surgery should have attempted a variety of nonsurgical weight-loss measures—such as dietary adjustments, exercise, medications, and behavior modification—prior to seeking surgery. Bariatric surgery patients should have realistic expectations about the amount of weight they are likely to lose, the diet they will need to follow, and the complications that may ensue. Some types of bariatric surgery can dramatically affect health and nutrition status, and many patients require lifelong management.

Bariatric Surgical Procedures Figure 17-3 illustrates the most popular surgical options for weight reduction, the gastric bypass and gastric banding procedures. The gastric bypass operation, (✚) which accounts for approximately two-thirds of bariatric surgeries,[23] constructs a small gastric pouch that reduces stomach capacity and thereby restricts meal size. In addition, the surgeon alters the digestive route by connecting the pouch directly to the jejunum; this reduces nutrient absorption because the nutrients bypass a significant portion of the small intestine. In the gastric banding procedure, a gastric pouch is created using a fluid-filled inflatable band. Adjusting the band's fluid level can tighten or loosen the band and alter the size of the opening between the pouch and the rest of the stomach. A smaller opening reduces the speed at which the pouch is emptied and prolongs the sense of fullness after a

✚ Bariatric surgery was introduced in Chapter 7 (see p. 176).

✚ The gastric bypass surgery is also known as a *Roux-en-Y gastric bypass* because the reconstructed small intestine resembles the letter *Y*.

> ### NURSING DIAGNOSIS
>
> Appropriate for the ideal bariatric surgery candidate may include *readiness for enhanced self health management* and *readiness for enhanced knowledge*.

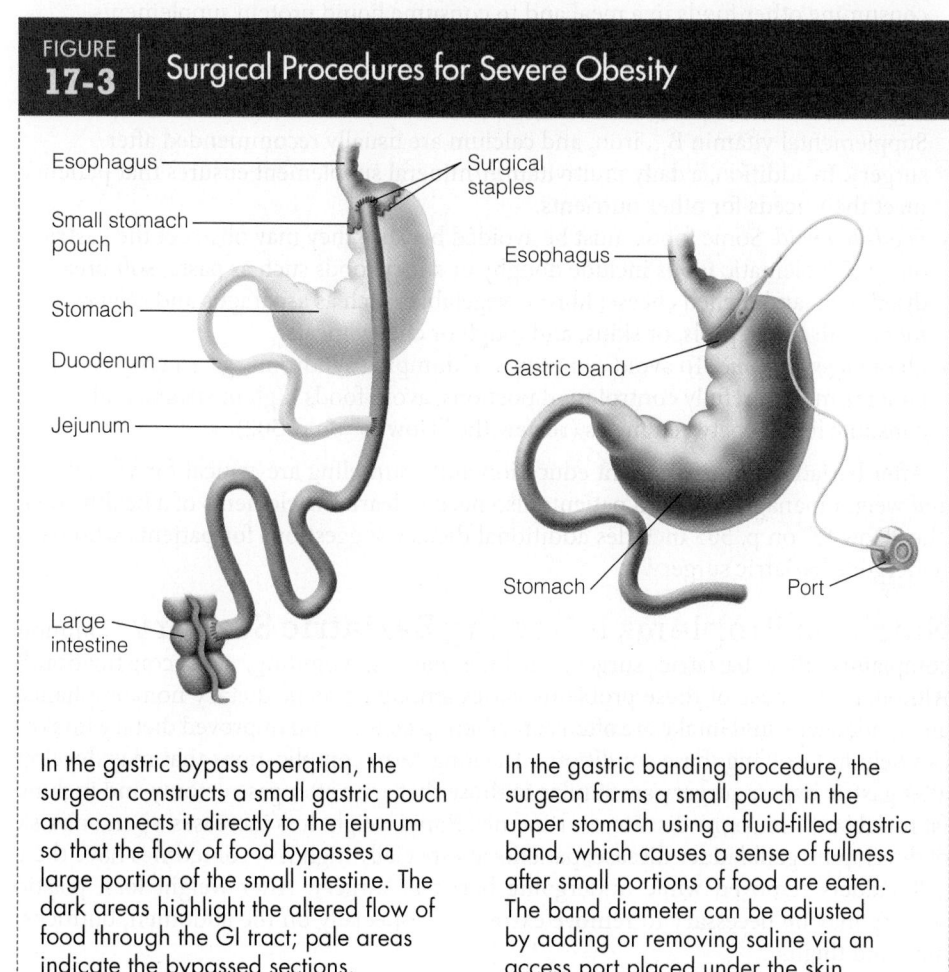

FIGURE 17-3 | Surgical Procedures for Severe Obesity

Esophagus
Small stomach pouch
Stomach
Duodenum
Jejunum
Large intestine

Surgical staples

Esophagus
Gastric band
Stomach
Port

In the gastric bypass operation, the surgeon constructs a small gastric pouch and connects it directly to the jejunum so that the flow of food bypasses a large portion of the small intestine. The dark areas highlight the altered flow of food through the GI tract; pale areas indicate the bypassed sections.

In the gastric banding procedure, the surgeon forms a small pouch in the upper stomach using a fluid-filled gastric band, which causes a sense of fullness after small portions of food are eaten. The band diameter can be adjusted by adding or removing saline via an access port placed under the skin.

meal. Whereas the gastric bypass operation is usually permanent, the gastric banding procedure is fully reversible.

Clinical studies indicate that both the short-term (1 year) and long-term (5 to 15 years) effectiveness of the gastric bypass surgery is better than that of the gastric banding procedure.[24] Although study results vary, gastric bypass patients typically lose 60 to 70 percent of their excess body weight, whereas those who undergo gastric banding lose about 50 percent of their excess weight.[25] Moreover, long-term complications and follow-up operations are more common after the gastric banding procedure.

Nutrition Care after Bariatric Surgery
The main objectives of nutrition care after bariatric surgery are to maximize and maintain weight loss, ensure appropriate nutrient intakes, maintain hydration, and avoid complications such as nausea and vomiting or dumping syndrome.[26] Although the gastric pouch created by surgery eventually expands to hold about ½ cup of food, its initial capacity is only a few tablespoons. Only sugar-free, noncarbonated clear liquids and low-fat broths are given on the day following bariatric surgery. Afterward, patients consume a liquid diet at first, followed by pureed foods and then a soft food diet; the diet is advanced as tolerated. Once the diet progresses to solid foods, patients often consume between three and six small meals per day. Only small portions of food should be consumed at each meal because overeating can stretch the gastric pouch. Similarly, fluids must be consumed separately from meals to avoid excessive distention. Nutrition-related concerns include the following:

- *Protein intake.* The protein recommendation for bariatric patients is 1.5 grams of protein per kilogram of body weight per day; however, intakes are often lower than recommended.[27] Patients are generally instructed to eat high-protein foods before consuming other foods in a meal and to consume liquid protein supplements regularly.
- *Vitamin and mineral deficiencies.* Bariatric patients have a high risk of developing nutrient deficiencies due to reduced food intake and nutrient malabsorption. Supplemental vitamin B_{12}, iron, and calcium are usually recommended after surgery. In addition, a daily multivitamin/mineral supplement ensures that patients meet their needs for other nutrients.
- *Foods to avoid.* Some foods must be avoided because they may obstruct the gastric outlet. Problematic foods include doughy or sticky foods such as pasta, soft breads, dried fruit, and melted cheese; fibrous vegetables such as asparagus and celery; foods with seeds, peels, or skins; and tough or chewy meats.
- *Dumping syndrome.* To avoid symptoms of dumping syndrome, gastric bypass patients must carefully control food portions, avoid foods high in sugars, and consume liquids between meals (review the "How to" on p. 502).

After bariatric surgery, patient education and counseling are critical for weight loss and weight management, and patients also need to learn the elements of a healthy diet. The "How to" on p. 505 includes additional dietary suggestions for patients who have undergone bariatric surgery.

Nutrition Problems following Bariatric Surgery
Common complaints after bariatric surgery include nausea, vomiting, and constipation.[28] Although the cause of these problems varies among patients, dietary noncompliance and inadequate fluid intake are often contributing factors, and improved dietary intakes can help in resolving these conditions. The long-term complications that may develop after gastric bypass surgery are similar to those that arise after gastrectomy and include fat malabsorption, bone disease, and anemia. Rapid weight loss increases a person's risk of developing gallbladder disease; patients at especially high risk sometimes have their gallbladders removed while undergoing bariatric surgery. After weight loss, plastic surgery may be necessary to remove extra skin, especially on the abdomen, buttocks, hips, and thighs.

Patients need to learn new dietary habits after bariatric surgery. The following recommendations may help:

- Consume only small portions of food, and chew food thoroughly. Use a small spoon, and take small bites. Relax and enjoy the meal, taking at least 20 minutes to eat.

- Understand that, at first, the appropriate amount of each food served at mealtime may be only a few spoonfuls. Learn to recognize the sensations that occur when the gastric pouch is full. Signs of fullness may include pressure in the stomach region, a slight feeling of nausea, or pain in the upper chest or shoulder.

- To control vomiting, try eating smaller volumes of food, eating more slowly, and avoiding foods known to cause difficulty. Continued vomiting may be a sign that some food choices or amounts are inappropriate.

- Consume food only during designated mealtimes (usually three to six small meals per day), and avoid consuming foods at other times of the day. Snacking throughout the day can become a bad habit that causes weight to be regained.

- Avoid consuming liquids within 45 minutes of mealtime. Avoid high-kcalorie drinks like sweetened soda, milk shakes, and alcoholic beverages. Avoid drinking carbonated beverages or using a straw, as these practices can increase stomach gas and cause bloating.

- Sip water and other beverages throughout the day to obtain sufficient fluids. Generally, between 6 and 8 cups of water and other noncaloric beverages should be consumed daily. Remember that most people can meet a significant fraction of their fluid needs by eating food, but a person who has undergone bariatric surgery has a limited food intake.

- Engage in regular physical activity. Activity is a valuable aid to weight maintenance and can help to maintain lean tissue while weight is being lost.

Review Notes

- Gastric surgeries are used to treat cancer, peptic ulcer complications, and obesity. These surgeries may alter stomach size or function, and therefore dietary adjustments are required afterward.

- After a gastrectomy procedure, dietary measures depend on the size of the remaining stomach and the stomach emptying rate. Complications may include dumping syndrome, fat malabsorption, bone disease, and anemia.

- Dumping syndrome, characterized by a group of symptoms caused by rapid gastric emptying, is managed by controlling food portions, avoiding foods high in sugars, and consuming liquids between meals.

- After bariatric surgery, patients must learn to consume appropriate food portions; use dietary supplements to prevent nutrient deficiencies; and choose foods that are unlikely to cause abdominal discomfort, vomiting, or dumping syndrome.

Nutrition Assessment | CHECKLIST FOR PEOPLE WITH UPPER GI TRACT DISORDERS

MEDICAL HISTORY

Check the medical history to uncover conditions or treatments that may:

- Interfere with chewing or swallowing
- Lead to dry mouth
- Lead to dyspepsia, nausea, or vomiting

Check for a medical diagnosis of:

- Gastritis or peptic ulcer
- GERD
- Hiatal hernia
- Pernicious anemia

For a patient who has undergone gastric surgery, check for the following complications:

- Anemia
- Bone disease
- Dumping syndrome
- Fat malabsorption

MEDICATIONS

Record all medications and note:

- ❍ Aspirin or NSAID use in patients with gastritis or peptic ulcer disease
- ❍ Medications that may cause dry mouth
- ❍ Medications that may cause nausea and vomiting

To help alleviate nausea, suggest that medications be taken with food, when possible.

DIETARY INTAKE

To devise an acceptable meal plan, obtain:

- ❍ An accurate and thorough record of food intake
- ❍ A record of foods that provoke symptoms of GERD, dyspepsia, gastritis, peptic ulcers, or dumping syndrome

For patients on long-term dysphagia diets, monitor:

- ❍ Appetite
- ❍ Food tolerances
- ❍ Variety of foods regularly consumed

ANTHROPOMETRIC DATA

Measure baseline height and weight. Address weight loss early to prevent malnutrition in patients with:

- ❍ Dumping syndrome
- ❍ Dyspepsia or long-term nausea

- ❍ Dysphagia or difficulty chewing
- ❍ Malabsorption

LABORATORY TESTS

Check laboratory tests for signs of dehydration for patients with:

- ❍ Constipation
- ❍ Dumping syndrome
- ❍ Persistent vomiting

Check laboratory tests for nutrition-related anemia in patients with:

- ❍ Gastritis
- ❍ Long-term use of antisecretory drugs
- ❍ Previous gastric surgeries

PHYSICAL SIGNS

Look for physical signs of:

- ❍ Dehydration—in patients with persistent vomiting, dumping syndrome, or constipation
- ❍ Iron and vitamin B_{12} deficiencies—in patients with hypochlorhydria or achlorhydria

Self Check

1 • If a patient with dysphagia has difficulty swallowing solids but can easily swallow liquids:
   a. the problem is probably a motility disorder.
   b. the patient most likely has achalasia.
   c. the problem is probably an esophageal obstruction.
   d. the problem is most likely oropharyngeal dysphagia.

2 • The nurse working with a patient with dysphagia should recognize that:
   a. only pureed foods should be given to minimize the risk of aspiration.
   b. the patient can have any food that can be comfortably and safely chewed and swallowed.
   c. highly seasoned foods are often restricted.
   d. conventional diets are unable to meet total nutrient needs, so supplements are required.

3 • Gastroesophageal reflux disease (GERD) is:
   a. characterized by frequent backflow of the stomach's gastric secretions into the esophagus.
   b. a protuberance of a portion of the stomach above the lower esophageal sphincter.
   c. an open sore in the GI mucosa caused by the destructive effects of gastric secretions.
   d. an obstruction of the lower esophagus that results in dysphagia.

4 • Conditions associated with an increased risk of developing GERD include:
   a. hiatal hernia.
   b. asthma.
   c. pregnancy.
   d. all of the above.

5 • For the patient with persistent vomiting, the major nutrition-related concern(s) is/are:
   a. dehydration and malnutrition.
   b. reflux esophagitis.
   c. dyspepsia.
   d. peptic ulcers.

6 • Chronic gastritis frequently leads to:
   a. dumping syndrome.
   b. bone disease.
   c. iron and vitamin B_{12} deficiencies.
   d. excessive hydrochloric acid secretion.

7 • The primary cause of most peptic ulcers is:
   a. consumption of spicy foods.
   b. hypochlorhydria.
   c. smoking cigarettes.
   d. *Helicobacter pylori* infection.

8 • Foods discouraged for patients with gastritis or active ulcers include those that:
   a. are high in fiber.
   b. irritate the gastric mucosa.
   c. are easy to swallow.
   d. contain simple sugars.

9 • People at risk of dumping syndrome should generally avoid:
   a. high-fiber foods.
   b. sweets and sugars.
   c. beverages.
   d. bread and potatoes.

10• The nurse assessing a patient who underwent a gastrectomy several years ago should be alert to signs of:
   a. dysphagia.
   b. GERD.
   c. anemia.
   d. gastritis.

Answers to these questions appear in Appendix H.

Clinical Applications

1 • Although some individuals require a mechanically altered diet for just a few weeks, others have medical problems that require long-term use of such diets. Consider the difference between working with a person who has had a swallowing problem for years and a person who recently had mouth surgery and is just beginning to eat again.

   • Explain how the needs of these individuals may differ. What nutrition-related problems may develop if a person has been following a restrictive dysphagia diet for several years?
   • Using Table 17-3 and the "How to" on p. 491, create a day's worth of menus for a person who requires long-term use of a pureed dysphagia diet and tolerates only liquids that have a honeylike consistency.

2 • Jillian, a 35-year-old woman who is 5 feet 4 inches tall and weighs 227 pounds, has had severe hip and knee osteoarthritis for several years and was recently diagnosed with type 2 diabetes. After trying numerous diet programs without success, she finally visits a bariatric surgeon to learn about the surgical options for treating her obesity.

   • Calculate Jillian's BMI, and explain why or why not Jillian would be a good candidate for bariatric surgery.
   • Should Jillian decide to undergo gastric bypass surgery, she will need to permanently change her dietary habits. Outline the diet progression typically recommended after bariatric surgery, and describe the dietary measures necessary for preventing vomiting, distention of the gastric pouch, gastric outlet obstruction, and dumping syndrome.
   • Explain why dehydration is a frequent complication following bariatric surgery. What tips can you give Jillian to help her avoid this problem?

Nutrition on the Net
For further study of topics covered in this chapter, access these websites.

• Find updates and quick links to these and other nutrition-related sites at our website: www.cengage.com/nutrition/whitney/nhhc4e
• Visit the websites of these organizations to find information that is helpful both for health practitioners and patients with gastrointestinal problems:
American College of Gastroenterology: www.acg.gi.org
American Gastroenterological Association: www.gastro.org
Digestive Health Center of Excellence, University of Virginia Health System: www.healthsystem.virginia.edu/internet/digestive-health

International Foundation for Functional Gastrointestinal Disorders: www.iffgd.org
National Institute of Diabetes and Digestive and Kidney Diseases, a division of the National Institutes of Health: www2.niddk.nih.gov
• Learn more about *Helicobacter pylori* from the Helicobacter Foundation: www.helico.com
• The Consumer Guide to Bariatric Surgery provides general information about bariatric surgeries at this website: www.yourbariatricsurgeryguide.com

Notes

1. T. E. Daniels, Diseases of the mouth and salivary glands, in L. Goldman and D. Ausiello, eds., *Cecil Medicine* (Philadelphia: Saunders, 2008), pp. 2867–2874; D. P. DePaola and coauthors, Nutrition and dental medicine, in M. E. Shils and coeditors, *Modern Nutrition in Health and Disease* (Baltimore: Lippincott Williams & Wilkins, 2006), pp. 1152–1178.

2. J. J. Heidelbaugh and coauthors, Gastroenterology, in R. E. Rakel, ed., *Textbook of Family Medicine* (Philadelphia: Saunders, 2007), pp. 1115–1171.

3. R. K. Goyal, A. Chaudhury, and H. Mashimo, Oropharyngeal and esophageal motility disorders, in N. J. Greenberger, ed., *Current Diagnosis and Treatment: Gastroenterology, Hepatology, and Endoscopy* (New York: McGraw-Hill Companies, 2009), pp. 155–171.

4. R. C. Orlando, Diseases of the esophagus, in L. Goldman and D. Ausiello, eds., *Cecil Medicine* (Philadelphia: Saunders, 2008), pp. 998–1009.

5. The National Dysphagia Diet Task Force, *The National Dysphagia Diet: Standardization for Optimal Care* (Chicago: American Dietetic Association, 2002).

6. American Dietetic Association, *Nutrition Care Manual* (Chicago: American Dietetic Association, 2009).

7. J. R. Agrawal and S. Friedman, Gastrointestinal and biliary complications of pregnancy, in N. J. Greenberger, ed., *Current Diagnosis and Treatment: Gastroenterology, Hepatology, and Endoscopy* (New York: McGraw-Hill Companies, 2009), pp. 75–97.

8. Agrawal and Friedman, 2009; Orlando, 2008.

9. N. J. Talley, Functional gastrointestinal disorders: Irritable bowel syndrome, dyspepsia, and noncardiac chest pain, in L. Goldman and D. Ausiello, eds., *Cecil Medicine* (Philadelphia: Saunders, 2008), pp. 990–998.

10. V. S. Wang and R. Burakoff, Functional (nonulcer) dyspepsia, in N. J. Greenberger, ed., *Current Diagnosis and Treatment: Gastroenterology, Hepatology, and Endoscopy* (New York: McGraw-Hill Companies, 2009), pp. 189–199.

11. Talley, 2008.

12. Wang and Burakoff, 2009; S. Escott-Stump, *Nutrition and Diagnosis-Related Care* (Baltimore: Lippincott Williams & Wilkins, 2008).

13. American Dietetic Association, 2009; Escott-Stump, 2008.

14. B. Cryer and S. J. Spechler, Peptic ulcer disease, in M. Feldman, L. S. Friedman, and L. J. Brandt, eds., *Sleisenger and Fordtran's Gastrointestinal and Liver Disease* (Philadelphia: Saunders, 2006), pp. 1089–1110.

15. K. Ramakrishnan and R. C. Salinas, Peptic ulcer disease, *American Family Physician* 76 (2007): 1005–1012.

16. E. Lew, Peptic ulcer disease, in N. J. Greenberger, ed., *Current Diagnosis and Treatment: Gastroenterology, Hepatology, and Endoscopy* (New York: McGraw-Hill Companies, 2009), pp. 175–183.

17. American Dietetic Association, 2009.

18. F. F. Ferri, *Ferri's Clinical Advisor 2009: Instant Diagnosis and Treatment* (Philadelphia: Mosby, 2009), pp. 693–694; W. F. Stenson, The esophagus and stomach, in M. E. Shils and coeditors, *Modern Nutrition in Health and Disease* (Baltimore: Lippincott Williams & Wilkins, 2006), pp. 1179–1188.

19. American Dietetic Association, 2009.

20. American Dietetic Association, 2009.

21. C. R. Parrish, Post-gastrectomy: Managing the nutrition fall-out, *Nutrition Issues in Gastroenterology* 18 (2004): 63–75.

22. M. K. Robinson and N. J. Greenberger, Treatment of obesity: The impact of bariatric surgery, in N. J. Greenberger, ed., *Current Diagnosis and Treatment: Gastroenterology, Hepatology, and Endoscopy* (New York: McGraw-Hill Companies, 2009), pp. 210–221.

23. Robinson and Greenberger, 2009.

24. Weight Management Dietetic Practice Group, *ADA Pocket Guide to Bariatric Surgery* (Chicago: American Dietetic Association, 2009), pp. 1–16; American Dietetic Association, 2009; J. A. Tice and coauthors, Gastric banding or bypass? A systematic review comparing the two most popular bariatric procedures, *American Journal of Medicine* 121 (2008): 885–893.

25. Weight Management Dietetic Practice Group, 2009.

26. American Dietetic Association, 2009.

27. American Dietetic Association, 2009.

28. Robinson and Greenberger, 2009.

Nutrition and Oral Health

Several aspects of nutrition and oral health were discussed earlier in this book. Chapter 3 described the relationship between carbohydrate-containing foods and dental caries. Chapter 9 explained how the fluoridation of water can help to prevent dental decay. Chapter 10 discussed the development of dental caries in babies who are given bottles for prolonged periods. This Nutrition in Practice provides additional information about dental caries and introduces other dental problems related to nutritional health. Related terms are defined in the accompanying glossary.

What is dental caries, and what factors influence its development?

Dental caries is an oral infectious disease that affects the structures and integrity of the teeth. Caries develops when the bacteria that reside in **dental plaque** metabolize dietary carbohydrates and produce acids that attack tooth enamel. If allowed to progress, the decay can penetrate the dentin and destroy other structures that support and maintain the tooth (see Figure NP17-1). The development of dental caries is influenced by the type of carbohydrate consumed,

| FIGURE NP17-1 | Development of Dental Caries |

Labels: Enamel, Caries, Dentin, Gum, Crown, Pulp (blood vessels, nerves), Bone, Root canal, Nerve, Blood vessel

Dental caries begins when acid dissolves the enamel that covers the tooth. If not repaired, the decay may penetrate the dentin and spread into the pulp of the tooth, causing inflammation, abscess, and possible loss of the tooth.

frequency of carbohydrate intake, stickiness of the foods that contain carbohydrate, and the availability of saliva to rinse the teeth and neutralize acid. Other factors include oral hygiene, fluoride intake, and the composition of tooth enamel, which together affect a person's susceptibility to caries. In addition, poor nutrition during pregnancy, infancy, or early childhood can impair the development of healthy teeth, increasing vulnerability to dental caries.[1] Table NP17-1 shows the effects of specific nutrient deficiencies on the development of dental caries.

Which foods promote caries development?

As mentioned, foods that contain sugars or starches can support the growth of bacteria in dental plaque. The most **cariogenic** foods are those that remain in contact with the teeth for prolonged periods, are difficult to clear from the mouth, or are consumed frequently or over an extended time period. Examples include hard candies or lozenges that dissolve slowly in the mouth; sticky or chewy foods such as dried fruits, jelly beans, or chewy breads; starchy snack foods such as pretzels or chips, and sweetened beverages that are

Glossary

cariogenic (KAH-ree-oh-JEN-ik): conducive to development of dental caries.

dental calculus: mineralized dental plaque, often associated with inflammation and bleeding.

dental caries (KAH-reez): infectious disease of the teeth that causes the gradual decay and disintegration of tooth structures.

dental plaque (PLACK): a film of bacteria and bacterial by-products that accumulates on the tooth surface.

gingiva (jin-JYE-va, JIN-jeh-va): the gums.

gingivitis (jin-jeh-VYE-tus): inflammation of the gums, characterized by redness, swelling, and bleeding.

periodontal disease: disease that involves the connective tissue that supports the teeth.

periodontitis: inflammation or degeneration of the tissues that support the teeth.

periodontium: the tissues that support the teeth, including the gums, cementum (bonelike material covering the dentin layer of the tooth), periodontal ligament, and underlying bone.

- *peri* = around, surrounding
- *odont* = tooth

TABLE NP17-1	Nutrient Deficiencies Affecting Development of Dental Caries	
Nutrient Deficiency	**Effect on Dental Tissues**	
Protein	Increased solubility of tooth enamel	
Vitamin A	Impaired formation of tooth enamel	
Vitamin D	Impaired formation of tooth enamel, reduced enamel mineralization	
Calcium	Reduced enamel mineralization	
Phosphorus	Reduced enamel mineralization	
Fluoride	Increased susceptibility to enamel demineralization, reduced protection against decay-causing bacteria	

repeatedly sipped. These foods can be eaten without provoking tooth decay if they are consumed quickly and removed from tooth surfaces promptly.

Acidic foods and beverages, such as cola drinks, citrus fruits and juices, pickles, and some herbal teas, also contribute to the erosion of tooth enamel.[2] Acidic food items are more cariogenic when consumed after or between meals because they are less likely to be rinsed away by saliva or neutralized by alkaline foods that may be consumed during the meal.

Do any foods help to prevent caries?

Yes. Foods that stimulate saliva flow, neutralize mouth acidity, or induce the clearance of food particles from the teeth can help to prevent caries formation. Examples include cheese, which increases salivary secretions and contains nutrients that neutralize acid; milk, which reduces mouth acidity due to its nearly neutral pH; and raw vegetables, which require vigorous chewing and therefore stimulate saliva flow. Some foods contain substances that reduce enamel solubility, such as the fluoride in tea and an unidentified compound in cocoa. The sequence in which foods are eaten influences caries development; for example, eating cheese after consuming an acidic fruit dessert can raise plaque pH and reduce caries risk, whereas drinking sugared coffee at the end of the meal can prolong plaque acidity. Chewing sugarless gum after or between meals can help to prevent caries by stimulating salivary flow, pushing saliva into hard-to-reach crevices in and around teeth, and removing food particles from the teeth.[3]

How does saliva protect against caries formation?

In addition to rinsing away the sugars and food particles that remain on the teeth, saliva contains substances—including proteins, bicarbonate, and phosphates—that dilute and neutralize mouth acidity. Furthermore, saliva contains antimicrobial proteins (immunoglobulins and lysozyme) that defend against bacteria and fungi. Finally, the calcium, phosphate, and fluoride ions in saliva help to prevent dissolution of enamel and promote remineralization. Therefore, if salivary secretions are low or absent, the risk of developing dental caries and other dental diseases greatly increases.

Does dental plaque contribute to other dental diseases?

Yes, the deposits of plaque can thicken and lead to a number of other dental problems. As plaque accumulates, it fills with calcium and phosphate, eventually forming **dental calculus**. Calculus may develop either at the gum surface or in the crevice between the gum and a tooth; its presence may lead to additional plaque retention. The buildup of plaque and calculus increases the likelihood of infection and subsequent inflammation.

Periodontal disease is the name given to inflammatory conditions that involve the **periodontium**, the structures that support the tooth in its bony socket. The periodontium includes the gums (called **gingiva**), other connective tissues surrounding the tooth, and the bone underneath. Inflammation of the gums, called **gingivitis**, is characterized by redness, bleeding, and swelling of gum tissue. **Periodontitis** is an inflammation of the other tissues surrounding the tooth. As plaque invades the space below the gum line, the combination of toxic bacterial by-products and the body's immune response can damage the tissues holding a tooth in place.

Periodontal disease destroys the tissues and bones that hold teeth in place.

Left untreated, the tissues and bone of the peridontium may ultimately be destroyed, leading to permanent tooth loss.

What are the risk factors for periodontal disease, and how is it treated?

Dental plaque is the major risk factor associated with periodontal disease, and the severity of disease is related to the amount of plaque present. Tobacco smoking is another factor, possibly because of its destructive effects on cellular immune responses.[4] The risk of developing periodontal disease is especially high if a person has a chronic illness that impairs immune status, such as diabetes mellitus or HIV infection. Other risk factors include stress, pregnancy, use of certain medications (including oral contraceptives, antiepileptic drugs, and anticancer drugs), and dental conditions that increase plaque accumulation, such as poorly aligned teeth or ill-fitting bridges.[5] Strategies for reducing risk focus on improving oral hygiene (proper brushing and flossing) and encouraging smoking cessation.

Treatment of periodontal disease depends on the extent of damage. In mild cases, deep cleaning and proper oral hygiene may reverse the condition. Antimicrobial mouth rinses and topical antibiotics are often prescribed to control infection. Surgical approaches are sometimes necessary to remove plaque or calculus deposits underneath gum tissue or to replace tissues that have been destroyed.

How do chronic illnesses influence a person's risk for dental diseases?

Maintaining dental health is especially challenging for people who have certain chronic illnesses. Some diseases can alter the structure and function of dental tissues, impair immune responses, or cause reduced salivary flow. Furthermore, many medications can reduce salivary secretions, along with the immune protection that saliva provides. Examples of conditions that increase risk for dental diseases include the following:

- *Diabetes mellitus.* Periodontal disease is more prevalent among people with diabetes mellitus, especially those whose diabetes is poorly controlled. People with diabetes often have impaired immune responses and a greater susceptibility to infections. Diabetes also favors the growth of bacteria that tend to infect periodontal tissues. People with diabetes tend to have higher plaque accumulations and dry mouth. In addition, the damaging effects of hyperglycemia weaken the collagen structure of dental tissues, making them more vulnerable to destruction.[6]
- *Human immunodeficiency virus (HIV)/AIDS.* HIV infection is characterized by compromised immunity, and the risk of developing periodontal disease is closely linked

to the extent of HIV infection. Those at greatest risk include smokers, individuals who decline therapy, and patients in the advanced stages of disease.[7] In untreated persons, fungal and viral infections are common and may cause burning in the mouth and painful ulcerations. HIV-infected individuals often have dry mouth as a result of medications or salivary gland dysfunction.[8]
- *Oral cancers.* Radiation treatment of oral cancers often causes serious oral and dental complications.[9] Inflammation and tissue damage can be so severe that the radiation treatment may need to be halted or the intensity significantly reduced. Dry mouth is a common side effect of radiation therapy. Other complications include fungal and viral infections, changes in taste sensation, and tissue and muscle scarring (which often reduces chewing ability). To minimize complications, dental care is often initiated before radiation therapy begins.

Can dental diseases have adverse effects on health beyond their effects on the teeth?

Yes, the bacteria that reside on dental tissues can enter the bloodstream and travel to other tissues; therefore, they may be able to trigger immune responses or cause infections elsewhere in the body.[10] Evidence supports a link between dental bacteria and other medical conditions, including the following:

- *Systemic inflammation.* The inflammatory process induced by periodontal disease increases levels of cytokines and other mediators that have systemic effects. Systemic inflammation may contribute to the development of certain chronic illnesses, including heart disease and diabetes.
- *Atherosclerosis and heart disease.* Oral bacteria are frequently found residing in the arteries of people with atherosclerosis, where they may induce the release of inflammatory mediators that promote atherosclerosis. Studies suggest that severe periodontal disease may increase the risk of cardiovascular disease by 25 to 90 percent.[11]
- *Diabetes mellitus.* The chronic inflammation caused by periodontal disease is a potential risk factor for the development of type 2 diabetes. Severe periodontal disease has also been linked to poor glycemic control in persons with diabetes.
- *Respiratory illnesses.* The teeth of hospital patients often become colonized with bacteria that cause respiratory illnesses. In one research study, only patients whose teeth were colonized by respiratory pathogens ended up with pneumonia.[12]

Research studies are in progress to confirm cause-and-effect relationships between oral bacteria and the medical conditions described above, as well as the specific mechanisms involved.

Nutrition status has a strong influence on oral health. Developing sound eating habits and maintaining good dental hygiene are practices that can promote dental health and possibly reduce the risk of developing other medical problems. Additional studies will help to clarify the complex interactions between dental disease and chronic illnesses.

Notes

1. D. P. DePaola and coauthors, Nutrition and dental medicine, in M. E. Shils and coeditors, *Modern Nutrition in Health and Disease* (Baltimore: Lippincott Williams & Wilkins, 2006), pp. 1152–1178.
2. S. Wongkhantee and coauthors, Effect of acidic food and drinks on surface hardness of enamel, dentine, and tooth-coloured filling materials, *Journal of Dentistry* 34 (2006): 214–220; J. Phelan and J. Rees, The erosive potential of some herbal teas, *Journal of Dentistry* 31 (2003): 241–246.
3. S. K. Stookey, The effect of saliva on dental caries, *Journal of the American Dental Association* 139 (2008): 11S–17S; DePaola and coauthors, 2006.
4. B. Loos and coauthors, Lymphocyte numbers and function in relation to periodontitis and smoking, *Journal of Periodontology* 75 (2004): 557–564.
5. J. Kim and S. Amar, Periodontal disease and systemic conditions: A bidirectional relationship, *Odontology* 94 (2006): 10–21; Y.-T. A. Teng and coauthors, Periodontal health and systemic disorders, *Journal of the Canadian Dental Association* 68 (2002): 188–192.
6. American Dietetic Association, Position of the American Dietetic Association: Oral health and nutrition, *Journal of the American Dietetic Association* (2007): 1418–1428; DePaola and coauthors, 2006.
7. T. Alpagot and coauthors, Risk factors for periodontitis in HIV patients, *Journal of Periodontal Research* 39 (2004): 149–157.
8. M. Navazesh and coauthors, A 4-year longitudinal evaluation of xerostomia and salivary gland hypofunction in the Women's Interagency HIV Study participants, *Oral Surgery Oral Medicine Oral Pathology Oral Radiology and Endodontics* 95 (2003): 693–698.
9. American Dietetic Association, 2007; J. B. Epstein and coauthors, Cancer-related oral health care services and resources: A survey of oral and dental care in Canadian cancer centres, *Journal of the Canadian Dental Association* 70 (2004): 302–304.
10. Kim and Amar, 2006; Teng and coauthors, 2002.
11. Kim and Amar, 2006.
12. Teng and coauthors, 2002.

CHAPTER 18 | Nutrition and Lower Gastrointestinal Disorders

© Istockphoto.com/ambaradan

CONTENTS

The fiber DRI for women and men aged 19 to 50 years are 25 and 38 grams, respectively. Recommendations for increasing fiber intake are described on p. 81, and Appendix A includes the fiber values of most common foods.

NURSING DIAGNOSIS

Perceived constipation may apply to people with adequate bowel movements who self-diagnose constipation.

NURSING DIAGNOSIS

Constipation and *risk for constipation* may apply to persons with medical problems that predispose them to constipation.

BECAUSE MOST DIGESTIVE AND ABSORPTIVE PROCESSES OCCUR IN THE small intestine, disorders of the lower gastrointestinal (GI) tract can interfere substantially with a patient's diet and lifestyle. Some of the diets required for these conditions are complicated and difficult to follow, and the foods that are tolerated can vary considerably. In visits with patients, nurses should ensure that patients understand the nutrition prescription and help to pinpoint difficult foods. They can also suggest ways to make restrictive diets more acceptable.

Common Intestinal Problems

Nearly all people experience occasional intestinal problems, which usually clear up without medical treatment. Intestinal discomfort can sometimes drive a person to seek medical attention, however, and the symptoms may be evidence of a serious intestinal disorder or other illness. The most common intestinal problems and their causes and treatments are discussed below.

CONSTIPATION

A medical diagnosis of constipation is based, in part, on a defecation frequency of fewer than three bowel movements per week. Other symptoms may include the passage of hard stool and excessive straining during defecation. In some cases, a person's perception of constipation may be due to a mistaken notion of what constitutes "normal" bowel habits, so the person's expectations about bowel function may need to be addressed.

Constipation is much more prevalent among women than men and is a common complaint during pregnancy. The incidence of constipation increases with aging, although elderly individuals tend to find straining during defecation to be a greater problem than infrequent defecation.[1]

Causes of Constipation In Western societies, the incidence of constipation often correlates with low-fiber diets, low food intake, inadequate fluid intake, and physical inactivity. All of these factors can extend transit time, leading to increased water reabsorption within the colon and dry, hard stools that are difficult to pass. Medical conditions often associated with constipation include diabetes mellitus, hypothyroidism, and chronic kidney disease. Neurological conditions such as multiple sclerosis, Parkinson's disease, and spinal cord injuries may cause motor problems that lead to constipation. During pregnancy, women can experience constipation because the enlarged uterus presses against the rectum and colon. Constipation is also a common side effect of several classes of medications and some dietary supplements, including opiate-containing analgesics, tricyclic antidepressants, anticonvulsants, calcium channel blockers, aluminum-containing antacids, and iron and calcium supplements.

Treatment of Constipation The primary treatment for constipation is a gradual increase in fiber intake to about 25 grams per day.[2] (✚) High-fiber diets increase stool weight and fecal water content and promote a more rapid transit of materials through the colon. Foods that increase stool weight the most are wheat bran, fruits, and vegetables.[3] Bran intake can be increased by adding bran cereals and whole-wheat bread to the diet or by mixing bran powder with beverages or foods. The transition to a high-fiber diet may be difficult for some people because it can increase intestinal gas, so high-fiber foods should be added gradually, as tolerated. Fiber supplements such as methylcellulose (Citrucel), psyllium (Metamucil, Fiberall), and polycarbophil (Fiber-Lax) are also effective (see Table 18-1); these supplements can be mixed with beverages and taken several times daily. Unlike other fibers, methylcellulose and polycarbophil do not increase intestinal gas.

Several other measures may also help constipation. Consuming adequate fluid (usually 1.5 to 2 liters daily) helps to increase stool frequency in people who are already consuming a high-fiber diet.[4] An appropriate fluid intake prevents excessive reabsorption of water from the colon, resulting in wetter stools. Adding prunes or prune juice to the diet is often recommended because prunes contain compounds that have a mild laxative effect. Increasing daily exercise can help to stimulate peristalsis.

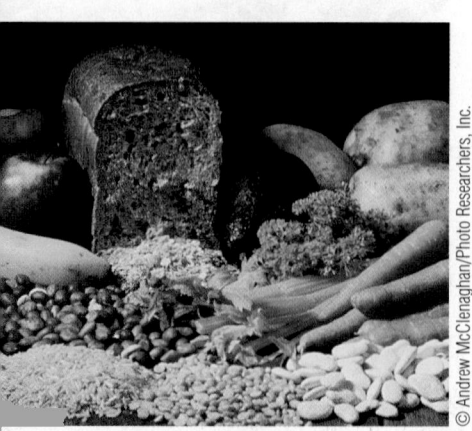

© Andrew McClenaghan/Photo Researchers, Inc.

High-fiber foods promote regular bowel movements.

TABLE
18-1 | Laxatives and Bulk-Forming Agents

Laxative Type	Active Ingredients	Product Examples	Method of Action	Cautions
Fiber (bulk-forming agents)	Malt soup extract, methylcellulose, polycarbophil, psyllium	Citrucel, Fiberall, Fiber-Lax, Metamucil	Fiber supplements increase stool weight and aid in formation of soft, bulky stools. Similar effects are achieved by adding bran to the diet. For mild constipation. Safe for long-term use.	Some fiber supplements may increase flatulence. Psyllium may cause an allergic reaction.
Osmotic laxatives: nonabsorbable salts	Magnesium citrate, magnesium hydroxide, sodium phosphate	Epsom salts, milk of magnesia	Unabsorbed salts attract and retain water in the large intestine and stimulate contractions.	May cause bloating and watery stools or diarrhea. Should be used with caution. Avoid using in renal patients and children.
Osmotic laxatives: nonabsorbable sugars	Lactulose, polyethylene glycol, sorbitol	Cephulac, Chronulac	Unabsorbed sugars attract water to the large intestine and promote softer stools. Must be used for several days to take effect. Safe for long-term use.	May cause flatulence and cramps. Can lose effectiveness over time.
Stimulant or irritant laxatives	Aloe, bisacodyl, cascara, castor oil, senna	Correctol, Dulcolax, Ex-Lax	Act as local irritants to colonic tissue; stimulate peristalsis and mucosal secretions. For moderate to severe constipation. Long-term use is discouraged.	Usually given only after milder treatments fail. May alter fluid and electrolyte balances. May lead to laxative dependency.
Stool surfactant agents (stool softeners)	Docusate sodium	Colace, Kaopectate, Surfak	Detergent action promotes the mixing of water with stools. Prevents formation of dry, hard stools.	Do not increase stool weight. Limited effectiveness.

Laxatives Many laxatives can be purchased without prescription. They work by increasing stool weight, increasing the water content of stool, or stimulating peristaltic contractions. Table 18-1 includes examples of common laxatives and describes their modes of action. Enemas and suppositories (chemicals introduced into the rectum) are also used to promote defecation; they work by distending and stimulating the rectum or by lubricating the stool.

Medical Interventions Patients with severe constipation who do not respond to dietary or laxative treatments may require medications that stimulate colonic contractions. Physical therapy and biofeedback techniques are sometimes successful in training patients to relax their pelvic muscles more effectively. Surgical interventions are a last resort and include colonic resections and colostomy operations, which are discussed later in the chapter.

INTESTINAL GAS

As mentioned in the previous section, excessive intestinal gas (**flatulence**) may be an unpleasant side effect of consuming a high-fiber diet. Because dietary fibers are not digested, they pass into the colon and are fermented by bacteria, which produce gas as a by-product. (✚) Other incompletely digested or poorly absorbed carbohydrates have similar effects; these include fructose, sugar alcohols (sorbitol and mannitol), the

✚ Reminder: The *soluble fibers* in foods are more readily fermented in the small intestine than the *insoluble fibers*.

flatulence: the condition of having excessive intestinal gas, which causes abdominal discomfort.

Apples

Asparagus

Beer

Broccoli

Brussels sprouts

Cabbage

Carbonated beverages

Cauliflower

Corn

Dried beans and peas

Fructose-sweetened products

Fruit juices

Leeks

Milk products (if lactose intolerant)

Onions

Peanuts

Pears

Potatoes

Turnips

✚ *Probiotics* are live bacteria provided in foods and dietary supplements for the purpose of preventing or treating disease. Nutrition in Practice 18 describes the potential health benefits of probiotics.

indigestible carbohydrates in beans (raffinose and stachyose), and some forms of resistant starch, found in grain products and potatoes. Table 18-2 lists examples of foods commonly associated with excessive gas production, although individual responses vary. Malabsorptive disorders (discussed later in this chapter) can cause considerable flatulence because the undigested nutrients can be metabolized by colonic bacteria. Swallowed air that is not expelled by belching may travel to the intestines and be a source of intestinal gas as well.

Many people blame abdominal bloating and pain on excessive gas, but these symptoms do not correlate well with an increase in intestinal gas.[5] In fact, most people who self-diagnose a flatulence problem have no more intestinal gas than others. Some individuals who experience frequent symptoms of abdominal bloating and pain may eventually be diagnosed with irritable bowel syndrome (see pp. 533–534) or dyspepsia (discussed in Chapter 17).

DIARRHEA

Diarrhea is characterized by the passage of frequent, watery stools. In most cases, it lasts for only a day or two and subsides without complication. Severe or persistent diarrhea, however, can cause dehydration and electrolyte imbalances. If chronic, it may lead to weight loss and malnutrition. Serious cases of diarrhea are often accompanied by other symptoms, such as fever, abdominal cramps, dyspepsia, or bleeding, which help in diagnosing the cause.

Causes of Diarrhea Diarrhea is a complication of many gastrointestinal disorders and may also be induced by infections, medications, or dietary substances. It results from inadequate fluid reabsorption in the intestines, sometimes in conjunction with an increase in intestinal secretions.[6] In *osmotic diarrhea,* unabsorbed nutrients or other substances attract water to the colon and increase fecal water content; the usual causes include high intakes of poorly absorbed sugars (such as sorbitol, mannitol, or fructose), lactase deficiency (which causes lactose malabsorption), and ingestion of laxatives that contain magnesium or phosphates. In *secretory diarrhea,* the fluid secreted by the intestines exceeds the amount that can be reabsorbed by intestinal cells. Secretory diarrhea is often due to bacterial food poisoning but can also be caused by chemical substances or intestinal diseases that induce intestinal inflammation. Motility disorders that hasten the transit of colonic residue can also result in diarrhea due to the reduced contact time available for fluid reabsorption.

Acute cases of diarrhea start abruptly and may persist for several weeks; they are frequently caused by viral, bacterial, or protozoal infections or occur as a side effect of medications. Chronic diarrhea, which persists for three weeks or longer,[7] can result from malabsorptive disorders, inflammatory diseases, motility disorders, infectious diseases, radiation treatment, and many other conditions. As mentioned in earlier chapters, diarrhea is a frequent complication of tube feedings, and it may also occur when enteral feedings are resumed after a period of bowel rest (see Chapter 15).

Medical Treatment of Diarrhea Correcting the underlying medical problem is the first step in treating diarrhea. For example, antibiotics can be prescribed for treating intestinal infections. If a medication is the cause of diarrhea, a different drug may be prescribed. If certain foods are responsible, they can be omitted from the diet. Bulk-forming agents such as psyllium (Metamucil) or methylcellulose (Citrucel) can help to reduce the liquidity of the stool. If chronic diarrhea does not respond to treatment, antidiarrheal drugs may be prescribed to slow GI motility or reduce intestinal secretions. Probiotics (✚) may be beneficial for certain types of diarrhea (especially diarrhea caused by infections), but standard treatment protocols have not been developed.[8] People with severe, **intractable** diarrhea sometimes require total parenteral nutrition.

Oral Rehydration Therapy

Severe diarrhea requires the replacement of lost fluid and electrolytes. Oral rehydration solutions can be purchased or easily mixed using water, salts, and glucose or sucrose (see the recipe in the margin). (✚) The addition of carbohydrate to the rehydration solution facilitates sodium and water absorption. Commercial sports drinks are not ideal remedies for rehydration because their sodium content is too low, but they can be used if accompanied by salty snack foods.[9] When diarrhea results in extreme dehydration, intravenous solutions are used to quickly replenish fluid and electrolytes.

Nutrition Therapy for Diarrhea

Because diarrhea can develop for numerous reasons, the nutrition prescription depends on the medical diagnosis and severity of the condition. The dietary treatment often recommended is a low-residue, low-fat, lactose-free diet.[10] The low-residue diet limits foods that contribute to colonic residue, such as those with significant amounts of fiber, resistant starch, lactose (in lactose-intolerant individuals), fructose, and sugar alcohols. Fructose and sugar alcohols, which are poorly absorbed, retain fluids in the colon and contribute to osmotic diarrhea. Similarly, milk products may worsen osmotic diarrhea in persons who are lactose intolerant. Avoidance of fatty foods is recommended because they can sometimes aggravate diarrhea. Gas-producing foods can increase intestinal distention and cause additional discomfort. Patients should avoid coffee and tea because caffeine stimulates GI motility and can thereby reduce water reabsorption. In the treatment of formula-fed infants, apple pectin or banana flakes are sometimes added to formulas to help thicken stool consistency. Table 18-3 lists examples of foods that may worsen diarrhea, although individual tolerances vary.

✚ An oral rehydration solution can be mixed from the following ingredients:
- ½ tsp sodium chloride (table salt)
- ⅓ tsp potassium chloride (salt substitute)
- ¾ tsp sodium bicarbonate (baking soda)
- 1⅓ tbs sugar
- 1 qt water

intractable: not easily managed or controlled.

TABLE 18-3	Foods That May Worsen Diarrhea[a]	
Foods to Avoid	**Rationale**	**Selected Examples**
High-fiber foods	They increase colonic residue.	Breads and cereals with more than 2 g fiber per serving, fruits and vegetables with peels or skins
Foods with indigestible carbohydrates	They contribute to osmotic diarrhea.	Artichokes, asparagus, brussels sprouts, cabbage, dried beans and peas, fruit, garlic, green beans, leeks, onions, wheat, zucchini
Foods that contain fructose or sugar alcohols	They contribute to osmotic diarrhea.	Dried fruits, fresh fruits (except bananas), fruit juices, fructose-sweetened soft drinks, sugar-free gums and candies
Milk products, if person is lactose intolerant	They contribute to osmotic diarrhea.	Milk and milk products
Gas-producing foods	They increase abdominal discomfort.	Foods with poorly digested or absorbed carbohydrates (including foods listed in the three rows directly above)
Caffeine-containing beverages	They increase intestinal motility.	Coffee, tea, colas, energy drinks

[a]Individual tolerances vary; the foods to avoid are best determined by trial and error.

Review Notes

- The most common intestinal problems include constipation, intestinal gas, and diarrhea.
- Constipation accompanies a wide range of conditions but generally correlates with low-fiber diets, low food intake, and physical inactivity.
- Intestinal gas is largely produced by bacteria that colonize the colon and is most frequently associated with nutrient malabsorption.
- Diarrhea can result from malabsorption, intestinal infections, motility disorders, medications, or dietary substances and may require oral rehydration therapy to replace fluid and electrolyte losses. Dietary modifications may help to improve bowel function and alleviate intestinal discomfort.

Malabsorption

To digest and absorb nutrients, we depend on normal digestive secretions and healthy intestinal mucosa. Malabsorption can therefore be caused by pancreatic disorders that lead to enzyme deficiencies, and inflammatory conditions or medical treatments that damage intestinal tissue. In some cases, the treatment of an intestinal disorder requires surgical removal of a section (**resection**) of the small intestine, leaving minimal absorptive capacity in the portion that remains. Table 18-4 lists examples of diseases and treatments that are frequently associated with malabsorption. Some of these conditions are described later in this chapter.

Malabsorption rarely involves a single nutrient. When malabsorption is caused by pancreatic enzyme deficiencies, all macronutrients—protein, carbohydrate, and fat—may be affected. Whenever fat is malabsorbed, fat-soluble nutrients and minerals are usually malabsorbed as well. Malabsorptive disorders and their treatments can tax nutrition status further by causing complications that alter food intake, raise nutrient needs, and incur additional nutrient losses.

FAT MALABSORPTION

Fat is the nutrient most frequently malabsorbed because both digestive enzymes and bile must be present for its digestion. Thus, fat malabsorption often develops when an illness reduces pancreatic secretions or bile production. For example, both pancreatitis and cystic fibrosis can reduce the secretion of pancreatic lipase, whereas severe liver disease can cause bile insufficiency. Motility disorders that accelerate gastric emptying or intestinal transit can cause fat malabsorption because they prevent the normal mixing of dietary fat with lipase and bile. Fat malabsorption can also be caused by conditions or treatments that damage the intestinal mucosa, such as inflammatory bowel diseases, AIDS, and radiation treatments for cancer.

Fat malabsorption is often evidenced by **steatorrhea**, the presence of excessive fat in the stools. Steatorrhea can be evaluated by placing the patient on a high-fat diet (100 grams per day), performing a 72-hour fecal collection, and measuring the stool's fat content. Healthy individuals generally excrete less than 7 grams of fat per day under these conditions.[11]

Consequences of Fat Malabsorption
Fat malabsorption is associated with losses of food energy, essential fatty acids, fat-soluble vitamins, and some minerals (see Figure 18-1). Weight loss may result if the individual does not consume alternative sources of energy. Deficiencies of fat-soluble vitamins and essential fatty acids are common in chronic conditions. Malabsorption of some minerals, including calcium, magnesium, and zinc, often occurs because the minerals form **soaps** with the unabsorbed

TABLE 18-4	Potential Causes of Malabsorption

Genetic disorders
- Enzyme deficiencies

Intestinal disorders
- AIDS-related enteropathy
- Bacterial overgrowth
- Celiac disease
- Crohn's disease
- Radiation enteritis

Intestinal infections
- Giardiasis
- Nematode (roundworm) infections

Liver disease (bile insufficiency)

Pancreatic disorders
- Chronic pancreatitis
- Cystic fibrosis

Surgeries
- Gastric bypass surgery
- Intestinal resection (short bowel syndrome)

FIGURE 18-1 | The Consequences of Fat Malabsorption

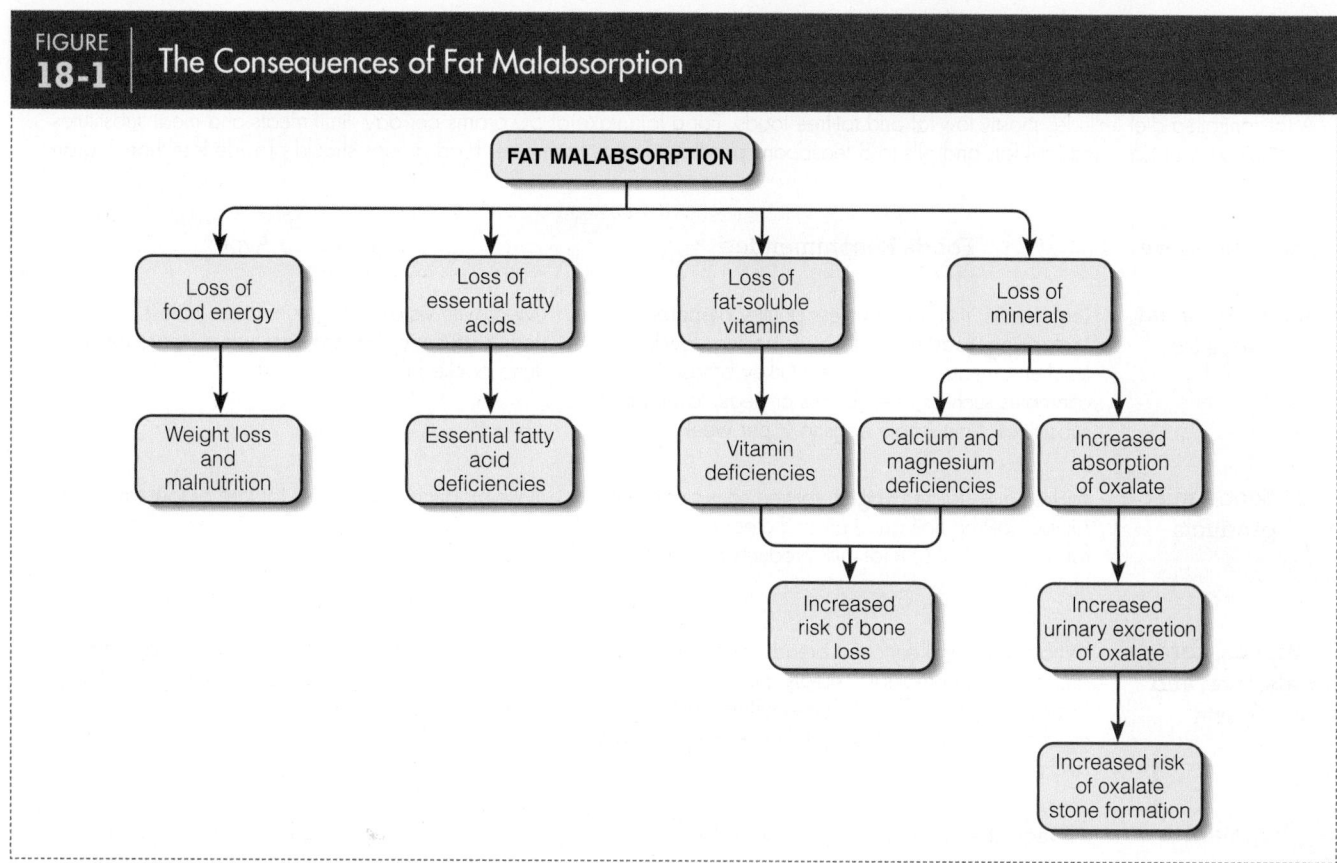

fatty acids. Calcium deficiency may lead to bone loss, which is further aggravated by the vitamin D deficiency that may be present due to fat malabsorption.

Another consequence of fat malabsorption is an increased risk of kidney stones, which are most often composed of calcium oxalate. (✚) The oxalates in foods ordinarily bind to calcium in the small intestine and are excreted in the stool. If calcium instead binds to fatty acids or bile acids, the oxalates are free to be absorbed into the blood and are ultimately excreted in the urine. The risk of developing oxalate stones increases when urinary oxalate levels are high. Kidney stones are discussed further in Chapter 22.

Nutrition Therapy for Fat Malabsorption If steatorrhea does not improve, a fat-controlled diet may be recommended (see Table 18-5). The objectives of the diet are to relieve intestinal symptoms that are aggravated by fat intake (usually diarrhea and flatulence) and to reduce vitamin and mineral losses. Fat should not be restricted more than necessary because fat is an important source of energy. Medium-chain triglycerides (MCT), which do not require lipase or bile for digestion and absorption, can be used as an alternative source of dietary fat, although MCT oil does not provide essential fatty acids. Figure 18-2 shows an example of a menu for a fat-controlled diet, and the "How to" on p. 521 offers suggestions for following the fat-controlled diet and for using MCT oil.

BACTERIAL OVERGROWTH

Ordinarily, the stomach and small intestine are protected from **bacterial overgrowth** by gastric acid, which destroys bacteria; peristalsis, which flushes bacteria through the small intestine before they multiply; and immunoglobulins secreted into the GI lumen.[12] When bacterial overgrowth does occur, it disrupts fat digestion and absorption, because excessive bacteria in the small intestine dismantle the bile acids needed for fat emulsification. Consequently, fat malabsorption and deficiencies of the

✚ Reminder: *Oxalates* are plant compounds that bind with some minerals to form complexes that the body cannot absorb. They are present in green leafy vegetables such as beet greens and spinach.

bacterial overgrowth: excessive bacterial colonization of the stomach and small intestine; may be due to low gastric acidity, altered GI motility, mucosal damage, or contamination.

TABLE 18-5 | Fat-Controlled Diet

A fat-controlled diet includes mostly low-fat and fat-free foods. For a fat intake of 50 grams per day, limit meats and meat substitutes to 6 ounces per day, and limit fats and oils to 8 teaspoons per day.[a] Foods from other food groups should provide less than 1 gram of fat per serving.

Food Category	Foods Recommended	Foods to Avoid
Meat and meat alternates	Lean meats, fish, and skinless poultry prepared by broiling, roasting, grilling, or boiling; low-fat luncheon meats such as sliced turkey breast; meat alternates such as dried beans or peas; low-fat egg substitutes. Limit whole eggs to 2 per week.	Meat with visible fat, ground beef (unless extra lean), sausage, bacon, frankfurters, spareribs, duck, tuna packed in oil
Milk and milk products	Fat-free milk, fat-free yogurt, fat-free sour cream substitutes, fat-free half and half and cream substitutes, fat-free cheeses. Low-fat milk products can be used in moderation.	Milk products that are not fat free or low fat
Breads, cereals, rice, and pasta	Whole-grain and enriched breads, cooked cereals and most cold breakfast cereals, plain tortillas, bagels, English muffins, fat-free muffins, saltine crackers, graham crackers, plain rice, plain noodles and pasta.	Biscuits, pancakes, waffles, granola, snack crackers made with fat, cornbread, doughnuts, corn chips, fried rice
Vegetables	All vegetables prepared without added fat.	Buttered, creamed, breaded, or fried vegetables; vegetables prepared au gratin style; french-fried potatoes; olives
Fruits	All fruits except avocado.	Avocado; fruits prepared with fats, nuts, or coconut
Desserts	Sherbet; fruit ices; flavored gelatin; angel food cake; meringue; fat-free puddings; fat-free bakery products; fat-free ice cream or frozen yogurt; fat-free candies such as marshmallows, jelly beans, and hard candy.	Cakes, cookies, pies, and pastries made with fat; puddings made with whole milk or eggs; ice cream; candies made with fat such as caramel and chocolates
Fats	For a total fat intake of 50 grams per day, limit intake of the following foods to 8 teaspoons daily: vegetable oil, butter, margarine, mayonnaise, lard (each has 3½ to 4½ grams of fat). These foods can replace the fat sources listed above, in the amounts specified: 1 tbs salad dressing, 2 tbs low-fat salad dressing, ½ tbs peanut butter, 1 tbs chopped nuts, 2 tbs mashed avocado.	Dietary fat that exceeds the amount specified in the nutrition prescription
Beverages	Fruit juices, soft drinks, fat-free milk, coffee, tea, coffee substitutes.	Beverages made with milk (unless fat free) or added cream, chocolate milk, eggnog, milk shakes

[a] For a fat intake of 25 grams per day, limit meats and meat substitutes to 4 ounces per day, and limit fats and oils to 2 teaspoons per day.

fat-soluble vitamins may eventually develop. The bacteria also produce enzymes and toxins that damage the intestinal mucosa, destroying mucosal enzymes (especially lactase) and reducing the absorptive surface area. In addition, the bacteria bind and metabolize vitamin B_{12}, impairing its absorption and increasing the risk of vitamin B_{12} deficiency. Although symptoms of bacterial overgrowth are often minor and nonspecific, severe cases may lead to chronic diarrhea, steatorrhea, flatulence, bloating, and weight loss.

FIGURE
18-2 | Sample Menu—Fat-Controlled Diet

The menu shown here contains approximately 50 grams of fat.

SAMPLE MENU

Breakfast
6 oz orange juice
1 c oatmeal with raisins, nonfat milk, and sugar
1 slice whole-wheat toast with 1 tsp margarine
Coffee with fat-free half and half

Lunch
Turkey breast sandwich (includes 2 slices whole-wheat bread,
    2 oz lean turkey breast, 2 tomato slices, lettuce leaf, and
    2 tsp mayonnaise)
2 c salad greens with 1 tbs salad dressing
Fruit cup (includes 1 c peaches and ½ c berries) with ½ c
    orange sherbet

Snack
6 oz nonfat fruit yogurt
6 saltine crackers with 1 tbs peanut butter and ½ tbs honey

Dinner
4 oz cod with sliced lemon and dill
1 slice French bread with 1 tsp butter
1 c steamed rice with herbs and walnut oil (includes ½ tsp oil)
1 c steamed broccoli and carrots with ½ tsp margarine
1 piece angel food cake with fat-free whipped cream

Causes of Bacterial Overgrowth Conditions that impair intestinal motility and allow material to stagnate can greatly increase susceptibility to bacterial overgrowth. For example, in some types of gastric surgery, a portion of the small intestine is bypassed, preventing the flow of material in the bypassed region and allowing bacteria to flourish (see the "blind loop" shown in Figure 17-2 on p. 500). Intestinal motility can also be reduced by strictures, obstructions, and diverticula (protrusions) in the small intestine, as well as by some chronic illnesses, including diabetes mellitus and scleroderma.

Reduced secretions of gastric acid may also lead to bacterial overgrowth. Possible causes include chronic gastritis, use of acid-suppressing medications, and some gastrectomy procedures.

Treatment for Bacterial Overgrowth Treatment may include antibiotics to suppress bacterial growth and surgical correction of the anatomical defects that contribute to a motility disorder. Medications may be given to stimulate peristalsis.

HOW TO | Follow a Fat-Controlled Diet

For some individuals, fat-controlled diets may be difficult to follow. Fats add flavors, aromas, and textures to foods—characteristics that make foods more enjoyable. Unlike some diets that can be introduced gradually, a fat-controlled diet is often implemented immediately, allowing little time for adaptation. These suggestions may help:

- Fat is better tolerated if provided in small portions. Divide the day's allotment into several servings that can be consumed throughout the day.

- Use variety to enhance enjoyment of meals: vary flavors, textures, colors, and seasonings.

- Look for fat-free items when grocery shopping. Incorporate fat-free ingredients when preparing favorite recipes.

- Try fat-free and low-fat condiments to improve the diet's palatability. Experiment with herbs and spices. Instead of butter, use fruit butters on toast. Use butter-flavored granules on vegetables. Replace mayonnaise in sandwiches with spicy mustard. Replace salad dressings with flavored vinegars.

- Avoid products that contain the fat substitute olestra, which may aggravate GI symptoms.

If patients are interested in using medium-chain triglyceride (MCT) oil:

- Explain that MCT products are expensive but that the cost is sometimes covered by medical insurance.

- Advise patients to add MCT oil to the diet gradually. Diarrhea and abdominal cramps may result if too much is used at once. Tolerance to MCT oil may improve in time.

- Advise patients that MCT oil may have an unpleasant taste when used alone. Suggest using MCT oil in recipes as a substitute for regular oil. MCT oil can replace oil in salad dressings, be incorporated into sauces, and be used in cooking or baking. It can also be added to fat-free milk products to make milk shakes.

- Point out that MCT oil should not be used to fry foods because it decomposes at lower temperatures than most cooking oils.

Most people with lactose intolerance can drink milk, especially if they drink it along with other foods and limit the amount they consume at any one time.

A lactose-restricted diet may help to reduce flatulence and diarrhea in some individuals.[13] Dietary supplements can help to correct nutrient deficiencies, especially deficiencies in the fat-soluble vitamins A, D, and E; calcium (which combines with malabsorbed fatty acids); and vitamin B_{12}.[14]

LACTOSE INTOLERANCE

Approximately 75 percent of people worldwide have some degree of lactose intolerance, which is caused by the loss or reduction of lactase, the intestinal enzyme that digests the lactose in milk products.[15] Lactose intolerance is especially prevalent among individuals of certain ethnic groups, including Asians, African Americans, Native Americans, Ashkenazi Jews, and Latinos. It can also result from GI disorders that damage the small intestinal mucosa. The primary symptoms of lactose intolerance are diarrhea and increased intestinal gas.

Lactose intolerance is rarely serious and is easily managed by simple dietary adjustments. Although people with the condition are sometimes reluctant to consume milk products, clinical studies have found that individuals with lactose intolerance can tolerate up to 2 cups of milk daily without significant symptoms.[16] People who avoid milk for fear of intestinal discomfort can be urged to gradually increase consumption of lactose-containing foods. They may more readily tolerate milk when intake is divided throughout the day and the milk is taken with food. Some people tolerate chocolate milk better than plain milk. Most aged cheeses are well tolerated because they contain little lactose. Yogurts that contain live bacterial cultures are usually acceptable because the bacteria contain lactase, which may aid in lactose digestion. Other options are to add a lactase preparation to milk or to take enzyme tablets before consuming lactose-containing foods. Lactose-free milk is also commercially available.

People who develop lactose intolerance as a result of intestinal illness are often advised to temporarily restrict milk and milk products. Foods that contain lactose can be reintroduced in small amounts once the condition improves. All individuals who restrict milk products should be encouraged to consume alternative food sources of calcium and vitamin D; dietary sources of these nutrients are discussed in Chapters 8 and 9 (see pp. 209 and 249).

Review Notes

- Malabsorption syndromes can be caused by reduced digestive secretions or damaged intestinal mucosa. Malabsorption often affects multiple nutrients and can lead to complications that impair nutrition status further.
- Fat malabsorption, usually indicated by the development of steatorrhea, is associated with the loss of food energy and deficiencies of essential fatty acids, fat-soluble vitamins, and some minerals.
- Bacterial overgrowth can result from impaired peristalsis or reduced gastric acidity and typically causes malabsorption of fat and vitamin B_{12}.
- Lactose intolerance, caused by lactase deficiency, can be managed by adjusting the amount and timing of lactose consumption.

Reminder: The digestive secretions of the pancreas include bicarbonate and digestive enzymes. The bicarbonate neutralizes the acidic gastric contents that enter the duodenum, and the digestive enzymes break down protein, carbohydrate, and fat.

Conditions Affecting the Pancreas

As mentioned previously, pancreatic disorders can lead to maldigestion and malabsorption due to the impaired secretion of digestive enzymes. (✚) This section describes several pancreatic illnesses that are characterized by widespread malabsorption.

PANCREATITIS

Pancreatitis is an inflammatory disease of the pancreas. Although mild cases may subside in a few days, other cases can persist for weeks or months. Chronic pancreatitis can lead to irreversible damage to pancreatic tissue and permanent loss of function.

Acute Pancreatitis In acute pancreatitis, the digestive enyzmes in pancreatic cells become prematurely activated, leading to destruction of pancreatic tissue and subsequent inflammation. The condition is most often caused by gallstones or alcohol abuse—factors that account for more than 70 to 80 percent of acute cases.[17] Less common causes include hypertriglyceridemia (triglyceride concentrations higher than 1000 milligrams per deciliter), exposure to toxins, and the use of some medications. Common symptoms include severe abdominal pain, nausea and vomiting, and abdominal distention. In most patients, the condition resolves within a week with no complications. More serious cases may lead to additional pancreatic damage, infection, the systemic inflammatory response syndrome (see p. 472), and kidney failure.

Nutrition Therapy for Acute Pancreatitis The initial treatment goal is to provide supportive care, including pain control and complete bowel rest. Oral fluids and food are withheld until pain and tenderness have subsided, and fluids and electrolytes are supplied intravenously. After several days, patients may be able to consume small amounts (½ to 1 cup) of fluids; water or other clear liquids may be provided initially. If tolerated, the diet progresses from liquid feedings to solid foods, given in small, frequent feedings. Because fat stimulates the pancreas more than other nutrients, a low-fat diet may be better tolerated at first. In severe pancreatitis, tube feedings are sometimes necessary; either standard formulas or elemental formulas (✚) may be used, depending on patient tolerance. Protein and energy needs are high in severe cases due to the catabolic and hypermetabolic effects of inflammation.[18]

Chronic Pancreatitis Chronic pancreatitis is characterized by permanent and progressive damage to pancreatic tissue, resulting in the impaired secretion of digestive enzymes. Although there are multiple causes, about 70 percent of chronic pancreatitis cases are caused by excessive alcohol consumption.[19] Unlike acute pancreatitis, chronic pancreatitis is not caused by gallstones. In children, most cases are attributable to cystic fibrosis, discussed in a later section.

In chronic pancreatitis, abdominal pain is often severe and unrelenting and worsens with eating. Analgesics or opiate drugs may be needed for pain control. Fat maldigestion develops sooner than maldigestion of protein or carbohydrate, and steatorrhea is common in advanced cases. Food avoidance (due to pain associated with eating) and malabsorption may lead to weight loss and malnutrition. Advanced cases are associated with reductions in both insulin and glucagon secretions, and diabetes eventually develops in up to 80 percent of patients.[20]

Nutrition Therapy for Chronic Pancreatitis The objectives of nutrition therapy are to improve nutrition status, reduce malabsorption, and prevent symptom recurrence. Protein and energy needs are high in patients who have lost weight or are malnourished. Dietary supplements are often needed to correct nutrient deficiencies, which may be due to malabsorption or to the alcohol abuse that caused the disease. Patients must avoid alcohol completely and quit smoking cigarettes, as these substances can exacerbate symptoms and interfere with healing.[21]

Steatorrhea is usually treated with pancreatic enzyme replacement. Pancreatic enzymes are often **enteric coated** to resist the acidity of the stomach and do not dissolve until the pH is above 5.5. If nonenteric-coated preparations are used, acid-suppressing drugs may be required. Fecal fat concentrations must be monitored to determine whether the enzyme treatment has been effective. If steatorrhea is resistant to treatment, a fat-controlled diet may help to reduce symptoms, and MCT oil can be used as an alternative source of fat kcalories.

✚ Reminder: An *elemental formula* contains hydrolyzed nutrients that require minimal digestion and are easily absorbed.

enteric coated: refers to medications or enzyme preparations that are coated to withstand stomach acidity and dissolve only at the higher pH of the small intestine.

> **NURSING DIAGNOSIS**
>
> Nursing diagnoses for people with acute pancreatitis may include *acute pain, nausea, diarrhea,* and *risk for deficient fluid volume.*

> **NURSING DIAGNOSIS**
>
> *Imbalanced nutrition: less than body requirements* may be appropriate for some individuals with chronic pancreatitis.

CYSTIC FIBROSIS

Cystic fibrosis is the most common life-threatening genetic disorder among Caucasians, with an incidence of approximately 1 in 2500 white births. In the United States, about 30,000 people are affected.[22] Cystic fibrosis is caused by a genetic mutation that disturbs the transport of chloride ions in **exocrine** glands. This defect results in thickened glandular secretions and a broad range of serious complications. Until a few decades ago, few infants born with cystic fibrosis survived to adulthood. Now, with early detection and advances in medical treatment, the median life span has extended beyond 35 years of age, with many patients surviving into their 50s.[23]

Consequences of Cystic Fibrosis
Cystic fibrosis is characterized by abnormal chloride and sodium levels in exocrine secretions. The secretions are unusually viscous and can obstruct the ducts that normally allow their passage. The blockages that develop can disrupt tissue function and cause tissue damage. The major complications of cystic fibrosis involve the lungs, pancreas, (✚) and sweat glands:

- *Lung disease.* The abnormally thick mucus secretions cause obstructions in many of the small airways of the lungs. The obstructions lead to chronic coughing and persistent respiratory infections, both of which contribute to progressive inflammation in bronchial tissues. The lung damage that eventually develops results in breathing difficulties and lower exercise tolerance. As with other obstructive airway diseases, nutrition status may become impaired due to hypermetabolism, the greater energy cost of labored breathing, and anorexia (loss of appetite). The chronic respiratory infections raise energy needs further. (Chapter 16 describes the nutrition problems associated with chronic obstructive lung diseases.)

- *Pancreatic disease.* Approximately 85 percent of cystic fibrosis patients develop thickened pancreatic secretions that obstruct the pancreatic ducts, causing digestive enzymes to accumulate in the pancreas and destroy pancreatic tissue.[24] Fewer pancreatic enzymes reach the small intestine, leading to malabsorption of protein, fat, and fat-soluble vitamins. Other problems that may develop over time include pancreatitis, hyperglycemia (due to destruction of the insulin-producing cells), and diabetes.

- *Other complications.* Because cystic fibrosis affects all exocrine secretions, complications typically develop in many other tissues or organs. Salt losses in sweat are usually excessive, increasing the risk of dehydration. Intestinal obstruction is a common symptom in newborn infants and may also occur in older patients. Gallbladder and liver diseases may result from bile duct obstructions. Abnormalities in genital tissues cause sterility in men and reduced fertility in women.

Nutrition Therapy for Cystic Fibrosis
Children with cystic fibrosis are chronically undernourished, grow poorly, and have difficulty maintaining normal body weight. Their energy and protein needs are high due to increased requirements and nutrient malabsorption. To achieve normal growth and maintain optimal nutrition status, energy intakes should be 20 to 50 percent higher than DRI values, and protein should provide 15 to 20 percent of kcalories.[25] To compensate for fat malabsorption, about 35 to 40 percent of kcalories should come from fat. A patient with cystic fibrosis is therefore encouraged to consume high-kcalorie and high-fat foods, eat frequent meals and snacks, and supplement meals with milk shakes or liquid dietary supplements. Supplemental tube feedings can help to improve nutrition status if energy intakes are inadequate.

Pancreatic enzyme replacement therapy is a central feature of cystic fibrosis treatment. Supplemental enzymes must be included with every meal or snack. For infants and small children, the contents of capsules are mixed in small amounts of liquid or a soft food (such as applesauce) and fed with a spoon. Enzyme dosages may need to be adjusted if malabsorption continues, as evidenced by poor growth or GI symptoms such as steatorrhea, intestinal gas, or abdominal pain.

✚ Reminder: The pancreas secretes digestive enzymes and bicarbonate into the digestive tract (*exocrine* secretions) and the hormones insulin and glucagon into the bloodstream (*endocrine* secretions).

cystic fibrosis: an inherited disease characterized by the presence of abnormally viscous exocrine secretions; often leads to respiratory illness and pancreatic insufficiency.

exocrine: pertains to external secretions, such as those of the mucous membranes or the skin. Opposite of *endocrine,* which pertains to hormonal secretions into the blood.
- *exo* = outside
- *krinein* = to secrete

Postural drainage, a type of physical therapy used in cystic fibrosis, helps to clear the thick, sticky secretions that block airways and increase infection risk.

© Mauro Fermariello/Photo Researchers, Inc.

The risk of nutrient deficiency depends on the degree of malabsorption. The nutrients of greatest concern include the fat-soluble vitamins, essential fatty acids, and calcium. Multivitamin and fat-soluble vitamin supplements are routinely recommended. The liberal use of table salt and salty foods is encouraged to make up for losses of sodium in sweat.

Review Notes

- Chronic pancreatic disorders can lead to widespread maldigestion and malabsorption due to the impaired secretion of digestive enzymes.
- Acute pancreatitis is short lived and does not cause permanent damage, but it requires the withholding of food and liquids until healing has occurred. Chronic pancreatitis leads to digestive enzyme deficiencies and is treated with pancreatic enzyme replacement therapy.
- Cystic fibrosis, a genetic disorder associated with thickened exocrine secretions, causes obstructive lung disease and pancreatic damage. Children with cystic fibrosis have high protein and energy requirements and must use pancreatic enzyme replacement therapy and dietary supplements to reverse malnutrition.

Conditions Affecting the Small Intestine

When the intestinal mucosa is damaged due to inflammation, infection, or other causes, malabsorption is the likely outcome. This section discusses *celiac disease; inflammatory bowel diseases,* which are intestinal illnesses that can impair mucosal function; and *short bowel syndrome,* the malabsorptive disorder that results when a substantial portion of the small intestine is surgically removed.

CELIAC DISEASE

Celiac disease is an immune disorder characterized by an abnormal immune response to **gluten**, a group of water-insoluble proteins found in wheat, barley, and rye. The reaction to gluten causes severe damage to the intestinal mucosa and subsequent malabsorption. Celiac disease is estimated to affect approximately 1 percent of individuals in the United States; current data suggest that the condition is approximately twice as prevalent in Caucasians as it is in other ethnic groups.[26]

Consequences of Celiac Disease The immune reaction to gluten can cause striking changes in intestinal tissue. In affected areas, the villi may be shortened or absent, resulting in a significant reduction in mucosal surface area (and, therefore, in intestinal digestive enzymes). The damage may be restricted to the duodenum or may involve the full length of the small intestine. Individuals with severe disease may malabsorb all nutrients to some degree, especially the macronutrients, calcium, iron, folate, the fat-soluble vitamins, and vitamin B_{12}.[27]

Symptoms of celiac disease include GI disturbances such as diarrhea, steatorrhea, and flatulence. Because lactase deficiency can result from mucosal damage, GI symptoms may be exacerbated by milk products. Due to nutrient malabsorption, children with celiac disease often have stunted growth and are severely underweight. Adults may develop anemia, bone disorders, chronic fatigue, and fertility problems. Individuals with celiac disease who do not eliminate gluten from the diet are at increased risk of developing intestinal and lymphatic cancers.[28]

Some gluten-sensitive individuals may have few GI symptoms but react to gluten by developing a severe rash. This condition is called **dermatitis herpetiformis** and requires dietary adjustments similar to those for celiac disease.

celiac (SEE-lee-ack) disease: an immune disorder characterized by an abnormal immune response to the dietary protein gluten; also called *gluten-sensitive enteropathy* or *celiac sprue.*

gluten (GLU-ten): a group of water-insoluble proteins in wheat, rye, and barley.

dermatitis herpetiformis (DERM-ah-TYE-tis HER-peh-tih-FOR-mis): a gluten-sensitive disorder characterized by a severe skin rash.

NURSING DIAGNOSIS

Nursing diagnoses for people with celiac disease may include *diarrhea, risk for disproportionate growth,* and *imbalanced nutrition: less than body requirements.*

Gluten-free products help people with celiac disease enjoy a wider variety of foods.

© Wadsworth, Cengage Learning

Nutrition Therapy for Celiac Disease
The treatment for celiac disease is lifelong adherence to a gluten-free diet. Improvement in symptoms is often evident within several weeks, although mucosal healing can sometimes take years. If lactase deficiency is suspected, patients should avoid lactose-containing foods until the intestine has recovered. Dietary supplements can be used to meet micronutrient needs and reverse deficiencies.

The gluten-free diet eliminates foods that contain wheat, barley, and rye (see Table 18-6). Because many foods contain ingredients derived from these grains, foods that are problematic are not always obvious. Even small amounts of gluten may cause symptoms in some people, so patients need to check ingredient lists on food labels carefully. Gluten-containing products that may be overlooked include beer, caramel coloring, coffee substitutes, communion wafers, imitation meats, malt syrup, medications, salad dressings, and soy sauce. Special gluten-free products can be purchased to replace common food items such as bread, pasta,

TABLE 18-6	Gluten-Free Diet	
Food Category	**Gluten-Free Choices**	**Potential Gluten Sources**
Meat and meat alternates	Fresh meat, fish, or poultry; shellfish; dried peas and beans; tofu; nuts and seeds; eggs	Luncheon meats, sandwich spreads, meatloaf, meatballs, frankfurters, sausages, poultry injected with broth, imitation meat products, imitation seafood, meat extenders, miso, egg substitutes, dried egg products, dry roasted nuts, peanut butter. *Avoid:* products made with hydrolyzed vegetable protein (HVP), marinades, and soy sauce; breaded foods; foods prepared with cream sauces or gravies.
Milk and milk products	Milk, buttermilk, half and half, cream, plain yogurt, cheese, cottage cheese, cream cheese	Chocolate milk, milk shakes, frozen yogurt, flavored yogurt, cheese spreads, cheese sauces. *Avoid:* malted milk, malted milk powders.
Breads, cereals, rice, and pasta	Breads, bakery products, and cereals made with amaranth, arrowroot, buckwheat, corn, flax, hominy grits, millet, potato flour or potato starch, quinoa, rice, sorghum, soybean flour, tapioca, and teff; pasta and noodles made with the grains or starches listed above; corn tacos and corn tortillas	Oatmeal and oat bran (due to contamination), rice crackers, rice cakes, corn cakes. *Avoid:* breads, bakery products, cereals, tortillas, pastas, and pancake or baking mixes made with wheat, rye, barley, and triticale. *Wheat products* include bulghur, cous cous, durum flour, einkorn, emmer, farina, graham flour, kamut, semolina, spelt, wheat bran, wheat germ. *Barley products* include malt, malt flavoring, and malt extract.
Fruits and vegetables	Any fresh, frozen, or canned fruits or vegetables	French fries from fast-food restaurants, commercial salad dressings, fruit pie fillings, dried fruits (may be dusted with flour). *Avoid:* scalloped potatoes (usually made with wheat flour), creamed vegetables, vegetables dipped in batters.
Desserts	Bakery products made with gluten-free flours, most ice creams, sherbet, sorbet, Italian ices, popsicles, gelatin desserts, egg custards, most chocolate bars, chocolate chips, hard candies, whipped toppings	Some ice creams (especially if made with cookie dough, brownies, nuts, and other added ingredients), icing or frosting, candies and candy bars, marshmallows. *Avoid:* bakery products or doughnuts made with wheat, rye, or barley; puddings made with wheat flour; ice cream or sherbets that contain gluten stabilizers; ice cream cones; licorice.
Beverages	Coffee; tea; cocoa made with pure cocoa powder; soft drinks; wine; distilled alcoholic beverages such as rum, gin, whiskey, and vodka	Instant tea or coffee, coffee substitutes, chocolate drinks, hot cocoa mixes. *Avoid:* beer, ale, lager, malted beverages, cereal beverages, beverages that contain nondairy cream substitutes.

FIGURE
18-3
Sample Menu—Gluten-Free Diet

SAMPLE MENU

Breakfast
Orange juice
Gluten-free pancake with maple syrup
Plain yogurt with banana and strawberries
Coffee with half and half

Lunch
Grilled chicken breast with cranberry chutney
Baked potato topped with grated cheddar
　　cheese
Sliced tomato with chopped basil
Raspberry sherbet

Snack
Tortilla chips and guacamole
Hot cocoa (made with cocoa powder)

Dinner
Sauteed catfish with sliced lemon and dill
Wild rice pilaf
Collard greens and garlic sauteed in
　　olive oil
Green salad with oil and vinegar dressing
Vanilla egg custard

and cereals. Although somewhat expensive, these foods increase food choices and allow celiac patients to enjoy foods that would otherwise be forbidden. Patients should also be instructed in food preparation methods that prevent cross-contamination from utensils, cutting boards, and toasters.

Although most people with celiac disease can safely consume moderate amounts of oats, most oats grown in the United States are contaminated with wheat, barley, or rye. Oats are usually grown in rotation with other grains and may become contaminated during harvesting or processing. However, several oat manufacturers in the United States produce oats in dedicated facilities and test the products to ensure they are gluten free.[29] Individuals who wish to include oats in their diet should be advised to purchase only uncontaminated oats and to limit intakes to the amounts found to be safe (about ½ cup of dry rolled oats per day).

A gluten-free diet may become monotonous unless care is taken to diversify food choices. The diet can also be a social liability by restricting food choices when individuals eat in restaurants, visit friends, or travel. Nonadherence is common when individuals eat away from home.[30] Nutrition education and dietetic counseling can help celiac patients learn how to meet their nutrient needs and expand meal options despite dietary constraints. Figure 18-3 shows an example of a menu for a gluten-free diet.

INFLAMMATORY BOWEL DISEASES

Inflammatory bowel diseases are chronic inflammatory illnesses characterized by abnormal immune responses in the GI tract. Although both genetic and environmental factors contribute to the development of these diseases, the exact triggers are unknown. Disease onset occurs most often in individuals between 15 and 25 years of age.[31]

Table 18-7 compares the two major forms of inflammatory bowel disease, **Crohn's disease** and **ulcerative colitis**. Crohn's disease usually involves the small intestine and can lead to nutrient malabsorption, whereas ulcerative colitis affects the large intestine, where little nutrient absorption occurs. (➕) Both diseases are characterized by periods of active disease interspersed with periods of remission. Nutrient losses can result from tissue damage, bleeding, and diarrhea.

Complications of Crohn's Disease Crohn's disease may occur in any region of the GI tract, but most cases involve the ileum and/or large intestine. Lesions may develop in different areas in the intestine, with normal tissue separating affected regions (called "skip" lesions). During exacerbations, the inflammation can extend deeply into intestinal tissue and be accompanied by ulcerations, fissures, and **fistulas** (abnormal passages between tissues). Loops of intestine may become matted together. Scar tissue eventually thickens and stiffens the intestinal wall, narrowing the lumen and sometimes causing strictures or obstructions. About 60 to 75 percent of patients require surgical resections during the course of illness, although disease often

➕ Although ulcerative colitis affects the large intestine, the condition is included in this section because it is one of the major subtypes of inflammatory bowel disease.

Crohn's disease: an inflammatory bowel disease that usually occurs in the lower portion of the small intestine and the colon. Inflammation may pervade the entire intestinal wall.

ulcerative colitis (ko-LY-tis): an inflammatory bowel disease that involves the colon. Inflammation affects the mucosa and submucosa of the intestinal wall.

fistulas (FIST-you-luz): abnormal passages between organs or tissues that permit the passage of fluids or secretions.

TABLE 18-7	Comparison of Crohn's Disease and Ulcerative Colitis	
	Crohn's Disease	**Ulcerative Colitis**
Location of inflammation	Approximately 40 percent of cases involve the ileum and cecum, 30 percent are in the small intestine only, and 20 percent are in the colon	Inflammation is confined to the rectum and colon; it begins at the rectum and spreads into the colon
Pattern of inflammation	Discrete areas separated by normal tissue ("skip" lesions)	Continuous inflammation that begins at the rectum and ends abruptly within the colon
Depth of damage	Damage throughout all layers of tissue; causes deep fissures that give intestinal tissue a "cobble-stone" appearance	Damage primarily in the mucosa and submucosa (layers of intestinal tissue closest to the lumen)
Fistulas	Common	Usually do not occur
Cancer risk	Increased	Greatly increased

✚ Reminder: Most of the bile used during digestion is eventually reabsorbed in the ileum and returned to the liver.

recurs in the remaining intestine.[32] Patients with Crohn's disease are at increased risk of developing intestinal cancers.

Malnutrition may result from malabsorption, nutrient losses (especially of protein) associated with the tissue damage, reduced food intake, and surgical resections that shorten the small intestine. If the ileum is affected, bile acids may become depleted, (✚) causing malabsorption of fat, fat-soluble vitamins, calcium, magnesium, and zinc (the minerals bind to the unabsorbed fatty acids). Because the ileum is the site of vitamin B_{12} absorption, deficiency can develop unless the patient is given vitamin B_{12} injections. Anemia may result from bleeding, inadequate absorption of the nutrients involved in blood cell formation, or the metabolic effects of chronic illness. Anorexia often develops due to abdominal discomfort and the effects of cytokines produced during the inflammatory process.[33]

Complications of Ulcerative Colitis Ulcerative colitis always involves the rectum and usually extends into the colon. Inflammation is continuous

The healthy colon has a smooth surface with a visible pattern of fine blood vessels.

In Crohn's disease, the mucosa has a "cobblestone" appearance due to deep fissuring in the inflamed mucosal tissue.

In ulcerative colitis, the colon appears inflamed and reddened, and ulcers are visible.

Nutrition and Lower Gastrointestinal Disorders

along the length of intestine affected, ending abruptly at the area where healthy tissue begins. Tissue erosion or ulceration develops primarily in the mucosa and submucosa (the layers of intestinal tissue closest to the lumen). During active episodes, patients have frequent, urgent bowel movements that are small in volume. Stools are often streaked with blood and contain mucus.

Although mild disease may cause few complications, weight loss, fever, and weakness are common when most of the colon is involved. Severe disease is often associated with anemia (due to blood loss), dehydration, and electrolyte imbalances. Protein losses from the inflamed tissue can be substantial. A **colectomy** (removal of the colon) is performed in 20 to 25 percent of patients and prevents future recurrence.[34] Colon cancer risk is substantially increased in ulcerative colitis patients.

Drug Treatment of Inflammatory Bowel Diseases

Medications help to reduce inflammation, control symptoms, and minimize complications. The drugs prescribed include antidiarrheal agents, immunosuppressants, anti-inflammatory drugs (usually corticosteroids and salicylates), and antibiotics. Although these medications may allow the patient to achieve and maintain remission, some may cause side effects that are detrimental to nutrition status. The Diet-Drug Interactions feature lists some nutrition-related effects of the medications used in inflammatory bowel diseases.

Nutrition Therapy for Crohn's Disease

Crohn's disease often requires aggressive dietary management because it can lead to protein-energy malnutrition (PEM), nutrient deficiencies, and growth failure in children. Specific dietary measures depend on the functional status of the GI tract and the symptoms and complications that develop; thus, nutrition care varies among patients and throughout the course of illness.

During disease exacerbations, a low-residue, low-fat diet provided in small, frequent feedings can minimize stool output and reduce symptoms of malabsorption. High-kcalorie, high-protein diets are prescribed to prevent or treat malnutrition or promote healing; the amount of protein recommended may be 50 percent higher than DRI levels. Enteral supplements can be used to increase energy intake and improve weight gain. Vitamin and mineral supplements are usually necessary, especially if nutrient

colectomy: removal of a portion or all of the colon.

DIET-DRUG INTERACTIONS

Check this table for notable nutrition-related effects of the medications discussed in this chapter.

	GASTROINTESTINAL EFFECTS	INTERACTIONS WITH DIETARY SUBSTANCES	METABOLIC EFFECTS
Antidiarrheals	Constipation	—	—
Anti-inflammatory drugs (sulfasalazine, corticosteroids)	Nausea, heartburn (sulfasalazine)	Sulfasalazine may decrease folate absorption; supplementation is recommended.	Anemia (sulfasalazine); fluid retention, hyperglycemia, hypocalcemia, hypokalemia, hypophosphatemia, increased appetite, protein catabolism (corticosteroids).
Laxatives	Diarrhea, flatulence, abdominal discomfort	—	Dehydration, electrolyte imbalances, laxative dependency
Pancreatic enzyme replacements	Diarrhea, nausea, stomach cramping, irritation of GI mucosa	—	—

TABLE 18-8	Management of Symptoms and Complications in Crohn's Disease

Symptom or Complication	Possible Dietary Measures
Growth failure or weight loss	• High-kcalorie diet • Enteral supplements • Elemental tube feedings
Anorexia or pain with eating	• Small, frequent meals • Enteral supplements • If long term (>5 to 7 days): elemental tube feedings
Malabsorption	• High-kcalorie diet • Nutrient supplementation
Steatorrhea (fat malabsorption)	• Fat restriction • Medium-chain triglycerides • Nutrient supplementation
Diarrhea	• Fluid and electrolyte replacement • Nutrient supplementation
Lactose intolerance	• Avoidance of lactose-containing foods
Nutrient deficiencies	• Nutrient-dense diet • Nutrient supplementation
Strictures or fistulas	• Low-fiber diet
Severe bowel obstruction, high-output fistulas, or severe exacerbations of disease	• Total parenteral nutrition

malabsorption is present; nutrients at risk include calcium, iron, magnesium, zinc, folate, vitamin B_{12}, and vitamin D.[35] In some instances, tube feedings may be used to supplement the diet or may be the sole means of providing nutrients; some patients may tolerate elemental formulas more easily than standard formulas. Table 18-8 includes examples of other dietary adjustments that may be beneficial for patients with Crohn's disease.

During periods of remission, dietary restrictions are unnecessary unless complications develop. Symptoms that may interfere with food intake include anorexia, pain, and diarrhea. A restricted intake of lactose, fructose, and sorbitol may improve symptoms of diarrhea and flatulence. Adequate fluid replacement should be encouraged in patients with diarrhea. Individuals with partial obstructions may need to restrict high-fiber foods. Although some research studies suggest that supplementation with fish oil, glutamine, or probiotics may be helpful, more research is necessary to confirm the benefits.[36]

Nutrition Therapy for Ulcerative Colitis In most cases, the diet for ulcerative colitis requires few adjustments. As in Crohn's disease, the symptoms and complications that arise are managed with the appropriate dietary measures (see Table 18-8). During disease exacerbations, the primary goals are to restore fluid and electrolyte balances and correct deficiencies that result from protein and blood losses; dietary adjustments are based on the extent of bleeding and diarrhea output. Thus, adequate protein, energy, fluid, and electrolytes need to be provided. A low-fiber diet may reduce irritation by minimizing fecal volume. If colon function becomes severely impaired, food and fluids may be withheld and fluids and electrolytes supplied intravenously until colon function is restored.[37]

SHORT BOWEL SYNDROME

The treatment of Crohn's disease, cancers of the small intestine, and other intestinal disorders may include the surgical resection (removal) of a major portion of the small intestine. **Short bowel syndrome** is the malabsorption syndrome that results when the absorptive capacity of the remaining intestine is insufficient for meeting nutritional needs. Without appropriate dietary adjustments, short bowel syndrome can result in fluid and electrolyte imbalances and multiple nutrient deficiencies. Symptoms include diarrhea, steatorrhea, dehydration, weight loss, and growth impairment in children.

Figure 18-4 reviews nutrient absorption in the GI tract and describes how absorption is affected by surgical resections. Generally, up to 50 percent of the small intestine can be resected without serious nutritional consequences.[38] More extensive resections lead to generalized malabsorption, and patients may need lifelong parenteral nutrition to supplement oral intakes.

Intestinal Adaptation After an intestinal resection, the remaining intestine undergoes **intestinal adaptation**, an adaptive response that dramatically improves the intestine's absorptive capacity. Adaptation begins soon after surgery and continues for several years. During this period, the remaining section of intestine increases in diameter and develops taller villi, helping to compensate for the removed length of intestine. The ileum has a greater capacity for adaptation than the jejunum; thus, removal of the ileum has more severe consequences than removal of the jejunum. Loss of the ileum permanently disrupts both vitamin B_{12} and bile acid absorption. Depletion

short bowel syndrome: the malabsorption syndrome that follows resection of the small intestine, which results in inadequate absorptive capacity in the remaining intestine.

intestinal adaptation: the process of intestinal recovery following resection that leads to improved absorptive capacity.

FIGURE 18-4 | Nutrient Absorption and Consequences of Intestinal Surgeries

About 90 to 95 percent of nutrient absorption takes place in the first half of the small intestine. After a resection, nutrient absorption may be reduced.

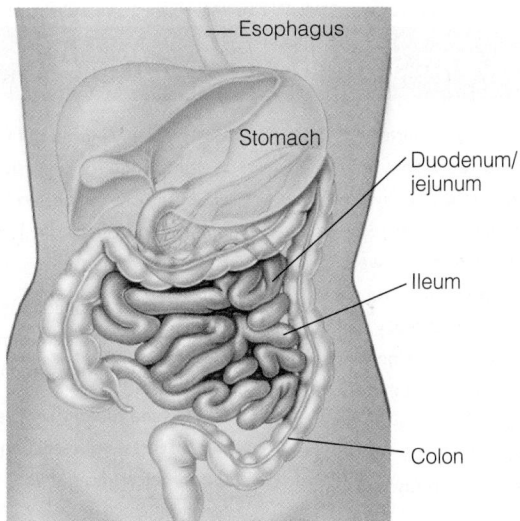

WHAT IS ABSORBED

Duodenum/jejunum
- Simple carbohydrates
- Fats
- Amino acids
- Vitamins[a]
- Minerals[a]
- Water

Ileum
- Bile salts
- Vitamin B_{12}
- Water
(Assumes absorptive function of duodenum and jejunum with adaptation)

Colon
- Water
- Electrolytes
- Short-chain fatty acids

— Esophagus

Stomach

Duodenum/jejunum

Ileum

Colon

POSSIBLE CONSEQUENCES OF RESECTION

Duodenum/jejunum
- Minimal consequences if the ileum remains intact
- Calcium and iron malabsorption if duodenum resected

Ileum
- Fat malabsorption
- Protein malabsorption
- Malabsorption of fat-soluble vitamins and vitamin B_{12}
- Reduced calcium, magnesium, and zinc absorption
- Fluid losses
- Diarrhea/steatorrhea

Colon
- Fluid and electrolyte losses
- Diarrhea
(Losses are compounded if ileum is also resected)

[a] The absorption of vitamins and minerals begins in the duodenum and continues throughout the length of the small intestine.

of bile acids exacerbates fat malabsorption, and the unabsorbed bile acids can worsen diarrhea because they irritate the colon walls. Adaptation is achieved more easily if the colon is present, because the colon's resident bacteria can metabolize unabsorbed carbohydrates and produce some usable nutrients. An intact colon also helps to reduce losses of fluids and electrolytes.

Nutrition Therapy for Short Bowel Syndrome

Immediately after a resection, fluids and electrolytes must be supplied intravenously. In the first few weeks after surgery, the fluid losses from diarrhea can be substantial (sometimes exceeding 2 liters per day), so appropriate rehydration therapy is critical to recovery. The diarrhea gradually lessens as intestinal adaptation progresses.

Total parenteral nutrition meets nutrient needs after surgery and is gradually reduced as oral feedings increase. To promote intestinal adaptation, (✚) oral feedings may be started just a few days after surgery, after diarrhea subsides somewhat and some bowel function is restored. Initial oral intake may consist of occasional sips of clear, sugar-free liquids, with intake progressing to larger amounts of liquid formulas and then to solid foods, as tolerated. Very small, frequent feedings can utilize the remaining intestine most efficiently. Parenteral infusions are tapered and gradually discontinued once oral intakes can supply adequate nourishment. Some patients require tube feedings in addition to oral feedings to successfully meet nutrient needs.

The exact diet prescribed for short bowel syndrome depends on the portion of intestine removed, the length of intestine that remains, and whether the colon is still intact; moreover, dietary readjustments may be required as intestinal adaptation progresses.[39] A high-kcalorie intake is typically recommended to compensate for malabsorption. To provide adequate kcalories, a high-fat, low-carbohydrate diet may be recommended if the fat is sufficiently tolerated. Conversely, a high-complex-carbohydrate, low-fat diet may be suggested for patients who have an intact colon, because the colon bacteria can metabolize the unabsorbed carbohydrates and produce usable nutrients, and the low fat intake can improve steatorrhea. Some patients may be lactose intolerant, but they can minimize symptoms by consuming small amounts of lactose-containing foods throughout the day. Patients should avoid concentrated sweets, which draw fluid into the intestines, if they cause additional diarrhea. Vitamin and mineral supplements can prevent deficiencies from developing due to malabsorption. The accompanying Case Study can help you review the material on Crohn's disease and short bowel syndrome.

CASE STUDY | Patient with Short Bowel Syndrome

Judi Morel is a 28-year-old economist with an eight-year history of Crohn's disease. Judi is 5 feet 7 inches tall. Three years ago, she underwent a small bowel resection and remained free of active disease for two years. During that time, her symptoms subsided; she was able to tolerate most foods without any problem and gained weight. Ten months ago, Judi experienced a severe flare-up of her Crohn's disease. Since that time, she has lost 15 pounds and currently weighs 118 pounds. She has experienced severe abdominal pain and fatigue that have persisted despite aggressive medical management that included intravenous nutrition. Five days ago, Judi finally underwent another resection, which left her with 40 percent of healthy small intestine. Her colon is intact. She is experiencing extensive diarrhea.

1. Describe the manifestations of Crohn's disease, and explain why surgery is sometimes performed as part of the treatment. Describe the complications of disease that may affect nutrient needs.

2. Using the BMI table in the back of the book, check the ideal weight range for a person of Judi's height. What nutrition-related concerns are suggested by Judi's recent weight loss? What other nutrition problems did Judi probably experience as a consequence of Crohn's disease?

3. Discuss the complications that may follow an extensive intestinal resection. What factors may affect a person's ability to meet nutrient needs with an oral diet?

4. Discuss the dietary progression that is recommended following an intestinal resection. After Judi is able to eat solid foods, what factors may affect the type of diet that is recommended for her?

Conditions Affecting the Large Intestine

The large intestine moves undigested substances to the rectum and has a central role in maintaining fluid and electrolyte balances. Its bacterial population ferments undigested nutrients and produces short-chain fatty acids and some vitamins that our bodies can absorb and use. This section describes several conditions that may upset the normal functioning of the large intestine.

IRRITABLE BOWEL SYNDROME

People with **irritable bowel syndrome** experience chronic and recurring intestinal symptoms that cannot be explained by specific physical abnormalities. The symptoms may include diarrhea and/or constipation, abdominal pain or discomfort, flatulence, and distention; the abdominal pain is generally aggravated by eating and relieved by defecation. In some patients, symptoms may be mild; in others, the disturbances in colon function can interfere with work and social activities and dramatically alter life-style and sense of well-being. Irritable bowel syndrome generally occurs in individuals between 20 and 40 years of age and affects twice as many women as men. About 30 percent of people with the disorder eventually become asymptomatic.[40]

Although the causes of irritable bowel syndrome remain elusive, people with the disorder tend to have excessive colonic responses to meals, GI hormones, and stress. Many individuals exhibit hypersensitivity to a normal degree of intestinal distention and may feel discomfort when experiencing normal meal transit or typical amounts of intestinal gas. Intestinal motility after meals may be excessive, leading to diarrhea, or be reduced, causing constipation. Symptoms often worsen during periods of psychological stress, and stressful life events may trigger the illness. Diagnosing irritable bowel syndrome is often difficult because its symptoms are typical of other GI disorders and laboratory tests for the condition are nonexistent.

Treatment of Irritable Bowel Syndrome Medical treatment of irritable bowel syndrome often includes dietary adjustments, stress management, and behavioral therapies. Medications may be prescribed to manage symptoms, but they are not always helpful. The drugs prescribed may include antidiarrheal agents, anticholinergics (which affect GI motility), antidepressants, and laxatives.

irritable bowel syndrome: an intestinal disorder of unknown cause that disturbs the functioning of the lower bowel; symptoms include abdominal pain, flatulence, diarrhea, and constipation.

NURSING DIAGNOSIS

Appropriate for people with irritable bowel syndrome may include *diarrhea, constipation, acute pain, chronic pain, ineffective health maintenance,* and *ineffective therapeutic regimen management.*

Hannah Trang is a 22-year-old recent college graduate who began her first professional job in a bank one month ago. As a college student, she occasionally experienced abdominal pain and cramping after eating. She also had frequent bouts of diarrhea and felt somewhat better after bowel movements. Once Hannah began her new job, her symptoms occurred more frequently. At first she attributed her symptoms to job stress, but when the symptoms continued for several months, she decided to see her physician. After taking a careful history and conducting tests to rule out other bowel disorders, the physician diagnosed irritable bowel syndrome. The physician prescribed bulk-forming fibers and advised Hannah to keep a record of her food intake and symptoms for one week. Hannah was then referred to a dietitian for a review of her dietary record. The dietitian noticed that Hannah routinely drank several cups of coffee in the morning and had

large meals for lunch and dinner. Hannah often ate out in Mexican restaurants and favored spicy foods, refried beans, and fatty desserts. Between meals, she snacked on low-carbohydrate foods sweetened with sugar alcohols and drank several cans of soda daily. Her dietary fiber intake, however, totaled only about 13 grams daily.

1. Describe the characteristics of irritable bowel syndrome to Hannah, and indicate the role that stress might play in her illness.

2. Explain how the record of food intake and symptoms might be helpful in devising an appropriate dietary plan for Hannah. Could any of the foods that are currently in Hannah's diet be aggravating her symptoms?

3. What dietary measures might benefit individuals with irritable bowel syndrome? What problems might the dietary changes cause?

diverticulosis (DYE-ver-tic-you-LOH-sis): an intestinal condition characterized by the presence of small herniations (called diverticula) in the intestinal wall.

diverticulitis (DYE-ver-tic-you-LYE-tis): an inflammation or infection involving diverticula.

Nutrition Therapy for Irritable Bowel Syndrome
Although dietary adjustments may be useful, measures that help one symptom can sometimes make another worse. The most common dietary recommendation is to gradually increase fiber intake to relieve constipation and improve stool bulk, although clinical studies suggest that additional fiber has limited effectiveness in improving symptoms and may worsen flatulence.[41] Some individuals have fewer symptoms when they consume small, frequent meals instead of larger ones. Foods that worsen symptoms often include fried or fatty foods, gas-producing foods (review pp. 515–516 and Table 18-2), milk products (not necessarily due to lactose intolerance), wheat products, coffee (with or without caffeine), and alcoholic beverages; however, individual tolerances vary and are best determined by trial and error.[42] Psychological associations have a strong influence on food tolerance, so foods that patients perceive to be problematic should be discussed so that the diet is not restricted unnecessarily. A careful evaluation of the dietary patterns that exacerbate symptoms may uncover the foods and habits most closely associated with intestinal discomfort.

Treatments under investigation for irritable bowel syndrome include peppermint oil, which relaxes smooth muscle within the GI tract, and various types of probiotics (see Nutrition in Practice 18).[43] The accompanying Case Study can help you apply your knowledge about irritable bowel syndrome to a clinical situation.

DIVERTICULAR DISEASE OF THE COLON

Diverticulosis refers to the presence of pebble-sized herniations (outpockets) in the intestinal wall, known as diverticula (see Figure 18-5). The prevalence of diverticulosis increases with age, occurring in 50 to 65 percent of 80-year-old individuals.[44] Most people with diverticulosis are symptom free and remain unaware of the condition until a complication develops.

Population studies suggest that the development of diverticula is strongly influenced by the amount of dietary fiber a person consumes. By increasing stool weight and bulk, high-fiber diets reduce the workload of the circular muscles that move wastes through the colon. Low-fiber diets require more vigorous muscle contractions, increasing pressure within the segments immediately adjacent to the circular muscles. This increase in pressure induces small areas of intestinal tissue to weaken and balloon outward over time.

Diverticulitis Inflammation or infection sometimes develops in the area around a diverticulum. This condition, called **diverticulitis**, is the most common complication of diverticulosis, affecting 10 to 25 percent

| FIGURE 18-5 | Diverticula in the Colon |

Diverticula (plural)

Diverticulum (singular)

Diverticula are small pouches that develop in weakened areas of the intestinal wall. The condition of having diverticula is known as diverticulosis.

of individuals with the condition.[45] It is thought to result from erosion of the diverticular wall due to high pressure within the lumen, causing inflammation and eventually a microperforation that leads to subsequent infection.[46] If the infection spreads to adjacent organs, fistulas may develop. Less frequently, the infection spreads to the peritoneal cavity, causing life-threatening illness. Symptoms of diverticulitis may include persistent abdominal pain, tenderness in the affected area, fever, constipation, and diarrhea. Anorexia, nausea, and vomiting may also occur.

Treatment for Diverticular Disease Treatment for diverticulosis is necessary only if symptoms develop. Because a high-fiber diet may prevent disease progression and the development of intestinal symptoms, patients are advised to increase fiber intake, with an emphasis on insoluble fiber sources. (✚) Fiber should be increased gradually to ensure tolerance. Bulk-forming agents, such as psyllium, can help to increase fiber intake if food sources are insufficient. Avoiding nuts, seeds, and popcorn is sometimes suggested to prevent complications, but no evidence is available to justify the recommendation.[47]

Patients with diverticulitis may need antibiotics to treat infections and, possibly, pain-control medications. In mild cases, a clear liquid diet may be advised initially, with progression to solid foods as symptoms resolve. In severe cases, bowel rest is necessary (oral fluids and food are withheld), and fluids are given intravenously. An oral diet is gradually reintroduced as the condition improves, beginning with clear liquids and progressing to a restricted-fiber, low-residue diet until inflammation and bleeding subside. After recovery, a high-fiber diet is recommended to prevent disease progression and symptom recurrence. Surgical interventions are sometimes necessary to treat complications of diverticulitis and may include removal of the affected portion of the colon.[48]

COLOSTOMIES AND ILEOSTOMIES

An *ostomy* is a surgically created opening (called a **stoma**) in the abdominal wall through which dietary wastes can be eliminated. A permanent ostomy is necessary after a partial or total colectomy. A temporary ostomy is sometimes constructed so that part or all of the colon can be bypassed after injury or extensive surgery. To create the stoma, the cut end of the remaining segment of functioning intestine is brought through an opening in the abdominal wall and stitched in place so that it empties to the exterior. The stoma can be formed from a section of the colon (**colostomy**) or ileum (**ileostomy**), as shown in Figure 18-6. Conditions that may require these procedures include inflammatory bowel diseases, diverticulitis, and colorectal cancers.

To collect wastes, a disposable bag is affixed to the skin around the stoma and emptied during the day as needed. Alternatively, an interior pouch can be surgically constructed behind the stoma using intestinal tissue, and the pouch can be emptied with a catheter when convenient. Stool consistency varies according to the length of colon that is functional. If a small portion of the colon is absent or bypassed, the stools may continue to be semisolid. If the entire colon has been removed or is bypassed, the ability to reabsorb fluid and electrolytes is substantially reduced, and the output is liquid.

Nutrition Therapy for Patients with Ostomies The nutrition care after an ostomy depends on the length of colon removed and the portion of ileum that remains, so dietary adjustments are individualized according to the surgical procedure and symptoms that develop afterward. Following surgery, the diet gradually progresses from clear liquids that are low in sugars to a normal meal plan, as tolerated. To reduce stool output, a low-residue diet is often recommended. Small, frequent meals may be more acceptable than larger ones. To determine food tolerances, patients should add questionable foods to the diet one at a time and in small amounts to assess their effects; a food that causes problems can be tried again later. Appropriate fluid and electrolyte intakes should be encouraged when a large portion of the colon has been removed.

People with ileostomies need to chew thoroughly to ensure that foods are adequately digested and to prevent obstructions, which are a common complication due to the

Diverticula are frequently seen during a colonoscopy, a procedure that uses a flexible, lighted tube to examine the inside of the colon.

✚ Recommendations for increasing fiber intake are described on p. 81, and Appendix A includes the fiber values of most common foods.

stoma (STOE-ma): a surgically created opening in a body tissue or organ.

colostomy (co-LAH-stoe-me): a surgical passage through the abdominal wall into the colon.

ileostomy (ill-ee-AH-stoe-me): a surgical passage through the abdominal wall into the ileum.

NURSING DIAGNOSIS

Nursing diagnoses that may apply to people with diverticulitis include *acute pain, constipation, diarrhea,* and *risk for deficient fluid volume.*

NURSING DIAGNOSIS

Appropriate for people with ostomies may include *disturbed body image, risk for diarrhea, risk for deficient fluid volume,* and *risk for impaired skin integrity.*

FIGURE 18-6 | Colostomy and Ileostomy

Colostomy

In a colostomy, a portion of the colon is removed or bypassed, and the stoma is formed from the remaining section of functional colon.

Ileostomy

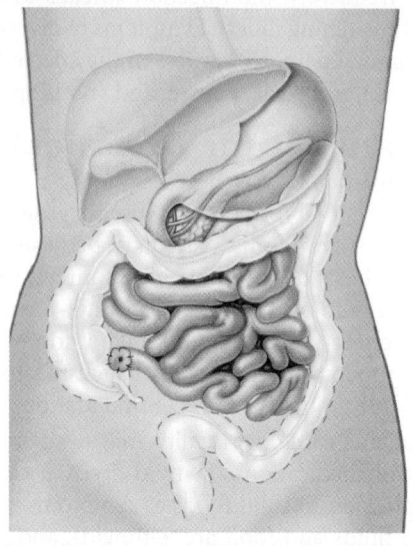

In an ileostomy, the entire colon is removed or bypassed, and the stoma is formed from the ileum.

small diameter of the ileal lumen. Foods high in insoluble fibers are sometimes avoided because they shorten intestinal transit time, may cause obstructions, and increase stool output. Because the colon is no longer available for water reabsorption, the diet should provide at least 8 cups of liquid daily to prevent dehydration. To ensure adequate electrolyte intakes, patients are encouraged to use salt liberally and to ingest beverages with added electrolytes (such as sports drinks and oral rehydration beverages), if necessary. If a large portion of the ileum has been removed, fat malabsorption may occur due to bile acid depletion, and vitamin B_{12} injections may be required.

Dietary concerns after colostomies depend on the length of colon remaining. Most patients have no dietary restrictions and can return to a regular diet.[49] Patient concerns may include stool odors, excessive gas production, and diarrhea. If a large portion of colon was removed, recommendations may be similar to those given to ileostomy patients.

Obstructions As mentioned, foods that are incompletely digested can cause obstructions, a primary concern of ileostomy patients. Although these patients can consume almost any food that is cut into small pieces and carefully chewed, the following foods may cause difficulty: celery, coconut, corn, dried fruit, grapes, nuts, raw cabbage (for example, in coleslaw), and unpeeled apples.[50]

Reducing Gas and Odors Persons with ostomies are often concerned about foods that may increase gas production or cause strong odors. Foods that may cause excessive gas include those listed in Table 18-2 on p. 516; practices that increase gas formation include smoking, gum or tobacco chewing, using drinking straws, and eating quickly. Foods that sometimes produce unpleasant odors include asparagus, beer, broccoli, brussels sprouts, cabbage, dried beans and peas, eggs, fish, garlic, and onions. Foods that may help to reduce odors include buttermilk, cranberry juice, parsley, and yogurt.[51]

Diarrhea Examples of foods that may aggravate diarrhea were listed in Table 18-3 on p. 517. Foods that may thicken stool include applesauce, banana, cheese, smooth peanut butter, pasta, potatoes, tapioca, and white rice.[52] What works may differ for each individual, however, and is best determined by trial and error.

Nutrition Assessment | CHECKLIST FOR PEOPLE WITH LOWER GI TRACT DISORDERS

MEDICAL HISTORY

Check the medical record for diseases that:

- ○ Cause chronic GI symptoms, such as irritable bowel syndrome or ulcerative colitis
- ○ Interfere with pancreatic enzyme secretion, such as chronic pancreatitis or cystic fibrosis
- ○ Interfere with nutrient absorption, such as Crohn's disease or celiac disease

Check for surgical procedures involving the lower GI tract, such as:

- ○ Intestinal resections
- ○ Ileostomy
- ○ Colostomy

Check for the following symptoms or complications:

- ○ Anemia
- ○ Bacterial overgrowth
- ○ Bone disease
- ○ Constipation
- ○ Diarrhea, dehydration
- ○ Fistulas
- ○ Lactose intolerance
- ○ Nutrient deficiencies
- ○ Obstructions
- ○ Oxalate kidney stones
- ○ Poor growth, in children
- ○ Steatorrhea

MEDICATIONS

Check for medications or dietary supplements that may:

- ○ Cause constipation or diarrhea
- ○ Interfere with food intake by causing nausea, vomiting, cramps, dry mouth, or drowsiness
- ○ Alter appetite or nutrient needs

DIETARY INTAKE

Note the following problems, and contact the dietitian if you suspect difficulties such as:

- ○ Poor appetite or food intake
- ○ Food intolerances
- ○ Inadequate fiber intake, in patients with constipation
- ○ Lactose intolerance, in patients with diarrhea
- ○ Inadequate fluid intake

ANTHROPOMETRIC DATA

Measure baseline height and weight. Address weight loss early to prevent malnutrition in patients with:

- ○ Severe or persistent diarrhea
- ○ Nutrient malabsorption

LABORATORY TESTS

Check laboratory tests for signs of dehydration, electrolyte imbalances, nutrient deficiencies, and anemia in patients with:

- ○ Severe or persistent diarrhea
- ○ Nutrient malabsorption
- ○ Intestinal resections

PHYSICAL SIGNS

Look for physical signs of:

- ○ Dehydration
- ○ Essential fatty acid and fat-soluble vitamin deficiencies
- ○ Folate and vitamin B_{12} deficiencies
- ○ Mineral deficiencies
- ○ Protein-energy malnutrition

Self Check

1. The nurse advising an elderly patient with constipation encourages the patient to:
   a. consume a low-fat diet low in sodium.
   b. consume a high-protein diet rich in calcium.
   c. eliminate gas-forming foods from the diet.
   d. gradually add high-fiber foods to the diet.

2. Osmotic diarrhea often results from:
   a. excessive colonic contractions.
   b. excessive fluid secretion by the intestines.
   c. nutrient malabsorption.
   d. viral, bacterial, or protozoal infections.

3. Nutrition problems that may result from fat malabsorption include all of the following *except*:
   a. weight loss.
   b. essential amino acid deficiencies.
   c. bone loss.
   d. oxalate kidney stones.

4. Common nutrition problems associated with bacterial overgrowth in the stomach and small intestine include:
   a. sensitivity to gluten.
   b. fat malabsorption and vitamin B_{12} deficiency.
   c. constipation.
   d. permanent loss of digestive enzymes.

5. The majority of chronic pancreatitis cases can be attributed to:
   a. bacterial and viral infections.
   b. gallstones.
   c. excessive alcohol use.
   d. elevated triglyceride levels.

6. Chronic pancreatitis and cystic fibrosis are both treated with:
   a. intestinal resection.
   b. postural drainage.
   c. enzyme replacement therapy.
   d. stool softeners.

7. A person on a gluten-free diet must avoid products containing:
   a. wheat, barley, and rye.
   b. barley, soybeans, and corn.
   c. wheat, corn, and rice.
   d. buckwheat, rice, and millet.

8. Symptoms of irritable bowel syndrome most often include:
   a. nausea and vomiting.
   b. weight loss and malnutrition.
   c. strong odors and obstructions.
   d. constipation, diarrhea, and flatulence.

9. Diverticulosis is most often associated with:
   a. a low-fiber diet.
   b. inadequate exercise.
   c. intestinal surgery.
   d. a high-fiber diet.

10. After an ileostomy, the most serious concern is that:
    a. the diet is too restrictive to meet nutrient needs.
    b. waste disposal causes frequent daily interruptions.
    c. fluid restrictions prevent patients from drinking beverages freely.
    d. incompletely digested foods may cause obstructions.

Answers to these questions appear in Appendix H.

Clinical Applications

1. A nurse working with a patient with a constipation problem provides him with detailed information about a high-fiber diet. At a follow-up appointment, the patient reports no change in symptoms. His food diary for that day shows that he consumed an omelet and toast for breakfast and a sandwich with juice for lunch.
   - Considering these two meals only, what additional information would help the nurse evaluate the man's compliance with the diet he was given?
   - Review the discussion about fiber in Chapter 3, and create a one-day menu that provides the DRI for fiber for an adult male, using the fiber values listed in Appendix A.

2. Using Table 18-5 on p. 520 as a guide, plan a day's menus for a diet containing approximately 50 grams of fat. Take care to make the meals both palatable and nutritious. How can these menus be improved using the suggestions in the "How to" on p. 521?

3 • As stated in this chapter, treatment of celiac disease is deceptively simple—eliminate wheat, barley, and rye, and possibly oats. Remaining on a gluten-free diet is more challenging than it appears, however.

- Randomly select 10 of your favorite snack and convenience foods. Take a trip to the grocery store, and check the labels of the products you selected to see if they would be allowed on a gluten-free diet. Keep in mind that the labels may not list all offending ingredients.
- Find acceptable substitutes for the products that are not allowed, either by substituting other foods or by checking for gluten-free products in the grocery store. If you have access to the Internet, you may want to investigate websites that advertise gluten-free products to get an idea of what's available.

Nutrition on the Net

For further study of topics covered in this chapter, access these websites.

Visit the websites of these organizations to find information that is helpful both for health practitioners and patients with gastrointestinal problems:

- Find updates and quick links to these and other nutrition-related sites at our website: www.cengage.com/nutrition/whitney/nhhc4e
- American College of Gastroenterology: www.acg.gi.org
- American Gastroenterological Association: www.gastro.org
- National Institute of Diabetes and Digestive and Kidney Diseases, a division of the National Institutes of Health: www2.niddk.nih.gov

Find additional information about cystic fibrosis at the website of the Cystic Fibrosis Foundation: www.cff.org/home

Find more information about celiac disease by visiting these websites:

- Celiac Disease Foundation: www.celiac.org
- Celiac Sprue Association: www.csaceliacs.org
- Gluten Intolerance Group: www.gluten.net

Learn more about inflammatory bowel diseases at the website of the Crohn's and Colitis Foundation of America: www.ccfa.org

Notes

1. S. M. Patel and A. J. Lembo, Constipation, in M. Feldman, L. S. Friedman, and L. J. Brandt, eds., *Sleisenger and Fordtran's Gastrointestinal and Liver Disease* (Philadelphia: Saunders, 2006), pp. 221–253.
2. C. A. Ternent and coauthors, Practice parameters for the evaluation and management of constipation, *Diseases of the Colon and Rectum* 50 (2007): 2013–2022.
3. Standing Committee on the Scientific Evaluation of Dietary Reference Intakes, Food and Nutrition Board, Institute of Medicine, *Dietary Reference Intakes for Energy, Carbohydrate, Fiber, Fat, Fatty Acids, Cholesterol, Protein, and Amino Acids* (Washington, D.C.: National Academies Press, 2002).
4. Ternent and coauthors, 2007.
5. H. Ohge and M. D. Levitt, Intestinal gas, in M. Feldman, L. S. Friedman, and L. J. Brandt, eds., *Sleisenger and Fordtran's Gastrointestinal and Liver Disease* (Philadelphia: Saunders, 2006), pp. 187–197.
6. L. R. Schiller and J. H. Sellin, Diarrhea, in M. Feldman, L. S. Friedman, and L. J. Brandt, eds., *Sleisenger and Fordtran's Gastrointestinal and Liver Disease* (Philadelphia: Saunders, 2006), pp. 159–186.
7. J. S. Trier, Acute diarrheal disorders, in N. J. Greenberger, ed., *Current Diagnosis and Treatment: Gastroenterology, Hepatology, and Endoscopy* (New York: McGraw-Hill Companies, 2009), pp. 45–63.
8. M. de Vrese and P. R. Marteau, Probiotics and prebiotics: Effects on diarrhea, *American Journal of Clinical Nutrition* 137 (2007): 803S–811S.
9. Schiller and Sellin, 2006.
10. American Dietetic Association, *Nutrition Care Manual* (Chicago: American Dietetic Association, 2009).
11. C. E. Semrad and D. W. Powell, Approach to the patient with diarrhea and malabsorption, in L. Goldman and D. Ausiello, eds., *Cecil Medicine* (Philadelphia: Saunders, 2008), pp. 1019–1042.
12. J. S. Trier, Intestinal malabsorption, in N. J. Greenberger, ed., *Current Diagnosis and Treatment: Gastroenterology, Hepatology, and Endoscopy* (New York: McGraw-Hill Companies, 2009), pp. 223–242.
13. J. K. DiBaise, Nutritional consequences of small intestinal bacterial overgrowth, *Practical Gastroenterology* 32 (December, 2008): 15–28.
14. Semrad and Powell, 2008.
15. S. Hertzler and coauthors, Nutrient considerations in lactose intolerance, in A. M. Coulston and C. J. Boushey, eds., *Nutrition in the Prevention and Treatment of Disease* (Burlington, MA: Elsevier, 2008), pp. 755–770.
16. Hertzler and coauthors, 2008.
17. V. Singh, D. L. Conwell, and P. A. Banks, Acute pancreatitis, in N. J. Greenberger, ed., *Current Diagnosis and Treatment: Gastroenterology, Hepatology, and Endoscopy* (New York: McGraw-Hill Companies, 2009), pp. 291–298.
18. American Dietetic Association, 2009; M. Raimondo and J. S. Scolapio, Nutrition in pancreatic disorders, in M. E. Shils and coeditors, *Modern Nutrition in Health and Disease* (Baltimore: Lippincott Williams & Wilkins, 2006), pp. 1227–1234.
19. C. Owyang, Pancreatitis, in L. Goldman and D. Ausiello, eds., *Cecil Medicine* (Philadelphia: Saunders, 2008), pp. 1070–1078.
20. C. E. Forsmark, Chronic pancreatitis, in M. Feldman, L. S. Friedman, and L. J. Brandt, eds., *Sleisenger and Fordtran's Gastrointestinal and Liver Disease* (Philadelphia: Saunders, 2006), pp. 1271–1308.
21. B. Wu, D. Conwell, and P. Banks, Chronic pancreatitis, in N. J. Greenberger, ed., *Current Diagnosis and Treatment: Gastroenterology, Hepatology, and Endoscopy* (New York: McGraw-Hill Companies, 2009), pp. 299–304; Owyang, 2008.
22. M. J. Welsh, Cystic fibrosis, in L. Goldman and D. Ausiello, eds., *Cecil Medicine* (Philadelphia: Saunders, 2008), pp. 627–631.
23. M. P. Boyle, Adult cystic fibrosis, *Journal of the American Medical Association* 298 (2007): 1787–1793.
24. Welsh, 2008.
25. K. M. Hayek, Medical nutrition therapy for cystic fibrosis: Beyond pancreatic enzyme replacement therapy, *Journal of the American Dietetic Association* 106 (2006): 1186–1188.

26. M. M. Niewinski, Advances in celiac disease and gluten-free diet, *Journal of the American Dietetic Association* (2008): 661–672.

27. Niewinski, 2008.

28. A. Di Sabatino and G. R. Corazza, Coeliac disease, *Lancet* 373 (2009): 1480–1493; J. J. Heidelbaugh and coauthors, Gastroenterology, in R. E. Rakel, ed., *Textbook of Family Medicine* (Philadelphia: Saunders, 2007), pp. 1115–1171.

29. N. Raymond, J. Heap, and S. Case, The gluten-free diet: An update for health professionals, *Practical Gastroenterology* 30 (September, 2006): 67–92.

30. Raymond, Heap, and Case, 2006.

31. W. F. Stenson, Inflammatory bowel disease, in L. Goldman and D. Ausiello, eds., *Cecil Medicine* (Philadelphia: Saunders, 2008), pp. 1042–1050.

32. Stenson, 2008; B. E. Sands, Crohn's disease, in M. Feldman, L. S. Friedman, and L. J. Brandt, eds., *Sleisenger and Fordtran's Gastrointestinal and Liver Disease* (Philadelphia: Saunders, 2006), pp. 2459–2498.

33. A. M. Griffiths, Inflammatory bowel disease, in M. E. Shils and coeditors, *Modern Nutrition in Health and Disease* (Baltimore: Lippincott Williams & Wilkins, 2006), pp. 1209–1218.

34. Stenson, 2008.

35. American Dietetic Association, 2009.

36. American Dietetic Association, 2009.

37. Stenson, 2008.

38. Trier, Intestinal malabsorption, 2009.

39. K. N. Jeejeebhoy, Short bowel syndrome, in M. E. Shils and coeditors, *Modern Nutrition in Health and Disease* (Baltimore: Lippincott Williams & Wilkins, 2006), pp. 1201–1208; C. R. Parrish, The clinician's guide to short bowel syndrome, *Practical Gastroenterology* (September 2005): 67–106.

40. S. Friedman, Irritable bowel syndrome, in N. J. Greenberger, ed., *Current Diagnosis and Treatment: Gastroenterology, Hepatology, and Endoscopy* (New York: McGraw-Hill Companies, 2009), pp. 279–290; N. J. Talley, Functional gastrointestinal disorders: Irritable bowel syndrome, dyspepsia, and noncardiac chest pain, in L. Goldman and D. Ausiello, eds., *Cecil Medicine* (Philadelphia: Saunders, 2008), pp. 990–998.

41. W. D. Heizer, S. Southern, and S. McGovern, The role of diet in symptoms of irritable bowel syndrome in adults: A narrative review, *Journal of the American Dietetic Association* 109 (2009): 1204–1214; A. Sanjeevi and D. F. Kirby, The role of food and dietary intervention in the irritable bowel syndrome, *Practical Gastroenterology* 32 (July 2008): 33–42.

42. Friedman, 2009; Heizer, Southern, and McGovern, 2009; Sanjeevi and Kirby, 2008.

43. Heizer, Southern, and McGovern, 2009.

44. A. C. Travis and R. S. Blumberg, Diverticular disease of the colon, in N. J. Greenberger, ed., *Current Diagnosis and Treatment: Gastroenterology, Hepatology, and Endoscopy* (New York: McGraw-Hill Companies, 2009), pp. 243–255.

45. C. Prather, Inflammatory and anatomic diseases of the intestine, peritoneum, mesentery, and omentum, in L. Goldman and D. Ausiello, eds., *Cecil Medicine* (Philadelphia: Saunders, 2008), pp. 1050–1061.

46. J. R. Turner, The gastrointestinal tract, in V. Kumar and coeditors, *Robbins and Cotran Pathologic Basis of Disease* (Philadelphia: Saunders, 2010), pp. 763–831; Travis and Blumberg, 2009.

47. Travis and Blumberg, 2009; Prather, 2008; L. L. Strate and coauthors, Nut, corn, and popcorn consumption and the incidence of diverticular disease, *Journal of the American Medical Association* 300 (2008): 907–914.

48. American Dietetic Association, 2009; Prather, 2008.

49. K. Willcutts, K. Scarano, and C. W. Eddins, Ostomies and fistulas: A collaborative approach, *Practical Gastroenterology* (December 2005): 63–79.

50. American Dietetic Association, 2009.

51. American Dietetic Association, 2009; Willcutts, Scarano, and Eddins, 2005.

52. American Dietetic Association, 2009; Willcutts, Scarano, and Eddins, 2005

Probiotics and Intestinal Health

Soon after birth, the warm, nutrient-rich environment within the gastrointestinal tract is colonized by a wide variety of bacterial species. The approximately 10 trillion bacterial cells inhabiting our bodies (**flora**) make up more than 90 percent of all our cells. Most bacterial cells reside in our colon, which harbors more than 400 different species.[1] Although the exact composition of intestinal bacteria varies among individuals, the pattern within an individual tends to remain constant over time, fluctuating somewhat due to illness, antibiotic treatment, and, to some extent, dietary factors. Table NP18-1 lists the predominant types of bacteria that colonize the human intestines, and Table NP18-2 shows how the bacterial populations vary within different regions of the GI tract.

Over the past several decades, nutritional scientists and microbiologists have tried to determine whether **probiotics**—live, **nonpathogenic** bacteria supplied in sufficient numbers to possibly benefit our health—can be useful for preventing or treating various medical conditions. Although the diseases of interest include gastrointestinal disorders, researchers have also been studying the effects of bacterial cells on cancer, immune system disorders, and other illnesses. This Nutrition in Practice discusses some of the research and explains some of the issues involved in selecting and consuming probiotic bacteria. The accompanying glossary defines the relevant terms.

TABLE NP18-1	Intestinal Flora	
Predominant Types	**Subdominant Types**
Bacteroides	Enterobacteria
Bifidobacteria	Enterococci
Clostridia	Escherichia
Eubacteria	Klebsiella
Peptococci	Lactobacilli
Peptostreptococci	Micrococci
Ruminococci	Staphylococci

TABLE NP18-2	Bacterial Populations in the Gastrointestinal Tract
Organ	**Total Bacteria (per mL of contents)**
Stomach	0 to 100
Small intestine: duodenum	0 to 1000
Small intestine: jejunum and ileum	10^5 to 10^8
Colon	10^{10} to 10^{12}

How do our intestinal bacteria influence health?

Intestinal bacteria can benefit our health in a number of different ways. First, the bacteria degrade much of our undigested or unabsorbed dietary carbohydrate, including dietary fibers, starch that is resistant to digestion, and poorly absorbed sugars and sugar alcohols. In turn, the bacteria produce some vitamins, as well as short-chain fatty acids that our cells can use as an energy source. Intestinal bacteria also stimulate our immune defenses and may prevent the overgrowth of **pathogenic** bacteria in the gastrointestinal tract. Healthy bacteria may help to prevent invasion of our tissues by pathogenic bacteria by creating a barrier on the intestinal walls.[2]

Certain nondigestible substances in food, called **prebiotics,** can stimulate the growth or activity of resident bacteria within the large intestine. Prebiotics include some of the carbohydrates found in asparagus, chicory root, garlic, Jerusalem artichokes, onions, and other foods.[3] Because the intestinal bacteria that degrade these substances produce gas as a by-product, people who consume high amounts of these foods may experience more flatulence than usual.

Glossary

flora: the bacteria that normally reside in a person's body.
nonpathogenic: not capable of causing disease.
pathogenic: capable of causing disease.
prebiotics: nondigestible substances in foods that stimulate the growth of nonpathogenic bacteria within the large intestine.
probiotics: live bacteria provided in foods and dietary supplements for the purpose of preventing or treating disease.

Why are certain types of bacteria considered "probiotic"?

For bacteria to be "probiotic"—that is, beneficial to health—they must be nonpathogenic when consumed. They must survive their transit through the digestive tract; therefore, they must be resistant to destruction by stomach acid, bile, and other digestive substances. They should be able to alter the intestinal environment in some way that is beneficial to the human host, either by producing antimicrobial substances, altering immune defenses, metabolizing undigested foodstuffs, or protecting the intestinal walls.[4]

Probiotic bacteria must be consumed in large amounts—between 100 million and 100 billion live bacteria per day—to survive in sufficient numbers to influence the bacterial populations in the large intestine; a serving of yogurt usually provides these amounts. Carefully controlled studies have not found that probiotic bacteria actually *colonize* the intestine, however, as they are no longer detected in fecal or intestinal samples once ingestion of the probiotic product stops.[5] Note that only a few different types of bacteria are used in foods, and the relatively small amounts consumed cannot compete with the huge populations that normally populate our digestive tract.

What types of medical problems are helped by probiotic bacteria?

Although the results of research studies vary, probiotic bacteria may help to prevent and treat some gastric and intestinal disorders, alter susceptibility to food allergens and alleviate some allergy symptoms, and improve the availability and digestibility of various nutrients.[6] Some evidence suggests that probiotics may help to prevent or reverse infections in the urethra and vagina.[7] Other potential benefits include improved immune responses, reduced symptoms of lactose intolerance, and reduced cancer risk.[8]

Much of the research investigating probiotics and intestinal illness has focused on the prevention and treatment of infectious diarrhea. For example, controlled trials have suggested that certain strains of probiotic bacteria may shorten the duration of diarrhea caused by rotavirus infection in infants and children, decrease the incidence of traveler's diarrhea in tourists visiting high-risk areas, and prevent the recurrence of infectious diarrhea in hospitalized patients.[9] In studies of children and adults using antibiotics, some strains of probiotic bacteria have been shown to reduce the incidence and duration of antibiotic-associated diarrhea. As another example, some studies have suggested that probiotic treatment may help to reduce the recurrence of *pouchitis,* an inflammation of the surgical pouch created in patients who have had an ileostomy or colostomy.[10]

Despite promising research results thus far, there are no clear conclusions about the appropriate probiotic

Various species of *Lactobacillus* are used in the production of fermented food products, such as the foods shown in this photo.

doses or durations of treatment for many of these conditions.[11] Moreover, the beneficial effects of one bacterial strain cannot be extrapolated to other strains of the same species.[12] Thus, individuals who decide to consume probiotic-containing foods and supplements to benefit their health cannot be certain that the substances they use will help their condition. At best, probiotics should be considered an adjunct therapy rather than a primary treatment for an illness.

What are the main dietary sources of probiotic bacteria?

Probiotics are provided mainly by fermented foods. In the United States, yogurt and acidophilus milk are produced using various species of lactobacilli and bifidobacteria, although the species are chosen for their ability to produce desirable food products rather than their potential health benefits. In Europe and Asia, food products containing probiotic bacteria include yogurt, milk, ice cream, oatmeal gruel, and soft drinks. Although lactobacilli are used to produce various other fermented food products, such as sauerkraut, pickles, brined olives, and sausages, these foods retain few, if any, live bacteria after they undergo typical food processing methods.[13]

A number of companies market probiotic supplements, which are available in capsules, tablets, and powders. Because probiotic bacteria are living organisms, storage conditions may affect their viability—heat, moisture, and oxygen can reduce survival times—and therefore consumers should check the expiration date before purchasing a product. When a consumer group (ConsumerLab.com) tested 13 probiotic supplements, they found that 5 of the products contained substantially fewer live bacteria than was claimed on the label.[14] Thus, there is no guarantee that a dietary supplement will contain the amount of bacteria expected.

Are there any potential problems associated with the use of probiotic bacteria?

Yes. One major concern is the possibility that probiotic bacteria may cause infection in immune-compromised individuals. Various species of probiotic bacteria, including *Lactobacillus* species, have been isolated from the infection sites of severely ill individuals who were consuming the probiotic orally.[15] The individuals most likely to be susceptible to infectious complications are those with reduced immunity, such as people with AIDS or cancer and those undergoing organ transplantation. Care should be taken to inquire about probiotic use in these patients.

Other concerns are related to the lack of industry standards for probiotics in foods and supplements: the concentrations and strains of probiotic bacteria in foods may vary substantially.[16] Thus, a consumer who wishes to try probiotics would find it difficult to determine how much of a product to consume in order to achieve the desired effect.

In recent years, the contributions of our intestinal flora to health have been increasingly recognized. Preliminary research suggests that altering our bacterial populations by consuming probiotics or prebiotics may help to improve our defenses against certain illnesses. Additional studies are needed to verify the beneficial effects of probiotics and prebiotics and to develop standard protocols that can be used for treating illness.

Notes

1. S. O'Mahony and F. Shanahan, Enteric bacterial flora and bacterial overgrowth, in M. Feldman, L. S. Friedman, and L. J. Brandt, eds., *Sleisenger and Fordtran's Gastrointestinal and Liver Disease* (Philadelphia: Saunders, 2006), pp. 2243–2256.
2. F. Guarner and J.-R. Malagelada, Gut flora in health and disease, *Lancet* 361 (2003): 512–519.
3. S. Kolida and G. R. Gibson, Prebiotic capacity of inulin-type fructans, *Journal of Nutrition* 137 (2007): 2503S–2506S.
4. P. Winkler and coauthors, Molecular and cellular basis of microflora-host interactions, *Journal of Nutrition* 137 (2007): 756S–772S.
5. B. Corthésy, H. R. Gaskins, and A. Mercenier, Cross-talk between probiotic bacteria and the host immune system, *Journal of Nutrition* 137 (2007): 781S–790S.
6. M. de Vrese and P. R. Marteau, Probiotics and prebiotics: Effects on diarrhea, *Journal of Nutrition* 137 (2007): 803S–811S; A. C. Ouwehand, Antiallergic effects of probiotics, *Journal of Nutrition* 137 (2007): 794S–797S.
7. G. Reid and J. Burton, Use of *Lactobacillus* to prevent infection by pathogenic bacteria, *Microbes and Infection* 4 (2002): 319–324.
8. S. Parvez and coauthors, Probiotics and their fermented food products are beneficial for health, *Journal of Applied Microbiology* 100 (2006): 1171–1185.
9. de Vrese and Marteau, 2007.
10. J. J. Jones and A. E. Foxx-Orenstein, Probiotics in inflammatory bowel disease, *Practical Gastroenterology* (March 2006): 44–50.
11. E. I. Benchimol and D. R. Mack, Safety issues of probiotic ingestion, *Practical Gastroenterology* (November 2005): 23–34; R. S. Carvalho and M. Oliva-Hemker, Clinical indications for the use of probiotics in the pediatric population, *Practical Gastroenterology* (October 2005): 51–64.
12. L. C. Douglas and M. E. Sanders, Probiotics and prebiotics in dietetics practice, *Journal of the American Dietetic Association* (2008): 510–521; Guarner and Malagelada, 2003.
13. Douglas and Sanders, 2008.
14. ConsumerLab.com, Product review: Probiotic supplements (including *Lactobacillus acidophilus*, *Bifidobacterium*, and others), available at **www.consumerlab.com;** site visited August 29, 2009.
15. Benchimol and Mack, 2005; N. Ishibashi and S. Yamazaki, Probiotics and safety, *American Journal of Clinical Nutrition* 73 (2001): 465S–470S.
16. E. R. Farnworth, The evidence to support health claims for probiotics, *Journal of Nutrition* 138 (2008): 1250S–1254S.

CHAPTER 19 | Nutrition and Liver Diseases

© Custom Medical Stock Photo/Alamy

CONTENTS

THE LIVER IS THE MOST METABOLICALLY ACTIVE ORGAN IN THE BODY. It plays a central role in processing, storing, and redistributing the nutrients provided by the foods we eat. As Chapter 2 described, the liver produces the bile that emulsifies fat during digestion. The liver manufactures most of the proteins that circulate in plasma, including albumin, clotting proteins, and transport proteins. In addition, the liver detoxifies drugs and alcohol and processes excess nitrogen so that it can be safely excreted as urea. If the liver's numerous roles are upset by liver damage or disease, the effects on health and nutrition status can be profound.

Liver disease progresses slowly. Its primary symptom, fatigue, often goes unnoticed. Other symptoms may be so mild that complications develop before a diagnosis is made. Once liver disease is recognized, preserving remaining liver function becomes a primary concern, because the liver can regenerate some healthy tissue, improving prognosis. Preventing additional damage is the principal means of avoiding liver failure or transplantation.

Fatty Liver and Hepatitis

Fatty liver and hepatitis are the two most common disorders affecting the liver. Although both conditions may be mild and are usually reversible, each may progress to more serious illness and eventually cause liver damage.

FATTY LIVER

Fatty liver is an accumulation of fat in liver tissue. Ordinarily, the liver's triglycerides are packaged into very low-density lipoproteins (VLDL) and exported to the bloodstream. Fatty liver represents an imbalance between the amount of fat synthesized in the liver or picked up from the blood and the amount exported to the blood via VLDL. Fatty liver is estimated to affect 20 percent or more of the adult population in the United States.[1]

Fatty liver is a clinical finding that is common to many conditions. It is present in the majority of patients who have alcoholic liver disease (described in Nutrition in Practice 19) and can also result from exposure to drugs and toxic metals. It often accompanies diabetes mellitus, metabolic syndrome, and obesity. Other potential causes of fatty liver include various inherited disorders, total parenteral nutrition, gastrointestinal bypass surgery, and diseases of malnutrition (such as kwashiorkor and marasmus).[2]

Consequences of Fatty Liver In many individuals, fatty liver is asymptomatic and causes no harm. In other cases, it may be accompanied by inflammation (**steatohepatitis**), liver enlargement (**hepatomegaly**), and fatigue. If liver damage and scarring develop, fatty liver may progress to cirrhosis (discussed in a later section), liver failure, or liver cancer.

Fatty liver is a frequent cause of abnormal liver enzyme levels in the blood. Laboratory findings may include elevated blood concentrations of the liver enzymes ALT and AST, as well as increased levels of triglycerides, cholesterol, and glucose. (✚) Table 19-2 on p. 549 provides normal ranges for these liver enzymes.

Treatment of Fatty Liver The usual treatment for fatty liver is to eliminate the factors that cause it. For example, if fatty liver is due to alcohol abuse or drug therapy, it may improve after the patient discontinues use of the substance. In patients with elevated blood lipids, fatty liver may improve after blood lipid levels are lowered. An appropriate treatment for obese or diabetic patients might be weight reduction, increased physical activity, or medications that improve insulin sensitivity. Rapid weight loss should be discouraged, however, because it may accelerate the progression of liver disease. Note that lifestyle modifications are not always successful in reversing fatty liver, especially in patients who lack the usual risk factors.[3]

HEPATITIS

Hepatitis, a condition of liver inflammation, can result from any factor that causes damage to liver tissue. Most often, the damage is caused by infection with specific viruses, which are designated by the letters A, B, C, D, and E. Hepatitis can also be caused by

✚ The liver enzymes ALT (alanine aminotransferase) and AST (aspartate aminotransferase) are involved in amino acid catabolism.

fatty liver: an accumulation of fat in liver tissue; also called *hepatic steatosis*.

steatohepatitis (STEE-ah-to-HEP-ah-TYE-tis): liver inflammation that is associated with fatty liver.

hepatomegaly (HEP-ah-toe-MEG-ah-lee): enlargement of the liver.

hepatitis (hep-ah-TYE-tis): inflammation of the liver.

Hepatitis is considered *acute* if it lasts less than six months; *chronic* cases are those that last six months or longer.

excessive alcohol intake, exposure to certain drugs and toxic chemicals, and fatty liver disease. A number of herbal remedies may lead to hepatitis; they include chaparral, germander, ma huang, jin bu huan, kava kava, and skullcap.[4] Less common causes of hepatitis include infection with other viruses and autoimmune disease. Chronic hepatitis can lead to cirrhosis (discussed in a later section) and liver cancer. (✚)

Viral Hepatitis Acute hepatitis is most often caused by infection with hepatitis viruses A, B, and C (see Table 19-1). Specific features of these viruses include the following:

- *Hepatitis A virus* (HAV) is primarily spread via fecal-oral transmission, which usually involves the ingestion of foods or beverages that have been contaminated with fecal material. Outbreaks of HAV infection are often associated with floods and other natural disasters, when inadequately treated sewage may contaminate water supplies with fecal matter. Less frequently, HAV infection is contracted by the consumption of undercooked shellfish obtained from contaminated waters. Individuals at highest risk of HAV infection include food handlers, child care workers, illicit drug users, and travelers to regions where the virus is endemic. In the United States, the incidence of HAV infection has declined 92 percent since 1995 as a result of routine vaccinations in children and high-risk individuals.[5] HAV infection usually resolves within a few months and does not cause chronic illness or permanent liver damage.
- *Hepatitis B virus* (HBV) is transmitted by infected blood or needles or by sexual contact. A major global health concern, HBV has infected one-third of the world population, although chronic illness develops in less than 10 percent of cases.[6] In the United States, HBV incidence has dropped 82 percent since 1990 due to routine screenings and vaccinations for at-risk individuals.[7] Vaccinations against HBV are currently recommended for newborn infants and children, health-care workers, recipients of blood products, dialysis patients, sexually active adults, and users of injected drugs.
- *Hepatitis C virus* (HCV) is spread via infected blood or needles but is not readily spread by sexual contact. Most HCV cases progress to chronic illness, and HCV is currently the most common cause of chronic liver disease in the United States.[8] No vaccine is available to protect against HCV infection. Preventive measures include blood donor screening, viral inactivation of blood products, and infection control practices in health-care settings. The incidence of HCV infection has declined markedly in recent years; newly diagnosed cases usually involve individuals with chronic infections who contracted hepatitis C decades ago.[9]

TABLE 19-1	Features of Hepatitis Viruses				
Hepatitis Virus	**Major Mode of Transmission**	**New Cases (United States, 2007)**	**Chronic Disease Rate (% of cases)**	**Chronic Cases (United States)**	**Vaccination Available**
A	Fecal-oral	25,000	None	0	Yes
B	Bloodborne, sexual transmission	43,000	2–7	1.25 million	Yes
C	Bloodborne	17,000	50–85	3.2 million	No

Note: There are fewer new cases of hepatitis C virus (HCV) infection than of hepatitis B virus (HBV) infection each year, but more HCV cases become chronic. Therefore, there are more HCV carriers than HBV carriers.

Sources: Centers for Disease Control and Prevention, Surveillance for acute viral hepatitis—United States, 2007, *Morbidity and Mortality Weekly Report* 58, No. SS03 (2009): 1–27; A. Rutherford and J. L. Dienstag, Viral hepatitis, in N. J. Greenberger, ed., *Current Diagnosis and Treatment: Gastroenterology, Hepatology, and Endoscopy* (New York: McGraw-Hill Companies, 2009), pp. 420–443; J. H. Hoofnagle, Acute viral hepatitis, in L. Goldman and D. Ausiello, eds., *Cecil Medicine* (Philadelphia: Saunders, 2008), pp. 1101–1108.

Symptoms of Hepatitis The effects of hepatitis depend on the cause and severity of the disease. Individuals with mild or chronic hepatitis are often asymptomatic. The onset of acute hepatitis may be accompanied by fatigue, nausea, anorexia, and pain in the liver area. The liver is often slightly enlarged and tender. **Jaundice** (yellow discoloration of tissues) may develop, causing yellowing of the skin, urine, and the whites of the eyes. (✚) Other symptoms of hepatitis include fever, muscle weakness, joint pain, and skin rashes. Serum levels of the liver enzymes ALT and AST are typically elevated. Chronic hepatitis may cause complications that are typical of liver cirrhosis.

Treatment of Hepatitis Hepatitis is treated with supportive care, such as bed rest (if necessary) and an appropriate diet. Hepatitis patients should avoid substances that irritate the liver, such as alcohol and drugs or dietary supplements that cause liver damage. Hepatitis A infection usually resolves without the use of medications. Antiviral agents may be used to treat HBV and HCV infections; examples include lamivudine and ribavirin, which block viral replication, and interferon, which both inhibits viral replication and enhances immune responses.[10] Nonviral forms of hepatitis may be treated with anti-inflammatory and immunosuppressant drugs. Hospitalization is not required for hepatitis unless other medical conditions or complications hamper recovery.

Nutrition Therapy for Hepatitis Nutrition care varies according to a patient's symptoms and nutrition status.[11] Most individuals require no dietary changes. Those with anorexia or gastrointestinal discomfort may find small, frequent meals easier to tolerate. Malnourished individuals should consume adequate protein and energy to replenish nutrient stores; the diet should include 1.0 to 1.2 grams of protein per kilogram of body weight each day. A low-fat diet, with fat limited to less than 30 percent of total kcalories, may be necessary for those with steatorrhea. Patients with persistent vomiting may require fluid and electrolyte replacement. Dietary supplements can be helpful for improving nutrient intakes.

© Dr. P. Marazzi/Science Photo Library/Photo Researchers, Inc.

Jaundice is a yellow discoloration of the tissues that is most easily seen in the whites of the eyes.

✚ Jaundice results when liver dysfunction impairs the metabolism of bilirubin, a breakdown product of hemoglobin that is normally eliminated in bile. Accumulation of bilirubin in the bloodstream leads to yellow discoloration of tissues.

> ### Review Notes
>
> - Fatty liver can result from excessive alcohol intake, drug toxicity, and chronic disorders such as diabetes and obesity. Hepatitis is frequently caused by viral infection but can also result from alcohol abuse, drug toxicity, and other causes.
> - Although fatty liver is often benign, hepatitis can become chronic and lead to cirrhosis and liver cancer.
> - Fatty liver may be treated by eliminating the factors that cause it. Hepatitis treatment involves supportive care and varies according to illness severity and symptoms. Hepatitis patients should avoid substances that cause liver damage, use antiviral medications if necessary, and follow a diet that maintains or improves nutrition status.

NURSING DIAGNOSIS

Appropriate for people with hepatitis may include *fatigue, acute pain, risk for deficient fluid volume* (due to vomiting and diarrhea), *risk for impaired liver function,* and *imbalanced nutrition: less than body requirements.*

Cirrhosis

Cirrhosis is the final phase of chronic liver disease. Long-term liver disease gradually destroys liver tissue, leading to scarring (fibrosis) in some regions and small areas of regenerated, healthy tissue in others. As the disease progresses, the scarring becomes more extensive, leaving fewer areas of healthy tissue. A cirrhotic liver is often shrunken and has an irregular, nodular appearance. Cirrhosis impairs liver function and can eventually lead to liver failure. It is the 12th leading cause of death in the United States.[12]

The chief causes of cirrhosis in the United States are alcoholic liver disease and chronic hepatitis C infection, followed by fatty liver disease and chronic hepatitis B infection.[13] Additional causes include other types of chronic hepatitis; bile duct blockages, which cause bile acids to accumulate to toxic levels in the liver; drug-induced liver injury; and inherited disorders that cause toxic substances to build up in the liver.

jaundice (JAWN-dis): yellow discoloration of the skin and eyes due to an accumulation of bilirubin, a breakdown product of hemoglobin that normally exits the body via bile secretions.

cirrhosis (sih-ROE-sis): an advanced stage of liver disease in which extensive scarring replaces healthy liver tissue, causing impaired liver function and eventual liver failure

Normal liver tissue is smooth and has a regular texture.

© Martin Rotker/Phototake

A cirrhotic liver has an irregular, nodular appearance. The nodules represent clusters of regenerating cells within the damaged liver tissue.

© Dr. Joseph William/Phototake

CONSEQUENCES OF CIRRHOSIS

About 40 percent of cirrhosis patients are asymptomatic.[14] Because liver damage progresses slowly, the effects of cirrhosis may be minimal at first. Initial symptoms are usually nonspecific and may include fatigue, weakness, anorexia, and weight loss. Later, the decline in liver function can lead to metabolic disturbances: patients may develop anemia, bruise easily, and be more susceptible to infections. If bile obstruction occurs, jaundice and fat malabsorption are likely. The physical changes in liver tissue may interfere with blood flow, causing fluid to accumulate in blood vessels and body tissues. Advanced cirrhosis can disrupt kidney and lung function. Figure 19-1 illustrates some of the clinical effects of liver cirrhosis, and later sections describe some of these complications in more detail.

Table 19-2 lists laboratory tests that are used to monitor the extent of liver damage. Liver enzyme levels are increased because the injured liver tissue releases enzymes into the bloodstream. Levels of bilirubin may be elevated if the liver is too damaged to process it or if bile ducts are blocked and prevent its excretion. The impaired synthesis of plasma proteins by the liver lowers albumin levels and extends blood-clotting time. Liver damage also reduces the conversion of ammonia to urea, causing ammonia levels in the blood to rise.

Portal Hypertension

A large volume of blood normally flows through the liver. The portal vein (✚) and hepatic artery together supply approximately 1500 milliliters (about 1.5 quarts) of blood each minute to the extensive network of vessels in the liver. The scarred tissue of a cirrhotic liver impedes the flow of blood, which is mostly supplied by the portal vein. The resistance to blood flow within the liver causes a rise in blood pressure within the portal vein, called **portal hypertension**.

Collaterals and Gastroesophageal Varices

When blood flow through the portal vein is impeded, the blood is diverted to the smaller blood vessels surrounding the liver. These **collaterals** develop throughout the gastrointestinal (GI) tract and in regions near the abdominal wall. As pressure builds, the collateral vessels become enlarged and engorged, forming abnormally dilated vessels called **varices** (see the photo). The varices that develop in the esophagus (*esophageal varices*) and stomach (*gastric varices*) are vulnerable to rupture because they have thin walls and often bulge into the lumen. If ruptured, they can cause massive bleeding that is sometimes fatal. The blood loss is exacerbated by the liver's reduced production of blood-clotting factors.

Ascites

Within 10 years of disease onset, about 50 percent of cirrhosis patients develop **ascites**, a large accumulation of fluid in the abdominal cavity. The development of ascites indicates that liver damage has reached a critical stage, as half of patients with ascites die within 5 years.[15] Ascites is primarily a consequence of portal hypertension, reduced albumin

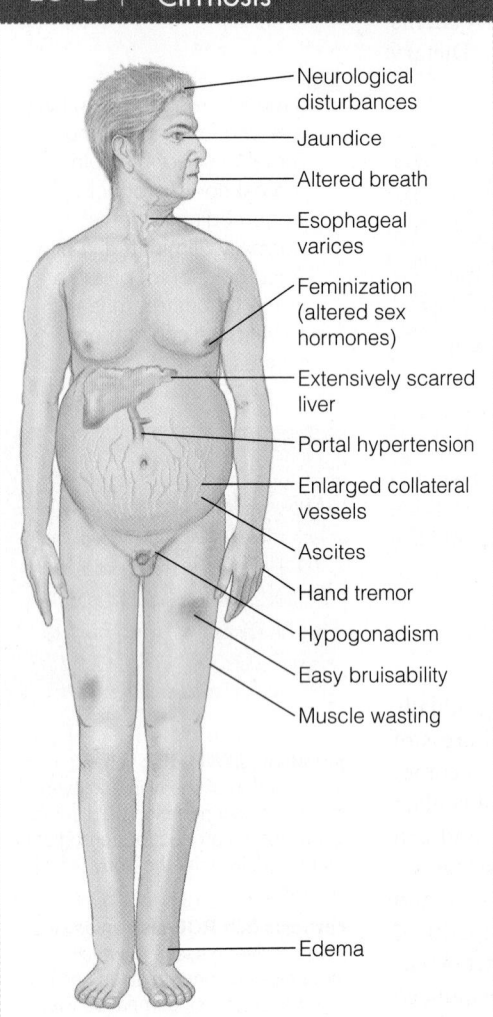

FIGURE 19-1 | Clinical Effects of Liver Cirrhosis

- Neurological disturbances
- Jaundice
- Altered breath
- Esophageal varices
- Feminization (altered sex hormones)
- Extensively scarred liver
- Portal hypertension
- Enlarged collateral vessels
- Ascites
- Hand tremor
- Hypogonadism
- Easy bruisability
- Muscle wasting
- Edema

TABLE 19-2	Laboratory Tests for Evaluation of Liver Disease	
Laboratory Test	**Normal Ranges (serum)**	**Values in Liver Disease**
Alanine aminotransferase (ALT)	Male: 10–40 U/L Female: 7–35 U/L	Elevated
Albumin	3.4–4.8 g/dL	Decreased
Alkaline phosphatase	25–100 U/L	Normal or elevated
Ammonia	15–45 µg N/dL	Elevated
Aspartate aminotransferase (AST)	10–30 U/L	Elevated
Bilirubin (total)	0.3–1.2 mg/dL	Elevated
Blood urea nitrogen (BUN)	6–20 mg/dL	Normal or decreased
Prothrombin time[a]	10–13 seconds	Prolonged

[a] The test for prothrombin time evaluates the clotting ability of blood.

Note: U/L = units per liter; dL = deciliter; µg = micrograms; N = nitrogen

+ Reminder: The *portal vein* is the large blood vessel that carries nutrient-rich blood from the digestive tract to the liver.

portal hypertension: elevated blood pressure in the portal vein due to obstructed blood flow through the liver.

collaterals: blood vessels that enlarge to allow an alternative pathway for diverted blood.

varices (VAH-rih-seez): abnormally dilated blood vessels (singular: *varix*).

ascites (ah-SIGH-teez): an abnormal accumulation of fluid in the abdominal cavity.

sinusoids: the small, capillary-like passages that carry blood through liver tissue.

hepatic encephalopathy (en-sef-ah-LOP-ah-thie): a condition that develops in advanced liver disease that is characterized by altered neurological functioning, including changes in personality and behavior, reduced mental abilities, and disturbances in motor function.
- *encephalo* = brain
- *pathy* = disease

hepatic coma: loss of consciousness resulting from severe liver disease.

synthesis by the diseased liver, and sodium and water retention in the kidneys. Portal hypertension raises pressure in the liver's **sinusoids**, forcing fluid to leak from the blood into the abdominal cavity. The fluid accumulation is exacerbated by low plasma albumin levels, because albumin helps to retain fluid in blood vessels. The increased pressure within the portal vein triggers the release of chemical factors (such as nitric oxide) that dilate local blood vessels and lower the blood volume elsewhere; these changes activate sodium and water retention in the kidneys and lead to additional water pooling. Ascites can cause abdominal discomfort and early satiety, which contribute to malnutrition. Because ascites can raise body weight considerably, weight changes may be difficult to interpret.

Hepatic Encephalopathy
Advanced liver disease sometimes leads to **hepatic encephalopathy**, a disorder characterized by abnormal neurological functioning. Symptoms of hepatic encephalopathy include changes in personality, behavior, mental abilities, and motor functions (see Table 19-3). At worst, amnesia, seizures, and **hepatic coma** may develop. Although hepatic encephalopathy is fully reversible with medical treatment, prognosis is poor when it progresses to the advanced stages.[16]

The exact causes of hepatic encephalopathy remain elusive, although elevated blood ammonia levels are thought to play a key role in its development due to ammonia's neurotoxicity.[17] A number of other compounds potentially toxic to brain tissue, such as sulfur compounds, short-chain fatty acids, and gamma-aminobutyric acid (GABA; a neurotransmitter), may also accumulate in brain cells and disturb brain function. Another theory is that the brain's neurotransmitters are altered by an increased ratio of aromatic amino acids to branched-chain amino acids in brain tissue, a result of disordered amino acid metabolism in the liver. (**+**) Most likely, a combination of metabolic abnormalities contributes to the disruption in neurological functioning.

© Hans Bjorknas/Gastrolab.net

Esophageal varices, such as the one shown here, may protrude into the lumen and be vulnerable to rupture and bleeding.

Ascites is caused by different diseases, but cirrhosis is the underlying cause in most patients with this condition.

TABLE 19-3	Symptoms of Hepatic Encephalopathy		
	Early Stages	**Middle Stages**	**Later Stages**
	Short attention span	Disorientation, impaired memory	Confusion, amnesia
	Depression, irritability	Anxiety, impaired judgment	Anger, paranoia
	Lack of coordination, tremor	Slurred speech, abnormal reflexes	Muscular rigidity, abnormal reflexes
	Sleep disorders	Lethargy	Semi-stupor

Elevated Blood Ammonia Levels
Much of the body's free ammonia is produced by bacterial action on unabsorbed dietary protein in the colon. Normally, the liver extracts this ammonia from portal blood and converts it to urea, which is then excreted by the kidneys. In advanced liver disease, the liver is unable to process the ammonia sufficiently. In addition, the ammonia-laden portal blood bypasses the liver by way of collateral vessels and reaches the general blood circulation, causing a substantial increase in the ammonia that reaches brain tissue. Although ammonia levels do not correlate well with the degree of neurological impairment in hepatic encephalopathy, ammonia-reducing medications can successfully reverse the neurological symptoms.[18]

Malnutrition and Wasting
Most patients with cirrhosis develop protein-energy malnutrition (PEM) and experience some degree of wasting. Malnutrition is usually caused by a combination of factors (see Table 19-4). Patients may consume less food due to reduced appetite, gastrointestinal symptoms, early satiety caused by ascites, or fatigue. If the diet is sodium restricted (to treat ascites), meals may seem monotonous or unpalatable. Fat malabsorption is common due to reduced bile flow, which leads to steatorrhea and deficiencies of the fat-soluble vitamins and some minerals. Additional nutrient losses may result from diarrhea, vomiting, and gastrointestinal bleeding. If cirrhosis is a consequence of alcohol abuse, multiple nutrient deficiencies may be present.

➕ The aromatic amino acids—phenylalanine, tyrosine, and tryptophan—have carbon rings in their side groups. The branched-chain amino acids are leucine, isoleucine, and valine; their side groups have a branched structure.

TABLE 19-4	Possible Causes of Malnutrition in Liver Disease	
	Mechanism	**Examples**
	Reduced nutrient intake	Abdominal discomfort, altered mental status, anorexia, early satiety (due to ascites), effects of medications (including gastrointestinal disturbances and taste changes), fasting for medical procedures, fatigue, nausea and vomiting, restrictive diets
	Malabsorption or nutrient losses	Diarrhea, effects of medications (including malabsorption and nutrient losses from diuretic use), fat malabsorption (due to reduced bile flow), gastrointestinal bleeding, vomiting
	Altered metabolism or increased nutrient needs	Hypermetabolism, impaired protein synthesis, infections or inflammation, muscle catabolism, reduced nutrient storage and metabolism in the liver

TREATMENT OF CIRRHOSIS

Medical treatment for cirrhosis aims to correct both the underlying cause of disease and the complications that arise during the course of illness. Antiviral medications may be prescribed to treat viral infections. Avoidance of alcohol and liver toxins is critical for preserving liver function and extending survival. Patients should be screened and treated for life-threatening complications, such as gastroesophageal varices and liver cancer. Liver transplantation may be necessary in advanced cirrhosis.

Medications can effectively treat many of the complications that accompany cirrhosis.[19] Individuals with portal hypertension and varices may be given propranolol or octreotide, which constrict blood vessels and reduce bleeding. Diuretics can help to control portal hypertension and ascites; common examples include spironolactone and furosemide. Lactulose, a nonabsorbable disaccharide, treats hepatic encephalopathy by reducing ammonia production and absorption in the colon. The antibiotic rifaximin is an alternative treatment for elevated ammonia that works by altering bacterial populations. To stimulate the appetite and promote weight gain, megestrol acetate or dronabinol may be prescribed. The Diet-Drug Interactions feature lists potential nutritional problems associated with these medications.

MEDICAL NUTRITION THERAPY FOR CIRRHOSIS

Nutrition therapy for cirrhosis is customized to each patient's needs, which vary considerably and depend on the accompanying complications. Patients with cirrhosis are at high risk of protein-energy malnutrition and muscle wasting; therefore, protein and energy intakes must be sufficient for maintaining nitrogen balance. Dietary substances that may cause additional liver injury must be avoided; examples include

DIET-DRUG INTERACTIONS

Check this table for notable nutrition-related effects of the medications discussed in this chapter.

	GASTROINTESTINAL EFFECTS	INTERACTIONS WITH DIETARY SUBSTANCES	METABOLIC EFFECTS
Appetite stimulants (megestrol acetate, dronabinol)	Nausea, vomiting, diarrhea	—	Hyperglycemia (megestrol acetate)
Diuretics (furosemide, spironolactone)[a]	Dry mouth, anorexia, decreased taste perception	Furosemide's bioavailability is reduced when taken with food.	Fluid and electrolyte imbalances,[a] hyperglycemia (spironolactone), hyperlipidemia (spironolactone), thiamin and zinc deficiencies
Immunosuppressants (cyclosporine, tacrolimus)	Nausea, vomiting, diarrhea, anorexia (tacrolimus)	Cyclosporine potentiates the effects of alcohol. The bioavailability of tacrolimus is reduced when the drug is taken with food. Grapefruit juice can raise serum concentrations of these drugs to toxic levels.	Electrolyte imbalances, hypertension, hyperglycemia, hyperlipidemia
Lactulose	Diarrhea	—	Fluid and electrolyte imbalances

[a] *Furosemide* is a "potassium-wasting" diuretic; patients should increase intakes of potassium-rich foods. *Spironolactone* is a "potassium-sparing" diuretic; patients should avoid supplemental potassium and potassium-containing salt substitutes.

TABLE 19-5	**Medical Nutrition Therapy for Liver Cirrhosis**

Energy	• Energy needs may be approximately 20 percent above resting metabolic rate (RMR); calculate or measure RMR and apply the stress factor 1.2 initially (see Table 14-3 and the "How to" on p. 411).
	• Use estimated dry body weight for RMR calculations in patients with ascites.
	• Energy requirements may be higher in patients with hypermetabolism, infection, malabsorption, or malnutrition. Energy requirements may be lower in patients who would benefit from weight loss.
Meal frequency	• To improve food intake, patients should consume small meals four to six times daily.
Protein	• Provide 0.8 to 1.2 g protein per kilogram of dry body weight per day to maintain nitrogen balance and prevent wasting.
Carbohydrate	• No carbohydrate restrictions unless the patient has insulin resistance or diabetes.
	• For persons with insulin resistance or diabetes, monitor carbohydrate intakes and provide a diet that maintains blood glucose control (see Chapter 20).
Fat	• No fat restrictions unless fat malabsorption is present.
	• If fat is malabsorbed, restrict fat to 30 percent of total kcalories or as necessary to control steatorrhea (see Chapter 18); use medium-chain triglycerides (MCT) to increase kcalories.
Sodium and fluid	• Restrict sodium as necessary to control ascites; 2000 mg sodium per day is adequate restriction in most cases.
	• If ascites is accompanied by low serum sodium levels (less than 128 mEq/L), restrict fluids to 1200 to 1500 mL per day. In severe cases (serum sodium less than 125 mEq/L), restrict fluids to 1000 to 1200 mL per day.
Vitamins and minerals	• Ensure adequate intake from diet or supplements based on individual needs.

alcohol, certain herbal supplements, and vitamin or mineral megadoses. Table 19-5 lists the general dietary guidelines for cirrhosis, which are discussed in the sections that follow.

Energy   To estimate energy requirements, health practitioners measure or calculate the resting metabolic rate (RMR) and then apply a stress factor, as described in the "How to" on p. 411 (Chapter 14). If possible, indirect calorimetry should be used to determine RMR. For most patients with cirrhosis, the stress factor 1.2 can be used initially and adjusted as necessary.[20] Hypermetabolism, infection, nutrient malabsorption, and recent unintentional weight loss can increase energy needs. For patients with ascites, RMR calculations should use either the patient's desirable weight or an estimated dry weight (weight without ascites). A value for dry weight can be obtained after diuretic therapy or after a medical procedure that directly removes excess abdominal fluid.

Many patients with cirrhosis have difficulty consuming enough food, and some individuals may find four to six small meals easier to tolerate than three large meals each day. Nutritional supplements, including liquid formulas and energy bars, can be used to improve energy intakes. The "How to" on p. 553 offers additional suggestions that can help a patient meet energy needs.

Protein   The protein recommendation is 0.8 to 1.2 grams of protein per kilogram of body weight per day, based on dry weight or an appropriate weight for height. (✚) Patients with hepatic encephalopathy should avoid excessive protein consumption, and their protein intake should be spread throughout the day so that they consume only modest amounts at each meal. Protein restriction is not helpful, however, because an inadequate protein intake can worsen malnutrition and wasting.

✚ Reminder: The protein RDA for healthy adults is 0.8 g/kg.

In an attempt to normalize plasma amino acid ratios and possibly improve the mental status of patients with hepatic encephalopathy, some health care providers may prescribe enteral formulas enriched with branched-chain amino acids. Clinical studies testing the use of these formulas have yielded mixed results, however, and their use is recommended only in patients who do not respond to conventional treatment.[21]

Carbohydrate and Fat Carbohydrate provides a substantial proportion of energy needs. Many patients with cirrhosis are insulin resistant, however, and require medications or insulin to manage their hyperglycemia. These individuals should follow the dietary guidelines for diabetes: monitor carbohydrate intakes and consume a diet that maintains blood glucose levels within a normal range (see Chapter 20). Carbohydrate intakes should be fairly consistent from day to day for improved blood glucose control.

Fat provides both energy and essential fatty acids. In patients with fat malabsorption, fat intake may be restricted to less than 30 percent of total kcalories or as necessary to control steatorrhea. Medium-chain triglycerides (MCT) may be used to provide additional energy, although essential fatty acids cannot be obtained from MCT oils and may need to be supplemented. Severe steatorrhea warrants supplementation of the fat-soluble vitamins, calcium, magnesium, and zinc (see Chapter 18).

Sodium and Fluid Patients with ascites are typically advised to restrict sodium. Ascites is partly caused by sodium and water retention in the kidneys, and treatment usually includes both a moderate sodium restriction (to no more than 2000 milligrams of sodium per day) and diuretic therapy to promote fluid loss. (✚) Potassium intake should be monitored if a potassium-wasting diuretic (such as furosemide) is used.

✚ Table 22-1 (p. 625) and the "How to" on p. 609 provide information about following a sodium-controlled diet.

Many patients find low-sodium diets unpalatable, so some health practitioners may allow a more liberal sodium intake and depend on diuretics to mobilize excess fluids. If patients do not respond to sodium restriction and diuretic therapy, fluid may be removed from the abdomen by surgical puncture (**paracentesis**) or may be diverted to the bloodstream using a catheter (**peritoneovenous shunt**).

Fluid restriction may be necessary when ascites is accompanied by a low concentration of serum sodium. If the sodium level falls below 128 milliequivalents per liter, the fluid intake should be limited to 1200 to 1500 milliliters daily; with a sodium level below 125 milliequivalents per liter, fluids should be restricted to 1000 to 1200 milliliters per day.[22]

Vitamins and Minerals Vitamin and mineral deficiencies are common in patients with cirrhosis due to the effects of illness, disease complications, or the alcohol abuse that may have induced liver disease. Thus, multivitamin supplementation is often necessary. If steatorrhea is present, fat-soluble nutrients can be provided in a water-soluble form. Patients with esophageal varices may find it easier to ingest supplements in liquid form.

Food Safety As mentioned, individuals with cirrhosis are susceptible to infections. They should therefore avoid foods that may increase risk of foodborne illness, such as unpasteurized milk products; undercooked meat, fish, poultry, and eggs; unwashed fruits and vegetables; raw vegetable sprouts; and unpasteurized juices.[23] Nutrition in Practice 2 provides additional information about safe food practices (pp. 54–62).

Enteral and Parenteral Nutrition Support In patients who are unable to consume enough food, tube feedings may be infused overnight as a supplement to oral intakes or may replace oral feedings entirely. Although standard formulas are often appropriate, an energy-dense, moderate-protein, low-electrolyte formula may be necessary for patients with ascites or fluid restrictions. In patients with esophageal varices, the feeding tube should be as narrow and flexible as possible to prevent rupture and bleeding. Parenteral nutrition support should be considered for patients who are unable to tolerate enteral feedings due to intestinal obstruction, gastrointestinal bleeding, or uncontrollable vomiting. To avoid excessive fluid delivery, patients with ascites typically require concentrated parenteral solutions, which are infused into central veins. The Case Study allows you to apply your knowledge of cirrhosis to a clinical situation.

CASE STUDY | Patient with Cirrhosis

Marty Hamilton, a 49-year-old carpenter, has just been diagnosed with cirrhosis, which is a consequence of his alcohol abuse over the past 25 years. Although he recognizes that he has an alcohol problem and recently entered an alcohol rehabilitation program, he is still drinking. At 5 feet 8 inches tall, Mr. Hamilton, who formerly weighed 160 pounds, now weighs 130 pounds. According to family members, he is showing signs of mental deterioration, such as forgetfulness and an inability to concentrate. He is jaundiced and appears thin, although his abdomen is distended with ascites. Laboratory findings indicate elevated serum concentrations of AST, ALT, and ammonia; reduced albumin levels; and hyperglycemia.

1. Do Mr. Hamilton's laboratory values suggest liver disease? Compare the results of his laboratory tests with the values shown in Table 19-2.

2. From the limited information available, evaluate Mr. Hamilton's nutrition status. What medical problem makes it difficult to interpret his present weight? Describe the development of that type of problem in liver disease, and explain how the diet is usually adjusted for such a patient.

3. Calculate Mr. Hamilton's energy and protein needs. Describe the general diet you might recommend for him. What suggestions do you have for increasing his energy intake?

4. Explain the significance of Mr. Hamilton's elevated blood ammonia levels. What are some signs that would indicate that he is undergoing mental decline?

5. Describe each of the following complications of liver disease: portal hypertension, jaundice, and gastroesophageal varices. What complication may result if the esophageal varices are not treated?

Liver Transplantation

Acute or chronic liver disease can lead to liver failure, in which case liver transplantation is the only remaining treatment option. The most common illnesses that precede liver transplantation are chronic hepatitis C infection and alcoholic liver disease, which account for about 50 percent of liver transplant cases.[24] The five-year survival rate among transplant recipients ranges from 58 to 81 percent, depending on the cause of illness.[25] Complications such as ascites and hepatic encephalopathy worsen the prognosis.

NUTRITION STATUS OF TRANSPLANT PATIENTS

As mentioned earlier, advanced liver disease is usually associated with malnutrition, which can increase the risk of complications following a liver transplant. Evaluating nutrition status in transplant candidates can be difficult, however, because liver dysfunction and malnutrition often have similar metabolic effects. If fluid retention is present, it can mask weight loss and alter anthropometric and laboratory values. Correcting malnutrition prior to transplant surgery can help speed recovery after the surgery.

POSTTRANSPLANTATION CONCERNS

The immediate concerns following a transplant are organ rejection and infection. Immunosuppressive drugs, including prednisone, cyclosporine, and tacrolimus, help to reduce the immune responses that cause rejection, but they also raise the risk of infection. Infections are a potential cause of death following a liver transplant; therefore, antibiotics and antiviral medications are prescribed to reduce infection risk.

Immunosuppressive drugs can affect nutrition status in numerous ways. Gastrointestinal side effects include nausea, vomiting, diarrhea, abdominal pain, and mouth sores. Some medications may alter appetite and taste perception. Some of the drugs may cause hyperglycemia or outright diabetes, which may need to be controlled with insulin. Electrolyte and fluid imbalances are common. Other possible effects include hypertension, hyperlipidemias, protein catabolism, and increased osteoporosis risk.[26]

Protein and energy requirements are increased after transplantation due to the stress of surgery. High-kcalorie, high-protein snacks and enteral supplements can help the transplant patient meet postsurgical needs. Vitamin and mineral supplementation is also an integral part of nutrition care. To help transplant patients avoid developing foodborne illnesses, nurses can provide information about food safety measures, such as cooking foods adequately, washing fresh produce, and avoiding foods that may be contaminated. See Nutrition in Practice 2 (pp. 54–62) for additional information on food safety.

NURSING DIAGNOSIS

For people with liver transplants may include *ineffective protection, risk for infection,* and *imbalanced nutrition: less than body requirements.*

Nutrition Assessment | CHECKLIST FOR PEOPLE WITH DISORDERS OF THE LIVER

MEDICAL HISTORY

Check the medical record to determine:

- ○ Type of liver disorder
- ○ Cause of the liver disorder
- ○ If the patient has received a liver transplant

Review the medical record for complications that may alter nutritional needs, including:

- ○ Abdominal pain
- ○ Anemia
- ○ Ascites
- ○ Esophageal varices
- ○ Hepatic encephalopathy
- ○ Impaired kidney or lung function
- ○ Infections
- ○ Insulin resistance or diabetes mellitus
- ○ Malabsorption
- ○ Malnutrition
- ○ Pancreatitis

MEDICATIONS

In patients with liver dysfunction, the risk of diet-drug interactions is high because most drugs are metabolized in the liver. Risk of interactions is intensified for patients with:

- ○ Ascites (medications may take a long time to reach the liver)
- ○ Renal failure (medications are often metabolized further in the kidneys and excreted in the urine)
- ○ Malnutrition
- ○ Multiple prescriptions
- ○ Long-term medication use

DIETARY INTAKE

For patients with fatty liver, pay special attention to:

- ○ Energy intake, if the patient is overweight or malnourished, has diabetes, or is receiving total parenteral nutrition
- ○ Carbohydrate intake, if the patient has diabetes or is receiving total parenteral nutrition
- ○ Alcohol abuse

For patients with hepatitis, cirrhosis, or ascites:

- ○ Check appetite.
- ○ Ensure that energy and nutrient intakes are adequate.
- ○ Determine whether alcohol is being consumed.
- ○ Determine whether sodium or fluid restriction is warranted.
- ○ Base energy intakes on dry weight or an appropriate weight for height to avoid overfeeding.

ANTHROPOMETRIC DATA

Take baseline height and weight measurements, and monitor weight regularly. For patients with ascites and edema:

- ○ Monitor weight changes to evaluate the degree of fluid retention.
- ○ Remember that the patient may be malnourished, and weight may be deceptively high.

LABORATORY TESTS

Note that albumin and serum proteins are often reduced in people with liver disease and cannot always be used as indicators of nutrition status. Review the following laboratory test results to assess liver function:

- ○ Albumin
- ○ Alkaline phosphatase
- ○ ALT and AST
- ○ Ammonia
- ○ Bilirubin
- ○ Prothrombin time

Check laboratory test results for complications associated with liver failure, including:

- ○ Anemia
- ○ Decreased renal function
- ○ Fluid retention
- ○ Hyperglycemia

PHYSICAL SIGNS

Look for physical signs of:

- ○ Fluid retention (ascites and edema)
- ○ PEM (muscle wasting and unintentional weight loss)
- ○ Nutrient deficiencies

Self Check

1. Which of the following dietary strategies would be the most appropriate for reversing fatty liver associated with diabetes mellitus?
   a. Following a low-protein diet
   b. Following a fat-controlled diet
   c. Following a fluid- and sodium-controlled diet
   d. Modifying energy to achieve a desirable weight and modifying carbohydrates to attain blood glucose control

2. Which of the following statements about hepatitis is true?
   a. Chronic hepatitis can progress to cirrhosis.
   b. Whatever the cause of hepatitis, symptoms are typically severe.
   c. Vaccines are available to protect against hepatitis A, B, and C viruses.
   d. HCV infection can be spread through contaminated foods and water.

3. The most common causes of cirrhosis in the United States are:
   a. infection with hepatitis A and hepatitis C viruses.
   b. infection with hepatitis A virus and fatty liver disease.
   c. infection with hepatitis B and hepatitis C viruses.
   d. infection with hepatitis C virus and alcoholic liver disease.

4. Esophageal varices are a dangerous complication of liver disease primarily because they:
   a. interfere with food intake.
   b. can lead to massive bleeding.
   c. divert blood flow from the GI tract.
   d. contribute to hepatic encephalopathy.

5. A complication of liver disease that contributes to the development of ascites is:
   a. portal hypertension.
   b. rising blood ammonia levels.
   c. elevated serum albumin levels.
   d. insulin resistance.

6. A patient with cirrhosis may develop personality changes and motor dysfunction, which are signs of:
   a. jaundice.
   b. hepatic encephalopathy.
   c. hyperammonemia.
   d. hepatic coma.

7. With respect to protein intake, patients with cirrhosis should:
   a. consume no more than the protein RDA.
   b. restrict protein intake to 0.6 grams per kilogram of body weight.
   c. maintain nitrogen balance by consuming 0.8 to 1.2 grams of protein per kilogram of body weight per day.
   d. use formulas enriched with aromatic amino acids to meet their protein needs.

8. People with ascites must often restrict dietary intake of:
   a. fat.
   b. protein.
   c. sugars.
   d. sodium.

9. After a liver transplant, a major health concern is:
   a. jaundice.
   b. ascites.
   c. infection.
   d. hepatic coma.

10. Dietary concerns after a liver transplant include all of the following *except*:
    a. severe protein restrictions that are difficult to adhere to.
    b. increased risk of foodborne illness.
    c. gastrointestinal side effects of medications.
    d. altered appetite and taste perception from medications.

Answers to these questions appear in Appendix H.

Clinical Applications

1. Vijaya Reddy is a college student who visited relatives near her parents' birthplace in Anantapur, India, during summer vacation. Although her relatives provided boiled or purified water at their home, they occasionally took Vijaya to local restaurants, where she drank tap water. Several weeks after Vijaya returned home, she developed flu-like symptoms and started feeling extremely tired. She also experienced upper abdominal pain and felt nauseous after meals. After her roommate told her that her eyes and skin appeared yellow, she knew something was definitely wrong. A physician at the student health center diagnosed hepatitis.

   • Which type of hepatitis did Vijaya most likely have?
   • What additional symptoms may develop? Is Vijaya's condition likely to become chronic?
   • What medical treatment is suggested for Vijaya's condition? Describe the dietary modifications that may be necessary in some cases.

2 • As discussed in the section on cirrhosis, many patients develop protein-energy malnutrition and wasting during the course of illness. Review Table 19-4 to find examples of problems that may lead to malnutrition. Select three nutrition or medical problems (from the "Examples" column), and discuss the complications of liver disease that may cause the problems you selected. What dietary or medical treatments can help in managing these problems?

Nutrition on the Net

For further study of topics covered in this chapter, access these websites.

- Find updates and quick links to these and other nutrition-related sites at our website: www.cengage.com/nutrition/whitney/nhhc4e
- To obtain additional information about liver diseases, visit the American Liver Foundation and the Canadian Liver Foundation: www.liverfoundation.org and www.liver.ca
- The websites of the following organizations include information that is helpful for both health practitioners and patients with liver diseases:

- American College of Gastroenterology: www.acg.gi.org
- American Gastroenterological Association: www.gastro.org
- Learn more about hepatitis by visiting the Hepatitis Foundation International: www.hepfi.org
- To uncover more information about liver transplants, search the Center Span Transplant News Network: www.centerspan.org

Notes

1. A. M. Diehl, Alcoholic and nonalcoholic steatohepatitis, in L. Goldman and D. Ausiello, eds., *Cecil Medicine* (Philadelphia: Saunders, 2008), pp. 1135–1139.
2. D. E. Cohen and F. A. Anania, Nonalcoholic fatty liver disease, in N. J. Greenberger, ed., *Current Diagnosis and Treatment: Gastroenterology, Hepatology, and Endoscopy* (New York: McGraw-Hill Companies, 2009), pp. 467–472; Diehl, 2008.
3. Cohen and Anania, 2009; Diehl, 2008.
4. J. H. Lewis, Liver disease caused by anesthetics, toxins, and herbal preparations, in M. Feldman, L. S. Friedman, and L. J. Brandt, eds., *Sleisenger and Fordtran's Gastrointestinal and Liver Disease* (Philadelphia: Saunders, 2006), pp. 1793–1805.
5. Centers for Disease Control and Prevention, Surveillance for acute viral hepatitis—United States, 2007, *Morbidity and Mortality Weekly Report* 58, No. SS03 (2009): 1–27.
6. J. M. Crawford and C. Liu, Liver and biliary tract, in V. Kumar and coeditors, *Robbins and Cotran Pathologic Basis of Disease* (Philadelphia: Saunders, 2010), pp. 833–890.
7. Centers for Disease Control and Prevention, 2009.
8. Crawford and Liu, 2010.
9. A. Rutherford and J. L. Dienstag, Viral hepatitis, in N. J. Greenberger, ed., *Current Diagnosis and Treatment: Gastroenterology, Hepatology, and Endoscopy* (New York: McGraw-Hill Companies, 2009), pp. 420–443.
10. S. Safrin, Antiviral agents, in B. G. Katzung, ed., *Basic and Clinical Pharmacology* (New York: McGraw-Hill/Lange, 2007), pp. 790–818.
11. American Dietetic Association, *Nutrition Care Manual* (Chicago: American Dietetic Association, 2009).
12. G. Garcia-Tsao, Cirrhosis and its sequelae, in L. Goldman and D. Ausiello, eds., *Cecil Medicine* (Philadelphia: Saunders, 2008), pp. 1140–1147.
13. Garcia-Tsao, 2008.
14. J. J. Heidelbaugh and coauthors, Gastroenterology, in R. E. Rakel, ed., *Textbook of Family Medicine* (Philadelphia: Saunders, 2007), pp. 1115–1171.
15. N. J. Greenberger, Ascites and spontaneous bacterial peritonitis, in N. J. Greenberger, ed., *Current Diagnosis and Treatment: Gastroenterology, Hepatology, and Endoscopy* (New York: McGraw-Hill Companies, 2009), pp. 478–484.
16. J. G. Fitz, Hepatic encephalopathy, hepatopulmonary syndromes, hepatorenal syndrome, and other complications of liver disease, in M. Feldman, L. S. Friedman, and L. J. Brandt, eds., *Sleisenger and Fordtran's Gastrointestinal and Liver Disease* (Philadelphia: Saunders, 2006), pp. 1965–1991.
17. Garcia-Tsao, 2008; Fitz, 2006.
18. Fitz, 2006.
19. Garcia-Tsao, 2008.
20. American Dietetic Association, 2009.
21. S. A. McClave and coauthors, Guidelines for the provision and assessment of nutrition support therapy in the adult critically ill patient: Society of Critical Care Medicine (SCCM) and American Society for Parenteral and Enteral Nutrition (A.S.P.E.N.), *Journal of Parenteral and Enteral Nutrition* 33 (2009): 277–316; C. S. Lieber, Nutrition in liver disorders and the role of alcohol, in M. E. Shils and coeditors, *Modern Nutrition in Health and Disease* (Baltimore: Lippincott Williams & Wilkins, 2006), pp. 1235–1259.
22. American Dietetic Association, 2009.
23. American Dietetic Association, 2009.
24. E. B. Keeffe, Hepatic failure and liver transplantation, in L. Goldman and D. Ausiello, eds., *Cecil Medicine* (Philadelphia: Saunders, 2008), pp. 1147–1152.
25. Keeffe, 2008.
26. American Dietetic Association, 2009; M. J. Weiss, V. T. Armenti, and J. M. Hasse, Drug-nutrient interactions in transplantation, in J. I. Boullata and V. T. Armenti, eds., *Handbook of Drug-Nutrient Interactions* (Totowa, NJ: Humana Press, 2004), pp. 425–440.

Alcohol in Health and Disease

As Chapter 19 described, excessive alcohol consumption is a primary cause of liver disease. Alcohol can be toxic to other organs as well, including the brain, gastrointestinal tract, and pancreas. In addition, **alcohol abuse** can lead to a number of nutrient deficiencies. Moderate use of alcohol, however, has been shown to reduce deaths from coronary heart disease in middle-aged and older adults. This Nutrition in Practice discusses current recommendations concerning alcohol and the health problems and benefits associated with its use. The Glossary defines the relevant terms.

What are the current dietary guidelines for alcohol consumption?

For those who choose to drink alcoholic beverages, the *Dietary Guidelines for Americans* specify that women and men should limit their alcohol intakes to one drink and two drinks per day, respectively. One **drink** is equivalent to 12 ounces of beer, 5 ounces of wine, 10 ounces of wine cooler, or 1½ ounces of 80 proof distilled spirits such as gin, rum, vodka, and whiskey. Some individuals should not consume alcohol at all; these include pregnant and lactating women, women of childbearing age who may become pregnant, children and adolescents, people using medications that can interact with alcohol, and people who are unable to voluntarily restrict their alcohol intake. Alcohol should also be avoided by anyone who is involved in an activity that requires attention or coordination, such as driving or operating machinery.[1]

About 64 percent of adults in the United States drink alcoholic beverages.[2] The prevalence of alcohol abuse is estimated to be between 7.4 and 9.7 percent in the general population.

What happens to alcohol in the body?

Recall that alcohol is a source of food energy, providing 7 kcalories per gram. Although a small amount of alcohol is metabolized in the stomach, most of the alcohol that is consumed is quickly absorbed in the stomach or small intestine and passes readily into the body's cells, where alcohol concentrations reach levels similar to those in the blood. The liver is the site of most alcohol metabolism, although its ability to metabolize alcohol is somewhat limited: the average adult metabolizes only 7 to 10 grams of alcohol per hour, about the amount in one drink.[3] The main product of alcohol metabolism is **acetate**, which can be used as a source of energy by most tissues.

Because there is no storage pool for alcohol and it can be toxic to cells, the metabolism of alcohol in the liver takes priority over that of other substances. Thus, alcohol suppresses the breakdown of fat for energy, leading to fat accumulation in the liver and the increased release of triglyceride-carrying lipoproteins (VLDL). Excessive alcohol intakes inhibit both the storage of glycogen and the liver's production of glucose between meals. Heavy drinkers are at risk of developing hypoglycemia, an effect that is accentuated in people with diabetes who use insulin or medication to reduce glucose levels. Alcohol ingestion can also impair the synthesis and secretion of a number of liver proteins, including albumin and fibrinogen (a blood-clotting protein).

Glossary

acetaldehyde (ah-set-AL-deh-hide): an intermediate in alcohol metabolism that, in excess, can damage the body's tissues and interfere with cellular functions.

acetate (AH-seh-tate): the product of alcohol metabolism that is used as a source of energy by many tissues in the body.

alcohol abuse: the continued use of alcohol despite the development of social, legal, or health problems. Individuals who abuse alcohol are called *alcoholics.*

alcoholic liver disease: liver disease that is related to excessive alcohol consumption. Disorders that may develop include fatty liver, hepatitis, and cirrhosis, which may lead to liver failure.

drink: an alcoholic beverage that contains about half an ounce of pure alcohol. One drink is equivalent to 12 ounces of beer, 5 ounces of wine, 10 ounces of wine cooler, or 1½ ounces of 80 proof distilled spirits.

12oz beer

10oz wine cooler

1½oz hard liquor (80 proof whiskey, gin, brandy, rum, vodka)

© Polara Studios, Inc.

5 oz wine

Each of the amounts shown is equivalent to one drink.

How is alcohol toxic to cells?

Alcohol can damage cells either directly, or indirectly via the metabolite **acetaldehyde** that is created during alcohol metabolism. High alcohol concentrations change the structure of cell membranes, increasing membrane permeability. Cell membrane proteins may become damaged, interfering with the transport of substances across the membrane. The presence of alcohol also activates inflammatory responses in cells, which can eventually lead to cell death and tissue damage. Acetaldehyde can cause numerous adverse effects: it binds to proteins and interferes with their functions, prevents formation of microtubules within cells, alters immune responses, causes oxidative damage, and inhibits DNA repair.

How does alcohol affect brain function?

Alcohol acts as a central nervous system depressant. It can cause sedation, slow reaction times, and relieve anxiety. In excess, it impairs judgment, reduces inhibitions, and impairs speech and motor functions. Extremely high blood alcohol levels can lead to coma, respiratory depression, and death.

Chronic heavy drinking can cause certain types of neurological damage. The most common abnormality is injury to the peripheral nerves, which is evidenced by tingling in the hands and feet, lack of muscular coordination, and changes in a person's manner of walking. Visual impairments, such as blurred vision and optic nerve degeneration, can also occur.

Chronic drinkers who are forced to discontinue alcohol use may experience withdrawal symptoms, which include anxiety, irritability, and palpitations. In severe cases, symptoms may include nausea and vomiting, delirium, and seizures.[4]

What are some other long-term consequences of drinking too much alcohol?

Alcoholic liver disease is the most common complication of alcohol abuse, occurring in about 15 to 30 percent of chronic heavy drinkers.[5] The disease develops in a manner similar to the disease progression described in Chapter 19: fatty liver, hepatitis, and, eventually, cirrhosis and liver failure. In addition to liver damage, alcohol can cause damage to the GI tract, pancreas, and heart (see Figure NP19-1). In the GI tract, alcohol's eventual effects may include gastritis, ulcers, nutrient malabsorption, diarrhea, and GI cancers. Chronic alcohol ingestion frequently injures pancreatic tissue and may lead to chronic pancreatitis. Heavy drinking is also associated with heart arrhythmias, impaired heart muscle contractility, and hypertension.

What are the effects of excessive alcohol consumption on nutrition status?

An excessive intake of alcohol often causes multiple nutrient deficiencies. Because alcohol supplies 7 kcalories per gram, it displaces other energy sources along with the essential nutrients such foods would provide. As mentioned earlier, alcohol can cause nutrient malabsorption as a result of direct damage to the GI mucosa. Alcohol also interferes with the way the body processes nutrients. Examples of common deficiencies in persons who abuse alcohol include:[6]

- *Vitamin A.* Alcohol and vitamin A are metabolized by similar enzymes, so an increase in the enzymes that break down alcohol—induced by heavy drinking—can increase degradation of vitamin A.
- *Thiamin.* Alcohol abuse is the most common cause of thiamin deficiency in the United States. Heavy drinking is associated with low thiamin intakes, and alcohol ingestion dramatically reduces thiamin absorption.
- *Folate.* Alcohol reduces the absorption of folate in the small intestine, alters folate metabolism, and increases folate losses in urine. Because folate has a central role in cell division (and cells of the GI tract turn over rapidly), folate deficiency contributes to malabsorption of other nutrients as well.

Can alcohol have disruptive effects on the metabolism of medications?

Yes. Some of the liver enzymes that degrade alcohol have the additional role of metabolizing drugs (which prepares them for excretion). When alcohol is consumed, the enzymes involved in alcohol degradation are not available to metabolize drugs, and therefore the effects of the drugs may be prolonged. It is especially problematic to combine alcohol and drugs if they have similar effects in the body; examples of such drugs include sedatives and blood glucose–lowering medications.[7] Another effect of alcohol is to delay stomach emptying, which can reduce the rate and extent of drug absorption and result in undermedication.[8]

Does alcohol have any beneficial effects on health?

Yes, a moderate alcohol intake can reduce risk of heart disease. Alcohol's protective effects are seen mainly in older persons who have one or more classic risk factors for heart disease (see Chapter 21). Although the reasons that alcohol is beneficial are not entirely clear, alcohol increases levels of HDL cholesterol (protecting against further development of atherosclerosis) and also reduces the tendency for blood clotting. These effects occur when any type of

Brain and central nervous system
- Alters judgment
- Depresses inhibitions
- Impairs motor skills
- Slows breathing

Upper GI tract
- Acts as carcinogen to upper GI tract cells
- Stimulates secretion of gastric acid
- Inflames lining of stomach
- Raises the likelihood of nausea, reflux esophagitis, gastritis, and ulcers

Cardiovascular system
- Raises likelihood of hypertension and heart attacks
- Leads to deterioration of heart muscle
- Alters heart rhythm

Liver
- Acts as toxin to liver cells
- Alters metabolism of nutrients and drugs
- Impairs liver's ability to store nutrients

Lower GI tract
- Damages and inflames cells of the lower GI tract
- Delays GI motility
- Impairs absorption

Pancreas
- Acts as toxin to pancreatic cells
- Alters secretion of pancreatic hormones
- May raise risks of type 2 diabetes in men

alcoholic beverage is consumed and are seen most frequently when alcohol is consumed several times per week. Unlike other recommendations for heart disease, however, alcohol consumption is not recommended solely to reduce heart disease risk, due to the potential for addiction and the adverse effects caused by excessive intakes.[9]

The benefits or harm associated with alcohol consumption depend on a person's health status, age, and the amount consumed. Most people in the United States who consume alcoholic beverages are not heavy drinkers; however, health professionals should be alert to those who may be abusing alcohol and potentially endangering their health.

Notes

1. U.S. Department of Agriculture and U.S. Department of Health and Human Services, *Nutrition and Your Health: Dietary Guidelines for Americans 2005,* 6th ed. (Washington, D.C.: U.S. Government Printing Office, 2005).

2. P. G. O'Connor, Alcohol abuse and dependence, in L. Goldman and D. Ausiello, eds., *Cecil Medicine* (Philadelphia: Saunders, 2008), pp. 167–174.

3. S. B. Masters, The alcohols, in B. G. Katzung, ed., *Basic and Clinical Pharmacology* (New York: McGraw-Hill Companies, 2007), pp. 363–373.

4. O'Connor, 2008; Masters, 2007.

5. Masters, 2007.

6. C. S. Lieber, Nutrition in liver disorders and the role of alcohol, in M. E. Shils and coeditors, *Modern Nutrition in Health and Disease* (Baltimore: Lippincott Williams & Wilkins, 2006), pp. 1235–1266; K. E. Light and R. Hakkak, Alcohol and nutrition, in B. J. McCabe, E. H. Frankel, and J. J. Wolfe, eds., *Handbook of Food-Drug Interactions* (Boca Raton, FL: CRC Press, 2003), pp. 167–189.

7. Masters, 2007.

8. Light and Hakkak, 2003.

9. A. Lichtenstein and coauthors, Diet and lifestyle recommendations revision 2006: A scientific statement from the American Heart Association Nutrition Committee, *Circulation* 114 (2006): 82–96.

CHAPTER 20

Nutrition and Diabetes Mellitus

© Karen Kasmauski/CORBIS

CONTENTS

THE INCIDENCE OF **DIABETES MELLITUS** IS STEADILY INCREASING IN the United States and many other countries. The condition affects an estimated 10.2 percent of adults aged 20 and older in the United States, or approximately 24 million people.[1] About 25 percent of persons with diabetes are unaware that they have it,[2] a danger because its damaging effects often occur before symptoms develop. Diabetes ranks sixth among the leading causes of death in the United States. It also contributes to the development of other life-threatening diseases, including heart disease and kidney failure, which are discussed in the two chapters that follow. The glossary defines diabetes-related symptoms and complications.

Overview of Diabetes Mellitus

The term *diabetes mellitus* refers to metabolic disorders characterized by elevated blood glucose concentrations and disordered insulin metabolism. People with diabetes may be unable to secrete sufficient insulin or use insulin effectively, or they may have both types of abnormalities. (✚) These impairments lead to the reduced utilization of glucose in muscle and adipose cells and unrestrained glucose production in the liver. The result is **hyperglycemia**, a marked elevation in blood glucose levels that can ultimately cause damage to blood vessels, nerves, and tissues.

SYMPTOMS OF DIABETES MELLITUS

Symptoms of diabetes are usually related to the degree of hyperglycemia present (see Table 20-1). When the plasma glucose concentration rises above about 200 milligrams per deciliter (mg/dL), it exceeds the **renal threshold**, which is the concentration at which the kidneys begin to pass glucose into the urine (**glycosuria**). The presence of glucose in the urine draws additional water from the blood, increasing the amount of urine produced. Thus, the symptoms that arise in diabetes typically include frequent urination (**polyuria**), dehydration, and increased thirst (**polydipsia**). Some people lose weight and have an increased appetite (**polyphagia**) as a result of the nutrient depletion

diabetes (DYE-ah-BEE-teez) mellitus: a group of metabolic disorders characterized by hyperglycemia and disordered insulin metabolism.
- *diabetes* = siphon (in Greek), referring to the excessive passage of urine that is characteristic of untreated diabetes
- *mellitus* = sweet, honeylike

renal threshold: the blood concentration of a substance that exceeds the kidneys' capacity for reabsorption, causing the substance to be passed into the urine.

Glossary of Diabetes-Related Symptoms and Complications

acetone breath: a distinctive fruity odor on the breath of a person with ketosis.

claudication (CLAW-dih-KAY-shun): pain in the legs while walking; usually due to an inadequate supply of blood to muscles.

diabetic coma: a coma that occurs in uncontrolled diabetes; may be due to diabetic ketoacidosis, the hyperosmolar hyperglycemic syndrome, or severe hypoglycemia.

diabetic nephropathy (neh-FRAH-pah-thee): damage to the kidneys that results from long-term diabetes.

diabetic neuropathy (nur-RAH-pah-thee): complications of diabetes that cause damage to nerves.

diabetic retinopathy (REH-tih-NAH-pah-thee): retinal damage that results from long-term diabetes.

gangrene: death of tissue due to a deficient blood supply and/or infection.

gastroparesis (GAS-troe-pah-REE-sis): delayed stomach emptying.

glycosuria (GLY-co-SOOR-ee-ah): an abnormal amount of glucose in urine.

hyperglycemia: elevated blood glucose concentrations. Normal fasting plasma glucose levels are less than 100 mg/dL. Fasting plasma glucose levels between 100 and 125 mg/dL suggest prediabetes; values of 126 mg/dL and above suggest diabetes.

hyperosmolar hyperglycemic syndrome: extreme hyperglycemia associated with dehydration, hyperosmolar blood, and altered mental status; sometimes called the *hyperosmolar hyperglycemic nonketotic state.*

hypoglycemia: abnormally low concentrations of blood glucose. In diabetes, hypoglycemia is treated when plasma glucose levels fall below 70 mg/dL.

ketoacidosis (KEY-toe-ass-ih-DOE-sis): an acidosis (lowering of blood pH) that results from the excessive production of ketone bodies.

ketonuria (KEY-toe-NOOR-ee-ah): the presence of ketone bodies in the urine.

macrovascular complications: disorders that affect the large blood vessels, including the coronary arteries and arteries of the limbs.

microalbuminuria: the presence of albumin (a blood protein) in the urine, a sign of diabetic nephropathy.

microvascular complications: disorders that affect the small blood vessels and capillaries, including those in the retina and kidneys.

polydipsia (POL-ee-DIP-see-ah): excessive thirst.

polyphagia (POL-ee-FAY-jee-ah): excessive appetite or food intake.

polyuria (POL-ee-YOOR-ree-ah): excessive urine production.

TABLE 20-1	Symptoms of Diabetes Mellitus

Frequent urination (polyuria)

Dehydration, dry mouth

Increased thirst (polydipsia)

Weight loss

Increased hunger (polyphagia)

Blurred vision

Increased infections

Fatigue

that occurs when insulin is deficient. Another potential consequence of hyperglycemia is blurred vision, which is caused by the exposure of eye tissues to hyperosmolar fluids. (✚) Increased infections are common in individuals with diabetes and may be due to hyperglycemia, impaired circulation, or weakened immune function. In some cases, constant fatigue is the only symptom and may be related to altered energy metabolism, dehydration, or other effects of the disease.

DIAGNOSIS OF DIABETES MELLITUS

The diagnosis of diabetes is based primarily on plasma glucose levels, which may be measured under fasting conditions or at random times during the day. (✚) In some cases, an **oral glucose tolerance test** is given: the individual ingests a 50- or 75-gram glucose load, and plasma glucose is measured at one or more time intervals following glucose ingestion. **Glycated hemoglobin** (**HbA$_{1c}$**) levels, which reflect hemoglobin's exposure to glucose over prolonged periods, are an indirect assessment of blood glucose levels. The following criteria are currently used to diagnose diabetes:[3]

- The plasma glucose concentration of a blood sample obtained at a random time during the day (without regard to food intake) is 200 mg/dL or higher, and classic symptoms of diabetes (such as polyuria, polydipsia, and unexplained weight loss) are present.
- The plasma glucose concentration is 126 mg/dL or higher after a fast of at least eight hours.
- The plasma glucose concentration measured two hours after a 75-gram glucose load is 200 mg/dL or higher.
- The HbA$_{1c}$ level is 6.5 percent or higher.

Overt symptoms of hyperglycemia help to confirm the diagnosis. Otherwise, a diagnosis of diabetes is confirmed only if a subsequent test yields similar results.

The term **prediabetes** pertains to individuals with blood glucose levels between normal and diabetic, that is, between 100 and 125 mg/dL when fasting or between 140 and 200 mg/dL when measured two hours after ingesting a 75-gram glucose load. HbA$_{1c}$ levels between 5.7 and 6.4 percent also suggest prediabetes. Although people with prediabetes are usually asymptomatic, they are at increased risk of developing diabetes and cardiovascular diseases. Prediabetes has been estimated to affect approximately 26 percent of adults in the United States,[4] and it is especially prevalent among those who are overweight or obese.

TYPES OF DIABETES MELLITUS

Table 20-2 lists features of the two main types of diabetes, type 1 and type 2 diabetes. Pregnancy can lead to abnormal glucose tolerance and the condition known as *gestational diabetes* (discussed later in this chapter), which often resolves after pregnancy but is a risk factor for type 2 diabetes. Diabetes can also be caused by medical conditions that damage the pancreas or interfere with insulin function.

Type 1 Diabetes
Type 1 diabetes accounts for about 5 to 10 percent of diabetes cases. It is usually caused by **autoimmune** destruction of the pancreatic beta cells, which produce and secrete insulin. By the time symptoms develop, the damage to the beta cells has progressed so far that insulin must be supplied exogenously, most often by injection. Although the precise cause of the autoimmune attack is usually unknown, environmental toxins or infections are likely triggers. People with type 1 diabetes often have a genetic susceptibility for the disorder and are at increased risk of developing other autoimmune diseases.

TABLE 20-2 | Features of Type 1 and Type 2 Diabetes Mellitus

Feature	Type 1	Type 2
Prevalence in diabetic population	5 to 10 percent of cases	90 to 95 percent of cases
Age of onset	<30 years	>40 years[a]
Associated conditions	Autoimmune diseases, viral infection, inherited factors	Obesity, aging, inactivity, inherited factors
Major defect	Destruction of pancreatic beta cells; insulin deficiency	Insulin resistance; insulin deficiency relative to needs
Insulin secretion	Little or none	Varies; may be normal, increased, or decreased
Requirement for insulin therapy	Always	Sometimes
Other names	Juvenile-onset diabetes Insulin-dependent diabetes	Adult-onset diabetes Noninsulin-dependent diabetes

[a] Incidence of type 2 diabetes is increasing in children and adolescents; in more than 90 percent of these cases, it is associated with overweight or obesity and a family history of type 2 diabetes.

Type 1 diabetes usually develops during childhood or adolescence, and symptoms may appear abruptly in previously healthy children.[5] Classic symptoms are frequent urination, increased thirst, weight loss, and weakness or fatigue. **Ketoacidosis**—acidosis due to excessive production of ketone bodies—is sometimes the first sign of disease. (✚) Disease onset tends to be more gradual in individuals who develop type 1 diabetes in later years. Blood tests that detect antibodies to insulin, pancreatic islet cells, and pancreatic enzymes can confirm the diagnosis and help to predict development of the disease in close relatives.

Type 2 Diabetes

Type 2 diabetes is the most prevalent form of diabetes, accounting for 90 to 95 percent of cases, and it is often asymptomatic. A primary defect in type 2 diabetes is **insulin resistance**, the reduced sensitivity to insulin in muscle, adipose, and liver cells. To compensate, the pancreas increases its secretion of insulin, and plasma insulin concentrations may rise to abnormally high levels (**hyperinsulinemia**). Over time, the pancreas becomes less able to compensate for the cells' reduced sensitivity to insulin, and hyperglycemia worsens. The high demand for insulin can eventually exhaust the beta cells of the pancreas and lead to impaired insulin production and reduced plasma insulin concentrations. Type 2 diabetes is therefore associated with both insulin resistance and relative insulin deficiency; that is, the amount of insulin secreted is insufficient to compensate for insulin's diminished effect in cells.

Although the actual causes of type 2 diabetes are unknown, the risk is substantially increased by obesity (especially abdominal obesity), aging, and physical inactivity. An estimated 80 to 90 percent of individuals with type 2 diabetes are obese, and obesity itself can directly cause some degree of insulin resistance.[6] (✚) The prevalence of type 2 diabetes, which increases with age, is about 21 percent for persons over 60 years of age; however, many of these cases remain undiagnosed.[7] Inherited factors strongly influence risk, and type 2 diabetes is more common in certain ethnic populations, including African Americans, Asian Americans, Hispanic Americans, Mexican Americans, Native Americans, and Pacific Islanders.

✚ Reminder: *Ketone bodies* are products of fat metabolism that are produced in the liver; they accumulate in tissues when fatty acids are released in abnormally high amounts from adipose tissue.

✚ Nutrition in Practice 20 provides information about the relationship between obesity and insulin resistance.

type 2 diabetes: the type of diabetes that accounts for 90 to 95 percent of diabetes cases and usually results from insulin resistance coupled with insufficient insulin secretion.

insulin resistance: reduced sensitivity to insulin in muscle, adipose, and liver cells.

hyperinsulinemia: abnormally high levels of insulin in the blood.

Cross-sections of the pancreas reveal small clusters of cells known as the islets of Langerhans; these regions contain the beta cells that produce insulin.

Type 2 Diabetes in Children and Adolescents Although most cases of type 2 diabetes are diagnosed in individuals over 40 years old, children and teenagers who are overweight or obese or have a family history of diabetes are at increased risk. Because type 2 diabetes is frequently asymptomatic, it is generally identified in youths only when high-risk groups are screened for the disease. One multicenter study found that approximately half of the cases of newly diagnosed diabetes in African American and Hispanic individuals between 10 and 19 years old were due to type 2 diabetes.[8]

Increased rates of both type 1 and type 2 diabetes have been documented in children in past decades and correlate with the rise in childhood obesity. Type 1 and type 2 diabetes are sometimes difficult to distinguish in children, however, and some children exhibit features of both diseases. Although some studies indicate that obesity may drive the autoimmune beta-cell failure that underlies type 1 diabetes, other research suggests that some children who were diagnosed with type 1 diabetes may actually have had type 2 diabetes.[9] Type 2 diabetes is still relatively rare in children, but its increasing prevalence indicates that routine screening and diabetes prevention programs may be important safeguards for children at risk.

PREVENTION OF TYPE 2 DIABETES MELLITUS

Clinical studies suggest that lifestyle changes can prevent or delay the incidence of type 2 diabetes in individuals at risk. In the Diabetes Prevention Program, a multicenter trial of 3234 adults with impaired glucose tolerance, dietary changes and increased physical activity led to a 58 percent reduction in diabetes incidence.[10] Based on the results of this and similar studies, guidelines for diabetes prevention include the following strategies:[11]*

- *Weight management.* A sustained weight loss of 5 to 10 percent of body weight is recommended for overweight and obese individuals. If weight loss cannot be achieved, healthy eating behaviors should be encouraged to prevent additional weight gain.
- *Active lifestyle.* At least 150 minutes of moderate physical activity, such as brisk walking, is recommended weekly.
- *Dietary modifications.* An increased intake of whole grains and dietary fiber has been associated with a reduced risk for type 2 diabetes. Individuals who are overweight or obese should decrease their intake of dietary fat to avoid consuming excessive energy.
- *Regular monitoring.* Individuals at risk should be monitored every year to check for the possible development of type 2 diabetes. If necessary, they can be provided with additional counseling, education, or resources.

ACUTE COMPLICATIONS OF DIABETES MELLITUS

Untreated diabetes may result in life-threatening complications. Insulin deficiency can cause significant disturbances in energy metabolism, and severe hyperglycemia can lead to dehydration and electrolyte imbalances. In treated diabetes, hypoglycemia (low blood glucose) is a possible complication of inappropriate disease management.

Diabetic Ketoacidosis in Type 1 Diabetes A severe lack of insulin causes diabetic ketoacidosis. Without insulin, glucagon's effects become more pronounced, leading to the unrestrained breakdown of the triglycerides in adipose tissue and the protein in muscle. As a result, an increased supply of fatty acids and amino acids arrives in the liver, fueling the production of ketone bodies and glucose. Ketone bodies, which are acidic, can reach dangerously high levels in the bloodstream (ketoacidosis) and spill into the urine (**ketonuria**). Blood pH typically falls below 7.30 (blood pH normally ranges between 7.35 and 7.45). Blood glucose concentrations

---

*The antidiabetic medication metformin may be beneficial for preventing diabetes in high-risk individuals, such as those with obesity, a sedentary lifestyle, prediabetes, and a family history of diabetes.

exceed 250 mg/dL and rise above 1000 mg/dL in severe cases. The main features of diabetic ketoacidosis therefore include severe ketosis (abnormally high ketone body levels), acidosis, and hyperglycemia.[12]

Patients with ketoacidosis may exhibit symptoms of both acidosis and dehydration. Acidosis is partially corrected by exhalation of carbon dioxide, so rapid or deep breathing is characteristic. (✚) Ketone accumulation is sometimes evident by a fruity odor on a person's breath (**acetone breath**). Significant fluid loss (polyuria) accompanies the hyperglycemia, lowering blood volume and blood pressure and depleting electrolytes. In response, patients may demonstrate marked fatigue, lethargy, nausea, and vomiting. Mental state may vary from alert to comatose (**diabetic coma**). (✚) Treatment of diabetic ketoacidosis includes insulin therapy to correct hyperglycemia, intravenous fluid and electrolyte replacement, and, in some cases, bicarbonate therapy to treat acidosis.

Although diabetic ketoacidosis is sometimes the earliest sign that leads to diagnosis of type 1 diabetes, more often it results from inappropriate treatment (such as missed insulin injections), illness or infection, alcohol abuse, or other physiological stressors.[13] The condition usually develops quickly, within one to two days. The mortality rate is nearly 5 percent in individuals under 40 years of age but exceeds 20 percent in elderly individuals.[14] Although diabetic ketoacidosis can occur in type 2 diabetes—usually due to severe stressors such as infection, trauma, or surgery—it rarely develops because even relatively low insulin concentrations are able to suppress ketone body production.

Hyperosmolar Hyperglycemic Syndrome in Type 2 Diabetes

The **hyperosmolar hyperglycemic syndrome** is a condition of severe hyperglycemia and dehydration that develops in the absence of significant ketosis. As mentioned, the hyperglycemia that develops in poorly controlled diabetes leads to polyuria, which results in fluid and electrolyte losses. In the hyperosmolar hyperglycemic syndrome, patients typically are unable to recognize thirst or adequately replace fluid losses due to age, illness, sedation, or incapacity. The profound dehydration that eventually develops exacerbates the rise in blood glucose levels, which often exceed 600 mg/dL and may climb above 1000 mg/dL. Blood plasma may become so hyperosmolar as to cause neurological abnormalities, such as abnormal reflexes, motor impairments, reduced verbal ability, and seizures; about 10 percent of patients lapse into coma.[15] Treatment includes intravenous fluid and electrolyte replacement and insulin therapy.

The hyperosmolar hyperglycemic syndrome is sometimes the first sign of type 2 diabetes in older persons. It is usually precipitated by infection, illness, or a drug treatment that impairs insulin action or secretion. Unlike diabetic ketoacidosis, the condition often evolves slowly, over one week or longer; the lack of clinical symptoms can delay its diagnosis. The mortality rate in patients who develop the hyperosmolar hyperglycemic syndrome may be as high as 20 percent, in part because the condition occurs more often in older patients who have cardiovascular disease or other major illnesses.[16]

Hypoglycemia

Hypoglycemia, or low blood glucose, is the most frequent complication of type 1 diabetes and may occur in type 2 diabetes as well. It arises from the inappropriate management of diabetes rather than from the disease itself, and it usually results from excessive dosages of insulin or antidiabetic drugs, prolonged exercise, skipped or delayed meals, inadequate food intake, or the consumption of alcohol without food. Hypoglycemia is the most frequent cause of coma in insulin-treated patients and is believed to account for 3 to 4 percent of deaths in this population.[17]

Symptoms of hypoglycemia include sweating, shakiness, heart palpitations, slurred speech, double vision, and irritability. Mental confusion may prevent a person from recognizing the problem and taking such corrective action as ingesting glucose tablets, juice, or candy. If hypoglycemia occurs during the night, patients may be completely unaware of its presence.

✚ Bicarbonate is a buffer in the blood that corrects acidosis. Acid (H^+) combines with bicarbonate (HCO_3^-) to form carbonic acid (H_2CO_3), which breaks down to water (H_2O) and carbon dioxide (CO_2). The carbon dioxide is then exhaled.

✚ Diabetic coma was a frequent cause of death before insulin was routinely used to manage diabetes.

NURSING DIAGNOSIS

For people with diabetic ketoacidosis or the hyperosmolar hyperglycemic syndrome may include *ineffective self health management, deficient fluid volume, risk for electrolyte imbalance,* and *acute confusion.*

Foot ulcers are a common complication of diabetes because blood circulation is impaired, which slows healing, and nerve damage dampens foot pain, delaying recognition and treatment of cuts and bruises.

➕ People with type 2 diabetes frequently develop the *metabolic syndrome,* a cluster of symptoms associated with insulin resistance (including hyperglycemia, hypertension, and altered blood lipids) that substantially increase heart disease risk (see Nutrition in Practice 20).

advanced glycation end products (AGEs): reactive compounds formed after glucose combines with protein; AGEs can damage tissues and lead to diabetic complications.

NURSING DIAGNOSIS

For persons with chronic complications of diabetes may include *ineffective peripheral tissue perfusion, risk for infection, risk for impaired skin integrity, risk for injury,* and *disturbed sensory perception.*

CHRONIC COMPLICATIONS OF DIABETES MELLITUS

Prolonged exposure to high glucose concentrations can alter cellular functions and damage cells and tissues. Glucose nonenzymatically combines with proteins, producing molecules that eventually break down to form reactive compounds known as **advanced glycation end products** (AGEs); in diabetes, these AGEs accumulate to such high levels that they cause damage to cells and blood vessels. Excessive glucose also promotes the production and accumulation of sorbitol, which increases oxidative stress and alters molecular structures and functions.

Chronic complications of diabetes typically involve the large blood vessels (**macrovascular complications**), smaller vessels such as arterioles and capillaries (**microvascular complications**), and the nervous system (**diabetic neuropathy**). Other tissues adversely affected by diabetes include the lens of the eye and the skin; cataracts, glaucoma, and various types of skin lesions frequently develop. Infections are common in diabetes, a possible consequence of hyperglycemia, impaired circulation, or depressed immune responses. Many of these complications appear 15 to 20 years after diabetes onset.[18] In individuals with type 2 diabetes, complications often develop before diabetes is diagnosed.

Macrovascular Complications The damage caused by diabetes accelerates the development of atherosclerosis in the coronary arteries and the arteries of the limbs. Cardiovascular diseases are the leading cause of death in people with diabetes, accounting for up to 70 percent of deaths.[19] Moreover, type 2 diabetes is often accompanied by multiple risk factors for coronary heart disease, including hypertension, abnormal blood lipids, and obesity. (➕) People with diabetes also have increased tendencies for thrombosis (blood clot formation) and abnormal ventricle function, both of which can worsen the clinical course of heart disease.

Impaired blood flow in the arteries of the limbs increases the risk of **claudication** (pain while walking) and contributes to the development of foot ulcers (see the photo). Left untreated, foot ulcers can lead to **gangrene** (tissue death), and some patients require foot amputation, a major cause of disability in individuals with diabetes. About 15 percent of diabetic patients experience clinically significant foot ulcers during the course of illness.[20]

Microvascular Complications Long-term diabetes is associated with a thickening of the basement membrane of capillaries and small arterioles, which impairs the normal functioning of these blood vessels. The primary microvascular complications involve the retina of the eye and the kidneys. Diabetes is currently the leading cause of both adult blindness and kidney failure in the United States.[21]

In **diabetic retinopathy**, the weakened capillaries of the retina leak fluid, lipids, or blood, causing local edema or hemorrhaging. The defective blood flow also leads to damage and scarring within retinal tissue. New blood vessels eventually form, but they are fragile and bleed easily, releasing blood and proteins that obscure vision. The retinal changes usually occur after an individual has had diabetes for many years. Up to 80 percent of diabetes patients develop retinopathy 15 to 20 years after diabetes onset.[22]

In **diabetic nephropathy**, damage to the kidneys' specialized capillaries prevents adequate filtration of the blood, resulting in abnormal protein losses in the urine (**microalbuminuria**). As the kidney damage worsens, urine production decreases and nitrogenous wastes accumulate in the blood; eventually, the individual requires dialysis (artificial filtration of blood) to survive. Because the kidneys normally regulate blood volume and blood pressure, inadequate kidney function leads to high blood pressure in patients with nephropathy. Kidney failure eventually develops in about 30 to 35 percent of patients with type 1 diabetes and 20 percent of those with type 2 diabetes.[23] (Chapter 22 provides details about the progression and treatment of chronic kidney disease.)

Diabetic Neuropathy The extent of neuropathy (nerve damage) that develops in diabetes depends on the severity and duration of hyperglycemia. Symptoms of neuropathy vary and may be experienced as deep pain or burning in the legs and feet, weakness of the arms and legs, or numbness and tingling in the hands and feet. Pain and cramping, especially in the legs, are often severe during the night and may interrupt sleep. Neuropathy also contributes to the development of foot ulcers because cuts and bruises may go unnoticed until wounds are severe. Other manifestations of neuropathy include sweating abnormalities, disturbances in bladder and bowel function, sexual dysfunction, constipation, and delayed stomach emptying (**gastroparesis**). Neuropathy occurs in about 50 percent of diabetes cases.[24]

Review Notes

- Diabetes mellitus is a chronic condition characterized by inadequate insulin secretion and/or impaired insulin action.
- In type 1 diabetes, the pancreas secretes little or no insulin, and insulin therapy is necessary for survival. Type 2 diabetes is characterized by insulin resistance coupled with relative insulin deficiency, and disease risk is increased by obesity, aging, and physical inactivity.
- Acute complications of diabetes include diabetic ketoacidosis, in which hyperglycemia is accompanied by ketosis and acidosis, and the hyperosmolar hyperglycemic syndrome, which is characterized by severe hyperglycemia, dehydration, and possible mental impairments. Another acute complication, hypoglycemia, is usually a consequence of inappropriate disease management.
- Chronic complications of diabetes include macrovascular disorders such as cardiovascular diseases and peripheral vascular disease, microvascular conditions such as diabetic retinopathy and diabetic nephropathy, and diabetic neuropathy.

Treatment of Diabetes Mellitus

Diabetes is a chronic and progressive illness that requires lifelong treatment. Managing blood glucose levels is a delicate balancing act that involves meal planning, proper timing of medications, and physical exercise. Frequent adjustments in treatment are often necessary to establish good **glycemic** control. Individuals with type 1 diabetes require insulin therapy for survival. Type 2 diabetes is initially treated with diet therapy and exercise, but most patients eventually need antidiabetic medications or insulin. Diabetes management becomes even more difficult once complications develop. Although the health care team must determine the appropriate therapy, the individual with diabetes ultimately assumes much of the responsibility for treatment and therefore requires education in self-management of the disease.

TREATMENT GOALS

The main goal of diabetes treatment is to maintain blood glucose levels within a desirable range to prevent or reduce the risk of complications. Several multicenter clinical trials have shown that *intensive* diabetes treatment, which keeps blood glucose levels tightly controlled, can greatly reduce the incidence and severity of diabetic retinopathy, nephropathy, and neuropathy.*[25] (✚) Therefore, maintenance of near-normal glucose levels has become the fundamental objective of all diabetes care plans. Other goals of treatment include maintaining healthy blood lipid concentrations, controlling blood pressure, and managing weight—measures that can help to prevent or delay diabetes

✚ Studies that evaluated the benefits of intensive treatment include the Diabetes Control and Complications Trial and the United Kingdom Prospective Diabetes Study.

glycemic (gly-SEE-mic): pertaining to blood glucose.

---

*Intensive treatment may be inappropriate for some individuals with diabetes; examples include individuals with limited life expectancies or a history of hypoglycemia and middle-aged or older adults with previous heart disease or multiple heart disease risk factors.

TABLE 20-3	Comparison of Conventional and Intensive Therapies for Type 1 Diabetes	
	Conventional Therapy	**Intensive Therapy**
Blood glucose monitoring	Monitored daily	Monitored at least three times daily
Insulin therapy	One or two daily injections; no daily adjustments	Three or more daily injections or use of an external insulin pump; dosage adjusted according to the results of blood glucose monitoring and expected carbohydrate intake
Advantages	Fewer incidences of severe hypoglycemia; less weight gain	Delayed progression of retinopathy, nephropathy, and neuropathy
Disadvantages	More rapid progression of retinopathy, nephropathy, and neuropathy	Twofold to threefold increase in severe hypoglycemia; weight gain; increased risk of becoming overweight

Certified Diabetes Educator (CDE): a health care professional who specializes in diabetes management education. Certification is obtained from the National Certification Board for Diabetes Educators.

self-monitoring of blood glucose: home monitoring of blood glucose levels using a glucose meter.

Self-monitoring of blood glucose can help individuals with diabetes learn how to maintain blood glucose levels within a desirable range.

complications as well. Table 20-3 provides examples of the major differences between conventional and intensive therapies for type 1 diabetes. Although intensive therapy is associated with some risks, including an increased risk of hypoglycemia, its benefits outweigh these disadvantages.

Newly diagnosed patients and their families have much to learn about diabetes and its management. Diabetes education provides an individual with the knowledge and skills necessary to implement treatment. The primary instructor is often a **Certified Diabetes Educator** (CDE), a health care professional (often a nurse or dietitian) who has specialized knowledge about diabetes treatment and the health education process. To manage diabetes, patients need to learn about appropriate meal planning, medication administration, blood glucose monitoring, weight management, appropriate physical activity, and prevention and treatment of diabetic complications.

EVALUATING DIABETES TREATMENT

Diabetes treatment is largely evaluated by monitoring glycemic status. Good glycemic control requires frequent home monitoring of blood glucose levels using a glucose meter, referred to as **self-monitoring of blood glucose**. In this procedure, a drop of blood from a finger prick is applied to a chemically treated paper strip, which is then analyzed for glucose. Glucose testing provides valuable feedback when the patient adjusts food intake, medications, and physical activity and is helpful for preventing hypoglycemia. Ideally, patients with type 1 diabetes should monitor blood glucose levels three or more times daily—and more frequently when therapy is adjusted. Self-monitoring of blood glucose is also useful in type 2 diabetes, although the recommended frequency depends on the specific needs of individual patients.[26]

Long-Term Glycemic Control Health care providers periodically evaluate long-term glycemic control by measuring HbA_{1c} levels. The glucose in blood freely enters red blood cells and attaches to hemoglobin molecules in direct proportion to the amount of glucose present. Because the life span of red blood cells averages 120 days, the percentage of HbA_{1c} is a measure of glycemic control during the preceding two to three months (the average age of circulating red blood cells).[27] In people without diabetes, HbA_{1c} is typically less than 6 percent of total hemoglobin. The goal of diabetes treatment is an HbA_{1c} value under 7 percent,[28] but the concentration is often markedly higher in people with diabetes, even those who are maintaining near-normal blood glucose levels. Less stringent HbA_{1c} goals may be suitable for certain patients, including those with limited life expectancy, advanced diabetic complications, or a history of severe hypoglycemia.

The **fructosamine test** is sometimes conducted to determine glycemic control for the preceding two-week period. This test determines the nonenzymatic glycation of serum proteins (primarily albumin), which have a shorter half-life than hemoglobin. Most often, the fructosamine test is used to evaluate recent adjustments in diabetes treatment or glycemic control during pregnancy. The test cannot be interpreted correctly in patients with kidney or liver disease.

Monitoring for Long-Term Complications Individuals with diabetes are routinely monitored for signs of long-term complications. Blood pressure is measured at each checkup. Annual lipid screening is suggested for most adult patients. Routine checks for urinary protein (microalbuminuria) help to determine if nephropathy has developed. Physical examinations generally screen for signs of retinopathy, neuropathy, and foot problems.

Ketone Testing Ketone testing checks for the development of ketoacidosis if symptoms are present or if risk has increased due to acute illness, stress, or pregnancy. Both blood and urine tests are available for home use, although the blood tests are currently more reliable.[29] Ketone testing is most useful for patients who have type 1 diabetes or gestational diabetes. Individuals with type 2 diabetes may produce excessive ketone bodies when severely stressed by infection or trauma.

BODY WEIGHT CONCERNS

Whereas individuals with newly diagnosed type 1 diabetes are likely to be thin, most people with type 2 diabetes are overweight or obese. In children, body weight and growth patterns are monitored to evaluate whether energy intakes are appropriate.

Body Weight in Type 1 Diabetes In general, people with type 1 diabetes are less likely to be overweight than those in the general population. However, excessive weight gain is sometimes an unintentional side effect of improved glycemic control, especially in those undergoing intensive insulin therapy. Although the cause of the weight gain is unclear, it is possibly related to the insulin therapy, which may stimulate fat synthesis or induce energy intake in some way.[30] In addition, the insulin treatment eliminates urinary glucose losses and may indirectly contribute to energy excess.[31] Although patients should try to prevent excessive weight gain, concerns about weight should not discourage the use of intensive therapy, which is associated with longer life expectancy and fewer complications than occur with conventional therapy. It is also important to ensure that growing children receive sufficient energy for normal growth and development.

Body Weight in Type 2 Diabetes Because excessive body fat can worsen insulin resistance, weight loss is recommended for overweight or obese individuals who have diabetes.[32] Even moderate weight loss (10 to 20 pounds) can help to improve glycemic control, blood lipid levels, and blood pressure. Weight loss is most beneficial early in the course of diabetes, before insulin secretion has diminished.

Not all persons with type 2 diabetes are overweight or obese. Older adults and those in long-term care facilities are often underweight and may need to gain weight. Low body weight increases risks of morbidity and mortality in these individuals.

MEDICAL NUTRITION THERAPY: NUTRIENT RECOMMENDATIONS

Medical nutrition therapy has a considerable influence on diabetes outcome. The appropriate dietary choices can both improve blood glucose levels and slow the progression of diabetes complications. As always, the nutrition care plan must take personal preferences and lifestyle habits into account. Dietary intakes need to be modified to accommodate growth, lifestyle changes, aging, and any complications that develop. Although all members of the diabetes care team should understand the principles of dietary treatment, a registered dietitian is best suited to design and implement the

fructosamine test: a measurement of glycated serum proteins; used to analyze glycemic control over the preceding two weeks. Also known as the *glycated albumin test* or the *glycated serum protein test*.

medical nutrition therapy for diabetes patients. This section presents the nutrient recommendations for diabetes. Meal-planning strategies are described later in the chapter.

Total Carbohydrate Intake The amount of carbohydrate consumed has the greatest influence on blood glucose levels after meals—the more grams of carbohydrate ingested, the greater the glycemic response. The carbohydrate recommendation is based in part on the person's metabolic needs (which are related to the type of diabetes, degree of glucose tolerance, and blood lipid levels), the type of insulin or other medications used to manage the diabetes, and individual preferences. Low-carbohydrate diets, which restrict carbohydrate intake to less than 130 grams per day, are not recommended.[33]

Carbohydrate Sources Different carbohydrate-containing foods have different effects on blood glucose levels; for example, consuming a portion of white rice causes blood glucose to rise more than would a similar portion of barley. This *glycemic effect* of foods is influenced by the type of carbohydrate in a food, the food's fiber content, the preparation method, the other foods included in a meal, and individual tolerances. (✚) A food's glycemic effect is not a primary consideration when treating diabetes, however, because clinical studies investigating the potential benefits of low-glycemic index diets on glycemic control have had mixed results.[34] Nonetheless, high-fiber, minimally processed foods—which typically have more moderate effects on blood glucose than do highly processed, starchy foods—are among the foods frequently recommended for persons with diabetes.

Fiber Fiber recommendations for individuals with diabetes are similar to those for the general population; (✚) thus, people with diabetes are encouraged to include fiber-rich foods such as legumes, whole-grain cereals, fruits, and vegetables in their diet. Although some studies have suggested that very high fiber intakes (50 grams or more per day) may improve glycemic control, many individuals have difficulty enjoying or tolerating such large amounts of fiber.[35]

Sugars A common misperception is that people with diabetes need to avoid sugar and sugar-containing foods. In reality, table sugar (sucrose), made up of glucose and fructose, has a lower glycemic effect than starch. Because moderate consumption of sugar has not been shown to adversely affect glycemic control,[36] sugar recommendations for people with diabetes are similar to those for the general population, which suggest minimizing foods and beverages that contain added sugars. However, sugars and sugary foods must be counted as part of the daily carbohydrate allowance.

Although fructose has a minimal glycemic effect, its use as an added sweetener is not advised because excessive dietary fructose may adversely affect blood lipid levels. (Note that it is not necessary to avoid the naturally occurring fructose in fruits and vegetables.) Sugar alcohols (such as sorbitol and maltitol) have lower glycemic effects than glucose, fructose, or sucrose, but their use has not been found to significantly improve long-term glycemic control. Artificial sweeteners (such as aspartame, saccharin, and sucralose) contain no digestible carbohydrate and can be safely used in place of sugar.

Dietary Fat As mentioned earlier, people with diabetes are at high risk of developing cardiovascular diseases. Guidelines for dietary fat are similar to those for other persons at risk: saturated fat intake should be limited to less than 7 percent of total kcalories, *trans* fat intake should be minimized, and cholesterol intake should be limited to less than 200 milligrams daily.[37] In addition, two or more servings of fish are recommended weekly because fish supplies omega-3 fatty acids that improve heart disease risk and can also help to displace foods that are high in saturated fat from the diet. Dietary strategies for cardiovascular disease are discussed further in Chapter 21.

Protein The protein recommendations for people with diabetes are similar to those for the general population. (✚) In the United States, protein intakes usually range between 15 and 20 percent of the energy intake. Although small, short-term

✚ Reminder: The *glycemic index* ranks foods according to their glycemic effect (see Nutrition in Practice 3). The website **www.glycemicindex.com** provides glycemic index values for a wide variety of common foods.

✚ The fiber DRI for adult women and men ranges from 21 to 38 g; check the DRI table on the inside front cover of this text for specific values.

✚ The protein RDA for adults is 0.8 g/kg body weight.

studies have suggested that diets with higher protein intakes may improve glycemic control, increase satiety, and help with weight loss, the long-term effects of such diets on diabetes management are unknown.[38] In addition, high protein intakes are discouraged because they may be detrimental to kidney function in some individuals.

Alcohol Use in Diabetes Guidelines for alcohol intake are similar to those for the general population, which advise a daily limit of one drink for women and two drinks for men. (✚) However, individuals using insulin or medications that promote insulin secretion should consume food when they ingest alcoholic beverages to avoid hypoglycemia. Alcohol can cause hypoglycemia by interfering with glucose production in the liver. Conversely, an excessive alcohol intake (three or more drinks per day) can worsen hyperglycemia and raise triglyceride levels in susceptible persons. People who should avoid alcohol include pregnant women and individuals with pancreatitis, advanced neuropathy, abnormally high triglyceride levels, or a history of alcohol abuse.[39]

Micronutrients Micronutrient recommendations for people with diabetes are the same as for the general population. Vitamin and mineral supplementation is not recommended unless nutrient deficiencies develop; those at risk include the elderly, pregnant or lactating women, strict vegetarians, and individuals on kcalorie-restricted diets. Although some studies have suggested that supplemental chromium can improve glycemic control in type 2 diabetes, results have not been consistent.[40] At present, chromium supplementation is not recommended for those with type 2 diabetes.

MEDICAL NUTRITION THERAPY: MEAL-PLANNING STRATEGIES

Dietitians provide a number of meal-planning strategies to help people with diabetes maintain glycemic control. These strategies emphasize control of carbohydrate intake and portion sizes. Initial dietary instructions may include a discussion of the *Dietary Guidelines for Americans* or other recommendations designed for the general population (see Chapter 2), as well as guidelines for improving blood lipids and other cardiovascular risk factors. Sample menus that include commonly eaten foods can help to illustrate general principles.

Carbohydrate Counting Carbohydrate-counting techniques are simpler and more flexible than other menu-planning approaches and are widely used for planning diabetes diets. Carbohydrate counting works as follows: After a dietitian determines a person's nutrient and energy needs, the individual is given a daily carbohydrate allowance, often divided into a pattern of meals and snacks according to individual preferences. The carbohydrate allowance can be expressed in grams or as the number of carbohydrate portions allowed per meal (see Table 20-4, p. 574). The user of the plan need only be concerned about meeting carbohydrate goals and can select from any of the carbohydrate-containing food groups when planning meals (see Table 20-5 and Figure 20-1). Although encouraged to make healthy food choices, the individual has the freedom to choose the foods desired at each meal without risking loss of glycemic control. Some people may also need guidance about noncarbohydrate foods to help them choose a healthy diet that improves blood lipids or energy intakes. The "How to" on pp. 574–575 includes additional information about using carbohydrate counting in clinical practice.

Carbohydrate counting is taught at different levels of complexity depending on a person's needs and abilities. The basic carbohydrate-counting method just described can be helpful for most people, although it requires a consistent carbohydrate intake from day to day to match the medication or insulin regimen. Advanced carbohydrate counting allows more flexibility but is best suited for patients using intensive insulin therapy. With this method, a person can determine the specific dose of insulin needed to cover the amount of carbohydrate consumed at a meal. The person is then free to choose the types and portions of food desired without sacrificing glycemic control. Advanced carbohydrate counting requires some training and should be attempted only after an individual has mastered more basic methods.

✚ Reminder: One drink is equivalent to 12 ounces of beer; 5 ounces of wine; 10 ounces of wine cooler; or 1½ ounces of 80 proof distilled spirits such as gin, rum, vodka, and whiskey.

1. The first step in basic carbohydrate counting is to determine an appropriate carbohydrate intake and suitable distribution pattern; an example is shown in Table 20-4. A nutrition assessment can help to estimate a person's usual energy and carbohydrate intakes. The carbohydrate level should be acceptable to the person using the plan. Frequent monitoring of blood glucose levels can help determine whether additional carbohydrate restriction would be helpful.

   The example given in Table 20-4 illustrates a meal pattern for a person consuming 2000 kcalories daily with a carbohydrate allowance of 50 percent of kcalories. This is calculated as follows:

   $$50\% \times 2000 \text{ kcal} = 1000 \text{ kcal of carbohydrate}$$

   $$\frac{1000 \text{ kcal carbohydrate}}{4 \text{ kcal/g carbohydrate}} = 250 \text{ g carbohydrate/day}$$

   $$\frac{250 \text{ g carbohydrate}}{15 \text{ g/1 carbohydrate portion}} = 16.7 \text{ carbohydrate portion/day}$$

2. The distribution of carbohydrates among meals and snacks is based on both individual preferences and metabolic needs. In type 1 diabetes, the insulin regimen must coordinate with the individual's dietary and lifestyle choices. People using conventional insulin therapy must maintain a consistent carbohydrate intake from day to day to match their particular insulin prescription, whereas those using intensive therapy can alter insulin dosages when carbohydrate intakes change. People with type 2 diabetes are encouraged to develop dietary patterns that suit their lifestyle and medication schedules. For all types of diabetes, the carbohydrate recommendation may need to be altered periodically to improve blood glucose control.

3. Carbohydrate counting can be done in one of two ways:

   - Count the grams of carbohydrate provided by foods.
   - Count carbohydrate portions, expressed in terms of servings that contain approximately 15 grams each.

   Success with carbohydrate counting requires knowledge about the food sources of carbohydrates and an understanding of portion control. As shown in Table 20-5, food selections that contain about 15 grams of carbohydrate are interchangeable.

TABLE 20-5	Carbohydrate-Containing Food Groups and Sample Portion Sizes

Bread, cereal, rice, and pasta: 1 portion = 15 g carbohydrate
1 slice of bread or 1 tortilla
½ English muffin
¾ c unsweetened, ready-to-eat cereal
½ c cooked oatmeal
⅓ c cooked rice or pasta

Starchy vegetables: 1 portion = 15 g carbohydrate
1 small (3 oz) potato
½ c canned or frozen corn
½ c cooked beans
1 c winter squash, cubed

Fruit: 1 portion = 15 g carbohydrate
1 medium apple, orange, or peach
1 small banana
¾ c blueberries or chopped pineapple
½ c apple or orange juice

Milk products: 1 portion = 12 g carbohydrate; may be rounded up to 15 g for ease in counting carbohydrate portions
1 c milk (whole, low fat, or fat free)
1 c buttermilk
6 oz plain yogurt

Sweets and desserts: Considerable variation in carbohydrate content; portions listed contain approximately 15 g
½ c ice cream
2 sandwich cookies (with cream filling)
½ frosted cupcake
1 granola bar (1 oz)
1 tbs honey

Nonstarchy vegetables: 1 portion = 3 to 6 g carbohydrate; 3 servings are equivalent to 1 carbohydrate portion; can be disregarded if less than 3 servings are consumed
½ c cooked cauliflower
½ c cooked cabbage, collards, or kale
½ c cooked okra
½ c diced or raw tomatoes

Note: Unprocessed meats, fish, and poultry contain negligible amounts of carbohydrate.

TABLE 20-4	Sample Carbohydrate Distribution for a 2000-kCalorie Diet

| | Carbohydrate Allowance | |
Meals	Grams	Portions[a]
Breakfast	60	4
Lunch	60	4
Afternoon snack	30	2
Dinner	75	5
Evening snack	30	2
Totals	255 g	17

Note: The carbohydrate allowance in this example is approximately 50 percent of total kcalories.

[a] 1 portion = 15 g carbohydrate = 1 portion of starchy food, milk, or fruit.

The portions of foods that contain 15 grams may vary substantially, however, even among foods in a single food group. Accurate carbohydrate counting often requires instruction and practice in portion control using measuring cups, spoons, and a food scale. Food lists that indicate the carbohydrate contents of common foods are available from the American Diabetes Association and the American Dietetic Association; these are helpful resources for learning carbohydrate-counting methods.

When using packaged foods, individuals should check the Nutrition Facts panel of food labels to find the carbohydrate content of a serving. If the fiber content is greater than 5 grams per serving, it should be subtracted from the *Total Carbohydrate* value, as fiber does not contribute to blood glucose. If the sugar alcohol content is greater than 5 grams per serving, half of the grams of sugar alcohol can be subtracted from the *Total Carbohydrate* value.

4. Once they have learned the basic carbohydrate counting method, individuals can select whatever foods they wish as long as they do not exceed their carbohydrate goals. Figure 20-1 shows a day's menu that provides the carbohydrate allowance shown in Table 20-4. Although carbohydrate counting focuses on a single macronutrient, people using this technique should be encouraged to follow a healthy eating plan that meets other dietary objectives as well.

FIGURE 20-1 | Translating Carbohydrate Portions into a Day's Meals

SAMPLE MENU

	Carbohydrate Portions			Carbohydrate Portions
Breakfast:		**Afternoon snack:**		
Carbohydrate goal = 4 portions or 60 g.		Carbohydrate goal = 2 portions or 30 g.		
¾ c unsweetened, ready-to-eat cereal	1	2 sandwich cookies		1
½ c low-fat milk	½	1 c low-fat millk		1
1 scrambled egg	—	**Dinner:**		
1 slice whole-wheat toast (with margarine or butter)	1	Carbohydrate goal = 5 portions or 75 g.		
6 oz orange juice	1 ½	4 oz grilled steak		—
Coffee (without milk or sugar)	—	1 small baked potato (with margarine or butter)		1
Lunch:		Corn on cob, 1 large ear		2
Carbohydrate goal = 4 portions or 60 g.		½ c steamed collard greens[a]		
1 tuna salad sandwich (includes 2 slices whole-grain bread, mayonnaise)	2	1 c sliced, raw tomatoes[a]		1
6 oz yogurt (plain) with ¾ c blueberries and artificial sweetener	2	½ c ice cream		1
Diet cola	—	**Evening snack:**		
		Carbohydrate goal = 2 portions or 30 g.		
		1 medium apple		1
		1 oz granola bar		1

[a] Three servings of nonstarchy vegetables are equivalent to 1 carbohydrate portion.

Exchange Lists for Diabetes The exchange list system is an alternative meal-planning method, although it is more complex and difficult for patients to learn than carbohydrate counting. The exchange system sorts foods according to their proportions of carbohydrate, fat, and protein so that each item in a food group (or "exchange list") has a similar macronutrient and energy content (see pp. C-1 to C-2). Thus, any food on a list can be exchanged, or traded, for any other food on the same list without affecting the macronutrient balance in a day's meals. Although the exchange list system can be helpful for individuals who want a structured dietary plan that provides specific percentages of protein, carbohydrate, and fat, it offers no advantages for maintaining glycemic control and is less flexible than carbohydrate counting. This system of meal planning is described further in Appendix C (Appendix B for Canadians).

The exchange lists can be helpful resources for individuals using carbohydrate-counting methods because the portions in the exchange lists are interchangeable with the portions used in carbohydrate counting. Foods listed in the starch, fruit, and milk lists, for example, are equivalent to carbohydrate "portions," as each item contains approximately 15 grams of carbohydrate (see pp. C-3 to C-6; note that the carbohydrate in the milk exchanges can be rounded up to 15 grams). In the list labeled "Sweets, Desserts, and Other Carbohydrates" (p. C-7), the number of carbohydrate portions per serving is indicated in the far-right column.

INSULIN THERAPY

Insulin therapy is necessary for individuals who cannot produce enough insulin to meet their metabolic needs. It is therefore required by people with type 1 diabetes and those with type 2 diabetes who cannot maintain glycemic control with antidiabetic medications, diet, and exercise. The pancreas normally secretes insulin in relatively low amounts between meals and during the night (called *basal insulin*) and in much higher amounts when meals are ingested. Ideally, the insulin treatment should reproduce the natural pattern of insulin secretion as closely as possible.

Insulin Preparations The forms of insulin that are commercially available differ by their onset of activity, timing of peak activity, and duration of effects. Table 20-6 and Figure 20-2 show how insulin preparations are classified: they may be rapid acting (lispro, aspart, and glulisine), short acting (regular), intermediate acting (NPH), or long acting (glargine and detemir), thereby allowing substantial flexibility in establishing a suitable insulin regimen.[41] The rapid- and short-acting insulins are used at mealtimes, whereas the intermediate- and long-acting insulins provide basal insulin for the periods between meals and during the night. Thus, mixtures of several types of insulin can produce greater glycemic control than any one type alone. Several premixed formulations are also available; several examples are listed in Table 20-6.

TABLE 20-6	Insulin Preparations			
Form of Insulin	Common Preparations	Onset of Action	Peak Activity	Duration of Action
Rapid-acting	Lispro Aspart Glulisine	5 to 15 minutes	60 to 90 minutes	3 to 5 hours
Short-acting	Regular	30 minutes	2 to 3 hours	5 to 8 hours
Intermediate-acting	NPH	2 to 4 hours	6 to 10 hours	10 to 16 hours
Long-acting	Glargine Detemir	1 to 2 hours	Steady effects	24 hours
Insulin mixtures (with sample ratios)	NPH/regular (70:30) NPH/regular (50:50)	Variable; depends on formulation	Variable; depends on formulation	Variable; depends on formulation

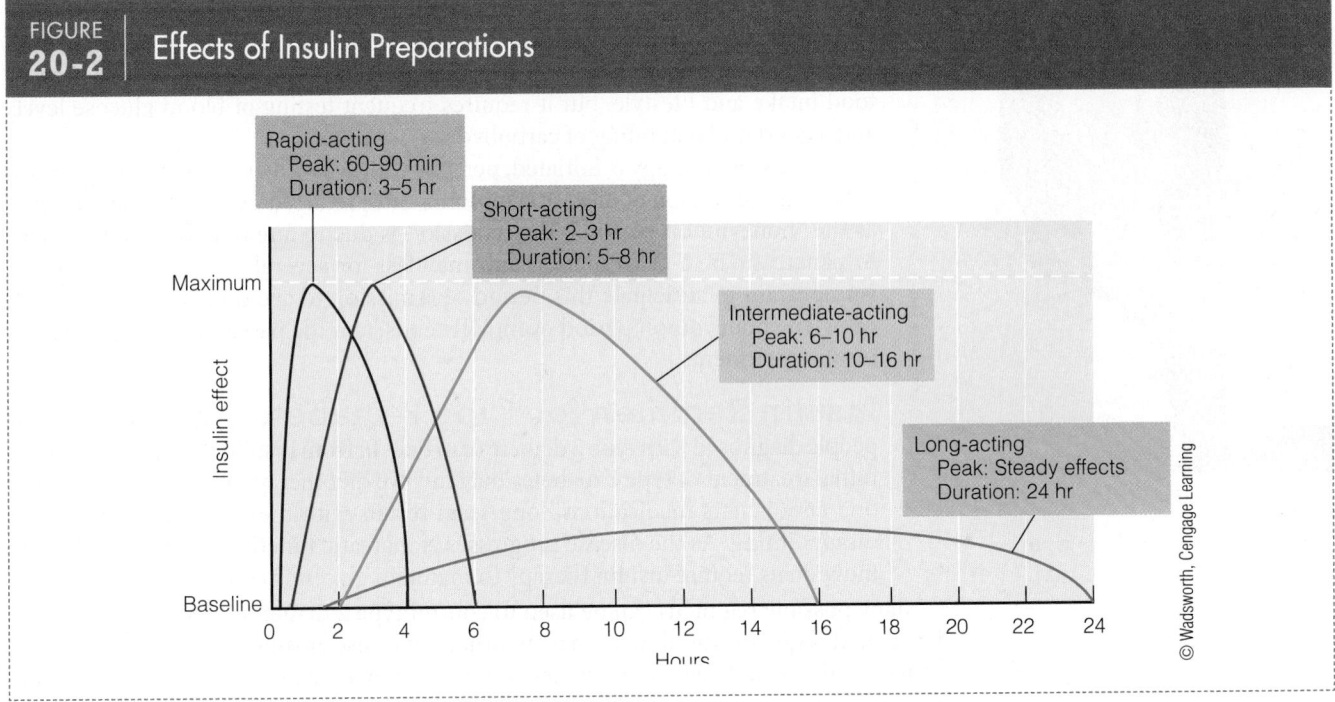

FIGURE 20-2 | Effects of Insulin Preparations

Rapid-acting
Peak: 60–90 min
Duration: 3–5 hr

Short-acting
Peak: 2–3 hr
Duration: 5–8 hr

Intermediate-acting
Peak: 6–10 hr
Duration: 10–16 hr

Long-acting
Peak: Steady effects
Duration: 24 hr

Maximum

Insulin effect

Baseline

0 2 4 6 8 10 12 14 16 18 20 22 24
Hours

© Wadsworth, Cengage Learning

Insulin Delivery Insulin is most often administered by **subcutaneous** injection, either self-administered or provided by caregivers. (✚) Disposable **syringes**, which are filled from vials that contain multiple doses of insulin, are the most common devices used for injecting insulin. Another option is to use insulin pens, injection devices that resemble permanent marking pens. Disposable insulin pens are prefilled with insulin and used one time only, whereas reusable pens can be fitted with prefilled insulin cartridges and replaceable needles. Some individuals use insulin pumps, computerized devices that can be programmed to deliver basal insulin continuously and bolus doses at mealtimes. These pumps infuse insulin through thin, flexible tubing that remains in the skin. An insulin pump can be worn under clothes, attached to a belt, or kept in a pocket.

✚ Because insulin is a protein, it would be destroyed by digestive processes if taken orally.

✚ Rapid-acting insulin begins working within 15 minutes, so it can be injected right before a meal. Short-acting insulin requires a half-hour wait before the meal can begin.

Insulin Regimen for Type 1 Diabetes

Type 1 diabetes is best managed with intensive insulin therapy, which involves multiple daily injections of several types of insulin or the use of an insulin pump (review Table 20-3). Usually, intermediate- or long-acting insulin meets basal insulin needs, and rapid- or short-acting insulin is injected before meals. (✚) Three or more daily injections are required for good glycemic control. Simpler regimens involve twice-daily injections of a mixture of intermediate- and short-acting insulin. Regimens that include three or more injections allow for greater flexibility in carbohydrate intake and meal timing. With fewer injections, the timing of both meals and injections must be similar from day to day to avoid periods of insulin deficiency or excess.

A person using intensive therapy must learn to accurately determine the amount of insulin to inject before each meal. The amount required depends on the premeal blood glucose level, the carbohydrate content of the meal, and the person's body weight and sensitivity to insulin. To determine insulin sensitivity, a person keeps careful records of food intake, insulin dosages, and blood glucose levels. Eventually,

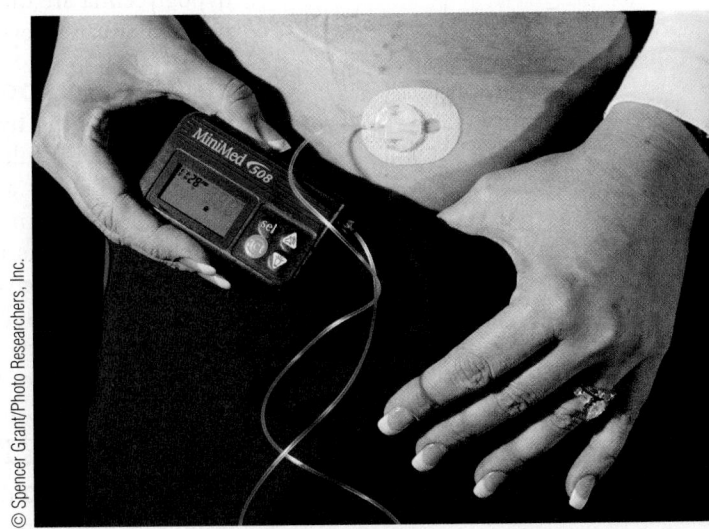

© Spencer Grant/Photo Researchers, Inc.

External insulin pumps deliver insulin continuously through thin, flexible tubing inserted into the skin.

Children often become adept at administering the insulin they require.

these records are analyzed by medical personnel to determine the appropriate **carbohydrate-to-insulin ratio** for that individual, which assists in calculating insulin doses at mealtime. Intensive therapy allows for substantial variation in food intake and lifestyle, but it requires frequent testing of blood glucose levels and a good understanding of carbohydrate counting.

After insulin therapy is initiated, persons with type 1 diabetes may experience a temporary remission of disease symptoms and a reduced need for insulin, known as the "honeymoon period." The remission is due to a temporary improvement in pancreatic beta-cell function and may last for several weeks or months.[42] It is important to anticipate this period of remission to avoid insulin excess. In all cases, the honeymoon period eventually ends, and the patient must reinstate full insulin treatment.

Insulin Regimen for Type 2 Diabetes

About 30 percent of people diagnosed with type 2 diabetes can benefit from insulin therapy.[43] Although initial treatment of type 2 diabetes may involve diet therapy, physical activity, and oral antidiabetic medications, long-term results with these treatments are often disappointing. As the disease progresses, pancreatic function worsens, and many individuals require insulin therapy to maintain glycemic control.

Many possible regimens can be used to control type 2 diabetes.[44] Some persons may be treated with insulin alone, whereas others may use insulin in combination with other antidiabetic drugs. Many patients need only one or two daily injections. Some regimens involve a mixture of rapid- and intermediate-acting insulin in the morning and an injection of intermediate- or long-acting insulin at dinner or before bedtime. In other cases, only a single injection of intermediate- or long-acting insulin may be needed at bedtime.[45] Doses and timing are adjusted according to the results of blood glucose self-monitoring.

Insulin Therapy and Hypoglycemia

Hypoglycemia is the most common complication of insulin treatment, although it may also result from the use of some oral antidiabetic drugs. It most often results from intensive insulin therapy, because the attempt to attain near-normal blood glucose levels increases the risk of overtreatment. Hypoglycemia can be corrected with the immediate intake of glucose or a carbohydrate-containing food. Usually, 15 to 20 grams of carbohydrate (✚) can relieve hypoglycemia in about 15 minutes, although patients should retest their blood glucose levels after 15 minutes in case additional treatment is necessary.[46] Foods that provide pure glucose yield a better response than foods that contain other sugars, such as sucrose or fructose. Persons using insulin are usually advised to carry glucose tablets or a source of carbohydrate that can be readily ingested. Those at risk of severe hypoglycemia are often given prescriptions for the hormone glucagon, which can be injected by caregivers in case of unconsciousness.

Fasting Hyperglycemia

Insulin therapy must sometimes be adjusted to prevent **fasting hyperglycemia**, which has three possible causes. The usual cause is a waning of insulin action during the night due to insufficient insulin. A second possibility, known as the **dawn phenomenon**, occurs when blood glucose levels increase in the morning due to the early morning secretion of growth hormone, which counteracts insulin's actions. Less frequently, fasting hyperglycemia develops as a result of nighttime hypoglycemia, which causes hormonal responses that stimulate glucose production; the resulting condition is known as **rebound hyperglycemia** (also called the **Somogyi effect**). Whatever the cause, fasting hyperglycemia can be treated by adjusting the dose or formulation of insulin administered in the evening.

ANTIDIABETIC DRUGS

Treatment of type 2 diabetes often requires the use of oral medications and injectable drugs other than insulin. These drugs can improve hyperglycemia by several modes of action: they can stimulate insulin secretion, suppress glucagon secretion, decrease insulin resistance, improve glucose utilization in tissues, reduce glucose production

✚ Each of the following sources provides approximately 15 g of carbohydrate:

- Glucose tablets: 2 to 3 tablets
- Table sugar: 4 tsp
- Honey: 1 tbs
- Jelly beans: 15 small
- Grape juice, unsweetened: ½ c
- Orange juice, canned: ½ c

carbohydrate-to-insulin ratio: the amount of carbohydrate that can be handled per unit of insulin. On average, every 15 grams of carbohydrate requires about 1 unit of rapid- or short-acting insulin.

fasting hyperglycemia: hyperglycemia that develops after an overnight fast of at least eight hours.

dawn phenomenon: morning hyperglycemia that is caused by the early-morning release of growth hormone, which counteracts insulin's glucose-lowering effects.

rebound hyperglycemia: hyperglycemia that results from the release of counterregulatory hormones following nighttime hypoglycemia; also called the **Somogyi effect.**

Nutrition and Diabetes Mellitus

c. following menus and recipes provided by a registered dietitian.

d. any approach that best helps the patient control blood glucose levels.

8 • A patient using intensive insulin therapy is likely to follow a regimen that involves:

a. twice-daily injections that combine short-, intermediate-, and long-acting insulin in each injection.

b. a mixture of intermediate- and long-acting insulin injected between meals.

c. multiple daily injections that supply basal insulin and precise insulin doses at each meal.

d. the use of both insulin and oral antidiabetic agents.

9 • In a person who has previously maintained good glycemic control, hyperglycemia can be precipitated by:

a. infections or illnesses.

b. chronic alcohol ingestion.

c. undertreatment of hypoglycemia.

d. prolonged exercise.

10• Women with pregnancies complicated by diabetes:

a. generally benefit from larger meals and a snack at bedtime.

b. often need less carbohydrate at breakfast.

c. need more carbohydrate than women with diabetes who are not pregnant.

d. need more kcalories to support the pregnancy than women without diabetes.

Answers to these questions appear in Appendix H.

Clinical Applications

1 • Using the carbohydrate-counting method described in the "How to" on pp. 574–575, determine an appropriate carbohydrate intake (in both grams and portions) for a man with type 2 diabetes who requires approximately 2600 kcalories daily. Assume he would benefit from a carbohydrate allowance that is 50 percent of his energy intake. Using information from Tables 20-4 and 20-5, develop a one-day sample menu that is likely to meet his carbohydrate goals. Use the exchange lists in Appendix C to find additional examples of foods to include in your menu.

2 • Take a trip to a pharmacy or use information from an online drugstore to price these items: blood glucose meter, test strips for the glucose meter selected, lancets, insulin, and syringes. Determine the approximate cost of insulin and syringes for a person who uses 12 units of short-acting insulin (regular) and 18 units of intermediate-acting insulin (NPH) taken in three injections daily (thus, the insulin requirement is 30 units per day). Also estimate the cost of testing blood glucose three times daily. Approximately how much would these supplies cost per month?

Nutrition on the Net

For further study of topics covered in this chapter, access these websites.

- Find updates and quick links to these and other nutrition-related sites at our website: www.cengage.com/nutrition/whitney/nhhc4e
- Visit the American Diabetes Association and the Joslin Diabetes Center to find information on a wide range of topics related to diabetes: www.diabetes.org and www.joslin.org
- Comprehensive and reliable information about diabetes for both health practitioners and consumers is available

from the National Institute of Diabetes and Digestive and Kidney Diseases and the Centers for Disease Control and Prevention: www2.niddk.nih.gov and www.cdc.gov/diabetes

- Find out how to become a diabetes educator by visiting the website of the American Association of Diabetes Educators: www.diabeteseducator.org

Notes

1. National Center for Health Statistics, *Health, United States, 2008—With Chartbook* (Hyattsville, MD: author, 2009), p. 276.
2. National Center for Health Statistics, 2009.
3. American Diabetes Association, Diagnosis and classification of diabetes mellitus, *Diabetes Care* 33 (2010): S62–S69.
4. D. Lloyd-Jones and coauthors, Heart disease and stroke statistics—2009 update: A report from the American Heart Association Statistics Committee and Stroke Statistics Subcommittee, *Circulation* 119 (2009): 480–486.
5. S. E. Inzucchi and R. S. Sherwin, Type 1 diabetes mellitus, in L. Goldman and D. Ausiello, eds., *Cecil Medicine* (Philadelphia: Saunders, 2008), pp. 1727–1747.
6. *Diabetes Mellitus: A Guide to Patient Care* (Philadelphia: Lippincott Williams & Wilkins, 2007), p. 12.
7. National Center for Health Statistics, 2009.
8. The Writing Group for the SEARCH for Diabetes in Youth Study Group, Incidence of diabetes in youth in the United States, *Journal of the American Medical Association* 297 (2007): 2716–2724.
9. R. B. Lipton, Incidence of diabetes in children and youth—tracking a moving target, *Journal of the American Medical Association* 297 (2007): 2760–2762.
10. *Diabetes Mellitus: A Guide to Patient Care*, 2007, pp. 37–49; J. Wylie-Rosett and L. M. Delahanty, Diabetes prevention, in T. A. Ross, J. L. Boucher, and B. S. O'Connell, eds., *American Dietetic Association Guide to Diabetes: Medical Nutrition Therapy and Education* (Chicago: American Dietetic Association, 2005), pp. 49–58.
11. American Diabetes Association, Standards of medical care in diabetes—2010, *Diabetes Care* 33 (2010): S11–S61; *Diabetes Mellitus: A Guide to Patient Care*, 2007, pp. 37–49.
12. U. Masharani and M. S. German, Pancreatic hormones and diabetes mellitus, in D. G. Gardner and D. Shoback, eds., *Greenspan's Basic and Clinical Endocrinology* (New York: McGraw-Hill/Lange, 2007), pp. 661–747.
13. Inzucchi and Sherwin, Type 1 diabetes mellitus, 2008.
14. Masharani and German, 2007.
15. S. E. Inzucchi and R. S. Sherwin, Type 2 diabetes mellitus, in L. Goldman and D. Ausiello, eds., *Cecil Medicine* (Philadelphia: Saunders, 2008), pp. 1748–1760.
16. D. G. Gardner, Endocrine emergencies, in D. G. Gardner and D. Shoback, eds., *Greenspan's Basic and Clinical Endocrinology* (New York: McGraw-Hill/Lange, 2007), pp. 868–893.
17. Inzucchi and Sherwin, Type 1 diabetes mellitus, 2008.
18. A. Maitra, The endocrine system, in V. Kumar and coeditors, *Robbins and Cotran Pathologic Basis of Disease* (Philadelphia: Saunders, 2010), pp. 1097–1164.
19. Inzucchi and Sherwin, Type 2 diabetes mellitus, 2008.
20. Inzucchi and Sherwin, Type 1 diabetes mellitus, 2008.
21. Inzucchi and Sherwin, Type 1 diabetes mellitus, 2008.
22. Maitra, The endocrine system, 2010.
23. Inzucchi and Sherwin, Type 1 diabetes mellitus, 2008.
24. Inzucchi and Sherwin, Type 1 diabetes mellitus, 2008.
25. American Diabetes Association, Implications of the United Kingdom Prospective Diabetes Study, *Diabetes Care* 21 (1998): 2180–2184; Diabetes Control and Complications Trial Research Group, The effect of intensive treatment of diabetes on the development and progression of long-term complications in insulin-dependent diabetes mellitus, *New England Journal of Medicine* 329 (1993): 977–986.
26. American Diabetes Association, Standards of medical care in diabetes—2009, *Diabetes Care* 32 (2009): S13–S61.
27. Masharani and German, 2007.
28. American Diabetes Association, Standards of medical care in diabetes, 2009.
29. A. Fischl, Monitoring, in T. A. Ross, J. L. Boucher, and B. S. O'Connell, eds., *American Dietetic Association Guide to Diabetes: Medical Nutrition Therapy and Education* (Chicago: American Dietetic Association, 2005), pp. 106–115.
30. M. Ryan and coauthors, Is a failure to recognize an increase in food intake a key to understanding insulin-induced weight gain? *Diabetes Care* epub 17 December 2007 (DOI 10.2337/dc07-1171); A. N. Jacob and coauthors, Potential causes of weight gain in type 1 diabetes mellitus, *Diabetes, Obesity and Metabolism* 8 (2006): 404–411.
31. A. Daly, Use of insulin and weight gain: Optimizing diabetes nutrition therapy, *Journal of the American Dietetic Association* 107 (2007): 1386–1393.
32. American Diabetes Association, Standards of medical care in diabetes, 2009.
33. American Diabetes Association, Standards of medical care in diabetes, 2009; American Diabetes Association, Nutrition recommendations and interventions for diabetes, *Diabetes Care* 31 (2008): S61–S78.
34. American Diabetes Association, Nutrition recommendations and interventions for diabetes, 2008; T. M. S. Wolever and coauthors, The Canadian Trial of Carbohydrates in Diabetes (CCD), a 1-y controlled trial of low-glycemic-index dietary carbohydrate in type 2 diabetes: No effect on glycated hemoglobin but reduction in C-reactive protein, *American Journal of Clinical Nutrition* 87 (2008): 114–125.
35. American Diabetes Association, Nutrition recommendations and interventions for diabetes, 2008.
36. American Diabetes Association, Nutrition recommendations and interventions for diabetes, 2008.
37. American Diabetes Association, Nutrition recommendations and interventions for diabetes, 2008.
38. American Diabetes Association, Nutrition recommendations and interventions for diabetes, 2008.
39. American Diabetes Association, Nutrition recommendations and interventions for diabetes, 2008.
40. American Diabetes Association, Nutrition recommendations and interventions for diabetes, 2008.
41. M. S. Nolte and J. H. Karam, Pancreatic hormones and antidiabetic drugs, in B. G. Katzung, ed., *Basic and Clinical Pharmacology* (New York: McGraw-Hill/Lange, 2007), pp. 683–705; Masharani and German, 2007.
42. Inzucchi and Sherwin, Type 1 diabetes mellitus, 2008.
43. Nolte and Karam, 2007.
44. Nolte and Karam, 2007.
45. Inzucchi and Sherwin, Type 2 diabetes mellitus, 2008.
46. American Diabetes Association, Standards of medical care in diabetes, 2009.
47. American Diabetes Association, Standards of medical care in diabetes, 2009.
48. Inzucchi and Sherwin, Type 1 diabetes mellitus, 2008; *Diabetes Mellitus: A Guide to Patient Care*, 2007, p. 74.
49. American Diabetes Association, Physical activity/exercise and diabetes, *Diabetes Care* 27 (2004): S58–S62.
50. *Diabetes Mellitus: A Guide to Patient Care*, 2007, pp. 248–249.
51. American Diabetes Association, Standards of medical care in diabetes, 2009.
52. A. Maitra, Diseases of infancy and childhood, in V. Kumar and coeditors, *Robbins and Cotran Pathologic Basis of Disease* (Philadelphia: Saunders, 2010), pp. 447–483.
53. American Diabetes Association, Preconception care of women with diabetes, *Diabetes Care* 27 (2004): S76–S78.
54. Z. Hussain and L. Jovanovic, Nutritional strategies in pregestational, gestational, and postpartum diabetic patients, in J. I. Mechanick and E. M. Brett, eds., *Nutritional Strategies for the Diabetic and Prediabetic Patient* (Boca Raton, FL: CRC Press, 2006), pp. 133–148.
55. American Diabetes Association, Nutrition recommendations and interventions for diabetes, 2008.
56. American Dietetic Association, *Nutrition Care Manual* (Chicago: American Dietetic Association, 2009).
57. O. Langer, Oral antidiabetic drugs in pregnancy: The other alternative, *Diabetes Spectrum* 20 (2007): 101–105.

Metabolic Syndrome

Chapter 20 described how insulin resistance—a reduced sensitivity to insulin in muscle, adipose, and liver cells—can contribute to hyperglycemia and hyperinsulinemia and, eventually, to type 2 diabetes. Insulin resistance is also a central feature of several other conditions, including the **metabolic syndrome,** a cluster of metabolic abnormalities that raise the risk of developing cardiovascular diseases (CVD) and type 2 diabetes. This Nutrition in Practice describes how the metabolic syndrome is diagnosed, how and why it might develop, its consequences, and current treatment approaches. The accompanying glossary defines the relevant terms.

How is the metabolic syndrome diagnosed, and how many people in the United States does it affect?

Table NP20-1 lists the laboratory values used to identify the metabolic syndrome, which is diagnosed when at least three of the following disorders are present: hyperglycemia, obesity, **hypertriglyceridemia** (high blood triglyceride levels), low HDL cholesterol levels, and hypertension (high blood pressure). Note that the metabolic syndrome is not a disease *per se*, but the diagnosis may help to focus treatment on the interrelated risk factors that typically lead to heart disease and diabetes.

Glossary

adiponectin (AH-dih-poe-NECK-tin): a hormone produced by adipose cells that improves insulin sensitivity.

fibrinogen (fye-BRIN-oh-jen): a liver protein that promotes blood clot formation.

hypertriglyceridemia (HYE-per-try-gliss-er-rye-DEE-me-ah): high blood triglyceride levels.

metabolic syndrome: a cluster of interrelated clinical disorders, including obesity, insulin resistance, high blood pressure, and abnormal blood lipids, which together increase risk of diabetes and cardiovascular disease; also known as *syndrome X* or *insulin resistance syndrome*.

nitric oxide: a compound produced by blood vessel cells that helps to regulate blood vessel function, including dilation and constriction.

plasminogen activator inhibitor-1: a protein that promotes blood clotting by inhibiting blood clot degradation within blood vessels.

resistin (re-ZIST-in): a hormone produced by adipose cells that induces insulin resistance.

TABLE NP20-1	Features of the Metabolic Syndrome

Metabolic syndrome is diagnosed when three or more of the following abnormalities are present.

Measure	Diagnostic Cut Point
Hyperglycemia	Fasting plasma glucose ≥100 mg/dL
Abdominal obesity	Waist circumference >40" in men, >35" in women
Hypertriglyceridemia	≥150 mg/dL
Reduced HDL cholesterol	<40 mg/dL in men, <50 mg/dL in women
Hypertension	≥130/85 mm Hg

An estimated 34 percent of adults in the United States may meet the criteria for the metabolic syndrome.[1] As Figure NP20-1 shows, prevalence increases with age. Risk also varies among ethnic groups: Mexican Americans have the highest incidence of the metabolic syndrome in the United States, with an overall prevalence of about 37 percent.[2]

What causes the metabolic syndrome?

The precise causes of the metabolic syndrome are unknown and still under investigation. Because different combinations of metabolic abnormalities can result in diagnosis of the metabolic syndrome, its actual causes may vary somewhat among individuals. In most cases, both genetic and environmental factors probably contribute to its development.[3]

The close relationship between abdominal obesity and insulin resistance suggests that the current obesity crisis may be partly responsible for the high prevalence of the metabolic syndrome. Obesity is thought to induce a number of metabolic changes that lead to insulin resistance, which then leads to hyperglycemia and other abnormalities. Note that overweight individuals (BMI from 25 to 29.9) have about a sixfold increased risk of developing metabolic syndrome compared with underweight and normal-weight persons (BMI less than 25).[4]

How can obesity lead to insulin resistance?

Various theories have been proposed to explain the relationship between obesity and insulin resistance, although the exact mechanisms are still unclear. Much of the research suggests that obesity leads to an increase in fatty acid concentrations in the blood, resulting in the abnormal deposition of triglycerides in the muscle, liver, and abdominal region.[5] The abnormally high fat content of these tissues may alter cellular responses to insulin and result in insulin resistance. In addition, adipose cells produce hormones and proteins that influence metabolic processes and fuel use in the body.[6] Obesity is associated with the reduced secretion of **adiponectin**, a hormone involved in sensitivity to insulin. Conversely, the hormone **resistin**, which promotes insulin resistance, is released in greater amounts. The enlarged adipose cells also secrete a variety of cytokines (signaling proteins) that induce inflammation and blood coagulation. The inflammatory process activates multiple metabolic changes that antagonize insulin responsiveness.

Can obesity lead to other problems related to the metabolic syndrome?

Obesity increases the risk of developing high blood pressure, a common component of the metabolic syndrome. Both the insulin resistance and hyperinsulinemia that develop in obesity may be implicated in raising blood pressure. Insulin resistance interferes with the normal relaxation and dilation of blood vessels. Hyperinsulinemia promotes reabsorption of sodium in the kidneys, resulting in fluid retention and increased blood volume.[7] These effects contribute to an increase in blood pressure.

Abdominal obesity is frequently associated with blood lipid abnormalities.[8] Increases in body weight are linked with higher triglyceride and LDL cholesterol levels and lower HDL cholesterol levels. As a result of obesity, the adipose cells are less responsive to insulin and release more fatty acids into the blood. At the same time, they are less able to extract and store triglycerides from chylomicrons and VLDL. To keep up with the greater influx of fatty acids from the bloodstream, the liver must accelerate its production of VLDL, and hypertriglyceridemia develops.

How does the metabolic syndrome contribute to cardiovascular disease risk?

The disorders that characterize the metabolic syndrome—obesity, lipid abnormalities, and hypertension—are all independent risk factors for CVD. In addition, both insulin resistance and elevated lipoprotein levels can cause damage to blood vessels, promoting inflammation and accelerating the progression of atherosclerosis.[9] Blood vessel inflammation induces liver secretion of **fibrinogen**, a protein that promotes blood clot formation (note that blood clotting in arteries can lead to a heart attack or stroke). C-reactive protein, which is elevated by both inflammation and obesity, inhibits **nitric oxide** production by blood vessel cells, an effect that impairs blood vessel activity and also promotes blood clotting.[10] Another procoagulant factor—**plasminogen activator inhibitor-1**— is overproduced as a consequence of both obesity and hyperinsulinemia. The combined effect of these multiple abnormalities can worsen atherosclerosis and increase the risks of developing heart attack and stroke. Individuals with the metabolic syndrome are also at increased risk of developing diabetes, which is another major risk factor for CVD.

What is the treatment for the metabolic syndrome?

The metabolic syndrome is primarily treated with dietary and lifestyle changes, with the goal of correcting the abnormalities that increase CVD risk.[11] In most individuals, a combination of weight loss and physical activity can improve insulin resistance, blood pressure, and blood lipid levels. Even a moderate weight loss (about 7 percent of body weight) can improve symptoms, although many people find this difficult to achieve. Additional dietary strategies depend on a patient's specific symptoms. If dietary and lifestyle changes are not successful, medications may be prescribed. Because effective treatment requires lifelong commitment, health care providers should work with patients to develop a treatment plan that they are willing to adopt.

What dietary strategies, other than weight loss, are suggested for people with the metabolic syndrome?

In individuals with hypertriglyceridemia, the general recommendation is to reduce intake of added sugars and refined grain products (soda, juices, white bread, sweetened cereal, and desserts) and increase servings of whole grains and foods high in fiber (whole-wheat bread, oatmeal, legumes, fruits, and vegetables). In some people, carbohydrate restriction may help to reduce blood triglyceride levels and improve hyperglycemia.[12] Including fish in the diet each week may also improve triglyceride levels. Individuals with hypertension are encouraged to reduce sodium intake and increase consumption of fruits and vegetables and low-fat milk products. A diet low in saturated fat, *trans* fats, and cholesterol can help to reduce LDL cholesterol levels. Chapter 21 includes additional information about dietary modifications that can reduce CVD risk.

Why is physical activity recommended for people with the metabolic syndrome?

Regular physical activity helps with weight management and may also improve blood lipid concentrations, hypertension, and insulin resistance—all changes that can reduce the risk of developing CVD. A regular exercise program can also prevent or delay the onset of diabetes in persons at risk.[13] A program that includes both aerobic exercise and strength training is best. A minimum of 30 minutes of moderate aerobic activity (brisk walking, jogging, or cycling) daily is suggested, although longer periods (1 hour daily) are recommended for weight control. A sedentary lifestyle can worsen the progression of metabolic syndrome and should be discouraged.

Are medications used to treat the metabolic syndrome?

If dietary and lifestyle changes are unsuccessful, medications may be prescribed to correct hypertriglyceridemia and hypertension (Chapter 21 provides details). Obese

Regular exercise can reduce the risks of developing the metabolic syndrome, cardiovascular diseases, and type 2 diabetes.

patients may be provided with medications to help with weight loss (see Chapter 7). At present, antidiabetic drugs are not routinely used to treat insulin resistance in patients with the metabolic syndrome due to insufficient evidence that the drugs can improve long-term outcomes better than lifestyle changes.

As explained in this Nutrition in Practice, the metabolic syndrome consists of a cluster of interrelated disorders that increase the risk for developing CVD and type 2 diabetes. Whereas individually the features of the metabolic syndrome are risk factors for CVD, in combination they may raise risk twofold to threefold. Treatment of the metabolic syndrome emphasizes dietary and lifestyle changes. The following chapter provides additional information about the dietary and lifestyle changes that can reduce CVD risk.

Notes

1. R. B. Ervin, Prevalence of metabolic syndrome among adults 20 years of age and over, by sex, age, race and ethnicity, and body mass index: United States, 2003–2006, *National Health Statistics Reports,* no. 13 (Hyattsville, MD: National Center for Health Statistics, 2009).

2. Ervin, 2009.

3. Z. T. Bloomgarden, The 6th Annual World Congress on the Insulin Resistance Syndrome, *Diabetes Care* 32 (2009): e104–e111; R. L. Pollex and R. A. Hegele, Genetic determinants of the metabolic syndrome, *Nature Clinical Practice Cardiovascular Medicine* 3 (2006): 482–489.

4. Ervin, 2009.

5. J.-P. Després and I. Lemieux, Abdominal obesity and metabolic syndrome, *Nature* 444 (2006): 881–887.

6. A. Maitra, The endocrine system, in V. Kumar and coeditors, *Robbins and Cotran Pathologic Basis of Disease* (Philadelphia: Saunders, 2010), pp. 1097–1164; M. D. Jensen, Obesity, in L. Goldman and D. Ausiello, eds., *Cecil Medicine* (Philadelphia: Saunders, 2008), pp. 1643–1652.

7. V. Kumar and coauthors, Environmental and nutritional diseases, in V. Kumar and coeditors, *Robbins and Cotran Pathologic Basis of Disease* (Philadelphia: Saunders, 2010), pp. 399–445.

8. Jensen, 2008.

9. R. F. Kushner and J. L. Roth, Nutritional strategies for patients with obesity and the metabolic syndrome, in J. I. Mechanick and E. M. Brett, eds., *Nutritional Strategies for the Diabetic and Prediabetic Patient* (Boca Raton, FL: CRC Press, 2006), pp. 55–80.

10. S. M. Grundy and coauthors, Clinical management of metabolic syndrome: Report of the American Heart Association/National Heart, Lung, and Blood Institute/American Diabetes Association Conference on Scientific Issues Related to Management, *Circulation* 109 (2004): 551–556.

11. F. Magkos and coauthors, Management of the metabolic syndrome and type 2 diabetes through lifestyle modification, *Annual Review of Nutrition* 29 (2009): 223–256; Kushner and Roth, 2006.

12. Kushner and Roth, 2006.

13. Magkos and coauthors, 2009; *Diabetes Mellitus: A Guide to Patient Care* (Philadelphia: Lippincott Williams & Wilkins, 2007), pp. 37–49.

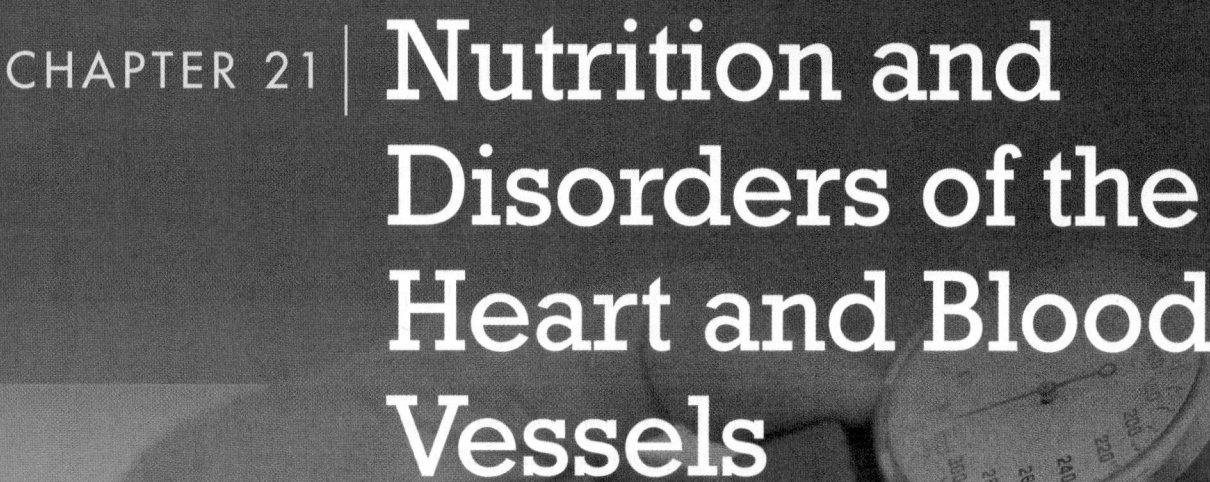

CHAPTER 21 | # Nutrition and Disorders of the Heart and Blood Vessels

© Royalty-Free/Corbis

CONTENTS

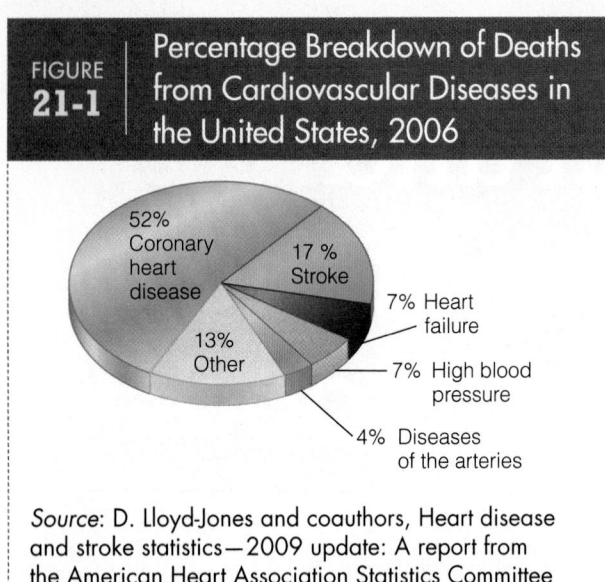

FIGURE 21-1 Percentage Breakdown of Deaths from Cardiovascular Diseases in the United States, 2006

52% Coronary heart disease
17% Stroke
7% Heart failure
13% Other
7% High blood pressure
4% Diseases of the arteries

Source: D. Lloyd-Jones and coauthors, Heart disease and stroke statistics—2009 update: A report from the American Heart Association Statistics Committee and Stroke Statistics Subcommittee, *Circulation* 119 (2009):480–486.

CARDIOVASCULAR DISEASE (CVD) IS A GENERAL term describing diseases of the heart and blood vessels. **Coronary heart disease (CHD)**, the most common form of CVD, is caused by **atherosclerosis** in the coronary arteries that supply blood to the heart muscle. If atherosclerosis interferes with blood flow in these arteries, the resulting deprivation of oxygen and nutrients can destroy heart tissue and cause a **myocardial infarction (MI)**—a **heart attack**. When the blood supply to brain tissue is blocked, a **stroke** occurs. Both heart attack and stroke may result in disablement or death. This chapter describes these and other cardiovascular disorders. Figure 21-1 shows the percentages of deaths resulting from all types of CVD. The glossary below defines some common terms related to CVD.

Cardiovascular disease is responsible for approximately 35 percent of deaths in the United States, claiming about as many lives as the next four leading causes of death combined.[1] Although many people assume that heart conditions are men's diseases, more women than men die each year from the various types of CVD. Furthermore, CVD is a global health issue; it is the leading cause of death in Europe and contributes to 30 percent of deaths worldwide.[2]

Atherosclerosis

In atherosclerosis, (✚) sometimes called "hardening of the arteries," the artery walls become progressively thickened due to an accumulation of fatty deposits, smooth muscle cells, and fibrous connective tissue, collectively known as **plaque**.

Glossary

aneurysm (AN-you-rih-zum): an abnormal enlargement or bulging of a blood vessel (usually an artery) caused by weakness in the blood vessel wall.

angina (an-JYE-nah or AN-ji-nah) pectoris: a condition caused by ischemia in the heart muscle that results in discomfort or dull pain in the chest region. The pain often radiates to the left shoulder and arm or to the back, neck, and lower jaw.

atherosclerosis (ATH-er-oh-scler-OH-sis): a type of artery disease characterized by accumulations of fatty material on the inner walls of arteries.

cardiovascular disease (CVD): a general term describing diseases of the heart and blood vessels.
- *cardio* = heart
- *vascular* = blood vessels

coronary heart disease (CHD): a chronic, progressive disease characterized by obstructed blood flow in the coronary arteries; also called *coronary artery disease.*

embolism (EM-boh-lizm): the obstruction of a blood vessel by an embolus, causing sudden tissue death.
- *embol* = to insert, plug

embolus (EM-boh-lus): an abnormal particle, such as a blood clot or air bubble, that travels in the blood.

intermittent claudication (claw-dih-KAY-shun): severe pain and weakness in the legs (especially the calves) caused by inadequate blood supply to the muscles; it usually occurs with walking and subsides during rest.

ischemia (iss-KEE-mee-a): inadequate blood supply within tissues due to obstructed blood flow in the arteries.

myocardial (MY-oh-CAR-dee-al) infarction (in-FARK-shun), or MI: death of heart muscle caused by a sudden reduction in coronary blood flow; also called a **heart attack** or *cardiac arrest.*
- *myo* = muscle
- *cardial* = heart
- *infarct* = tissue death

plaque (PLACK): an accumulation of fatty deposits, smooth muscle cells, and fibrous connective tissue in blood vessels.

stroke: a sudden injury to brain tissue resulting from impaired blood flow through an artery that supplies blood to the brain; also called a *cerebrovascular accident.*
- *cerebro* = brain

thrombosis (throm-BOH-sis): the formation or presence of a blood clot in blood vessels. A *coronary thrombosis* occurs in a coronary artery, and a *cerebral thrombosis* occurs in an artery that supplies blood to the brain.
- *thrombo* = clot

thrombus: a blood clot formed within a blood vessel that remains attached to its place of origin.

Atherosclerosis initially arises in response to minimal but chronic injuries that damage the inner arterial wall. The first lesions tend to develop in regions where the arteries branch or bend because the blood flow is disturbed in those areas (see Figure 21-2). Eventually, the plaque thickens and hardens as additional lipids, connective tissue, and calcium accumulate. Plaque begins to develop as early as childhood or adolescence and usually progresses over several decades before symptoms develop.

FIGURE 21-2 | Plaque Formation in Atherosclerosis

1 The coronary arteries deliver oxygen and nutrients to the heart muscle.

Plaque

2 Plaque often develops at regions where arteries branch or bend.

3 When arteries become blocked by plaque or a blood clot, the part of the muscle that the arteries supply with blood may die.

CONSEQUENCES OF ATHEROSCLEROSIS

As atherosclerosis worsens, it can eventually narrow the lumen of an artery and interfere with blood flow. Some types of plaque are highly susceptible to rupture, which promotes blood clotting within the artery (**thrombosis**). A blood clot (**thrombus**) may enlarge in time and ultimately obstruct blood flow. A portion of a clot can also break free (**embolus**) and travel through the circulatory system until it lodges in a narrowed artery and shuts off blood flow to the surrounding tissue (**embolism**). Most complications of atherosclerosis result from the deficiency of blood and oxygen within the tissue served by an artery (**ischemia**).

Atherosclerosis can affect almost any organ or tissue in the body and, accordingly, is a major cause of disablement or death. Obstructed blood flow in the coronary arteries can cause pain or discomfort in the chest and surrounding regions (**angina pectoris**) or lead to a heart attack. Obstructed blood flow to the brain can cause injury or destruction to brain tissue, or a stroke. Inadequate blood circulation in the legs can cause fatigue and pain while walking, known as **intermittent claudication**. Blockage of the arteries that supply the kidneys can result in kidney disease or even acute kidney failure.

Atherosclerosis is the most common cause of an **aneurysm**—a saclike distention in a weakened blood vessel. Plaque can weaken the blood vessel wall, and eventually the pressure of blood flow may cause the weakened region to stretch and balloon outward. Aneurysms can rupture and lead to massive bleeding and death, particularly when a large vessel such as the aorta is affected. In the arteries of the brain, an aneurysm may lead to bleeding within the brain, a coma, or a stroke.

CAUSES OF ATHEROSCLEROSIS

The reasons why atherosclerosis develops and progresses are complex. Generally, the factors that initiate atherosclerosis either cause direct damage to the artery wall or allow lipid materials to penetrate its surface. Factors that worsen atherosclerosis are those that lead to plaque rupture or blood coagulation.

Inflammation and Infection The formation of plaque is an inflammatory response to an injury on the artery wall, so the body's immune system is directly involved in its development.[3] (✚) There is also evidence that a persistent infection within the body may contribute to plaque formation. A number of different bacterial and viral antigens have been identified in plaque.[4]

Shear Stress/Hypertension The stress of blood flow along the artery walls—called *shear stress*—can cause physical damage to arteries. The resulting inflammatory response can initiate the development of plaque.[5] Hypertension (high blood pressure) intensifies the stress of blood flow on arterial tissue and also induces the production of proinflammatory cytokines in artery cells.[6]

✚ Atherosclerosis is the most common form of *arteriosclerosis*, a more general term for arterial diseases that are characterized by abnormally thickened walls and lost elasticity.

✚ C-reactive protein, an acute-phase protein secreted during the inflammatory response (see Chapter 16), is associated with increased heart disease risk.

Plaques form along the artery's inner wall reducing blood flow. Clots can form, aggravating the problem.

Cigarette Smoking

Chemicals in cigarette smoke (including nicotine) are toxic to blood vessel cells, and the resulting damage can initiate plaque development. Smoking also promotes chronic inflammation, raises low-density lipoprotein (LDL) cholesterol, and lowers high-density lipoprotein (HDL) cholesterol—effects that can promote the progression of atherosclerosis. Other consequences of smoking include vasoconstriction and blood coagulation, which increase the risk of heart attack and stroke in arteries already narrowed by atherosclerosis. Passive smoking can have these effects as well.[7]

Elevated LDL and VLDL

High blood levels of LDL and very-low-density lipoproteins (VLDL) (✚) promote atherosclerosis, particularly if the lipoproteins are oxidized.[8] Oxidized LDL and VLDL are actively taken up and retained in the artery wall. Oxidation may result from free-radical generation by macrophages and blood vessel cells or various enzyme reactions. HDL help to prevent the oxidation of LDL and also remove cholesterol from circulation, so low levels of HDL contribute to the development of atherosclerosis. (✚) It is not yet known whether the oxidation of dietary lipids contributes significantly to the levels of oxidized LDL and VLDL in the blood.

LDL vary in size and density, and these LDL subtypes have differing effects on heart disease risk. The smallest, most dense LDL are the most **atherogenic** (and more likely to become oxidized), whereas larger, less dense LDL are less atherogenic.[9] People who have small, dense LDL frequently have elevated VLDL and low HDL levels as well. This lipoprotein profile is especially prevalent in individuals with metabolic syndrome and type 2 diabetes.

Elevated concentrations of a variant form of LDL called *lipoprotein(a)* have been found to speed the progression of atherosclerosis and to raise the risk of various types of CVD.[10] Lipoprotein(a) levels are primarily genetically determined and are influenced to only a minor degree by age and environmental factors.

Diabetes Mellitus

Diabetes can both initiate and accelerate the development of atherosclerosis. Chronic hyperglycemia leads to the formation of advanced glycation end products (AGEs) (✚), reactive compounds that disturb the functioning of proteins in blood vessel cells and ultimately disrupt blood vessel function. AGEs also promote inflammation and oxidative stress, which contribute to plaque's progression.[11] Various other effects of diabetes worsen atherosclerosis by inducing plaque rupture and blood clotting.[12]

Age and Gender

Advancing age promotes atherosclerosis due to the cumulative exposure to risk factors and the degeneration of arterial cells with age. Risk of atherosclerosis increases substantially in men aged 45 or older and women aged 55 or older. After menopause, women's risk increases because the loss of estrogen reduces the arteries' defenses against atherosclerosis and causes a rise in LDL cholesterol levels.[13] (✚) Levels of the amino acid homocysteine, which may damage artery walls and promote blood clotting, rise with age and are generally higher in men; however, researchers have not determined whether homocysteine is a cause or an effect of the disease process.[14] (✚)

✚ Reminder: VLDL transport triglycerides in the blood. In clinical practice, VLDL levels are commonly referred to as *blood triglycerides*.

✚ Disorders characterized by abnormal levels of blood lipids are called *hyperlipidemias* or *dyslipidemias*.

✚ Reminder: *Advanced glycation end products* are compounds formed after glucose nonenzymatically attaches to proteins (see Chapter 20).

✚ Estrogen replacement therapy after menopause has mixed effects on heart disease risk; it can improve blood vessel function, lower LDL, and raise HDL, but it also promotes blood clotting.

✚ Reminder: Blood homocysteine levels are influenced by intakes of folate, vitamin B_{12}, and vitamin B_6 (see Chapter 8).

atherogenic: able to initiate or promote atherosclerosis.

Review Notes

- Atherosclerosis, which is characterized by the buildup of arterial plaque, can lead to complications such as angina pectoris, heart attack, stroke, intermittent claudication, kidney disease, and aneurysms.
- Plaque is caused by factors that damage the artery wall and promote blood coagulation. Leading causes of plaque formation and progression include inflammation, shear stress, hypertension, cigarette smoking, elevated LDL and VLDL cholesterol, reduced HDL cholesterol, diabetes, and aging.

Coronary Heart Disease

Coronary heart disease (CHD), also called *coronary artery disease,* is the most common type of cardiovascular disease and the leading cause of death in the United States.[15] As discussed earlier, CHD is characterized by impaired blood flow through the coronary arteries, which may lead to angina pectoris, heart attack, or sudden death. CHD is most often caused by atherosclerosis but occasionally results from a **spasm** or inflammatory condition that causes narrowing of the coronary arteries.

SYMPTOMS OF CORONARY HEART DISEASE

Symptoms of CHD usually arise only after many years of disease progression. In angina pectoris and heart attacks, pain or discomfort usually occurs in the chest region and may be perceived as a feeling of heaviness, pressure, or squeezing. The pain may radiate to the left arm, shoulders, back, throat, jaws, or teeth. In angina pectoris, the symptoms are often triggered by exertion and subside with rest. In a heart attack, the pain may be severe, last longer, and occur without exertion. Other symptoms of CHD include shortness of breath, nausea, vomiting, sweating, lightheadedness, weakness, and anxiety. In some cases, a feeling of indigestion or lower abdominal pain may occur.[16]

EVALUATING RISK FOR CORONARY HEART DISEASE

Because CHD develops over many years, prevention should begin well before symptoms appear. Population studies have suggested that about 90 percent of people with CHD have at least one of the four classic risk factors: smoking, high LDL cholesterol, hypertension, and diabetes.[17] These and other major risk factors for CHD are listed in Table 21-1; most of the risk factors listed can be modified by changes in diet and lifestyle.

CHD Risk Assessment
Risk assessment requires several key laboratory measures (see Table 21-2) and a thorough medical history. A complete lipoprotein profile (also called a *blood lipid profile*), which includes measures of total cholesterol, LDL and HDL cholesterol, and blood triglycerides, should be obtained every five years starting at 20 years of age. Sometimes the ratio of total cholesterol to HDL cholesterol is used to predict CHD risk: a high total cholesterol value suggests elevated LDL cholesterol levels, and a low HDL value is often linked with other lipid abnormalities, such as small, dense LDL and elevated VLDL. Overweight and obesity predispose to CHD, particularly when abdominal obesity is present. Hypertension is a major risk factor; for people over 50 years of age, a high systolic blood pressure is more predictive of CHD risk than is high diastolic blood pressure. Finally, cigarette smoking and the presence of diabetes strongly contribute to CHD risk. The "How to" on p. 597 presents a screening method for assessing a person's 10-year risk of developing CHD that includes some of these risk factors.

Blood Cholesterol Levels and CHD Risk
Once a person's level of risk has been identified, treatment focuses on lowering LDL cholesterol. Elevated LDL cholesterol levels are directly related to the development of atherosclerosis, and clinical studies have confirmed that LDL-lowering treatments can successfully reduce CHD mortality rates. CHD is seldom seen in populations that maintain desirable LDL levels.

As mentioned earlier, HDL help to protect against atherosclerosis, and low HDL levels often coexist with other lipid abnormalities;

TABLE 21-1	Risk Factors for CHD

Major Risk Factors for CHD (not modifiable)
- Increasing age
- Male gender
- Family history of premature heart disease

Major Risk Factors for CHD (modifiable)
- High blood LDL cholesterol
- Low blood HDL cholesterol
- Hypertension (high blood pressure)
- Diabetes
- Obesity (especially abdominal obesity)
- Physical inactivity
- Cigarette smoking
- An "atherogenic" diet (high in saturated fats and low in vegetables, fruits, and whole grains)

Note: Risk factors highlighted in yellow have relationships with diet.

Source: Expert Panel on Detection, Evaluation, and Treatment of High Blood Cholesterol in Adults (Adult Treatment Panel III), *Third Report of the National Cholesterol Education Program (NCEP),* NIH publication no. 02-5215 (Bethesda, MD: National Heart, Lung, and Blood Institute, 2002), pp. II-15 to II-20.

| TABLE 21-2 | Standards for CHD Risk Assessment |

Clinical Measures	Desirable	Borderline Risk	High Risk
Total blood cholesterol (mg/dL)	<200	200–239	≥240
LDL cholesterol (mg/dL)	<100[a]	130–159	160–189[b]
HDL cholesterol (mg/dL)	≥60	40–59	<40
Triglycerides, fasting (mg/dL)	<150	150–199	200–499[c]
Body mass index (BMI)[d]	18.5–24.9	25–29.9	≥30
Blood pressure (systolic and diastolic pressure)	<120/<80	120–139/80–89[e]	≥140/≥90[f]

[a] LDL levels of 100–129 mg/dL indicate a near or above optimal level; <70 mg/dL is a desirable goal for very high-risk persons.

[b] LDL levels ≥190 mg/dL indicate a very high risk.

[c] Triglyceride levels ≥500 mg/dL indicate a very high risk.

[d] Body mass index (BMI) was defined in Chapter 6; BMI standards are found on the inside back cover.

[e] These values indicate prehypertension.

[f] These values indicate stage one hypertension; ≥160/≥100 indicates stage two hypertension. Physicians use these classifications to determine medical treatment.

thus, a low HDL value is highly predictive of CHD risk. In addition, some risk factors for CHD—obesity, smoking, inactivity, and male gender—can also reduce HDL levels. It is not known whether raising HDL will help to reduce CHD risk, but weight loss, smoking cessation, and physical activity can all independently help to lower risk.

THERAPEUTIC LIFESTYLE CHANGES FOR LOWERING CHD RISK

People who have CHD or multiple risk factors for CHD are often advised to make dietary and lifestyle changes before considering drug treatment. An approach to risk reduction promoted by the National Cholesterol Education Program, (✚) known as Therapeutic Lifestyle Changes (TLC), is summarized in Table 21-3.[18] The main features of the TLC plan include a cholesterol-lowering diet, regular physical activity, and weight reduction. If the TLC recommendations are followed carefully, substantial progress may be seen after six weeks. People with a high risk of CHD should try to lower LDL cholesterol with at least a three-month trial of TLC before starting drug therapy. This section describes the elements of the TLC plan in detail.

Saturated Fat
Of the dietary lipids, saturated fat has the strongest effect on blood cholesterol levels, and replacing saturated fat with monounsaturated and polyunsaturated fats can generally lower LDL levels. The TLC recommendation is to consume less than 7 percent of total kcalories as saturated fat. Currently, the average saturated fat intake in the United States is about 11.4 percent of total kcalories consumed.[19]

For most people, cutting down on saturated fat involves more than just switching from butter to vegetable oil, as the main sources of saturated fat in the United States are whole-milk products, high-fat meats, and baked goods. Choosing lean meats or fish, using fat-free or low-fat milk products, and avoiding certain types of bakery products are usually more effective ways of reducing saturated fat.

Replacing saturated fat with carbohydrate can also lower LDL cholesterol, but such a change may lower HDL cholesterol as well and also raise blood triglyceride (VLDL) levels. (✚) The effect on triglyceride levels can be minimized by limiting added sugars

✚ The National Cholesterol Education Program was developed by a division of the National Institutes of Health.

✚ Diets high in carbohydrate—especially those high in added sugars—can raise blood triglyceride levels in some people.

NURSING DIAGNOSIS

Readiness for enhanced self health management applies to people who wish to alter their health behaviors to reduce risk of CHD.

HOW TO | Assess a Person's Risk of Heart Disease

This assessment estimates a person's 10-year risk for developing a major coronary event associated with CHD, such as a heart attack.[a] A high score does not mean that the person *will* develop a heart attack, but it warns of the possibility and suggests the need to consult a physician. To use this tool, you need to know a person's age, total and HDL cholesterol levels, and blood pressure.

Age (years):	Men	Women
20–34	–9	–7
35–39	–4	–3
40–44	0	0
45–49	3	3
50–54	6	6
55–59	8	8
60–64	10	10
65–69	11	12
70–74	12	14
75–79	13	16

HDL (mg/dL):	Men	Women
≥60	–1	–1
50–59	0	0
40–49	1	1
<40	2	2

Systolic Blood Pressure (mm Hg):	Untreated		Treated	
	Men	Women	Men	Women
<120	0	0	0	0
120–129	0	1	1	3
130–139	1	2	2	4
140–159	1	3	2	5
≥160	2	4	3	6

Total Cholesterol (mg/dL):

	Age 20–39		Age 40–49		Age 50–59		Age 60–69		Age 70–79	
	Men	Women	Men	Women	Men	Women	Men	Women	Men	Women
<160	0	0	0	0	0	0	0	0	0	0
160–199	4	4	3	3	2	2	1	1	0	1
200–239	7	8	5	6	3	4	1	2	0	1
240–279	9	11	6	8	4	5	2	3	1	2
≥280	11	13	8	10	5	7	3	4	1	2

Smoking (any cigarette smoking in the past month):

	Men	Women	Men	Women	Men	Women	Men	Women	Men	Women
Smoker	8	9	5	7	3	4	1	2	1	1
Nonsmoker	0	0	0	0	0	0	0	0	0	0

Scoring Heart Disease Risk

Add up the total points: _____. Using the table at the right, find the total in the first column for the appropriate gender, and then check the second column to learn the percentage risk of developing severe CHD within the next 10 years. A person's risk for an acute coronary event (such as a heart attack) may be identified as low (less than 10 percent), moderate (10 to 20 percent), or high (more than 20 percent). Treatment strategies vary according to a person's risk category.

Men		Women	
Total	Risk (%)	Total	Risk (%)
<0	<1	<9	<1
0–4	1	9–12	1
5–6	2	13–14	2
7	3	15	3
8	4	16	4
9	5	17	5
10	6	18	6
11	8	19	8
12	10	20	11
13	12	21	14
14	16	22	17
15	20	23	22
16	25	24	27
≥17	≥30	≥25	≥30

[a] A link to the electronic version of this assessment is available on the ATP III page of the National Heart, Lung, and Blood Institute's website (www.nhlbi.nih.gov/guidelines/cholesterol).
Source: Adapted from Expert Panel on Detection, Evaluation, and Treatment of High Blood Cholesterol in Adults (Adult Treatment Panel III), *Third Report of the National Cholesterol Education Program (NCEP)*, NIH publication no. 02-5216 (Bethesda, MD: National Heart, Lung, and Blood Institute, 2002), section III.

TABLE
21-3 | Reducing Risk of CHD with Therapeutic Lifestyle Changes

Dietary Strategies

- Limit saturated fat to less than 7 percent of total kcalories and cholesterol to less than 200 milligrams per day. Maintaining a fat intake that is 25 to 35 percent of total kcalories may help with this goal.
- Replace saturated fats with carbohydrates from whole grains, legumes, fruits, and vegetables or with unsaturated fats from fish, vegetable oils, and nuts.
- Avoid food products that contain *trans*-fatty acids. The *trans* fat content in packaged foods is shown on the Nutrition Facts panel.
- Choose foods high in soluble fibers, including oats, barley, legumes, and fruit. Psyllium seed husks can be used as a food supplement to help lower LDL cholesterol levels.
- Regularly consume food products that contain added plant sterols or stanols.
- To reduce blood pressure, limit sodium intake to 2400 milligrams per day,[a] and choose a diet that is high in fruits and vegetables, low-fat milk products, nuts, and whole grains.
- Fish can be consumed regularly as part of a CHD risk-reduction diet.
- If alcohol is consumed, it should be limited to one drink daily for women and two drinks daily for men.

Lifestyle Choices

- Physical activity: At least 30 minutes of moderate-intensity endurance activity should be undertaken on most days of the week. The eventual goal should be an expenditure of at least 2000 kcalories weekly.
- Smoking cessation: Exposure to any form of tobacco smoke should be minimized.

Weight Reduction

- Weight reduction may improve other CHD risk factors. The general goals of a weight-management program should be to prevent weight gain, reduce body weight, and maintain a lower body weight over the long term. The initial goal of a weight-loss program should be to lose no more than 10 percent of original body weight.

[a] According to DRI recommendations, sodium intake should be limited to 2300 milligrams daily.

and including fiber-rich foods; ideally, the diet should include generous amounts of whole grains, legumes, fruits, and vegetables. The TLC diet recommends a carbohydrate intake in the range of 50 to 60 percent of total kcalories.

Polyunsaturated and Monounsaturated Fat

As described in the previous section, replacing saturated fat with either monounsaturated or polyunsaturated fat helps to lower LDL levels. A switch to polyunsaturated fat tends to have the greater effect, but it also promotes a slight reduction in HDL cholesterol.[20] Other concerns are that high intakes of polyunsaturated fat may contribute to oxidative stress (✚) or increase inflammation within the body. (✚) Therefore, TLC guidelines limit polyunsaturated fat to 10 percent of total kcalories, whereas up to 20 percent of kcalories from monounsaturated fat are allowed. Note that most polyunsaturated fat in the diet consists of omega-6 fatty acids such as linoleic acid; omega-3 fatty acids may have beneficial effects on heart disease risk, as described in a later section.

Total Fat

For people whose fat intake includes substantial saturated fat, limiting total fat may indirectly reduce saturated fat. Therefore, the TLC recommendation for total fat is an intake of 25 to 35 percent of kcalories. Individuals with elevated blood triglycerides may benefit from a fat intake at the upper end of this range (30 to 35 percent) so that their carbohydrate intakes are not excessive. Fat intakes higher than 35 percent of kcalories are discouraged because they may promote weight gain in some people.

Dietary Cholesterol

A high cholesterol intake can raise LDL levels, and reducing dietary cholesterol lowers LDL cholesterol in most people. The TLC recommendation is a cholesterol intake of less than 200 milligrams per day. Currently, the daily cholesterol intake in the United States averages about 278 milligrams, although it is higher in men (358 milligrams) than in women (237 milligrams).[21] Eggs contribute

✚ Polyunsaturated fats are more susceptible to oxidation than saturated fats, although the clinical significance of consuming high amounts is still unknown.

✚ Reminder: Polyunsaturated fatty acids are precursors for the eicosanoids, which mediate inflammation (see pp. 471–472).

about one-third of the cholesterol in the American diet, followed by beef, poultry, and milk products.

Trans Fat *Trans*-fatty acids can raise LDL cholesterol levels, and when they replace saturated fats in the diet (as when stick margarine replaces butter), they may also cause a reduction in HDL cholesterol. Most sources of *trans* fats are foods made with partially hydrogenated vegetable oils; examples include baked goods such as crackers, cookies, and doughnuts; snack foods such as potato chips and corn chips; and fried foods such as french fries and fried chicken. The TLC recommendation is to keep *trans* fat intake as low as possible.

In the past few years, many food manufacturers have reformulated food products so that they contain minimal amounts of *trans* fat. Thus, margarine, vegetable shortening, and many baked goods and snack foods are now available with little or no *trans* fat.

Soluble Fibers

Soluble, viscous fibers can reduce LDL cholesterol levels by inhibiting cholesterol and bile absorption in the small intestine and reducing cholesterol synthesis in the liver. Dietary sources of soluble fibers include oats, barley, legumes, and fruits. The soluble fiber in psyllium seed husks, frequently used to treat constipation, is effective for lowering cholesterol levels when used as a dietary supplement.

Plant Sterols and Stanols

Foods or supplements that contain significant amounts of plant sterols or plant stanols can help to lower LDL cholesterol levels. (✚) Plant sterols and stanols are added to various food products, such as margarine or cheese, or supplied in dietary supplements. These plant compounds work by interfering with cholesterol and bile absorption. Clinical trials have shown that about 2 grams of plant sterols daily (provided by 2 to 2½ tablespoons of sterol-enriched margarines) can lower LDL cholesterol by up to 15 percent without lowering HDL cholesterol.[22]

Sodium and Potassium Intakes

Excessive dietary sodium can raise blood pressure, whereas potassium can help to lower blood pressure. A low-sodium diet that contains generous amounts of fruits and vegetables, low-fat milk products, nuts, and whole grains has been found to substantially reduce blood pressure, largely due to the diet's content of potassium and several other minerals that have blood pressure–lowering effects. This diet (the *DASH Eating Plan*) and other factors that influence blood pressure are discussed in a later section (see pp. 607–609).

Fish and Omega-3 Fatty Acids

The omega-3 fatty acids in fish, known as EPA and DHA (see p. 96), may benefit people who have had a heart attack by suppressing inflammation, reducing blood clotting, stabilizing heart rhythm, and lowering blood triglyceride levels. In addition, including fish in the diet can reduce CHD risk because fish is low in saturated fat and often replaces entrées that contain animal fats. The American Heart Association recommends consuming two servings of fish per week, with an emphasis on fatty fish.[23] Fish oil supplements (providing 1 gram of EPA and DHA daily) may be helpful for individuals with documented CHD, and they are particularly useful for treating individuals with elevated triglyceride levels (see p. 602).[24]

The 18-carbon omega-3 fatty acids found in flaxseed and other land plants have lesser or different effects than the omega-3 fatty acids from marine sources. Although some evidence suggests that moderate increases in these plant sources of omega-3 fatty acids may improve CHD risk, additional research is needed to confirm their benefits.[25]

Alcohol

Moderate consumption of alcohol—from beer, wine, or liquor—has favorable effects on atherosclerosis, blood-clotting activity, HDL cholesterol levels, inflammation, and insulin resistance.[26] These benefits are most apparent in men and women who are at least 45 and 55 years old, respectively. Of note, only low or moderate amounts of alcohol—no more than one drink daily for women and two for men—have been found to lower CHD risk, and higher intakes are associated with higher mortality rates. One "drink" is equivalent to 12 ounces of beer, 5 ounces of wine, 10 ounces of wine cooler, or 1½ ounces of 80 proof distilled spirits such as gin, rum, vodka, and whiskey.

✚ Plant sterols are extracted from soybeans and pine tree oils and are hydrogenated to produce the plant stanols that are added to commercial products.

Regular aerobic exercise can strengthen the cardiovascular system, promote weight loss, reduce blood pressure, and improve blood glucose and lipid levels.

For some people, alcohol's negative effects can offset its health advantages. Alcohol consumption is associated with cancers of the gastrointestinal (GI) tract and several other cancers, including liver cancer and breast cancer.[27] Alcohol is destructive to the liver and male reproductive system, and high alcohol intakes can elevate blood pressure and triglyceride levels. For these reasons, nondrinkers are not encouraged to start drinking in an effort to decrease their risk for CHD.

Regular Physical Activity

Regular physical activity reverses a number of risk factors for CHD: it can lower triglycerides, raise HDL, lower blood pressure, promote weight loss, improve insulin sensitivity, strengthen heart muscle, and increase coronary artery size and tone. The American Heart Association recommends that all adults participate in at least 30 minutes of moderate-intensity physical activity on most days of the week.[28] Aerobic activities that use large muscle groups have the greatest benefits; such activities include brisk walking, running, swimming, cycling, stair-stepping, and cross-country skiing. If preferred, physical activity can be divided into several sessions during the day.

Smoking Cessation

Cigarette smoking is a major risk factor for CHD as well as other types of cardiovascular disease. (✚) In addition to promoting atherosclerosis, cigarette smoking decreases the oxygen-carrying capacity of the blood, raises the heart rate, reduces exercise tolerance, and interferes with vasodilator medications used for treating angina and hypertension.[29] Even one or two cigarettes daily can increase CHD risk, and cigarettes that have low tar and nicotine do not lower the risk. Quitting smoking improves CHD risk quickly; the incidence of CHD drops to levels near those of nonsmokers in just two years.[30]

Weight Reduction

Obesity, especially abdominal obesity, is an independent risk factor for CHD.[31] In obesity, the enlarged adipose cells increase their production and release of inflammatory mediators and blood clotting factors; these compounds raise the risks of both atherosclerosis and heart attack. Obesity also strains the heart and blood vessels because **cardiac output** is greater, thus increasing the workload of the left ventricle, which pumps blood to the major arteries. Moreover, obesity leads to metabolic abnormalities that increase CHD risk, such as insulin resistance, hypertension, elevated triglycerides, and low HDL levels (recall that these disorders characterize the metabolic syndrome, which was described in Nutrition in Practice 20).

Weight reduction can improve such CHD risk factors as insulin resistance, hypertension, and blood lipid abnormalities. However, individuals should focus on weight reduction only *after* they have adopted other dietary measures to lower LDL.[32] This approach ensures that LDL reduction is given priority and that the individual does not receive a multitude of dietary suggestions at one time. The initial goal of a weight-loss program should be no more than 10 percent of a person's original body weight. For some, avoiding additional weight gain may be a desirable starting point.

Successful Adherence to Lifestyle Changes

Incorporating many lifestyle changes at once can be difficult, and instruction and counseling are critical for success. Nurses can help to motivate patients by explaining the reasons for each change, setting obtainable goals, and providing practical suggestions. In some individuals, high LDL cholesterol levels may persist despite adherence to a TLC program, and drug therapy may be the only effective treatment. Review Table 21-3 (p. 598) for a summary of the Therapeutic Lifestyle Changes discussed in this section. The "How to" offers suggestions for implementing a heart-healthy diet.

LIFESTYLE CHANGES FOR HYPERTRIGLYCERIDEMIA

Hypertriglyceridemia (elevated blood triglycerides) (✚) is common in people with diabetes and the metabolic syndrome and may also result from other disorders. Elevated triglyceride levels may coexist with elevated LDL cholesterol or occur

✚ Cigar and pipe smoking can also increase the risk of CHD, but the risk may be lower because the smoke is less likely to be inhaled.

✚ Blood triglycerides:
- Borderline high: 150–199 mg/dL
- High: 200–499 mg/dL
- Very high: ≥500 mg/dL

cardiac output: the volume of blood pumped by the heart within a specified period of time.

For some people, following a heart-healthy diet may require significant changes in food choices. It is often easier to adopt a new diet if only a few changes are made at a time. Discussing positive choices (what to eat) first, rather than negative ones (what not to eat), may improve compliance. These suggestions can help patients implement their diet:

Breads, Cereals, and Pasta

- Choose whole-grain breads and cereals. Make sure the first ingredient on bread and cereal labels is "whole wheat" rather than "enriched wheat flour." Consume oats and barley regularly, as they are good sources of soluble fibers.

- Bakery products and snack foods often contain *trans*-fatty acids. Choose products whose labels do not list *trans* fat in the Nutrition Facts panel or "hydrogenated vegetable oil" in the ingredients list.

- Avoid products that contain tropical oils (coconut, palm, and palm kernel oil), which are high in saturated fat.

Fruits and Vegetables

- Incorporate at least one or two servings of fruits and vegetables into each meal. Keep the refrigerator stocked with a variety of colorful fruits and vegetables (baby carrots, blueberries, grapes) that can be eaten when the urge to nibble arises.

- Check food labels on canned products carefully. Canned vegetables (especially tomato-based products) are often high in sodium. Fruits that are canned in juice are higher in nutrient density than those canned in syrup.

- Avoid french fries from fast-food restaurants, which are often prepared with *trans* fats. Restrict high-sodium foods such as pickles, olives, sauerkraut, and kimchee.

Lunch and Dinner Entrées

- Limit meat, fish, and poultry intakes to 5 ounces per day. Plan to eat fish twice a week, preferably fatty fish such as salmon, tuna, and mackerel.

- Select lean cuts of beef, such as sirloin tip and round steak; lean cuts of pork, such as loin chops and tenderloin; and skinless poultry pieces. Trim visible fat before cooking.

- Select extra-lean ground meat and drain well after cooking. Use lean ground turkey, without skin added, in place of ground beef.

- Prepare pasta and vegetable stir-fry dishes several times weekly to help reduce meat intake and increase vegetable intake. Use soybean products and other legumes as sources of protein.

- Limit cholesterol-rich organ meats (liver, brain, sweetbreads) and shrimp. Limit intake of whole eggs to two per week, as the yolks are high in cholesterol (about 210 milligrams per yolk). Replace whole eggs in recipes with egg whites or commercial egg substitutes or similar reduced-cholesterol products.

- Restrict these high-sodium foods: cured or smoked meats such as beef jerky, bologna, corned beef, frankfurters, ham, luncheon meats, salt pork, and sausage; salty or smoked fish such as anchovies, caviar, salted or dried cod, herring, and smoked salmon; and canned, frozen, or packaged soups, sauces, and entrées.

Milk Products

- Select fat-free or low-fat milk products only. Use yogurt or fat-free sour cream to make dips or salad dressings. Substitute evaporated fat-free milk for heavy cream.

- Restrict foods high in saturated fat or sodium, such as cheese, processed cheeses, and ice cream or other milk-based desserts.

Fats and Oils

- Prepare salad dressings and other foods with vegetable oils rich in omega-3 fatty acids, such as canola, soybean, flaxseed, and walnut oils. Select other unsaturated vegetable oils, such as corn, olive, peanut, safflower, sesame, and sunflower oils, instead of saturated fat sources such as butter and lard.

- Select margarines that do not list *trans* fat in the Nutrition Facts panel or "hydrogenated vegetable oil" in the ingredients list. Tub margarines are less likely to contain *trans* fat than stick margarines. To lower LDL cholesterol levels, use margarines with added plant sterols or stanols.

- Add unsalted nuts or avocados to meals to make meals more appetizing; these foods are good sources of unsaturated fats.

- Avoid tropical oils (coconut, palm, and palm kernel oil), which are high in saturated fat.

Spices and Seasonings

- Use salt only at the end of cooking, and you will need to add much less. Use salt substitutes at the table.

- Spices and herbs can improve food flavor without adding sodium. Try using more garlic, ginger, basil, curry or chili powder, cumin, pepper, lemon, mint, oregano, rosemary, and thyme.

- Check the sodium content on food labels. Flavorings and sauces that are usually high in sodium include bouillon cubes, soy sauce, steak and barbecue sauces, relishes, mustard, and catsup.

Snacks and Desserts

- Select low-sodium and low–saturated fat snacks such as unsalted pretzels and nuts, plain popcorn, and unsalted chips and crackers. Check labels on snack foods and desserts to ensure that they do not include *trans* fats.

- Enjoy angel food cake, which is made without egg yolks and added fat. Select low-fat frozen desserts such as sherbet, sorbet, fruit bars, and some low-fat ice creams.

- Choose canned or dried fruits and crunchy raw vegetables to boost fruit and vegetable intake.

separately. Whereas mild or moderate hypertriglyceridemia is often associated with increased risk of CHD and fatty liver disease, severe hypertriglyceridemia can cause additional complications, including fatty deposits in the skin and soft tissues and acute pancreatitis.[33]

Medical Nutrition Therapy for Hypertriglyceridemia

Dietary and lifestyle changes can improve most cases of hypertriglyceridemia.[34] Overweight and obesity, a sedentary lifestyle, and cigarette smoking all can raise triglyceride levels. Dietary factors that increase triglyceride levels include high intakes of alcohol and refined carbohydrates; sucrose and fructose are the carbohydrates with the strongest effect. Thus, controlling body weight, being physically active, quitting smoking, restricting alcohol, and limiting intakes of refined carbohydrates (especially foods made with white flour or added sugars) are basic treatments for hypertriglyceridemia. As mentioned earlier, high triglyceride levels are often associated with low HDL, and the lifestyle changes listed here are likely to improve HDL levels as well.

Severe Hypertriglyceridemia Medications are usually necessary for lowering blood triglyceride levels that exceed 500 milligrams per deciliter. Although dietary and lifestyle changes are still recommended, a very-low-fat diet, providing less than 15 percent of kcalories from fat, may be required if blood triglycerides exceed 1000 milligrams per deciliter.[35] Patients must also eliminate consumption of alcoholic beverages.

Fish Oil Supplements and Hypertriglyceridemia Fish oil supplements are sometimes recommended for treating hypertriglyceridemia. Clinical trials have shown that a daily intake of 2 to 4 grams of EPA and DHA (combined) can lower triglyceride levels by 30 to 50 percent.[36] Fish oil therapy should be monitored by a physician due to the potential for adverse effects.

VITAMIN SUPPLEMENTATION AND CHD RISK

People often ask about the potential benefits of using certain types of vitamin supplements for reducing CHD risk, particularly B vitamin and antioxidant supplements. Most clinical trials have not been able to confirm any benefits from using these supplements, as described in this section.

B Vitamin Supplements and Homocysteine As mentioned earlier, elevated blood homocysteine levels are a known risk factor for CHD, but whether homocysteine itself is directly damaging or is simply an indicator of other abnormalities remains unknown. Possibly, homocysteine has harmful effects on the artery wall, causes oxidative stress, or heightens blood-clotting activity that worsens atherosclerosis.[37] Although increased intakes of folate, vitamin B_6, and vitamin B_{12} can lower homocysteine levels, clinical research trials have not demonstrated that supplementation with these vitamins can reduce the incidence of heart attacks in those at risk.[38] Hence, B vitamin supplements are not currently recommended for patients at risk for CHD.

Antioxidant Vitamin Supplements Because oxidized LDL promote atherosclerosis, researchers have hypothesized that antioxidant supplementation may help to prevent atherosclerosis and reduce CHD risk. Several epidemiological studies have suggested that antioxidant-rich diets may protect against CHD, but because persons who consume such diets usually maintain a healthy lifestyle and body weight as well, it has been difficult to determine whether the antioxidants are responsible for the effect. Most studies that tested supplementation with single antioxidants (such as vitamins C or E), combinations of antioxidants, or multivitamins have produced weak or inconsistent results, and several studies suggested possible harm.[39] Until more data are available, there is no recommendation to use antioxidant supplements for heart disease prevention.[40]

DIET-DRUG INTERACTIONS

Check this table for notable nutrition-related effects of the medications discussed in this chapter.

	GASTROINTESTINAL EFFECTS	INTERACTIONS WITH DIETARY SUBSTANCES	METABOLIC EFFECTS
Anticoagulants (warfarin)	—	Requires consistent vitamin K intake to maintain effectiveness. Drug effects are enhanced with supplementation of vitamin E, dong quai, danshen, fish oils, garlic, and ginkgo. Drug effects are reduced with coenzyme Q, ginseng, and green tea. Avoid alcohol.	—
Antihypertensives Beta-blockers	—	—	Elevated serum potassium levels, hypoglycemia
Calcium channel blockers	Nausea, constipation	Avoid herbal supplements that contain natural licorice. Avoid grapefruit juice, which may enhance drug effects.	—
ACE inhibitors[a]	Reduced taste sensation	Avoid herbal supplements that contain natural licorice. Avoid potassium supplements and salt substitutes that contain potassium.	Elevated serum potassium levels
Antilipimics Statins	Constipation, flatulence, GI discomfort	Avoid grapefruit juice, which may enhance drug effects.	Elevated serum liver enzymes
Bile acid sequestrants	Constipation, flatulence, diarrhea	Cause reduced absorption of fat-soluble vitamins.	Electrolyte imbalances, iron deficiency
Nicotinic acid	GI discomfort	Avoid alcoholic beverages, coffee, and tea, which may increase side effects.	Elevated serum liver enzymes, elevated uric acid levels, hyperglycemia, low blood pressure
Digoxin	Anorexia, nausea, stomach cramps, diarrhea	High-fiber foods and magnesium supplements can reduce drug absorption. St. John's wort may reduce drug efficacy.	Elevated serum potassium and reduced serum magnesium levels. Drug toxicity can develop if body potassium levels are low.
Diuretics (furosemide, spironolactone)[b]	Dry mouth, anorexia, decreased taste perception	Furosemide bioavailability is reduced when the drug is taken with food.	Fluid and electrolyte imbalances,[b] hyperglycemia (spironolactone), hyperlipidemia (spironolactone), thiamin and zinc deficiencies
Nitroglycerin	Decreased taste perception	Increases effects of alcohol.	—

[a] ACE is an abbreviation for *angiotensin-converting enzyme*. An ACE inhibitor interferes with the conversion of angiotensin I to angiotensin II, a peptide that helps to regulate blood pressure.

[b] *Furosemide* is a "potassium-wasting" diuretic; patients taking furosemide should increase intakes of potassium-rich foods. *Spironolactone* is a "potassium-sparing" diuretic; patients taking spironolactone should avoid supplemental potassium and salt substitutes that contain potassium.

DRUG THERAPIES FOR CHD PREVENTION

Individuals who cannot reach LDL goals with dietary and lifestyle changes alone may be prescribed one or more medications. The most common LDL-lowering drugs are statins, which reduce cholesterol synthesis in the liver. Bile acid sequestrants lower LDL cholesterol by interfering with bile reabsorption in the small intestine, but their side effects (constipation and intestinal gas) may cause difficulty with compliance.

For lowering triglyceride levels and increasing HDL, both fibrates and nicotinic acid (a form of niacin) are effective; nicotinic acid can also reduce LDL and lipoprotein(a) levels. Individuals using medications for CHD prevention should continue the TLC program so that they can use the lowest possible doses of the drugs.[41]

In addition to lipid-lowering medications, some people may benefit from drugs that suppress blood clotting (such as anticoagulants and aspirin) or reduce blood pressure. Nitroglycerin may be given to alleviate angina as needed. Some medications may affect nutrition status or food intake (see the Diet-Drug Interactions feature); the interactions can be even more complicated when multiple medications are used.

TREATMENT OF HEART ATTACK

As explained earlier, a heart attack occurs when the blood supply to heart muscle is blocked, causing damage or death to heart tissue. If the blood flow within the artery is restored quickly, the heart muscle may be saved; if not, the muscle tissue dies. Drug therapies given immediately after a heart attack may include thrombolytic drugs (clot-busting drugs), anticoagulants, aspirin, painkillers, and medications that regulate heart rhythm and reduce blood pressure.[42] Patients are not given food or beverages, except for sips of water or clear liquids, until their condition stabilizes. Once able to eat, they are initially offered small portions of foods that are low in sodium, saturated fat, and cholesterol. The sodium restriction helps to limit fluid retention but may be lifted after several days if the patient shows no signs of heart failure.

A heart attack patient needs to regain strength and learn strategies that can reduce the risk of a future heart attack; such strategies are similar to the Therapeutic Lifestyle Changes (TLC) described earlier. Thus, the cardiac rehabilitation programs in hospitals and outpatient clinics include exercise therapy, instruction about a heart-healthy diet, help with smoking cessation, and medication counseling. The programs often last several months. Home-based rehabilitation programs are also beneficial, but they are more limited in scope and lack the benefit of group interaction.

Review Notes

- Long-term CHD management emphasizes risk reduction. Modifiable risk factors include elevated LDL and triglyceride levels, low HDL levels, hypertension, diabetes, obesity, a sedentary lifestyle, cigarette smoking, and various dietary factors.
- Therapeutic Lifestyle Changes (TLC) can help patients reduce LDL levels and eliminate other risk factors. Dietary recommendations are to reduce saturated fat, *trans* fats, and cholesterol; increase soluble fiber; and incorporate plant sterols, plant stanols, and fish into the diet. Other recommendations include regular physical activity, smoking cessation, and weight reduction.
- Treatment for mild hypertriglyceridemia emphasizes weight control, regular physical activity, smoking cessation, alcohol restriction, and avoiding a high carbohydrate intake. Severe hypertriglyceridemia requires drug therapies and dietary fat restriction.
- Medications given after a heart attack suppress blood clotting, regulate heart rhythm, and reduce blood pressure. To reduce the risk of a future heart attack, patients must learn strategies similar to the TLC approach.

Blood pressure is measured both when heart muscle contracts (*systolic* blood pressure) and when it relaxes (*diastolic* blood pressure). Measurements are expressed as millimeters of mercury (mm Hg).

	Systolic	Diastolic
• Desirable blood pressure	<120	<80
• Prehypertension	120–139	80–89
• Hypertension	≥140	≥90

NURSING DIAGNOSIS

For persons who experience a heart attack may include *decreased cardiac output, risk for decreased cardiac tissue perfusion, acute pain,* and *activity intolerance.*

Hypertension

Hypertension (high blood pressure) affects about one-third of adults in the United States.[43] Prevalence is especially high among African Americans, who develop hypertension earlier in life and sustain higher average blood pressures throughout their lives than other ethnic groups. An estimated 21 percent of people with hypertension are unaware that they have it.[44] (✚)

Although people cannot feel the physical effects of hypertension, it is a primary risk factor for atherosclerosis and cardiovascular diseases. For each 20/10 mm Hg increase above normal blood pressure (an increase of 20 mm Hg in systolic blood pressure and 10 mm Hg in diastolic blood pressure), the risk of death from CVD doubles.[45] Elevated blood pressure forces the heart to work harder to eject blood into the arteries; this effort weakens heart muscle and increases the risk of developing heart arrhythmias, heart failure, and even sudden death. Hypertension is also a primary cause of stroke and kidney failure. Reducing blood pressure can dramatically reduce the incidence of these diseases.

FACTORS THAT INFLUENCE BLOOD PRESSURE

Although the underlying causes of most cases of hypertension are not fully understood, much is known about the physiological factors that affect blood pressure (the force exerted by the blood on artery walls). As shown in Figure 21-3, blood pressure depends on the volume of blood pumped by the heart (cardiac output) and the resistance the blood encounters in the arterioles (peripheral resistance). (✚) When either

✚ The equation describing this relationship is blood pressure (BP) = cardiac output (CO) × peripheral resistance (PR).

FIGURE 21-3 | Determinants of Blood Pressure

Cardiac output is the volume of blood pumped by the heart within a specified period of time.

Peripheral resistance refers to the resistance to pumped blood by the small arterial branches (arterioles) that carry blood to tissues.

Screening people for hypertension is a first step toward early detection and prevention of complications.

© 2010/Jupiterimages Corporation

cardiac output or peripheral resistance increases, blood pressure rises. Cardiac output is raised when heart rate or blood volume increases; peripheral resistance is affected mostly by the diameters of the arterioles and blood viscosity. Blood pressure is therefore influenced by the nervous system, which regulates heart muscle contractions and the arterioles' diameters, and hormonal signals, which may cause fluid retention or blood vessel constriction. The kidneys also play a role in regulating blood pressure by controlling the secretion of the hormones involved in vasoconstriction and retention of sodium and water.

FACTORS THAT CONTRIBUTE TO HYPERTENSION

In 90 to 95 percent of hypertension cases, the cause is unknown (called **primary or essential hypertension**).[46] In other cases, hypertension is caused by a known physical or metabolic disorder (**secondary hypertension**), such as an abnormality in an organ or hormone involved in blood pressure regulation. For example, chronic kidney disease interferes with the removal of sodium and water from blood, directly increasing blood volume and thus blood pressure. Atherosclerosis in renal arteries may cause increased production of the hormones that stimulate water retention and vasoconstriction. Stiffness and thickening of the aorta or arteries (arteriosclerosis) due to age, diabetes, or other reasons can increase resistance to blood flow, thereby raising blood pressure.

A number of risk factors have been identified in the development of hypertension. These include the following:

- *Aging.* Hypertension risk increases with age. More than two-thirds of persons older than 65 years have hypertension.[47] Moreover, individuals who have normal blood pressure at age 55 still have a 90 percent risk of developing high blood pressure during their lifetimes.[48]
- *Genetic factors.* Risk of hypertension is similar among family members. It is also more prevalent and severe in certain ethnic groups; for example, the prevalence of hypertension in African American adults is about 44 percent, compared with a prevalence of about 32 percent in whites and 27 percent in Mexican Americans.[49]
- *Obesity.* Of people with hypertension, most—an estimated 60 percent—are obese.[50] Obesity may raise blood pressure, in part, by increasing blood volume, promoting vasoconstriction, and increasing activity of the sympathetic nervous system.[51]
- *Salt sensitivity.* (✚) Among those with hypertension, approximately 30 to 50 percent are sensitive to salt and can improve blood pressure by reducing salt consumption.[52]
- *Alcohol.* Heavy drinking (an alcohol intake of three or more drinks daily) increases the incidence and severity of hypertension by stimulating the sympathetic nervous system.[53] Reducing alcohol consumption reverses this effect.
- *Dietary factors.* A person's diet may increase risk for hypertension. As explained later, dietary modifications that increase intakes of potassium, calcium, and magnesium have been shown to reduce blood pressure.

TREATMENT OF HYPERTENSION

As mentioned, controlling hypertension improves CVD risk considerably. The goal of hypertension treatment is to reduce blood pressure to <140/<90 mm Hg; for people with diagnosed CHD, diabetes, or kidney disease, the blood pressure goal is <130/<80 mm Hg. Both lifestyle modifications and drug therapies are used to treat hypertension. For people with prehypertension (120–139/80–89 mm Hg), changes in diet and lifestyle alone may lower blood pressure to a normal level.

Table 21-4 describes the lifestyle modifications recommended for reducing blood pressure and the expected reduction in systolic blood pressure for each change. The

✚ *Salt sensitivity* is also known as *sodium sensitivity*. Salt is the main source of sodium in the diet.

primary hypertension: hypertension with an unknown cause; also known as **essential hypertension.**

secondary hypertension: hypertension that results from a known physiological abnormality.

NURSING DIAGNOSIS

For some individuals with hypertension may include *imbalanced nutrition: more than body requirements* and *ineffective self health management.*

Nutrition and Disorders of the Heart and Blood Vessels

TABLE
21-4

Lifestyle Modifications for Blood Pressure Reduction

Modification	Recommendation	Expected Reduction in Systolic Blood Pressure
Weight reduction	Maintain healthy body weight (BMI below 25).	5–20 mm Hg/10 kg weight loss
DASH Eating Plan[a]	Adopt a diet rich in fruits, vegetables, and low-fat milk products with reduced saturated fat intake.	8–14 mm Hg
Sodium restriction	Reduce dietary sodium intake to less than 2400 milligrams sodium (less than 6 grams salt) per day.[b]	2–8 mm Hg
Physical activity	Perform aerobic physical activity for at least 30 minutes per day, most days of the week.	4–9 mm Hg
Moderate alcohol consumption	Men: Limit to two drinks per day. Women and lighter-weight men: Limit to one drink per day.	2–4 mm Hg

[a] The DASH Eating Plan was tested in a study called Dietary Approaches to Stop Hypertension.

[b] According to DRI recommendations, sodium intake should be limited to 2300 milligrams daily.

Source: Adapted from *Reference Card from the Seventh Report of the Joint National Committee on Prevention, Detection, Evaluation, and Treatment of High Blood Pressure (JNC 7)*, NIH publication no. 03-5231 (Bethesda, MD: National Institutes of Health, National Heart, Lung, and Blood Institute, and National High Blood Pressure Education Program, May 2003).

recommendations include weight reduction if overweight or obese; a diet low in sodium and rich in potassium, calcium, and magnesium; regular physical activity; and a moderate alcohol intake, if one chooses to drink.[54] Combining two or more of these modifications can enhance results.

Dietary Approaches for Reducing Blood Pressure

Several research studies have shown that a significant reduction in blood pressure can be achieved by following a diet that emphasizes fruits, vegetables, and low-fat dairy products and includes whole grains, poultry, fish, and nuts.[55] The diet tested in these studies, now known as the *DASH Eating Plan,* (✚) provides more fiber, potassium, magnesium, and calcium than the typical American diet. The diet also limits red meat, sweets, sugar-containing beverages, saturated fat (to 7 percent of kcalories), and cholesterol (to 150 milligrams per day), so it is beneficial for reducing CHD risk as well. During the eight-week study period when hypertensive subjects consumed the DASH diet, their systolic blood pressures fell by 11.4 mm Hg more than the blood pressures of subjects who remained on the standard American control diet.[56] The DASH Eating Plan, shown in Table 21-5, is a dietary pattern that meets the goals specified in the *Dietary Guidelines for Americans.*[57]

The DASH Eating Plan is even more effective when accompanied by a low sodium intake. In a research study that tested the blood pressure–lowering effects of the DASH dietary pattern in combination with sodium restriction, the best results were achieved when sodium was reduced to 1500 milligrams daily—a lower level than the maximum intake of 2400 milligrams* recommended for people with hypertension.[58] These results suggest that the optimal sodium intake for people with hypertension may be far lower than is typically recommended.

✚ The DASH Eating Plan is based on the test diet used in a study called Dietary Approaches to Stop Hypertension.

---

* The maximum sodium intake recommended for people with hypertension (2400 mg) is similar to the tolerable upper intake level (UL) for sodium, which was set at 2300 mg to prevent the adverse effects of high sodium intakes on blood pressure in the general population.

TABLE
21-5 | The DASH Eating Plan

Food Group	Recommended Servings for Different Energy Intakes (servings per day except as noted)			
	1600 kcal	2000 kcal	2600 kcal	3100 kcal
Grains and grain products[a] (1 serving = 1 slice bread, 1 oz dry cereal,[b] or ½ c cooked rice, pasta, or cereal)	6	6–8	10–11	12–13
Vegetables (1 serving = ½ c cooked vegetables, 1 c raw leafy vegetables, or ½ c vegetable juice)	3–4	4–5	5–6	6
Fruits (1 serving = 1 medium fruit; ½ c fresh, frozen, or canned fruit; ¼ c dried fruit; or ½ c fruit juice)	4	4–5	5–6	6
Milk products (low fat or fat free) (1 serving = 1 c milk or yogurt, or 1½ oz cheese)	2–3	2–3	3	3–4
Meat, poultry, and fish (1 serving = 3 oz cooked lean meat, poultry, or fish)	1–2	1–2	2	2–3
Nuts, seeds, and legumes (1 serving = ⅓ c nuts, 2 tbs peanut butter, 2 tbs seeds, or ½ c cooked dry beans or peas)	3 per week	4–5 per week	1	1
Fats and oils (1 serving = 1 tsp vegetable oil or soft margarine, ½ tbs mayonnaise, or 1 tbs salad dressing)	2	2–3	3	4
Sweets (1 serving = 1 tbs sugar, jelly, or jam; ½ c sorbet; or 1 c lemonade)	0	up to 5 per week	≤ 2	≤ 2

[a] Whole grains are recommended for most servings consumed.

[b] One ounce of dry cereal may be equivalent to ½ to 1¼ cups, depending on the cereal. Check the food label for the portion size.

Source: National Heart, Lung, and Blood Institute, National Institutes of Health, *Your Guide to Lowering Your Blood Pressure with DASH*, NIH publication no. 06-4082 (Bethesda, MD: National Heart, Lung, and Blood Institute, 2006).

Sodium restriction by itself can have a modest blood pressure–lowering effect (review Table 21-4), but some people are more responsive than others. Although a low-sodium diet may improve blood pressure to some extent, it should be combined with other lifestyle modifications for greater effect. The "How to" lists practical suggestions for restricting sodium intake; additional detail is provided in Table 22-1 on p. 625.

Weight Reduction Weight reduction may reduce blood pressure considerably. Clinical studies suggest that systolic blood pressure can be reduced by 1 mm Hg for each kilogram of weight loss and that the blood pressure reduction may be sustained for several years.[59] The long-term benefits of weight loss in people with hypertension are still under investigation.

- Select fresh, unprocessed foods. Packaged foods, canned goods, and frozen meals are often high in sodium.

- Do not use salt at the table or while cooking. Salt substitutes may be useful for some people. Salt substitutes often contain potassium, however, and are not appropriate for people using diuretics that promote potassium retention in the blood.

- Avoid eating in fast-food restaurants; most menu choices are very high in sodium.

- Check food labels. The labeling term *low sodium* is a better guide than the terms *reduced sodium* (contains 25 percent less sodium than the regular product) or *light in sodium* (contains 50 percent less sodium). To be labeled *low sodium*, a food product must contain less than 140 milligrams of sodium per serving. Keep your goal sodium level in mind when you read labels.

- Recognize the high-sodium foods in each food category, and purchase only unsalted or low-sodium varieties of these products if they are available. High-sodium foods include the following:

  - Snack foods made with added salt, such as tortilla chips, popcorn, and nuts.

- Processed meats, such as ham, corned beef, bologna, salami, sausage, bacon, frankfurters, and pastrami.

- Processed fish, such as salted fish and canned fish.

- Tomato-based products, such as tomato sauce, tomato juice, pizza, canned tomatoes, and catsup.

- Canned soups and broths; note that even reduced-sodium varieties may contain excessive sodium.

- Cheese, such as cottage cheese, American cheese, and Parmesan and most other hard cheeses.

- Bakery products made with baking powder or baking soda (sodium bicarbonate), such as cakes, cookies, doughnuts, and muffins.

- Condiments and relishes, such as bouillon cubes, olives, and pickled vegetables.

- Flavoring sauces, such as soy sauce, barbecue sauce, and steak sauce.

- Check for the word *sodium* on medication labels. Sodium is often an ingredient in some types of antacids and laxatives.

Drug Therapies for Reducing Blood Pressure

People with hypertension usually require two or more medications to meet their blood pressure goals. Using a combination of drugs with different modes of action can reduce the doses of each drug needed and minimize side effects. Most treatments include diuretics, which lower blood pressure by reducing blood volume. (✚) Other medications commonly prescribed include ACE inhibitors, beta-blockers, and calcium channel blockers; these drugs are also used to treat various heart conditions. The Diet-Drug Interactions feature lists nutrition-related side effects of these medications (see p. 603).

✚ Some diuretics may cause potassium depletion. When these diuretics are used, serum potassium levels are monitored several times yearly and supplements are prescribed when necessary.

CASE STUDY | Patient with Cardiovascular Disease

Andrew Reid, a 48-year-old African American computer programmer, is 5 feet 9 inches tall and weighs 240 pounds. He sits for long hours at work and is too tired to exercise when he gets home at night. His meals usually include fatty meats, eggs, and cheese, and he likes dairy desserts such as pudding and ice cream. He has a family history of CHD and hypertension. His recent laboratory tests show that his blood pressure is 160/100 mm Hg, and his LDL and HDL levels are 160 mg/dL and 35 mg/dL, respectively. He smokes a pack of cigarettes each day and usually has two glasses of wine at both lunch and dinner.

1. Name Mr. Reid's major risk factors for CHD and hypertension. Which can be modified? What complications might occur if he doesn't seek treatment for his blood lipids and blood pressure?

2. What dietary changes would you recommend that could help to improve Mr. Reid's blood pressure and his LDL and HDL cholesterol? Explain the rationale for each dietary change. Prepare a day's menu for Mr. Reid using the DASH Eating Plan as an outline for your choices.

3. What other laboratory tests or measurements would you need to better assess Mr. Reid's condition? Why?

4. Describe several benefits that Mr. Reid might obtain from a program that includes weight reduction and regular physical activity. Explain why the use of alcohol can be both a protective and a damaging lifestyle habit.

5. Assuming that Mr. Reid does not make any changes in his diet and lifestyle and suffers a heart attack, identify the elements of a cardiac rehabilitation program that would be critical for his long-term survival.

heart failure: a condition with various causes that is characterized by the heart's inability to pump adequate blood to the body's cells, resulting in fluid accumulation in the tissues; also called *congestive heart failure.*

cardiac cachexia: a condition of severe malnutrition that develops in heart failure patients; characterized by weight loss and tissue wasting.

Review Notes

- About one in three persons in the United States has hypertension, which increases the risk of developing CHD, heart failure, stroke, and kidney failure.
- Blood pressure is elevated by factors that increase blood volume, heart rate, and resistance to blood flow. Although the underlying cause of most cases of hypertension is unknown, major risk factors include aging, family history, ethnicity, obesity, and various dietary factors.
- Treatment of hypertension usually includes a combination of lifestyle modifications and drug therapies. The Case Study on p. 609 provides an opportunity to review the risk factors and treatments for CHD and hypertension.

Heart Failure

Heart failure, also called *congestive heart failure,* is characterized by the heart's inability to pump adequate blood, resulting in a buildup of fluids in the veins and tissues. Heart failure has various causes, but it is often a consequence of disorders that create extra work for the heart muscle, such as hypertension and CHD. To accommodate the extra workload, the heart enlarges or pumps faster or harder, but it eventually may weaken enough to fail completely. Heart failure develops mostly in older adults and the elderly: approximately 75 percent of persons with heart failure in the United States are age 65 or older.[60]

CONSEQUENCES OF HEART FAILURE

The symptoms and consequences of heart failure depend on the side of the heart that fails. The right side of the heart normally receives blood from the peripheral tissues and pumps the blood to the lungs. With impaired pumping, blood can back up in the peripheral tissues and abdominal organs. Fluid may accumulate in the lower extremities and in the liver and abdomen, causing chest pain, difficulty with digestion and absorption, and swelling in the legs, ankles, and feet. In contrast, the left side of the heart receives blood from the lungs and pumps it to the peripheral tissues. A weakened left heart can cause a buildup of fluid in the lungs (called *pulmonary edema*), resulting in extreme shortness of breath and limited oxygen for activity; in severe cases, it can lead to respiratory failure. The inadequate blood flow to tissues can also impair the functions of various organs, such as the liver and kidneys. Note that the effects of heart failure depend on the seriousness of the illness: mild cases may be asymptomatic, but severe cases may cause significant damage to health.

Heart failure can dramatically affect a person's food intake and level of physical activity. Right-sided heart failure may cause abdominal bloating and an enlarged liver, and pain and discomfort may worsen with meals. Left-sided failure can limit physical activity substantially due to limb weakness and fatigue. End-stage heart failure is often accompanied by **cardiac cachexia,** a condition of severe malnutrition characterized by weight loss and tissue wasting. Cardiac cachexia is brought about by changes in body chemistry that promote catabolism and is worsened by the reduced appetite and food intake

An overburdened heart enlarges in an effort to supply blood to the body's tissues.

© Susan Leavines/Photo Researchers, Inc.

common to heart failure patients. The resultant weakness further lowers the person's strength, functional capacity, and activity levels.

MEDICAL MANAGEMENT OF HEART FAILURE

Heart failure is a chronic, progressive illness that may require frequent hospitalizations. Many patients face a combination of debilitating symptoms, complex treatments, and an uncertain outcome. Important goals of medical therapy are to slow disease progression and enhance the patient's quality of life. Successful treatment depends on patient participation and compliance with medications and dietary restrictions.

The specific treatment for heart failure depends on the nature and severity of the illness. In general, medications help to manage fluid retention and improve heart function. Dietary sodium and fluid restrictions may help to prevent fluid accumulation. Vaccinations for influenza and pneumonia reduce the risk of developing respiratory infections. Treatment of CHD risk factors, such as hypertension and lipid disorders, may help to slow disease progression. Heart failure patients are also encouraged to participate in exercise programs to avoid becoming physically disabled and to improve endurance.

Drug Therapies for Heart Failure The medications prescribed for heart failure include diuretics, ACE inhibitors, angiotensin receptor blockers, beta-blockers, vasodilators, and digitalis.[61] The diuretics are given to reverse or prevent fluid retention. The patient must monitor fluid fluctuations with daily weight measurements and can make small adjustments in the diuretic dose as needed. The other drugs listed help to improve heart and blood vessel functioning and blood flow.

Nutrition Therapy for Heart Failure The main dietary recommendation for heart failure is a moderate sodium restriction of 2000 milligrams or less daily, depending on the severity of the illness.[62] (➕) The sodium restriction reduces the likelihood of fluid retention. In patients with persistent or recurrent fluid retention, fluid intakes may be restricted to 2 liters per day.[63] Individuals who have difficulty eating due to abdominal or chest pain may tolerate small, frequent meals better than large meals.

Other Dietary Recommendations Patients with heart failure may be prone to constipation due to diuretic use and reduced physical activity. Maintaining an adequate fiber intake can help to minimize constipation problems. Because of alcohol's deleterious effects on blood pressure and heart function, most patients need to restrict or avoid alcoholic beverages.

Cardiac Cachexia No known therapies can reverse cardiac cachexia, and prognosis is poor. For some patients, liquid supplements, tube feedings, or parenteral nutrition support can be supportive additions to treatment.

Review Notes

- Heart failure is usually a chronic, progressive condition that results from other cardiovascular illnesses.
- In heart failure, the heart is unable to pump adequate blood to tissues. Consequences may include fluid accumulation in the veins, lungs, and other organs and impaired organ function.
- Treatment of heart failure includes drug therapies that reduce fluid accumulation and improve heart function. The main dietary recommendation is a moderate sodium restriction.

➕ The recommendation of 2000 mg of sodium is not very restrictive. The current DRI recommendation is to limit sodium intake to 2300 mg daily.

Stroke

Stroke is the third most common cause of death in the United States after heart disease and cancer, and it is a leading cause of serious long-term disability in adults.[64] About 87 percent of strokes are **ischemic strokes**, caused by the obstruction of blood flow to brain tissue. **Hemorrhagic strokes** occur in 13 percent of cases and result from bleeding within the brain, which damages brain tissue.[65] Most ischemic strokes are a result of ruptured atherosclerotic plaque and subsequent blood clot formation, but an embolism (✚) may also cause a stroke. Hemorrhagic strokes often result from the rupture of a blood vessel that has been weakened by atherosclerosis and chronic hypertension. Hemorrhagic strokes are generally more deadly: 38 percent result in death within 30 days.[66]

Strokes that occur suddenly and are short-lived (lasting several minutes to several hours) are called **transient ischemic attacks (TIAs)**. These brief strokes are a warning sign that a heart attack or a more severe stroke may follow, and they need to be evaluated and treated quickly.[67] TIAs typically cause short-term neurological symptoms, such as confusion, slurred speech, numbness, paralysis, or difficulty speaking. Treatment includes the use of aspirin and other drugs that inhibit blood clotting.

STROKE PREVENTION

Stroke is largely preventable by recognizing risk factors and making lifestyle choices that reduce risk. Many of the risk factors are similar to those for heart disease; they include hypertension, cigarette smoking, diabetes mellitus, elevated LDL cholesterol levels, and a history of cardiovascular disease. Medications that suppress blood clotting reduce the risk of ischemic stroke, especially in people who have suffered a first stroke or a transient ischemic attack. The drugs typically prescribed include antiplatelet drugs (such as aspirin and clopidogrel) and anticoagulants (such as warfarin). (✚) Anticoagulant therapy requires regular follow-up and occasional adjustments in dosage to prevent excessive bleeding.

STROKE MANAGEMENT

The consequences of a stroke vary according to the area of the brain that has been injured. Body movements, senses, and speech are often impaired, and one side of the body may be weakened or paralyzed. Early diagnosis and treatment are necessary to preserve brain tissue and minimize long-term disability. Thrombolytic (clot-busting) drugs are given within the first few hours following an ischemic stroke to prevent additional brain damage.[68]

The focus of nutrition care is to help patients maintain nutrition status and overall health despite the disabilities caused by the stroke. Some patients may need to learn about dietary treatments that improve blood lipid levels and blood pressure. Dysphagia (difficulty swallowing) is a frequent complication of stroke and is associated with a poorer prognosis. Difficulty with speech prevents patients from describing the problems they may be having with eating and from communicating their food preferences. Coordination problems can make it hard for stroke patients to grasp utensils or bring food from table to mouth. In some cases, tube feedings may be necessary until the patient has regained these skills. Nutrition in Practice 21 describes additional options for feeding people with disabilities, such as those that follow stroke.

✚ Reminder: An *embolism* is the obstruction of a blood vessel by a traveling blood clot or air bubble (an *embolus*).

✚ Warfarin acts by interfering with vitamin K's blood-clotting function (see Chapter 14).

NURSING DIAGNOSIS

For stroke patients may include *impaired physical mobility, impaired swallowing, risk for aspiration, impaired verbal communication,* and *feeding self-care deficit.*

ischemic strokes: strokes caused by the obstruction of blood flow to brain tissue.

hemorrhagic strokes: strokes caused by bleeding within the brain, which destroys or compresses brain tissue.

transient ischemic attacks (TIAs): brief ischemic strokes that cause short-term neurological symptoms.

Review Notes

- The two major types of strokes, ischemic and hemorrhagic stroke, can be a consequence of atherosclerosis, hypertension, or both. Transient ischemic attacks, which are short-lived ischemic strokes, are a warning sign that a heart attack or a more severe stroke may follow.

- Strokes are largely preventable by reversing modifiable risk factors, such as hypertension, cigarette smoking, diabetes mellitus, and elevated LDL cholesterol.

- Treatment of a stroke includes the use of anticlotting drugs such as antiplatelet drugs and anticoagulants. A patient who has had a major stroke may have problems eating normally due to difficulty swallowing or lack of coordination.

MEDICAL HISTORY

Check the medical record for a diagnosis of:

- ○ Coronary heart disease
- ○ Hypertension
- ○ Heart failure
- ○ Stroke

Review the medical record for complications related to cardiovascular diseases:

- ○ Heart attack
- ○ Transient ischemic attack
- ○ Cardiac cachexia

Note risk factors for CHD related to diet, including:

- ○ Elevated LDL or triglyceride levels
- ○ Obesity or overweight
- ○ Diabetes
- ○ Hypertension

MEDICATIONS

For patients using drug treatments for cardiovascular diseases, note:

- ○ Side effects that may alter food intake
- ○ Medications that may interact with grapefruit juice
- ○ Use of warfarin, which requires a consistent vitamin K intake
- ○ Use of diuretics or other drugs associated with potassium imbalances
- ○ Potential diet-drug or herb-drug interactions

DIETARY INTAKE

For patients with CHD or hypertension, assess the diet for:

- ○ Energy intake
- ○ Saturated fat, *trans* fat, cholesterol, and sodium content
- ○ Soluble fiber and plant sterol or plant stanol content
- ○ Intake of whole grains, fruits, vegetables, legumes, and nuts
- ○ Alcohol content

For patients with complications resulting from cardiovascular diseases:

- ○ Check adequacy of food intake in patients with heart failure.
- ○ Check physical disabilities that may interfere with food preparation or consumption following a stroke.

ANTHROPOMETRIC DATA

Measure baseline height and weight, and reassess weight at each medical checkup. Note whether patients are meeting weight goals, including:

- ○ Weight loss or maintenance in patients who are overweight
- ○ Weight maintenance in patients with advanced heart failure

Remember that weight may be deceptively high in people who are retaining fluids, especially individuals with heart failure.

LABORATORY TESTS

Monitor the following laboratory tests in people with cardiovascular diseases:

- ○ LDL cholesterol, blood triglycerides, and HDL cholesterol
- ○ Blood glucose in patients with diabetes
- ○ Serum potassium in patients using diuretics, antihypertensive medications, or digoxin
- ○ Indicators of fluid retention in patients with heart failure
- ○ Blood-clotting times in patients using anticoagulants

PHYSICAL SIGNS

Blood pressure measurement is routine in physical exams but is especially important for people who:

- ○ Have cardiovascular diseases
- ○ Have experienced a heart attack or stroke
- ○ Have risk factors for CHD or hypertension

Look for signs of:

- ○ Potassium imbalances (muscle weakness, numbness and tingling, irregular heartbeat) in those using diuretics, antihypertensive medications, or digoxin
- ○ Fluid overload in patients with heart failure

Self Check

1 ● Ischemia in the coronary arteries is a frequent cause of:
   - a. angina pectoris.
   - b. hemorrhagic stroke.
   - c. aneurysm.
   - d. hypertension.

2 ● Risk factors for atherosclerosis include all of the following *except*:
   - a. smoking.
   - b. hypertension.
   - c. diabetes mellitus.
   - d. elevated HDL cholesterol.

3 ● The dietary lipids with the strongest LDL cholesterol-raising effects are:
   - a. monounsaturated fats.
   - b. polyunsaturated fats.
   - c. saturated fats.
   - d. plant sterols.

4 • The omega-3 fatty acids EPA and DHA, which may improve some risk factors for heart disease, are obtained by consuming:
   a. fatty fish.
   b. soy products.
   c. egg yolks and organ meats.
   d. nuts and seeds.

5 • Moderate alcohol consumption can improve heart disease risk, in part, because it:
   a. lowers blood pressure.
   b. improves nutrition status.
   c. offsets the damage from smoking.
   d. increases HDL cholesterol levels.

6 • Patients with mild hypertriglyceridemia may improve their triglyceride levels by:
   a. reducing sodium intake.
   b. consuming moderate amounts of alcohol.
   c. avoiding a high carbohydrate intake.
   d. reducing cholesterol intake.

7 • In most cases of hypertension, the cause is:
   a. excessive alcohol use.
   b. atherosclerosis.
   c. hormonal imbalances.
   d. unknown.

8 • Hypertensive patients can benefit from all of the following dietary and lifestyle modifications *except*:
   a. including fat-free or low-fat milk products in the diet.
   b. reducing total fat intake.
   c. consuming generous amounts of fruits, vegetables, legumes, and nuts.
   d. reducing sodium intake.

9 • Nutrition therapy for a patient with heart failure usually includes:
   a. weight loss.
   b. reducing total fat intake.
   c. sodium restriction.
   d. cholesterol restriction.

10 • Hemorrhagic stroke:
   a. is the most common type of stroke.
   b. results from obstructed blood flow within brain tissue.
   c. comes on suddenly and usually lasts for up to 30 minutes.
   d. results from bleeding within the brain, which damages brain tissue.

Answers to these questions appear in Appendix H.

Clinical Applications

1 • List risk factors for coronary heart disease, and identify possible interrelationships among the factors. For example, a woman over age 55 is also at risk for diabetes; a person with diabetes is more likely to have hypertension.

2 • Review the DASH Eating Plan shown in Table 21-5. As the chapter described, the DASH dietary pattern is helpful for lowering blood pressure and for reducing CHD risk as well.
   • List elements of the DASH Eating Plan that are consistent with the TLC recommendations.
   • Suggest ways in which a person following the DASH Eating Plan might accomplish the following additional dietary modifications: consume a higher percentage of fat from monounsaturated sources, reduce intake of *trans*-fatty acids, and include EPA/DHA and plant sterols in the diet.

Nutrition on the Net

For further study of topics covered in this chapter, access these websites.

- Find updates and quick links to these and other nutrition-related sites at our website: www.cengage.com/nutrition/whitney/nhhc4e
- To search for additional information about cardiovascular diseases, obtain the American Heart Association dietary guidelines, or find links to other relevant materials, visit the website of the American Heart Association: www.americanheart.org
- Information about cardiovascular diseases, the DASH Eating Plan, and implementation of heart-healthy diets is available at the websites of the National Heart, Lung, and Blood Institute and the Heart and Stroke Foundation of Canada: www.nhlbi.nih.gov and ww2.heartandstroke.ca
- To learn about improving health care and life expectancy of ethnic minority populations at high risk for cardiovascular diseases, visit the website of the International Society on Hypertension in Blacks: www.ishib.org
- Learn more about the prevention and treatment of stroke at the website of the National Stroke Association: www.stroke.org

Notes

1. D. Lloyd-Jones and coauthors, Heart disease and stroke statistics—2009 update: A report from the American Heart Association Statistics Committee and Stroke Statistics Subcommittee, *Circulation* 119 (2009):480–486.

2. American Heart Association, *International Cardiovascular Disease Statistics* (2009), available at **www.americanheart.org/presenter.jhtml?identifier=3001008**; site visited October 30, 2009.

3. V. Fuster, Atherosclerosis, thrombosis, and vascular biology, in L. Goldman and D. Ausiello, coeditors, *Cecil Medicine* (Philadelphia: Saunders, 2008), pp. 472–477; P. Bloomfield and coauthors, Cardiovascular disease, in N. A. Boon and coeditors, *Davidson's Principles and Practice of Medicine* (Philadelphia: Churchill Livingstone/Elsevier, 2006), pp. 519–646.

4. M. H. Criqui, Epidemiology of cardiovascular disease, in L. Goldman and D. Ausiello, eds., *Cecil Medicine* (Philadelphia: Saunders, 2008), pp. 301–305.

5. C. Cheng and coauthors, Atherosclerotic lesion size and vulnerability are determined by patterns of fluid shear stress, *Circulation* 113 (2006): 2744–2753.

6. M. H. Beers and coeditors, *The Merck Manual of Diagnosis and Therapy* (Whitehouse Station, NJ: Merck Research Laboratories, 2006), pp. 570–772.

7. N. L. Benowitz, Tobacco, in L. Goldman and D. Ausiello, eds., *Cecil Medicine* (Philadelphia: Saunders, 2008), pp. 162–166; Beers and coeditors, 2006.

8. S. M. Grundy, Nutrition in the management of disorders of serum lipids and lipoproteins, in M. E. Shils and coeditors, *Modern Nutrition in Health and Disease* (Baltimore: Lippincott Williams & Wilkins, 2006), pp. 1076–1094; Beers and coeditors, 2006.

9. M. J. Chapman, Metabolic syndrome and type 2 diabetes: Lipid and physiological consequences, *Diabetes and Vascular Disease Research* 4 (2007): S5–S8.

10. G. T. Jones and coauthors, Plasma lipoprotein(a) indicates risk for 4 distinct forms of vascular disease, *Clinical Chemistry* 53 (2007): 679–685.

11. S. Vasdev, V. Gill, and P. Singal, Role of advanced glycation end products in hypertension and atherosclerosis: Therapeutic implications, *Cell Biochemistry and Biophysics* 49 (2007): 48–63; Beers and coeditors, 2006.

12. M. A. Creager and coauthors, Diabetes and vascular disease: Pathophysiology, clinical consequences, and medical therapy: Part I, *Circulation* 108 (2003): 1527–1532.

13. M. A. Maturana, M. C. Irigoyen, and P. M. Spritzer, Menopause, estrogens, and endothelial dysfunction: Current concepts, *Clinics* 62 (2007): 77–86; Grundy, 2006.

14. K. S. McCully, Homocysteine, vitamins, and vascular disease prevention, *American Journal of Clinical Nutrition* 86 (2007): 1563S–1568S.

15. Lloyd-Jones and coauthors, 2009.

16. P. P. Toth and coauthors, Cardiovascular disease, in R. E. Rakel, ed., *Textbook of Family Medicine* (Philadelphia: Saunders, 2007), pp. 735–805; Beers and coeditors, 2006.

17. Lloyd-Jones and coauthors, 2009.

18. National Cholesterol Education Program, *Third Report of the National Cholesterol Education Program (NCEP) Expert Panel on Detection, Evaluation, and Treatment of High Blood Cholesterol in Adults (Adult Treatment Panel III): Final Report*, NIH publication no. 02-5215 (Bethesda, MD: National Heart, Lung, and Blood Institute, 2002).

19. U.S. Department of Agriculture, Agricultural Research Service, *Nutrient Intakes from Food: Mean Amounts and Percentages of Calories from Protein, Carbohydrate, Fat, and Alcohol, One Day, 2005–2006* (2008), available at **www.ars.usda.gov/ba/bhnrc/fsrg**; site visited November 11, 2009.

20. American Dietetic Association, Position of the American Dietetic Association and Dietitians of Canada: Dietary fatty acids, *Journal of the American Dietetic Association* 107 (2007): 1599–1611.

21. U.S. Department of Agriculture, 2008.

22. A. H. Lichtenstein and coauthors, Diet and lifestyle recommendations revision 2006: A scientific statement from the American Heart Association Nutrition Committee, *Circulation* 114 (2006): 82–96.

23. Lichtenstein and coauthors, 2006.

24. Lichtenstein and coauthors, 2006.

25. Lichtenstein and coauthors, 2006; C. Wang and coauthors, n-3 Fatty acids from fish or fish-oil supplements, but not alpha-linolenic acid, benefit cardiovascular disease outcomes in primary- and secondary-prevention studies: A systematic review, *American Journal of Clinical Nutrition* 84 (2006): 5–17.

26. Lichtenstein and coauthors, 2006; I. Gigleux and coauthors, Moderate alcohol consumption is more cardioprotective in men with the metabolic syndrome, *Journal of Nutrition* 136 (2006): 3027–3032.

27. World Cancer Research Fund/American Institute for Cancer Research, *Food, Nutrition, Physical Activity, and the Prevention of Cancer: A Global Perspective* (Washington, D.C.: American Institute for Cancer Research, 2007), pp. 157–171.

28. Lichtenstein and coauthors, 2006.

29. Benowitz, 2008.

30. Criqui, 2008.

31. P. Poirier and coauthors, Obesity and cardiovascular disease: Pathophysiology, evaluation, and effect of weight loss, *Circulation* 113 (2006): 898–918; D. M. Mann and coauthors, Independent effect and population impact of obesity on fatal coronary heart disease in adults, *Preventive Medicine* 42 (2006): 66–72.

32. National Cholesterol Education Program, 2002.

33. G. Yuan, K. Z. Al-Shali, and R. A. Hegele, Hypertriglyceridemia: Its etiology, effects, and treatment, *Canadian Medical Association Journal* 176 (2007): 1113–1120; M. J. Malloy and J. P. Kane, Disorders of lipoprotein metabolism, in D. G. Gardner and D. Shoback, eds., *Greenspan's Basic and Clinical Endocrinology* (New York: McGraw-Hill/Lange, 2007), pp. 770–795.

34. American Dietetic Association, *Nutrition Care Manual* (Chicago: American Dietetic Association, 2009); Yuan, Al-Shali, and Hegele, 2007.

35. R. C. Oh and J. B. Lanier, Management of hypertriglyceridemia, in *American Family Physician* 75 (2007): 1365–1371.

36. Oh and Lanier, 2007.

37. McCully, 2007; E. Lonn and coauthors, Homocysteine lowering with folic acid and B vitamins in vascular disease, *New England Journal of Medicine* 354 (2006): 1567–1577.

38. A. J. Martí-Carvajal and coauthors, Homocysteine lowering interventions for preventing cardiovascular events, *Cochrane Database of Systematic Reviews* Oct 7 (2009): CD006612; McCully, 2007; K. H. Bonaa and coauthors, Homocysteine lowering and cardiovascular events after acute myocardial infarction, *New England Journal of Medicine* 35 (2006): 1578–1588.

39. E. R. Miller and coauthors, Meta-analysis: High-dosage vitamin E supplementation may increase all-cause mortality, *Annals of Internal Medicine* 142 (2005): 37–46; D. H. Lee and coauthors, Does supplemental vitamin C increase cardiovascular disease risk in women with diabetes? *American Journal of Clinical Nutrition* 80 (2004): 1194–1200.

40. L. Mosca and coauthors, Evidence-based guidelines for cardiovascular disease prevention in women: 2007 update, *Circulation* 115 (2007): 1481–1501; Lichtenstein and coauthors, 2006.

41. Toth and coauthors, 2007.

42. J. L. Anderson, ST segment elevation acute myocardial infarction and complications of myocardial infarction, in L. Goldman and D. Ausiello, eds., *Cecil Medicine* (Philadelphia: Saunders, 2008), pp. 500–518.

43. Lloyd-Jones and coauthors, 2009.

44. Lloyd-Jones and coauthors, 2009.

45. C. Rosendorff and coauthors, Treatment of hypertension in the prevention and management of ischemic heart disease: A scientific statement from the American Heart Association Council for High Blood Pressure Research and the Councils on Clinical Cardiology and Epidemiology and Prevention, *Circulation* 115 (2007): 2761–2788.

46. R. G. Victor, Arterial hypertension, in L. Goldman and D. Ausiello, eds., *Cecil Medicine* (Philadelphia: Saunders, 2008), pp. 430–450.

47. Lloyd-Jones and coauthors, 2009.

48. Beers and coeditors, 2006.

49. Lloyd-Jones and coauthors, 2009.

50. T. A. Kotchen and J. M. Kotchen, Nutrition, diet, and hypertension, in M. E. Shils and coeditors, *Modern Nutrition in Health and Disease* (Philadelphia: Lippincott Williams & Wilkins, 2006), pp. 1095–1107.

51. M. D. Jensen, Obesity, in L. Goldman and D. Ausiello, eds., *Cecil Medicine* (Philadelphia: Saunders, 2008), pp.1643–1652.

52. Kotchen and Kotchen, 2006.

53. Victor, 2008.

54. National High Blood Pressure Education Program/National Institutes of Health, *The Seventh Report of the Joint National Committee on Prevention, Detection, Evaluation, and Treatment of High Blood Pressure (JNC 7)*, NIH publication no. 03-5233 (Bethesda, MD: National Heart, Lung, and Blood Institute, 2003).

55. F. M. Sacks and coauthors, Effects on blood pressure of reduced dietary sodium and the Dietary Approaches to Stop Hypertension (DASH) diet, *New England Journal of Medicine* 344 (2001): 3–10; L. J. Appel and coauthors, A clinical trial on the effects of dietary patterns on blood pressure, *New England Journal of Medicine* 336 (1997): 1117–1124.

56. Appel and coauthors, 1997.

57. U.S. Department of Agriculture and U.S. Department of Health and Human Services, *Dietary Guidelines for Americans, 2005* (Washington, D.C.: Government Printing Office, January 2005).

58. Sacks and coauthors, 2001.

59. L. Aucott and coauthors, Long-term weight loss from lifestyle intervention benefits blood pressure? A systematic review, *Hypertension* 54 (2009): 756–762.

60. B. M. Massie, Heart failure: Pathophysiology and diagnosis, in L. Goldman and D. Ausiello, eds., *Cecil Medicine* (Philadelphia: Saunders, 2008), pp. 345–354.

61. B. G. Katzung and W. W. Parmley, Drugs used in heart failure, in B. G. Katzung, ed., *Basic and Clinical Pharmacology* (New York: McGraw-Hill/Lange, 2007), pp. 198–210.

62. American Dietetic Association, 2009.

63. S. A. Hunt and coauthors, ACC/AHA 2005 guideline update for the diagnosis and management of chronic heart failure in the adult: A report of the American College of Cardiology/American Heart Association Task Force on Practice Guidelines, *Circulation* 105 (2005): e154–e234.

64. Lloyd-Jones and coauthors, 2009.

65. Lloyd-Jones and coauthors, 2009.

66. Lloyd-Jones and coauthors, 2009.

67. B. T. Vanderhoff and W. Carroll, Neurology, in R. E. Rakel, ed., *Textbook of Family Medicine* (Philadelphia: Saunders, 2007), pp. 1283–1334.

68. J. A. Zivin, Ischemic cerebrovascular disease, in L. Goldman and D. Ausiello, eds., *Cecil Medicine* (Philadelphia: Saunders, 2008), pp. 2708–2719.

Helping People with Feeding Disabilities

Chapter 21 referred to difficulties following a stroke that can interfere with the ability to eat independently. This Nutrition in Practice discusses the problems faced by individuals who must cope with various disabilities that interfere with the process of eating, such as those that interfere with chewing and swallowing. These obstacles can arise at any time during a person's life and from any number of causes. An infant may be born with a physical impairment such as cleft palate; an adolescent may lose motor control following injuries sustained in an automobile accident; an older adult may struggle with the pain of arthritis or the mental deterioration of dementia. Table NP21-1 lists some of the conditions that may lead to feeding problems.

In what ways can disabilities impair a person's ability to eat?

Eating and drinking require a considerable number of individual coordinated motions. Consider an infant learning the skills required for feeding: each step—sitting, grasping cups and utensils, bringing food to the mouth, biting, chewing, and swallowing—requires coordinated movements. An injury or disability that interferes with any of these movements can lead to feeding problems and inadequate food intake. Total food intake is often significantly reduced when individuals with inefficient motor function take a long time to eat.[1] Difficulties that affect procurement of food, such as the inability to drive, walk, or carry groceries, can also lower food intake and lead to malnutrition and weight loss.

How may disease symptoms or medications alter food intake or nutrition status?

Examples of disease symptoms that can alter food intake include nausea, frequent coughing or choking, difficulty breathing, and gastroesophageal reflux. Individuals with speech and hearing problems may have a difficult time communicating with caregivers about thirst and hunger. Mobility problems can influence nutrition status by leading to bone demineralization and pressure sores.

Conditions that require the use of multiple medications can also have a significant impact on nutrition status (see Chapter 14).[2] Medications may increase or decrease appetite, interfere with nutrient metabolism, or have gastrointestinal effects that cause pain or discomfort with eating.

Can disabilities alter a person's energy needs?

Yes, certain disabilities can either increase or decrease energy requirements. Disabilities that affect muscle tension and mobility can reduce physical activity and, consequently, energy requirements. Other disabilities, such as certain forms of cerebral palsy, cause involuntary muscle activity that raises energy requirements.[3] Loss of a limb due to amputation reduces energy needs in proportion to the weight and metabolism represented by the missing limb, but energy needs may be greater if an individual increases activity to compensate for the loss, such as by propelling a wheelchair. Because the effects of disabilities are often unpredictable, the health care practitioner may find it difficult to assess energy requirements until weight gain or loss has occurred.

Overweight and obesity often accompany conditions that limit mobility or result in short stature; examples include Down syndrome and spina bifida. Obesity may also develop because the family or caregiver provides an inappropriate amount of food, sometimes out of sympathy for the disabled individual.[4] In these cases, the health practitioner may need to counsel the family or caregiver about appropriate food choices and portion sizes.

TABLE NP21-1	Conditions That May Lead to Feeding Problems

The following conditions may lead to feeding problems by interfering with a person's ability to suck, bite, chew, swallow, or coordinate hand-to-mouth movements.

- Accidents
- Amputations
- Arthritis
- Birth defects
- Cerebral palsy
- Cleft palate
- Down syndrome
- Head injuries
- Huntington's chorea
- Language, visual, or hearing impairments
- Multiple sclerosis
- Muscle weakness
- Muscular dystrophy
- Neuromotor dysfunction
- Parkinson's disease
- Polio
- Spinal cord injuries
- Stroke

Which health professionals typically work with people who have feeding problems?

Evaluating and treating feeding problems often involve the joint efforts of health care professionals from a variety of disciplines, including nurses, dietitians, occupational and physical therapists, speech-language pathologists, and dentists. Together, these professionals evaluate each patient's dietary needs and assess abilities to chew, sip, swallow, grasp utensils, use utensils to pick up foods, and bring foods from the plate to the mouth. A speech-language pathologist most often evaluates chewing and swallowing abilities and trains patients to use lips, tongue, and throat for eating and speaking. An occupational therapist can demonstrate alternate feeding strategies, including changes in body position that improve feeding, techniques for handling utensils and food, and use of special feeding devices.

Direct observation of a patient during mealtimes allows health care professionals to assess current eating behaviors, demonstrate feeding techniques, monitor the patient's and caregiver's understanding of the techniques, and evaluate how well the care plan is working. To illustrate, consider a child with a feeding problem caused by hypersensitivity to oral stimulation. The health care professional may start by teaching the caregiver to gently and playfully stroke the child's face with a hand, washcloth, or soft toy. Once the child tolerates touch on less sensitive areas of the face, the health care professional may encourage the caregiver to slowly begin to rub the child's lips, gums, palate, and tongue. With time, the child may be better able to tolerate the presence

Adaptive feeding equipment can help patients with feeding disabilities gain independence.

© Wadsworth, Cengage Learning

TABLE NP21-2 | Interventions for Feeding-Related Problems

Inability to Suck
- Use squeeze bottles, which do not require sucking, to express liquids into the mouth.
- Place a spoon on the center of the tongue, and apply downward pressure to stimulate sucking.
- Apply rhythmic, slow strokes on the tongue to alter tongue position and improve the sucking response.

Inability to Chew
- Place foods between gums and teeth to promote chewing.
- Improve chewing skills with foods of different textures; for example, fruit leathers stimulate jaw movements but dissolve quickly enough to minimize choking.
- Provide soft foods that require minimal chewing or are easily chewed.

Inability to Swallow
- Provide thickened liquids, pureed foods, and moist foods that form boluses easily.
- Provide cold formulas, frozen fruit juice bars, and ice; cold substances promote swallowing movements by the tongue and soft palate.
- Make sure the patient's jaw and lips are closed to facilitate swallowing action.
- Correct posture and head position if they interfere with swallowing ability.

Inability to Grasp or Coordinate Movements
- Provide utensils that have modified handles, or are smaller or larger as necessary.
- Encourage the use of hands for feeding if utensils are difficult to maneuver.
- Provide plates with food guards to prevent spilling.
- Supply clothing protection.

Impaired Vision
- Place foods (meats, vegetables) in similar locations on the plate at each meal.
- Provide plates with food guards to prevent spilling.

of food in the mouth. Examples of other strategies that can help feeding problems are listed in Table NP21-2.

Can special equipment be used to help people with certain feeding difficulties?

Yes. Adaptive feeding devices can make a remarkable difference in a person's ability to eat independently. Figure NP21-1

Nutrition and Disorders of the Heart and Blood Vessels

Utensils

Rocker knife

Roller knife

People with only one arm or hand may have difficulty cutting foods and may appreciate using a *rocker knife* or a *roller knife.*

People with a limited range of motion can feed themselves better when they use *flatware with built-up handles.*

People with extreme muscle weakness may be able to eat with a *utensil holder.*

For people with tremors, spasticity, and uneven jerky movements, *weighted utensils* can aid the feeding process.

Battery-powered feeding machines enable people with severe limitations to eat with less assistance from others.

Plates

People who have limited dexterity and difficulty maneuvering food find *scoop dishes* or *food guards* useful.

People with uncontrolled or excessive movements might move dishes around while eating and may benefit from using *unbreakable dishes with suction cups.*

Cups

People with limited neck motion can use a *cutout plastic cup.*

Two-handed cups enable people with moderate muscle weakness to lift a cup with two hands.

People with uncontrolled or excessive movements might prefer to drink liquids from a *covered cup* or glass with a *slotted opening* or spout.

A soft, flexible long plastic straw may also ease the task of drinking.

shows a few of the many special feeding devices that are available and describes their uses. Other examples of adaptive equipment include specialized chairs to improve posture, bolsters inserted under arms to improve elbow stability, and raised trays or eating surfaces to simplify hand-to-mouth movements.[5]

Sometimes, despite the best efforts of all involved, a patient is unable to consume enough food by mouth. In these cases, tube feedings can help to improve nutrition status. Tube feedings are also recommended for patients who have severe dysphagia (difficulty swallowing) or aspiration pneumonia.[6]

In what ways can feeding difficulties affect family life?

Mealtimes are a critical time for social interaction, and therefore individuals with feeding problems may encounter emotional and social problems if they are unable to participate. Children may fail to develop social skills, whereas adults may miss the social stimulation that mealtimes provide. Individuals should be encouraged to sit with family and friends during meals so that they are not deprived of the social and cultural aspects of eating.

The responsibility of caring for a person with a feeding problem can frequently overwhelm a caregiver. Caring for a person with disabilities requires time and patience—and many new therapies to be learned and administered. The caregiver may spend many hours preparing special foods, monitoring the use of adaptive feeding equipment, and helping with feedings. Moreover, a person with disabilities may need help with other tasks as well, and all may require a considerable amount of time. In many cases, a caregiver receives little or no assistance. These conditions may lead to strained interactions between caregiver and patient and cause frustration and depression.[7] Psychologists can offer counseling to patients or caregivers to help them adjust, and all members of the health care team can offer emotional support and practical suggestions to ease caregivers' responsibilities and frustrations.

Successful therapy for people with feeding disabilities requires the involvement of many health care professionals and depends on accurate identification of impaired feeding skills and determination of appropriate interventions. Ideally, with training, people with disabilities attain total independence—they are able to prepare, serve, and eat nutritionally adequate food daily without help. In some cases, these goals can be met with the help of caregivers. The combined efforts of the health care team can support both patients and caregivers in enhancing quality of life and in achieving independence to the greatest degree possible.

Notes

1. E. B. Fung and coauthors, Feeding dysfunction is associated with poor growth and health status in children with cerebral palsy, *Journal of the American Dietetic Association* 102 (2002): 361–368.
2. Position of the American Dietetic Association: Providing nutrition services for infants, children, and adults with developmental disabilities and special health care needs, *Journal of the American Dietetic Association* 104 (2004): 97–107.
3. Position of the American Dietetic Association, 2004.
4. H. H. Cloud, Expanding roles for dietitians working with persons with developmental disabilities, *Journal of the American Dietetic Association* 97 (1997): 129–130.
5. J. Case-Smith and R. Humphry, Feeding and oral motor skills, in J. Case-Smith, A. S. Allen, and P. N. Pratt, eds., *Occupational Therapy for Children* (St. Louis: Mosby–Year Book, 1996), pp. 430–460.
6. Position of the American Dietetic Association, 2004.
7. Fung and coauthors, 2002.

CONTENTS

nephron (NEF-ron): the functional unit of the kidneys, consisting of a glomerulus and tubules.
- *nephros* = kidney

glomerulus (gloh-MEHR-yoo-lus): a tuft of capillaries within the nephron that filters water and solutes from blood as urine production begins (plural: *glomeruli*).

filtrate: the substances that pass through the glomerulus and travel through the nephron's tubules, eventually forming urine.

Bowman's (BOE-minz) capsule: a cuplike component of the nephron that surrounds the glomerulus and collects the filtrate that is passed to the tubules.

tubules: tubelike structures of the nephron that process filtrate during urine production. The tubules are surrounded by capillaries that reabsorb substances retained by tubule cells.

erythropoietin (eh-RITH-ro-POY-eh-tin): a hormone made by the kidneys that stimulates red blood cell production.

renal (REE-nal): pertaining to the kidneys.

THE TWO KIDNEYS SIT JUST ABOVE THE WAIST ON EACH SIDE OF THE spinal column. As part of the urinary system, they are responsible for filtering the blood and removing excess fluid and wastes for elimination in urine. Because the kidneys are so proficient at this task, disturbances in body fluids that result from food intake, physical activity, and metabolism are normally corrected within hours.

Figure 22-1 shows the kidneys' placement and structure and one of their functional units, the **nephron**. Within each nephron, the **glomerulus**, a ball-shaped tuft of capillaries, serves as a gateway through which the blood components must pass to form **filtrate**. The glomerulus and surrounding **Bowman's capsule** function like a sieve, retaining blood cells and plasma proteins in blood while allowing fluid and small solutes to enter the nephron's system of **tubules**. As the filtrate passes through the tubules, its composition changes as some of its components are reabsorbed and returned to the blood via capillaries surrounding each tubule. Eventually, the remaining filtrate enters a duct shared by several nephrons, and additional water is reabsorbed to form the final urine product. By filtering the blood and forming urine, the kidneys regulate the extracellular fluid volume and osmolarity, electrolyte concentrations, and acid-base balance. They also excrete metabolic waste products such as urea and creatinine, as well as various drugs and toxins. Other roles of the kidney include the following:

- Secretion of the enzyme *renin*, which helps to regulate blood pressure
- Production of the hormone **erythropoietin**, which stimulates the production of red blood cells in the bone marrow
- Conversion of vitamin D to its active form, thereby playing a primary role in calcium regulation and bone formation

Subsequent sections of this chapter explain how **renal** diseases can interfere with the kidneys' various functions and severely disrupt health.

FIGURE 22-1 | The Kidneys and Nephron Function

A nephron (a working unit of the kidney). Each kidney contains about one million nephrons.

Blood vessel — Glomerulus

Capillaries of glomerulus

Tubule

1 Blood flows into the glomerulus, and some of its fluid, with dissolved substances, is absorbed into the tubule.

Kidney
Ureter
Pelvis
Bladder

To the body

Renal artery
Renal vein

2 Then the fluid and substances needed by the body are returned to the blood in vessels alongside the tubule.

3 The tubule passes waste materials on to the bladder.

To the bladder

Kidney, sectioned to show location of nephrons

The Nephrotic Syndrome

The **nephrotic syndrome** is not a specific disease; rather, the term refers to kidney disorders that result in urinary protein losses (**proteinuria**) exceeding 3 grams per day.[1] The condition arises when damage to the glomeruli increases their permeability to plasma proteins, allowing protein to escape into the urine. The nephrotic syndrome can occur at any age, but it is seen most often in children between 1½ and 4 years of age.[2] Although various diseases involving the glomeruli are often the cause, the nephrotic syndrome may also be a complication of diabetes mellitus, immunological and hereditary disorders, infections (involving the kidneys or elsewhere in the body), chemical damage (from medications or illicit drugs), and some cancers. Along with proteinuria, typical clinical findings include low serum albumin levels, edema, elevated blood lipids, and blood coagulation disorders. The nephrotic syndrome can sometimes progress to renal failure.

CONSEQUENCES OF THE NEPHROTIC SYNDROME

In the nephrotic syndrome, urinary protein losses generally average about 8 grams daily, but additional protein is lost due to protein catabolism within the kidney tubules.[3] The liver attempts to compensate for these losses by increasing its synthesis of certain plasma proteins, but the excessive production of some of the proteins leads to various complications.

Edema Because albumin is the most abundant plasma protein, it is also the protein with the most significant losses in urine. Consequently, blood levels of albumin are markedly reduced, contributing to a fluid shift from blood plasma to the interstitial spaces and, thus, edema. (✚) Impaired sodium excretion also contributes to edema: the kidney tubules reabsorb sodium in greater amounts than usual, causing sodium and water retention within the body.[4]

Risk of Cardiovascular Disease Individuals with the nephrotic syndrome frequently have elevated levels of low-density lipoproteins (LDL), very-low-density lipoproteins (VLDL), and the more damaging LDL variant known as lipoprotein(a). Furthermore, the risk of blood clotting is increased due to urinary losses of proteins that inhibit blood clotting and elevated levels of plasma proteins that favor clotting. These factors raise the risks of developing heart disease and stroke.[5]

Other Effects of the Nephrotic Syndrome The proteins lost in urine include immunoglobulins (antibodies) and vitamin D–binding protein. Depletion of immunoglobulins increases susceptibility to infection. Loss of vitamin D–binding protein results in lower vitamin D and calcium levels and increases the risk of rickets in children. Patients with the nephrotic syndrome frequently develop protein-energy malnutrition (PEM) and muscle wasting from the continued proteinuria. Figure 22-2 summarizes the effects of urinary protein losses in the nephrotic syndrome.

TREATMENT OF THE NEPHROTIC SYNDROME

Medical treatment of the nephrotic syndrome requires diagnosis and management of the underlying disorder responsible for the proteinuria. Complications are managed with medications and medical nutrition therapy. The drugs prescribed may include diuretics, ACE inhibitors (which reduce protein losses), lipid-lowering drugs, anticoagulants, antiinflammatory drugs (usually corticosteroids), and immunosuppressants (such as cyclosporine).[6] Nutrition therapy helps to alleviate edema, prevent PEM, and slow the progression of atherosclerosis.

✚ Reminder: Plasma proteins, such as albumin, help to maintain fluid balance within the blood.

nephrotic (neh-FROT-ik) syndrome: a syndrome associated with kidney disorders that cause urinary protein losses exceeding 3 g/day; symptoms include low serum albumin, elevated blood lipids, and edema.

proteinuria (PRO-teen-NOO-ree-ah): loss of protein, mostly albumin, in the urine; also known as *albuminuria*.

> NURSING DIAGNOSIS
>
> *Excess fluid volume, risk for infection, and imbalanced nutrition: less than body requirements* may apply to people with the nephrotic syndrome.

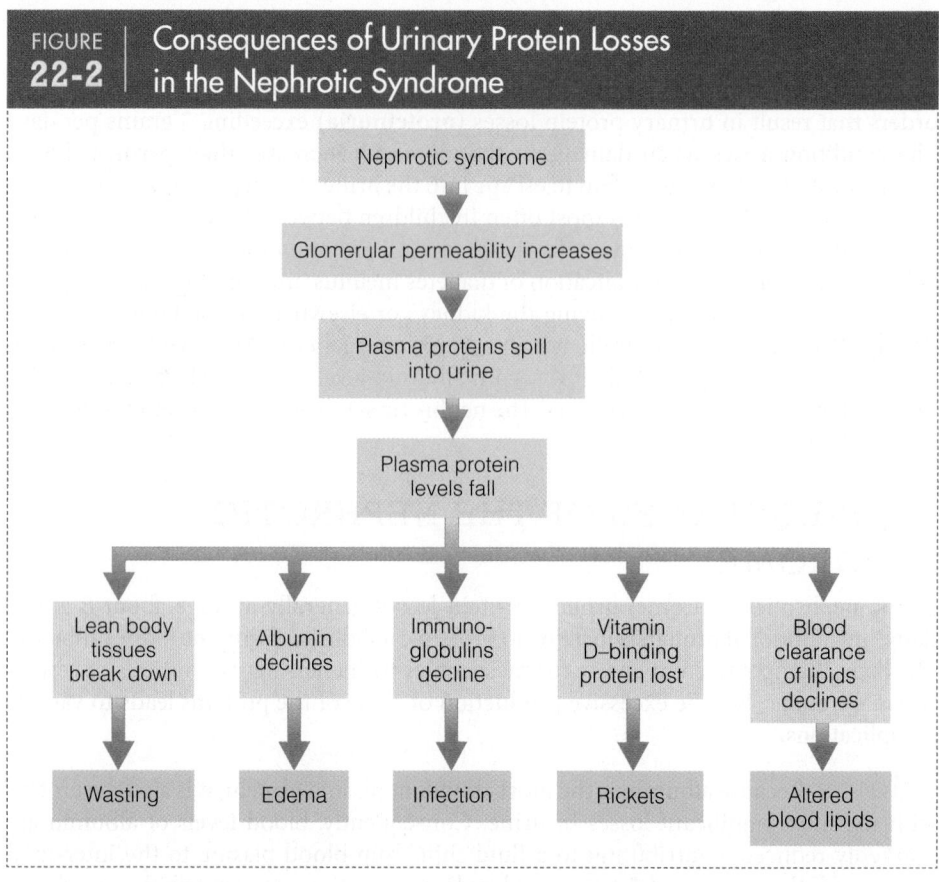

FIGURE
22-2

FIGURE 22-2 | Consequences of Urinary Protein Losses in the Nephrotic Syndrome

Nephrotic syndrome

Glomerular permeability increases

Plasma proteins spill into urine

Plasma protein levels fall

Lean body tissues break down	Albumin declines	Immuno-globulins decline	Vitamin D–binding protein lost	Blood clearance of lipids declines
Wasting	Edema	Infection	Rickets	Altered blood lipids

Protein and Energy Meeting protein and energy needs helps to minimize losses of muscle tissue. High-protein diets are not advised, however, because they can exacerbate urinary protein losses and result in further damage to the kidneys.[7] Instead, the protein intake should fall between 0.8 and 1.0 gram per kilogram of body weight per day. At least half of the protein consumed should be from high-quality sources, such as milk products, meat, fish, poultry, eggs, and soy products. An adequate energy intake (about 35 kcalories per kilogram of body weight daily) sustains weight and spares protein. Weight loss or infections suggest the need for additional kcalories.

Fat As Chapter 21 explained, a diet low in saturated fat, *trans* fats, cholesterol, and refined sugars helps to control elevated blood lipids. Thus, patients with the nephrotic syndrome should limit saturated fat intake to 7 percent of total kcalories, avoid foods that contain *trans* fats, and limit cholesterol intake to 200 milligrams per day. Dietary measures are usually inadequate for controlling blood lipids, however, so physicians usually prescribe lipid-lowering medications as well.

Sodium and Potassium Controlling sodium intake helps to control edema; therefore, sodium intake is often restricted to 1 to 2 grams daily.[8] Table 22-1 provides guidelines for following a diet restricted to 2 grams of sodium. If diuretics prescribed for the edema cause potassium losses, patients are encouraged to select foods rich in potassium (see Chapter 9).

Vitamins and Minerals Multivitamin/mineral supplementation is often advised to avoid nutrient deficiencies; nutrients at risk include vitamin B_6, vitamin B_{12}, folate, iron, copper, and zinc.[9] (✚) Patients with the nephrotic syndrome also require calcium and vitamin D supplementation to help prevent bone loss and rickets.

✚ Nutrient deficiencies may develop if the carrier proteins for nutrients are lost in the urine.

| TABLE 22-1 | Sodium-Controlled Diet |

General Guidelines

About 75 percent of the sodium in a typical diet comes from processed foods, about 10 percent from unprocessed natural foods, and about 15 percent from table salt. With this in mind:

- Whenever possible, select fresh foods, which are usually low in sodium.
- Select frozen and canned food products that have been prepared without added salt.
- Avoid adding salt to foods while cooking or at the table.
- When dining in restaurants, ask that meals be prepared without salt.

Sodium in Foods

All foods contain sodium, but some contain more than others. Use the information in the table below to plan meals that are low in sodium.

Food Group	Serving Size	Sodium per Serving (mg)
Milk products	1 cup milk or yogurt; 1 oz hard cheese (cheddar, Swiss, jack)	150–200
	Avoid: buttermilk, cottage cheese, cheese spreads, prepared cheeses (such as American cheese)	
Meat, fish, poultry, and eggs	3 oz fresh meat, fish, or poultry; 1 large egg	60
	Avoid: luncheon meats, corned beef, salt pork, sausage, frankfurters, bacon, canned meats or fish, fresh meats prepared with injected broth	
Fruits and vegetables	½ cup fresh vegetables, ½ cup fresh or frozen fruit, 6 oz fruit juice; 6 oz tomato or vegetable juice without added salt	10–20
	Avoid: pickled vegetables, olives, tomato or vegetable juices with added salt; dried fruits with added sodium sulfite	
Breads and cereals	½–⅔ cup dry or cooked cereal without added salt, ½ cup cooked rice or pasta	0–10
	1 slice bread, 1 roll or tortilla, ½–⅔ cup dry or cooked cereal prepared with salt	150
	Avoid: pancakes, waffles, muffins, biscuits, and quick breads made with baking powder or baking soda; instant and ready-to-eat cereals with >175 mg sodium; salted snack foods	
Condiments	Unsalted butter; low-sodium salad dressings, mayonnaise, sauces, and gravies; low-sodium catsup, mustard, and hot sauces; garlic or onion powders without added salt; lemon or lime juice, vinegar	Varies; check labels
	Avoid: commercial salad dressings, gravy mixes, barbeque sauces, soy sauce, steak sauces, and spices or herb products made with salt; bouillon, meat tenderizers, monosodium glutamate	

A Sample Diet Restricted to 2 Grams (2000 mg) of Sodium

Using the information above, an individual can develop many sample menus. A possible plan for a day might look like this:

Food Group	Sodium (mg)
Meat, 6 oz (2 servings × 60 mg)	120
Milk, 3 c (3 servings × 150 mg)	450
Fruit, 2 servings	negligible
Vegetables, 3 servings	45
Whole-grain bread, 4 slices (4 × 150 mg)	600
Salt, ¼ tsp (used lightly at meals)	600
Total	**1815**

Individuals can use the remainder of the sodium allowance for whatever foods they choose. The sodium content of most foods can be determined by reading food labels or using food composition tables.

Review Notes

- The nephrotic syndrome is characterized by urinary protein losses exceeding 3 grams per day. Complications include edema, lipid abnormalities, blood coagulation disorders, reduced immunity, rickets, and PEM.
- Individuals with the nephrotic syndrome are prescribed medications to treat the underlying cause of proteinuria and manage complications. The diet should provide sufficient protein and energy to maintain health, but patients should avoid consuming excess protein. Other dietary adjustments can help to correct edema, lipid disorders, and nutrient deficiencies.

Acute Kidney Injury

In **acute kidney injury**, kidney function declines rapidly, over hours or days. The loss of kidney function reduces urine output and allows nitrogenous wastes to build up in blood. The degree of renal dysfunction varies from mild to severe. With prompt treatment, acute kidney injury is often reversible, although mortality rates are high, ranging from 36 to 86 percent.[10]

CAUSES OF ACUTE KIDNEY INJURY

Many different disorders can lead to acute kidney injury, and it often develops as a consequence of severe illness, injury, or surgery. To aid in diagnosis and treatment, its causes are commonly classified as prerenal, intrarenal, or postrenal. *Prerenal* factors are those that cause a sudden reduction in blood flow to the kidneys; they often involve a severe stressor such as heart failure, shock, or blood loss. Factors that damage kidney tissue, such as infections, toxins, drugs, or direct trauma, are classified as *intrarenal* causes of acute kidney injury. *Postrenal* factors are those that prevent excretion of urine due to urinary tract obstructions. Table 22-2 provides examples of specific disorders that may cause acute kidney injury.

CONSEQUENCES OF ACUTE KIDNEY INJURY

A decline in renal function alters the composition of blood and urine. The kidneys may become unable to regulate the levels of electrolytes, acid, and nitrogenous wastes in the blood. Urine may be diminished in quantity or absent, leading to fluid retention. Diagnosis is often a complex task because the clinical effects can be subtle and vary according to the underlying cause of disease.

TABLE 22-2	Causes of Acute Kidney Injury	
Prerenal Factors (60 to 70% of cases)	**Intrarenal Factors** (25 to 40% of cases)	**Postrenal Factors** (5 to 10% of cases)
• **Low blood volume or pressure:** hemorrhage, burns, sepsis or shock, anaphylactic reactions, nephrotic syndrome, gastrointestinal losses, diuretics, antihypertensive medications • **Renal artery disorders:** blood clots or emboli, stenosis, aneurysm, trauma • **Heart disorders:** heart failure, heart attack, arrhythmias	• **Vascular disorders:** sickle-cell disease, diabetes mellitus, transfusion reactions • **Obstructions (within kidney):** inflammation, tumors, stones, scar tissue • **Renal injury:** infections, environmental contaminants, drugs, medications, *E. coli* food poisoning	• **Obstructions (ureter or bladder):** strictures, tumors, stones, trauma • **Prostate disorders:** cancer or hyperplasia • **Renal vein thrombosis** • **Bladder disorders:** neurological conditions, bladder rupture • **Pregnancy**

Fluid and Electrolyte Imbalances About half of patients with acute kidney injury experience **oliguria**, producing less than 400 milliliters of urine per day (normal urine volume typically exceeds 800 milliliters, or about 3.4 cups, daily).[11] The reduced excretion of fluids and electrolytes results in sodium retention and elevated levels of potassium, phosphate, and magnesium in the blood. Elevated potassium (**hyperkalemia**) is of particular concern because potassium imbalances can alter heart rate and lead to heart failure. Elevated serum phosphate levels (**hyperphosphatemia**) (✚) promote excessive secretion of parathyroid hormone, leading to losses in bone calcium. Due to the sodium retention and reduced urine production, edema is a common symptom of acute kidney injury and may be apparent as puffiness in the face and hands and swelling of the feet and ankles.

Uremia As a result of impaired kidney function, nitrogen-containing waste products—blood urea nitrogen (BUN), creatinine, and uric acid—accumulate in the blood (refer to Table 13-9 on pp. 395–396 for normal laboratory values). Furthermore, the tissue catabolism that accompanies illness generates more nitrogenous waste than usual. The clinical outcome, called **uremia**, includes symptoms such as fatigue, lethargy, confusion, headache, anorexia, a metallic taste in the mouth, nausea and vomiting, and diarrhea. In more serious cases, elevated blood pressure, rapid heartbeat, seizures, and delirium or coma may occur. It is sometimes difficult to distinguish the symptoms of uremia from those of the underlying illness.

TREATMENT OF ACUTE KIDNEY INJURY

Treatment of acute kidney injury involves a combination of drug therapy, **dialysis**, (✚) and medical nutrition therapy to restore fluid and electrolyte balances and minimize blood concentrations of toxic waste products. Both medical care and dietary recommendations are highly individualized to suit each patient's needs. Correcting the underlying illness is necessary to prevent further damage to the kidneys.

In oliguric patients (those with reduced urine production), recovery from kidney injury sometimes begins with a period of **diuresis**, in which large amounts of fluid are excreted. Because tubular function is minimal at this stage, electrolytes may not be sufficiently reabsorbed; consequently, both fluid depletion and electrolyte imbalances become a concern. Patients with this pattern of recovery (generally those with tubular injury) must be monitored closely in case they require fluid and electrolyte replacement.[12]

Drug Treatment in Acute Kidney Injury Because kidney function is required for drug excretion, patients may need to use lower doses of their usual medications to compensate for limited urine output. Conversely, dialysis treatment may increase losses of some drugs, and doses may need to be increased. Drugs that are **nephrotoxic** (including some antibiotics and nonsteroidal antiinflammatory drugs) must be avoided until kidney function improves.

The medications prescribed for acute kidney injury depend on the underlying cause of illness and the complications that develop. For patients with edema, diuretics may be used to mobilize fluids; furosemide (Lasix) is the usual choice. Immunosuppressants may be prescribed for patients with inflammatory conditions. Patients with hyperkalemia are given potassium-exchange resins that bind potassium ions in the gastrointestinal (GI) tract, ensuring the elimination of potassium in the stool. Rapid correction of hyperkalemia requires the use of insulin, which causes a temporary shift of extracellular potassium into the cells. (Glucose must be supplied along with insulin to prevent hypoglycemia.) If acidosis is present, bicarbonate may be administered orally or intravenously.[13]

Protein and Energy Although its effects are highly variable, acute kidney injury is often a catabolic condition associated with hypermetabolism and muscle wasting. Thus, sufficient protein and energy must be ingested to preserve muscle mass. Initially, the patient may be provided with about 30 to 35 kcalories per kilogram of body weight per day, while body weight is monitored to ensure that energy intake is adequate. If available, indirect calorimetry provides the best estimate of energy needs.

✚ To measure serum phosphate levels, the phosphorus content of the blood is analyzed; thus, the terms *serum phosphate* and *serum phosphorus* are often used interchangeably.

✚ Nutrition in Practice 22 describes common dialysis procedures, including *continuous renal replacement therapy*, the approach usually used for treating acute kidney injury.

oliguria (OL-lih-GOO-ree-ah): an abnormally low amount of urine, often less than 400 mL/day.

hyperkalemia (HIGH-per-ka-LEE-me-ah): elevated serum potassium levels.

hyperphosphatemia (HIGH-per-fos-fa-TEE-me-ah): elevated serum phosphate levels.

uremia (you-REE-me-ah): the abnormal accumulation of nitrogen-containing substances, especially urea, in the blood; also called *azotemia* (AZE-oh-TEE-me-ah).

dialysis (dye-AH-lih-sis): a treatment that removes wastes and excess fluid from the blood after the kidneys have stopped functioning. The most common types of dialysis are *hemodialysis* and *peritoneal dialysis* (see Nutrition in Practice 22).

diuresis (DYE-uh-REE-sis): increased urine production.

nephrotoxic: toxic to the kidneys.

Protein contributes nitrogen, increasing the kidneys' workload, but intake should be sufficient to prevent negative nitrogen balance and additional wasting. Protein recommendations are influenced by kidney function, the degree of catabolism, and the use of dialysis (dialysis removes nitrogenous wastes).[14] Protein restriction to about 0.6 to 0.8 grams per kilogram of body weight per day may be necessary for patients with limited kidney function who are not treated with dialysis. Higher intakes (up to 2.0 grams per kilogram daily) may be recommended if kidney function improves or the treatment includes dialysis. Patients who are catabolic or septic typically have high protein needs, but they require dialysis to accommodate the additional nitrogen load.

Fluids Health practitioners can assess fluid status by monitoring weight fluctuations, blood pressure, pulse rates, and the appearance of the skin and mucous membranes. Another method is to measure serum sodium concentrations: a low level of sodium often indicates excessive fluid intake, and a high level suggests inadequate intake.

Fluid balance must be restored in patients who are either overhydrated or dehydrated. Thereafter, fluid needs can be estimated by measuring urine output and adding about 500 milliliters to account for the water lost from skin, lungs, and perspiration. An individual with fever, vomiting, or diarrhea requires additional fluid. Patients undergoing dialysis can ingest fluids more freely.

Electrolytes Serum electrolyte levels are monitored closely to determine appropriate electrolyte intakes. Generally, the potassium intake is restricted to 2000 to 3000 milligrams daily. A phosphorus restriction may be necessary if hyperphosphatemia is present. The sodium intake should match urinary sodium losses unless edema is present; the recommended intake is usually between 1100 and 3300 milligrams sodium per day.[15] Patients undergoing dialysis can consume electrolytes more freely. As mentioned previously, oliguric patients who experience diuresis at the beginning of the recovery period may need electrolyte replacement to compensate for urinary losses.

Enteral and Parenteral Nutrition Some patients need enteral or parenteral nutrition support to obtain adequate energy. Enteral nutrition (tube feeding) is generally preferred over parenteral nutrition because it is less likely to cause infection and sepsis. Enteral formulas for patients with renal failure are more kcalorically dense and have lower protein and electrolyte concentrations than standard formulas. Total parenteral nutrition is necessary only if patients are severely malnourished or cannot consume food for more than 14 days.

CASE STUDY | Woman with Acute Kidney Injury

Catherine Garber is a 42-year-old office manager admitted to the hospital's intensive care unit. She was first seen in the emergency room with severe edema, headache, nausea and vomiting, and a rapid heart rate. She reported an inability to pass more than minimal amounts of urine in the past two days. Her son, who drove her to the emergency room, reported that she had missed work for several days and seemed confused and unusually tired. Laboratory tests revealed elevated serum creatinine, BUN, and potassium levels. After learning from her medical history that Mrs. Garber had begun taking penicillin earlier in the week, the physician diagnosed acute kidney injury, probably caused by a reaction to the medication. Mrs. Garber is 5 feet 3 inches tall and weighs 125 pounds.

1. Describe the probable reason for Mrs. Garber's inability to produce urine. Is her reaction to penicillin considered a prerenal, intrarenal, or postrenal cause of kidney injury? Give examples of other medical problems that can cause acute kidney injury.

2. What medications can the physician prescribe to treat Mrs. Garber's edema and hyperkalemia? What recommendation is likely regarding her continued use of penicillin?

3. What concerns should be kept in mind when determining Mrs. Garber's energy, protein, fluid, and electrolyte needs during acute kidney injury? How would dialysis treatment alter recommendations?

4. After treatment begins, Mrs. Garber suddenly begins producing copious amounts of urine. How should this development alter dietary treatment?

As you read through the discussion of chronic kidney disease, consider how Mrs. Garber's diet should change if her kidney problems become chronic.

➕ The kidneys' ability to function despite loss of nephrons is referred to as *renal reserve*.

➕ Reminder: *Creatinine* is a waste product of creatine, a nitrogen-containing compound in muscle cells.

➕ Reminder: *Aldosterone* promotes sodium (and therefore water) retention and potassium excretion.

Chronic Kidney Disease

Unlike acute kidney injury, in which kidney function declines suddenly and rapidly, **chronic kidney disease** is characterized by gradual, irreversible deterioration. Because the kidneys have a large functional reserve, (➕) the disease typically progresses over many years without causing symptoms. Patients are typically diagnosed late in the course of illness, after most kidney function has been lost.[16]

The most common causes of chronic kidney disease are diabetes mellitus and hypertension, which are estimated to cause 45 and 27 percent of cases, respectively.[17] Other conditions that lead to chronic kidney disease include inflammatory, immunological, and hereditary diseases that directly involve the kidneys. **Polycystic kidney disease**, characterized by the formation of multiple cysts in both kidneys, is a common hereditary condition that accounts for about 5 to 10 percent of chronic kidney disease cases.[18] Chronic kidney disease sometimes follows acute kidney injury.

chronic kidney disease: a kidney disease characterized by gradual, irreversible deterioration of the kidneys; also known as *chronic renal failure.*

polycystic kidney disease: a hereditary disorder characterized by the formation of multiple cysts in the kidneys.

end-stage renal disease (ESRD): an advanced stage of chronic kidney disease in which dialysis or a kidney transplant is necessary to sustain life.

CONSEQUENCES OF CHRONIC KIDNEY DISEASE

In the early stages of chronic kidney disease, the nephrons compensate by enlarging so that they can handle the extra workload. As the nephrons deteriorate, however, there is additional work for the remaining nephrons. The overburdened nephrons continue to degenerate until finally the kidneys are unable to function adequately, resulting in kidney failure. Once the extent of kidney damage necessitates active treatment—either dialysis or a kidney transplant—the condition is classified as **end-stage renal disease (ESRD)**.[19] Without intervention at this stage, an individual cannot survive. Table 22-3 lists the common clinical effects of the early and advanced stages of chronic kidney disease. Symptoms of chronic kidney disease may not appear until more than 75 percent of kidney function is lost.[20]

Renal disease is evaluated using the **glomerular filtration rate (GFR)**, the rate at which the kidneys form filtrate. The GFR can be estimated using predictive equations that are based on serum creatinine levels, (➕) age, gender, race, and body size. Table 22-4 shows how chronic kidney disease is classified according to estimated GFR. Other laboratory measures used to assess kidney function include urinary protein levels, BUN, and the ratio of albumin to creatinine in a urine sample.[21]

Altered Electrolytes and Hormones As GFR falls, the increased activity by the remaining nephrons is often sufficient to maintain electrolyte excretion. Therefore, fluid and electrolyte disturbances may not develop until the third or fourth stage of chronic kidney disease (see Table 22-4).[22] A number of hormonal adaptations also help to regulate electrolyte levels, but these changes may cause complications of their own. The increased secretion of aldosterone (➕) helps to prevent increases in

TABLE 22-3	Clinical Effects of Chronic Kidney Disease

Early Stages

- Anorexia
- Fatigue
- Headache
- Hypertension
- Itching
- Kidney inflammation or nephrotic syndrome
- Nausea and vomiting
- Proteinuria, hematuria (blood in urine)

Advanced Stages

- Anemia, bleeding tendency
- Cardiovascular disease
- Confusion, mental impairments
- Electrolyte abnormalities
- Fluid retention
- Hormonal abnormalities
- Metabolic acidosis
- Peripheral neuropathy
- Protein-energy malnutrition
- Reduced immunity
- Renal osteodystrophy

TABLE 22-4	Evaluation of Chronic Kidney Disease	
Stage of Disease	Description	GFR[a] (mL/min per 1.73 m²)
1	Kidney damage with normal or increased GFR	≥90
2	Kidney damage with mildly decreased GFR	60–89
3	Moderately decreased GFR	30–59
4	Severely decreased GFR	15–29
5	Kidney failure	<15 (or undergoing dialysis)

[a] Glomerular filtration rate, or GFR, is estimated from the Modification of Diet in Renal Disease study equation and is based on age, gender, race, and calibration for serum creatinine. Normal GFR is approximately 125 milliliters per minute.

Source: A. S. Levey and coauthors, National Kidney Foundation practice guidelines for chronic kidney disease: Evaluation, classification, and stratification, *Annals of Internal Medicine* 139 (2003): 137–147.

✚ Reminder: *Parathyroid hormone* helps to regulate serum concentrations of calcium and phosphorus. Elevated parathyroid hormone stimulates bone turnover and the release of calcium from bone into blood.

glomerular filtration rate (GFR): the rate at which filtrate is formed within the kidneys, normally approximately 125 mL/min.

renal osteodystrophy: a bone disorder that develops in patients with chronic kidney disease as a consequence of increased secretion of parathyroid hormone, reduced serum calcium, acidosis, and impaired vitamin D activation by the kidneys.

uremic syndrome: the cluster of symptoms associated with a GFR below 15 mL/min, including uremia, anemia, bone disease, hormonal imbalances, bleeding impairment, increased cardiovascular disease risk, and reduced immunity.

serum potassium but contributes to the development of hypertension (in patients who were not previously hypertensive). Increased secretion of parathyroid hormone (✚) helps to prevent elevations in serum phosphorus but contributes to bone loss and the development of **renal osteodystrophy**, a bone disorder common in renal patients. Electrolyte imbalances are likely when GFR becomes extremely low (less than 5 milliliters per minute), when hormonal adaptations are inadequate, or when intakes of water and electrolytes are either very restricted or excessive.

Because the kidneys are responsible for maintaining acid-base balance, acidosis often develops in chronic kidney disease. Although usually mild, the acidosis exacerbates renal bone disease because compounds in bone (for example, protein and phosphates) are released to buffer the acid in blood.

Uremic Syndrome Uremia usually develops during the final stages of chronic renal failure, when GFR is below 15 milliliters per minute and BUN exceeds 60 milligrams per deciliter.[23] The many symptoms and complications that develop during this stage of illness are collectively known as the **uremic syndrome**. The uremia itself can cause subtle mental dysfunctions and neuromuscular changes such as muscle cramping, twitching, and restless leg syndrome. Other complications include:

- *Impaired hormone synthesis.* Diseased kidneys are unable to produce erythropoietin, causing anemia. Reduced production of active vitamin D contributes to bone disease.
- *Impaired hormone degradation.* Imbalances develop in hormones involved in growth, reproduction, fluid balance, blood glucose regulation, and nutrient metabolism.
- *Bleeding abnormalities.* Defects in platelet function and clotting factors prolong bleeding time and contribute to bruising, gastrointestinal bleeding, and anemia.
- *Increased cardiovascular disease risk.* Chronic kidney disease worsens risk factors such as hypertension, insulin resistance, and homocysteinemia. Elevated parathyroid hormone levels lead to calcification of blood vessels and heart tissue. Patients are at increased risk of stroke, heart attack, and heart failure.
- *Reduced immunity.* Patients with uremia have poor immune responses and are at high risk of developing infections, which are a frequent cause of death.

Protein-Energy Malnutrition Patients with chronic kidney disease often develop PEM and wasting. Many patients have inadequate protein and energy intakes, even during the early stages of disease. Anorexia is thought to contribute to poor food intake and may result from hormonal disturbances, nausea and vomiting, restrictive diets, uremia, and medications. Nutrient losses also contribute to malnutrition and may be a consequence of vomiting, diarrhea, gastrointestinal bleeding, and dialysis. In addition, many of the illnesses that lead to chronic kidney disease can induce a catabolic state that contributes to protein losses.[24]

TREATMENT OF CHRONIC KIDNEY DISEASE

The goals of treatment for patients with chronic kidney disease are to slow disease progression and prevent or alleviate symptoms. Dietary measures help to prevent PEM and weight loss. Once kidney disease reaches the final stages, dialysis or a kidney transplant is necessary to sustain life.

Drug Therapy for Chronic Kidney Disease

Drug therapies help to control some of the complications associated with chronic kidney disease. Treatment of hypertension is critical for slowing disease progression and reducing cardiovascular disease risk; thus, antihypertensive drugs are usually prescribed (see Chapter 21). Some antihypertensive drugs (such as ACE inhibitors) can reduce proteinuria, helping to prevent additional kidney damage. Anemia is usually treated by injection or intravenous administration of erythropoietin (epoetin). Other common drug treatments include the administration of phosphate binders (taken with food) to reduce serum phosphorus levels, sodium bicarbonate to reverse acidosis, and cholesterol-lowering medications. Supplementation with active vitamin D (called *calcitriol*) helps to raise serum calcium and reduce parathyroid hormone levels.

Dialysis

Dialysis replaces kidney function by removing excess fluid and wastes from the blood. In **hemodialysis**, the blood is circulated through a **dialyzer** (artificial kidney), where it is bathed by a **dialysate**, a solution that selectively removes fluid and wastes. In **peritoneal dialysis**, the dialysate is infused into a person's peritoneal cavity, and blood is filtered by the peritoneum (the membrane that surrounds the abdominal cavity). After several hours, the dialysate is drained, removing unneeded fluid and wastes. Nutrition in Practice 22 provides additional information about dialysis.

Medical Nutrition Therapy for Chronic Kidney Disease

The patient's diet strongly influences disease progression, the development of complications, and serum levels of nitrogenous wastes and electrolytes. Because the dietary measures for chronic kidney disease are complex and nutrient needs change frequently during the course of illness, a dietitian who specializes in renal disease is best suited to provide medical nutrition therapy. Table 22-5 summarizes the dietary guidelines for patients in the different stages of chronic kidney disease. The predialysis guidelines apply to patients in stages 1 through 4; by stage 5, either hemodialysis or peritoneal dialysis is necessary. Because patients' needs can vary considerably, actual recommendations should be based on the results of a nutrition assessment.

Energy

The energy intake should be high enough to allow patients to maintain a healthy weight and to prevent wasting. Foods and beverages with a high energy density are typically recommended. (✚) Malnourished patients may require oral supplements or tube feedings to maintain weight.

The dialysate used in peritoneal dialysis contains glucose in order to draw fluid from the blood to the peritoneal cavity by osmosis. Thus, patients using this treatment can absorb a substantial amount of glucose, which can contribute as many as 800 kcalories daily. These kcalories must be included in estimates of energy intake. Weight gain is sometimes a problem when peritoneal dialysis continues for a long period.

Protein

A low-protein diet is usually prescribed to help slow the progression of kidney disease. During the predialysis period, the recommended protein intake is 0.60 to 0.75 grams per kilogram of body weight per day.[25] (✚) Low-protein diets produce fewer nitrogenous wastes and therefore reduce the risk of uremia. In addition, low-protein diets supply less phosphorus than high-protein diets, reducing the risks associated with hyperphosphatemia. Because renal patients often develop PEM,

✚ Reminder: Foods with high energy density contain a high number of kcalories per unit weight; these foods are generally high in fat and low in water content.

✚ The protein RDA for adults is 0.8 g/kg body weight.

hemodialysis (HE-moe-dye-AL-ih-sis): a treatment that removes fluids and wastes from the blood by passing the blood through a dialyzer.

dialyzer (DYE-ah-LYE-zer): a machine used in hemodialysis to filter the blood; also called an *artificial kidney*.

dialysate (dye-AL-ih-sate): the solution used in dialysis to draw wastes and fluids from the blood.

peritoneal (PEH-rih-toe-NEE-al) dialysis: a treatment that removes fluids and wastes from the blood by using the body's peritoneal membrane as a filter.

TABLE
22-5 Dietary Recommendations for Chronic Kidney Disease

Nutrient	Predialysis	Hemodialysis	Peritoneal Dialysis
Energy[a] (kcal/kg body weight)	35 for <60 years old 30–35 for ≥60 years old	35 for <60 years old 30–35 for ≥60 years old	35 for <60 years old 30–35 for ≥60 years old (total energy intake includes kcalories absorbed from the dialysate)
Protein (g/kg body weight)	0.60–0.75 (≥50% high-quality proteins)	≥1.2 (≥50% high-quality proteins)	≥1.2–1.3 (≥50% high-quality proteins)
Fat	As necessary to maintain a healthy lipid profile	As necessary to maintain a healthy lipid profile	As necessary to maintain a healthy lipid profile
Fluid (mL/day)	Unrestricted if urine output is normal	500–1000 plus daily urine output	As necessary to maintain fluid balance
Sodium (mg/day)	1000–3000	1000–3000	2000–4000
Potassium (mg/day)	Unrestricted unless hyperkalemia is present	2000–3000; adjust according to serum potassium levels	3000–4000; adjust according to serum potassium levels
Calcium (mg/day)	1000–1500	≤2000 from diet and medications	≤2000 from diet and medications
Phosphorus (mg/day)	800–1000 if serum phosphorus or parathyroid hormone is elevated	800–1000 if serum phosphorus or parathyroid hormone is elevated	800–1000 if serum phosphorus or parathyroid hormone is elevated

[a] Values listed apply to adults; recommendations for children should not fall below DRI levels.

Sources: D. J. Goldstein-Fuchs and C. M. Goeddeke-Merickel, Nutrition and kidney disease, in A. Greenberg, ed., *Primer on Kidney Diseases* (Philadelphia: Saunders, 2009), pp. 479–486; American Dietetic Association, *Nutrition Care Manual* (Chicago: American Dietetic Association, 2009).

however, their diet must provide enough protein to meet needs and prevent wasting. Thus, at least 50 percent of the protein consumed should be from high-quality protein sources (such as eggs, milk products, meat, poultry, fish, and soybeans) to ensure that the patient consumes adequate amounts of the essential amino acids. Low-protein breads, pastas, and other grain-based products are commercially available to help renal patients improve energy intakes without increasing protein consumption.

Because of the high risk of wasting and compliance difficulties associated with low-protein diets, some dietitians suggest that patients consume higher amounts of protein to preserve health.[26] Another option is to encourage patients to undergo a resistance training program, which can improve protein utilization, nitrogen retention, and muscle strength despite adherence to a low-protein diet.[27] Once dialysis has begun, protein restrictions can be relaxed, because dialysis removes nitrogenous wastes and results in some amino acid losses as well.

Lipids Patients with chronic kidney disease are at increased risk of coronary heart disease and are therefore advised to restrict their intakes of saturated fat, *trans* fat, and cholesterol to help control elevated blood lipids. Although patients are often encouraged to consume high-fat foods to improve their energy intakes, the foods they select should provide mostly unsaturated fats. Good choices include nuts and seeds, oil-based salad dressings, mayonnaise, (✚) avocados, and soybean products (Nutrition in Practice 4 provides additional suggestions).

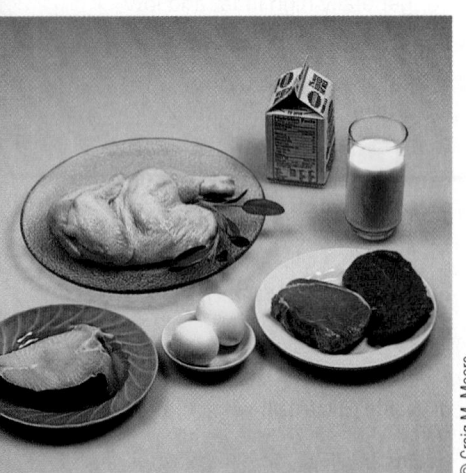

© Craig M. Moore

In a renal diet, at least half of the protein consumed should be from high-quality protein sources such as eggs, milk, meat, poultry, and fish.

Sodium and Fluids As kidney disease progresses, the patient excretes less urine and cannot handle normal intakes of sodium and fluids. Recommendations depend on the total urine output, changes in body weight and blood pressure, and serum sodium levels. A rise in body weight and blood pressure suggests that the person is retaining sodium and fluid; conversely, declines in these measurements indicate fluid loss. Most people with kidney disease tend to retain sodium and may benefit from mild restriction; less frequently, a patient may have a salt-wasting condition that requires additional dietary sodium.

Fluids are not restricted until urine output decreases. For a person who is neither dehydrated nor overhydrated, the daily fluid intake should match the daily urine output. (Obligatory water losses—from skin and lungs—are replaced from the water contained in solid foods.) Once a person is on dialysis, sodium and fluid intakes should be controlled so that only about 2 pounds of water weight is gained daily—this excess fluid is then removed during the next dialysis treatment.[28] Patients on fluid-restricted diets should be advised that foods such as flavored gelatin, soups, fruit ices, frozen fruit juice bars, and ice milk contribute to the fluid allowance.

Potassium Before dialysis treatments begin, most renal patients can handle typical intakes of potassium. Potassium restrictions are usually necessary only in patients with elevated potassium levels. Individuals with diabetic nephropathy are at high risk of hyperkalemia and may need to limit dietary potassium during the early stages of disease. Conversely, potassium supplementation may be necessary for persons using potassium-wasting diuretics.

Dialysis patients must control potassium intakes to prevent hyperkalemia or, more rarely, **hypokalemia**. Restriction is usually necessary for people treated with hemodialysis, whereas those undergoing peritoneal dialysis can consume potassium more freely. Recommended intakes are based on serum potassium levels, renal function, medications, and the dialysis procedure used.

All fresh foods provide potassium, but some fruits and vegetables contain such high amounts that their regular use is discouraged in patients at risk of hyperkalemia; Table 22-6 shows the potassium content of some common fruits and vegetables. Foods in other food groups may be high in potassium as well; examples include dried beans, fish, milk and milk products, molasses, nuts and nut butters, and wheat bran; patients with potassium restrictions must limit these foods as well. Patients should be cautioned that salt substitutes and other low-sodium products often contain potassium chloride, which people on a potassium-restricted diet should avoid.

Calcium, Phosphorus, and Vitamin D To prevent bone disease, calcium and phosphorus intakes may need adjustment, even during the early stages of kidney disease. Laboratory values usually help to guide dietary recommendations for these nutrients. Serum calcium levels must be monitored to guard against **hypercalcemia**, which can develop in response to simultaneous calcium and vitamin D supplementation. Elevated serum phosphorus levels indicate the need for dietary phosphorus restriction. Vitamin D supplementation is standard treatment for many renal patients, (✚) but the amount prescribed depends on the serum levels of calcium, phosphorus, and parathyroid hormone.

High-protein foods are also high in phosphorus, so the protein-restricted diets consumed by predialysis patients curb phosphorus intakes as well. After dialysis treatments begin and protein intakes are liberalized, phosphate binders (taken with meals) become essential for phosphorus control. Because foods that are rich in calcium (such as milk and milk products) are usually high in phosphorus and are therefore restricted, patients must rely on calcium supplements to meet their calcium needs.

Vitamins and Minerals The restrictive renal diet interferes with vitamin and mineral intakes, increasing the risk of deficiencies. In addition, patients treated with dialysis lose water-soluble vitamins and some trace minerals into the dialysate. Dietary supplements for renal patients typically supply generous amounts of folate and vitamin B$_6$—1 milligram and 10 milligrams per day, respectively—along with

hypokalemia (HIGH-po-ka-LEE-me-ah): low serum potassium levels.

hypercalcemia (HIGH-per-kal-SEE-me-ah): elevated serum calcium levels.

People on a renal diet can consume most fruits and vegetables in limited amounts.

TABLE
22-6 | Potassium Guide—Fruits and Vegetables

This table lists common fruits and vegetables according to their potassium content. One serving is ½ cup raw fruit or cooked vegetable unless otherwise noted. Keep in mind that the portion size may determine how a food is categorized. Check Appendix A for additional information about the potassium content of foods.

High Potassium (>250 mg per serving)	Medium Potassium (150–250 mg per serving)	Low Potassium (<150 mg per serving)
Avocado	Apple (1 medium)	Blueberries
Banana	Apricots (2 whole)	Cabbage
Beets	Asparagus	Carrots (1 medium)
Chard	Broccoli	Cauliflower
Dates (3 whole)	Cantaloupe	Cucumbers
Nectarine (1 small)	Celery	Eggplant
Orange (1 medium)	Corn	Grapes
Parsnips	Grapefruit (½ fruit)	Green beans
Potatoes	Honeydew melon	Green pepper
Pumpkin	Kale	Lettuce (4 leaves, raw)
Raisins	Kiwi (1 small)	Mushrooms, shiitake
Rutabagas	Peach (1 small)	Onions (1 small)
Spinach	Pear (1 medium)	Plum (1 small)
Sweet potatoes	Peas	Strawberries
Tomato	Zucchini	Watermelon

recommended amounts of the other water-soluble vitamins.[29] Supplemental vitamin C should be limited to 100 milligrams per day, because excessive intakes can contribute to kidney stone formation in individuals at risk (see p. 638). Supplements containing vitamins A and E are not recommended because these vitamins sometimes accumulate in patients with renal disease.[30]

Iron deficiency is common in hemodialysis patients and may be due to inadequate erythropoietin, gastrointestinal bleeding, reduced iron absorption, or blood losses associated with the dialysis treatment.[31] Intravenous administration of iron, in conjunction with erythropoietin therapy, is more effective than oral iron supplementation for improving iron status.

Enteral and Parenteral Nutrition

Enteral and parenteral nutrition support can provide nutrients to renal patients who cannot consume adequate amounts of food. The enteral formulas suitable for chronic kidney disease are more kcalorically dense and have lower protein and electrolyte concentrations than standard formulas. **Intradialytic parenteral nutrition** is an option for supplying supplemental nutrients to dialysis patients; this technique combines parenteral feedings with hemodialysis treatments. An advantage of this approach is that the volume of parenteral solution infused can be simultaneously removed (recall that fluid intake is controlled in dialysis patients). However, clinical studies have not shown intradialytic parenteral nutrition to be more successful than oral supplementation in improving nutrition status or mortality rates in malnourished dialysis patients.[32]

Dietary Compliance Adhering to a renal diet is probably the most difficult aspect of treatment for patients with renal disease. These patients often require extensive counseling once multiple dietary restrictions become necessary. Depending on the stage of illness and the patient's laboratory values, the renal diet may limit protein, fluids, sodium, potassium, and phosphorus, thereby affecting food selections from all major food groups. Because these diets have so many restrictions, patient compliance is often a problem.[33] The "How to" on this page provides suggestions to help patients comply with renal diets. The Case Study (p. 636) allows you to apply your knowledge about chronic kidney disease and hemodialysis.

KIDNEY TRANSPLANTS

A preferred alternative to dialysis in patients with end-stage renal disease is kidney transplantation.[34] A successful kidney transplant restores kidney function, allows a more liberal diet, and frees the patient from routine dialysis. Given the choice, many patients would prefer transplants, but the demand for suitable kidneys far exceeds the supply. Other barriers to transplantation include advanced age, poor health, financial difficulties, and abnormalities of the urinary tract. Approximately 30 percent of patients who develop end-stage renal disease receive a kidney transplant.[35]

HOW TO | Help Patients Comply with a Renal Diet

Patients with renal disease and their caregivers face considerable challenges as they learn to manage a renal diet. The following suggestions may help:

1. *To keep track of fluid intake:*
   - Fill a container with an amount of water equal to your total fluid allowance. Each time you use a liquid food or beverage, discard an equivalent amount of water from the container. The amount remaining in the container will show you how much fluid you have left for the day.
   - Be sure to save enough fluid to take medications.

2. *To help control thirst:*
   - Chew gum or suck hard candy.
   - Freeze beverages to a semisolid state so that they take longer to consume.
   - Add lemon juice or crumpled mint leaves to water to make it more refreshing.
   - Gargle with refrigerated mouthwash.

3. *To increase the energy content of meals:*
   - Add extra margarine or butter to rice, noodles, breads, crackers, and cooked vegetables. Add extra salad dressing or oil to salads.
   - Add nondairy whipped toppings to desserts.
   - Include fried foods in your diet.

4. *To include more of your favorite vegetables in meals:*
   - Consult your nurse or dietitian to learn whether you can safely use the process of leaching to remove some of the potassium from vegetables.
   - To leach potassium from vegetables: Cut the vegetables into ⅛-inch slices and rinse. Soak the vegetables in a large amount of warm water for two hours—about 10 parts of water to 1 part of vegetables. Cook the vegetables using 5 parts of water to 1 part of vegetables.

5. *To prevent the diet from becoming monotonous:*
   - Experiment with new combinations of allowed foods.
   - Substitute nondairy products for milk products. Nondairy products, which are lower in protein, phosphorus, and potassium, can substitute for milk and add energy to the diet.
   - Add flavor to foods by seasoning with garlic, onion, chili powder, curry powder, oregano, mint, basil, parsley, pepper, or lemon juice.
   - Consult a nurse or dietitian when you want to eat restricted foods. Many restricted foods can be used occasionally and in small amounts if the menu is carefully adjusted.

Thomas Stone is a 55-year-old banker who developed chronic kidney disease as a result of hypertension. His condition was discovered several years ago, when routine laboratory tests revealed elevated serum creatinine and BUN levels. Since then, he has been taking antihypertensive medications and restricting dietary sodium; he reported difficulty following the low-protein diet that was also prescribed. Mr. Stone recently visited his doctor with complaints of low urine output and reduced sensation in his hands and feet. He also reported feeling drowsy at work and mentioned that he was bruising more than usual. The examination revealed a 9-pound weight gain since his last visit and swelling in his ankles and feet. Tests revealed that his GFR had fallen to 10 milliliters per minute. Mr. Stone is 5 feet 8 inches tall and normally weighs 160 pounds.

1. Explain how chronic kidney disease progresses. What happens to GFR, serum creatinine levels, and BUN as renal function declines?

2. Describe the clinical effects you would expect during the final stage of disease, when kidney failure develops. Explain the significance of each of Mr. Stone's physical complaints.

3. Explain why a low-sodium, low-protein diet was prescribed for Mr. Stone at a former visit. What energy and protein intakes were probably recommended at that time?

4. The physician determines that Mr. Stone's kidney disease has reached the final stage and prescribes hemodialysis. How will dialysis alter Mr. Stone's diet? Calculate his new protein recommendation, and compare it to the amount of protein recommended before dialysis. What other changes in nutrient intake may be necessary?

Immunosuppressive Drug Therapy To prevent tissue rejection following transplant surgery, patients require high doses of immunosuppressive drugs such as corticosteroids, cyclosporine, tacrolimus, sirolimus, and azathioprine. These drugs have multiple effects that can alter nutrition status, including nausea, vomiting, diarrhea, glucose intolerance, altered blood lipids, fluid retention, hypertension, and infection. Because immunosuppressive drug therapy increases the

DIET-DRUG INTERACTIONS

Check this table for notable nutrition-related effects of the medications discussed in this chapter.

	GASTROINTESTINAL EFFECTS	INTERACTIONS WITH DIETARY SUBSTANCES	METABOLIC EFFECTS
Anti-inflammatory/ immunosuppressive drugs			
Corticosteroids	–	–	Glucose intolerance, sodium retention, negative nitrogen balance, appetite stimulation, weight gain, growth suppression in children
Cyclosporine	–	Grapefruit juice raises drug levels and increases risk of toxicity. Avoid potassium supplements and salt substitutes with potassium. St. John's wort can alter drug efficacy.	Hyperkalemia, hypomagnesia, hyperglycemia, hyperlipidemia
Phosphate binders (calcium-containing)	Constipation	–	Electrolyte imbalances
Potassium-exchange resins (sodium polystyrene sulfonate)	–	–	Fluid retention, hypokalemia, hypocalcemia
Potassium citrate	Nausea, vomiting, stomach pain, diarrhea	–	Hyperkalemia

TABLE 22-7	Dietary Guidelines Following a Kidney Transplant

- **Energy:** Initially, 30–35 kcal/kg body weight per day; reduce to 25–30 kcal/kg body weight per day to maintain healthy body weight, and adjust as necessary.

- **Protein:** Initially, 1.5 to 2.0 g/kg body weight per day; reduce to 0.8 to 1.0 g/kg per day after 6–8 weeks.

- **Carbohydrate:** For hyperglycemia, maintain consistent carbohydrate intake at meals and snacks, emphasize complex carbohydrates, and limit refined carbohydrates and concentrated sweets.

- **Fat:** Limit saturated fat to 7–10 percent of total kcalories and cholesterol to 300 mg/day to help control serum lipids; emphasize omega-3 and monounsaturated fats.

- **Fluid:** Generally unrestricted; monitor serum levels, and adjust if necessary.

- **Sodium:** Generally unrestricted. Restrict to 2–3 grams/day if fluid retention and hypertension are present.

- **Potassium:** Generally unrestricted. Adjust according to serum potassium levels if necessary.

- **Calcium:** 1200–1500 mg/day to minimize bone loss associated with drug therapy.

- **Phosphorus:** Generally unrestricted; monitor serum levels and adjust if necessary.

Sources: American Dietetic Association, *Nutrition Care Manual* (Chicago: American Dietetic Association, 2009); J. A. Beto and V. K. Bansal, Medical nutrition therapy in chronic kidney failure: Integrating clinical practice guidelines, *Journal of the American Dietetic Association* 104 (2004): 404–409.

risk of foodborne infection, food safety guidelines should be provided to patients and caregivers. The Diet-Drug Interactions feature summarizes the nutrition-related effects of immunosuppressants and other drugs mentioned in this chapter.

Nutrition Therapy after Kidney Transplant Protein and energy requirements increase after surgery due to stress and the catabolic effects of drug therapy. Once recovery is under way, the side effects of drugs can strongly influence dietary treatment. Typical dietary modifications are shown in Table 22-7.[36] Hyperglycemia (due to drug treatment) may be improved by controlling carbohydrate intake, although oral medications or insulin therapy may also be required. Because blood lipids are frequently elevated, patients should limit saturated fat and cholesterol intakes. Sodium, potassium, and phosphorus intakes are often liberalized following a transplant, but serum electrolyte levels must be monitored closely because some drug therapies can cause hyperkalemia or hypophosphatemia. Calcium supplementation is advised due to urinary calcium losses associated with corticosteroids (which are often used as immunosuppressants). To avoid foodborne illness, patients should avoid raw or undercooked meat, fish, poultry, and eggs; unpasteurized milk and juices; cheese made with unpasteurized milk; fresh bean sprouts; and food that is spoiled or moldy.[37]

Review Notes

- Chronic kidney disease causes gradual loss of kidney function and often results from long-standing diabetes mellitus or hypertension.
- Depending on the stage of chronic kidney disease, its complications may include fluid and electrolyte disturbances, hypertension, renal osteodystrophy, mental impairments, bleeding abnormalities, anemia, increased risk for cardiovascular disease, and reduced immunity.

- Treatment of chronic kidney disease can slow disease progression and correct complications; it includes drug therapies, dialysis, and medical nutrition therapy. Dietary measures usually feature a low-protein diet, controlled fluid and sodium intakes, phosphorus restrictions, and calcium and vitamin D supplementation; potassium restrictions are usually necessary after dialysis treatment begins.
- In patients with chronic kidney disease, kidney transplantation can restore renal function and liberalize dietary restrictions.

Kidney Stones

Approximately 12 percent of men and 6 percent of women in the United States develop one or more **kidney stones** during their lifetimes.[38] A kidney stone is a crystalline mass that forms within the urinary tract. Although stones are often asymptomatic, their passage can cause severe pain or block the urinary tract. Stones tend to recur but can be prevented with dietary measures and medical treatment.

FORMATION OF KIDNEY STONES

Kidney stones develop when stone constituents become concentrated in urine, allowing crystals to form and grow. About 70 percent of kidney stones are made up primarily of calcium oxalate. Less commonly, stones are composed of uric acid, the amino acid cystine, calcium phosphate, or magnesium ammonium phosphate (the latter are known as *struvite* stones). Factors that predispose an individual to stone formation include the following:

- *Dehydration* or *low urine volume,* which promotes the crystallization of minerals and other compounds in urine.
- *Obstruction,* which prevents the flow of urine and encourages salt precipitation.
- *Urine acidity,* which affects the dissolution of urinary constituents. Some stones form more readily in acidic urine, whereas others form in alkaline urine.
- *Metabolic factors,* which affect the presence of compounds that either promote or inhibit crystal growth.
- *Renal disease,* which is associated with calcification of tissues and phosphate accumulation.

The most common types of kidney stones are described in this section.

Calcium Oxalate Stones The most common abnormality in people with calcium oxalate stones is **hypercalciuria** (elevated urinary calcium levels). Hypercalciuria can result from excessive calcium absorption, impaired calcium reabsorption in kidney tubules, or elevated serum levels of parathyroid hormone or vitamin D. However, some people with calcium oxalate stones excrete normal amounts of calcium in the urine, and the reason they form stones is unknown.

Elevated urinary oxalate levels, or **hyperoxaluria**, also promote the formation of calcium oxalate crystals. Oxalate is a normal product of metabolism that readily binds to calcium. Hyperoxaluria may reflect an increase in the body's synthesis of oxalate or increased absorption from dietary sources. (✛) People who form calcium oxalate stones are advised to reduce their dietary intake of oxalate (see Table 22-8) and to avoid supplementation with vitamin C, which degrades to oxalate in the body.[39]

Uric Acid Stones Uric acid stones develop when the urine is abnormally acidic, contains excessive uric acid, or both. These stones are frequently associated with **gout**, a metabolic disorder characterized by elevated uric acid levels in the blood and urine. Other diseases that increase the risk of uric acid stones include leukemia, lymphoma, and glycogen storage disease: these conditions are associated with the overproduction of **purines**, which degrade to uric acid in the body. A diet rich in purines also contributes to high uric acid levels (see Table 22-9).

The most common type of kidney stone is composed of calcium oxalate crystals, as shown here.

TABLE 22-8	Foods High in Oxalate	
Vegetables	**Fruits**	**Other**
Beans, green and wax	Blackberries	Chocolate*
Beets*	Blueberries	Cocoa
Chard	Currants, red	Coffee
Collard greens	Figs	Draft beer
Dandelion greens	Grapes, Concord	Fruit cake
Eggplant	Kiwi	Grits
Endive	Lemon peel	Nuts, nut butters*
Escarole	Oranges, orange peel	Peanut butter*
Leeks	Raspberries	Sesame seeds, tahini
Legumes	Rhubarb*	Soy milk, soy burgers
Okra	Strawberries*	Tea*
Parsley		Tofu
Spinach*		Wheat bran*
Sweet potatoes		Wheat germ
Zucchini		

Note: The oxalate content of many foods has not been analyzed, and few studies have been conducted to determine which foods raise urinary oxalate levels.

* The foods marked with an asterisk have been documented to raise urinary oxalate levels and should be avoided by people who form calcium oxalate stones.

Cystine and Struvite Stones Cystine stones can form in people with the inherited disorder **cystinuria**, in which the renal tubules are unable to reabsorb the amino acid cystine. The abnormality results in abnormally high concentrations of cystine in the urine, leading to subsequent crystallization and stone formation. **Struvite** stones, composed primarily of magnesium ammonium phosphate, form in alkaline urine as a result of the bacterial degradation of urea to ammonia. The ammonia elevates urinary pH to a level that favors struvite formation. Struvite stones can accompany chronic urinary infections or disorders that interfere with urinary flow.

CONSEQUENCES OF KIDNEY STONES

In most cases, kidney stones do not pose serious medical problems. Small stones can readily pass through the ureters and out of the body with minimal treatment.

TABLE 22-9	Foods High in Purines	
Organ Meats	**Meat and Meat Products**	**Seafood**
Brains	Game meat	Anchovies
Kidney	Gravies	Herring
Liver	Meat extracts	Mackerel
Sweetbreads		Sardines
		Scallops

Source: J. A. T. Pennington, *Bowes and Church's Food Values of Portions Commonly Used* (Philadelphia: J. B. Lippincott, 1994), p. 387.

cystinuria (SIS-tin-NOO-ree-ah): an inherited disorder characterized by elevated urinary excretion of several amino acids, including cystine.

struvite (STROO-vite): crystals of magnesium ammonium phosphate.

Drinking plenty of water throughout the day is the most important measure for preventing kidney stones.

Renal Colic A stone passing through the ureter can produce severe, stabbing pain, called **renal colic**. Generally, the pain begins in the back and intensifies as the stone travels toward the bladder (review Figure 22-1 on p. 622). The pain can be severe enough to cause nausea and vomiting and sometimes requires medication. When the stone reaches the bladder, the pain abruptly stops. Blood may appear in the urine (**hematuria**) as a result of damage to the kidney or ureter lining.

Urinary Tract Complications Depending on the location of the stone, symptoms may include urination urgency, frequent urination, or inability to urinate. Stones that are unable to pass through the ureter can cause a urinary tract obstruction and possibly lead to infection.

PREVENTION AND TREATMENT OF KIDNEY STONES

Solutes are less likely to crystallize and form stones in dilute urine. Therefore, people who form kidney stones are advised to drink 12 to 16 cups of fluids daily to maintain urine volumes of least 2½ liters (about 10½ cups) per day.[40] Additional fluid may be needed in hot weather or if an individual is extremely active. Acceptable fluid sources include tea, coffee, wine, and beer, but apple and grapefruit juices should be limited because they may increase the risk of stones.[41]

Calcium Oxalate Stones Dietary measures and drug treatments aim to reduce urinary calcium and oxalate levels. Furthermore, the uric acid content of urine must be kept low, because uric acid reduces the solubility of calcium oxalate.[42] Thiazide diuretics are a mainstay of drug therapy and help to reduce urinary calcium by enhancing calcium reabsorption in the kidney tubules.[43] Other medications include cholestyramine, which reduces oxalate absorption, and allopurinol, which reduces uric acid production in the body. Potassium citrate can inhibit the formation and growth of crystals but may cause stomach upset and diarrhea.

Medical nutrition therapy includes adjustments in calcium, oxalate, protein, and sodium intakes.[44] Patients should consume adequate calcium from food sources (800 to 1200 milligrams per day) because dietary calcium combines with oxalate in the intestines, reducing oxalate absorption and helping to control hyperoxaluria. (✚) Conversely, low-calcium diets promote oxalate absorption and higher urinary oxalate levels. Foods high in oxalate should be restricted, because dietary oxalate contributes to urinary oxalate content (review Table 22-8). High protein and sodium intakes increase urinary calcium excretion, so moderate protein consumption (about 0.8 to 1.0 gram per kilogram of body weight per day) and controlled sodium intake (no more than 3450 milligrams daily) are also advised. Vitamin C intake should be limited to the DRI (75 and 90 milligrams per day for women and men, respectively).

Uric Acid Stones Drug treatments for uric acid stones include allopurinol to reduce urinary uric acid and potassium citrate to reduce urine acidity. Diets restricted in purines may also help to control urinary uric acid levels (review Table 22-9). Because all meats, poultry, fish, and shellfish contain considerable amounts of purines, strict dietary control over a long period may be difficult to achieve. In addition, the benefits of purine restriction are unknown.

Cystine and Struvite Stones High fluid intakes may prevent the formation of cystine stones in some patients, whereas other individuals require drug therapy to reduce cystine production in the body. Medications frequently prescribed include penicillamine and tiopronin, which reduce cystine levels, and potassium citrate, which reduces urine acidity. Preventing urinary tract infections is an important strategy for preventing struvite stones. Patients with these stones may require antibiotic therapy to prevent further stone formation.

✚ Because calcium supplements can elevate urinary calcium levels, they are not as helpful as food sources of calcium.

renal colic: the intense pain that occurs when a kidney stone passes through the ureter.

hematuria (HE-mah-TOO-ree-ah): blood in the urine.

NURSING DIAGNOSIS

For patients with kidney stones may include *acute pain, risk for infection,* and *impaired urinary elimination.*

Nutrition and Renal Diseases

Review Notes

- Kidney stones form when stone constituents—calcium oxalate, calcium phosphate, uric acid, cystine, or magnesium ammonium phosphate—crystallize in urine. Complications include renal colic, difficulty with urination, and obstruction.
- Kidney stones may be prevented by maintaining urine volumes of at least 2½ liters daily. Other dietary measures include consumption of enough calcium to control oxalate absorption, dietary oxalate and purine restrictions, a moderate protein intake, and controlled sodium intake.

Nutrition Assessment | CHECKLIST FOR PEOPLE WITH RENAL DISORDERS

MEDICAL HISTORY

Check the medical record to determine:

- Degree of renal function
- Cause of the nephrotic syndrome or kidney disease
- Type of dialysis, if appropriate
- Whether the patient has received a kidney transplant
- Type of kidney stone

Review the medical record for complications that may alter nutritional needs:

- Anemia
- Diabetes mellitus
- Edema or oliguria
- Hyperlipidemia
- Hypertension
- Metabolic stress or infection
- Protein-energy malnutrition

MEDICATIONS

Assess risks for medication-related malnutrition related to:

- Long-term use of medications
- Multiple medication use, especially if medications affect nutrition status

For all patients with renal diseases, note:

- Whether medications or supplements contain electrolytes that must be controlled
- Use of drugs or herbs that may be toxic to the kidneys

DIETARY INTAKE

For patients with the nephrotic syndrome, kidney disease, or kidney transplant, assess intakes of:

- Protein and energy
- Fluid
- Vitamins, especially vitamin D
- Minerals, especially calcium, phosphorus, iron, and electrolytes

For patients with kidney stones or a history of kidney stones:

- Stress the need to drink plenty of fluids throughout the day.
- Assess intake of calcium, oxalate, sodium, protein, purines, or vitamin C, as appropriate for the type of stone.

ANTHROPOMETRIC DATA

Take accurate baseline height and weight measurements. Keep in mind that:

- Fluid retention due to the nephrotic syndrome or kidney failure can mask malnutrition.
- For dialysis patients, the weight measured immediately after the dialysis treatment (called the *dry weight*) most accurately reflects the person's true weight. Rapid weight gain between dialysis treatments reflects fluid retention. If fluid retention is excessive, review fluid intake to determine if the patient understands and is complying with diet recommendations.

LABORATORY TESTS

Note that serum protein levels are often low in patients with nephrotic syndrome or kidney failure. Review the following laboratory test results to assess the degree of renal function and response to treatments:

- Blood urea nitrogen (BUN)
- Creatinine
- Glomerular filtration rate (GFR)
- Serum electrolytes
- Urinary protein

Check laboratory test results for complications associated with kidney disease, including:

- Anemia
- Hyperglycemia
- Hyperlipidemia
- Hyperparathyroidism (related to bone disease)

PHYSICAL SIGNS

For patients with nephrotic syndrome or kidney disease, look for physical signs of:

○ Bone disease
○ Dehydration or fluid retention
○ Hyperkalemia
○ Iron deficiency
○ Uremia

Self Check

1 ● Which of the following is *not* a function of the kidneys?
   a. Activation of vitamin K
   b. Maintenance of acid-base balance
   c. Elimination of metabolic waste products
   d. Maintenance of fluid and electrolyte balances

2 ● The nephrotic syndrome frequently results in:
   a. the uremic syndrome.
   b. oliguria.
   c. edema.
   d. renal colic.

3 ● Dietary recommendations for patients with the nephrotic syndrome include:
   a. a high-protein intake.
   b. sodium restriction.
   c. potassium and phosphorus restrictions.
   d. fluid restriction.

4 ● Hyperkalemia is often treated by:
   a. eliminating potassium from the diet.
   b. using diuretics to increase potassium losses.
   c. increasing fluid consumption.
   d. using potassium-exchange resins, which bind potassium in the GI tract.

5 ● Fluid requirements for oliguric patients are estimated by adding about ____ milliliters to the volume of urine output.
   a. 100
   b. 300
   c. 500
   d. 750

6 ● The most common cause of chronic kidney disease is:
   a. diabetes mellitus.
   b. hypertension.
   c. autoimmune disease.
   d. exposure to toxins.

7 ● A person with chronic kidney disease who has been following a renal diet for several years begins hemodialysis treatment. An appropriate dietary adjustment would be to:
   a. reduce protein intake.
   b. consume protein more liberally.
   c. increase intakes of sodium and water.
   d. consume potassium and phosphorus more liberally.

8 ● Which of the following nutrients may be unintentionally restricted when a patient restricts phosphorus intake?
   a. Fluid
   b. Calcium
   c. Potassium
   d. Sodium

9 ● Most kidney stones are made primarily from:
   a. struvite.
   b. uric acid.
   c. calcium oxalate.
   d. cystine.

10● Treatment for all kidney stones includes:
   a. dietary oxalate restriction.
   b. dietary protein restriction.
   c. vitamin C supplementation.
   d. a fluid intake that maintains a urine volume of at least 2½ liters per day.

Answers to these questions appear in Appendix H.

Clinical Applications

1 ● A person with chronic kidney disease may need multiple medications to control disease progression and treat symptoms and complications. For people with diabetes and hyperlipidemias who develop chronic kidney disease, medications might include insulin, oral hypoglycemic drugs, antihypertensives, diuretics, lipid-lowering medications, and phosphate binders. Review the nutrition-related side effects of these medications. Describe the ways in which these medications may make it harder for people to maintain nutrition status.

2. • Because the diet for chronic kidney disease is so restrictive, patients often find the diet difficult to manage and maintain over the long term. Review the suggestions in the "How to" on p. 635. Can you think of additional suggestions that may help? List ideas that may help patients adjust to each of the different aspects of their renal diets.

Nutrition on the Net

For further study of topics covered in this chapter, access these websites.

- Find updates and quick links to these and other nutrition-related sites at our website: www.cengage.com/nutrition/whitney/nhhc4e
- To search for specific topics related to kidney diseases, dialysis, and kidney transplants, visit these sites:
- Kidney Foundation of Canada: www.kidney.ca
- National Institute of Diabetes and Digestive and Kidney Diseases: www2.niddk.nih.gov

- National Kidney Foundation: www.kidney.org
- To find materials for patients with kidney diseases, visit the American Association of Kidney Patients: www.aakp.org
- To find more information about kidney stones, visit the Oxalosis and Hyperoxaluria Foundation: www.ohf.org
- To see photographs of kidney stones, visit the website of the Louis C. Herring and Company Laboratory: www.herringlab.com

Notes

1. J. C. Jennette and R. J. Falk, Glomerular clinicopathologic syndromes, in A. Greenberg, ed., *Primer on Kidney Diseases* (Philadelphia: Saunders, 2009), pp. 148–159.
2. M. H. Beers and coeditors, *The Merck Manual of Diagnosis and Therapy* (Whitehouse Station, NJ: Merck Research Laboratories, 2006), pp. 2004–2006.
3. G. B. Appel, Glomerular disorders and nephrotic syndromes, in L. Goldman and D. Ausiello, eds., *Cecil Medicine* (Philadelphia: Saunders, 2008), pp. 866–876.
4. J. Goddard and coauthors, Kidney and urinary tract disease, in N. A. Boon, N. R. Colledge, and B. R. Walker, eds., *Davidson's Principles and Practice of Medicine* (Philadelphia: Churchill Livingstone/Elsevier, 2006), pp. 455–518.
5. Goddard and coauthors, 2006.
6. Appel, 2008; J. A. Charlesworth, D. M. Gracey, and B. A. Pussell, Adult nephrotic syndrome: Non-specific strategies for treatment, *Nephrology* 13 (2008): 45–50.
7. American Dietetic Association, *Nutrition Care Manual* (Chicago: American Dietetic Association, 2009).
8. American Dietetic Association, 2009.
9. American Dietetic Association, 2009; G. M. Podda and coauthors, Abnormalities of homocysteine and B vitamins in the nephrotic syndrome, *Thrombosis Research* 120 (2007): 647–652.
10. B. A. Molitoris, Acute kidney injury, in L. Goldman and D. Ausiello, eds., *Cecil Medicine* (Philadelphia: Saunders, 2008), pp. 862–866.
11. C. L. Edelstein and R. W. Schrier, Acute renal failure: Pathogenesis, diagnosis, and management, in R. W. Schrier, ed., *Renal and Electrolyte Disorders* (Philadelphia: Lippincott Williams & Wilkins, 2003), pp. 401–455.
12. Goddard and coauthors, 2006.
13. Molitoris, 2008; Goddard and coauthors, 2006.
14. American Dietetic Association, 2009.
15. American Dietetic Association, 2009.
16. R. G. Luke, Chronic renal failure, in L. Goldman and D. Ausiello, eds., *Cecil Textbook of Medicine* (Philadelphia: Saunders, 2004), pp. 708–716.
17. W. E. Mitch, Chronic kidney disease, in L. Goldman and D. Ausiello, eds., *Cecil Medicine* (Philadelphia: Saunders, 2008), pp. 921–930.
18. Beers and coeditors, 2006, pp. 1978–1979.
19. L. A. Stevens, N. Stoycheff, and A. S. Levey, Staging and management of chronic kidney disease, in A. Greenberg, ed., *Primer on Kidney Diseases* (Philadelphia: Saunders, 2009), pp. 436–445.
20. Goddard and coauthors, 2006.
21. Mitch, 2008.
22. Mitch, 2008; Beers and coeditors, 2006, pp. 1978–1979.
23. Luke, 2004.
24. J. D. Kopple, Nutrition, diet, and the kidney, in M. E. Shils and coeditors, *Modern Nutrition in Health and Disease* (Baltimore, MD: Lippincott Williams & Wilkins, 2006), pp. 1475–1511.

25. American Dietetic Association, 2009.
26. J. A. Beto and V. K. Bansal, Medical nutrition therapy in chronic kidney failure: Integrating clinical practice guidelines, *Journal of the American Dietetic Association* 104 (2004): 404–409.
27. C. Castaneda and coauthors, Resistance training to counteract the catabolism of a low-protein diet in patients with chronic renal insufficiency, *Annals of Internal Medicine* 135 (2001): 965–976.
28. Beto and Bansal, 2004.
29. D. J. Goldstein-Fuchs and C. M. Goeddeke-Merickel, Nutrition and kidney disease, in A. Greenberg, ed., *Primer on Kidney Diseases* (Philadelphia: Saunders, 2009), pp. 478–486.
30. Beto and Bansal, 2004.
31. N. Tolkoff-Rubin, Treatment of irreversible renal failure, in L. Goldman and D. Ausiello, eds., *Cecil Medicine* (Philadelphia: Saunders, 2008), pp. 936–947.
32. N. J. Cano and coauthors, Intradialytic parenteral nutrition does not improve survival in malnourished hemodialysis patients: A 2-year multicenter, prospective, randomized study, *Journal of the American Society of Nephrology* 18 (2007): 2583–2591; L. B. Pupim and coauthors, Intradialytic oral nutrition improves protein homeostasis in chronic hemodialysis patients with deranged nutritional status, *Journal of the American Society of Nephrology* 17 (2006): 149–157.
33. C. L. Durose and coauthors, Knowledge of dietary restrictions and the medical consequences of noncompliance by patients on hemodialysis are not predictive of dietary compliance, *Journal of the American Dietetic Association* 104 (2004): 35–41.
34. Tolkoff-Rubin, 2008.
35. S. Beddhu, Outcome of end-stage renal disease therapies, in A. Greenberg, ed., *Primer on Kidney Diseases* (Philadelphia: Saunders, 2009), pp. 472–477.
36. Beto and Bansal, 2004.
37. American Dietetic Association, 2009.
38. G. C. Curhan, Nephrolithiasis, in L. Goldman and D. Ausiello, eds., *Cecil Medicine* (Philadelphia: Saunders, 2008), pp. 897–903.
39. L. K. Massey, M. Liebman, and S. A. Kynast-Gales, Ascorbate increases human oxaluria and kidney stone risk, *Journal of Nutrition* 135 (2005): 1673–1677.
40. American Dietetic Association, 2009.
41. S. Escott-Stump, *Nutrition and Diagnosis-Related Care* (Baltimore, MD: Lippincott Williams & Wilkins, 2008), pp. 800–804.
42. F. L. Coe, A. Evan, and E. Worcester, Kidney stone disease, *Journal of Clinical Investigation* 115 (2005): 2598–2608.
43. Curhan, 2008.
44. American Dietetic Association, 2009.

Dialysis

Although there is no perfect substitute for one's own kidneys, dialysis offers a life-sustaining treatment option for people with chronic kidney disease who develop renal failure. Dialysis can serve as a permanent treatment or as a temporary measure to sustain life until a suitable kidney donor can be found. Dialysis can also restore fluid and electrolyte balances in patients with acute kidney injury. Clinicians who routinely work with renal patients should understand how dialysis procedures work. This Nutrition in Practice describes the process of dialysis and outlines the various types of procedures that are available. The accompanying glossary defines the relevant terms.

How does dialysis work?

Dialysis removes excess fluids and wastes from the blood by employing the processes of **diffusion**, **osmosis**, and **ultrafiltration** (see Figure NP22-1). The dialysate, a solution similar in composition to normal blood plasma, is delivered to a compartment beside a **semipermeable membrane**; the person's blood flows along the other side of the membrane. The semipermeable membrane acts like a filter: small molecules such as urea and glucose can pass through microscopic pores in the membrane, whereas large molecules are unable to cross.

In *hemodialysis,* the tiny tubes that carry blood through the dialyzer are made of materials that serve as semipermeable membranes. In *peritoneal dialysis,* the body's peritoneal membrane, rich with blood vessels, is used to filter blood.

Glossary

continuous ambulatory peritoneal dialysis (CAPD): the most common method of peritoneal dialysis; involves frequent exchanges of dialysate, which remains in the peritoneal cavity throughout the day.

continuous renal replacement therapy (CRRT): a slow, continuous method of removing solutes and/or fluids from blood by gently pumping blood across a filtration membrane over a prolonged time period.

diffusion: movement of solutes from an area of high concentration to one of low concentration.

hemofiltration: removal of fluid and solutes by pumping blood across a membrane; no osmotic gradients are created during the process.

oncotic pressure: the pressure exerted by fluid on one side of a membrane as a result of osmosis.

osmosis: movement of water across a membrane toward the side where solutes are more concentrated.

peritonitis: inflammation of the peritoneal membrane.

pressure gradient: the change in pressure over a given distance. In dialysis, a pressure gradient is created between the blood and the dialysate.

semipermeable membrane: a membrane that allows some particles to pass through but not others.

ultrafiltration: removal of fluids and solutes from blood by using pressure to transfer the blood across a semipermeable membrane.

urea kinetic modeling: a method of determining the adequacy of dialysis treatment by calculating the urea clearance from blood.

FIGURE NP22-1 | Diffusion, Osmosis, and Ultrafiltration

Diffusion

Small molecules (electrolytes and waste products) move from an area of high concentration to an area of low concentration by diffusion.

Osmosis

Water moves from an area of high water concentration to an area of low water concentration. In other words, water moves toward the side where solutes are more concentrated.

Ultrafiltration

Pressure squeezes water and small molecules through the pores of a semipermeable membrane during ultrafiltration.

How are solutes separated from the blood in dialysis?

The chemical composition of the dialysate affects the movement of solutes across the semipermeable membrane. When the concentration of a substance is lower in the dialysate than in the blood, the substance—provided it can cross the membrane—will diffuse out of the blood. For example, the goal is to remove as much as possible of the waste product urea from the blood, so the dialysate contains no urea. For many other solutes, the dialysate is adjusted so that only excesses will be removed. Potassium can be removed from the blood, for example, by providing a dialysate that has a lower concentration of potassium than is found in the person's blood. The dialysate must contain some potassium, however; otherwise, the blood potassium would fall too low.

The dialysate can also be used to add needed components back into the blood. For a person with acidosis, for example, bases such as bicarbonate are added to the dialysate; the bases then move by diffusion into the blood to alleviate the acidosis.

How is fluid removed from the blood?

Because albumin and other plasma proteins are so adept at retaining fluids in blood, osmosis alone is not an efficient process for removing fluid. In hemodialysis, a **pressure gradient** is created between the blood and the dialysate. Most modern dialyzers produce *positive* pressure in the blood compartment and *negative* pressure in the dialysate compartment, establishing a pressure gradient that "pushes" water (and accompanying solutes) through the pores of the membrane.[1] This process, called ultrafiltration, relies on pumps to establish an appropriate flow rate between the blood and the dialysate.

How does the health practitioner know if the dialysis treatment has been effective?

A number of methods have been devised for gauging the adequacy of dialysis treatment. The most common method is **urea kinetic modeling**, a technique that evaluates the amount of urea cleared from the blood. The formula used most often is Kt/V, where K is the amount of urea cleared, t is the time spent on dialysis, and V is the blood volume. The value obtained indicates whether the patient has undergone sufficient dialysis; the goal is a Kt/V result of approximately 1.2. Because technical data (such as dialyzer clearance data, blood flow rate, and dialysate flow rate) need to be incorporated into the calculation, the computation is usually done by computer analysis. Current treatment guidelines recommend that hemodialysis adequacy be evaluated at least monthly, or more often if problems develop or patients are noncompliant.[2]

How long does a hemodialysis treatment last?

As described previously, hemodialysis utilizes a dialyzer to cleanse the patient's blood. Although dialyzers vary in efficiency, the treatment usually lasts 3 to 4 hours and is required at least three times weekly. Other options include short daily dialysis, performed for about 2 hours per day, and daily nocturnal hemodialysis, in which dialysis is done at home overnight while the patient is sleeping. Although some studies have reported improved outcomes in patients who undergo daily dialysis, these approaches have not been widely adopted.[3] Note that most patients must visit dialysis centers to obtain treatment; few patients have access to a dialysis machine at home.

Are any complications associated with hemodialysis?

Yes. Although lifesaving, hemodialysis is associated with a substantial number of complications.[4] Problems at the vascular access site include infections and blood clotting. Hypotension can develop while blood is circulated through the dialyzer. Muscle cramping often occurs during the procedure, especially in the hands, legs, and feet. Blood losses can worsen anemia, which is already severe in two-thirds of patients beginning hemodialysis treatment.[5] Patients may also experience headaches, weakness, nausea, vomiting, restlessness, and agitation.

How does peritoneal dialysis work?

In peritoneal dialysis, the peritoneal membrane surrounding the abdominal organs serves as a semipermeable membrane. The dialysate is infused into a catheter that empties into the peritoneal space—the space within the abdomen near the intestines (see Figure NP22-2). In the most common procedure, **continuous ambulatory**

During hemodialysis, blood passes through a dialyzer where wastes are extracted, and the cleansed blood is returned to the body.

In peritoneal dialysis, dialysate is infused into the peritoneal cavity.

Peritoneum

Peritoneal cavity

Catheter

Dialysate in

Four to six hours later, the fluid is drained and replaced with new dialysate. This process is repeated several times daily.

Waste out

Dialysate

Internal organs

Drain line

Waste solution

peritoneal dialysis (CAPD), the dialysate remains in the peritoneal cavity for 4 to 6 hours, after which it is drained and replaced with fresh dialysate (about 2 to 3 liters in adults). Generally, the dialysate solution is exchanged four times daily and requires only about 30 minutes to drain and replace.

Because a pressure gradient cannot be created in the peritoneal cavity as it can in a dialyzer, the glucose concentration in the dialysate must be high enough to create enough **oncotic pressure** to draw fluid from the blood. As indicated in Chapter 22, a substantial amount of glucose can be absorbed into the patient's blood and may contribute to weight gain over time. The high glucose load may also cause hyperglycemia and hypertriglyceridemia in some patients.

What are the advantages and disadvantages of peritoneal dialysis?

Peritoneal dialysis offers a number of advantages over hemodialysis: vascular access is not required, dietary restrictions are fewer, and the procedure can be scheduled when convenient. The most common complication is infection, which can occur at the catheter site or within the peritoneal cavity (**peritonitis**). Other problems that may arise include blood clotting in the catheter, catheter migration, and abdominal hernia due to the dialysate volume.

What are the features of continuous renal replacement therapy?

In people with acute kidney injury, **continuous renal replacement therapy (CRRT)** removes fluids and wastes. CRRT utilizes the process of **hemofiltration**, in which blood is gently pumped across a filtration membrane over a prolonged time period. (This process differs from dialysis treatments that rely on the diffusion of wastes across a membrane into the dialysate.) Either a pump or the patient's own blood pressure moves the blood across the membrane. The procedure can be used to remove fluids, solutes, or both. Some patients require fluid replacement during the procedure to maintain adequate blood volume, so hydration status must be closely monitored.

The use of CRRT is advantageous in acute care situations because it corrects imbalances without causing sudden shifts in blood volume, which are poorly tolerated in acute care patients. In addition, replacement fluids can include parenteral feedings without upsetting fluid balance. Complications include clotting problems, damage to arteries, and inadequate blood flow rates in hypotensive patients.

Dialysis and CRRT help to remove the wastes and fluids that are normally removed by healthy kidneys. Although these procedures cannot restore the kidneys' hormonal functions, they provide a lifesaving means of alleviating symptoms of uremia, hypertension, and edema.

Notes

1. J. Z. Kallenbach and coauthors, *Review of Hemodialysis for Nurses and Dialysis Personnel* (St. Louis: Elsevier/Mosby, 2005), pp. 61–70.
2. National Kidney Foundation, K/DOQI clinical practice guidelines for hemodialysis adequacy: Update 2006, available at **www.kidney.org/PROFESSIONALS/kdoqi/guideline_upHD_PD_VA/hd_guide2.htm**; site visited December 12, 2009.
3. K. L. Johansen and coauthors, Survival and hospitalization among patients using nocturnal and short daily compared to conventional hemodialysis: A USRDS study, *Kidney International* 76 (2009): 984–990.
4. N. Tolkoff-Rubin, Treatment of irreversible renal failure, in L. Goldman and D. Ausiello, eds., *Cecil Medicine* (Philadelphia: Saunders, 2008), pp. 936–947.
5. Tolkoff-Rubin, 2008.

CHAPTER 23 | # Nutrition, Cancer, and HIV Infection

Will & Deni McIntyre/Stone/Getty Images

CONTENTS

ALTHOUGH **CANCERS** AND **HUMAN IMMUNODEFICIENCY VIRUS (HIV)** infections are distinct disorders, from a nutritional standpoint they share some similarities. Both disorders have debilitating effects that influence nutritional needs, and both can lead to severe wasting in advanced cases. These illnesses require medical nutrition therapy that is highly individualized based on the symptoms manifested and the organ systems involved.

Cancer

Cancer, the growth of **malignant** tissue, is the second most common cause of death in the United States, ranking just below cardiovascular disease. Cancer is not a single disorder, however; there are many different kinds of malignant growths. The different types of cancer have different characteristics, occur in different locations in the body, take different courses, and require different treatments. (✚) Whereas an isolated, nonspreading type of skin cancer may be removed in a physician's office with no effect on nutrition status, advanced cancers—especially those of the gastrointestinal (GI) tract and pancreas—can seriously impair nutrition status.

HOW CANCER DEVELOPS

The development of cancer, called **carcinogenesis**, often proceeds slowly and continues for several decades. A cancer arises from mutations in the genes that control cell division in a single cell.[1] These mutations may promote cellular growth, interfere with growth restraint, or prevent cellular death. The affected cell thereby loses its built-in capacity for halting cell division and produces daughter cells with the same genetic defects. As the abnormal mass of cells, called a **tumor** (or *neoplasm*), grows, blood vessels form to supply the tumor with the nutrients it needs to support its growth. The tumor can disrupt the functioning of the normal tissue around it, and some tumor cells may **metastasize**, spreading to another region in the body. In leukemia (cancer affecting the white blood cells), the abnormal cells do not form a tumor but rather accumulate in the blood and other tissues. Figure 23-1 illustrates the steps in cancer development. (Note that an abnormal mass of cells that is noncancerous is called a *benign* tumor.)

The reasons why cancers develop are numerous and varied. Vulnerability to cancer is sometimes inherited, as when a person is born with a genetic defect that alters DNA structure, function, or repair. Certain metabolic processes may initiate carcinogenesis, as when phagocytes (immune cells) produce oxidants that cause DNA damage, or when chronic inflammation increases the rate of cell division, increasing the risk of a damaging mutation. More often, cancers are caused by interactions between a

✚ Cancers are classified by the tissues or cells from which they develop:

- *Adenomas* (ADD-eh-NO-muz) arise from glandular tissues.
- *Carcinomas* (CAR-sih-NO-muz) arise from epithelial tissues.
- *Gliomas* (gly-OH-muz) arise from glial cells of the central nervous system.
- *Leukemias* (loo-KEY-mee-uz) arise from white blood cell precursors.
- *Lymphomas* (lim-FOE-muz) arise from lymphoid tissues.
- *Melanomas* (MEL-ah-NO-muz) arise from pigmented skin cells.
- *Myelomas* (MY-ah-LOE-muz) arise from plasma cells in the bone marrow.
- *Sarcomas* (sar-KO-muz) arise from connective tissues, such as muscle or bone.

cancers: diseases characterized by the uncontrolled growth of a group of cells, which can destroy adjacent tissues and spread to other areas of the body via lymph or blood.

human immunodeficiency virus (HIV): the virus that causes acquired immune deficiency syndrome (AIDS). HIV destroys immune cells and progressively impedes the body's ability to fight infections and certain cancers.

FIGURE
23-1 Cancer Development

Normal cells

Initiation

Mutations alter the DNA in one of the cells and induce abnormal cell division.

Promotion

Proliferation of the altered cells results in formation of a tumor.

Further tumor development

Malignant cells   Normal cells

The cancerous tumor releases cells into the bloodstream or lymphatic system (metastasis).

TABLE 23-1 | Environmental Factors That Increase Cancer Risk

Environmental Factors	Cancer Sites
Aflatoxins (toxins in moldy peanuts or grains)	Liver
Alcohol[a]	Mouth, pharynx, larynx, esophagus, colon, rectum, liver, breast
Asbestos[b]	Lung, pleura, peritoneum
Chromium (hexavalent) compounds	Nasal cavity, lung
Estrogen-progesterone replacement therapy	Breast
Immunosuppressive medications	Lymphoid tissues, liver
Infection with *Helicobacter pylori*	Stomach
Infection with hepatitis B and hepatitis C viruses	Liver
Infection with human papillomavirus (HPV)	Cervix
Ionizing radiation (X-rays, radioactive isotopes, and other sources)	White blood cells (leukemia), esophagus, stomach, colon, thyroid, lung, bladder, breast
Tobacco[a]	Nasal cavity, lung, mouth, pharynx, larynx, esophagus, stomach, colon, rectum, liver, pancreas, kidney, renal pelvis, bladder
Ultraviolet radiation (sun exposure)	Skin

[a] A combined exposure to alcohol and tobacco multiplies the risks of developing cancers of the oral cavity, pharynx, larynx, and esophagus.

[b] Risk is greatly increased in cigarette smokers.

Sources: M. J. Thun, Epidemiology of cancer, in L. Goldman and D. Ausiello, eds., *Cecil Medicine* (Philadelphia: Saunders, 2008), pp. 1335–1340; World Cancer Research Fund/American Institute for Cancer Research, *Food, Nutrition, Physical Activity, and the Prevention of Cancer: A Global Perspective* (Washington, D.C.: American Institute for Cancer Research, 2007), pp. 157–171.

malignant (ma-LIG-nent): describes a cancerous cell or tumor, which can injure healthy tissue and spread cancer to other regions of the body.

carcinogenesis (CAR-sin-oh-JEN-eh-sis): the process of cancer development.

tumor: an abnormal tissue mass that has no physiological function; also called a *neoplasm* (NEE-oh-plazm).

metastasize (meh-TAS-tah-size): to spread from one part of the body to another; refers to cancer cells.

carcinogens (CAR-sin-oh-jenz or car-SIN-oh-jenz): substances that can cause cancer (the adjective is *carcinogenic*).

person's genes and environmental agents. Exposure to cancer-causing substances, or **carcinogens**, may either induce genetic mutations that lead to cancer or promote the proliferation of cancerous cells. Table 23-1 provides examples of environmental factors that increase cancer risk.

NUTRITION AND CANCER RISK

Like other environmental factors, diet and lifestyle strongly influence cancer risk. Certain food components may directly damage DNA, alter the metabolism of carcinogens by liver enzymes, or inhibit the formation of carcinogens in the body.[2] In addition, energy balance and growth rates affect the rate of cell division and consequently influence the rates at which mutations form and are replicated. Table 23-2 lists examples of nutrition-related factors that may increase or decrease the risk of developing cancer.

Nutrition and Increased Cancer Risk As shown in Table 23-2, obesity is a risk factor for a number of different cancers, including some relatively common cancers such as colon cancer and postmenopausal breast cancer. Obesity increases cancer risk, in part, by altering levels of hormones that influence cell growth, such as the sex hormones, insulin, and several kinds of growth factors. For example,

Nutrition, Cancer, and HIV Infection

TABLE 20-7	Antidiabetic Drugs		
Drug Category	**Common Examples**	**Mode of Action**	
Alpha-glucosidase inhibitors	Acarbose Miglitol	Delay carbohydrate digestion and absorption	
Amylin analogs (injected)	Pramlintide	Suppress glucagon secretion, delay stomach emptying, suppress appetite	
Biguanides	Metformin	Inhibit liver glucose production, improve glucose utilization	
DPP-4 inhibitors	Sitagliptin	Improve insulin secretion, suppress glucagon secretion, delay stomach emptying	
Incretin mimetics (injected)	Exenatide	Improve insulin secretion, suppress glucagon secretion, delay stomach emptying	
Meglitinides	Nateglinide Repaglinide	Stimulate insulin secretion by the pancreas	
Sulfonylureas	Glipizide Glyburide	Stimulate insulin secretion by the pancreas	
Thiazolidinediones	Pioglitazone Rosiglitazone	Decrease insulin resistance	

in the liver, delay stomach emptying, or delay carbohydrate digestion and absorption. Treatment may involve the use of a single medication (monotherapy) or a combination of several medications (combination therapy). By utilizing several mechanisms at once, combination therapy achieves more rapid and sustained glycemic control than is possible with monotherapy. Table 20-7 lists examples of antidiabetic drugs, and the Diet-Drug Interactions feature lists some of their nutrition-related effects. Because medications cannot replace the benefits offered by dietary modifications and physical activity, persons with diabetes should be advised to continue both.

PHYSICAL ACTIVITY AND DIABETES MANAGEMENT

Regular physical activity can improve glycemic control considerably and is therefore a central feature of diabetes management. A regular exercise program improves insulin sensitivity, which reduces insulin requirements. Physical activity also benefits other aspects of health, including blood lipid levels, blood pressure, body weight, and cardiovascular functioning. People with diabetes are advised to perform at least 150 minutes of moderate-intensity activity each week. In addition, those with type 2 diabetes should be encouraged to participate in a resistance exercise program three times per week, unless contraindicated by a medical condition that increases risk of injury.[47]

Physical Activity in Type 1 Diabetes People with type 1 diabetes must carefully adjust food intake and insulin therapy to prevent hypoglycemia during physical activity. Insulin doses that precede exercise often need to be reduced substantially. Blood glucose levels need to be checked both before and after an activity. If blood glucose is below 100 mg/dL, the individual should

	GASTROINTESTINAL EFFECTS	INTERACTIONS WITH DIETARY SUBSTANCES	METABOLIC EFFECTS
Sulfonylureas	Nausea, vomiting, cramps, diarrhea	Avoid using with alcohol due to a toxic reaction that causes flushing, throbbing head and neck pain, shortness of breath, palpitations, and sweating. Avoid using with dietary supplements that contain ginseng, garlic, fenugreek, coriander, and celery, as they may increase risk of hypoglycemia.	Hypoglycemia, weight gain, allergic skin reactions
Biguanides (metformin)	Abdominal pain and cramps, nausea, vomiting, gas, diarrhea, metallic taste, anorexia	—	Asymptomatic vitamin B_{12} deficiency
Thiazolidinediones	—	—	Hypoglycemia, weight gain, fluid retention, edema, anemia
Alpha-glucosidase inhibitors	Abdominal pain and cramps, nausea, gas, diarrhea	—	Elevated liver enzymes, hyperbilirubinemia

consume carbohydrate before beginning the activity. Additional carbohydrate may be needed during or after prolonged activity or even several hours after the activity is completed. The individual should avoid strenuous exercise if fasting blood glucose levels are 250 mg/dL or higher and should avoid all types of physical activity when blood glucose levels are 300 mg/dL or higher or ketosis is present.[48] Predicting the precise adjustments in diet and insulin becomes easier as a person gains experience in maintaining glycemic control.

Physical Activity in Type 2 Diabetes People with type 2 diabetes are often overweight and sedentary, and many develop complications during the course of disease. Before an exercise program is planned, a medical evaluation should screen for problems that may be aggravated by certain activities. Complications involving the heart and blood vessels, eyes, kidneys, feet, and nervous system may limit the types of activity recommended.

Only mild or moderate exercise may be prescribed at first. For obese, inactive persons, a short walk at a comfortable pace may be the first activity suggested. Individuals with retinopathy should avoid heavy lifting or straining, which may raise blood pressure and damage eye tissue. Persons with nephropathy often have reduced capacity for physical activity, and strenuous exercise is discouraged. Peripheral neuropathy precludes repetitive weight-bearing exercises such as jogging and step exercises because these activities may lead to foot ulcerations. The use of protective foot gear, such as gel soles or air midsoles and socks that prevent blisters, can help to prevent foot trauma. To prevent dehydration, which can adversely affect blood glucose levels and heart function, proper hydration should be encouraged before and during exercise.[49]

SICK-DAY MANAGEMENT

Illness, infection, or injury can cause hormonal changes that raise blood glucose levels and increase the risk of developing diabetic ketoacidosis or the hyperosmolar hyperglycemic syndrome. Hence, individuals with diabetes are counseled about sick-day

NURSING DIAGNOSIS

Risk for unstable blood glucose level may apply to an individual with diabetes who has an illness or injury.

Nora is a 12-year-old girl who was diagnosed with type 1 diabetes two years ago. She practices intensive therapy and has had the support of her parents and an excellent diabetes management team. With their help, Nora has been able to assume the bulk of the responsibility for her diabetes care and has managed to control her blood glucose remarkably well. In the past few months, however, Nora has been complaining bitterly about the impositions diabetes has placed on her life and her interactions with friends. Sometimes she refuses to monitor her blood glucose levels, and she has skipped insulin injections a few times. Recently, Nora was admitted to the emergency room complaining of fever, nausea, vomiting, and intense thirst. The physician noted that Nora was confused and lethargic. A urine test was positive for ketones, and her blood glucose levels were 400 mg/dL. The diagnosis was diabetic ketoacidosis.

1. Describe the metabolic events that lead to ketoacidosis. Were Nora's symptoms and laboratory tests consistent with the diagnosis?

2. Review Table 20-3, and consider the advantages and disadvantages that intensive therapy might have for Nora.

3. Discuss how Nora's age might influence her ability to cope with and manage her diabetes. Why might she feel that diabetes is disrupting her life? What suggestions may help?

4. Review the complications associated with long-term diabetes. How might you explain the importance of glycemic control to a 12-year-old girl?

management along with other self-care measures for diabetes. During illness, patients with diabetes should measure blood glucose levels and ketone levels in blood or urine several times daily. They should continue to take antidiabetic drugs, including insulin, as prescribed; some individuals may require medication adjustments if hyperglycemia persists. Some over-the-counter drugs may affect blood glucose levels or interact with oral antidiabetic drugs, so patients should check with health care providers before using an unfamiliar drug.[50]

During illness, individuals with diabetes should consume their usual diet, if possible. If appetite is poor, they should choose easy-to-manage foods and beverages that provide the prescribed amount of carbohydrate at each meal. Foods that are easily tolerated include toast, crackers, soup, yogurt, fruit, fruit juices, frozen juice bars, and carbohydrate-sweetened beverages. To prevent dehydration, especially if vomiting or diarrhea is present, liquids should be ingested in adequate amounts throughout the day.

Review Notes

- Diabetes treatment includes medical nutrition therapy, the use of insulin or other antidiabetic medications, and appropriate physical activity. Glycemic control is most often evaluated by monitoring blood glucose levels and glycated hemoglobin.

- The quantity of carbohydrate consumed has the greatest influence on blood glucose levels after meals. The total amount of carbohydrate ingested is more important than the type of carbohydrate consumed.

- Carbohydrate counting is widely used in menu planning and can be taught at different levels of complexity, depending on individual needs and abilities.

- Insulin therapy is required for patients who are unable to produce sufficient insulin and may be used in both type 1 and type 2 diabetes. Antidiabetic drugs can improve insulin secretion and effectiveness, suppress glucagon secretion, reduce glucose production by the liver, and delay carbohydrate absorption.

- Physical activity can improve glycemic control and enhance various aspects of general health. Illness can worsen glycemic control and may necessitate adjustments in medications and careful attention to dietary and fluid requirements. The Case Study provides an opportunity to review the factors that influence treatment of type 1 diabetes.

Glycemic control during pregnancy offers the best chance of a safe delivery and a healthy infant.

Diabetes Management in Pregnancy

Women with diabetes face new challenges during pregnancy. Due to hormonal changes, pregnancy increases insulin resistance and the need for insulin, so maintaining glycemic control may be more difficult. In addition, approximately 7 percent of nondiabetic women develop gestational diabetes and require treatment during pregnancy.[51] Women with gestational diabetes are at greater risk of developing type 2 diabetes later in life, and their children are at increased risk of developing obesity and type 2 diabetes as they enter adulthood. (Gestational diabetes was introduced in Chapter 10.)

A pregnancy complicated by diabetes increases health risks for both mother and fetus. Uncontrolled diabetes is linked with increased incidences of miscarriage, birth defects, and fetal deaths. Newborns are more likely to suffer from respiratory distress and to develop metabolic problems such as hypoglycemia, jaundice, and hypocalcemia. Women with diabetes often deliver babies with **macrosomia** (abnormally large bodies), which makes delivery more difficult and can result in birth trauma or the need for a cesarean section. Macrosomia results because maternal hyperglycemia induces excessive insulin production by the fetal pancreas, which stimulates growth and fat deposition.[52]

PREGNANCY IN TYPE 1 OR TYPE 2 DIABETES

Women with diabetes who achieve glycemic control at conception and during the first trimester of their pregnancy substantially reduce the risks of birth defects and spontaneous abortion. For this reason, it is recommended that women contemplating pregnancy receive preconception care to avoid the complications associated with poorly controlled diabetes.[53] Maintaining glycemic control during the second and third trimesters can minimize the risks of macrosomia and morbidity in newborn infants.

Nutrient requirements during pregnancy are generally similar for women with and without diabetes. The dietary adjustments suggested for improving glycemic control should be based on a woman's dietary habits and the results of blood glucose monitoring. Regular meals and snacks help to avoid hypoglycemia, which is more likely to occur during pregnancy because glucose is continuously supplied to the fetus. An evening snack is usually required to prevent overnight hypoglycemia and ketosis. Insulin and medication changes are often needed during pregnancy, and the woman may have to adjust her dietary habits further as a result.

GESTATIONAL DIABETES

Risk of gestational diabetes is highest in women who have a family history of diabetes, are obese, are in a high-risk ethnic group (Hispanic American, Native American, Asian American, African American, or Pacific Islander), or have previously given birth to an infant weighing over 9 pounds. To ensure that problems are dealt with promptly, physicians routinely test all women for gestational diabetes between 24 and 28 weeks of gestation. In high-risk women, screening should begin prior to pregnancy or soon after conception. Even mild hyperglycemia can have adverse effects on a developing fetus and may lead to complications during pregnancy.[54]

Women with gestational diabetes who are overweight or obese may need to adjust their energy intakes during pregnancy. Although adequate energy is needed for fetal development, a modest kcaloric reduction (about 30 percent less than total energy needs) may improve glycemic control without increasing the risk of ketosis.[55] Restricting carbohydrate to 40 to 45 percent of total energy intake may improve blood glucose levels after meals. Carbohydrate is usually poorly tolerated in the morning; therefore, restricting carbohydrate (to about 30 grams) at breakfast is often necessary.[56] The remaining carbohydrate intake should be spaced throughout the day in several meals and snacks, including an evening snack to prevent ketosis during the night.

macrosomia (MAK-roh-SOH-mee-ah): the condition of having an abnormally large body; in infants, refers to birth weights of 4000 grams (8 pounds 13 ounces) and above.

> **NURSING DIAGNOSIS**
>
> For diabetic pregnancies may include *risk for disturbed maternal/fetal dyad; risk for delayed development: fetal;* and *risk for disproportionate growth: fetal.*

Regular aerobic activity is often recommended because it can help to improve glycemic control. Women who fail to achieve glycemic goals by diet and exercise alone may need to use insulin or an antidiabetic drug that is safe during pregnancy.[57] The Case Study reviews the connections between gestational diabetes and type 2 diabetes.

Review Notes

- Careful management of blood glucose levels before and during pregnancy may reduce complications in mother and infant.
- Most nutrient requirements during pregnancy are similar for women with and without diabetes.
- Carbohydrate intake should be distributed into several meals and snacks, including an evening snack to prevent overnight ketosis. Carbohydrate restriction may be recommended, especially in women with gestational diabetes.
- Moderate energy restriction may help to improve glycemic control in overweight and obese women with gestational diabetes.

Nutrition Assessment | CHECKLIST FOR PEOPLE WITH DIABETES

MEDICAL HISTORY

Check the medical record to determine:

- ❍ Type of diabetes
- ❍ Duration of diabetes
- ❍ Acute and chronic complications
- ❍ Conditions, including pregnancy, that may alter treatment

MEDICATIONS

For people with preexisting diabetes who use antidiabetic drugs (including insulin), note:

- ❍ Type of medication
- ❍ Administration schedule

Check for use of other medications, including:

○ Medications that affect blood glucose levels
○ Cholesterol- and triglyceride-lowering medications
○ Antihypertensive medications

DIETARY INTAKE

To devise an acceptable meal plan and coordinate medications, obtain:

○ An accurate and thorough record of food intake and meal patterns
○ An account of usual physical activities

At medical checkups, reassess the person's ability to:

○ Maintain an appropriate carbohydrate intake
○ Maintain an appropriate energy intake
○ Monitor blood glucose levels at home
○ Adjust insulin and diet to accommodate sick days
○ Use appropriate foods to treat hypoglycemia

ANTHROPOMETRIC DATA

Take accurate baseline height and weight measurements as a basis for:

○ Appropriate energy intake
○ Initial insulin therapy

Periodically reassess height and weight for children and weight for adults and pregnant women to ensure that the meal plan provides an appropriate energy intake.

LABORATORY TESTS

Monitor the success of diabetes treatment using these tests:

○ Blood lipid concentrations
○ Blood or urinary ketones
○ Fructosamine, if necessary
○ Glycated hemoglobin
○ Urinary protein (microalbuminuria)

PHYSICAL SIGNS

Look for physical signs of:

○ Dehydration, especially in older adults
○ Foot ulcers
○ Nerve damage
○ Vision problems

Self Check

1 • Which of the following is characteristic of type 1 diabetes?
   a. Abdominal obesity increases risk.
   b. The pancreas makes little or no insulin.
   c. It is the predominant form of diabetes.
   d. It often arises during pregnancy.

2 • Which of the following describes type 2 diabetes?
   a. It is usually an autoimmune disease.
   b. The pancreas makes little or no insulin.
   c. Diabetic ketoacidosis is a common complication.
   d. Chronic complications may develop before it is diagnosed.

3 • Most chronic complications associated with diabetes result from:
   a. altered kidney function.
   b. infections that deplete nutrient reserves.
   c. weight gain and hypertension.
   d. damage to blood vessels and nerves.

4 • Long-term glycemic control is usually evaluated by:
   a. self-monitoring of blood glucose.
   b. testing urinary ketone levels.
   c. measuring glycated hemoglobin.
   d. testing urinary protein levels (microalbuminuria).

5 • Regarding dietary carbohydrate, a patient with diabetes should be most concerned about:
   a. consuming the correct quantity of carbohydrate at each meal or snack.
   b. consuming the correct proportion of sugars, starches, and fiber in meals.
   c. avoiding added sugars and kcaloric sweeteners.
   d. choosing meals with ideal proportions of protein, carbohydrate, and fat.

6 • Which of the following is true regarding the general use of alcohol in diabetes?
   a. A serving of alcohol is considered part of the carbohydrate allowance.
   b. Alcohol contributes to hyperglycemia and should be avoided completely.
   c. Alcohol can cause hypoglycemia and should therefore be consumed with food if patients use insulin or medications that stimulate insulin secretion.
   d. Patients can use alcohol in unlimited quantities unless they are pregnant.

7 • The meal-planning strategy best suited to all people with diabetes is:
   a. carbohydrate counting.
   b. the exchange list system.

TABLE 23-2 | Nutrition-Related Factors That Influence Cancer Risk

Nutrition-Related Factors[a]	Cancer Sites
Factors that increase cancer risk:	
Obesity	Esophagus, colon, rectum, pancreas, gallbladder, kidney, breast (postmenopausal), endometrium
Red meat, processed meats	Colon, rectum
Salted and salt-preserved foods	Stomach
Beta-carotene supplements	Lung[b]
High-calcium diets (over 1500 mg daily)	Prostate
Low level of physical activity[c]	Colon, breast (postmenopausal), endometrium
Factors that decrease cancer risk:	
Fruits and nonstarchy vegetables	Lung, mouth, pharynx, larynx, esophagus, stomach
Carotenoid-containing foods	Lung, mouth, pharynx, larynx, esophagus
Tomato products	Prostate
Allium vegetables (onion, garlic)	Stomach, colon, rectum
Vitamin C–containing foods	Esophagus
Folate-containing foods	Pancreas
Fiber-containing foods	Colon, rectum
Milk and calcium supplements	Colon, rectum
High level of physical activity[c]	Colon, breast (postmenopausal), endometrium

[a] Altered cancer risk is associated with high intakes of the dietary substances listed. The cancer sites associated with alcohol are included in Table 23-1.

[b] Cancer risk is increased in tobacco smokers and may not apply to other groups.

[c] Physical activity may influence cancer risk by altering body fatness, intestinal transit time, insulin sensitivity, hormone levels, enzyme activities, and immune responses.

Source: World Cancer Research Fund/American Institute for Cancer Research, *Food, Nutrition, Physical Activity, and the Prevention of Cancer: A Global Perspective* (Washington, D.C.: American Institute for Cancer Research, 2007).

in the case of breast cancer in postmenopausal women, the hormone estrogen is likely involved: obese women have higher estrogen levels than do lean women, because adipose tissue produces estrogen.

Although studies in animals have suggested that high-fat diets can promote tumor growth, studies of humans have not proved that the effects of fat are independent of

Cruciferous vegetables, such as cauliflower, broccoli, and brussels sprouts, contain nutrients and phytochemicals that inhibit cancer development.

© Polara Studios, Inc.

the effects of energy intake and physical activity.[3] Evidence from population studies is mixed: high-fat diets often, but not always, correlate with high cancer rates. Within single populations, cancer rates do not reliably reflect fat intakes. In addition, the type of fat consumed may be critical: studies of colon and rectal cancers implicate animal fats but not vegetable fat, and a number of studies suggest that consuming fatty fish may be protective.[4]

Food preparation methods are responsible for producing certain types of carcinogens. Cooking meat, poultry, and fish at high temperatures causes carcinogens to form in these foods.[5] Carcinogens also accompany the smoke that adheres to food during grilling, and they are present in the charred surfaces of grilled meat and fish. The cancer risk from eating such foods is unclear, however, because the biological actions of these carcinogens are modulated by other dietary components, including compounds in vegetables and other plant foods. In several population studies, consumption of well-cooked meats was linked to cancers of the stomach, colon, breast, and prostate.[6]

Nutrition and Decreased Cancer Risk A considerable number of human studies have found a link between the consumption of fruits and vegetables and reduced incidences of certain cancers (review Table 23-2). Fruits and vegetables contain both nutrients and phytochemicals with antioxidant activity, and these substances may prevent or reduce the oxidative reactions in cells that cause DNA damage. Phytochemicals may also help to inhibit carcinogen production in the body, enhance immune functions that protect against cancer development, and promote enzyme reactions that inactivate carcinogens.[7] In addition, certain fruits and vegetables provide the B vitamin folate, which plays roles in DNA synthesis and repair; thus, inadequate folate intakes may allow DNA damage to accumulate.

Although research reports originally suggested that a fiber-rich diet could protect against colon cancer, recent studies have cast doubt on the earlier analyses.[8] The earlier studies depended on the ability of colon cancer patients to recall the foods they had consumed during the preceding years, whereas more recent studies—considered more reliable—tracked the subjects' health behaviors and cancer outcomes for extended periods (10 to 20 years). Moreover, some studies that had found fiber to be protective did not analyze factors such as physical activity, smoking, or folate intake, all of which can influence cancer outcome. A fiber-rich diet may be protective, in part, because high-fiber foods usually contain high levels of nutrients and phytochemicals that are protective against cancer. Table 23-3 summarizes the dietary and lifestyle practices that may help to reduce the risk of developing cancer.

CONSEQUENCES OF CANCER

Once cancer develops, its consequences depend on the location of the tumor, its severity, and the treatment. The complications that develop are often due to the tumor's impingement on surrounding tissues. Nonspecific effects of cancer include anorexia, lethargy, weight loss, night sweats, and fever.[9] During the early stages, many cancers produce no symptoms, and the person may be unaware of the threat to health.

Wasting Associated with Cancer Anorexia, muscle wasting, weight loss, and fatigue typify **cancer cachexia**, which eventually affects more than 80 percent of people with terminal cancer.[10] Weight loss is often evident at the time that cancer is diagnosed, and severe malnutrition, typically seen in the later stages of cancer, is the ultimate cause of death in many cases. Without adequate energy and nutrients, the body is poorly equipped to maintain organ function, support immune defenses, and mend damaged tissues. An involuntary weight loss of more than 10 percent, which indicates significant malnutrition, is cause for concern.[11]

Many factors play a role in the wasting associated with cancer. Cytokines, (✚) released by both tumor cells and immune cells, induce a catabolic state. The combined effects of a poor appetite, accelerated and abnormal metabolism, and the diversion of nutrients to support tumor growth result in a lower supply of energy and nutrients at a time when demands are high. Appetite and food intake are further disturbed by the effects of treatments and medications prescribed for cancer patients.

✚ The cytokines that induce cachexia include tumor necrosis factor-α, interleukin-1, interleukin-6, and γ-interferon.

cancer cachexia (ka-KEK-see-ah): a wasting syndrome associated with cancer that is characterized by anorexia, muscle wasting, weight loss, and fatigue.

NURSING DIAGNOSIS

Imbalanced nutrition: less than body requirements, adult failure to thrive, and *ineffective protection* may apply to those with cancer cachexia.

TABLE 23-3 | Recommendations for Reducing Cancer Risk

Maintain a healthy body weight.
- Balance energy intake with appropriate physical activity.
- Avoid weight gain and increases in waist circumference throughout adulthood.
- If overweight or obese, achieve a healthy body weight.

Be physically active.
- For adults: engage in moderate to vigorous activity for 30 minutes on at least five days of the week; 45 to 60 minutes is preferable.
- For children and adolescents: engage in moderate to vigorous activity for 60 minutes on at least five days of the week.

Choose a healthy diet that emphasizes plant sources.
- Consume five or more servings of a variety of vegetables and fruits daily.
- Choose whole-grain products instead of processed (refined) grains.
- Limit consumption of red meats and processed meats.
- Avoid salt-preserved and salty foods.
- Avoid moldy grains and legumes.

Limit consumption of alcoholic beverages.
- For women: drink no more than one drink daily.
- For men: drink no more than two drinks daily.

Avoid using tobacco in any form.

Sources: World Cancer Research Fund/American Institute for Cancer Research, *Food, Nutrition, Physical Activity, and the Prevention of Cancer: A Global Perspective* (Washington, D.C.: American Institute for Cancer Research, 2007); L. H. Kushi and coauthors, American Cancer Society guidelines on nutrition and physical activity for cancer prevention: Reducing the risk of cancer with healthy food choices and physical activity, *CA: A Cancer Journal for Clinicians* 56 (2006): 254–281.

Metabolic Changes The metabolic changes that arise in cancer exacerbate the wasting described in the previous section.[12] Cancer patients exhibit an increased rate of protein turnover (✚) but reduced muscle protein synthesis. Muscle contributes amino acids for glucose production, further depleting the body's supply of protein. Triglyceride breakdown increases, elevating serum lipids. Many patients develop insulin resistance. These metabolic abnormalities help to explain why people with cancer fail to regain lean tissue or maintain healthy body weights even when they are consuming adequate energy and nutrients.

Anorexia and Reduced Food Intake Anorexia is a major contributor to the wasting associated with cancer. Some factors that contribute to anorexia or otherwise reduce food intake include:

- *Chronic nausea and early satiety.* People with cancer frequently experience nausea and a premature feeling of fullness after eating small amounts of food.
- *Fatigue.* People with cancer often tire easily and lack the energy to prepare and eat meals. Once cachexia develops, these tasks become even more difficult.
- *Pain.* People in pain may have little interest in eating, particularly if eating makes the pain worse.
- *Mental stress.* A cancer diagnosis can cause distress, anxiety, and depression, all of which may reduce appetite. Facing and undergoing cancer treatments induces additional psychological stress.
- *Effects of cancer therapies.* Therapies for cancer (including medications, chemotherapy, radiation therapy, surgery, and bone marrow transplants) can reduce food

✚ Reminder: *Protein turnover* refers to the continuous degradation and synthesis of the body's proteins.

TABLE 23-4	Nutrition-Related Side Effects of Cancer Surgeries

Head and Neck Surgeries

Aspiration

Dry or sore mouth

Reduced chewing or swallowing ability

Reduced sense of taste or smell

Esophageal Resection

Acid reflux

Altered gastric motility

Reduced swallowing ability

Gastric Resection

Dumping syndrome

Early satiety

Inadequate gastric acid secretion

Malabsorption of iron, folate, and vitamin B_{12}

Intestinal Resection

Bile insufficiency

Diarrhea

Fluid and electrolyte imbalances

General malabsorption

Pancreatic Resection

Diabetes mellitus

General malabsorption

✚ One drug that inhibits cell division is *methotrexate,* which closely resembles the B vitamin folate (see Figure 14-3 on p. 422). Folate is required for cell division because it is needed for DNA synthesis. Methotrexate works by blocking activity of the enzyme that converts folate to its active form.

chemotherapy: the use of drugs to arrest or destroy cancer cells; these drugs are called *antineoplastic agents.*

intake by causing nausea, vomiting, altered taste perceptions, food aversions, inflammation of the mouth and esophagus, dry mouth, mouth sores, difficulty swallowing, intestinal cramping, diarrhea, and constipation.

- *Gastrointestinal obstructions.* A tumor may partially or completely obstruct a portion of the GI tract, causing complications such as nausea and vomiting, early satiety, delayed gastric emptying, and bacterial overgrowth. Some patients with obstructions are unable to tolerate oral diets.

TREATMENTS FOR CANCER

The primary medical treatments for cancer—surgery, chemotherapy, radiation therapy, or any combination of the three—aim to remove cancer cells, prevent further tumor growth, and alleviate symptoms.[13] The likelihood of effective treatment is highest with early detection and intervention. Because treatment decisions are difficult and cancer therapies have considerable side effects, patients rely on health care providers to help them make informed decisions.

Surgery Surgery is performed to remove tumors, determine the extent of cancer, and protect nearby tissues. Often, surgery must be followed by other cancer treatments to prevent growth of new tumors. The acute metabolic stress caused by surgery raises protein and energy needs and can exacerbate wasting. Surgery also contributes to pain, fatigue, and anorexia, all of which can reduce food intake at a time when nutritional needs are substantial. Blood loss contributes to nutrient losses and further exacerbates malnutrition. Some surgeries can have long-term effects on nutrition status (see Table 23-4).

Chemotherapy **Chemotherapy** relies on the use of drugs to treat cancer; it is used to inhibit tumor growth, shrink tumors before surgery, and prevent or eradicate metastasis. Some cancer drugs interfere with the process of cell division; (✚) others sterilize cells that are in a resting phase and are not actively dividing. Ideally, chemotherapy would wipe out cancer cells without destroying healthy ones. Unfortunately, most of these drugs have toxic effects on normal cells as well and are especially damaging to rapidly dividing cells, such as those of the GI tract, skin, and bone marrow. Some of the newer drugs are able to target properties specific to cancer cells and are better tolerated by the body's tissues. Table 23-5 includes a summary of the nutrition-related side effects that may result from chemotherapy.

Radiation Therapy **Radiation therapy** treats cancer by bombarding cancer cells with X-rays, gamma rays, or various atomic particles. These treatments generate reactive forms of oxygen, such as superoxide and hydroxyl radicals, which can damage cellular DNA and cause cell death. Newer techniques are able to focus radiation directly at tumors and minimize damage to nearby tissues. An advantage of radiation therapy over surgery is that it can shrink tumors while preserving organ structure and function. Compared with chemotherapy, radiation therapy is better able to target specific regions of the body, rather than involving all body cells. Nonetheless, radiation therapy can damage healthy tissues and sometimes has long-term detrimental effects on nutrition status. Radiation to the head and neck area can damage the salivary glands and taste buds, causing inflammation, dry mouth, and a reduced sense of taste; in severe cases, damage may be permanent. Radiation treatment in the lower abdominal area can cause **radiation enteritis**, an inflammatory condition of the small intestine that causes nausea, vomiting, malabsorption, and diarrhea. Table 23-5 includes additional side effects of radiation treatment that affect nutrition status.

Bone Marrow Transplant A **bone marrow transplant** replaces bone marrow that has been destroyed by chemotherapy or radiation therapy, and it is one of the

TABLE 23-5	Nutrition-Related Side Effects of Chemotherapy and Radiation Therapy		
	Reduced Nutrient Intake	**Accelerated Nutrient Losses**	**Altered Metabolism**
Chemotherapy	Abdominal pain Anorexia Mouth ulcers Nausea and vomiting Reduced taste sensation	Diarrhea Intestinal inflammation Malabsorption Vomiting	Fluid and electrolyte imbalances as a consequence of vomiting, diarrhea, or malabsorption Hyperglycemia Interference with vitamins or body compounds Negative nitrogen and micro-nutrient balances Secondary effects of malnutrition, infection, or inflammation
Radiation therapy	Anorexia Damage to teeth, jaws, or salivary glands Dysphagia Esophagitis Mouth sores Nausea and vomiting Reduced salivary secretions Reduced taste sensation	Blood loss from intestine and bladder Diarrhea Fistulas Intestinal obstructions Malabsorption Radiation enteritis Vomiting	Fluid and electrolyte imbalances as a consequence of vomiting, diarrhea, or malabsorption Secondary effects of malnutrition, infection, or inflammation

primary treatments for leukemia, lymphomas, and multiple myeloma.[14] If possible, bone marrow cells are collected from the patient before chemotherapy or radiation treatment begins so that it is not necessary to find a separate donor. If another person's cells are used, the patient must take immunosuppressant drugs to prevent **tissue rejection**.

The treatments that bone marrow transplant patients undergo have a substantial impact on their food intake and nutrition status. The chemotherapy or radiation therapy preceding the transplant and the immunosuppressant drugs required afterward can impair immune function substantially and increase the risk of foodborne illness. Other common complications include anorexia, dry mouth, altered taste sensations, inflamed mucous membranes, malabsorption, nausea, vomiting, and diarrhea. Patients are often unable to consume adequate food and may require nutrition support, as described in a later section.

Medications to Combat Anorexia and Wasting
To help cancer patients combat anorexia, medications may be prescribed to stimulate the appetite and promote weight gain. Examples include megestrol acetate (Megace), a synthetic compound similar in structure to the hormone progesterone, and dronabinol (Marinol), which resembles the psychoactive ingredient in marijuana and stimulates the appetite at doses that have minimal mental effects. Under investigation are medications that may help to restore lean tissue, such as anabolic steroids, growth hormone, and insulin-like growth factor.[15]

Alternative Therapies
Many patients turn to *complementary and alternative medicine (CAM)* (✚) to assist them in their fight against cancer. Patients may turn to CAM because they wish to gain more control over treatment or because they are concerned about the effectiveness of conventional approaches. Although few abandon conventional medicine, up to 80 percent of cancer patients combine one or more CAM approaches with standard treatment.[16] Many patients do not discuss their use of CAM with physicians.

Dietary supplements and herbal remedies are among the most frequently used CAM therapies. Although many supplements can be used without risk, some may have adverse effects or interfere with conventional treatments. Use of the herbal remedy St. John's wort, for example, can reduce the effectiveness of some anticancer drugs.[17]

✚ Reminder: *Complementary and alternative medicine (CAM)* refers to health care practices that have not been proved to be effective and consequently are not included as part of conventional treatment. Nutrition in Practice 14 provides additional information about CAM.

radiation therapy: the use of X-rays, gamma rays, or atomic particles to destroy cancer cells.

radiation enteritis: inflammation of intestinal tissue caused by radiation therapy.

bone marrow transplant: a procedure that replaces bone marrow that has been destroyed by cancer treatment; it is also used to treat certain types of cancers and blood disorders. Also called *hematopoietic stem cell transplantation.*

tissue rejection: destruction of donor tissue by the recipient's immune system, which recognizes the donor cells as foreign.

✚ Reminder: The high-kcalorie, high-protein diet, which is appropriate for some individuals with cancer, was described in Chapter 14 (see p. 414).

As another example, some studies suggest that antioxidant supplements interfere with chemotherapy and radiation treatments.[18] Clinical trials of several popular supplements are in progress and are expected to reveal more about their potential effects and interactions with cancer treatments.

MEDICAL NUTRITION THERAPY FOR CANCER

The objectives of medical nutrition therapy for cancer patients are to minimize loss of weight and muscle tissue, correct nutrient deficiencies, and provide a diet that patients can tolerate and enjoy despite the complications of illness. Appropriate nutrition care helps patients preserve their strength and improves recovery after stressful cancer treatments. Moreover, malnourished cancer patients develop more complications and have shorter survival times than patients who maintain good nutrition status.[19]

Because there are many forms of cancer and a variety of potential treatments, nutritional needs among cancer patients vary considerably. Furthermore, a person's needs may change at different stages of illness. Patients should be screened for malnutrition when cancer is diagnosed and be reassessed during the treatment and recovery periods.

Protein and Energy For patients at risk of weight loss and wasting, the focus of nutrition care is to ensure appropriate intakes of protein and energy. Health practitioners regularly monitor weight changes and adjust intake recommendations as necessary. Patients who cannot eat adequate food may be able to meet their needs by supplementing the diet with nutrient-dense formulas. The "How to" below provides suggestions that can help to increase the energy and protein content of meals. (✚)

Although weight loss is a problem for many cancer patients, breast cancer patients often gain weight.[20] The weight gain occurs during the first two years after breast cancer diagnosis and is associated with an increase in total body fat. By discussing weight maintenance soon after diagnosis and encouraging physical activity, health practitioners can help patients avoid unnecessary weight gain.

Managing Symptoms and Complications A thorough nutrition assessment often uncovers specific problems or symptoms that interfere with food

HOW TO | Increase kCalories and Protein in Meals

To increase the energy content of a meal, try these suggestions:

- *Butter or margarine.* Melt on pasta, potatoes, rice, and cooked vegetables. Add to hot cereals, casseroles, and soups. Spread liberally on bread, crackers, and rolls.

- *Mayonnaise or salad dressings.* Add to pasta, tuna, and potato salads. Use as dressings for raw or cooked vegetables.

- *Cream cheese.* Spread on raw vegetables, toast, and crackers. Mix into chopped fruit. Use as a spread in sandwiches made with luncheon meats.

- *Half-and-half and cream.* Replace milk or water with half-and-half or cream in soups, sauces, hot chocolate, desserts, mashed potatoes, and cold and cooked cereals. Use sour cream on potato dishes and soups. Add whipped cream to fruit salads and desserts.

- *Nuts.* Add chopped nuts to pasta dishes, stir-fried vegetables, fruit salads, and green salads. Use nut meats in baked products. Spread nut butters on bread and crackers.

- *Beverages.* Replace water and nonkcaloric beverages with sweetened drinks, fruit juices, and milk shakes. Drink whole milk instead of low-fat or nonfat milk. Add strawberry or chocolate syrup to plain milk to boost kcalories.

These suggestions can help to add protein to a meal:

- *Milk.* Use in place of water when preparing cereals and cream soups. Use cream sauces (which are made with milk) to flavor vegetable and pasta dishes.

- *Powdered milk (use full-fat milk powder if available).* Add to recipes that include milk. Dissolve extra milk powder into milk-containing beverages. Stir into hot cereals, potato dishes, casseroles, and sauces. Add to scrambled eggs, hamburger, and meat loaf.

- *Cheese.* Melt on burgers, meat loaf, cooked vegetables, scrambled eggs, casseroles, and potatoes. Add cottage cheese to casseroles, egg dishes, pasta recipes, and salad dressings. Grate hard cheeses and sprinkle on soups, salads, and cooked vegetable dishes.

- *Eggs.* Add raw eggs when preparing casseroles, meatballs, and hamburgers. Add chopped hard-cooked eggs to salads, vegetable dishes, sandwich fillings, and pasta and potato salads.

- *Meats.* Add small chunks of meat to soups, egg dishes, casseroles, bean dishes, and pasta sauces. Add minced meats to vegetable dishes. Add chunks of cooked chicken or turkey to salads. To improve kcalorie intakes, make sure you choose higher-fat meats instead of lean meats.

TABLE
23-6 | Dietary Considerations for Specific Cancers

Cancer Sites	Common Complications[a]	Possible Dietary Measures
Brain and nervous system	Chewing and swallowing difficulties, headache, altered taste or smell sensation, difficulty feeding oneself	Mechanically altered diet, use of adaptive feeding devices (see Nutrition in Practice 21)
Head and neck[b]	Swallowing difficulty, aspiration, inflamed mucosa, dry mouth, altered taste or smell sensation	Tube feeding, mechanically altered diet
Esophagus	Swallowing difficulty, aspiration, obstruction, acid reflux, inflamed mucosa	Tube feeding, mechanically altered diet
Stomach	Anorexia, early satiety, reduced secretion of gastric acid and intrinsic factor, delayed stomach emptying, dumping syndrome, malabsorption, nutrient deficiencies	Tube feeding (for obstruction or unmanageable dumping syndrome); postgastrectomy diet; small, frequent meals; limited sugars and insoluble fibers (see Chapter 17); nutrient supplementation
Intestine	Inflamed mucosa, bacterial overgrowth, obstruction, lactose intolerance, general malabsorption, bile insufficiency, nutrient deficiencies, short bowel syndrome (if resected), altered bowel function, fluid and electrolyte imbalances	Tube feeding or total parenteral nutrition for obstruction, enteritis, or short bowel syndrome; fat- and lactose-restricted diet (see Chapter 18); nutrient supplementation
Pancreas	Reduced secretion of digestive enzymes, bile insufficiency, general malabsorption, nutrient deficiencies, hyperglycemia	Fat-restricted diet; enzyme replacement (see Chapter 18); small, frequent meals; carbohydrate-controlled diet (Chapter 20); nutrient supplementation

[a] Actual complications depend on the exact location of the cancer and the specific methods used for treating the cancer.

[b] Includes cancers of the salivary glands, oral and nasal cavities, pharynx, and larynx.

consumption. Table 23-6 lists dietary considerations related to cancers affecting different sites in the body. The "How to" on pp. 657–658 outlines a variety of dietary strategies that may improve food intake and alleviate symptoms. Patients' responses to these strategies can vary considerably, and in some cases a number of adjustments may be necessary.

Enteral and Parenteral Nutrition Support
Nutrition support is used in limited situations during cancer treatment. Generally, tube feedings and

HOW TO | Help Patients Handle Food-Related Problems

In people with cancer or HIV infection, various complications can interfere with food intake. Nurses can try to identify a patient's specific problems and offer appropriate solutions. Not every suggestion will work for each patient; encourage patients to experiment and find strategies that work best.

- **I just don't have an appetite.**

  - Eat small meals and snacks at regular times each day.

  - Eat the largest meal at the time of day when you feel the best.

  - Include nutrient-dense foods in meals, and consume them before other foods.

- Indulge in favorite foods throughout the day. Serve foods attractively.

- Avoid drinking large amounts of liquids before or with meals.

- Eat in a pleasant and relaxed environment. Eat with family and friends when possible.

- Listen to your favorite music or enjoy a TV or radio program while you eat.

- Ask your doctor about appetite-enhancing medications.

- **I am too tired to fix meals and eat.**
  - Let family members and friends prepare food for you.
  - Obtain foods that are easy to prepare and easy to eat, such as sandwiches, frozen dinners, take-out meals from restaurants, instant breakfast drinks, liquid formulas, and energy bars.
  - Find time to rest before you attempt to prepare a large meal.
  - Prepare soups, stews, and casserole dishes in sufficient quantity to provide enough for several meals, so that you will have enough to eat at times when you are too tired to cook.

- **Foods just don't taste right.**
  - Brush your teeth or use mouthwash before you eat.
  - Consume foods chilled or at room temperature. Use plastic, rather than metal, eating utensils.
  - Choose eggs, fish, poultry, and milk products instead of meats.
  - Experiment with sauces, seasonings, herbs, spices, and sweeteners to improve food taste and flavor.
  - Save your favorite foods for times when you are not feeling nauseated.

- **I am nauseated a lot of the time, and sometimes I need to vomit.**
  - Consume liquids throughout the day to replace fluids.
  - If you become nauseated from chemotherapy treatments, avoid eating for at least two hours before treatments.
  - Consume your largest meal at a time when you are least likely to feel nauseous.
  - Try consuming smaller meals, and eat slowly. Experiment with foods to see if some foods cause nausea more than others.
  - Avoid foods and meals that have strong odors or are fatty, greasy, or gas forming.

- **I have problems chewing and swallowing food.**
  - Experiment with food consistencies to find the ones you can manage best. Thin liquids, dry foods, and sticky foods (such as peanut butter) are often difficult to swallow.
  - Add sauces and gravies to dry foods.
  - Drink fluids during meals to ease chewing and swallowing.
  - Try using a straw to drink liquids. Experiment with beverage thickeners if you cannot tolerate thin beverages.
  - Tilt your head forward and backward to see if you can swallow more easily when your head is positioned differently.

- **I have sores in my mouth, and they hurt when I eat.**
  - Use cold or frozen foods; they are often soothing.
  - Try soft foods such as ice cream, milk shakes, bananas, applesauce, mashed potatoes, cottage cheese, and macaroni and cheese. Mix dry foods with sauces or gravies.
  - Cut foods into smaller pieces, so they are less likely to irritate the mouth.

- Avoid foods that irritate mouth sores, such as citrus fruits and juices, tomatoes and tomato-based products, spicy foods, foods that are very salty, foods with seeds (such as poppy seeds and sesame seeds) that can scrape the sores, and coarse foods such as raw vegetables, crackers, corn chips, and toast.
- Ask your doctor about using a local anesthetic solution such as lidocaine before eating to reduce pain.
- Use a straw for drinking liquids, in order to bypass the sores.

- **My mouth is really dry.**
  - Rinse your mouth with warm salt water or mouthwash frequently. Avoid using mouthwash that contains alcohol.
  - Drink small amounts of liquid frequently between meals.
  - Ask your doctor or pharmacist about medications or saliva substitutes that can help a dry mouth condition.
  - Use sour candy or gum to stimulate the flow of saliva.
  - Sip fluids frequently while eating. Add broth, sauces, gravies, mayonnaise, butter, or margarine to dry foods.
  - Make sure you brush your teeth and floss regularly to prevent tooth decay and oral infections.

- **I am having trouble with constipation.**
  - Drink plenty of fluids. Try warm fluids, especially in the morning.
  - Eat whole-grain breads and cereals, nuts, fresh fruits and vegetables, prunes, and prune juice. Avoid refined carbohydrate foods such as white bread, white rice, and pasta.
  - Engage in physical activity regularly.
  - Try an over-the-counter bulk-forming agent, such as methylcellulose (Citrucel), psyllium (Metamucil or Fiberall), or polycarbophil (Fiber-Lax).

- **I am having trouble with diarrhea.**
  - Drink plenty of fluids. Salty broths and soups, diluted fruit juices, and sports drinks are good choices. Avoid caffeine- and alcohol-containing beverages. For severe diarrhea, try oral rehydration formulas that are commercially prepared.
  - Avoid foods and beverages that increase gas, such as legumes, onions, vegetables of the cabbage family, foods that contain sorbitol or mannitol, and carbonated beverages.
  - Try using lactase enzyme replacements when you use milk products in case you are experiencing lactose intolerance. Yogurt and aged cheeses may be easier to tolerate than milk and fresh cheeses.
  - Avoid fatty foods if you are fat intolerant. Try reducing your intake of whole-grain breads and cereals if they worsen the diarrhea.
  - Eat small, frequent meals instead of large ones. Try consuming cool or lukewarm foods instead of very cold or hot foods.
  - Ask your doctor about using a bulk-forming agent or antidiarrhea medication.

parenteral nutrition are provided to patients who have long-term or permanent gastrointestinal impairment or are experiencing complications that interfere with food intake.[21] For example, many patients undergoing radiation therapy for head and neck cancers require long-term tube feeding and may need to continue tube feedings at home. (✚) Parenteral nutrition is reserved for individuals who have inadequate GI function, such as those with chronic radiation enteritis. Whenever possible, enteral nutrition is strongly preferred over parenteral nutrition, to preserve GI function and avoid infection.

✚ Irradiation to the head and neck regions often causes dysphagia and mouth sores.

Nutrition Therapy for Bone Marrow Transplant Patients

Patients who undergo bone marrow transplants may require total parenteral nutrition (TPN) before and after the transplant, because the GI tract is often severely damaged by the chemotherapy or radiation treatment required beforehand. When GI function returns, the patient can begin consuming small amounts of food along with TPN. As oral intake improves, TPN is gradually tapered. Some patients may require a high-kcalorie, high-protein diet to reverse malnutrition. Because recipients of bone marrow transplants are severely immunocompromised, they should be instructed to follow safe food-handling practices to minimize the risk of foodborne illness (see Nutrition in Practice 2). In addition, they must avoid foods that are likely to contain unsafe levels of bacteria, such as unwashed raw fruits and vegetables; undercooked meat, poultry, and eggs; leftover luncheon meats and meat spreads; leftover foods that have not been adequately reheated; unpasteurized dairy products, juices, honey, and beer; blue-veined cheeses; and foods from salad bars or street vendors.[22]

Review Notes

- Cancer arises from mutations in the genes that control cell division. Some dietary substances promote carcinogenesis, while others may help to prevent cancer.
- Cancer's effects on nutrition status depend on the type of cancer a person has, its severity, and the methods used to treat the cancer. Cancer cachexia is a frequent complication of cancer and may be related to anorexia, altered metabolism, and responses to cancer treatment.
- Medical treatments for cancer include surgery, chemotherapy, and radiation therapy, which remove cancer cells, prevent tumor growth, and alleviate symptoms. Medical nutrition therapy aims to minimize weight loss and wasting, correct deficiencies, and manage complications that impair food intake. The accompanying Case Study allows you to apply information about nutrition and cancer to a clinical situation.

CASE STUDY | Woman with Cancer

Janet Woodhouse is a 58-year-old public relations consultant who was recently diagnosed with colon cancer after a routine colonoscopy, a procedure in which the colon is examined using a flexible tube attached to an optical device. Mrs. Woodhouse is scheduled to have surgery to remove the segment of colon that contains the tumor and to determine if the cancer has spread to the surrounding lymph nodes and, possibly, other organs. The nurse completing the nutrition assessment finds that Mrs. Woodhouse is 5 feet 5 inches tall and weighs 178 pounds. Mrs. Woodhouse usually spends most of the day sitting and has little time to engage in recreational exercise. Her diet is high in fat and typically includes red meat at both lunch and dinner. She eats two or three servings of fruits and vegetables each day, although she does not like green leafy vegetables very much. She rarely drinks milk or consumes milk products.

1. Review Table 23-2 on p. 651, and describe the factors in Mrs. Woodhouse's diet and lifestyle that may have contributed to the development of colon cancer.

2. What symptoms and complications may arise after colon surgery and impair nutrition status? If the cancer team decides that Mrs. Woodhouse needs follow-up chemotherapy, how might the chemotherapy affect her nutrition status?

3. If Mrs. Woodhouse is unresponsive to treatment and her cancer progresses, she may develop cancer cachexia. Describe this syndrome, its causes, and its consequences.

4. Provide suggestions that may help Mrs. Woodhouse handle the following problems should they develop: poor appetite, fatigue, taste alterations, nausea and vomiting, chewing and swallowing difficulties, mouth sores, dry mouth, diarrhea, constipation, and weight loss.

NURSING DIAGNOSIS

Appropriate for those with HIV infection may include *ineffective protection, risk for infection, impaired oral mucous membrane, risk for impaired skin integrity, chronic pain, diarrhea, risk for deficient fluid volume, fatigue, imbalanced nutrition: less than body requirements, hopelessness,* and *death anxiety.*

HIV Infection

Possibly, the most infamous infectious disease today is **acquired immune deficiency syndrome (AIDS)**. AIDS develops from infection with human immunodeficiency virus (HIV), which attacks the immune system and disables a person's defenses against other diseases, including infections and certain cancers. Then these diseases—which would cause few, if any, symptoms in people with healthy immune systems—destroy health and life.

The HIV/AIDS epidemic continues to sweep across countries, especially in sub-Saharan Africa (see Table 23-7). For many years, the destructive effects of HIV infection seemed unstoppable, but in the mid- to late 1990s the death rate from AIDS began to decline in the United States, and the progression from HIV infection to AIDS slowed dramatically. Though AIDS is still incurable, remarkable progress has been made in understanding and treating HIV infection.

Without a cure for AIDS, the best course is prevention. HIV is most often sexually transmitted and can be spread by direct contact with contaminated body fluids, such as blood, semen, vaginal secretions, and breast milk. Because many people remain symptom-free during the early stages of infection, they may not realize that they can pass the infection to others. To reduce the spread of HIV infection, individuals at risk (see Table 23-8) are encouraged to undergo testing. A blood test can usually detect HIV antibodies within several months after exposure and, often, after two or three weeks. An estimated 21 percent of persons in the United States who have HIV infection are unaware that they are infected.[23]

CONSEQUENCES OF HIV INFECTION

HIV infection destroys immune cells that have a protein called CD4 on their surfaces. The cells most affected are the **helper T cells**, also called *CD4+ T cells* because the presence of CD4 is a primary characteristic (T cells are lymphocytes that develop in the thymus gland). Other cells that have the CD4 protein (and are infected by HIV) include tissue macrophages, blood monocytes, and certain cells of the central nervous system.[24] Early symptoms of HIV infection are nonspecific and may include fever, sore throat, malaise, swollen lymph nodes, skin rashes, muscle and joint pain, and diarrhea. After these symptoms subside, many people remain symptom-free for 5 to 10 years or even longer. If the HIV infection is not treated, however, the depletion of T cells eventually increases the person's susceptibility to **opportunistic infections**—that is, infections caused by microorganisms that normally do not cause disease in healthy individuals.

The term *AIDS* applies to the advanced stages of HIV infection, in which the inability to fight illness allows a number of serious diseases and complications to develop; such **AIDS-defining illnesses** include severe infections, certain cancers, and wasting of muscle tissue. Health practitioners evaluate disease progression by measuring the concentrations of helper T cells and circulating virus (called the *viral load*) and by

TABLE 23-7	The HIV and AIDS Epidemic at a Glance, 2008		
Stage of Epidemic	World	Sub-Saharan Africa	North America
Individuals living with HIV infection or AIDS	33,400,000	22,400,000	1,400,000
Individuals newly infected with HIV	2,700,000	1,900,000	55,000
AIDS-related deaths	2,000,000	1,400,000	25,000

Source: Joint United Nations Programme on HIV/AIDS and World Health Organization, *AIDS epidemic update: December 2009,* available at http://data.unaids.org/pub/Report/2009/2009_epidemic_update_en.pdf; site visited December 29, 2009.

monitoring clinical symptoms. Although current drug therapies can dramatically slow the progression of HIV infection, the drugs' side effects may make it difficult for patients to adhere to treatments, as discussed in several of the following sections.

Lipodystrophy About one-third or more of patients using drug therapies to suppress HIV infection develop abnormalities in glucose and fat metabolism.[25] These complications, collectively known as the **HIV-lipodystrophy syndrome**, include body fat redistribution, abnormal blood lipid levels, and insulin resistance. Patients may accumulate abdominal fat, lose fat from the face and extremities, or both.[26] Also observed are breast enlargement (in both men and women), fat accumulation at the base of the neck (called a **buffalo hump**), and benign growths composed of fat tissue (called **lipomas**). The changes in body composition are often disfiguring and may cause physical discomfort; moreover, patients often develop hypertriglyceridemia, elevated low-density lipoprotein (LDL) cholesterol levels, low high-density lipoprotein (HDL) cholesterol levels, glucose intolerance, and hyperinsulinemia. The reasons for the development of lipodystrophy are unknown.

Weight Loss and Wasting Even with effective treatment of HIV infection, weight loss and wasting are ongoing problems for many HIV-infected patients. *HIV-associated wasting* is diagnosed in patients who unintentionally lose 7.5 percent of body weight within 6 months, or 10 percent of body weight within 12 months.[27] The wasting has been linked with accelerated disease progression, reduced strength, and fatigue. In the later stages of AIDS, the wasting is severe and increases the risk of death. Much as in cancer, wasting associated with HIV infection has many causes: anorexia and inadequate food intake, altered metabolism, malabsorption, chronic diarrhea, and diet-drug interactions.

Anorexia and Reduced Food Intake As mentioned, inadequate food intake is a key factor in the development of wasting. Poor food intake may result from various factors, including the following:

- *Emotional distress, pain, and fatigue.* The physical and social problems that accompany chronic illness may cause fear, anxiety, and depression, which contribute to anorexia. Pain and fatigue, which may be associated with some disease complications, can cause anorexia and difficulty with eating.
- *Oral infections.* The oral infections associated with HIV infection can cause discomfort and interfere with food consumption. Common infections include thrush and herpes simplex virus infection. **Thrush** can cause mouth pain, dysphagia (difficulty swallowing), and altered taste sensation; infection with **herpes simplex virus** may cause painful lesions around the lips and in the mouth.
- *Respiratory disorders.* Respiratory infections, including pneumonia and tuberculosis, are common in people with HIV infection. Symptoms often include chest pain, shortness of breath, and cough, which interfere with eating and contribute to anorexia.
- *Cancer.* As described earlier in this chapter, cancer leads to anorexia for numerous reasons. In addition, **Kaposi's sarcoma**, a type of cancer frequently associated with HIV infection, can cause lesions in the mouth and throat that make eating painful.
- *Medications.* The medications given to treat HIV infection, other infections, and cancer often cause anorexia, nausea and vomiting, altered taste sensation, food aversions, and diarrhea.

GI Tract Complications Complications of HIV infection involving the GI tract may result from opportunistic infections, medications, or the HIV infection itself.[28] In addition to the oral infections described previously, infections may develop in the esophagus, stomach, and intestines. Furthermore, advanced AIDS is often accompanied by characteristic changes in the small intestinal lining: the villi appear shortened and flattened, and the absorptive area is substantially reduced. These changes

TABLE 23-8 Risk Factors for HIV Infection

- History of receiving blood transfusions or blood components before 1985
- Infant born to mother with HIV infection
- Intravenous drug use in which syringes are shared among users
- Sexual contact with intravenous drug users, prostitutes, or individuals with a history of HIV or other sexually transmitted diseases
- Sexual contact with multiple partners
- Unsafe sexual practices

HIV-lipodystrophy (LIP-oh-DIS-tro-fee) syndrome: a group of abnormalities in fat and glucose metabolism that may result from drug treatments for HIV infection; changes include body fat redistribution, abnormal blood lipid levels, and insulin resistance. The accumulation of abdominal fat is sometimes called *protease paunch.*

buffalo hump: the accumulation of fatty tissue at the base of the neck.

lipomas (lih-POE-muz): benign tumors composed of fatty tissue.

thrush: a fungal infection of the mouth and throat, most often caused by *Candida albicans.*

© Visuals Unlimited

HIV-lipodystrophy is sometimes evident by the accumulation of fatty tissue at the base of the neck, referred to as buffalo hump.

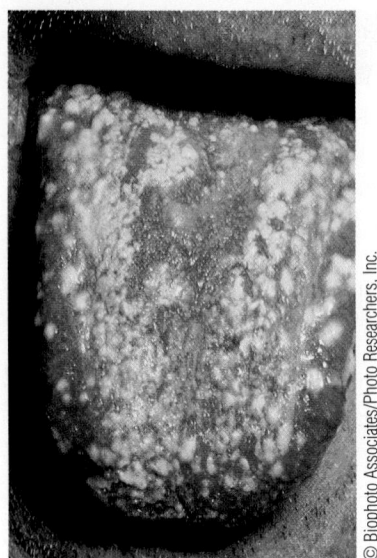

The oral infection *thrush* is easily identified by the characteristic milky white patches that appear on the tongue.

herpes simplex virus: a common virus that can cause blisterlike lesions on the lips and in the mouth.

Kaposi's (kah-POH-seez) sarcoma: a common cancer in HIV-infected persons that is characterized by lesions in the skin, lungs, and GI tract.

can cause malabsorption, steatorrhea, and diarrhea. The abnormalities that develop in the intestinal mucosa are sometimes referred to as *AIDS enteropathy.*

As described earlier, many patients are unable to tolerate the medications used to suppress HIV and develop nausea, vomiting, and diarrhea. In addition, the medications that treat the viral, parasitic, and fungal infections in the GI tract contribute to bacterial overgrowth. Thus, HIV-infected patients face an extremely high risk of malnutrition due to the combination of intestinal discomfort, bacterial overgrowth, malabsorption, and nutrient losses from vomiting, steatorrhea, and diarrhea.

Neurological Complications Neurological complications may be a consequence of HIV infection, immune suppression, or cancers and infections that target brain tissue.[29] Clinical features include mild to severe dementia; muscle weakness and gait disturbances; and pain, numbness, and tingling in the legs and feet. Neurological impairments are usually more pronounced in the advanced stages of AIDS.

Other Complications Patients with HIV infection can develop anemia due to nutrient malabsorption, blood loss, disturbances in bone marrow function, or medication side effects. HIV infection may also lead to skin disorders (rashes, infections, and cancers), eye diseases (retinal infection and detachment), kidney diseases (nephrotic syndrome and chronic kidney disease), and coronary heart disease.[30]

TREATMENTS FOR HIV INFECTION

Although there is no cure for HIV infection, treatments can help to slow its progression, reduce complications, and alleviate pain. The standard treatment for suppressing HIV infection, called *highly active antiretroviral therapy (HAART),* combines three or more antiretroviral drugs.[31] Table 23-9 lists the major drug categories included in antiretroviral therapy and describes the drugs' modes of action. These antiretroviral agents have multiple adverse effects that make their long-term use difficult to tolerate. In addition to the GI effects discussed previously, side effects include skin rashes, headache, anemia, tingling

TABLE 23-9	Antiretroviral Drugs for Treatment of HIV Infection	
Category	**Examples**	**Mode of Action**
CCR5 antagonist	Maraviroc	CCR5 antagonists prevent HIV from entering cells by blocking a membrane receptor on the host cell.
Fusion inhibitor	Enfuvirtide	Fusion inhibitors prevent HIV from entering cells by binding a viral protein needed for its entry.
Integrase inhibitor	Raltegravir	Integrase inhibitors impair the function of HIV's integrase enzyme, which incorporates viral DNA into the host cell's genome.
Non-nucleoside reverse transcriptase inhibitor (NNRTI)	Delavirdine, efavirenz, nevirapine	NNRTI bind active sites on HIV's reverse transcriptase enzyme, blocking the ability of HIV to produce DNA copies of its genetic material.
Nucleoside reverse transcriptase inhibitor (NRTI)	Didanosine, lamivudine, zidovudine	As analogs of the nucleosides needed for DNA synthesis, NRTI impair the ability of HIV's reverse transcriptase enzyme to produce usable copies of DNA.
Protease inhibitor (PI)	Saquinavir, ritonavir, indinavir	PI inhibit HIV's protease enzyme, which cleaves HIV's gene products into usable structural proteins.

Sources: U.S. Department of Health and Human Services, Panel on Antiretroviral Guidelines for Adult and Adolescents, *Guidelines for the Use of Antiretroviral Agents in HIV-1-Infected Adults and Adolescents,* December 1, 2009, pp 1–168, available at http://aidsinfo.nih.gov/contentfiles/AdultandAdolescentGL.pdf; site visited December 31, 2009; S. Safrin, Antiviral agents, in B. G. Katzung, ed., *Basic and Clinical Pharmacology* (New York: Lange/McGraw-Hill, 2007), pp. 790–818.

DIET-DRUG INTERACTIONS

Check this table for notable nutrition-related effects of the medications discussed in this chapter.

	GASTROINTESTINAL EFFECTS	INTERACTIONS WITH DIETARY SUBSTANCES	METABOLIC EFFECTS
Appetite stimulants (megestrol acetate, dronabinol)	Nausea, vomiting, diarrhea	–	Hyperglycemia (megestrol acetate)
Didanosine	Nausea, vomiting, dry mouth, altered taste perception, anorexia, diarrhea, constipation	Take medication either one-half hour before or two hours after a meal; avoid alcohol and aluminum- and magnesium-containing antacids.	Pancreatitis; anemia; reduced serum copper, zinc, and vitamin B_{12} levels
Enfuvirtide	Nausea, vomiting, anorexia, diarrhea, constipation	–	Pancreatitis, increased blood triglycerides
Methotrexate	Nausea, vomiting, diarrhea, reduced absorption of vitamin B_{12} and calcium	Milk may reduce methotrexate absorption if the milk and methotrexate are ingested together.	Increased serum uric acid levels, anemia, liver toxicity
Ritonavir	Nausea, vomiting, altered taste perception, anorexia, diarrhea	Take medication with food.	Pancreatitis, hyperglycemia, reduced serum copper and zinc levels; increased levels of blood triglycerides, LDL cholesterol, uric acid, liver enzymes, and creatine kinase
Zidovudine	Nausea, vomiting, altered taste perception, anorexia, mouth sores, constipation	Do not take medication with a high-fat meal.	Anemia; reduced serum copper, zinc, and vitamin B_{12} levels

Note: Other antiretroviral drugs that treat HIV infection have gastrointestinal and metabolic side effects; only a few are listed here as examples.

and numbness, hepatitis, pancreatitis, and kidney stones. Thus, although HAART has improved life span and quality of life for many patients, the drug regimens are difficult to adhere to and cause complications that require continual management. The Diet-Drug Interactions feature summarizes the nutrition-related effects of some of the antiretroviral agents and other drugs mentioned in this chapter.

Control of Lipodystrophy
Treatment strategies for lipodystrophy are under investigation. Both aerobic activity and resistance training may help to reduce abdominal fat, although some patients opt for cosmetic surgery. Patients may be given alternative antiretroviral drugs to alleviate symptoms. Medications may be prescribed to treat abnormal blood lipid levels and insulin resistance.

Control of Anorexia and Wasting
Anabolic hormones, appetite stimulants, and regular physical activity have been successful in reversing weight loss and increasing muscle mass in HIV-infected patients. Testosterone and human growth hormone have demonstrated positive effects on nitrogen balance and lean tissue content, especially in combination with resistance training. A regular program of resistance exercise improves muscle mass and strength and corrects some of the metabolic abnormalities (altered blood lipids and insulin resistance) that are common in HIV-infected patients. The medications megestrol acetate and dronabinol (described on p. 655) are sometimes prescribed to stimulate appetite and improve weight gain, although much of the weight increase is attributable to a gain of fat rather than lean tissue.[32]

Alternative Therapies
Like cancer patients, people with HIV infection and AIDS are frequently tempted to try unconventional methods of treatment. Although many alternative therapies are harmless, they can be expensive at a time when financial

Resistance training can help a person with HIV infection maintain muscle mass and strength.

security is of concern. Monitoring patients' use of dietary supplements is essential to reduce the possibility of nutrient-drug and herb-drug interactions.

MEDICAL NUTRITION THERAPY FOR HIV INFECTION

HIV-infected individuals must learn how to maintain body weight and muscle mass, prevent malnutrition, cope with nutrition-related side effects of medications, and manage other medical problems that accompany HIV infection. Therefore, nutrition assessment and counseling should begin soon after a patient is diagnosed with HIV infection. The initial assessment provides baseline data with which to monitor progress throughout the course of the disease, and it should include an evaluation of body weight and body composition. Nutrition reassessments and additional counseling may be required every three to six months.[33]

Protein and Energy To help prevent weight loss and wasting, HIV-infected individuals must obtain adequate amounts of protein and energy. Protein recommendations for asymptomatic persons with HIV infections are similar to those for healthy adults (0.8 grams per kilogram per day).[34] Energy needs are influenced by the stage and severity of illness, malabsorption problems, and infectious complications. Although intake levels have not been established for individuals with HIV infection, initial estimates may be made by using the energy recommendations for healthy individuals (see Chapter 6) and adjusting as necessary to maintain a healthy body weight.

Weight Management Individuals who experience weight loss and wasting may benefit from a high-kcalorie, high-protein diet. Daily energy needs may be 30 to 40 kcalories per kilogram body weight, and protein requirements may be as high as 1.2 to 2.0 grams per kilogram body weight.[35] The addition of nutrient-dense snacks, protein or energy bars, and oral supplements can improve intakes. Liquid formulas may be useful for the person who is too tired to eat or prepare meals. If food consumption is difficult, small, frequent feedings may be better tolerated than several large meals. The "How to" on p. 656 provides suggestions for adding energy and protein to the diet, and the "How to" on pp. 657–658 includes strategies for improving appetite and dealing with complications that interfere with eating.

Overweight/Obesity and HIV Infection Since the development of successful drug therapies for HIV infection, obesity and overweight have become more prevalent than wasting among HIV-infected individuals.[36] Because excessive body weight can increase risks for cardiovascular disease and diabetes, moderate weight loss is recommended for patients with HIV infection who are overweight and obese.

Metabolic Complications As mentioned, individuals who are using antiretroviral drugs frequently develop insulin resistance and elevated triglyceride and LDL cholesterol levels. Treating these conditions often requires both medications and dietary adjustments. Patients should be advised to achieve or maintain a desirable weight, replace saturated fats with monounsaturated and polyunsaturated fats, increase fiber intake, and limit intakes of *trans*-fatty acids, cholesterol, added sugars, and alcohol. Regular physical activity can improve both insulin resistance and blood lipid levels. (✚) If problems persist, alternative antiretroviral medications may be prescribed in an attempt to improve the metabolic abnormalities.

Vitamins and Minerals Vitamin and mineral needs of people with HIV infections are highly variable, and little information is available concerning specific needs. Because nutrient deficiencies are likely to result from reduced food intake, malabsorption, diet-drug interactions, and nutrient losses, multivitamin-mineral supplements are often recommended. Patients should be cautioned to maintain intakes that are close to DRI recommendations, however, due to the risk of adverse interactions between excessive amounts of vitamins and minerals, and antiretroviral drugs.[37]

Symptom Management The discomfort associated with antiretroviral therapy, opportunistic GI infections, and malabsorption symptoms can make food

✚ Additional suggestions for managing insulin resistance and hyperlipidemias are available in Chapters 20 and 21, respectively.

consumption difficult, and problems such as vomiting and diarrhea contribute to fluid and electrolyte losses. The "How to" on pp. 657–658 describes measures that can improve food and fluid intakes and alleviate discomfort in individuals with these problems.

cryptosporidiosis (KRIP-toe-spor-ih-dee-OH-sis): a foodborne illness caused by the parasite *Cryptosporidium parvum*.

Food Safety The depressed immunity of people with HIV infections places them at extremely high risk of developing foodborne infections. Health practitioners should caution patients about their high susceptibility to foodborne illness and provide detailed instructions about the safe handling and preparation of foods (see Nutrition in Practice 2). Water can also be a source of foodborne illness and is a common cause of **cryptosporidiosis** in HIV-infected individuals. Because water quality varies throughout the United States, patients should consult their local health departments to determine whether the local tap water is safe to drink. If not, or to take additional safety measures, they should boil drinking water for one minute. Some, but not all, types of filtered and bottled waters are safe.

Enteral and Parenteral Nutrition Support In later stages of illness, people with HIV infections may be unable to consume enough food and may need aggressive nutrition support. Tube feedings are preferred whenever the GI tract is functional; they can be provided at night to supplement oral diets consumed during the day. Parenteral nutrition is reserved for patients who are unable to tolerate enteral nutrition, such as those with GI obstructions that prevent food intake. For individuals with severe malabsorption, orally administered hydrolyzed formulas containing medium-chain triglycerides may be as effective as parenteral nutrition for reversing weight loss and wasting. For either type of feeding, careful measures are necessary to avoid bacterial contamination of nutrient formulas and feeding equipment.

Review Notes

- By attacking immune cells, HIV causes progressive damage to immune function and may eventually lead to AIDS.
- Improved drug therapies have slowed the progression of HIV infection; however, these drugs may promote the HIV-lipodystrophy syndrome, which is characterized by body fat redistribution, abnormal lipid levels, and insulin resistance.
- HIV infection is often associated with weight loss and wasting, anorexia, and various complications that affect food intake. Dietary adjustments, resistance training, and medications can help patients maintain their weight and prevent wasting.
- People with HIV infection must pay strict attention to food safety guidelines to prevent foodborne illnesses. The Case Study provides an opportunity to review the nutritional concerns of a person with HIV infection.

CASE STUDY | Patient with HIV Infection

Three years ago, Darrell Meckler, a 34-year-old financial planner, sought medical help when he began feeling run-down and developed a painful white fungal infection over his mouth and tongue. The presence of thrush, recent weight loss, and anemia alerted Mr. Meckler's physician to the possibility of an HIV infection. When Mr. Meckler tested positive for HIV, he and his family and friends were devastated by the news, but those close to him have remained supportive. During the three years since Mr. Meckler began antiretroviral drug therapy, he has maintained his weight but has also developed lipodystrophy and hypertriglyceridemia. Mr. Meckler is 6 feet tall and currently weighs 185 pounds. He occasionally develops diarrhea and sometimes anorexia.

1. Describe lipodystrophy, and discuss its typical pattern in people who have an HIV infection. What adjustments in treatment and lifestyle may be helpful for Mr. Meckler?

2. Describe an appropriate diet for Mr. Meckler. What strategies may improve his problems with diarrhea and anorexia? Suggest reasons why diarrhea and anorexia may develop in people with HIV infections.

3. Explain why an HIV infection can lead to wasting as the disease progresses to the later stages. What recommendations may be helpful for maintaining weight and health if wasting becomes a problem?

Nutrition Assessment | CHECKLIST FOR PEOPLE WITH CANCER OR HIV INFECTIONS

MEDICAL HISTORY

Check the medical record to determine:

- ○ Type and stage of cancer
- ○ Stage of HIV infection

Review the medical record for complications that may alter medical nutrition therapy, including:

- ○ Altered organ function
- ○ Altered taste perception
- ○ Anorexia
- ○ Dry mouth and oral infections
- ○ GI symptoms and infections
- ○ Hyperlipidemias
- ○ Insulin resistance
- ○ Malnutrition and wasting

MEDICATIONS

For patients with cancer or HIV infections:

- ○ Check medications to identify potential diet-drug interactions.
- ○ Recommend the use of antinauseants at mealtime, if needed.
- ○ Ask about the use of dietary supplements, including herbal remedies.

For cancer patients who require chemotherapy:

- ○ Recommend strategies to prevent food aversions.
- ○ Offer suggestions for managing drug-related complications.

For HIV-infected patients using antiretroviral drug therapy:

- ○ Remind patients that some drugs are better absorbed with foods and that others must be taken on an empty stomach.
- ○ Help patients work out a medication schedule that suits their lifestyle and is timed appropriately in regard to food intake.
- ○ Offer suggestions for managing drug-related complications.

DIETARY INTAKE

For patients with poor food intakes and weight loss:

- ○ Determine the reasons for reduced food intake.
- ○ Offer appropriate suggestions to improve food intake.
- ○ Provide interventions before weight loss progresses too far.

For patients with HIV infections who experience weight gain, elevated triglyceride or LDL cholesterol levels, or hyperglycemia:

- ○ Assess the diet for energy, total fat, types of fat, carbohydrates, fiber, and sugars.
- ○ For patients with hyperlipidemias, recommend a diet low in saturated fat, *trans*-fatty acids, and sugars.
- ○ For patients with hyperglycemia, recommend a consistent carbohydrate intake at meals and snacks that emphasizes complex carbohydrates and limits concentrated sweets.
- ○ Recommend regular physical activity for weight control and for improving blood lipid levels and insulin resistance.

ANTHROPOMETRIC DATA

Take baseline height and weight measurements, monitor weight regularly, and suggest dietary adjustments for weight maintenance, if necessary. Remember that body composition may change without affecting body weight. Perform baseline and periodic body composition measurements in HIV-infected patients who are using antiretroviral drug therapy.

LABORATORY TESTS

Note that albumin and other serum proteins may be reduced in patients with cancer or HIV infections, especially in those experiencing wasting. Check laboratory tests for indications of:

- ○ Anemia
- ○ Dehydration
- ○ Elevated LDL cholesterol levels
- ○ Elevated triglyceride levels
- ○ Hyperglycemia

For patients with HIV infections, evaluate disease progression by checking:

- ○ Helper T cell counts
- ○ Viral load

PHYSICAL SIGNS

Look for physical signs of:

- ○ Dehydration (especially for patients with fever, vomiting, or diarrhea)
- ○ Kaposi's sarcoma
- ○ Oral infections
- ○ Protein-energy malnutrition and wasting

Self Check

1 • Which of these dietary substances may help to protect against cancer?
   a. Alcohol
   b. Well-cooked meats, poultry, and fish
   c. Animal fats
   d. Phytochemicals from fruits and vegetables

2 • The metabolic changes that often accompany cancer include all of the following *except:*
   a. increased triglyceride breakdown.
   b. increased protein turnover.
   c. increased muscle protein synthesis.
   d. insulin resistance.

3 • An advantage of radiation therapy over chemotherapy is that:
   a. radiation is not damaging to rapidly dividing cells.
   b. side effects of radiation therapy do not include malnutrition.
   c. radiation can be directed toward the regions affected by cancer.
   d. the radiation used is too weak to damage GI tissues.

4 • Although many cancer patients lose weight, which type of cancer is often associated with weight gain?
   a. Kidney cancer
   b. Breast cancer
   c. Colon cancer
   d. Lung cancer

5 • Oral diets after bone marrow transplants may restrict:
   a. fiber.
   b. carbohydrates.
   c. high-protein foods.
   d. raw fruits and vegetables.

6 • HIV can enter and destroy these cells:
   a. epithelial cells.
   b. helper T cells.
   c. liver cells.
   d. intestinal cells.

7 • HIV-lipodystrophy syndrome may result in all of these changes *except:*
   a. increased abdominal fat.
   b. increased fat in the arms and legs.
   c. fat accumulation at the base of the neck.
   d. hypertriglyceridemia.

8 • Mouth sores in people with HIV infections are most frequently due to:
   a. oral infections.
   b. dehydration.
   c. nutrient deficiency.
   d. foodborne illnesses.

9 • Megestrol acetate and dronabinol are:
   a. medications used to promote weight gain.
   b. protease inhibitors that fight HIV infection.
   c. medications that treat common opportunistic infections.
   d. anabolic hormones that promote gain of muscle tissue.

10• To prevent cryptosporidiosis, a person with HIV infection may need to:
   a. wash hands carefully before meals.
   b. avoid consuming undercooked meat, poultry, and eggs.
   c. consume a high-kcalorie, high-protein diet.
   d. boil drinking water for one minute.

Answers to these questions appear in Appendix H.

Clinical Applications

1 • Consider the nutrition problems that may develop in a 36-year-old woman with a malignant brain tumor that affects her ability to move the right side of her body (including the tongue) and to speak coherently. She is taking a pain medication that makes her nauseated and sleepy. Her expected survival time is only about six months.
   • If she is right-handed, how might her impairment interfere with eating? What suggestions do you have for overcoming this problem?
   • How might her nutrition status be affected by her inability to communicate effectively? What suggestions may help?
   • In what ways might the pain medication she is taking affect her nutrition status?

2 • Various types of chronic conditions can lead to weight loss and wasting. For some of these conditions, such as Crohn's disease or celiac disease (Chapter 18), diet is a cornerstone of treatment. For others, such as cancer and HIV infection, nutrition plays a supportive role. What determines whether nutrition plays a primary role or a supportive role in the treatment of disease?

Nutrition on the Net

For further study of topics covered in this chapter, access these websites.

- Find updates and quick links to these and other nutrition-related sites at our website: www.cengage.com/nutrition/whitney/nhhc4e
- To learn more about cancer, including risk factors, prevention, screening, detection, treatments (including nutrition), and support networks, visit these sites:

  American Association for Cancer Research: www.aacr.org

  American Cancer Society: www.cancer.org

  American Institute for Cancer Research: www.aicr.org

  National Cancer Institute: www.cancer.gov

- To find additional information about HIV infection and AIDS, visit these sites:

  AIDS Education Global Information System: www.aegis.com

  AIDSinfo, an information service provided by the U.S. Department of Health and Human Services: aidsinfo.nih.gov

  HIV InSite, a project of the UCSF Center for HIV Information: hivinsite.ucsf.edu

  The Body: www.thebody.com

- To review information about safe food handling, visit a website sponsored by several agencies of the federal government: www.foodsafety.gov

Notes

1. R. S. K. Chaganti, Genetics of cancer, in L. Goldman and D. Ausiello, eds., *Cecil Medicine* (Philadelphia: Saunders, 2008), pp. 1340–1344.
2. W. C. Willett and E. Giovannucci, Epidemiology of diet and cancer risk, in M. E. Shils and coeditors, *Modern Nutrition in Health and Disease* (Philadelphia: Lippincott Williams & Wilkins, 2006), pp. 1267–1279.
3. Willett and Giovannucci, 2006.
4. World Cancer Research Fund/American Institute for Cancer Research, *Food, Nutrition, Physical Activity, and the Prevention of Cancer: A Global Perspective* (Washington, D.C.: American Institute for Cancer Research, 2007), pp. 280–288.
5. R. J. Turesky, Formation and biochemistry of carcinogenic heterocyclic aromatic amines in cooked meats, *Toxicology Letters* 168 (2007): 219–227; T. Sugimura and coauthors, Heterocyclic amines: Mutagens/carcinogens produced during cooking of meat and fish, *Cancer Science* 95 (2004): 290–299.
6. S. Koutros and coauthors, Meat and meat mutagens and risk of prostate cancer in the agricultural health study, *Cancer Epidemiology, Biomarkers, and Prevention* 17 (2008): 80–87; World Cancer Research Fund/American Institute for Cancer Research, 2007, pp. 116–128; Turesky, 2007.
7. R. H. Liu, Potential synergy of phytochemicals in cancer prevention: Mechanism of action, *Journal of Nutrition* 134 (2004): 3479S–3485S.
8. Willett and Giovannucci, 2006.
9. H. S. Rugo, Paraneoplastic syndromes and other non-neoplastic effects of cancer, in L. Goldman and D. Ausiello, eds., *Cecil Medicine* (Philadelphia: Saunders, 2008), pp. 1353–1362.
10. American Dietetic Association, *Nutrition Care Manual* (Chicago: American Dietetic Association, 2009).
11. M. Schattner and M. Shike, Nutrition support of the patient with cancer, in M. E. Shils and coeditors, *Modern Nutrition in Health and Disease* (Philadelphia: Lippincott Williams & Wilkins, 2006), pp. 1290–1313.
12. T. Agustsson and coauthors, Mechanism of increased lipolysis in cancer cachexia, *Cancer Research* 67 (2007): 5531–5537; L. G. Melstrom and coauthors, Mechanisms of skeletal muscle degradation and its therapy in cancer cachexia, *Histology and Histopathology* 22 (2007): 805–814; A. Lelbach, G. Muzes, and J. Feher, Current perspectives of catabolic mediators of cancer cachexia, *Medical Science Monitor* 13 (2007): RA168–173.
13. M. C. Perry, Principles of cancer therapy, in L. Goldman and D. Ausiello, eds., *Cecil Medicine* (Philadelphia: Saunders, 2008), pp. 1370–1387.
14. J. M. Vose and S. Z. Pavletic, Hematopoietic stem cell transplantation, in L. Goldman and D. Ausiello, eds., *Cecil Medicine* (Philadelphia: Saunders, 2008), pp. 1328–1332.
15. Schattner and Shike, 2006.
16. C. S. Roberts, Patient-physician communication regarding use of complementary therapies during cancer treatment, *Journal of Psychosocial Oncology* 23 (2005): 35–60.
17. S. Marchetti and coauthors, Concise review: Clinical relevance of drug–drug and herb–drug interactions mediated by the ABC transporter ABCB1 (MDR1, P-glycoprotein), *The Oncologist* 12 (2007): 927–941; I. Meijerman, J. H. Beijnen, and J. H. M. Schellens, Herb-drug interactions in oncology: Focus on mechanisms of induction, *The Oncologist* 11 (2006): 742–752.
18. B. Bruemmer and coauthors, The association between vitamin C and vitamin E supplement use before hematopoietic stem cell transplant and outcomes to two years, *Journal of the American Dietetic Association* 103 (2003): 982–990; H. E. Seifried and coauthors, The antioxidant conundrum in cancer, *Cancer Research* 63 (2003): 4295–4298.
19. Schattner and Shike, 2006.
20. N. Saquib and coauthors, Weight gain and recovery of pre-cancer weight after breast cancer treatments: Evidence from the women's healthy eating and living (WHEL) study, *Breast Cancer Research and Treatment* 105 (2007): 177–186; G. Makari-Judson, C. H. Judson, and W. C. Mertens, Longitudinal patterns of weight gain after breast cancer diagnosis: Observations beyond the first year, *Breast Journal* 13 (2007): 258–265.
21. Schattner and Shike, 2006.
22. American Dietetic Association, 2009.
23. UNAIDS/WHO, *AIDS Epidemic Update: December 2009,* available at http://data.unaids.org/pub/Report/2009/2009_epidemic_update_en.pdf; site visited December 29, 2009.
24. G. M. Shaw, Biology of human immunodeficiency viruses, in L. Goldman and D. Ausiello, eds., *Cecil Medicine* (Philadelphia: Saunders, 2008), pp. 2557–2561.
25. H. Masur, L. Healey, and C. Hadigan, Treatment of human immunodeficiency virus infection and acquired immunodeficiency syndrome, in L. Goldman and D. Ausiello, eds., *Cecil Medicine* (Philadelphia: Saunders, 2008), pp. 2571–2582.
26. K. R. Dong, HIV-associated fat deposition, in K. M. Hendricks, K. R. Dong, and J. L. Gerrior, eds., *Nutrition Management of HIV and AIDS* (Chicago: American Dietetic Association, 2009), pp. 57–65; Masur, Healey, and Hadigan, 2008.
27. J. L. Gerrior, Unintentional weight loss and wasting in HIV infection, in K. M. Hendricks, K. R. Dong, and J. L. Gerrior, eds., *Nutrition Management of HIV and AIDS* (Chicago: American Dietetic Association, 2009), pp. 41–55.
28. J. G. Bartlett, Gastrointestinal manifestations of human immunodeficiency virus and acquired immunodeficiency syndrome, in L. Goldman and D. Ausiello, eds., *Cecil Medicine* (Philadelphia: Saunders, 2008), pp. 2582–2585.
29. J. R. Berger and A. Nath, Neurologic complications of human immunodeficiency virus infection, in L. Goldman and D. Ausiello, eds., *Cecil Medicine* (Philadelphia: Saunders, 2008), pp. 2607–2611.
30. E. G. L. Wilkins, Human immunodeficiency virus infection and the human acquired immunodeficiency syndrome, in N. A. Boon, N. R. Colledge, and B. R. Walker, eds., *Davidson's Principles and Practice of Medicine* (Philadelphia: Churchill Livingstone/Elsevier, 2006), pp. 377–402.

31. U.S. Department of Health and Human Services, Panel on Antiretroviral Guidelines for Adult and Adolescents, *Guidelines for the Use of Antiretroviral Agents in HIV-1-Infected Adults and Adolescents,* December 1, 2009, pp. 1–168, available at http://aidsinfo.nih.gov/contentfiles/AdultandAdolescentGL.pdf; site visited December 31, 2009; S. Safrin, Antiviral agents, in B. G. Katzung, ed., *Basic and Clinical Pharmacology* (New York: Lange/McGraw-Hill, 2007), pp. 790–818.

32. K. Mulligan and coauthors, Testosterone supplementation of megestrol therapy does not enhance lean tissue accrual in men with human immunodeficiency virus-associated weight loss: A randomized, double-blind, placebo-controlled, multicenter trial, *Journal of Clinical Endocrinology and Metabolism* 92 (2007): 563–570.

33. American Dietetic Association, 2009.

34. L. Vining, General nutrition issues for healthy living with HIV infection, in K. M. Hendricks, K. R. Dong, and J. L. Gerrior, eds., *Nutrition Management of HIV and AIDS* (Chicago: American Dietetic Association, 2009), pp. 23–40.

35. Gerrior, 2009.

36. Vining, 2009.

37. A. Howard, K. M. Hendricks, and J. Dwyer, Dietary supplement use in HIV infection, in K. M. Hendricks, K. R. Dong, and J. L. Gerrior, eds., *Nutrition Management of HIV and AIDS* (Chicago: American Dietetic Association, 2009), pp. 109–127; P. K. Drain and coauthors, Micronutrients in HIV-positive persons receiving highly active antiretroviral therapy, *American Journal of Clinical Nutrition* 85 (2007).

Ethical Issues in Nutrition Care

As with other medical technologies, the availability of specialized nutrition support forces health care professionals and members of our society to face difficult **ethical** issues. When medical treatments prolong life by merely delaying death, the lifetime that remains may be of extremely low quality. This Nutrition in Practice examines the ethical dilemmas that clinicians must face when dealing with patients in critical care. The accompanying glossary defines the relevant terms.

If providing nutrition care can do little to promote recovery, is it appropriate to withhold or withdraw nutrition support?

In attempting to answer questions such as these, health professionals must consider the following ethical principles:[1]

- A patient has the right to make decisions concerning his or her own well-being (**patient autonomy**), even if refusing treatment could result in death. It is generally accepted that a patient's preferences should take precedence over the desires of others.[2]
- A patient should be fully informed of a treatment's benefits and risks in a fair and honest manner (**disclosure**). A patient's acceptance of a treatment that has been adequately disclosed is considered **informed consent**.
- A patient must have the mental capacity to make appropriate health care decisions (**decision-making capacity**). If a patient is mentally incapable of doing so, a person designated by the patient should serve as a **surrogate** decision maker.
- The potential benefits (**beneficence**) of any treatment should outweigh its potential harm (**maleficence**).
- Health care providers must determine whether the provision of health care to one patient would unfairly limit the care of other patients (**distributive justice**).

Although these principles may seem simple and logical, it is often difficult to determine the appropriate action to take

Glossary

advance directive: written or oral instruction regarding one's preferences for medical treatment to be used in the event of becoming incapacitated.

beneficence (be-NEF-eh-sense): the act of performing beneficial services rather than harmful ones.

cardiopulmonary resuscitation (CPR): life-sustaining treatment that supplies oxygen and restores a person's ability to breathe and pump blood.

decision-making capacity: the ability to understand pertinent information and make appropriate decisions; known as *decision-making competency* within the legal system.

defibrillation: life-sustaining treatment in which an electronic device is used to shock the heart and reestablish a pattern of normal contractions. Defibrillation is used when the heart has arrhythmias or has experienced arrest.

dialysis: life-sustaining treatment in which a patient's blood is filtered using selective diffusion through a semipermeable membrane; substitutes for kidney function.

disclosure: the act of revealing pertinent information. For example, clinicians should accurately describe proposed tests and procedures, their benefits and risks, and alternative approaches.

distributive justice: the equitable distribution of resources.

do-not-resuscitate (DNR) order: a request by a patient or surrogate to withhold cardiopulmonary resuscitation.

durable power of attorney: a legal document (sometimes called a *health care proxy)* that gives legal authority to another

(a health care agent) to make medical decisions in the event of incapacitation.

ethical: in accordance with accepted principles of right and wrong.

futile: medical care that will not improve the medical circumstances of a patient.

health care agent: a person given legal authority to make medical decisions for another in the event of incapacitation.

informed consent: a patient's or caregiver's agreement to undergo a treatment that has been adequately disclosed. Persons must be mentally competent in order to make the decision.

living will: a written statement that specifies the medical procedures desired or not desired in the event that a person is unable to communicate or is incapacitated; also called a *medical directive.*

maleficence (mah-LEF-eh-sense): the act of doing evil or harm.

mechanical ventilation: life-sustaining treatment in which a mechanical ventilator is used to substitute for a patient's failing lungs.

patient autonomy: a principle of self-determination, such that patients (or surrogate decision makers) are free to choose the medical interventions that are acceptable to them, even if they choose to refuse interventions that may extend their lives.

persistent vegetative state: a vegetative mental state resulting from brain injury that persists for at least one month. Individuals lose awareness and the ability to think but retain noncognitive brain functions, such as motor reflexes and normal sleep patterns.

surrogate: a substitute; a person who takes the place of another.

during intensive care.[3] When clinicians and families disagree, the courts may be asked to decide.

What kinds of treatments can help to sustain a patient's life?

Nutrition support and hydration are both considered life-sustaining treatments because withholding or withdrawing either can result in death. Other life-sustaining treatments include **cardiopulmonary resuscitation (CPR)**, which supplies oxygen and restores a person's ability to breathe and pump blood; **defibrillation**, in which an electronic device shocks the heart and reestablishes normal contractions; **mechanical ventilation**, which substitutes for lung function; and **dialysis**, which substitutes for kidney function.

Do patients have a right to life-sustaining treatments?

Although life-sustaining treatments are readily provided to patients who have a reasonable chance of recovering from illness, it is sometimes difficult to determine the best course of action for patients who are dying or who are unlikely to regain consciousness. Under such circumstances, such treatments may be considered **futile** because they are unable to improve the outcome of disease or increase the patient's comfort and well-being. If patients or caregivers demand treatment that health practitioners have determined to be useless, a legal resolution may be required. Conversely, medical personnel may find it objectionable to withdraw life support when they know that the inevitable consequence will be the patient's death.

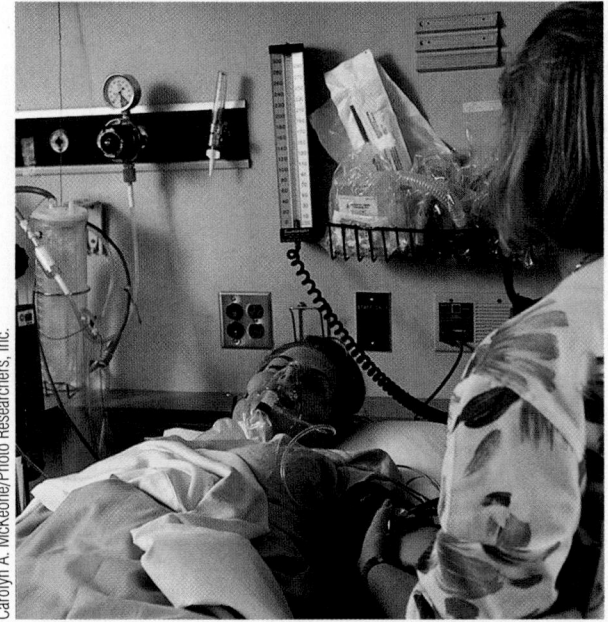

Carolyn A. McKeone/Photo Researchers, Inc.

Is it ever morally and legally appropriate to withhold or withdraw nutrition support?

How have the courts resolved conflicts involving nutrition support?

One of the landmark cases involving nutrition support concerned Nancy Cruzan, who suffered permanent and irreversible brain damage after a car crash in 1983, when she was 26 years of age.[4] After she had been in a **persistent vegetative state** for five years, her parents requested permission to discontinue tube feeding, but hospital staff refused to honor the request, and the matter was taken to court. The Missouri Supreme Court determined that Nancy had never definitively stated her "right to die" wishes and that her parents were unable to make such a request for her. The court also stated that preserving life, no matter what its quality, should take precedence over all other considerations. Nancy's parents appealed the ruling, but in 1990, the U.S. Supreme Court upheld the Missouri Supreme Court in a five-to-four decision. Three witnesses were eventually found who could testify that Nancy would not desire life-sustaining treatment under the circumstances, and the court finally granted permission to remove the feeding tube. This case illustrates the importance of having an **advance directive** (discussed in a later section) that clearly indicates one's preferences for medical treatment in the event of incapacitation.

In a more recent case that received widespread media attention, the spouse and parents of a patient in a persistent vegetative state fought a 10-year legal battle over her medical care. In 1990, at the age of 25, Terri Schiavo suffered a full cardiac arrest.[5] She initially fell into a coma, but her condition evolved into a persistent vegetative state that was considered irreversible. Despite the neurologists' diagnosis and a series of computed tomography (CT) and magnetic resonance imaging (MRI) scans showing extensive brain atrophy, her parents maintained that she was minimally conscious and could improve somewhat with rigorous treatment. Her husband, who was legally responsible for her care, insisted that she would never have wanted to be kept alive in a vegetative state. Like Nancy Cruzan, Terri had never expressed her wishes in an advance directive.

In 1998, Terri's husband filed a petition to have her feeding tube removed, and a Florida court approved the motion in February 2000. Although Terri's parents appealed, an appeals court affirmed the decision, and the Florida Supreme Court declined to review the case. In April 2001, Terri's physicians removed her feeding tube, but within days, a federal circuit court judge ordered it to be reinserted and reopened the case. Eventually, the various motions filed by the parents were dismissed, and Terri's feeding tube was removed for the second time in October 2003. Within days, the Florida legislature passed a bill known as "Terri's Law" that gave the governor the authority to intervene, and Governor Jeb Bush ordered the feeding tube reinserted. A year later, Florida's Supreme Court declared Terri's Law to be unconstitutional. Although the governor appealed the decision, his appeal was rejected in January 2005. Terri's feeding tube was removed for the third time in March 2005. Despite emergency petitions by her parents and an attempt by the U.S. Congress to have her case reconsidered, the courts refused to grant a restraining order, and Terri died 13 days after her feeding tube was removed.

How can people ensure that their wishes will be considered in the event that they become incapacitated?

People can declare their preferences about medical treatments in a **living will**, sometimes called a *medical directive*. Living wills can include detailed instructions about life-sustaining procedures that a person does or does not want. These directives are incorporated into the medical record and updated when appropriate. They take effect only if a physician determines that a patient lacks the ability to understand and make decisions about available treatments. If a person's preferences are unknown, decisions are usually based on a patient's best interests as determined by a caregiver or family member.[6]

Another important directive is a **durable power of attorney** (sometimes called a *health care proxy*), in which another person (a **health care agent**) is appointed to act as decision maker in the event of incapacitation. The agent should understand one's medical preferences and be absolutely trustworthy. Only one person can be designated, although one or two alternates may also be listed. If an agent is given comprehensive power to supervise care, he or she may make decisions about medical staff, health care facilities, and medical procedures.

Laws regarding advance directives vary from state to state. In some states, nutrition and hydration are not considered life-sustaining treatments, and a person's instructions about them may need to be indicated separately. Some states restrict the use of advance directives to terminal illness or disallow them if a woman is pregnant. State statutes also specify characteristics of people who may serve as health care agents and witnesses. Generally, advance directives created in one state are honored in another.

How does a "do-not-resuscitate" order differ from other advance directives?

A **do-not-resuscitate (DNR) order** is frequently used to withhold CPR in the event of cardiopulmonary arrest, which occurs too suddenly for deliberate decision-making.[7] A DNR order is written in the medical record as other directives are, but it does not exclude the use of other life-prolonging measures. A DNR order is most often used in patients with serious illnesses or advanced age. Some institutions allow a physician to write a DNR order for a patient who has a poor prognosis, but the physician must inform the patient or surrogate if this is done.

Have advance directives changed the way that medical care is provided?

Not really. Despite the availability of advance directives, only about 20 percent of people in the United States have completed one.[8] Furthermore, advance directives are often unavailable when intensive care decisions are made: one study found that only 57.5 percent of patient charts indicating the existence of an advance directive actually contained a copy.[9] In addition, advance directives are sometimes too general or vague to guide specific treatment decisions.

Physicians must often provide patient care before they have a chance to discuss treatments with patients or caregivers.[10] In many cases, life-sustaining treatments are begun without the prior knowledge of patients or their decision makers, or the treatments continue even if patients want them stopped. Patients who are fully aware of treatment options and clearly state their preferences are more likely to be successful at obtaining the care they desire.

Medical decisions that are planned in advance and discussed with close friends and family can help to prevent decision-making dilemmas during emergency situations. Health practitioners should strive to provide the best information possible so that patients can consider all of the medical options available and make their preferences known to medical personnel.

Notes

1. M. A. Grippi, Ethics in critical care, in A. P. Fishman and coeditors, *Fishman's Manual of Pulmonary Diseases and Disorders* (New York: McGraw-Hill, 2002), pp. 1111–1114.
2. E. J. Emanuel, Bioethics in the practice of medicine, in L. Goldman and D. Ausiello, eds., *Cecil Medicine* (Philadelphia: Saunders, 2008), pp. 6–11.
3. Emanuel, 2008.
4. J. O. Maillet, Position of the American Dietetic Association: Ethical and legal issues in nutrition, hydration, and feeding, *Journal of the American Dietetic Association* 108 (2008): 873–882.
5. R. Cranford, Facts, lies, and videotapes: The permanent vegetative state and the sad case of Terri Schiavo, *Journal of Law, Medicine, and Ethics* 33 (2005): 363–372.
6. L. Snyder and C. Leffler, Position paper: Ethics manual, *Annals of Internal Medicine* (2005): 560–582.
7. Snyder and Leffler, 2005.
8. Emanuel, 2008.
9. Institute of Medicine, *Approaching Death: Improving Care at the End of Life* (Washington, D.C.: National Academy Press, 1997), pp. 202–203.
10. Emanuel, 2008.

CONTENTS

Table of Food Composition

This edition of the table of food composition includes a wide variety of foods. It is updated with each edition to reflect current nutrient data for foods, to remove outdated foods, and to add foods that are new to the marketplace.*˙ The nutrient database for this appendix is compiled from a variety of sources, including the USDA Nutrient Database and manufacturers' data. The USDA database provides data for a wider variety of foods and nutrients than other sources. Because laboratory analysis for each nutrient can be quite costly, manufacturers tend to provide data only for those nutrients mandated on food labels. Consequently, data for their foods are often incomplete; any missing information on this table is designated as a dash. Keep in mind that a dash means only that the information is unknown and should not be interpreted as a zero. A zero means that the nutrient is not present in the food.

Whenever using nutrient data, remember that many factors influence the nutrient contents of foods. These factors include the mineral content of the soil, the diet fed to the animal or the fertilizer used on the plant, the season of harvest, the method of processing, the length and method of storage, the method of cooking, the method of analysis, and the moisture content of the sample analyzed. With so many influencing factors, users should view nutrient data as a close approximation of the actual amount.

For updates, corrections, and a list of more than 8000 foods and codes found in the diet analysis software that accompanies this text, visit **www.cengage.com/nutrition** and click on Diet Analysis Plus.

- **Fats** Total fats, as well as the breakdown of total fats to saturated, monounsaturated, polyunsaturated, and *trans* fats, are listed in the table. The fatty acids seldom add up to the total in part due to rounding but also because values may include some non-fatty acids, such as glycerol, phosphate, or sterols.
- **Trans Fats** *Trans* fat data have been listed in the table. Because food manufacturers have only been required to report *trans* fats on food labels since January 2006, much of the data is incomplete. Missing *trans* fat data are designated with a dash. As additional *trans* fat data become available, the table will be updated.
- **Vitamin A and Vitamin E** In keeping with the 2001 RDA for vitamin A, this appendix presents data for vitamin A in micrograms (μg) RAE. Similarly, because the 2000 RDA for vitamin E is based only on the alpha-tocopherol form of vitamin E, this appendix reports vitamin E data in milligrams (mg) alpha-tocopherol, listed on the table as Vit E (mg α).
- **Bioavailability** Keep in mind that the availability of nutrients from foods depends not only on the quantity provided by a food, but also on the amount absorbed and used by the body—the bioavailability. The bioavailability of folate from fortified foods, for example, is greater than from naturally occurring sources. Similarly, the body can make niacin

---

˙This food composition table has been prepared by Cengage Learning. The nutritional data are supplied by Axxya Systems.

+ A GRAS substance is one that is "generally recognized as safe."

from the amino acid tryptophan, but niacin values in this table (and most databases) report preformed niacin only. Chapter 8 provides conversion factors and additional details.

- *Using the Table* The foods and beverages in this table are organized into several categories, which are listed at the head of each right-hand page. Page numbers are provided, and each group is color-coded to make it easier to find individual foods.
- *Caffeine Sources* Caffeine occurs in several plants, including the familiar coffee bean, the tea leaf, and the cocoa bean from which chocolate is made. Most human societies use caffeine regularly, most often in beverages, for its stimulant effect and flavor. Caffeine contents of beverages vary depending on the plants they are made from, the climates and soils where the plants are grown, the grind or cut size, the method and duration of brewing, and the amounts served. The accompanying table shows that, in general, a cup of coffee contains the most caffeine; a cup of tea, less than half as much; and cocoa or chocolate, less still. As for cola beverages, they are made from kola nuts, which contain caffeine, but most of their caffeine is added, using the purified compound obtained from decaffeinated coffee beans. The FDA lists caffeine as a multipurpose GRAS substance (+) that may be added to foods and beverages. Drug manufacturers use caffeine in many products.

TABLE **Caffeine Content of Selected Beverages, Foods, and Medications**

Beverages and Foods	Serving Size	Average (mg)	Beverages and Foods	Serving Size	Average (mg)
Coffee			**Soft Drinks**		
Brewed	8 oz	95	A&W Creme Soda	12 oz	29
Decaffeinated	8 oz	2	Barq's Root Beer	12 oz	18
Instant	8 oz	64	Coca-Cola	12 oz	30
Tea			Dr. Pepper, Mr. Pibb, Sunkist Orange	12 oz	36
Brewed, green	8 oz	30	A&W Root Beer, club soda, Fresca, ginger ale, 7-Up, Sierra Mist, Sprite, Squirt, tonic water, caffeine-free soft drinks	12 oz	0
Brewed, herbal	8 oz	0			
Brewed, leaf or bag	8 oz	47			
Instant	8 oz	26	Mello Yello	12 oz	51
Lipton Brisk iced tea	12 oz	7	Mountain Dew	12 oz	45
Nestea Cool iced tea	12 oz	12	Pepsi	12 oz	32
Snapple iced tea (all flavors)	16 oz	42			

TABLE Caffeine Content of Selected Beverages, Foods, and Medications (*continued*)

Beverages and Foods	Serving Size	Average (mg)
Energy Drinks		
Amp	8.4 oz	70
Aqua Blast	.5 L	90
Aqua Java	.5 L	55
E Maxx	8.4 oz	74
Java Water	.5 L	125
KMX	8.4 oz	33
Krank	.5 L	100
Red Bull	8.3 oz	67
Red Devil	8.4 oz	42
Sobe Adrenaline Rush	8.3 oz	77
Sobe No Fear	16 oz	141
Water Joe	.5 L	65
Other Beverages		
Chocolate milk or hot cocoa	8 oz	5
Starbucks Frappuccino Mocha	9.5 oz	72
Starbucks Frappuccino Vanilla	9.5 oz	64
Yoohoo chocolate drink	9 oz	3
Candies		
Baker's chocolate	1 oz	26
Dark chocolate covered coffee beans	1 oz	235
Dark chocolate, semisweet	1 oz	18
Milk chocolate	1 oz	6
Milk chocolate covered coffee beans	1 oz	224
White chocolate	1 oz	0

Beverages and Foods	Serving Size	Average (mg)
Foods		
Frozen yogurt, Ben & Jerry's coffee fudge	1 cup	85
Frozen yogurt, Häagen-Dazs coffee	1 cup	40
Ice cream, Starbucks coffee	1 cup	50
Ice cream, Starbucks Frappuccino bar	1 bar	15
Yogurt, Dannon coffee flavored	1 cup	45

Drugs[a]	Serving Size	Average (mg)
Cold Remedies		
Coryban-D, Dristan	1 tablet	30
Diuretics		
Aqua-Ban	1 tablet	100
Pre-Mens Forte	1 tablet	100
Pain Relievers		
Anacin, BC Fast Pain Reliever	1 tablet	32
Excedrin, Midol, Midol Max Strength	1 tablet	65
Stimulants		
Awake, NoDoz	1 tablet	100
Awake Maximum Strength, Caffedrine, NoDoz Maximum Strength, Stay Awake, Vivarin	1 tablet	200
Weight-Control Aids		
Dexatrim	1 tablet	200

[a]A pharmacologically active dose of caffeine is defined as 200 milligrams.

NOTE: The FDA suggests a maximum of 65 milligrams per 12-ounce cola beverage but does not regulate the caffeine contents of other beverages. Because products change, contact the manufacturer for an update on products you use regularly.

SOURCE: Adapted from USDA database Release 18 (www.nal.usda.gov/fnic/foodcomp/Data/), Caffeine content of foods and drugs, Center for Science and the Public Interest (www.cspinet.org/new/cafchart.htm), and R. R. McCusker, B. A. Goldberger, and E. J. Cone, Caffeine content of energy drinks, carbonated sodas, and other beverages, *Journal of Analytical Toxicology* 30 (2006): 112–114.

TABLE A-1 Table of Food Composition

(Computer code is for Cengage Diet Analysis program)   (For purposes of calculations, use "0" for t, <1, <.1, <.01, etc.)

DA+ Code	Food Description	Quantity	Measure	Wt (g)	H₂O (g)	Ener (kcal)	Prot (g)	Carb (g)	Fiber (g)	Fat (g)	Sat	Mono	Poly	Trans
											Fat Breakdown (g)			

Breads, Baked Goods, Cakes, Cookies, Crackers, Chips, Pies

DA+ Code	Food Description	Quantity	Measure	Wt (g)	H₂O (g)	Ener (kcal)	Prot (g)	Carb (g)	Fiber (g)	Fat (g)	Sat	Mono	Poly	Trans
	Bagels													
8534	Cinnamon and raisin	1	item(s)	71	22.7	194	7.0	39.2	1.6	1.2	0.2	0.1	0.5	—
14395	Multi-grain	1	item(s)	61	—	170	6.0	35.0	1.0	1.5	0.5	0.1	0.4	—
8538	Oat bran	1	item(s)	71	23.4	181	7.6	37.8	2.6	0.9	0.1	0.2	0.3	—
4910	Plain, enriched	1	item(s)	71	25.8	182	7.1	35.9	1.6	1.2	0.3	0.4	0.5	0
4911	Plain, enriched, toasted	1	item(s)	66	18.7	190	7.4	37.7	1.7	1.1	0.2	0.3	0.6	0
	Biscuits													
25008	Biscuits	1	item(s)	41	15.8	121	2.6	16.4	0.5	4.9	1.4	1.4	1.8	—
16729	Scone	1	item(s)	42	11.5	148	3.8	19.1	0.6	6.2	2.0	2.5	1.3	—
25166	Wheat biscuits	1	item(s)	55	21.0	162	3.6	21.9	1.4	6.7	1.9	1.9	2.5	—
	Bread													
325	Boston brown, canned	1	slice(s)	45	21.2	88	2.3	19.5	2.1	0.7	0.1	0.1	0.3	—
8716	Bread sticks, plain	4	item(s)	24	1.5	99	2.9	16.4	0.7	2.3	0.3	0.9	0.9	—
25176	Cornbread	1	piece(s)	55	25.9	141	4.7	18.3	0.9	5.4	2.1	1.4	1.5	0
327	Cracked wheat	1	slice(s)	25	9.0	65	2.2	12.4	1.4	1.0	0.2	0.5	0.2	—
9079	Croutons, plain	¼	cup(s)	8	0.4	31	0.9	5.5	0.4	0.5	0.1	0.2	0.1	—
8582	Egg	1	slice(s)	40	13.9	113	3.8	19.1	0.9	2.4	0.6	0.9	0.4	—
8585	Egg, toasted	1	slice(s)	37	10.5	117	3.9	19.5	0.9	2.4	0.6	1.1	0.4	—
329	French	1	slice(s)	32	8.9	92	3.8	18.1	0.8	0.6	0.2	0.1	0.3	—
8591	French, toasted	1	slice(s)	23	4.7	73	3.0	14.2	0.7	0.5	0.1	0.1	0.2	—
42096	Indian fry, made with lard (Navajo)	3	ounce(s)	85	26.9	281	5.7	41.0	—	10.4	3.9	3.8	0.9	—
332	Italian	1	slice(s)	30	10.7	81	2.6	15.0	0.8	1.1	0.3	0.2	0.4	—
1393	Mixed grain	1	slice(s)	26	9.6	69	3.5	11.3	1.9	1.1	0.2	0.2	0.5	0
8604	Mixed grain, toasted	1	slice(s)	24	7.6	69	3.5	11.3	1.9	1.1	0.2	0.2	0.5	0
8605	Oat bran	1	slice(s)	30	13.2	71	3.1	11.9	1.4	1.3	0.2	0.5	0.5	—
8608	Oat bran, toasted	1	slice(s)	27	10.4	70	3.1	11.8	1.3	1.3	0.2	0.5	0.5	—
8609	Oatmeal	1	slice(s)	27	9.9	73	2.3	13.1	1.1	1.2	0.2	0.4	0.5	—
8613	Oatmeal, toasted	1	slice(s)	25	7.8	73	2.3	13.2	1.1	1.2	0.2	0.4	0.5	—
1409	Pita	1	item(s)	60	19.3	165	5.5	33.4	1.3	0.7	0.1	0.1	0.3	—
7905	Pita, whole wheat	1	item(s)	64	19.6	170	6.3	35.2	4.7	1.7	0.3	0.2	0.7	—
338	Pumpernickel	1	slice(s)	32	12.1	80	2.8	15.2	2.1	1.0	0.1	0.3	0.4	—
334	Raisin, enriched	1	slice(s)	26	8.7	71	2.1	13.6	1.1	1.1	0.3	0.6	0.2	—
8625	Raisin, toasted	1	slice(s)	24	6.7	71	2.1	13.7	1.1	1.2	0.3	0.6	0.2	—
10168	Rice, white, gluten free, wheat free	1	slice(s)	38	—	130	1.0	18.0	0.5	6.0	0	—	—	0
8653	Rye	1	slice(s)	32	11.9	83	2.7	15.5	1.9	1.1	0.2	0.4	0.3	—
8654	Rye, toasted	1	slice(s)	29	9.0	82	2.7	15.4	1.9	1.0	0.2	0.4	0.3	—
336	Rye, light	1	slice(s)	25	9.3	65	2.0	12.0	1.6	1.0	0.2	0.3	0.3	—
8588	Sourdough	1	slice(s)	25	7.0	72	2.9	14.1	0.6	0.5	0.1	0.1	0.2	—
8592	Sourdough, toasted	1	slice(s)	23	4.7	73	3.0	14.2	0.7	0.5	0.1	0.1	0.2	—
491	Submarine or hoagie roll	1	item(s)	135	40.6	400	11.0	72.0	3.8	8.0	1.8	3.0	2.2	—
8596	Vienna, toasted	1	slice(s)	23	4.7	73	3.0	14.2	0.7	0.5	0.1	0.1	0.2	—
8670	Wheat	1	slice(s)	25	8.9	67	2.7	11.9	0.9	0.9	0.2	0.2	0.4	—
8671	Wheat, toasted	1	slice(s)	23	5.6	72	3.0	12.8	1.1	1.0	0.2	0.2	0.4	—
340	White	1	slice(s)	25	9.1	67	1.9	12.7	0.6	0.8	0.2	0.2	0.3	—
1395	Whole wheat	1	slice(s)	46	15.0	128	3.9	23.6	2.8	2.5	0.4	0.5	1.4	—
	Cakes													
386	Angel food, prepared from mix	1	piece(s)	50	16.5	129	3.1	29.4	0.1	0.2	0	0	0.1	—
8772	Butter pound, ready to eat, commercially prepared	1	slice(s)	75	18.5	291	4.1	36.6	0.4	14.9	8.7	4.4	0.8	—
28517	Carrot	1	slice(s)	131	56.6	339	4.8	56.5	1.9	11.1	1.0	5.7	3.8	—
4931	Chocolate with chocolate icing, commercially prepared	1	slice(s)	64	14.7	235	2.6	34.9	1.8	10.5	3.1	5.6	1.2	—
8756	Chocolate, prepared from mix	1	slice(s)	95	23.2	352	5.0	50.7	1.5	14.3	5.2	5.7	2.6	—
393	Devil's food cupcake with chocolate frosting	1	item(s)	35	8.4	120	2.0	20.0	0.7	4.0	1.8	1.6	0.6	—
8757	Fruitcake, ready to eat, commercially prepared	1	piece(s)	43	10.9	139	1.2	26.5	1.6	3.9	0.5	1.8	1.4	—
1397	Pineapple upside down, prepared from mix	1	slice(s)	115	37.1	367	4.0	58.1	0.9	13.9	3.4	6.0	3.8	—
411	Sponge, prepared from mix	1	slice(s)	63	18.5	187	4.6	36.4	0.3	2.7	0.8	1.0	0.4	—
8817	White with coconut frosting, prepared from mix	1	slice(s)	112	23.2	399	4.9	70.8	1.1	11.5	4.4	4.1	2.4	—
8819	Yellow with chocolate frosting, ready to eat, commercially prepared	1	slice(s)	64	14.0	243	2.4	35.5	1.2	11.1	3.0	6.1	1.4	—

PAGE KEY: A-6 = Breads/Baked Goods A-12 = Cereal/Rice/Pasta A-16 = Fruit A-20 = Vegetables/Legumes A-30 = Nuts/Seeds A-32 = Vegetarian A-34 = Dairy A-42 = Eggs A-42 = Seafood A-44 = Meats A-48 = Poultry A-48 = Processed Meats A-50 = Beverages A-54 = Fats/Oils A-56 = Sweets A-58 = Spices/Condiments/Sauces A-62 = Mixed Foods/Soups/Sandwiches A-66 = Fast Food A-86 = Convenience A-88 = Baby Foods

Chol (mg)	Calc (mg)	Iron (mg)	Magn (mg)	Pota (mg)	Sodi (mg)	Zinc (mg)	Vit A (µg)	Thia (mg)	Vit E (mg α)	Ribo (mg)	Niac (mg)	Vit B$_6$ (mg)	Fola (µg)	Vit C (mg)	Vit B$_{12}$ (µg)	Sele (µg)
0	13	2.69	19.9	105.1	228.6	0.80	14.9	0.27	0.22	0.19	2.18	0.04	78.8	0.5	0	22.0
0	60	1.08	—	—	310.0	—	0	—	—	—	—	—	—	0	—	—
0	9	2.18	22.0	81.7	360.0	0.63	0.7	0.23	0.23	0.24	2.10	0.03	69.6	0.1	0	24.3
0	63	4.29	15.6	53.3	318.1	1.34	0	0.42	0.07	0.18	2.82	0.04	103.0	0.7	0	16.2
0	65	2.97	15.8	56.1	316.8	0.85	0	0.39	0.07	0.17	2.88	0.04	86.5	0	0	16.6
0	38	0.94	6.0	47.4	206.0	0.20	—	0.16	0.01	0.12	1.20	0.01	31.7	0.1	0.1	7.1
49	79	1.35	7.1	48.7	277.2	0.29	64.7	0.14	0.42	0.15	1.19	0.02	32.3	0	0.1	10.9
0	57	1.21	16.1	81.0	321.1	0.42	—	0.19	0.01	0.14	1.65	0.03	35.3	0.1	0.1	0
0	32	0.94	28.4	143.1	284.0	0.22	11.3	0.01	0.14	0.05	0.50	0.03	5.0	0	0	9.9
0	5	1.02	7.7	29.8	157.7	0.21	0	0.14	0.24	0.13	1.26	0.01	38.9	0	0	9.0
21	94	0.91	10.5	71.5	209.8	0.48	—	0.14	0.32	0.15	1.03	0.04	34.6	1.7	0.2	6.2
0	11	0.70	13.0	44.3	134.5	0.31	0	0.09	—	0.06	0.92	0.08	15.3	0	0	6.3
0	6	0.30	2.3	9.3	52.4	0.06	0	0.04	—	0.02	0.40	0.00	9.9	0	0	2.8
20	37	1.21	7.6	46.0	196.8	0.31	25.2	0.17	0.10	0.17	1.93	0.02	42.0	0	0	12.0
21	38	1.23	7.8	46.6	199.8	0.31	25.5	0.14	0.10	0.16	1.77	0.02	36.3	0	0	12.2
0	14	1.16	9.0	41.0	208.0	0.29	0	0.13	0.05	0.09	1.52	0.03	47.4	0.1	0	8.7
0	11	0.89	7.1	32.2	165.6	0.24	0	0.10	0.04	0.09	1.24	0.02	32.2	0	0	6.8
6	48	3.43	15.3	65.5	279.8	0.29	0	0.36	0.00	0.18	3.91	0.03	103.8	—	0	15.8
0	23	0.88	8.1	33.0	175.2	0.25	0	0.14	0.08	0.08	1.31	0.01	57.3	0	0	8.2
0	27	0.65	20.3	59.8	109.2	0.44	0	0.07	0.09	0.03	1.05	0.06	19.5	0	0	8.6
0	27	0.65	20.4	60.0	109.7	0.44	0	0.06	0.10	0.03	1.05	0.07	16.8	0	0	8.6
0	20	0.93	10.5	44.1	122.1	0.26	0.6	0.15	0.13	0.10	1.44	0.02	24.3	0	0	9.0
0	19	0.92	9.2	33.2	121.0	0.28	0.5	0.12	0.13	0.09	1.29	0.01	18.6	0	0	8.9
0	18	0.72	10.0	38.3	161.7	0.27	1.4	0.10	0.13	0.06	0.84	0.01	16.7	0	0	6.6
0	18	0.74	10.3	38.5	162.8	0.28	1.3	0.09	0.13	0.06	0.77	0.02	13.3	0.1	0	6.7
0	52	1.57	15.6	72.0	321.6	0.50	0	0.35	0.18	0.19	2.77	0.02	64.2	0	0	16.3
0	10	1.95	44.2	108.8	340.5	0.97	0	0.21	0.39	0.05	1.81	0.17	22.4	0	0	28.2
0	22	0.91	17.3	66.6	214.7	0.47	0	0.10	0.13	0.09	0.98	0.04	29.8	0	0	7.8
0	17	0.75	6.8	59.0	101.4	0.18	0	0.08	0.07	0.10	0.90	0.01	27.6	0	0	5.2
0	17	0.76	6.7	59.0	101.8	0.19	0	0.07	0.07	0.09	0.81	0.02	23.5	0.1	0	5.2
0	100	1.08	—	—	140	—	—	0.15	—	0.10	1.20	—	32.0	0	—	—
0	23	0.90	12.8	53.1	211.2	0.36	0	0.13	0.10	0.10	1.21	0.02	35.2	0.1	0	9.9
0	23	0.89	12.5	53.1	210.3	0.36	0	0.11	0.10	0.09	1.09	0.02	29.9	0.1	0	9.9
0	20	0.70	3.9	51.0	175.0	0.18	0	0.10	—	0.08	0.80	0.01	5.3	0	0	8.0
0	11	0.91	7.0	32.0	162.5	0.23	0	0.11	0.05	0.07	1.19	0.03	37.0	0.1	0	6.8
0	11	0.89	7.1	32.2	165.6	0.24	0	0.10	0.04	0.09	1.24	0.02	32.2	0	0	6.8
0	100	3.80	—	128.0	683.0	—	0	0.54	—	0.33	4.50	0.04	—	0	—	42.0
0	11	0.89	7.1	32.2	165.6	0.24	0	0.10	0.04	0.09	1.24	0.02	32.2	0	0	6.8
0	36	0.87	12.0	46.0	130.3	0.30	0	0.09	0.05	0.08	1.30	0.03	21.3	0.1	0	7.2
0	38	0.94	13.6	51.3	140.5	0.34	0	0.10	0.06	0.09	1.44	0.04	19.8	0	0	7.7
0	38	0.94	5.8	25.0	170.3	0.19	0	0.11	0.06	0.08	1.10	0.02	27.8	0	0	4.3
0	15	1.42	37.3	144.4	159.2	0.69	0	0.13	0.35	0.10	1.83	0.09	29.9	0	0	17.8
0	42	0.11	4.0	67.5	254.5	0.06	0	0.04	0.01	0.10	0.08	0.00	9.5	0	0	7.7
166	26	1.03	8.3	89.3	298.5	0.34	111.8	0.10	—	0.17	0.98	0.03	30.8	0	0.2	6.6
0	65	2.18	23.0	279.6	367.7	0.44	—	0.25	0.01	0.19	1.73	0.10	43.4	4.6	0	14.7
27	28	1.40	21.8	128.0	213.8	0.44	16.6	0.01	0.62	0.08	0.36	0.02	10.9	0.1	0.1	2.1
55	57	1.53	30.4	133.0	299.3	0.65	38.0	0.13	—	0.20	1.08	0.03	25.7	0.2	0.2	11.3
19	21	0.70	—	46.0	92.0	—	—	0.04	—	0.05	0.30	—	2.1	0	—	2.0
2	14	0.89	6.9	65.8	116.1	0.11	3.0	0.02	0.38	0.04	0.34	0.02	8.6	0.2	0	0.9
25	138	1.70	15.0	128.8	366.9	0.35	71.3	0.17	—	0.17	1.36	0.03	29.9	1.4	0.1	10.8
107	26	0.99	5.7	88.8	143.6	0.37	48.5	0.10	—	0.19	0.75	0.03	24.6	0	0.2	11.7
1	101	1.29	13.4	110.9	318.1	0.37	13.4	0.14	0.13	0.21	1.19	0.03	34.7	0.1	0.1	12.0
35	24	1.33	19.2	113.9	215.7	0.39	21.1	0.07	—	0.10	0.79	0.02	14.1	0	0.1	2.2

TABLE A-1 Table of Food Composition (*continued*) (Computer code is for Cengage Diet Analysis program) (For purposes of calculations, use "0" for t, <1, <.1, <.01, etc.)

DA+ Code	Food Description	Quantity	Measure	Wt (g)	H₂O (g)	Ener (kcal)	Prot (g)	Carb (g)	Fiber (g)	Fat (g)	Sat	Mono	Poly	Trans
												Fat Breakdown (g)		

Breads, Baked Goods, Cakes, Cookies, Crackers, Chips, Pies—*continued*

DA+ Code	Food Description	Quantity	Measure	Wt (g)	H₂O (g)	Ener (kcal)	Prot (g)	Carb (g)	Fiber (g)	Fat (g)	Sat	Mono	Poly	Trans
8822	Yellow with vanilla frosting, ready to eat, commercially prepared	1	slice(s)	64	14.1	239	2.2	37.6	0.2	9.3	1.5	3.9	3.3	—
	Snack cakes													
8791	Chocolate snack cake, creme filled, with frosting	1	item(s)	50	9.3	200	1.8	30.2	1.6	8.0	2.4	4.3	0.9	—
25010	Cinnamon coffee cake	1	piece(s)	72	22.6	231	3.6	35.8	0.7	8.3	2.2	2.6	3.0	—
16777	Funnel cake	1	item(s)	90	37.6	276	7.3	29.1	0.9	14.4	2.7	4.7	6.1	—
8794	Sponge snack cake, creme filled	1	item(s)	43	8.6	155	1.3	27.2	0.2	4.8	1.1	1.7	1.4	—
	Snacks, chips, pretzels													
29428	Bagel chips, plain	3	item(s)	29	—	130	3.0	19.0	1.0	4.5	0.5	—	—	—
29429	Bagel chips, toasted onion	3	item(s)	29	—	130	4.0	20.0	1.0	4.5	0.5	—	—	—
38192	Chex traditional snack mix	1	cup(s)	45	—	197	3.0	33.3	1.5	6.1	0.8	—	—	—
654	Potato chips, salted	1	ounce(s)	28	0.6	155	1.9	14.1	1.2	10.6	3.1	2.8	3.5	—
8816	Potato chips, unsalted	1	ounce(s)	28	0.5	152	2.0	15.0	1.4	9.8	3.1	2.8	3.5	—
5096	Pretzels, plain, hard, twists	5	item(s)	30	1.0	114	2.7	23.8	1.0	1.1	0.2	0.4	0.4	—
4632	Pretzels, whole wheat	1	ounce(s)	28	1.1	103	3.1	23.0	2.2	0.7	0.2	0.3	0.2	—
4641	Tortilla chips, plain	6	item(s)	11	0.2	53	0.8	7.1	0.6	2.5	0.3	0.8	0.5	0.3
	Cookies													
8859	Animal crackers	12	item(s)	30	1.2	134	2.1	22.2	0.3	4.1	1.0	2.3	0.6	—
8876	Brownie, prepared from mix	1	item(s)	24	3.0	112	1.5	12.0	0.5	7.0	1.8	2.6	2.3	—
25207	Chocolate chip cookies	1	item(s)	30	3.7	140	2.0	16.2	0.6	7.9	2.1	3.3	2.1	—
8915	Chocolate sandwich cookie with extra creme filling	1	item(s)	13	0.2	65	0.6	8.9	0.4	3.2	0.7	2.1	0.3	1.1
14145	Fig Newtons cookies	1	item(s)	16	—	55	0.5	11.0	0.5	1.3	0	—	—	0
8920	Fortune cookie	1	item(s)	8	0.6	30	0.3	6.7	0.1	0.2	0.1	0.1	0	—
25208	Oatmeal cookies	1	item(s)	69	12.3	234	5.7	45.1	3.1	4.2	0.7	1.3	1.8	—
25213	Peanut butter cookies	1	item(s)	35	4.1	163	4.2	16.9	0.9	9.2	1.7	4.7	2.3	—
33095	Sugar cookies	1	item(s)	16	4.1	61	1.1	7.4	0.1	3.0	0.6	1.3	0.9	—
9002	Vanilla sandwich cookie with creme filling	1	item(s)	10	0.2	48	0.5	7.2	0.2	2.0	0.3	0.8	0.8	—
	Crackers													
9012	Cheese cracker sandwich with peanut butter	4	item(s)	28	0.9	139	3.5	15.9	1.0	7.0	1.2	3.6	1.4	—
9008	Cheese crackers (mini)	30	item(s)	30	0.9	151	3.0	17.5	0.7	7.6	2.8	3.6	0.7	—
33362	Cheese crackers, low sodium	1	serving(s)	30	0.9	151	3.0	17.5	0.7	7.6	2.9	3.6	0.7	—
8928	Honey graham crackers	4	item(s)	28	1.2	118	1.9	21.5	0.8	2.8	0.4	1.1	1.1	—
9016	Matzo crackers, plain	1	item(s)	28	1.2	112	2.8	23.8	0.9	0.4	0.1	0	0.2	—
9024	Melba toast	3	item(s)	15	0.8	59	1.8	11.5	0.9	0.5	0.1	0.1	0.2	—
9028	Melba toast, rye	3	item(s)	15	0.7	58	1.7	11.6	1.2	0.5	0.1	0.1	0.2	—
14189	Ritz crackers	5	item(s)	16	0.5	80	1.0	10.0	0	4.0	1.0	—	—	0
9014	Rye crispbread crackers	1	item(s)	10	0.6	37	0.8	8.2	1.7	0.1	0	0	0.1	—
9040	Rye wafer	1	item(s)	11	0.6	37	1.1	8.8	2.5	0.1	0	0	0	—
432	Saltine crackers	5	item(s)	15	0.8	64	1.4	10.6	0.5	1.7	0.2	1.1	0.2	0.5
9046	Saltine crackers, low salt	5	item(s)	15	0.6	65	1.4	10.7	0.5	1.8	0.4	1.0	0.3	—
9052	Snack cracker sandwich with cheese filling	4	item(s)	28	1.1	134	2.6	17.3	0.5	5.9	1.7	3.2	0.7	—
9054	Snack cracker sandwich with peanut butter filling	4	item(s)	28	0.8	138	3.2	16.3	0.6	6.9	1.4	3.9	1.3	—
9048	Snack crackers, round	10	item(s)	30	1.1	151	2.2	18.3	0.5	7.6	1.1	3.2	2.9	—
9050	Snack crackers, round, low salt	10	item(s)	30	1.1	151	2.2	18.3	0.5	7.6	1.1	3.2	2.9	—
9044	Soda crackers	5	tem(s)	15	0.8	64	1.4	10.6	0.5	1.7	0.2	1.1	0.2	0.5
9059	Wheat cracker sandwich with cheese filling	4	item(s)	28	0.9	139	2.7	16.3	0.9	7.0	1.2	2.9	2.6	—
9061	Wheat cracker sandwich with peanut butter filling	4	item(s)	28	1.0	139	3.8	15.1	1.2	7.5	1.3	3.3	2.5	—
9055	Wheat crackers	10	item(s)	30	0.9	142	2.6	19.5	1.4	6.2	1.6	3.4	0.8	—
9057	Wheat crackers, low salt	10	item(s)	30	0.9	142	2.6	19.5	1.4	6.2	1.6	3.4	0.8	—
9022	Whole wheat crackers	7	item(s)	28	0.8	124	2.5	19.2	2.9	4.8	1.0	1.6	1.8	—
	Pastry													
16754	Apple fritter	1	item(s)	17	6.4	61	1.0	5.5	0.2	3.9	0.9	1.7	1.1	—
41565	Cinnamon rolls with icing, refrigerated dough	1	serving(s)	44	12.3	145	2.0	23.0	0.5	5.0	1.5	—	—	2.0
4945	Croissant, butter	1	item(s)	57	13.2	231	4.7	26.1	1.5	12.0	6.6	3.1	0.6	—
9096	Danish, nut	1	item(s)	65	13.3	280	4.6	29.7	1.3	16.4	3.8	8.9	2.8	—
9115	Doughnut with creme filling	1	item(s)	85	32.5	307	5.4	25.5	0.7	20.8	4.6	10.3	2.6	—

PAGE KEY: A-6 = Breads/Baked Goods A-12 = Cereal/Rice/Pasta A-16 = Fruit A-20 = Vegetables/Legumes A-30 = Nuts/Seeds A-32 = Vegetarian A-34 = Dairy A-42 = Eggs A-42 = Seafood A-44 = Meats A-48 = Poultry A-48 = Processed Meats A-50 = Beverages A-54 = Fats/Oils A-56 = Sweets A-58 = Spices/Condiments/Sauces A-62 = Mixed Foods/Soups/Sandwiches A-66 = Fast Food A-86 = Convenience A-88 = Baby Foods

Chol (mg)	Calc (mg)	Iron (mg)	Magn (mg)	Pota (mg)	Sodi (mg)	Zinc (mg)	Vit A (µg)	Thia (mg)	Vit E (mg α)	Ribo (mg)	Niac (mg)	Vit B_6 (mg)	Fola (µg)	Vit C (mg)	Vit B_{12} (µg)	Sele (µg)
35	40	0.68	3.8	33.9	220.2	0.16	12.2	0.06	—	0.04	0.32	0.01	17.3	0	0.1	3.5
0	58	1.80	18.0	88.0	194.5	0.52	0.5	0.01	0.54	0.03	0.46	0.07	13.0	1.0	0	1.7
26	55	1.36	9.9	91.9	277.6	0.30	—	0.17	0.23	0.16	1.29	0.02	36.1	0.3	0.1	9.6
62	126	1.90	16.2	152.1	269.1	0.65	49.5	0.23	1.54	0.32	1.86	0.04	50.4	0	0.3	17.7
7	19	0.54	3.4	37.0	155.1	0.12	2.1	0.06	0.50	0.05	0.52	0.01	17.0	0	0	1.3
0	0	0.72	—	45.0	70.0	—	0	—	—	—	—	—	—	0	0	—
0	0	0.72	—	50.0	300.0	—	0	—	—	—	—	—	—	0	0	—
0	0	0.55	—	75.8	621.2	—	0	0.09	—	0.05	1.21	—	12.1	0	—	—
0	7	0.45	19.8	465.5	148.8	0.67	0	0.01	1.91	0.06	1.18	0.20	21.3	5.3	0	2.3
0	7	0.46	19.0	361.5	2.3	0.30	0	0.04	2.58	0.05	1.08	0.18	12.8	8.8	0	2.3
0	11	1.29	10.5	43.8	514.5	0.25	0	0.13	0.10	0.18	1.57	0.03	51.3	0	0	1.7
0	8	0.76	8.5	121.9	57.6	0.17	0	0.12	—	0.08	1.85	0.07	15.3	0.3	0	—
0	19	0.25	15.8	23.2	45.5	0.26	0	0.00	0.46	0.01	0.13	0.02	2.2	0	0	0.7
0	13	0.82	5.4	30.0	117.9	0.19	0	0.10	0.03	0.09	1.04	0.01	30.9	0	0	2.1
18	14	0.44	12.7	42.2	82.3	0.23	42.2	0.03	—	0.05	0.24	0.02	7.0	0.1	0	2.8
13	11	0.69	12.4	62.1	108.8	0.24	—	0.08	0.54	0.06	0.87	0.01	17.8	0	0	4.1
0	2	1.01	4.7	17.8	45.6	0.10	0	0.02	0.25	0.02	0.25	0.00	6.0	0	0	1.1
0	10	0.36	—	—	57.5	—	0	—	—	—	—	—	—	0	—	—
0	1	0.12	0.6	3.3	21.9	0.01	0.1	0.01	0.00	0.01	0.15	0.00	5.3	0	0	0.2
0	26	1.93	48.8	176.7	311.1	1.42	—	0.26	0.23	0.13	1.35	0.09	34.9	0.3	0	17.4
13	27	0.65	21.1	112.8	154.1	0.46	—	0.08	0.73	0.09	1.85	0.05	23.5	0.1	0.1	4.8
18	5	0.30	1.7	12.2	49.4	0.08	—	0.04	0.28	0.05	0.31	0.01	9.5	0	0	3.1
0	3	0.22	1.4	9.1	34.9	0.04	0	0.02	0.16	0.02	0.27	0.00	5.0	0	0	0.3
0	14	0.76	15.7	61.0	198.8	0.29	0.3	0.15	0.66	0.08	1.63	0.04	26.3	0	0.1	2.3
4	45	1.43	10.8	43.5	298.5	0.33	8.7	0.17	0.01	0.12	1.40	0.16	45.6	0	0.1	2.6
4	45	1.43	10.8	31.8	137.4	0.33	5.1	0.17	0.09	0.12	1.40	0.16	26.7	0	0.1	2.6
0	7	1.04	8.4	37.8	169.4	0.22	0	0.06	0.09	0.08	1.15	0.01	12.9	0	0	2.9
0	4	0.89	7.1	31.8	0.6	0.19	0	0.11	0.01	0.08	1.10	0.03	4.8	0	0	10.5
0	14	0.55	8.9	30.3	124.4	0.30	0	0.06	0.06	0.04	0.61	0.01	18.6	0	0	5.2
0	12	0.55	5.9	29.0	134.9	0.20	0	0.07	—	0.04	0.70	0.01	12.8	0	0	5.8
0	20	0.72	—	10.0	135.0	—	—	—	—	—	—	—	—	0	—	—
0	3	0.24	7.8	31.9	26.4	0.23	0	0.02	0.08	0.01	0.10	0.02	4.7	0	0	3.7
0	4	0.65	13.3	54.5	87.3	0.30	0	0.04	0.08	0.03	0.17	0.03	5.0	0	0	2.6
0	10	0.84	3.3	23.1	160.8	0.12	0	0.01	0.14	0.06	0.78	0.01	20.9	0	0	1.5
0	18	0.81	4.1	108.6	95.4	0.11	0	0.08	0.01	0.06	0.78	0.01	18.6	0	0	2.9
1	72	0.66	10.1	120.1	392.3	0.17	4.8	0.12	0.06	0.19	1.05	0.01	28.0	0	0	6.0
0	23	0.77	15.4	60.2	201.0	0.31	0.3	0.13	0.57	0.07	1.71	0.04	24.1	0	0	3.0
0	36	1.08	8.1	39.9	254.1	0.20	0	0.12	0.60	0.10	1.21	0.01	27.0	0	0	2.0
0	36	1.08	8.1	106.5	111.9	0.20	0	0.12	0.60	0.10	1.21	0.01	27.0	0	0	2.0
0	10	0.84	3.3	23.1	160.8	0.12	0	0.01	0.14	0.06	0.78	0.01	20.9	0	0	1.5
2	57	0.73	15.1	85.7	255.6	0.24	4.8	0.10	—	0.12	0.89	0.07	17.9	0.4	0	6.8
0	48	0.74	10.6	83.2	226.0	0.23	0	0.10	—	0.08	1.64	0.03	19.6	0	0	6.1
0	15	1.32	18.6	54.9	238.5	0.48	0	0.15	0.15	0.09	1.48	0.04	35.1	0	0	1.9
0	15	1.32	18.6	60.9	84.9	0.48	0	0.15	0.15	0.09	1.48	0.04	15.0	0	0	10.1
0	14	0.86	27.7	83.2	184.5	0.60	0	0.05	0.24	0.02	1.26	0.05	7.8	0	0	4.1
14	9	0.26	2.2	22.4	6.8	0.09	7.1	0.03	0.07	0.04	0.23	0.01	6.3	0.2	0.1	2.6
0	—	0.72	—	—	340.1	—	0	—	—	—	—	—	—	—	—	—
38	21	1.15	9.1	67.3	424.1	0.42	117.4	0.22	0.47	0.13	1.24	0.03	50.2	0.1	0.1	12.9
30	61	1.17	20.8	61.8	236.0	0.56	5.9	0.14	0.53	0.15	1.49	0.06	54.0	1.1	0.1	9.2
20	21	1.55	17.0	68.0	262.7	0.68	9.4	0.28	0.24	0.12	1.90	0.05	59.5	0	0.1	9.2

TABLE A-1 Table of Food Composition (*continued*) (Computer code is for Cengage Diet Analysis program) (For purposes of calculations, use "0" for t, <1, <.1, <.01, etc.)

DA+ Code	Food Description	Quantity	Measure	Wt (g)	H₂O (g)	Ener (kcal)	Prot (g)	Carb (g)	Fiber (g)	Fat (g)	Sat	Mono	Poly	Trans
											\<Fat Breakdown (g)\>			

Breads, Baked Goods, Cakes, Cookies, Crackers, Chips, Pies—*continued*

DA+ Code	Food Description	Quantity	Measure	Wt (g)	H₂O (g)	Ener (kcal)	Prot (g)	Carb (g)	Fiber (g)	Fat (g)	Sat	Mono	Poly	Trans
9117	Doughnut with jelly filling	1	item(s)	85	30.3	289	5.0	33.2	0.8	15.9	4.1	8.7	2.0	—
4947	Doughnut, cake	1	item(s)	47	9.8	198	2.4	23.4	0.7	10.8	1.7	4.4	3.7	—
9105	Doughnut, cake, chocolate glazed	1	item(s)	42	6.8	175	1.9	24.1	0.9	8.4	2.2	4.7	1.0	—
437	Doughnut, glazed	1	item(s)	60	15.2	242	3.8	26.6	0.7	13.7	3.5	7.7	1.7	—
10617	Toaster pastry, brown sugar cinnamon	1	item(s)	50	5.3	210	3.0	35.0	1.0	6.0	1.0	4.0	1.0	—
30928	Toaster pastry, cream cheese	1	item(s)	54	—	200	3.0	23.0	0	11.0	4.5	—	—	1.5
Muffins														
25015	Blueberry	1	item(s)	63	29.7	160	3.4	23.0	0.8	6.0	0.9	1.5	3.3	—
9189	Corn, ready to eat	1	item(s)	57	18.6	174	3.4	29.0	1.9	4.8	0.8	1.2	1.8	—
9121	English muffin, plain, enriched	1	item(s)	57	24.0	134	4.4	26.2	1.5	1.0	0.1	0.2	0.5	—
29582	English muffin, toasted	1	item(s)	50	18.6	128	4.2	25.0	1.5	1.0	0.1	0.2	0.5	—
9145	English muffin, wheat	1	item(s)	57	24.1	127	5.0	25.5	2.6	1.1	0.2	0.2	0.5	—
8894	Oat bran	1	item(s)	57	20.0	154	4.0	27.5	2.6	4.2	0.6	1.0	2.4	—
Granola bars														
38161	Kudos milk chocolate granola bars w/fruit and nuts	1	item(s)	28	—	90	2.0	15.0	1.0	3.0	1.0	—	—	—
38196	Nature Valley banana nut crunchy granola bars	2	item(s)	42	—	190	4.0	28.0	2.0	7.0	1.0	—	—	—
38187	Nature Valley fruit 'n' nut trail mix bar	1	item(s)	35	—	140	3.0	25.0	2.0	4.0	0.5	—	—	—
1383	Plain, hard	1	item(s)	25	1.0	115	2.5	15.8	1.3	4.9	0.6	1.1	3.0	—
4606	Plain, soft	1	item(s)	28	1.8	126	2.1	19.1	1.3	4.9	2.1	1.1	1.5	—
Pies														
454	Apple pie, prepared from home recipe	1	slice(s)	155	73.3	411	3.7	57.5	2.3	19.4	4.7	8.4	5.2	—
470	Pecan pie, prepared from home recipe	1	slice(s)	122	23.8	503	6.0	63.7	—	27.1	4.9	13.6	7.0	—
33356	Pie crust mix, prepared, baked	1	slice(s)	20	2.1	100	1.3	10.1	0.4	6.1	1.5	3.5	0.8	—
9007	Pie crust, ready to bake, frozen, enriched, baked	1	slice(s)	16	1.8	82	0.7	7.9	0.2	5.2	1.7	2.5	0.6	—
472	Pumpkin pie, prepared from home recipe	1	slice(s)	155	90.7	316	7.0	40.9	—	14.4	4.9	5.7	2.8	—
Rolls														
8555	Crescent dinner roll	1	item(s)	28	9.7	78	2.7	13.8	0.6	1.2	0.3	0.3	0.6	—
489	Hamburger roll or bun, plain	1	item(s)	43	14.9	120	4.1	21.3	0.9	1.9	0.5	0.5	0.8	—
490	Hard roll	1	item(s)	57	17.7	167	5.6	30.0	1.3	2.5	0.3	0.6	1.0	—
5127	Kaiser roll	1	item(s)	57	17.7	167	5.6	30.0	1.3	2.5	0.3	0.6	1.0	—
5130	Whole wheat roll or bun	1	item(s)	28	9.4	75	2.5	14.5	2.1	1.3	0.2	0.3	0.6	—
Sport bars														
37026	Balance original chocolate bar	1	item(s)	50	—	200	14.0	22.0	0.5	6.0	3.5	—	—	—
37024	Balance original peanut butter bar	1	item(s)	50	—	200	14.0	22.0	1.0	6.0	2.5	—	—	—
36580	Clif Bar chocolate brownie energy bar	1	item(s)	68	—	240	10.0	45.0	5.0	4.5	1.5	—	—	0
36583	Clif Bar crunchy peanut butter energy bar	1	item(s)	68	—	250	12.0	40.0	5.0	6.0	1.5	—	—	0
36589	Clif Luna Nutz over Chocolate energy bar	1	item(s)	48	—	180	10.0	25.0	3.0	4.5	2.5	—	—	0
12005	PowerBar apple cinnamon	1	item(s)	65	—	230	9.0	45.0	3.0	2.5	0.5	1.5	0.5	0
16078	PowerBar banana	1	item(s)	65	—	230	9.0	45.0	3.0	2.5	0.5	1.0	0.5	0
16080	PowerBar chocolate	1	item(s)	65	6.4	230	10.0	45.0	3.0	2.0	0.5	0.5	1.0	0
29092	PowerBar peanut butter	1	item(s)	65	—	240	10.0	45.0	3.0	3.5	0.5	—	—	0
Tortillas														
1391	Corn tortillas, soft	1	item(s)	26	11.9	57	1.5	11.6	1.6	0.7	0.1	0.2	0.4	—
1669	Flour tortilla	1	item(s)	32	9.7	100	2.7	16.4	1.0	2.5	0.6	1.2	0.5	—
Pancakes, waffles														
8926	Pancakes, blueberry, prepared from recipe	3	item(s)	114	60.6	253	7.0	33.1	0.8	10.5	2.3	2.6	4.7	—
5037	Pancakes, prepared from mix with egg and milk	3	item(s)	114	60.3	249	8.9	32.9	2.1	8.8	2.3	2.4	3.3	—
1390	Taco shells, hard	1	item(s)	13	1.0	62	0.9	8.3	0.6	2.8	0.6	1.6	0.5	0.6
30311	Waffle, 100% whole grain	1	item(s)	75	32.3	200	6.9	25.0	1.9	8.4	2.3	3.3	2.1	—
9219	Waffle, plain, frozen, toasted	2	item(s)	66	20.2	206	4.7	32.5	1.6	6.3	1.1	3.2	1.5	—
500	Waffle, plain, prepared from recipe	1	item(s)	75	31.5	218	5.9	24.7	1.7	10.6	2.1	2.6	5.1	—

PAGE KEY: A-6 = Breads/Baked Goods A-12 = Cereal/Rice/Pasta A-16 = Fruit A-20 = Vegetables/Legumes A-30 = Nuts/Seeds A-32 = Vegetarian A-34 = Dairy A-42 = Eggs A-42 = Seafood A-44 = Meats A-48 = Poultry
A-48 = Processed Meats A-50 = Beverages A-54 = Fats/Oils A-56 = Sweets A-58 = Spices/Condiments/Sauces A-62 = Mixed Foods/Soups/Sandwiches A-66 = Fast Food A-86 = Convenience A-88 = Baby Foods

Chol (mg)	Calc (mg)	Iron (mg)	Magn (mg)	Pota (mg)	Sodi (mg)	Zinc (mg)	Vit A (µg)	Thia (mg)	Vit E (mg α)	Ribo (mg)	Niac (mg)	Vit B$_6$ (mg)	Fola (µg)	Vit C (mg)	Vit B$_{12}$ (µg)	Sele (µg)
22	21	1.49	17.0	67.2	249.1	0.63	14.5	0.26	0.36	0.12	1.81	0.08	57.8	0	0.2	10.6
17	21	0.91	9.4	59.7	256.6	0.25	17.9	0.10	0.90	0.11	0.87	0.02	24.4	0.1	0.1	4.4
24	89	0.95	14.3	44.5	142.8	0.23	5.0	0.01	0.08	0.02	0.19	0.01	18.9	0	0	1.7
4	26	0.36	13.2	64.8	205.2	0.46	2.4	0.53	—	0.04	0.39	0.03	13.2	0.1	0.1	5.0
0	0	1.80	—	70.0	190.0	—	—	0.15	—	0.17	2.00	0.20	40.0	0	0	—
10	100	1.80	—	—	220.0	—	—	0.15	—	0.17	2.00	—	40.0	0	0.6	—
20	56	1.02	7.8	70.2	289.4	0.28	—	0.17	0.75	0.15	1.25	0.02	34.0	0.4	0.1	8.8
15	42	1.60	18.2	39.3	297.0	0.30	29.6	0.15	0.45	0.18	1.16	0.04	45.6	0	0.1	8.7
0	30	1.42	12.0	74.7	264.5	0.39	0	0.25	—	0.16	2.21	0.02	42.2	0	0	—
0	95	1.36	11.0	71.5	252.0	0.38	0	0.19	0.16	0.14	1.90	0.02	43.5	0.1	0	13.5
0	101	1.63	21.1	106.0	217.7	0.61	0	0.24	0.25	0.16	1.91	0.05	36.5	0	0	16.6
0	36	2.39	89.5	289.0	224.0	1.04	0	0.14	0.37	0.05	0.23	0.09	50.7	0	0	6.3
0	200	0.36	—	—	60.0	—	0	—	—	—	—	—	—	0	0	—
0	20	1.08	—	120.0	160.0	—	0	—	—	—	—	—	—	0	—	—
0	0	0.00	—	—	95.0	—	0	—	—	—	—	—	—	0	—	—
0	15	0.72	23.8	82.3	72.0	0.50	0	0.06	—	0.03	0.39	0.02	5.6	0.2	0	4.0
0	30	0.72	21.0	92.3	79.0	0.42	0	0.08	—	0.04	0.14	0.02	6.8	0	0.1	4.6
0	11	1.73	10.9	122.5	327.1	0.29	17.1	0.22	—	0.16	1.90	0.05	37.2	2.6	0	12.1
106	39	1.80	31.7	162.3	319.6	1.24	100.0	0.22	—	0.22	1.03	0.07	31.7	0.2	0.2	14.6
0	12	0.43	3.0	12.4	145.8	0.07	0	0.06	—	0.03	0.47	0.01	14.0	0	0	4.4
0	3	0.36	2.9	17.6	103.5	0.05	0	0.04	0.42	0.06	0.39	0.01	8.8	0	0	0.5
65	146	1.96	29.5	288.3	348.8	0.71	660.3	0.14	—	0.31	1.21	0.07	32.6	2.6	0.1	11.0
0	39	0.93	5.9	26.3	134.1	0.18	0	0.11	0.02	0.09	1.16	0.02	31.1	0	0.1	5.5
0	59	1.42	9.0	40.4	206.0	0.28	0	0.17	0.03	0.13	1.78	0.03	47.7	0	0.1	8.4
0	54	1.87	15.4	61.6	310.1	0.53	0	0.27	0.23	0.19	2.41	0.02	54.2	0	0	22.3
0	54	1.86	15.4	61.6	310.1	0.53	0	0.27	0.23	0.19	2.41	0.01	54.2	0	0	22.3
0	30	0.69	24.1	77.1	135.5	0.57	0	0.07	0.26	0.04	1.04	0.06	8.5	0	0	14.0
3	100	4.50	40.0	160.0	180.0	3.75	—	0.37	—	0.42	5.00	0.50	100.0	60.0	1.5	17.5
3	100	4.50	40.0	130.0	230.0	3.75	—	0.37	—	0.42	5.00	0.50	100.0	60.0	1.5	17.5
0	250	4.50	100.0	370.0	150.0	3.00	—	0.37	—	0.25	3.00	0.40	80.0	60.0	0.9	14.0
0	250	4.50	100.0	230.0	250.0	3.00	—	0.37	—	0.25	3.00	0.40	80.0	60.0	0.9	14.0
0	350	5.40	80.0	190.0	190.0	5.25	—	1.20	—	1.36	16.00	2.00	400.0	60.0	6.0	24.5
0	300	6.30	140.0	125.0	100.0	5.25	—	1.50	—	1.70	20.00	2.00	400.0	60.0	6.0	—
0	300	6.30	140.0	190.0	100.0	5.25	0	1.50	—	1.70	20.00	2.00	400.0	60.0	6.0	—
0	300	6.30	140.0	200.0	95.0	5.25	0	1.50	—	1.70	20.00	2.00	400.0	60.0	6.0	5.1
0	300	6.30	140.0	130.0	120.0	5.25	0	1.50	—	1.70	20.00	2.00	400.0	60.0	6.0	—
0	21	0.32	18.7	48.4	11.7	0.34	0	0.02	0.07	0.02	0.39	0.06	1.3	0	0	1.6
0	41	1.06	7.0	49.6	203.5	0.17	0	0.17	0.06	0.08	1.14	0.01	33.3	0	0	7.1
64	235	1.96	18.2	157.3	469.7	0.61	57.0	0.22	—	0.31	1.73	0.05	41.0	2.5	0.2	16.0
81	245	1.48	25.1	226.9	575.7	0.85	82.1	0.22	—	0.35	1.40	0.12	104.6	0.7	0.4	—
0	13	0.25	11.3	29.7	51.7	0.21	0.1	0.03	0.09	0.01	0.25	0.03	9.2	0	0	0.6
71	194	1.60	28.5	171.0	371.3	0.87	48.8	0.15	0.32	0.25	1.47	0.08	28.5	0	0.4	20.0
10	203	4.56	15.8	95.0	481.8	0.35	262.7	0.34	0.64	0.46	5.86	0.68	49.5	0	1.9	8.3
52	191	1.73	14.3	119.3	383.3	0.51	48.8	0.19	—	0.26	1.55	0.04	34.5	0.3	0.2	34.7

TABLE A-1 Table of Food Composition (*continued*) (Computer code is for Cengage Diet Analysis program) (For purposes of calculations, use "0" for t, <1, <.1, <.01, etc.)

DA+ Code	Food Description	Quantity	Measure	Wt (g)	H₂O (g)	Ener (kcal)	Prot (g)	Carb (g)	Fiber (g)	Fat (g)	Sat	Mono	Poly	Trans
											\ Fat Breakdown (g)			

Cereal, Flour, Grain, Pasta, Noodles, Popcorn

DA+ Code	Food Description	Quantity	Measure	Wt (g)	H₂O (g)	Ener (kcal)	Prot (g)	Carb (g)	Fiber (g)	Fat (g)	Sat	Mono	Poly	Trans
	Grain													
2861	Amaranth, dry	½	cup(s)	98	9.6	365	14.1	64.5	9.1	6.3	1.6	1.4	2.8	—
1953	Barley, pearled, cooked	½	cup(s)	79	54.0	97	1.8	22.2	3.0	0.3	0.1	0	0.2	—
1956	Buckwheat groats, cooked, roasted	½	cup(s)	84	63.5	77	2.8	16.8	2.3	0.5	0.1	0.2	0.2	—
1957	Bulgur, cooked	½	cup(s)	91	70.8	76	2.8	16.9	4.1	0.2	0	0	0.1	—
1963	Couscous, cooked	½	cup(s)	79	57.0	88	3.0	18.2	1.1	0.1	0	0	0.1	—
1967	Millet, cooked	½	cup(s)	120	85.7	143	4.2	28.4	1.6	1.2	0.2	0.2	0.6	—
1969	Oat bran, dry	½	cup(s)	47	3.1	116	8.1	31.1	7.2	3.3	0.6	1.1	1.3	—
1972	Quinoa, dry	½	cup(s)	85	11.3	313	12.0	54.5	5.9	5.2	0.6	1.4	2.8	—
	Rice													
129	Brown, long grain, cooked	½	cup(s)	98	71.3	108	2.5	22.4	1.8	0.9	0.2	0.3	0.3	—
2863	Brown, medium grain, cooked	½	cup(s)	98	71.1	109	2.3	22.9	1.8	0.8	0.2	0.3	0.3	—
37488	Jasmine, saffroned, cooked	½	cup(s)	280	—	340	8.0	78.0	0	0	0	0	0	0
30280	Pilaf, cooked	½	cup(s)	103	74.0	129	2.1	22.2	0.6	3.3	0.6	1.5	1.0	—
28066	Spanish, cooked	½	cup(s)	244	184.2	241	5.7	50.2	3.3	1.9	0.4	0.6	0.7	0
2867	White glutinous, cooked	½	cup(s)	87	66.7	84	1.8	18.3	0.9	0.2	0	0.1	0.1	—
484	White, long grain, boiled	½	cup(s)	79	54.1	103	2.1	22.3	0.3	0.2	0.1	0.1	0.1	—
482	White, long grain, enriched, instant, boiled	½	cup(s)	83	59.4	97	1.8	20.7	0.5	0.4	0	0.1	0	—
486	White, long grain, enriched, parboiled, cooked	½	cup(s)	79	55.6	97	2.3	20.6	0.7	0.3	0.1	0.1	0.1	—
1194	Wild brown, cooked	½	cup(s)	82	60.6	83	3.3	17.5	1.5	0.3	0	0	0.2	—
	Flour and grain fractions													
505	All purpose flour, self-rising, enriched	½	cup(s)	63	6.6	221	6.2	46.4	1.7	0.6	0.1	0	0.2	—
503	All purpose flour, white, bleached, enriched	½	cup(s)	63	7.4	228	6.4	47.7	1.7	0.6	0.1	0	0.2	—
1643	Barley flour	½	cup(s)	56	5.5	198	4.2	44.7	2.1	0.8	0.2	0.1	0.4	—
383	Buckwheat flour, whole groat	½	cup(s)	60	6.7	201	7.6	42.3	6.0	1.9	0.4	0.6	0.6	—
504	Cake wheat flour, enriched	½	cup(s)	69	8.6	248	5.6	53.5	1.2	0.6	0.1	0.1	0.3	—
426	Cornmeal, degermed, enriched	½	cup(s)	69	7.8	255	5.0	54.6	2.8	1.2	0.1	0.2	0.5	0
424	Cornmeal, yellow whole grain	½	cup(s)	61	6.2	221	4.9	46.9	4.4	2.2	0.3	0.6	1.0	—
1978	Dark rye flour	½	cup(s)	64	7.1	207	9.0	44.0	14.5	1.7	0.2	0.2	0.8	—
1644	Masa corn flour, enriched	½	cup(s)	57	5.1	208	5.3	43.5	5.5	2.1	0.3	0.6	1.0	—
1976	Rice flour, brown	½	cup(s)	79	9.4	287	5.7	60.4	3.6	2.2	0.4	0.8	0.8	—
1645	Rice flour, white	½	cup(s)	79	9.4	289	4.7	63.3	1.9	1.1	0.3	0.3	0.3	—
1980	Semolina, enriched	½	cup(s)	84	10.6	301	10.6	60.8	3.2	0.9	0.1	0.1	0.4	—
2827	Soy flour, raw	½	cup(s)	42	2.2	185	14.7	14.9	4.1	8.8	1.3	1.9	4.9	—
1990	Wheat germ, crude	2	tablespoon(s)	14	1.6	52	3.3	7.4	1.9	1.4	0.2	0.2	0.9	—
506	Whole wheat flour	½	cup(s)	60	6.2	203	8.2	43.5	7.3	1.1	0.2	0.1	0.5	—
	Breakfast bars													
39230	Atkins Morning Start apple crisp breakfast bar	1	item(s)	37	—	170	11.0	12.0	6.0	9.0	4.0	—	—	—
10571	Nutri-Grain apple cinnamon cereal bar	1	item(s)	37	—	140	2.0	27.0	1.0	3.0	0.5	2.0	0.5	—
10647	Nutri-Grain blueberry cereal bar	1	item(s)	37	5.4	140	2.0	27.0	1.0	3.0	0.5	2.0	0.5	—
10648	Nutri-Grain raspberry cereal bar	1	item(s)	37	5.4	140	2.0	27.0	1.0	3.0	0.5	2.0	0.5	—
10649	Nutri-Grain strawberry cereal bar	1	item(s)	37	5.4	140	2.0	27.0	1.0	3.0	0.5	2.0	0.5	—
	Breakfast cereals, hot													
1260	Cream of Wheat, instant, prepared	½	cup(s)	121	—	388	12.9	73.3	4.3	0	0	0	0	0
365	Farina, enriched, cooked w/water and salt	½	cup(s)	117	102.4	56	1.7	12.2	0.3	0.1	0	0	0	—
363	Grits, white corn, regular and quick, enriched, cooked w/water and salt	½	cup(s)	121	103.3	71	1.7	15.6	0.4	0.2	0	0.1	0.1	—
8636	Grits, yellow corn, regular and quick, enriched, cooked w/salt	½	cup(s)	121	103.3	71	1.7	15.6	0.4	0.2	0	0.1	0.1	—
8657	Oatmeal, cooked w/water	½	cup(s)	117	97.8	83	3.0	14.0	2.0	1.8	0.4	0.5	0.7	0
5500	Oatmeal, maple and brown sugar, instant, prepared	1	item(s)	198	150.2	200	4.8	40.4	2.4	2.2	0.4	0.7	0.8	—
5510	Oatmeal, ready to serve, packet, prepared	1	item(s)	186	158.7	112	4.1	19.8	2.7	2.0	0.4	0.7	0.8	—
	Breakfast cereals, ready to eat													
1197	All-Bran	1	cup(s)	62	1.3	160	8.1	46.0	18.2	2.0	0.4	0.4	1.3	—
1200	All-Bran Buds	1	cup(s)	91	2.7	212	6.4	72.7	39.1	1.9	0.4	0.5	1.2	0

PAGE KEY: A-6 = Breads/Baked Goods A-12 = Cereal/Rice/Pasta A-16 = Fruit A-20 = Vegetables/Legumes A-30 = Nuts/Seeds A-32 = Vegetarian A-34 = Dairy A-42 = Eggs A-42 = Seafood A-44 = Meats A-48 = Poultry A-48 = Processed Meats A-50 = Beverages A-54 = Fats/Oils A-56 = Sweets A-58 = Spices/Condiments/Sauces A-62 = Mixed Foods/Soups/Sandwiches A-66 = Fast Food A-86 = Convenience A-88 = Baby Foods

Chol (mg)	Calc (mg)	Iron (mg)	Magn (mg)	Pota (mg)	Sodi (mg)	Zinc (mg)	Vit A (µg)	Thia (mg)	Vit E (mg α)	Ribo (mg)	Niac (mg)	Vit B$_6$ (mg)	Fola (µg)	Vit C (mg)	Vit B$_{12}$ (µg)	Sele (µg)
0	149	7.40	259.3	356.8	20.5	3.10	0	0.06	—	0.20	1.24	0.20	47.8	4.1	0	—
0	9	1.04	17.3	73.0	2.4	0.64	0	0.06	0.01	0.04	1.61	0.09	12.6	0	0	6.8
0	6	0.67	42.8	73.9	3.4	0.51	0	0.03	0.07	0.03	0.79	0.06	11.8	0	0	1.8
0	9	0.87	29.1	61.9	4.6	0.51	0	0.05	0.01	0.02	0.91	0.07	16.4	0	0	0.5
0	6	0.30	6.3	45.5	3.9	0.20	0	0.05	0.10	0.02	0.77	0.04	11.8	0	0	21.6
0	4	0.75	52.8	74.4	2.4	1.09	0	0.12	0.02	0.09	1.59	0.13	22.8	0	0	1.1
0	27	2.54	110.5	266.0	1.9	1.46	0	0.55	0.47	0.10	0.43	0.07	24.4	0	0	21.2
0	40	3.88	167.4	478.5	4.2	2.62	0.8	0.30	2.06	0.26	1.28	0.40	156.4	0	0	7.2
0	10	0.41	41.9	41.9	4.9	0.61	0	0.09	0.02	0.02	1.49	0.14	3.9	0	0	9.6
0	10	0.51	42.9	77.0	1.0	0.60	0	0.09	—	0.01	1.29	0.14	3.9	0	0	38.0
0	—	2.16	—	—	780.0	—	—	—	—	—	—	—	—	—	—	—
0	11	1.16	9.3	54.6	390.4	0.37	33.0	0.13	0.28	0.02	1.23	0.06	44.3	0.4	0	4.3
0	37	1.52	95.4	330.5	97.1	1.40	—	0.27	0.12	0.05	3.24	0.38	19.0	22.6	0	14.3
0	2	0.12	4.4	8.7	4.4	0.35	0	0.01	0.03	0.01	0.25	0.02	0.9	0	0	4.9
0	8	0.94	9.5	27.7	0.8	0.38	0	0.12	0.03	0.01	1.16	0.07	45.8	0	0	5.9
0	7	1.46	4.1	7.4	3.3	0.40	0	0.06	0.01	0.01	1.43	0.04	57.8	0	0	4.0
0	15	1.43	7.1	44.2	1.6	0.29	0	0.16	0.01	0.01	1.82	0.12	64.0	0	0	7.3
0	2	0.49	26.2	82.8	2.5	1.09	0	0.04	0.19	0.07	1.05	0.11	21.3	0	0	0.7
0	211	2.90	11.9	77.5	793.7	0.38	0	0.42	0.02	0.24	3.64	0.02	122.5	0	0	21.5
0	9	2.90	13.7	66.9	1.2	0.42	0	0.48	0.02	0.30	3.68	0.02	114.4	0	0	21.2
0	16	0.70	45.4	185.9	4.5	1.04	0	0.06	—	0.02	2.56	0.14	12.9	0	0	2.0
0	25	2.42	150.6	346.2	6.6	1.86	0	0.24	0.18	0.10	3.68	0.34	32.4	0	0	3.4
0	10	5.01	11.0	71.9	1.4	0.42	0	0.61	0.01	0.29	4.65	0.02	127.4	0	0	3.4
0	2	2.98	24.1	104.9	4.8	0.48	7.6	0.42	0.10	0.28	3.66	0.12	148.3	0	0	8.0
0	4	2.10	77.5	175.1	21.3	1.10	6.7	0.22	0.24	0.12	2.20	0.18	15.2	0	0	9.4
0	36	4.12	158.7	467.2	0.6	3.58	0.6	0.20	0.90	0.16	2.72	0.28	38.4	0	0	22.8
0	80	4.10	62.7	169.9	2.8	1.00	0	0.80	0.08	0.42	5.60	0.20	132.8	0	0	8.5
0	9	1.56	88.5	228.3	6.3	1.92	0	0.34	0.94	0.06	5.00	0.58	12.6	0	0	—
0	8	0.26	27.6	60.0	0	0.62	0	0.10	0.08	0.02	2.04	0.34	3.2	0	0	11.9
0	14	3.64	39.2	155.3	0.8	0.86	0	0.66	0.20	0.46	5.00	0.08	152.8	0	0	74.6
0	87	2.70	182.0	1067.0	5.5	1.65	2.5	0.24	0.82	0.48	1.83	0.18	146.4	0	0	3.2
0	6	0.90	34.4	128.2	1.7	1.76	0	0.27	—	0.07	0.97	0.18	40.4	0	0	11.4
0	20	2.32	82.8	243.0	3.0	1.74	0	0.26	0.48	0.12	3.82	0.20	26.4	0	0	42.4
0	200	—	—	90.0	70.0	—	—	0.22	—	0.25	3.00	—	—	9.0	—	—
0	200	1.80	8.0	75.0	110.0	1.50	—	0.37	—	0.42	5.00	0.50	40.0	0	—	—
0	200	1.80	8.0	75.0	110.0	1.50	—	0.37	—	0.42	5.00	0.50	40.0	0	0	—
0	200	1.80	8.0	70.0	110.0	1.50	—	0.37	—	0.42	5.00	0.50	40.0	0	0	—
0	200	1.80	8.0	55.0	110.0	1.50	—	0.37	—	0.42	5.00	0.50	40.0	0	0	—
0	862	34.91	21.4	150.8	732.6	0.86	—	1.59	—	1.47	21.55	2.15	431.0	0	0	—
0	5	0.58	2.3	15.1	383.3	0.09	0	0.07	0.01	0.05	0.57	0.01	39.6	0	0	10.6
0	4	0.73	6.1	25.4	269.8	0.08	0	0.10	0.02	0.07	0.87	0.03	39.9	0	0	3.8
0	4	0.73	6.1	25.4	269.8	0.08	2.4	0.10	0.02	0.07	0.87	0.03	39.9	0	0	3.3
0	11	1.05	31.6	81.9	4.7	1.17	0	0.09	0.09	0.02	0.26	0.01	7.0	0	0	6.3
0	26	6.83	49.9	126.4	403.5	1.03	0	1.02	—	0.05	1.56	0.30	42.2	0	0	11.1
0	21	3.96	44.7	112.4	240.9	0.92	0	0.60	—	0.04	0.77	0.18	18.7	0	0	3.8
0	241	10.90	224.4	632.4	150.0	3.00	300.1	1.40	—	1.68	9.16	7.44	800.0	12.4	12.0	5.8
0	57	13.64	186.4	909.1	614.5	4.55	464.5	1.09	1.42	1.27	15.45	6.09	1222.7	18.2	18.2	26.3

TABLE A-1 Table of Food Composition (*continued*) (Computer code is for Cengage Diet Analysis program)   (For purposes of calculations, use "0" for t, <1, <.1, <.01, etc.

DA+ Code	Food Description	Quantity	Measure	Wt (g)	H₂O (g)	Ener (kcal)	Prot (g)	Carb (g)	Fiber (g)	Fat (g)	Fat Breakdown (g)			
											Sat	Mono	Poly	*Trans*
Cereal, Flour, Grain, Pasta, Noodles, Popcorn—*continued*														
1199	Apple Jacks	1	cup(s)	33	0.9	130	1.0	30.0	0.5	0.5	0	—	—	0
1204	Cap'n Crunch	1	cup(s)	36	0.9	147	1.3	30.7	1.3	2.0	0.5	0.4	0.3	—
1205	Cap'n Crunch Crunchberries	1	cup(s)	35	0.9	133	1.3	29.3	1.3	2.0	0.5	0.4	0.3	—
1206	Cheerios	1	cup(s)	30	1.0	110	3.0	22.0	3.0	2.0	0	0.5	0.5	—
3415	Cocoa Puffs	1	cup(s)	30	0.6	120	1.0	26.0	0.2	1.0	—	—	—	—
1207	Cocoa Rice Krispies	1	cup(s)	41	1.0	160	1.3	36.0	1.3	1.3	0.7	0	0	—
5522	Complete wheat bran flakes	1	cup(s)	39	1.4	120	4.0	30.7	6.7	0.7	—	—	—	0
1211	Corn Flakes	1	cup(s)	28	0.9	100	2.0	24.0	1.0	0	0	0	0	0
1247	Corn Pops	1	cup(s)	31	0.9	120	1.0	28.0	0.3	0	0	0	0	0
1937	Cracklin' Oat Bran	1	cup(s)	65	2.3	267	5.3	46.7	8.0	9.3	4.0	4.7	1.3	0
1220	Froot Loops	1	cup(s)	32	0.8	120	1.0	28.0	1.0	1.0	0.5	0	0	—
38214	Frosted Cheerios	1	cup(s)	37	—	149	2.5	31.1	1.2	1.2	—	—	—	—
372	Frosted Flakes	1	cup(s)	41	1.1	160	1.3	37.3	1.3	0	0	0	0	0
38215	Frosted Mini Chex	1	cup(s)	40	—	147	1.3	36.0	0	0	0	0	0	0
10268	Frosted Mini-Wheats	1	cup(s)	59	3.1	208	5.8	47.4	5.8	1.2	0	0	0.6	—
38216	Frosted Wheaties	1	cup(s)	40	—	147	1.3	36.0	0.3	0	0	0	0	0
1223	Granola, prepared	½	cup(s)	61	3.3	298	9.1	32.5	5.5	14.7	2.5	5.8	5.6	0
2415	Honey Bunches of Oats honey roasted	1	cup(s)	40	0.9	160	2.7	33.3	1.3	2.0	0.7	1.2	0.1	—
1227	Honey Nut Cheerios	1	cup(s)	37	0.9	149	3.7	29.9	2.5	1.9	0	0.6	0.6	—
2424	Honeycomb	1	cup(s)	22	0.3	83	1.5	19.5	0.8	0.4	0	—	—	—
10286	Kashi whole grain puffs	1	cup(s)	19	—	70	2.0	15.0	1.0	0.5	0	—	—	—
41142	Kellogg's Mueslix	1	cup(s)	83	7.2	298	7.6	60.8	6.1	4.6	0.7	2.4	1.5	0
1231	Kix	1	cup(s)	24	0.5	96	1.6	20.8	0.8	0.4	—	—	—	—
30569	Life	1	cup(s)	43	1.7	160	4.0	33.3	2.7	2.0	0.3	0.6	0.6	—
1233	Lucky Charms	1	cup(s)	24	0.6	96	1.6	20.0	0.8	0.8	—	—	—	—
38220	Multi Grain Cheerios	1	cup(s)	30	—	110	3.0	24.0	3.0	1.0	—	—	—	—
1201	Multi-Bran Chex	1	cup(s)	63	1.3	216	4.3	52.9	8.6	1.6	0	0	0.5	0
13633	Post Bran Flakes	1	cup(s)	40	1.5	133	4.0	32.0	6.7	0.7	0	—	—	—
1241	Product 19	1	cup(s)	30	1.0	100	2.0	25.0	1.0	0	0	0	0	0
32432	Puffed rice, fortified	1	cup(s)	14	0.4	56	0.9	12.6	0.2	0.1	0	—	—	—
32433	Puffed wheat, fortified	1	cup(s)	12	0.4	44	1.8	9.6	0.5	0.1	0	—	—	—
13334	Quaker 100% natural granola oats and honey	½	cup(s)	48	—	220	5.0	31.0	3.0	9.0	3.8	4.1	1.2	—
13335	Quaker 100% natural granola oats, honey, and raisins	½	cup(s)	51	—	230	5.0	34.0	3.0	9.0	3.6	3.8	1.1	—
2420	Raisin Bran	1	cup(s)	59	5.0	190	4.0	46.0	8.0	1.0	0	0.1	0.4	—
1244	Rice Chex	1	cup(s)	31	0.8	120	2.0	27.0	0.3	0	0	0	0	0
1245	Rice Krispies	1	cup(s)	26	0.8	96	1.6	23.2	0	0	0	0	0	0
5593	Shredded Wheat	1	cup(s)	49	0.4	177	5.8	40.9	6.9	1.1	0.1	0	0.2	0
1248	Smacks	1	cup(s)	36	1.1	133	2.7	32.0	1.3	0.7	—	—	—	—
1246	Special K	1	cup(s)	31	0.9	110	7.0	22.0	0.5	0	0	0	0	0
3428	Total corn flakes	1	cup(s)	23	0.6	83	1.5	18.0	0.6	0	0	0	0	0
1253	Total whole grain	1	cup(s)	40	1.1	147	2.7	30.7	4.0	1.3	—	—	—	—
1254	Trix	1	cup(s)	30	0.6	120	1.0	27.0	1.0	1.0	—	—	—	—
382	Wheat germ, toasted	2	tablespoon(s)	14	0.8	54	4.1	7.0	2.1	1.5	0.3	0.2	0.9	—
1257	Wheaties	1	cup(s)	36	1.2	132	3.6	28.8	3.6	1.2	—	—	—	—
	Pasta, noodles													
449	Chinese chow mein noodles, cooked	½	cup(s)	23	0.2	119	1.9	12.9	0.9	6.9	1.0	1.7	3.9	—
1995	Corn pasta, cooked	½	cup(s)	70	47.8	88	1.8	19.5	3.4	0.5	0.1	0.1	0.2	—
448	Egg noodles, enriched, cooked	½	cup(s)	80	54.2	110	3.6	20.1	1.0	1.7	0.3	0.5	0.4	0
1563	Egg noodles, spinach, enriched, cooked	½	cup(s)	80	54.8	106	4.0	19.4	1.8	1.3	0.3	0.4	0.3	—
440	Macaroni, enriched, cooked	½	cup(s)	70	43.5	111	4.1	21.6	1.3	0.7	0.1	0.1	0.2	0
2000	Macaroni, tricolor vegetable, enriched, cooked	½	cup(s)	67	45.8	86	3.0	17.8	2.9	0.1	0	0	0	—
1996	Plain pasta, fresh-refrigerated, cooked	½	cup(s)	64	43.9	84	3.3	16.0	—	0.7	0.1	0.1	0.3	—
1725	Ramen noodles, cooked	½	cup(s)	114	94.5	104	3.0	15.4	1.0	4.3	0.2	0.2	0.2	—
2878	Soba noodles, cooked	½	cup(s)	95	69.4	94	4.8	20.4	—	0.1	0	0	0	—
2879	Somen noodles, cooked	½	cup(s)	88	59.8	115	3.5	24.2	—	0.2	0	0	0.1	—
493	Spaghetti, al dente, cooked	½	cup(s)	65	41.6	95	3.5	19.5	1.0	0.5	0.1	0.1	0.2	—
2884	Spaghetti, whole wheat, cooked	½	cup(s)	70	47.0	87	3.7	18.6	3.2	0.4	0.1	0.1	0.1	—
	Popcorn													
476	Air popped	1	cup(s)	8	0.3	31	1.0	6.2	1.2	0.4	0	0.1	0.2	—
4619	Caramel	1	cup(s)	35	1.0	152	1.3	27.8	1.8	4.5	1.3	1.0	1.6	

Chol (mg)	Calc (mg)	Iron (mg)	Magn (mg)	Pota (mg)	Sodi (mg)	Zinc (mg)	Vit A (µg)	Thia (mg)	Vit E (mg α)	Ribo (mg)	Niac (mg)	Vit B₆ (mg)	Fola (µg)	Vit C (mg)	Vit B₁₂ (µg)	Sele (µg)
0	0	4.50	8.0	30.0	130.0	1.50	150.2	0.37	—	0.42	5.00	0.50	100.0	15.0	1.5	2.4
0	5	6.80	20.0	73.3	266.7	5.00	2.5	0.51	—	0.57	6.68	0.67	133.5	0	0	6.7
0	7	6.53	18.7	73.3	240.0	5.13	2.4	0.51	—	0.57	6.68	0.67	133.7	0	0	6.7
0	100	8.10	40.0	95.0	280.0	3.75	150.3	0.37	—	0.42	5.00	0.50	200.0	6.0	1.5	11.3
0	100	4.50	8.0	50.0	170.0	3.75	0	0.37	—	0.42	5.00	0.50	100.0	6.0	1.5	2.0
0	53	6.00	10.7	66.7	253.3	2.00	200.1	0.49	—	0.56	6.67	0.67	133.3	20.0	2.0	5.8
0	0	24.00	53.3	226.7	280.0	20.00	300.1	2.00	—	2.27	26.67	2.67	533.3	80.0	8.0	4.1
0	0	8.10	3.4	25.0	200.0	0.16	149.8	0.37	—	0.42	5.00	0.50	100.0	6.0	1.5	1.4
0	0	1.80	2.5	25.0	120.0	1.50	150.0	0.37	—	0.42	5.00	0.50	100.0	6.0	1.5	2.0
0	27	2.40	80.0	293.3	200.0	2.00	299.9	0.49	—	0.56	6.67	0.67	133.3	20.0	2.0	14.4
0	0	4.50	8.0	35.0	150.0	1.50	150.1	0.37	—	0.42	5.00	0.50	100.0	15.0	1.5	2.3
0	124	5.60	19.9	68.4	261.3	4.67	—	0.46	—	0.52	6.22	0.62	124.4	7.5	1.9	—
0	0	6.00	3.7	26.7	200.0	0.20	200.1	0.49	—	0.56	6.67	0.67	133.3	8.0	2.0	1.8
0	133	12.00	—	33.3	266.7	4.00	—	0.49	—	0.56	6.67	0.67	266.7	8.0	2.0	—
0	0	16.66	69.4	196.7	5.8	1.74	0	0.43	—	0.49	5.78	0.58	115.7	0	1.7	2.4
0	133	10.80	0	46.7	266.7	10.00	—	1.00	—	1.13	13.33	1.33	533.3	8.0	4.0	—
0	48	2.58	106.8	329.4	15.3	2.45	0.6	0.44	6.77	0.17	1.30	0.17	50.0	0.7	0	17.0
0	0	10.80	21.3	0	253.3	0.40	—	0.49	—	0.56	6.67	0.67	133.0	0	2.0	—
0	124	5.60	39.8	112.0	336.0	4.67	—	0.46	—	0.52	6.22	0.62	248.9	7.5	1.9	8.8
0	0	2.03	6.0	26.3	165.4	1.13	—	0.28	—	0.32	3.74	0.37	75.0	0	1.1	—
0	0	0.36	—	60.0	0	—	0	0.03	—	0.03	0.80	0.00	—	0	—	—
0	48	6.83	74.2	363.3	257.5	5.67	136.7	0.67	6.00	0.67	8.33	3.08	615.0	0.3	9.2	14.4
0	120	6.48	6.4	28.0	216.0	3.00	120.2	0.30	—	0.34	4.00	0.40	160.0	4.8	1.2	4.8
0	149	11.87	41.3	120.0	213.3	5.33	0.9	0.53	—	0.60	7.12	0.71	142.4	0	0	10.7
0	80	3.60	12.8	48.0	168.0	3.00	—	0.30	—	0.34	4.00	0.40	160.0	4.8	1.2	4.8
0	100	18.00	24.0	85.0	200.0	15.00	—	1.50	—	1.70	20.00	2.00	400.0	15.0	6.0	—
0	108	17.50	64.8	237.7	410.6	4.05	171.1	0.40	—	0.45	5.40	0.54	432.2	6.5	1.6	4.9
0	0	10.80	80.0	266.7	280.0	2.00	—	0.49	—	0.56	6.67	0.67	133.3	0	2.0	—
0	0	18.00	16.0	50.0	210.0	15.00	225.3	1.50	—	1.70	20.00	2.00	400.0	60.0	6.0	3.6
0	1	4.43	3.5	15.8	0.4	0.14	0	0.36	—	0.25	4.94	0.01	2.7	0	0	1.5
0	3	3.80	17.4	41.8	0.5	0.28	0	0.31	—	0.21	4.23	0.02	3.8	0	0	14.8
0	61	1.20	51.0	220.0	20.0	1.05	0.5	0.13	—	0.12	0.82	0.07	15.0	0.2	0.1	8.3
0	59	1.20	49.0	250.0	20.0	0.99	0.5	0.13	—	0.12	0.80	0.08	14.1	0.4	0.1	8.8
0	20	10.80	80.0	360.0	360.0	2.25	—	0.37	—	0.42	5.00	0.50	100.0	0	2.1	—
0	100	9.00	9.3	35.0	290.0	3.75	—	0.37	—	0.42	5.00	0.50	200.0	6.0	1.5	1.2
0	0	1.44	12.8	32.0	256.0	0.48	120.1	0.30	—	0.34	4.80	0.40	80.0	4.8	1.2	4.1
0	18	2.90	60.3	179.3	1.1	1.37	0	0.14	—	0.12	3.47	0.18	21.1	0	0	2.0
0	0	0.48	10.7	53.3	66.7	0.40	200.2	0.49	—	0.56	6.67	0.67	133.3	8.0	2.0	17.5
0	0	8.10	16.0	60.0	220.0	0.90	225.1	0.52	—	0.59	7.00	2.00	400.0	21.0	6.0	7.0
0	752	13.53	0	22.6	157.9	11.28	112.8	1.13	22.56	1.28	15.04	1.50	300.8	45.1	4.5	1.2
0	1333	24.00	32.0	120.0	253.3	20.00	200.4	2.00	31.32	2.27	26.67	2.67	533.3	80.0	8.0	1.9
0	100	4.50	0	15.0	190.0	3.75	150.3	0.37	—	0.42	5.00	0.50	100.0	6.0	1.5	6.0
0	6	1.28	45.2	133.8	0.6	2.35	0.7	0.23	2.25	0.11	0.79	0.13	49.7	0.8	0	9.2
0	24	9.72	38.4	126.0	264.0	9.00	180.4	0.90	—	1.02	12.00	1.20	240.0	7.2	3.6	1.7
0	5	1.06	11.7	27.0	98.8	0.31	0	0.13	0.78	0.09	1.33	0.02	20.3	0	0	9.7
0	1	0.18	25.2	21.7	0	0.44	2.1	0.04	—	0.02	0.39	0.04	4.2	0	0	2.0
23	10	1.17	16.8	30.4	4.0	0.52	4.8	0.23	0.13	0.11	1.66	0.03	67.2	0	0.1	19.1
26	15	0.87	19.2	29.6	9.6	0.50	8.0	0.19	0.46	0.09	1.17	0.09	51.2	0	0.1	17.4
0	5	0.90	12.6	30.8	0.7	0.36	0	0.19	0.04	0.10	1.18	0.03	51.1	0	0	18.5
0	7	0.33	12.7	20.8	4.0	0.30	3.4	0.08	0.14	0.04	0.72	0.02	43.6	0	0	13.3
21	4	0.73	11.5	15.4	3.8	0.36	3.8	0.13	—	0.10	0.64	0.02	41.0	0	0.1	—
18	9	0.89	8.5	34.5	414.5	0.30	—	0.08	—	0.04	0.71	0.03	4.0	0.1	0	—
0	4	0.45	8.5	33.2	57.0	0.11	0	0.09	—	0.02	0.48	0.03	6.6	0	0	—
0	7	0.45	1.8	25.5	141.7	0.19	0	0.01	—	0.03	0.08	0.01	1.8	0	0	—
0	7	1.00	12.4	51.5	0.5	0.35	0	0.12	0.04	0.07	0.90	0.04	7.8	0	0	40.0
0	11	0.74	21.0	30.8	2.1	0.57	0	0.08	0.21	0.03	0.50	0.06	3.5	0	0	18.1
0	1	0.25	11.5	26.3	0.6	0.25	0.8	0.01	0.02	0.01	0.18	0.01	2.5	0	0	0
2	15	0.61	12.3	38.4	72.5	0.20	0.7	0.02	0.42	0.02	0.77	0.01	1.8	0	0	1.3

TABLE A-1 Table of Food Composition (*continued*) (Computer code is for Cengage Diet Analysis program) (For purposes of calculations, use "0" for t, <1, <.1, <.01, etc.)

DA+ Code	Food Description	Quantity	Measure	Wt (g)	H₂O (g)	Ener (kcal)	Prot (g)	Carb (g)	Fiber (g)	Fat (g)	Sat	Mono	Poly	Trans
											Fat Breakdown (g)			

DA+ Code	Food Description	Quantity	Measure	Wt (g)	H₂O (g)	Ener (kcal)	Prot (g)	Carb (g)	Fiber (g)	Fat (g)	Sat	Mono	Poly	Trans
Cereal, Flour, Grain, Pasta, Noodles, Popcorn—*continued*														
4620	Cheese flavored	1	cup(s)	36	0.9	188	3.3	18.4	3.5	11.8	2.3	3.5	5.5	—
477	Popped in oil	1	cup(s)	11	0.1	64	0.8	5.0	0.9	4.8	0.8	1.1	2.6	—
Fruit and Fruit Juices														
	Apples													
952	Juice, prepared from frozen concentrate	½	cup(s)	120	105.0	56	0.2	13.8	0.1	0.1	0	0	0	—
225	Juice, unsweetened, canned	½	cup(s)	124	109.0	58	0.1	14.5	0.1	0.1	0	0	0	—
224	Slices	½	cup(s)	55	47.1	29	0.1	7.6	1.3	0.1	0	0	0	—
946	Slices without skin, boiled	½	cup(s)	86	73.1	45	0.2	11.7	2.1	0.3	0	0	0.1	—
223	Raw medium, with peel	1	item(s)	138	118.1	72	0.4	19.1	3.3	0.2	0	0	0.1	—
948	Dried, sulfured	¼	cup(s)	22	6.8	52	0.2	14.2	1.9	0.1	0	0	0	—
226	Applesauce, sweetened, canned	½	cup(s)	128	101.5	97	0.2	25.4	1.5	0.2	0	0	0.1	—
227	Applesauce, unsweetened, canned	½	cup(s)	122	107.8	52	0.2	13.8	1.5	0.1	0	0	0	—
38492	Crabapples	1	item(s)	35	27.6	27	0.1	7.0	0.9	0.1	0	0	0	
	Apricot													
228	Fresh without pits	4	item(s)	140	120.9	67	2.0	15.6	2.8	0.5	0	0.2	0.1	—
229	Halves with skin, canned in heavy syrup	½	cup(s)	129	100.1	107	0.7	27.7	2.1	0.1	0	0	0	
230	Halves, dried, sulfured	¼	cup(s)	33	10.1	79	1.1	20.6	2.4	0.2	0	0	0	—
	Avocado													
233	California, whole, without skin or pit	½	cup(s)	115	83.2	192	2.2	9.9	7.8	17.7	2.4	11.3	2.1	—
234	Florida, whole, without skin or pit	½	cup(s)	115	90.6	138	2.5	9.0	6.4	11.5	2.2	6.3	1.9	—
2998	Pureed	⅛	cup(s)	28	20.2	44	0.5	2.4	1.8	4.0	0.6	2.7	0.5	—
	Banana													
4580	Dried chips	¼	cup(s)	55	2.4	285	1.3	32.1	4.2	18.5	15.9	1.1	0.3	—
235	Fresh whole, without peel	1	item(s)	118	88.4	105	1.3	27.0	3.1	0.4	0.1	0	0.1	—
	Blackberries													
237	Raw	½	cup(s)	72	63.5	31	1.0	6.9	3.8	0.4	0	0	0.2	—
958	Unsweetened, frozen	½	cup(s)	76	62.1	48	0.9	11.8	3.8	0.3	0	0	0.2	—
	Blueberries													
959	Canned in heavy syrup	½	cup(s)	128	98.3	113	0.8	28.2	2.0	0.4	0	0.1	0.2	—
238	Raw	½	cup(s)	73	61.1	41	0.5	10.5	1.7	0.2	0	0	0.1	—
960	Unsweetened, frozen	½	cup(s)	78	67.1	40	0.3	9.4	2.1	0.5	0	0.1	0.2	—
	Boysenberries													
961	Canned in heavy syrup	½	cup(s)	128	97.6	113	1.3	28.6	3.3	0.2	0	0	0.1	—
962	Unsweetened, frozen	½	cup(s)	66	56.7	33	0.7	8.0	3.5	0.2	0	0	0.1	—
35576	**Breadfruit**	1	item(s)	384	271.3	396	4.1	104.1	18.8	0.9	0.2	0.1	0.3	—
	Cherries													
967	Sour red, canned in water	½	cup(s)	122	109.7	44	0.9	10.9	1.3	0.1	0	0	0	—
3000	Sour red, raw	½	cup(s)	78	66.8	39	0.8	9.4	1.2	0.2	0.1	0.1	0.1	—
3004	Sweet, canned in heavy syrup	½	cup(s)	127	98.2	105	0.8	26.9	1.9	0.2	0	0.1	0.1	—
969	Sweet, canned in water	½	cup(s)	124	107.9	57	1.0	14.6	1.9	0.2	0	0	0	—
240	Sweet, raw	½	cup(s)	73	59.6	46	0.8	11.6	1.5	0.1	0	0	0	—
	Cranberries													
3007	Chopped, raw	½	cup(s)	55	47.9	25	0.2	6.7	2.5	0.1	0	0	0	—
1717	Cranberry apple juice drink	½	cup(s)	123	102.6	77	0	19.4	0	0.1	0	0	0.1	—
1638	Cranberry juice cocktail	½	cup(s)	127	109.0	68	0	17.1	0	0.1	0	0	0.1	—
241	Cranberry juice cocktail, low calorie, with saccharin	½	cup(s)	119	112.8	23	0	5.5	0	0	0	0	0	—
242	Cranberry sauce, sweetened, canned	¼	cup(s)	69	42.0	105	0.1	26.9	0.7	0.1	0	0	0	—
	Dates													
244	Domestic, chopped	¼	cup(s)	45	9.1	125	1.1	33.4	3.6	0.2	0	0	0	—
243	Domestic, whole	¼	cup(s)	45	9.1	125	1.1	33.4	3.6	0.2	0	0	0	—
	Figs													
975	Canned in heavy syrup	½	cup(s)	130	98.8	114	0.5	29.7	2.8	0.1	0	0	0.1	—
974	Canned in water	½	cup(s)	124	105.7	66	0.5	17.3	2.7	0.1	0	0	0.1	—
973	Raw, medium	2	item(s)	100	79.1	74	0.7	19.2	2.9	0.3	0.1	0.1	0.1	—
	Fruit cocktail and salad													
245	Fruit cocktail, canned in heavy syrup	½	cup(s)	124	99.7	91	0.5	23.4	1.2	0.1	0	0	0	—
978	Fruit cocktail, canned in juice	½	cup(s)	119	103.6	55	0.5	14.1	1.2	0	0	0	0	—
977	Fruit cocktail, canned in water	½	cup(s)	119	107.6	38	0.5	10.1	1.2	0.1	0	0	0	—
979	Fruit salad, canned in water	½	cup(s)	123	112.1	37	0.4	9.6	1.2	0.1	0	0	0	—

PAGE KEY: A-6 = Breads/Baked Goods   A-12 = Cereal/Rice/Pasta   A-16 = Fruit   A-20 = Vegetables/Legumes   A-30 = Nuts/Seeds   A-32 = Vegetarian   A-34 = Dairy   A-42 = Eggs   A-42 = Seafood   A-44 = Meats   A-48 = Poultry
A-48 = Processed Meats   A-50 = Beverages   A-54 = Fats/Oils   A-56 = Sweets   A-58 = Spices/Condiments/Sauces   A-62 = Mixed Foods/Soups/Sandwiches   A-66 = Fast Food   A-86 = Convenience   A-88 = Baby Foods

Chol (mg)	Calc (mg)	Iron (mg)	Magn (mg)	Pota (mg)	Sodi (mg)	Zinc (mg)	Vit A (µg)	Thia (mg)	Vit E (mg α)	Ribo (mg)	Niac (mg)	Vit B$_6$ (mg)	Fola (µg)	Vit C (mg)	Vit B$_{12}$ (µg)	Sele (µg)
4	40	0.79	32.5	93.2	317.4	0.71	13.6	0.04	—	0.08	0.52	0.08	3.9	0.2	0.2	4.3
0	0	0.22	8.7	20.0	116.4	0.34	0.9	0.01	0.27	0.00	0.13	0.01	2.8	0	0	0.2
0	7	0.31	6.0	150.6	8.4	0.05	0	0.00	0.01	0.02	0.05	0.04	0	0.7	0	0.1
0	9	0.46	3.7	147.6	3.7	0.04	0	0.03	0.01	0.02	0.12	0.04	0	1.1	0	0.1
0	3	0.06	2.7	58.8	0.5	0.02	1.6	0.01	0.10	0.01	0.05	0.02	1.6	2.5	0	0
0	4	0.16	2.6	75.2	0.9	0.03	1.7	0.01	0.04	0.01	0.08	0.04	0.9	0.2	0	0.3
0	8	0.16	6.9	147.7	1.4	0.05	4.1	0.02	0.24	0.03	0.12	0.05	4.1	6.3	0	0
0	3	0.30	3.4	96.8	18.7	0.04	0	0.00	0.11	0.03	0.20	0.03	0	0.8	0	0.3
0	5	0.44	3.8	77.8	3.8	0.05	1.3	0.01	0.26	0.03	0.24	0.03	1.3	2.2	0	0.4
0	4	0.14	3.7	91.5	2.4	0.03	1.2	0.01	0.25	0.03	0.22	0.03	1.2	1.5	0	0.4
0	6	0.12	2.5	67.9	0.4	—	0.7	0.01	0.20	0.01	0.03	—	2.0	2.8	0	—
0	18	0.54	14.0	362.6	1.4	0.28	134.4	0.04	1.24	0.05	0.84	0.07	12.6	14.0	0	0.1
0	12	0.38	9.0	180.6	5.2	0.14	80.0	0.02	0.77	0.02	0.48	0.07	2.6	4.0	0	0.1
0	18	0.87	10.5	381.5	3.3	0.12	59.1	0.00	1.42	0.02	0.85	0.05	3.3	0.3	0	0.7
0	15	0.66	33.3	583.0	9.2	0.78	8.0	0.08	2.23	0.16	2.19	0.31	102.3	10.1	0	0.4
0	12	0.19	27.6	403.6	2.3	0.45	8.0	0.02	3.03	0.04	0.76	0.08	40.3	20.0	0	—
0	3	0.14	8.0	134.1	1.9	0.17	1.9	0.01	0.57	0.03	0.48	0.07	22.4	2.8	0	0.1
0	10	0.69	41.8	294.8	3.3	0.40	2.2	0.04	0.13	0.01	0.39	0.14	7.7	3.5	0	0.8
0	6	0.30	31.9	422.4	1.2	0.17	3.5	0.03	0.11	0.08	0.78	0.43	23.6	10.3	0	1.2
0	21	0.45	14.4	116.6	0.7	0.38	7.9	0.01	0.84	0.02	0.47	0.02	18.0	15.1	0	0.3
0	22	0.60	16.6	105.7	0.8	0.19	4.5	0.02	0.88	0.03	0.91	0.05	25.7	2.3	0	0.3
0	6	0.42	5.1	51.2	3.8	0.09	2.6	0.04	0.49	0.07	0.14	0.05	2.6	1.4	0	0.1
0	4	0.20	4.4	55.8	0.7	0.12	2.2	0.03	0.41	0.03	0.30	0.04	4.4	7.0	0	0.1
0	6	0.14	3.9	41.9	0.8	0.05	1.6	0.03	0.37	0.03	0.40	0.05	5.4	1.9	0	0.1
0	23	0.55	14.1	115.2	3.8	0.24	2.6	0.03	—	0.04	0.29	0.05	43.5	7.9	0	0.5
0	18	0.56	10.6	91.7	0.7	0.15	2.0	0.04	0.57	0.02	0.51	0.04	41.6	2.0	0	0.1
0	65	2.07	96.0	1881.6	7.7	0.46	0	0.42	0.38	0.11	3.45	0.38	53.8	111.4	0	2.3
0	13	1.67	7.3	119.6	8.5	0.09	46.4	0.02	0.28	0.05	0.22	0.05	9.8	2.6	0	0
0	12	0.25	7.0	134.1	2.3	0.08	49.6	0.02	0.05	0.03	0.31	0.03	6.2	7.8	0	0
0	11	0.44	11.4	183.4	3.8	0.12	10.1	0.02	0.29	0.05	0.50	0.03	5.1	4.6	0	0
0	14	0.45	11.2	162.4	1.2	0.10	9.9	0.03	0.29	0.05	0.51	0.04	5.0	2.7	0	0
0	9	0.26	8.0	161.0	0	0.05	2.2	0.02	0.05	0.02	0.11	0.04	2.9	5.1	0	0
0	4	0.13	3.3	46.8	1.1	0.05	1.7	0.01	0.66	0.01	0.05	0.03	0.6	7.3	0	0.1
0	4	0.09	1.2	20.8	2.5	0.02	0	0.00	0.15	0.00	0.00	0.00	0	48.4	0	0
0	4	0.13	1.3	17.7	2.5	0.04	0	0.00	0.28	0.00	0.05	0.00	0	53.5	0	0.3
0	11	0.05	2.4	29.6	3.6	0.02	0	0.00	0.06	0.00	0.00	0.00	0	38.2	0	0
0	3	0.15	2.1	18.0	20.1	0.03	1.4	0.01	0.57	0.01	0.06	0.01	0.7	1.4	0	0.2
0	17	0.45	19.1	291.9	0.9	0.12	0	0.02	0.02	0.02	0.56	0.07	8.5	0.2	0	1.3
0	17	0.45	19.1	291.9	0.9	0.12	0	0.02	0.02	0.02	0.56	0.07	8.5	0.2	0	1.3
0	35	0.36	13.0	128.2	1.3	0.14	2.6	0.03	0.16	0.05	0.55	0.09	2.6	1.3	0	0.3
0	35	0.36	12.4	127.7	1.2	0.15	2.5	0.03	0.10	0.05	0.55	0.09	2.5	1.2	0	0.1
0	35	0.36	17.0	232.0	1.0	0.14	7.0	0.06	0.10	0.04	0.40	0.10	6.0	2.0	0	0.2
0	7	0.36	6.2	109.1	7.4	0.09	12.4	0.02	0.49	0.02	0.46	0.06	3.7	2.4	0	0.6
0	9	0.25	8.3	112.6	4.7	0.11	17.8	0.01	0.47	0.02	0.48	0.06	3.6	3.2	0	0.6
0	6	0.30	8.3	111.4	4.7	0.11	15.4	0.02	0.47	0.01	0.43	0.06	3.6	2.5	0	0.6
0	9	0.37	6.1	95.6	3.7	0.10	27.0	0.02	—	0.03	0.46	0.04	3.7	2.3	0	1.0

TABLE A-1 Table of Food Composition (*continued*) (Computer code is for Cengage Diet Analysis program) (For purposes of calculations, use "0" for t, <1, <.1, <.01, etc.

DA+ Code	Food Description	Quantity	Measure	Wt (g)	H₂O (g)	Ener (kcal)	Prot (g)	Carb (g)	Fiber (g)	Fat (g)	Sat	Mono	Poly	Trans
												Fat Breakdown (g)		
Fruit and Fruit Juices—*continued*														
	Gooseberries													
982	Canned in light syrup	½	cup(s)	126	100.9	92	0.8	23.6	3.0	0.3	0	0	0.1	—
981	Raw	½	cup(s)	75	65.9	33	0.7	7.6	3.2	0.4	0	0	0.2	—
	Grapefruit													
251	Juice, pink, sweetened, canned	½	cup(s)	125	109.1	57	0.7	13.9	0.1	0.1	0	0	0	—
249	Juice, white	½	cup(s)	124	111.2	48	0.6	11.4	0.1	0.1	0	0	0	—
3022	Pink or red, raw	½	cup(s)	114	100.8	48	0.9	12.2	1.8	0.2	0	0	0	—
248	Sections, canned in light syrup	½	cup(s)	127	106.2	76	0.7	19.6	0.5	0.1	0	0	0	—
983	Sections, canned in water	½	cup(s)	122	109.6	44	0.7	11.2	0.5	0.1	0	0	0	—
247	White, raw	½	cup(s)	115	104.0	38	0.8	9.7	1.3	0.1	0	0	0	—
	Grapes													
255	American, slip skin	½	cup(s)	46	37.4	31	0.3	7.9	0.4	0.2	0.1	0	0.1	—
256	European, red or green, adherent skin	½	cup(s)	76	60.8	52	0.5	13.7	0.7	0.1	0	0	0	—
3159	Grape juice drink, canned	½	cup(s)	125	106.6	71	0	18.2	0.1	0	0	0	0	0
259	Grape juice, sweetened, with added vitamin C, prepared from frozen concentrate	½	cup(s)	125	108.6	64	0.2	15.9	0.1	0.1	0	0	0	—
3060	Raisins, seeded, packed	¼	cup(s)	41	6.8	122	1.0	32.4	2.8	0.2	0.1	0	0.1	—
987	**Guava, raw**	1	item(s)	55	44.4	37	1.4	7.9	3.0	0.5	0.2	0	0.2	—
35593	**Guavas, strawberry**	1	item(s)	6	4.8	4	0	1.0	0.3	0	0	0	0	—
3027	**Jackfruit**	½	cup(s)	83	60.4	78	1.2	19.8	1.3	0.2	0	0	0.1	—
990	**Kiwi fruit or Chinese gooseberries**	1	item(s)	76	63.1	46	0.9	11.1	2.3	0.4	0	0	0.2	—
	Lemon													
262	Juice	1	tablespoon(s)	15	13.8	4	0.1	1.3	0.1	0	0	0	0	0
993	Peel	1	teaspoon(s)	2	1.6	1	0	0.3	0.2	0	0	0	0	—
992	Raw	1	item(s)	108	94.4	22	1.3	11.6	5.1	0.3	0	0	0.1	—
	Lime													
269	Juice	1	tablespoon(s)	15	14.0	4	0.1	1.3	0.1	0	0	0	0	—
994	Raw	1	item(s)	67	59.1	20	0.5	7.1	1.9	0.1	0	0	0	—
995	**Loganberries, frozen**	½	cup(s)	74	62.2	40	1.1	9.6	3.9	0.2	0	0	0.1	—
	Mandarin orange													
1038	Canned in juice	½	cup(s)	125	111.4	46	0.8	11.9	0.9	0	0	0	0	—
1039	Canned in light syrup	½	cup(s)	126	104.7	77	0.6	20.4	0.9	0.1	0	0	0	—
999	**Mango**	½	cup(s)	83	67.4	54	0.4	14.0	1.5	0.2	0.1	0.1	0	—
1005	**Nectarine, raw, sliced**	½	cup(s)	69	60.4	30	0.7	7.3	1.2	0.2	0	0.1	0.1	—
	Melons													
271	Cantaloupe	½	cup(s)	80	72.1	27	0.7	6.5	0.7	0.1	0	0	0.1	—
1000	Casaba melon	½	cup(s)	85	78.1	24	0.9	5.6	0.8	0.1	0	0	0	—
272	Honeydew	½	cup(s)	89	79.5	32	0.5	8.0	0.7	0.1	0	0	0	—
318	Watermelon	½	cup(s)	76	69.5	23	0.5	5.7	0.3	0.1	0	0	0	—
	Orange													
14412	Juice with calcium and vitamin D	½	cup(s)	120	—	55	1.0	13.0	0	0	0	0	0	0
29630	Juice, fresh squeezed	½	cup(s)	124	109.5	56	0.9	12.9	0.2	0.2	0	0	0	—
14411	Juice, not from concentrate	½	cup(s)	120	—	55	1.0	13.0	0	0	0	0	0	0
278	Juice, unsweetened, prepared from frozen concentrate	½	cup(s)	125	109.7	56	0.8	13.4	0.2	0.1	0	0	0	—
3040	Peel	1	teaspoon(s)	2	1.5	2	0	0.5	0.2	0	0	0	0	—
273	Raw	1	item(s)	131	113.6	62	1.2	15.4	3.1	0.2	0	0	0	—
274	Sections	½	cup(s)	90	78.1	42	0.8	10.6	2.2	0.1	0	0	0	—
	Papaya, raw													
16830	Dried, strips	2	item(s)	46	12.0	119	1.9	29.9	5.5	0.4	0.1	0.1	0.1	—
282	Papaya	½	cup(s)	70	62.2	27	0.4	6.9	1.3	0.1	0	0	0	—
35640	**Passion fruit, purple**	1	item(s)	18	13.1	17	0.4	4.2	1.9	0.1	0	0	0.1	—
	Peach													
285	Halves, canned in heavy syrup	½	cup(s)	131	103.9	97	0.6	26.1	1.7	0.1	0	0	0.1	—
286	Halves, canned in water	½	cup(s)	122	113.6	29	0.5	7.5	1.6	0.1	0	0	0.1	—
290	Slices, sweetened, frozen	½	cup(s)	125	93.4	118	0.8	30.0	2.3	0.2	0	0.1	0.1	—
283	Raw, medium	1	item(s)	150	133.3	59	1.4	14.3	2.3	0.4	0	0.1	0.1	—
	Pear													
8672	Asian	1	item(s)	122	107.7	51	0.6	13.0	4.4	0.3	0	0.1	0.1	—
293	D'Anjou	1	item(s)	200	168.0	120	1.0	30.0	5.2	1.0	0	0.2	0.2	—
294	Halves, canned in heavy syrup	½	cup(s)	133	106.9	98	0.3	25.5	2.1	0.2	0	0	0	—
1012	Halves, canned in juice	½	cup(s)	124	107.2	62	0.4	16.0	2.0	0.1	0	0	0	—
291	Raw	1	item(s)	166	139.0	96	0.6	25.7	5.1	0.2	0	0	0	—

PAGE KEY: A-6 = Breads/Baked Goods A-12 = Cereal/Rice/Pasta A-16 = Fruit A-20 = Vegetables/Legumes A-30 = Nuts/Seeds A-32 = Vegetarian A-34 = Dairy A-42 = Eggs A-42 = Seafood A-44 = Meats A-48 = Poultry A-48 = Processed Meats A-50 = Beverages A-54 = Fats/Oils A-56 = Sweets A-58 = Spices/Condiments/Sauces A-62 = Mixed Foods/Soups/Sandwiches A-66 = Fast Food A-86 = Convenience A-88 = Baby Foods

Chol (mg)	Calc (mg)	Iron (mg)	Magn (mg)	Pota (mg)	Sodi (mg)	Zinc (mg)	Vit A (µg)	Thia (mg)	Vit E (mg α)	Ribo (mg)	Niac (mg)	Vit B_6 (mg)	Fola (µg)	Vit C (mg)	Vit B_{12} (µg)	Sele (µg)
0	20	0.42	7.6	97.0	2.5	0.14	8.8	0.03	—	0.07	0.19	0.02	3.8	12.6	0	0.5
0	19	0.23	7.5	148.5	0.8	0.09	11.3	0.03	0.28	0.02	0.23	0.06	4.5	20.8	0	0.5
0	10	0.45	12.5	202.2	2.5	0.08	0	0.05	0.05	0.03	0.40	0.03	12.5	33.6	0	0.1
0	11	0.25	14.8	200.1	1.2	0.06	1.2	0.05	0.27	0.02	0.25	0.05	12.4	46.9	0	0.1
0	25	0.09	10.3	154.5	0	0.07	66.4	0.04	0.14	0.03	0.23	0.06	14.9	35.7	0	0.1
0	18	0.50	12.7	163.8	2.5	0.10	0	0.04	0.11	0.02	0.30	0.02	11.4	27.1	0	1.1
0	18	0.50	12.2	161.0	2.4	0.11	0	0.05	0.11	0.03	0.30	0.02	11.0	26.6	0	1.1
0	14	0.07	10.4	170.2	0	0.08	2.3	0.04	0.15	0.02	0.30	0.05	11.5	38.3	0	1.6
0	6	0.13	2.3	87.9	0.9	0.02	2.3	0.04	0.09	0.02	0.14	0.05	1.8	1.8	0	0
0	8	0.27	5.3	144.2	1.5	0.05	2.3	0.05	0.14	0.05	0.14	0.07	1.5	8.2	0	0.1
0	9	0.16	7.5	41.3	11.3	0.04	0	0.28	0.00	0.44	0.18	0.04	1.3	33.1	0	0.1
0	5	0.13	5.0	26.3	2.5	0.05	0	0.02	0.00	0.03	0.16	0.05	1.3	29.9	0	0.1
0	12	1.06	12.4	340.3	11.6	0.07	0	0.04	—	0.07	0.46	0.07	1.2	2.2	0	0.2
0	10	0.14	12.1	229.4	1.1	0.12	17.1	0.03	0.40	0.02	0.59	0.06	27.0	125.6	0	0.3
0	1	0.01	1.0	17.5	2.2	—	0.3	0.00	—	0.00	0.03	0.00	—	2.2	0	
0	28	0.49	30.5	250.0	2.5	0.35	12.4	0.02	—	0.09	0.33	0.09	11.5	5.5	0	0.5
0	26	0.23	12.9	237.1	2.3	0.10	3.0	0.02	1.11	0.01	0.25	0.04	19.0	70.5	0	0.2
0	1	0.00	0.9	18.9	0.2	0.01	0.2	0.00	0.02	0.00	0.02	0.01	2.0	7.0	0	0
0	3	0.01	0.3	3.2	0.1	0.01	0.1	0.00	0.01	0.00	0.01	0.00	0.3	2.6	0	0
0	66	0.75	13.0	156.6	3.2	0.10	2.2	0.05	—	0.04	0.21	0.11	—	83.2	0	1.0
0	2	0.02	1.2	18.0	0.3	0.01	0.3	0.00	0.03	0.00	0.02	0.01	1.5	4.6	0	0
0	22	0.40	4.0	68.3	1.3	0.07	1.3	0.02	0.14	0.01	0.13	0.02	5.4	19.5	0	0.3
0	19	0.47	15.4	106.6	0.7	0.25	1.5	0.04	0.64	0.03	0.62	0.05	19.1	11.2	0	0.1
0	14	0.34	13.7	165.6	6.2	0.64	53.5	0.10	0.12	0.04	0.55	0.05	6.2	42.6	0	0.5
0	9	0.47	10.1	98.3	7.6	0.30	52.9	0.07	0.13	0.06	0.56	0.05	6.3	24.9	0	0.5
0	8	0.10	7.4	128.7	1.7	0.03	31.4	0.05	0.92	0.04	0.48	0.11	11.6	22.8	0	0.5
0	4	0.19	6.2	138.7	0	0.12	11.7	0.02	0.53	0.02	0.78	0.02	3.5	3.7	0	0
0	7	0.17	9.6	213.6	12.8	0.14	135.2	0.03	0.04	0.01	0.59	0.05	16.8	29.4	0	0.3
0	9	0.29	9.4	154.7	7.7	0.06	0	0.01	0.04	0.03	0.20	0.14	6.8	18.5	0	0.3
0	5	0.15	8.8	201.8	15.9	0.07	2.7	0.03	0.01	0.01	0.37	0.07	16.8	15.9	0	0.6
0	5	0.18	7.6	85.1	0.8	0.07	21.3	0.02	0.04	0.01	0.13	0.02	2.3	6.2	0	0.3
0	175	0.00	12.0	225.0	0	—	0	0.08	—	0.03	0.40	0.06	30.0	36.0	0	—
0	14	0.25	13.6	248.0	1.2	0.06	12.4	0.11	0.05	0.04	0.50	0.05	37.2	62.0	0	0.1
0	10	0.00	12.5	225.0	0	0.06	0	0.08	—	0.03	0.40	0.06	30.0	36.0	0	0.1
0	11	0.12	12.5	236.6	1.2	0.06	6.2	0.10	0.25	0.02	0.25	0.06	54.8	48.4	0	0.1
0	3	0.01	0.4	4.2	0.1	0.01	0.4	0.00	0.01	0.00	0.01	0.00	0.6	2.7	0	0
0	52	0.13	13.1	237.1	0	0.09	14.4	0.11	0.23	0.05	0.36	0.07	39.3	69.7	0	0.7
0	36	0.09	9.0	162.9	0	0.06	9.9	0.07	0.16	0.03	0.25	0.05	27.0	47.9	0	0.4
0	73	0.30	30.4	782.9	9.2	0.21	83.7	0.06	2.22	0.08	0.93	0.05	58.0	37.7	0	1.8
0	17	0.07	7.0	179.9	2.1	0.05	38.5	0.02	0.51	0.02	0.24	0.01	26.6	43.3	0	0.4
0	2	0.28	5.2	62.6	5.0	0.01	11.5	0.00	0.00	0.02	0.27	0.01	2.5	5.4	0	0.1
0	4	0.35	6.6	120.5	7.9	0.11	22.3	0.01	0.64	0.03	0.80	0.02	3.9	3.7	0	0.4
0	2	0.39	6.1	120.8	3.7	0.11	32.9	0.01	0.59	0.02	0.63	0.02	3.7	3.5	0	0.4
0	4	0.46	6.3	162.5	7.5	0.06	17.5	0.04	0.77	0.04	0.81	0.02	3.8	117.8	0	0.5
0	9	0.37	13.5	285.0	0	0.25	24.0	0.03	1.09	0.04	1.20	0.03	6.0	9.9	0	0.2
0	5	0.00	9.8	147.6	0	0.02	0	0.01	0.14	0.01	0.26	0.02	9.8	4.6	0	0.1
0	22	0.50	12.0	250.0	0	0.24	—	0.04	1.00	0.08	0.20	0.03	14.6	8.0	0	1.0
0	7	0.29	5.3	86.5	6.7	0.10	0	0.01	0.10	0.02	0.32	0.01	1.3	1.5	0	0
0	11	0.36	8.7	119.0	5.0	0.11	0	0.01	0.10	0.01	0.25	0.02	1.2	2.0	0	0
0	15	0.28	11.6	197.5	1.7	0.16	1.7	0.02	0.19	0.04	0.26	0.04	11.6	7.0	0	0.2

TABLE A-1 Table of Food Composition (*continued*) (Computer code is for Cengage Diet Analysis program)   (For purposes of calculations, use "0" for t, <1, <.1, <.01, etc.)

DA+ Code	Food Description	Quantity	Measure	Wt (g)	H₂O (g)	Ener (kcal)	Prot (g)	Carb (g)	Fiber (g)	Fat (g)	Sat	Mono	Poly	*Trans*
												Fat Breakdown (g)		

Fruit and Fruit Juices—*continued*

DA+ Code	Food Description	Quantity	Measure	Wt (g)	H₂O (g)	Ener (kcal)	Prot (g)	Carb (g)	Fiber (g)	Fat (g)	Sat	Mono	Poly	*Trans*
1017	**Persimmon**	1	item(s)	25	16.1	32	0.2	8.4	—	0.1	0	0	0	—
	Pineapple													
3053	Canned in extra heavy syrup	½	cup(s)	130	101.0	108	0.4	28.0	1.0	0.1	0	0	0	—
1019	Canned in juice	½	cup(s)	125	104.0	75	0.5	19.5	1.0	0.1	0	0	0	—
296	Canned in light syrup	½	cup(s)	126	108.0	66	0.5	16.9	1.0	0.2	0	0	0.1	—
1018	Canned in water	½	cup(s)	123	111.7	39	0.5	10.2	1.0	0.1	0	0	0	—
299	Juice, unsweetened, canned	½	cup(s)	125	108.0	66	0.5	16.1	0.3	0.2	0	0	0.1	—
295	Raw, diced	½	cup(s)	78	66.7	39	0.4	10.2	1.1	0.1	0	0	0	—
1024	Plantain, cooked	½	cup(s)	77	51.8	89	0.6	24.0	1.8	0.1	0.1	0	0	—
300	Plum, raw, large	1	item(s)	66	57.6	30	0.5	7.5	0.9	0.2	0	0.1	0	—
1027	Pomegranate	1	item(s)	154	124.7	105	1.5	26.4	0.9	0.5	0.1	0.1	0.1	—
	Prunes													
5644	Dried	2	item(s)	17	5.2	40	0.4	10.7	1.2	0.1	0	0	0	—
305	Dried, stewed	½	cup(s)	124	86.5	133	1.2	34.8	3.8	0.2	0	0.1	0	—
306	Juice, canned	1	cup(s)	256	208.0	182	1.6	44.7	2.6	0.1	0	0.1	0	—
	Raspberries													
309	Raw	½	cup(s)	62	52.7	32	0.7	7.3	4.0	0.4	0	0	0.2	—
310	Red, sweetened, frozen	½	cup(s)	125	90.9	129	0.9	32.7	5.5	0.2	0	0	0.1	—
311	**Rhubarb, cooked with sugar**	½	cup(s)	120	81.5	140	0.5	37.5	2.7	0.1	0	0	0.1	—
	Strawberries													
313	Raw	½	cup(s)	72	65.5	23	0.5	5.5	1.4	0.2	0	0	0.1	—
315	Sweetened, frozen, thawed	½	cup(s)	128	99.5	99	0.7	26.8	2.4	0.2	0	0	0.1	—
16828	**Tangelo**	1	item(s)	95	82.4	45	0.9	11.2	2.3	0.1	0	0	0	—
	Tangerine													
1040	Juice	½	cup(s)	124	109.8	53	0.6	12.5	0.2	0.2	0	0	0	—
316	Raw	1	item(s)	88	74.9	47	0.7	11.7	1.6	0.3	0	0.1	0.1	—

Vegetables, Legumes

DA+ Code	Food Description	Quantity	Measure	Wt (g)	H₂O (g)	Ener (kcal)	Prot (g)	Carb (g)	Fiber (g)	Fat (g)	Sat	Mono	Poly	*Trans*
	Amaranth													
1043	Leaves, boiled, drained	½	cup(s)	66	60.4	14	1.4	2.7	—	0.1	0	0	0.1	—
1042	Leaves, raw	1	cup(s)	28	25.7	6	0.7	1.1	—	0.1	0	0	0	—
8683	**Arugula leaves, raw**	1	cup(s)	20	18.3	5	0.5	0.7	0.3	0.1	0	0	0.1	—
	Artichoke													
1044	Boiled, drained	1	item(s)	120	100.9	64	3.5	14.3	10.3	0.4	0.1	0	0.2	—
2885	Hearts, boiled, drained	½	cup(s)	84	70.6	45	2.4	10.0	7.2	0.3	0.1	0	0.1	—
	Asparagus													
566	Boiled, drained	½	cup(s)	90	83.4	20	2.2	3.7	1.8	0.2	0	0	0.1	—
568	Canned, drained	½	cup(s)	121	113.7	23	2.6	3.0	1.9	0.8	0.2	0	0.3	—
565	Tips, frozen, boiled, drained	½	cup(s)	90	84.7	16	2.7	1.7	1.4	0.4	0.1	0	0.2	—
	Bamboo shoots													
1048	Boiled, drained	½	cup(s)	60	57.6	7	0.9	1.2	0.6	0.1	0	0	0.1	—
1049	Canned, drained	½	cup(s)	66	61.8	12	1.1	2.1	0.9	0.3	0.1	0	0.1	—
	Beans													
1801	Adzuki beans, boiled	½	cup(s)	115	76.2	147	8.6	28.5	8.4	0.1	0	—	—	—
511	Baked beans with franks, canned	½	cup(s)	130	89.8	184	8.7	19.9	8.9	8.5	3.0	3.7	1.1	—
513	Baked beans with pork in sweet sauce, canned	½	cup(s)	127	89.3	142	6.7	26.7	5.3	1.8	0.6	0.6	0.5	0
512	Baked beans with pork in tomato sauce, canned	½	cup(s)	127	93.0	119	6.5	23.6	5.1	1.2	0.5	0.7	0.3	—
1805	Black beans, boiled	½	cup(s)	86	56.5	114	7.6	20.4	7.5	0.5	0.1	0	0.2	—
14597	Chickpeas, garbanzo beans or bengal gram, boiled	½	cup(s)	82	49.4	134	7.3	22.5	6.2	2.1	0.2	0.5	0.9	—
569	Fordhook lima beans, frozen, boiled, drained	½	cup(s)	85	62.0	88	5.2	16.4	4.9	0.3	0.1	0	0.1	—
1806	French beans, boiled	½	cup(s)	89	58.9	114	6.2	21.3	8.3	0.7	0.1	0	0.4	—
2773	Great northern beans, boiled	½	cup(s)	89	61.1	104	7.4	18.7	6.2	0.4	0.1	0	0.2	—
2736	Hyacinth beans, boiled, drained	½	cup(s)	44	37.8	22	1.3	4.0	—	0.1	0.1	0.1	0	—
570	Lima beans, baby, frozen, boiled, drained	½	cup(s)	90	65.1	95	6.0	17.5	5.4	0.3	0.1	0	0.1	—
515	Lima beans, boiled, drained	½	cup(s)	85	57.1	105	5.8	20.1	4.5	0.3	0.1	0	0.1	—
579	Mung beans, sprouted, boiled, drained	½	cup(s)	62	57.9	13	1.3	2.6	0.5	0.1	0	0	0	—
510	Navy beans, boiled	½	cup(s)	91	58.1	127	7.5	23.7	9.6	0.6	0.1	0.1	0.4	0
32816	Pinto beans, boiled, drained, no salt added	½	cup(s)	63	58.8	14	1.2	2.6	—	0.2	0	0	0.1	—

PAGE KEY: A-6 = Breads/Baked Goods A-12 = Cereal/Rice/Pasta A-16 = Fruit A-20 = Vegetables/Legumes A-30 = Nuts/Seeds A-32 = Vegetarian A-34 = Dairy A-42 = Eggs A-42 = Seafood A-44 = Meats A-48 = Poultry A-48 = Processed Meats A-50 = Beverages A-54 = Fats/Oils A-56 = Sweets A-58 = Spices/Condiments/Sauces A-62 = Mixed Foods/Soups/Sandwiches A-66 = Fast Food A-86 = Convenience A-88 = Baby Foods

Chol (mg)	Calc (mg)	Iron (mg)	Magn (mg)	Pota (mg)	Sodi (mg)	Zinc (mg)	Vit A (µg)	Thia (mg)	Vit E (mg α)	Ribo (mg)	Niac (mg)	Vit B$_6$ (mg)	Fola (µg)	Vit C (mg)	Vit B$_{12}$ (µg)	Sele (µg)
0	7	0.62	—	77.5	0.3	—	0	—	—	—	—	—	—	16.5	0	—
0	18	0.49	19.5	132.6	1.3	0.14	1.3	0.11	—	0.03	0.36	0.09	6.5	9.5	0	—
0	17	0.35	17.4	151.9	1.2	0.12	2.5	0.12	0.01	0.02	0.35	0.09	6.2	11.8	0	0.5
0	18	0.49	20.2	132.3	1.3	0.15	2.5	0.11	0.01	0.03	0.36	0.09	6.3	9.5	0	0.5
0	18	0.49	22.1	156.2	1.2	0.15	2.5	0.11	0.01	0.03	0.37	0.09	6.2	9.5	0	0.5
0	16	0.39	15.0	162.5	2.5	0.14	0	0.07	0.03	0.03	0.25	0.13	22.5	12.5	0	0.1
0	10	0.22	9.3	84.5	0.8	0.09	2.3	0.06	0.02	0.03	0.39	0.09	14.0	37.0	0	0.1
0	2	0.45	24.6	358.1	3.9	0.10	34.7	0.04	0.10	0.04	0.58	0.19	20.0	8.4	0	1.1
0	4	0.11	4.6	103.6	0	0.06	11.2	0.02	0.17	0.02	0.27	0.02	3.3	6.3	0	0
0	5	0.46	4.6	398.9	4.6	0.18	7.7	0.04	0.92	0.04	0.46	0.16	9.2	9.4	0	0.9
0	7	0.16	6.9	123.0	0.3	0.07	6.6	0.01	0.07	0.03	0.32	0.03	0.7	0.1	0	0
0	24	0.51	22.3	398.0	1.2	0.24	21.1	0.03	0.24	0.12	0.90	0.27	0	3.6	0	0.1
0	31	3.02	35.8	706.6	10.2	0.53	0	0.04	0.30	0.17	2.01	0.55	0	10.5	0	1.5
0	15	0.42	13.5	92.9	0.6	0.26	1.2	0.02	0.54	0.02	0.37	0.03	12.9	16.1	0	0.1
0	19	0.81	16.3	142.5	1.3	0.22	3.8	0.02	0.90	0.05	0.28	0.04	32.5	20.6	0	0.4
0	174	0.25	16.2	115.0	1.0	—	—	0.02	—	0.03	0.25	—	—	4.0	0	—
0	12	0.30	9.4	110.2	0.7	0.10	0.7	0.02	0.21	0.02	0.28	0.03	17.3	42.3	0	0.3
0	14	0.59	7.7	125.0	1.3	0.06	1.3	0.01	0.30	0.09	0.37	0.03	5.1	50.4	0	0.9
0	38	0.09	9.5	172.0	0	0.06	10.5	0.08	0.17	0.03	0.26	0.05	28.5	50.5	0	0.5
0	22	0.25	9.9	219.8	1.2	0.04	16.1	0.07	0.16	0.02	0.12	0.05	6.2	38.3	0	0.1
0	33	0.13	10.6	146.1	1.8	0.06	29.9	0.05	0.18	0.03	0.33	0.07	14.1	23.5	0	0.1
0	138	1.49	36.3	423.1	13.9	0.58	91.7	0.01	—	0.09	0.37	0.12	37.6	27.1	0	0.6
0	60	0.65	15.4	171.1	5.6	0.25	40.9	0.01	—	0.04	0.18	0.05	23.8	12.1	0	0.3
0	32	0.29	9.4	73.8	5.4	0.09	23.8	0.01	0.09	0.02	0.06	0.01	19.4	3.0	0	0.1
0	25	0.73	50.4	343.2	72.0	0.48	1.2	0.06	0.22	0.10	1.33	0.09	106.8	8.9	0	0.2
0	18	0.51	35.3	240.2	50.4	0.33	0.8	0.04	0.16	0.07	0.93	0.06	74.8	6.2	0	0.2
0	21	0.81	12.6	201.6	12.6	0.54	45.0	0.14	1.35	0.12	0.97	0.07	134.1	6.9	0	5.5
0	19	2.21	12.1	208.1	347.3	0.48	49.6	0.07	1.47	0.12	1.15	0.13	116.2	22.3	0	2.1
0	16	0.50	9.0	154.8	2.7	0.36	36.0	0.05	1.08	0.09	0.93	0.01	121.5	22.0	0	3.5
0	7	0.14	1.8	319.8	2.4	0.28	0	0.01	—	0.03	0.18	0.06	1.2	0	0	0.2
0	5	0.21	2.6	52.4	4.6	0.43	0.7	0.02	0.41	0.02	0.09	0.09	2.0	0.7	0	0.3
0	32	2.30	59.8	611.8	9.2	2.03	0	0.13	—	0.07	0.82	0.11	139.2	0	0	1.4
8	62	2.24	36.3	304.3	556.9	2.42	5.2	0.08	0.21	0.07	1.17	0.06	38.9	3.0	0.4	8.4
9	75	2.08	41.7	326.4	422.5	1.73	0	0.05	0.03	0.07	0.44	0.07	10.1	3.5	0	6.3
9	71	4.09	43.0	373.2	552.8	6.93	5.1	0.06	0.12	0.05	0.62	0.08	19.0	3.8	0	5.9
0	23	1.80	60.2	305.3	0.9	0.96	0	0.21	—	0.05	0.43	0.05	128.1	0	0	1.0
0	40	2.36	39.4	238.6	5.7	1.25	0.8	0.09	0.28	0.05	0.43	0.11	141.0	1.1	0	3.0
0	26	1.54	35.7	258.4	58.7	0.62	8.5	0.06	0.24	0.05	0.90	0.10	17.9	10.9	0	0.5
0	56	0.95	49.6	327.5	5.3	0.56	0	0.11	—	0.05	0.48	0.09	66.4	1.1	0	1.1
0	60	1.88	44.3	346.0	1.8	0.77	0	0.14	—	0.05	0.60	0.10	90.3	1.2	0	3.6
0	18	0.33	18.3	114.0	0.9	0.16	3.0	0.02	—	0.03	0.20	0.01	20.4	2.2	0	0.7
0	25	1.76	50.4	369.9	26.1	0.49	7.2	0.06	0.57	0.04	0.69	0.10	14.4	5.2	0	1.5
0	27	2.08	62.9	484.5	14.5	0.67	12.8	0.11	0.11	0.08	0.88	0.16	22.1	8.6	0	1.7
0	7	0.40	8.7	62.6	6.2	0.29	0.6	0.03	0.04	0.06	0.51	0.03	18.0	7.1	0	0.4
—	63	2.14	48.2	354.0	0	0.93	0	0.21	0.01	0.06	0.59	0.12	127.4	0.8	0	2.6
0	9	0.41	11.3	61.7	32.1	0.10	0	0.04	—	0.03	0.45	0.03	18.3	3.8	0	0.4

TABLE A-1 Table of Food Composition (*continued*) (Computer code is for Cengage Diet Analysis program) (For purposes of calculations, use "0" for t, <1, <.1, <.01, etc.)

DA+ Code	Food Description	Quantity	Measure	Wt (g)	H₂O (g)	Ener (kcal)	Prot (g)	Carb (g)	Fiber (g)	Fat (g)	Sat	Mono	Poly	Trans
											|← Fat Breakdown (g) →|			

Vegetables, Legumes—*continued*

DA+ Code	Food Description	Quantity	Measure	Wt (g)	H₂O (g)	Ener (kcal)	Prot (g)	Carb (g)	Fiber (g)	Fat (g)	Sat	Mono	Poly	Trans
1052	Pinto beans, frozen, boiled, drained	½	cup(s)	47	27.3	76	4.4	14.5	4.0	0.2	0	0	0.1	—
514	Red kidney beans, canned	½	cup(s)	128	99.0	108	6.7	19.9	6.9	0.5	0.1	0.2	0.2	—
1810	Refried beans, canned	½	cup(s)	127	96.1	119	6.9	19.6	6.7	1.6	0.6	0.7	0.2	—
1053	Shell beans, canned	½	cup(s)	123	111.1	37	2.2	7.6	4.2	0.2	0	0	0.1	—
1670	Soybeans, boiled	½	cup(s)	86	53.8	149	14.3	8.5	5.2	7.7	1.1	1.7	4.4	—
1108	Soybeans, green, boiled, drained	½	cup(s)	90	61.7	127	11.1	9.9	3.8	5.8	0.7	1.1	2.7	—
1807	White beans, small, boiled	½	cup(s)	90	56.6	127	8.0	23.1	9.3	0.6	0.1	0.1	0.2	—
575	Yellow snap, string or wax beans, boiled, drained	½	cup(s)	63	55.8	22	1.2	4.9	2.1	0.2	0	0	0.1	—
576	Yellow snap, string or wax beans, frozen, boiled, drained	½	cup(s)	68	61.7	19	1.0	4.4	2.0	0.1	0	0	0.1	—
	Beets													
584	Beet greens, boiled, drained	½	cup(s)	72	64.2	19	1.9	3.9	2.1	0.1	0	0	0.1	—
2730	Pickled, canned with liquid	½	cup(s)	114	92.9	74	0.9	18.5	3.0	0.1	0	0	0	—
581	Sliced, boiled, drained	½	cup(s)	85	74.0	37	1.4	8.5	1.7	0.2	0	0	0.1	—
583	Sliced, canned, drained	½	cup(s)	85	77.3	26	0.8	6.1	1.5	0.1	0	0	0	—
580	Whole, boiled, drained	2	item(s)	100	87.1	44	1.7	10.0	2.0	0.2	0	0	0.1	—
585	**Cowpeas or black-eyed peas, boiled, drained**	½	cup(s)	83	62.3	80	2.6	16.8	4.1	0.3	0.1	0	0.1	—
	Broccoli													
588	Chopped, boiled, drained	½	cup(s)	78	69.6	27	1.9	5.6	2.6	0.3	0.1	0	0.1	—
590	Frozen, chopped, boiled, drained	½	cup(s)	92	83.5	26	2.9	4.9	2.8	0.1	0	0	0.1	—
587	Raw, chopped	½	cup(s)	46	40.6	15	1.3	3.0	1.2	0.2	0	0	0	—
16848	**Broccoflower, raw, chopped**	½	cup(s)	32	28.7	10	0.9	1.9	1.0	0.1	0	0	0	—
	Brussels sprouts													
591	Boiled, drained	½	cup(s)	78	69.3	28	2.0	5.5	2.0	0.4	0.1	0	0.2	—
592	Frozen, boiled, drained	½	cup(s)	78	67.2	33	2.8	6.4	3.2	0.3	0.1	0	0.2	—
	Cabbage													
595	Boiled, drained, no salt added	1	cup(s)	150	138.8	35	1.9	8.3	2.8	0.1	0	0	0	—
35611	Chinese (pak choi or bok choy), boiled with salt, drained	1	cup(s)	170	162.4	20	2.6	3.0	1.7	0.3	0	0	0.1	—
16869	Kim chee	1	cup(s)	150	137.5	32	2.5	6.1	1.8	0.3	0	0	0.2	—
594	Raw, shredded	1	cup(s)	70	64.5	17	0.9	4.1	1.7	0.1	0	0	0	—
596	Red, shredded, raw	1	cup(s)	70	63.3	22	1.0	5.2	1.5	0.1	0	0	0.1	—
597	Savoy, shredded, raw	1	cup(s)	70	63.7	19	1.4	4.3	2.2	0.1	0	0	0	—
35417	**Capers**	1	teaspoon(s)	4	—	2	0	0	0	0	0	0	0	0
	Carrots													
8691	Baby, raw	8	item(s)	80	72.3	28	0.5	6.6	2.3	0.1	0	0	0.1	—
601	Grated	½	cup(s)	55	48.6	23	0.5	5.3	1.5	0.1	0	0	0.1	0
1055	Juice, canned	½	cup(s)	118	104.9	47	1.1	11.0	0.9	0.2	0	0	0.1	—
600	Raw	½	cup(s)	61	53.9	25	0.6	5.8	1.7	0.1	0	0	0.1	—
602	Sliced, boiled, drained	½	cup(s)	78	70.3	27	0.6	6.4	2.3	0.1	0	0	0.1	—
32725	**Cassava or manioc**	½	cup(s)	103	61.5	165	1.4	39.2	1.9	0.3	0.1	0.1	0	—
	Cauliflower													
606	Boiled, drained	½	cup(s)	62	57.7	14	1.1	2.5	1.4	0.3	0	0	0.1	—
607	Frozen, boiled, drained	½	cup(s)	90	84.6	17	1.4	3.4	2.4	0.2	0	0	0.1	—
605	Raw, chopped	½	cup(s)	50	46.0	13	1.0	2.6	1.2	0	0	0	0	—
	Celery													
609	Diced	½	cup(s)	51	48.2	8	0.3	1.5	0.8	0.1	0	0	0	—
608	Stalk	2	item(s)	80	76.3	13	0.6	2.4	1.3	0.1	0	0	0.1	—
	Chard													
1057	Swiss chard, boiled, drained	½	cup(s)	88	81.1	18	1.6	3.6	1.8	0.1	0	0	0	—
1056	Swiss chard, raw	1	cup(s)	36	33.4	7	0.6	1.3	0.6	0.1	0	0	0	—
	Collard greens													
610	Boiled, drained	½	cup(s)	95	87.3	25	2.0	4.7	2.7	0.3	0	0	0.2	—
611	Frozen, chopped, boiled, drained	½	cup(s)	85	75.2	31	2.5	6.0	2.4	0.3	0.1	0	0.2	—
	Corn													
29614	Yellow corn, fresh, cooked	1	item(s)	100	69.2	107	3.3	25.0	2.8	1.3	0.2	0.4	0.6	—
615	Yellow creamed sweet corn, canned	½	cup(s)	128	100.8	92	2.2	23.2	1.5	0.5	0.1	0.2	0.3	—
612	Yellow sweet corn, boiled, drained	½	cup(s)	82	57.0	89	2.7	20.6	2.3	1.1	0.2	0.3	0.5	—

PAGE KEY: A-6 = Breads/Baked Goods A-12 = Cereal/Rice/Pasta A-16 = Fruit A-20 = Vegetables/Legumes A-30 = Nuts/Seeds A-32 = Vegetarian A-34 = Dairy A-42 = Eggs A-42 = Seafood A-44 = Meats A-48 = Poultry A-48 = Processed Meats A-50 = Beverages A-54 = Fats/Oils A-56 = Sweets A-58 = Spices/Condiments/Sauces A-62 = Mixed Foods/Soups/Sandwiches A-66 = Fast Food A-86 = Convenience A-88 = Baby Foods

Chol (mg)	Calc (mg)	Iron (mg)	Magn (mg)	Pota (mg)	Sodi (mg)	Zinc (mg)	Vit A (µg)	Thia (mg)	Vit E (mg α)	Ribo (mg)	Niac (mg)	Vit B$_6$ (mg)	Fola (µg)	Vit C (mg)	Vit B$_{12}$ (µg)	Sele (µg)
0	24	1.27	25.4	303.6	39.0	0.32	0	0.12	—	0.05	0.29	0.09	16.0	0.3	0	0.7
0	32	1.62	35.8	327.7	330.2	2.09	0	0.13	0.02	0.11	0.57	0.10	25.6	1.4	0	0.6
10	44	2.10	41.7	337.8	378.2	1.48	0	0.03	0.00	0.02	0.39	0.18	13.9	7.6	0	1.6
0	36	1.21	18.4	133.5	409.2	0.33	13.5	0.04	0.04	0.07	0.25	0.06	22.1	3.8	0	2.6
0	88	4.42	74.0	442.9	0.9	0.98	0	0.13	0.30	0.24	0.34	0.20	46.4	1.5	0	6.3
0	131	2.25	54.0	485.1	12.6	0.82	7.2	0.23	—	0.14	1.13	0.05	99.9	15.3	0	1.3
0	65	2.54	60.9	414.4	1.8	0.97	0	0.21	—	0.05	0.24	0.11	122.6	0	0	1.2
0	29	0.80	15.6	186.9	1.9	0.23	2.5	0.05	0.28	0.06	0.38	0.04	20.6	6.1	0	0.3
0	33	0.59	16.2	85.1	6.1	0.32	4.1	0.02	0.03	0.06	0.26	0.04	15.5	2.8	0	0.3
0	82	1.36	49.0	654.5	173.5	0.36	275.8	0.08	1.30	0.20	0.35	0.09	10.1	17.9	0	0.6
0	12	0.46	17.0	168.0	299.6	0.29	1.1	0.01	—	0.05	0.28	0.05	30.6	2.6	0	1.1
0	14	0.67	19.6	259.3	65.5	0.30	1.7	0.02	0.03	0.03	0.28	0.05	68.0	3.1	0	0.6
0	13	1.54	14.5	125.8	164.9	0.17	0.9	0.01	0.02	0.03	0.13	0.04	25.5	3.5	0	0.4
0	16	0.79	23.0	305.0	77.0	0.35	2.0	0.02	0.04	0.04	0.33	0.06	80.0	3.6	0	0.7
0	106	0.92	42.9	344.9	3.3	0.85	33.0	0.08	0.18	0.12	1.15	0.05	104.8	1.8	0	2.1
0	31	0.52	16.4	228.5	32.0	0.35	60.1	0.04	1.13	0.09	0.43	0.15	84.2	50.6	0	1.2
0	30	0.56	12.0	130.6	10.1	0.25	46.9	0.05	1.21	0.07	0.42	0.12	51.5	36.9	0	0.6
0	21	0.33	9.6	143.8	15.0	0.19	14.1	0.03	0.36	0.05	0.29	0.08	28.7	40.6	0	1.1
0	11	0.23	6.4	96.0	7.4	0.20	2.6	0.02	0.01	0.03	0.23	0.07	18.2	28.2	0	0.2
0	28	0.93	15.6	247.3	16.4	0.25	30.4	0.08	0.33	0.06	0.47	0.13	46.8	48.4	0	1.2
0	20	0.37	14.0	224.8	11.6	0.18	35.7	0.08	0.39	0.08	0.41	0.22	78.3	35.4	0	0.5
0	72	0.24	22.5	294.0	12.0	0.30	6.0	0.08	0.20	0.04	0.36	0.16	45.0	56.2	0	0.9
0	158	1.76	18.7	630.7	459.0	0.28	360.4	0.04	0.14	0.10	0.72	0.28	69.7	44.2	0	0.7
0	144	1.26	27.0	379.5	996.0	0.36	288.0	0.06	0.36	0.10	0.80	0.32	88.5	79.6	0	1.5
0	28	0.33	8.4	119.0	12.6	0.12	3.5	0.04	0.10	0.02	0.16	0.08	30.1	25.6	0	0.2
0	31	0.56	11.2	170.1	18.9	0.15	39.2	0.04	0.07	0.05	0.29	0.14	12.6	39.9	0	0.4
0	24	0.28	19.6	161.0	19.6	0.18	35.0	0.05	0.11	0.02	0.21	0.13	56.0	21.7	0	0.6
0	0	0.00	—	—	140	—	0	—	—	—	—	—	—	0	—	—
0	26	0.71	8.0	189.6	62.4	0.13	552.0	0.02	—	0.02	0.44	0.08	21.6	2.1	0	0.7
0	18	0.16	6.6	176.0	37.9	0.13	459.2	0.03	0.36	0.03	0.54	0.07	10.4	3.2	0	0.1
0	28	0.54	16.5	344.6	34.2	0.21	1128.1	0.11	1.37	0.07	0.46	0.26	4.7	10.0	0	0.7
0	20	0.18	7.3	195.2	42.1	0.15	509.4	0.04	0.40	0.04	0.60	0.08	11.6	3.6	0	0.1
0	23	0.26	7.8	183.3	45.2	0.15	664.6	0.05	0.80	0.03	0.50	0.11	10.9	2.8	0	0.5
0	16	0.27	21.6	279.1	14.4	0.35	1.0	0.08	0.19	0.04	0.87	0.09	27.8	21.2	0	0.7
0	10	0.19	5.6	88.0	9.3	0.10	0.6	0.02	0.04	0.03	0.25	0.10	27.3	27.5	0	0.4
0	15	0.36	8.1	125.1	16.2	0.11	0	0.03	0.05	0.04	0.27	0.07	36.9	28.2	0	0.5
0	11	0.22	7.5	151.5	15.0	0.14	0.5	0.03	0.04	0.03	0.26	0.11	28.5	23.2	0	0.3
0	20	0.10	5.6	131.3	40.4	0.07	11.1	0.01	0.14	0.03	0.16	0.04	18.2	1.6	0	0.2
0	32	0.16	8.8	208.0	64.0	0.10	17.6	0.01	0.21	0.04	0.25	0.05	28.8	2.5	0	0.3
0	51	1.98	75.3	480.4	156.6	0.29	267.8	0.03	1.65	0.08	0.32	0.07	7.9	15.8	0	0.8
0	18	0.64	29.2	136.4	76.7	0.13	110.2	0.01	0.68	0.03	0.14	0.03	5.0	10.8	0	0.3
0	133	1.10	19.0	110.2	15.2	0.21	385.7	0.03	0.83	0.10	0.54	0.12	88.4	17.3	0	0.5
0	179	0.95	25.5	213.4	42.5	0.22	488.8	0.04	1.06	0.09	0.54	0.09	64.6	22.4	0	1.3
0	2	0.61	32.0	248.0	242.0	0.48	13.0	0.20	0.09	0.07	1.60	0.06	46.0	6.2	0	0.2
0	4	0.48	21.8	171.5	364.8	0.67	5.1	0.03	0.09	0.06	1.22	0.08	57.6	5.9	0	0.5
0	2	0.36	21.3	173.8	0	0.50	10.7	0.17	0.07	0.05	1.32	0.04	37.7	5.1	0	0.2

TABLE A-1 Table of Food Composition (*continued*) (Computer code is for Cengage Diet Analysis program) (For purposes of calculations, use "0" for t, <1, <.1, <.01, etc.

DA+ Code	Food Description	Quantity	Measure	Wt (g)	H₂O (g)	Ener (kcal)	Prot (g)	Carb (g)	Fiber (g)	Fat (g)	Sat	Mono	Poly	*Trans*
											Fat Breakdown (g)			

DA+ Code	Food Description	Quantity	Measure	Wt (g)	H₂O (g)	Ener (kcal)	Prot (g)	Carb (g)	Fiber (g)	Fat (g)	Sat	Mono	Poly	*Trans*
Vegetables, Legumes—*continued*														
614	Yellow sweet corn, frozen, boiled, drained	½	cup(s)	82	63.2	66	2.1	15.8	2.0	0.5	0.1	0.2	0.3	—
618	**Cucumber**	¼	item(s)	75	71.7	11	0.5	2.7	0.4	0.1	0	0	0	—
16870	**Cucumber, kim chee**	½	cup(s)	75	68.1	16	0.8	3.6	1.1	0.1	0	0	0	—
	Dandelion greens													
620	Chopped, boiled, drained	½	cup(s)	53	47.1	17	1.1	3.4	1.5	0.3	0.1	0	0.1	—
2734	Raw	1	cup(s)	55	47.1	25	1.5	5.1	1.9	0.4	0.1	0	0.2	—
1066	**Eggplant, boiled, drained**	½	cup(s)	50	44.4	17	0.4	4.3	1.2	0.1	0	0	0	—
621	**Endive or escarole, chopped, raw**	1	cup(s)	50	46.9	8	0.6	1.7	1.5	0.1	0	0	0	—
8784	**Jicama or yambean**	½	cup(s)	65	116.5	49	0.9	11.4	6.3	0.1	0	0	0.1	—
	Kale													
623	Frozen, chopped, boiled, drained	½	cup(s)	65	58.8	20	1.8	3.4	1.3	0.3	0	0	0.2	—
29313	Raw	1	cup(s)	67	56.6	33	2.2	6.7	1.3	0.5	0.1	0	0.2	—
	Kohlrabi													
1072	Boiled, drained	½	cup(s)	83	74.5	24	1.5	5.5	0.9	0.1	0	0	0	—
1071	Raw	1	cup(s)	135	122.9	36	2.3	8.4	4.9	0.1	0	0	0.1	—
	Leeks													
1074	Boiled, drained	½	cup(s)	52	47.2	16	0.4	4.0	0.5	0.1	0	0	0	—
1073	Raw	1	cup(s)	89	73.9	54	1.3	12.6	1.6	0.3	0	0	0.1	—
	Lentils													
522	Boiled	¼	cup(s)	50	34.5	57	4.5	10.0	3.9	0.2	0	0	0.1	—
1075	Sprouted	1	cup(s)	77	51.9	82	6.9	17.0	—	0.4	0	0.1	0.2	—
	Lettuce													
625	Butterhead leaves	11	piece(s)	83	78.9	11	1.1	1.8	0.9	0.2	0	0	0.1	—
624	Butterhead, Boston or Bibb	1	cup(s)	55	52.6	7	0.7	1.2	0.6	0.1	0	0	0.1	—
626	Iceberg	1	cup(s)	55	52.6	8	0.5	1.6	0.7	0.1	0	0	0	—
628	Iceberg, chopped	1	cup(s)	55	52.6	8	0.5	1.6	0.7	0.1	0	0	0	—
629	Looseleaf	1	cup(s)	36	34.2	5	0.5	1.0	0.5	0.1	0	0	0	—
1665	Romaine, shredded	1	cup(s)	56	53.0	10	0.7	1.8	1.2	0.2	0	0	0.1	—
	Mushrooms													
15585	Crimini (about 6)	3	ounce(s)	85	—	28	3.7	2.8	1.9	0	0	0	0	0
8700	Enoki	30	item(s)	90	79.7	40	2.3	6.9	2.4	0.3	0	0	0.1	—
1079	Mushrooms, boiled, drained	½	cup(s)	78	71.0	22	1.7	4.1	1.7	0.4	0	0	0.1	—
1080	Mushrooms, canned, drained	½	cup(s)	78	71.0	20	1.5	4.0	1.9	0.2	0	0	0.1	—
630	Mushrooms, raw	½	cup(s)	48	44.4	11	1.5	1.6	0.5	0.2	0	0	0.1	—
15587	Portabella, raw	1	item(s)	84	—	30	3.0	3.9	3.0	0	0	0	0	0
2743	Shiitake, cooked	½	cup(s)	73	60.5	41	1.1	10.4	1.5	0.2	0	0.1	0	—
	Mustard greens													
2744	Frozen, boiled, drained	½	cup(s)	75	70.4	14	1.7	2.3	2.1	0.2	0	0.1	0	—
29319	Raw	1	cup(s)	56	50.8	15	1.5	2.7	1.8	0.1	0	0	0	—
	Okra													
16866	Batter coated, fried	11	piece(s)	83	55.6	156	2.1	12.7	2.0	11.2	1.5	3.7	5.5	—
32742	Frozen, boiled, drained, no salt added	½	cup(s)	92	83.8	26	1.9	5.3	2.6	0.3	0.1	0	0.1	—
632	Sliced, boiled, drained	½	cup(s)	80	74.1	18	1.5	3.6	2.0	0.2	0	0	0	—
	Onions													
635	Chopped, boiled, drained	½	cup(s)	105	92.2	46	1.4	10.7	1.5	0.2	0	0	0.1	—
2748	Frozen, boiled, drained	½	cup(s)	106	97.8	30	0.8	7.0	1.9	0.1	0	0	0	—
1081	Onion rings, breaded and pan fried, frozen, heated	10	piece(s)	71	20.2	289	3.8	27.1	0.9	19.0	6.1	7.7	3.6	—
633	Raw, chopped	½	cup(s)	80	71.3	32	0.9	7.5	1.4	0.1	0	0	0	—
16850	Red onions, sliced, raw	½	cup(s)	57	50.7	24	0.5	5.8	0.8	0	0	0	0	—
636	Scallions, green or spring onions	2	item(s)	30	26.9	10	0.5	2.2	0.8	0.1	0	0	0	—
16860	**Palm hearts, cooked**	½	cup(s)	73	50.7	84	2.0	18.7	1.1	0.1	0	0	0.1	—
637	**Parsley, chopped**	1	tablespoon(s)	4	3.3	1	0.1	0.2	0.1	0	0	0	0	—
638	**Parsnips, sliced, boiled, drained**	½	cup(s)	78	62.6	55	1.0	13.3	2.8	0.2	0	0.1	0	—
	Peas													
639	Green peas, canned, drained	½	cup(s)	85	69.4	59	3.8	10.7	3.5	0.3	0.1	0	0.1	—
641	Green peas, frozen, boiled, drained	½	cup(s)	80	63.6	62	4.1	11.4	4.4	0.2	0	0	0.1	—
35694	Pea pods, boiled with salt, drained	½	cup(s)	80	71.1	32	2.6	5.2	2.2	0.2	0	0	0.1	—

PAGE KEY: A-6 = Breads/Baked Goods A-12 = Cereal/Rice/Pasta A-16 = Fruit A-20 = Vegetables/Legumes A-30 = Nuts/Seeds A-32 = Vegetarian A-34 = Dairy A-42 = Eggs A-42 = Seafood A-44 = Meats A-48 = Poultry A-48 = Processed Meats A-50 = Beverages A-54 = Fats/Oils A-56 = Sweets A-58 = Spices/Condiments/Sauces A-62 = Mixed Foods/Soups/Sandwiches A-66 = Fast Food A-86 = Convenience A-88 = Baby Foods

Chol (mg)	Calc (mg)	Iron (mg)	Magn (mg)	Pota (mg)	Sodi (mg)	Zinc (mg)	Vit A (µg)	Thia (mg)	Vit E (mg α)	Ribo (mg)	Niac (mg)	Vit B$_6$ (mg)	Fola (µg)	Vit C (mg)	Vit B$_{12}$ (µg)	Sele (µg)
0	2	0.38	23.0	191.1	0.8	0.51	8.2	0.02	0.05	0.05	1.07	0.08	28.7	2.9	0	0.6
0	12	0.20	9.8	110.6	1.5	0.14	3.8	0.01	0.01	0.01	0.07	0.03	5.3	2.1	0	0.2
0	7	3.61	6.0	87.8	765.8	0.38	—	0.02	—	0.02	0.34	0.08	17.3	2.6	0	—
0	74	0.95	12.6	121.8	23.1	0.15	179.6	0.07	1.28	0.09	0.27	0.08	6.8	9.5	0	0.2
0	103	1.70	19.8	218.3	41.8	0.22	279.4	0.10	1.89	0.14	0.44	0.13	14.8	19.2	0	0.3
0	3	0.12	5.4	60.9	0.5	0.06	1.0	0.04	0.20	0.01	0.30	0.04	6.9	0.6	0	0
0	26	0.41	7.5	157.0	11.0	0.39	54.0	0.04	0.22	0.03	0.20	0.01	71.0	3.2	0	0.1
0	16	0.78	15.5	194.0	5.2	0.20	1.3	0.02	0.59	0.04	0.25	0.05	15.5	26.1	0	0.9
0	90	0.61	11.7	208.7	9.8	0.11	477.8	0.02	0.59	0.07	0.43	0.05	9.1	16.4	0	0.6
0	90	1.14	22.8	299.5	28.8	0.29	515.2	0.07	—	0.08	0.66	0.18	19.4	80.4	0	0.6
0	21	0.33	15.7	280.5	17.3	0.26	1.7	0.03	0.43	0.02	0.32	0.13	9.9	44.6	0	0.7
0	32	0.54	25.7	472.5	27.0	0.04	2.7	0.06	0.64	0.02	0.54	0.20	21.6	83.7	0	0.9
0	16	0.56	7.3	45.2	5.2	0.02	1.0	0.01	—	0.01	0.10	0.04	12.5	2.2	0	0.3
0	53	1.86	24.9	160.2	17.8	0.10	73.9	0.05	0.81	0.02	0.35	0.20	57.0	10.7	0	0.9
0	9	1.65	17.8	182.7	1.0	0.63	0	0.08	0.05	0.04	0.52	0.09	89.6	0.7	0	1.4
0	19	2.47	28.5	247.9	8.5	1.16	1.5	0.17	—	0.09	0.86	0.14	77.0	12.7	0	0.5
0	29	1.02	10.7	196.4	4.1	0.16	137.0	0.04	0.14	0.05	0.29	0.06	60.2	3.1	0	0.5
0	19	0.68	7.1	130.9	2.7	0.11	91.3	0.03	0.09	0.03	0.19	0.04	40.1	2.0	0	0.3
0	10	0.22	3.8	77.5	5.5	0.08	13.7	0.02	0.09	0.01	0.07	0.02	15.9	1.5	0	0.1
0	10	0.22	3.8	77.5	5.5	0.08	13.7	0.02	0.09	0.01	0.07	0.02	15.9	1.5	0	0.1
0	13	0.31	4.7	69.8	10.1	0.06	133.2	0.02	0.10	0.02	0.13	0.03	13.7	6.5	0	0.2
0	18	0.54	7.8	138.3	4.5	0.13	162.4	0.04	0.07	0.03	0.17	0.04	76.2	13.4	0	0.2
0	0	0.67	—	—	32.6	—	0	—	—	—	—	—	—	0	0	—
0	1	0.98	14.4	331.2	2.7	0.54	0	0.16	0.01	0.14	5.31	0.07	46.8	0	0	2.0
0	5	1.35	9.4	277.7	1.6	0.67	0	0.05	0.01	0.23	3.47	0.07	14.0	3.1	0	9.3
0	9	0.61	11.7	100.6	331.5	0.56	0	0.06	0.01	0.01	1.24	0.04	9.4	0	0	3.2
0	1	0.24	4.3	152.6	2.4	0.25	0	0.04	0.01	0.19	1.73	0.05	7.7	1.0	0	4.5
0	39	0.35	—	—	9.9	—	0	—	—	—	—	—	—	0	0	—
0	2	0.31	10.2	84.8	2.9	0.96	0	0.02	0.02	0.12	1.08	0.11	15.2	0.2	0	18.0
0	76	0.84	9.8	104.3	18.8	0.15	265.5	0.03	1.01	0.04	0.19	0.08	52.5	10.4	0	0.5
0	58	0.81	17.9	198.2	14.0	0.11	294.0	0.04	1.12	0.06	0.45	0.10	104.7	39.2	0	0.5
2	54	1.13	32.2	170.8	109.7	0.44	14.0	0.16	1.50	0.12	1.29	0.11	39.6	9.2	0	3.6
0	88	0.61	46.9	215.3	2.8	0.57	15.6	0.09	0.29	0.11	0.72	0.04	134.3	11.2	0	0.6
0	62	0.22	28.8	108.0	4.8	0.34	11.2	0.10	0.21	0.04	0.69	0.15	36.8	13.0	0	0.3
0	23	0.24	11.5	174.3	3.1	0.21	0	0.03	0.02	0.02	0.17	0.12	15.7	5.5	0	0.6
0	17	0.32	6.4	114.5	12.7	0.06	0	0.02	0.01	0.02	0.14	0.06	13.8	2.8	0	0.4
0	22	1.20	13.5	91.6	266.3	0.29	7.8	0.19	—	0.09	2.56	0.05	46.9	1.0	0	2.5
0	18	0.16	8.0	116.8	3.2	0.13	0	0.03	0.01	0.02	0.09	0.09	15.2	5.9	0	0.4
0	13	0.10	5.7	82.4	1.7	0.09	0	0.02	0.01	0.01	0.04	0.08	10.9	3.7	0	0.3
0	22	0.44	6.0	82.8	4.8	0.11	15.0	0.01	0.16	0.02	0.15	0.01	19.2	5.6	0	0.2
0	13	1.23	7.3	1318.4	10.2	2.72	2.2	0.03	0.36	0.12	0.62	0.53	14.6	5.0	0	0.5
0	5	0.23	1.9	21.1	2.1	0.04	16.0	0.00	0.02	0.00	0.05	0.00	5.8	5.1	0	0
0	29	0.45	22.6	286.3	7.8	0.20	0	0.06	0.78	0.04	0.56	0.07	45.2	10.1	0	1.3
0	17	0.80	14.5	147.1	214.2	0.60	23.0	0.10	0.02	0.06	0.62	0.05	37.4	8.2	0	1.4
0	19	1.21	17.6	88.0	57.6	0.53	84.0	0.22	0.02	0.08	1.18	0.09	47.2	7.9	0	0.8
0	34	1.57	20.8	192.0	192.0	0.29	41.6	0.10	0.31	0.06	0.43	0.11	23.2	38.3	0	0.6

TABLE A-1 Table of Food Composition (*continued*) (Computer code is for Cengage Diet Analysis program) (For purposes of calculations, use "0" for t, <1, <.1, <.01, etc.)

DA+ Code	Food Description	Quantity	Measure	Wt (g)	H₂O (g)	Ener (kcal)	Prot (g)	Carb (g)	Fiber (g)	Fat (g)	Sat	Mono	Poly	Trans
												Fat Breakdown (g)		

Vegetables, Legumes—*continued*

DA+ Code	Food Description	Quantity	Measure	Wt (g)	H₂O (g)	Ener (kcal)	Prot (g)	Carb (g)	Fiber (g)	Fat (g)	Sat	Mono	Poly	Trans
1082	Peas and carrots, canned with liquid	½	cup(s)	128	112.4	48	2.8	10.8	2.6	0.3	0.1	0	0.2	—
1083	Peas and carrots, frozen, boiled, drained	½	cup(s)	80	68.6	38	2.5	8.1	2.5	0.3	0.1	0	0.2	—
2750	Snow or sugar peas, frozen, boiled, drained	½	cup(s)	80	69.3	42	2.8	7.2	2.5	0.3	0.10	0	0.1	—
640	Snow or sugar peas, raw	½	cup(s)	32	28.0	13	0.9	2.4	0.8	0.1	0	0	0	—
29324	Split peas, sprouted	½	cup(s)	60	37.4	77	5.3	16.9	—	0.4	0.1	0	0.2	—
	Peppers													
644	Green bell or sweet, boiled, drained	½	cup(s)	68	62.5	19	0.6	4.6	0.8	0.1	0	0	0.1	—
643	Green bell or sweet, raw	½	cup(s)	75	69.9	15	0.6	3.5	1.3	0.1	0	0	0	—
1664	Green hot chili	1	item(s)	45	39.5	18	0.9	4.3	0.7	0.1	0	0	0	—
1663	Green hot chili, canned with liquid	½	cup(s)	68	62.9	14	0.6	3.5	0.9	0.1	0	0	0	—
1086	Jalapeno, canned with liquid	½	cup(s)	68	60.4	18	0.6	3.2	1.8	0.6	0.1	0	0.3	—
8703	Yellow bell or sweet	1	item(s)	186	171.2	50	1.9	11.8	1.7	0.4	0.1	0	0.2	—
1087	**Poi**	½	cup(s)	120	86.0	134	0.5	32.7	0.5	0.2	0	0	0.1	—
	Potatoes													
1090	Au gratin mix, prepared with water, whole milk and butter	½	cup(s)	124	97.7	115	2.8	15.9	1.1	5.1	3.2	1.5	0.2	—
1089	Au gratin, prepared with butter	½	cup(s)	123	90.7	162	6.2	13.8	2.2	9.3	5.8	2.6	0.3	—
5791	Baked, flesh and skin	1	item(s)	202	151.3	188	5.1	42.7	4.4	0.3	0.1	0	0.1	—
645	Baked, flesh only	½	cup(s)	61	46.0	57	1.2	13.1	0.9	0.1	0	0	0	—
1088	Baked, skin only	1	item(s)	58	27.4	115	2.5	26.7	4.6	0.1	0	0	0	—
5795	Boiled in skin, flesh only, drained	1	item(s)	136	104.7	118	2.5	27.4	2.1	0.1	0	0	0.1	—
5794	Boiled, drained, skin and flesh	1	item(s)	150	115.9	129	2.9	29.8	2.5	0.2	0	0	0.1	—
647	Boiled, flesh only	½	cup(s)	78	60.4	67	1.3	15.6	1.4	0.1	0	0	0	—
648	French fried, deep fried, prepared from raw	14	item(s)	70	32.8	187	2.7	23.5	2.9	9.5	1.9	4.2	3.0	—
649	French fried, frozen, heated	14	item(s)	70	43.7	94	1.9	19.4	2.0	3.7	0.7	2.3	0.2	—
1091	Hashed brown	½	cup(s)	78	36.9	207	2.3	27.4	2.5	9.8	1.5	4.1	3.7	—
652	Mashed with margarine and whole milk	½	cup(s)	105	79.0	119	2.1	17.7	1.6	4.4	1.0	2.0	1.2	0.7
653	Mashed, prepared from dehydrated granules with milk, water, and margarine	½	cup(s)	105	79.8	122	2.3	16.9	1.4	5.0	1.3	2.1	1.4	—
2759	Microwaved	1	item(s)	202	145.5	212	4.9	49.0	4.6	0.2	0.1	0	0.1	—
2760	Microwaved in skin, flesh only	½	cup(s)	78	57.1	78	1.6	18.1	1.2	0.1	0	0	0	—
5804	Microwaved, skin only	1	item(s)	58	36.8	77	2.5	17.2	4.2	0.1	0	0	0	—
1097	Potato puffs, frozen, heated	½	cup(s)	64	38.2	122	1.3	17.8	1.6	5.5	1.2	3.9	0.3	—
1094	Scalloped mix, prepared with water, whole milk and butter	½	cup(s)	124	98.4	116	2.6	15.9	1.4	5.3	3.3	1.5	0.2	—
1093	Scalloped, prepared with butter	½	cup(s)	123	99.2	108	3.5	13.2	2.3	4.5	2.8	1.3	0.2	—
	Pumpkin													
1773	Boiled, drained	½	cup(s)	123	114.8	25	0.9	6.0	1.3	0.1	0	0	0	—
656	Canned	½	cup(s)	123	110.2	42	1.3	9.9	3.6	0.3	0.2	0	0	—
	Radicchio													
8731	Leaves, raw	1	cup(s)	40	37.3	9	0.6	1.8	0.4	0.1	0	0	0	—
2498	Raw	1	cup(s)	40	37.3	9	0.6	1.8	0.4	0.1	0	0	0	—
657	**Radishes**	6	item(s)	27	25.7	4	0.2	0.9	0.4	0	0	0	0	—
1099	**Rutabaga, boiled, drained**	½	cup(s)	85	75.5	33	1.1	7.4	1.5	0.2	0	0	0.1	—
658	**Sauerkraut, canned**	½	cup(s)	118	109.2	22	1.1	5.1	3.4	0.2	0	0	0.1	—
	Seaweed													
1102	Kelp	½	cup(s)	40	32.6	17	0.6	3.8	0.5	0.2	0.1	0	0	—
1104	Spirulina, dried	½	cup(s)	8	0.4	22	4.3	1.8	0.3	0.6	0.2	0.1	0.2	—
1106	**Shallots**	3	tablespoon(s)	30	23.9	22	0.8	5.0	—	0	0	0	0	—
	Soybeans													
1670	Boiled	½	cup(s)	86	53.8	149	14.3	8.5	5.2	7.7	1.1	1.7	4.4	—
2825	Dry roasted	½	cup(s)	86	0.7	388	34.0	28.1	7.0	18.6	2.7	4.1	10.5	—
2824	Roasted, salted	½	cup(s)	86	1.7	405	30.3	28.9	15.2	21.8	3.2	4.8	12.3	—
8739	Sprouted, stir fried	½	cup(s)	63	42.3	79	8.2	5.9	0.5	4.5	0.6	1.0	2.5	0
	Soy products													
1813	Soy milk	1	cup(s)	240	211.3	130	7.8	15.1	1.4	4.2	0.5	1.0	2.3	0
2838	Tofu, dried, frozen (koyadofu)	3	ounce(s)	85	4.9	408	40.8	12.4	6.1	25.8	3.7	5.7	14.6	—

PAGE KEY: A-6 = Breads/Baked Goods A-12 = Cereal/Rice/Pasta A-16 = Fruit A-20 = Vegetables/Legumes A-30 = Nuts/Seeds A-32 = Vegetarian A-34 = Dairy A-42 = Eggs A-42 = Seafood A-44 = Meats A-48 = Poultry A-48 = Processed Meats A-50 = Beverages A-54 = Fats/Oils A-56 = Sweets A-58 = Spices/Condiments/Sauces A-62 = Mixed Foods/Soups/Sandwiches A-66 = Fast Food A-86 = Convenience A-88 = Baby Foods

Chol (mg)	Calc (mg)	Iron (mg)	Magn (mg)	Pota (mg)	Sodi (mg)	Zinc (mg)	Vit A (µg)	Thia (mg)	Vit E (mg α)	Ribo (mg)	Niac (mg)	Vit B$_6$ (mg)	Fola (µg)	Vit C (mg)	Vit B$_{12}$ (µg)	Sele (µg)
0	29	0.96	17.9	127.5	331.5	0.74	368.5	0.09	—	0.07	0.74	0.11	23.0	8.4	0	1.1
0	18	0.75	12.8	126.4	54.4	0.36	380.8	0.18	0.41	0.05	0.92	0.07	20.8	6.5	0	0.9
0	47	1.92	22.4	173.6	4.0	0.39	52.8	0.05	0.37	0.09	0.45	0.13	28.0	17.6	0	0.6
0	14	0.65	7.6	63.0	1.3	0.08	17.0	0.04	0.12	0.02	0.19	0.05	13.2	18.9	0	0.2
0	22	1.34	33.6	228.6	12.0	0.62	4.8	0.12	—	0.08	1.84	0.14	86.4	6.2	0	0.4
0	6	0.31	6.8	112.9	1.4	0.08	15.6	0.04	0.34	0.02	0.32	0.15	10.9	50.6	0	0.2
0	7	0.25	7.5	130.4	2.2	0.09	13.4	0.04	0.27	0.02	0.35	0.16	7.5	59.9	0	0
0	8	0.54	11.3	153.0	3.2	0.13	26.6	0.04	0.31	0.04	0.42	0.12	10.4	109.1	0	0.2
0	5	0.34	9.5	127.2	797.6	0.10	24.5	0.01	0.46	0.02	0.54	0.10	6.8	46.2	0	0.2
0	16	1.28	10.2	131.2	1136.3	0.23	57.8	0.03	0.47	0.03	0.27	0.13	9.5	6.8	0	0.3
0	20	0.85	22.3	394.3	3.7	0.31	18.6	0.05	—	0.04	1.65	0.31	48.4	341.3	0	0.6
0	19	1.06	28.8	219.6	14.4	0.26	3.6	0.16	2.76	0.05	1.32	0.33	25.2	4.8	0	0.8
19	103	0.39	18.6	271.0	543.3	0.29	64.4	0.02	—	0.10	1.16	0.05	8.7	3.8	0	3.3
28	146	0.78	24.5	485.1	530.4	0.85	78.4	0.08	—	0.14	1.22	0.21	13.5	12.1	0	3.3
0	30	2.18	56.6	1080.7	20.2	0.72	2.0	0.12	0.08	0.09	2.84	0.62	56.6	19.4	0	0.8
0	3	0.21	15.3	238.5	3.1	0.18	0	0.06	0.02	0.01	0.85	0.18	5.5	7.8	0	0.2
0	20	4.08	24.9	332.3	12.2	0.28	0.6	0.07	0.02	0.06	1.77	0.35	12.8	7.8	0	0.4
0	7	0.42	29.9	515.4	5.4	0.40	0	0.14	0.01	0.02	1.95	0.40	13.6	17.7	0	0.4
0	13	1.27	34.1	572.0	7.4	0.46	0	0.14	0.01	0.03	2.13	0.44	15.0	18.4	0	—
0	6	0.24	15.6	255.8	3.9	0.21	0	0.07	0.01	0.01	1.02	0.21	7.0	5.8	0	0.2
0	16	1.05	30.8	567.0	8.4	0.39	0	0.08	0.09	0.03	1.34	0.37	16.1	21.2	0	0.4
0	8	0.51	18.2	315.7	271.6	0.26	0	0.09	0.07	0.02	1.55	0.12	19.6	9.3	0	0.1
0	11	0.43	27.3	449.3	266.8	0.37	0	0.13	0.01	0.03	1.80	0.37	12.5	10.1	0	0.4
1	23	0.27	19.9	344.4	349.6	0.31	43.0	0.09	0.44	0.04	1.23	0.25	9.4	11.0	0.1	0.8
2	36	0.21	21.0	164.8	179.5	0.26	49.3	0.09	0.53	0.09	0.90	0.16	8.4	6.8	0.1	5.9
0	22	2.50	54.5	902.9	16.2	0.72	0	0.24	—	0.06	3.46	0.69	24.2	30.5	0	0.8
0	4	0.31	19.4	319.0	5.4	0.25	0	0.10	—	0.01	1.26	0.25	9.3	11.7	0	0.3
0	27	3.44	21.5	377.0	9.3	0.29	0	0.04	0.01	0.04	1.28	0.28	9.9	8.9	0	0.3
0	9	0.41	10.9	199.7	307.2	0.21	0	0.08	0.15	0.02	0.97	0.08	9.0	4.0	0	0.4
14	45	0.47	17.4	252.2	423.7	0.31	43.5	0.02	—	0.06	1.28	0.05	12.4	4.1	0	2.0
15	70	0.70	23.3	463.1	410.4	0.49	0	0.08	—	0.11	1.29	0.22	13.5	13.0	0	2.0
0	18	0.69	11.0	281.8	1.2	0.28	306.3	0.03	0.98	0.09	0.50	0.05	11.0	5.8	0	0.2
0	32	1.70	28.2	252.4	6.1	0.20	953.1	0.02	1.29	0.06	0.45	0.06	14.7	5.1	0	0.5
0	8	0.23	5.2	120.8	8.8	0.25	0.4	0.01	0.90	0.01	0.10	0.02	24.0	3.2	0	0.4
0	8	0.23	5.2	120.8	8.8	0.25	0.4	0.01	0.90	0.01	0.10	0.02	24.0	3.2	0	0.4
0	7	0.09	2.7	62.9	10.5	0.07	0	0.00	0.00	0.01	0.06	0.01	6.8	4.0	0	0.2
0	41	0.45	19.6	277.1	17.0	0.30	0	0.07	0.27	0.04	0.61	0.09	12.8	16.0	0	0.6
0	35	1.73	15.3	200.6	780.0	0.22	1.2	0.03	0.17	0.03	0.17	0.15	28.3	17.3	0	0.7
0	67	1.12	48.4	35.6	93.2	0.48	2.4	0.02	0.32	0.04	0.16	0.00	72.0	1.2	0	0.3
0	9	2.14	14.6	102.2	78.6	0.15	2.2	0.18	0.38	0.28	0.96	0.03	7.1	0.8	0	0.5
0	11	0.36	6.3	100.2	3.6	0.12	18.0	0.02	—	0.01	0.06	0.09	10.2	2.4	—	0.4
0	88	4.42	74.0	442.9	0.9	0.98	0	0.13	0.30	0.24	0.34	0.20	46.4	1.5	0	6.3
0	120	3.39	196.1	1173.0	1.7	4.10	0	0.36	—	0.64	0.90	0.19	176.3	4.0	0	16.6
0	119	3.35	124.7	1264.2	140.2	2.70	8.6	0.08	0.78	0.12	1.21	0.17	181.5	1.9	0	16.4
0	52	0.25	60.4	356.6	8.8	1.32	0.6	0.26	—	0.12	0.69	0.10	79.9	7.5	0	0.4
0	60	1.53	60.0	283.2	122.4	0.28	0	0.14	0.26	0.16	1.23	0.18	43.2	0	0	11.5
0	310	8.27	50.2	17.0	5.1	4.16	22.1	0.42	—	0.27	1.01	0.24	78.2	0.6	0	46.2

TABLE A-1 Table of Food Composition (*continued*) <small>(Computer code is for Cengage Diet Analysis program) (For purposes of calculations, use "0" for t, <1, <.1, <.01, etc.)</small>

DA+ Code	Food Description	Quantity	Measure	Wt (g)	H₂O (g)	Ener (kcal)	Prot (g)	Carb (g)	Fiber (g)	Fat (g)	Fat Breakdown (g) Sat	Mono	Poly	Trans
Vegetables, Legumes—*continued*														
13844	Tofu, extra firm	3	ounce(s)	85	—	86	8.6	2.2	1.1	4.3	0.5	0.9	2.8	—
13843	Tofu, firm	3	ounce(s)	85	—	75	7.5	2.2	0.5	3.2	0	0.9	2.3	—
1816	Tofu, firm, with calcium sulfate and magnesium chloride (nigari)	3	ounce(s)	85	72.2	60	7.0	1.4	0.8	3.5	0.7	1.0	1.5	—
1817	Tofu, fried	3	ounce(s)	85	43.0	230	14.6	8.9	3.3	17.2	2.5	3.8	9.7	—
13841	Tofu, silken	3	ounce(s)	85	—	42	3.7	1.9	0	2.3	0.5	—	—	—
13842	Tofu, soft	3	ounce(s)	85	—	65	6.5	1.1	0.5	3.2	0.5	1.1	2.2	—
1671	Tofu, soft, with calcium sulfate and magnesium chloride (nigari)	3	ounce(s)	85	74.2	52	5.6	1.5	0.2	3.1	0.5	0.7	1.8	—
	Spinach													
663	Canned, drained	½	cup(s)	107	98.2	25	3.0	3.6	2.6	0.5	0.1	0	0.2	—
660	Chopped, boiled, drained	½	cup(s)	90	82.1	21	2.7	3.4	2.2	0.2	0	0	0.1	—
661	Chopped, frozen, boiled, drained	½	cup(s)	95	84.5	32	3.8	4.6	3.5	0.8	0.1	0	0.4	—
662	Leaf, frozen, boiled, drained	½	cup(s)	95	84.5	32	3.8	4.6	3.5	0.8	0.1	0	0.4	—
659	Raw, chopped	1	cup(s)	30	27.4	7	0.9	1.1	0.7	0.1	0	0	0	—
8470	Trimmed leaves	1	cup(s)	32	27.5	3	0.9	0	2.8	0.1	—	—	—	—
	Squash													
1662	Acorn winter, baked	½	cup(s)	103	85.0	57	1.1	14.9	4.5	0.1	0	0	0.1	—
29702	Acorn winter, boiled, mashed	½	cup(s)	123	109.9	42	0.8	10.8	3.2	0.1	0	0	0	—
29451	Butternut, frozen, boiled	½	cup(s)	122	106.9	47	1.5	12.2	1.8	0.1	0	0	0	—
1661	Butternut winter, baked	½	cup(s)	102	89.5	41	0.9	10.7	3.4	0.1	0	0	0	—
32773	Butternut winter, frozen, boiled, mashed, no salt added	½	cup(s)	121	106.4	47	1.5	12.2	—	0.1	0	0	0	—
29700	Crookneck and straightneck summer, boiled, drained	½	cup(s)	65	60.9	12	0.6	2.6	1.2	0.1	0	0	0.1	—
29703	Hubbard winter, baked	½	cup(s)	102	86.8	51	2.5	11.0	—	0.6	0.1	0	0.3	—
1660	Hubbard winter, boiled, mashed	½	cup(s)	118	107.5	35	1.7	7.6	3.4	0.4	0.1	0	0.2	—
29704	Spaghetti winter, boiled, drained, or baked	½	cup(s)	78	71.5	21	0.5	5.0	1.1	0.2	0	0	0.1	—
664	Summer, all varieties, sliced, boiled, drained	½	cup(s)	90	84.3	18	0.8	3.9	1.3	0.3	0.1	0	0.1	—
665	Winter, all varieties, baked, mashed	½	cup(s)	103	91.4	38	0.9	9.1	2.9	0.4	0.1	0	0.2	—
1112	Zucchini summer, boiled, drained	½	cup(s)	90	85.3	14	0.6	3.5	1.3	0	0	0	0	—
1113	Zucchini summer, frozen, boiled, drained	½	cup(s)	112	105.6	19	1.3	4.0	1.4	0.1	0	0	0.1	—
	Sweet potatoes													
666	Baked, peeled	½	cup(s)	100	75.8	90	2.0	20.7	3.3	0.2	0	0	0.1	—
667	Boiled, mashed	½	cup(s)	164	131.4	125	2.2	29.1	4.1	0.2	0.1	0	0.1	—
668	Candied, home recipe	½	cup(s)	91	61.1	132	0.8	25.4	2.2	3.0	1.2	0.6	0.1	—
670	Canned, vacuum pack	½	cup(s)	100	76.0	91	1.7	21.1	1.8	0.2	0	0	0.1	—
2765	Frozen, baked	½	cup(s)	88	64.5	88	1.5	20.5	1.6	0.1	0	0	0	—
1136	Yams, baked or boiled, drained	½	cup(s)	68	47.7	79	1.0	18.7	2.7	0.1	0	0	0	—
32785	**Taro shoots, cooked, no salt added**	½	cup(s)	70	66.7	10	0.5	2.2	—	0.1	0	0	0	—
	Tomatillo													
8774	Raw	2	item(s)	68	62.3	22	0.7	4.0	1.3	0.7	0.1	0.1	0.3	—
8777	Raw, chopped	½	cup(s)	66	60.5	21	0.6	3.9	1.3	0.7	0.1	0.1	0.3	—
	Tomato													
16846	Cherry, fresh	5	item(s)	85	80.3	15	0.7	3.3	1.0	0.2	0	0	0.1	—
671	Fresh, ripe, red	1	item(s)	123	116.2	22	1.1	4.8	1.5	0.2	0	0	0.1	—
675	Juice, canned	½	cup(s)	122	114.1	21	0.9	5.2	0.5	0.1	0	0	0	—
75	Juice, no salt added	½	cup(s)	122	114.1	21	0.9	5.2	0.5	0.1	0	0	0	—
1699	Paste, canned	2	tablespoon(s)	33	24.1	27	1.4	6.2	1.3	0.2	0	0	0.1	—
1700	Puree, canned	¼	cup(s)	63	54.9	24	1.0	5.6	1.2	0.1	0	0	0.1	—
1118	Red, boiled	½	cup(s)	120	113.2	22	1.1	4.8	0.8	0.1	0	0	0.1	—
3952	Red, diced	½	cup(s)	90	85.1	16	0.8	3.5	1.1	0.2	0	0	0.1	—
1120	Red, stewed, canned	½	cup(s)	128	116.7	33	1.2	7.9	1.3	0.2	0	0	0.1	—
1125	Sauce, canned	¼	cup(s)	61	55.6	15	0.8	3.3	0.9	0.1	0	0	0	—
8778	Sun dried	½	cup(s)	27	3.9	70	3.8	15.1	3.3	0.8	0.1	0.1	0.3	—
8783	Sun dried in oil, drained	¼	cup(s)	28	14.8	59	1.4	6.4	1.6	3.9	0.5	2.4	0.6	—
	Turnips													
678	Turnip greens, chopped, boiled, drained	½	cup(s)	72	67.1	14	0.8	3.1	2.5	0.2	0	0	0.1	—

PAGE KEY: A-6 = Breads/Baked Goods A-12 = Cereal/Rice/Pasta A-16 = Fruit A-20 = Vegetables/Legumes A-30 = Nuts/Seeds A-32 = Vegetarian A-34 = Dairy A-42 = Eggs A-42 = Seafood A-44 = Meats A-48 = Poultry
A-48 = Processed Meats A-50 = Beverages A-54 = Fats/Oils A-56 = Sweets A-58 = Spices/Condiments/Sauces A-62 = Mixed Foods/Soups/Sandwiches A-66 = Fast Food A-86 = Convenience A-88 = Baby Foods

Chol (mg)	Calc (mg)	Iron (mg)	Magn (mg)	Pota (mg)	Sodi (mg)	Zinc (mg)	Vit A (µg)	Thia (mg)	Vit E (mg α)	Ribo (mg)	Niac (mg)	Vit B$_6$ (mg)	Fola (µg)	Vit C (mg)	Vit B$_{12}$ (µg)	Sele (µg)
0	65	1.16	84.1	—	0	—	0	—	—	—	—	—	—	0	0	—
0	108	1.16	56.1	—	0	—	0	—	—	—	—	—	—	0	0	—
0	171	1.36	31.5	125.9	10.2	0.70	0	0.05	0.01	0.05	0.08	0.06	16.2	0.2	0	8.4
0	316	4.14	51.0	124.2	13.6	1.69	0.9	0.14	0.03	0.04	0.08	0.08	23.0	0	0	24.2
0	56	0.34	33.1	—	4.7	—	0	—	—	—	—	—	—	0	1.7	—
0	108	1.16	35.5	—	0	—	0	—	—	—	—	—	—	0	1.9	—
0	94	0.94	23.0	102.1	6.8	0.54	0	0.04	0.01	0.03	0.45	0.04	37.4	0.2	0	7.6
0	136	2.45	81.3	370.2	28.9	0.48	524.3	0.02	2.08	0.14	0.41	0.11	104.8	15.3	0	1.5
0	122	3.21	78.3	419.4	63.0	0.68	471.6	0.08	1.87	0.21	0.44	0.21	131.4	8.8	0	1.4
0	145	1.86	77.9	286.9	92.2	0.46	572.9	0.07	3.36	0.16	0.41	0.12	115.0	2.1	0	5.2
0	145	1.86	77.9	286.9	92.2	0.46	572.9	0.07	3.36	0.16	0.41	0.12	115.0	2.1	0	5.2
0	30	0.81	23.7	167.4	23.7	0.16	140.7	0.02	0.61	0.06	0.22	0.06	58.2	8.4	0	0.3
0	25	2.13	25.5	134.1	38.0	0.18	—	0.03	—	0.05	0.18	0.07	0	7.5	0	—
0	45	0.95	44.1	447.9	4.1	0.17	21.5	0.17	—	0.01	0.90	0.19	19.5	11.1	0	0.7
0	32	0.68	31.9	322.2	3.7	0.13	50.2	0.12	—	0.01	0.65	0.14	13.5	8.0	0	0.5
0	23	0.70	10.9	161.9	2.4	0.14	203.3	0.06	0.14	0.05	0.56	0.08	19.5	4.3	0	0.6
0	42	0.61	29.6	289.6	4.1	0.13	569.1	0.07	1.31	0.01	0.99	0.12	19.4	15.4	0	0.5
0	23	0.70	10.9	161.2	2.4	0.14	202.4	0.06	—	0.05	0.56	0.08	19.4	4.2	0	0.6
0	14	0.31	13.6	137.1	1.3	0.19	5.2	0.03	—	0.02	0.29	0.07	14.9	5.4	0	0.1
0	17	0.48	22.4	365.1	8.2	0.15	308.0	0.07	—	0.04	0.57	0.17	16.3	9.7	0	0.6
0	12	0.33	15.3	252.5	5.9	0.11	236.0	0.05	0.14	0.03	0.39	0.12	11.8	7.7	0	0.4
0	16	0.26	8.5	90.7	14.0	0.15	4.7	0.02	0.09	0.01	0.62	0.07	6.2	2.7	0	0.2
0	24	0.32	21.6	172.8	0.9	0.35	9.9	0.04	0.12	0.03	0.46	0.05	18.0	5.0	0	0.2
0	23	0.45	13.3	247.0	1.0	0.23	267.5	0.02	0.12	0.07	0.51	0.17	20.5	9.8	0	0.4
0	12	0.32	19.8	227.7	2.7	0.16	50.4	0.04	0.11	0.04	0.39	0.07	15.3	4.1	0	0.2
0	19	0.54	14.5	216.3	2.2	0.22	10	0.05	0.13	0.04	0.43	0.05	8.9	4.1	0	0.2
0	38	0.69	27.0	475.0	36.0	0.32	961.0	0.10	0.71	0.10	1.48	0.28	6.0	19.6	0	0.2
0	44	1.18	29.5	377.2	44.3	0.33	1290.7	0.09	1.54	0.08	0.88	0.27	9.8	21.0	0	0.3
7	24	1.03	10.0	172.6	63.9	0.13	0	0.01	—	0.03	0.36	0.03	10.0	6.1	0	0.7
0	22	0.89	22.0	312.0	53.0	0.18	399.0	0.04	1.00	0.06	0.74	0.19	17.0	26.4	0	0.7
0	31	0.47	18.4	330.1	7.0	0.26	913.3	0.05	0.67	0.04	0.49	0.16	19.3	8.0	0	0.5
0	10	0.35	12.2	455.6	5.4	0.13	4.1	0.06	0.23	0.01	0.37	0.15	10.9	8.2	0	0.5
0	10	0.28	5.6	240.8	1.4	0.37	2.1	0.02	—	0.03	0.56	0.07	2.1	13.2	0	0.7
0	5	0.42	13.6	182.2	0.7	0.15	4.1	0.03	0.25	0.02	1.25	0.03	4.8	8.0	0	0.3
0	5	0.41	13.2	176.9	0.7	0.15	4.0	0.03	0.25	0.02	1.22	0.04	4.6	7.7	0	0.3
0	9	0.22	9.4	201.5	4.3	0.14	35.7	0.03	0.45	0.01	0.50	0.06	12.8	10.8	0	0
0	12	0.33	13.5	291.5	6.2	0.20	51.7	0.04	0.66	0.02	0.73	0.09	18.5	15.6	0	0
0	12	0.52	13.4	278.2	326.8	0.18	27.9	0.06	0.39	0.04	0.82	0.14	24.3	22.2	0	0.4
0	12	0.52	13.4	278.2	12.2	0.18	27.9	0.06	0.39	0.04	0.82	0.14	24.3	22.2	0	0.4
0	12	0.97	13.8	332.6	259.1	0.20	24.9	0.02	1.41	0.05	1.00	0.07	3.9	7.2	0	1.7
0	11	1.11	14.4	274.4	249.4	0.22	16.3	0.01	1.23	0.05	0.91	0.07	6.9	6.6	0	0.4
0	13	0.82	10.8	261.6	13.2	0.17	28.8	0.04	0.67	0.03	0.64	0.10	15.6	27.4	0	0.6
0	9	0.24	9.9	213.3	4.5	0.15	37.8	0.03	0.48	0.01	0.53	0.07	13.5	11.4	0	0
0	43	1.70	15.3	263.9	281.8	0.22	11.5	0.06	1.06	0.04	0.91	0.02	6.4	10.1	0	0.8
0	8	0.62	9.8	201.9	319.6	0.12	10.4	0.01	0.87	0.04	0.59	0.06	6.7	4.3	0	0.1
0	30	2.45	52.4	925.3	565.7	0.53	11.9	0.14	0.00	0.13	2.44	0.09	18.4	10.6	0	1.5
0	13	0.73	22.3	430.4	73.2	0.21	17.6	0.05	—	0.10	0.99	0.08	6.3	28.0	0	0.8
0	99	0.58	15.8	146.2	20.9	0.10	274.3	0.03	1.35	0.05	0.30	0.13	85.0	19.7	0	0.6

TABLE A-1 Table of Food Composition (*continued*) <small>(Computer code is for Cengage Diet Analysis program) (For purposes of calculations, use "0" for t, <1, <.1, <.01, etc.)</small>

DA+ Code	Food Description	Quantity	Measure	Wt (g)	H₂O (g)	Ener (kcal)	Prot (g)	Carb (g)	Fiber (g)	Fat (g)	Fat Breakdown (g) Sat	Mono	Poly	Trans
Vegetables, Legumes—*continued*														
679	Turnip greens, frozen, chopped, boiled, drained	½	cup(s)	82	74.1	24	2.7	4.1	2.8	0.3	0.1	0	0.1	—
677	Turnips, cubed, boiled, drained	½	cup(s)	78	73.0	17	0.6	3.9	1.6	0.1	0	0	0	—
	Vegetables, mixed													
1132	Canned, drained	½	cup(s)	82	70.9	40	2.1	7.5	2.4	0.2	0	0	0.1	—
680	Frozen, boiled, drained	½	cup(s)	91	75.7	59	2.6	11.9	4.0	0.1	0	0	0.1	—
7489	V8 100% vegetable juice	½	cup(s)	120	—	25	1.0	5.0	1.0	0	0	0	0	0
7490	V8 low sodium vegetable juice	½	cup(s)	120	—	25	0	6.5	1.0	0	0	0	0	0
7491	V8 spicy hot vegetable juice	½	cup(s)	120	—	25	1.0	5.0	0.5	0	0	0	0	0
	Water chestnuts													
31073	Sliced, drained	½	cup(s)	75	70.0	20	0	5.0	1.0	0	0	0	0	0
31087	Whole	½	cup(s)	75	70.0	20	0	5.0	1.0	0	0	0	0	0
1135	**Watercress**	1	cup(s)	34	32.3	4	0.8	0.4	0.2	0	0	0	0	—
Nuts, Seeds, and Products														
	Almonds													
32940	Almond butter with salt added	1	tablespoon(s)	16	0.2	101	2.4	3.4	0.6	9.5	0.9	6.1	2.0	—
1137	Almond butter, no salt added	1	tablespoon(s)	16	0.2	101	2.4	3.4	0.6	9.5	0.9	6.1	2.0	—
32886	Blanched	¼	cup(s)	36	1.6	211	8.0	7.2	3.8	18.3	1.4	11.7	4.4	—
32887	Dry roasted, no salt added	¼	cup(s)	35	0.9	206	7.6	6.7	4.1	18.2	1.4	11.6	4.4	—
29724	Dry roasted, salted	¼	cup(s)	35	0.9	206	7.6	6.7	4.1	18.2	1.4	11.6	4.4	—
29725	Oil roasted, salted	¼	cup(s)	39	1.1	238	8.3	6.9	4.1	21.7	1.7	13.7	5.3	—
508	Slivered	¼	cup(s)	27	1.3	155	5.7	5.9	3.3	13.3	1.0	8.3	3.3	0
1138	**Beechnuts, dried**	¼	cup(s)	57	3.8	328	3.5	19.1	5.3	28.5	3.3	12.5	11.4	—
517	**Brazil nuts, dried, unblanched**	¼	cup(s)	35	1.2	230	5.0	4.3	2.6	23.3	5.3	8.6	7.2	—
1166	**Breadfruit seeds, roasted**	¼	cup(s)	57	28.3	118	3.5	22.8	3.4	1.5	0.4	0.2	0.8	—
1139	**Butternuts, dried**	¼	cup(s)	30	1.0	184	7.5	3.6	1.4	17.1	0.4	3.1	12.8	—
	Cashews													
32931	Cashew butter with salt added	1	tablespoon(s)	16	0.5	94	2.8	4.4	0.3	7.9	1.6	4.7	1.3	—
32889	Cashew butter, no salt added	1	tablespoon(s)	16	0.5	94	2.8	4.4	0.3	7.9	1.6	4.7	1.3	—
1140	Dry roasted	¼	cup(s)	34	0.6	197	5.2	11.2	1.0	15.9	3.1	9.4	2.7	—
518	Oil roasted	¼	cup(s)	32	1.1	187	5.4	9.6	1.1	15.4	2.7	8.4	2.8	—
	Coconut, shredded													
32896	Dried, not sweetened	¼	cup(s)	23	0.7	152	1.6	5.4	3.8	14.9	13.2	0.6	0.2	—
1153	Dried, shredded, sweetened	¼	cup(s)	23	2.9	116	0.7	11.1	1.0	8.3	7.3	0.4	0.1	—
520	Shredded	¼	cup(s)	20	9.4	71	0.7	3.0	1.8	6.7	5.9	0.3	0.1	—
	Chestnuts													
1152	Chinese, roasted	¼	cup(s)	36	14.6	87	1.6	19.0	—	0.4	0.1	0.2	0.1	—
32895	European, boiled and steamed	¼	cup(s)	46	31.3	60	0.9	12.8	—	0.6	0.1	0.2	0.2	—
32911	European, roasted	¼	cup(s)	36	14.5	88	1.1	18.9	1.8	0.8	0.1	0.3	0.3	—
32922	Japanese, boiled and steamed	¼	cup(s)	36	31.0	20	0.3	4.5	—	0.1	0	0	0	—
32923	Japanese, roasted	¼	cup(s)	36	18.1	73	1.1	16.4	—	0.3	0	0.1	0.1	—
4958	**Flax seeds or linseeds**	¼	cup(s)	43	3.3	225	8.4	12.3	11.9	17.7	1.7	3.2	12.6	0
32904	**Ginkgo nuts, dried**	¼	cup(s)	39	4.8	136	4.0	28.3	—	0.8	0.1	0.3	0.3	—
	Hazelnuts or filberts													
32901	Blanched	¼	cup(s)	30	1.7	189	4.1	5.1	3.3	18.3	1.4	14.5	1.7	—
32902	Dry roasted, no salt added	¼	cup(s)	30	0.8	194	4.5	5.3	2.8	18.7	1.3	14.0	2.5	—
1156	**Hickory nuts, dried**	¼	cup(s)	30	0.8	197	3.8	5.5	1.9	19.3	2.1	9.8	6.6	—
	Macadamias													
32905	Dry roasted, no salt added	¼	cup(s)	34	0.5	241	2.6	4.5	2.7	25.5	4.0	19.9	0.5	—
32932	Dry roasted, with salt added	¼	cup(s)	34	0.5	240	2.6	4.3	2.7	25.5	4.0	19.9	0.5	—
1157	Raw	¼	cup(s)	34	0.5	241	2.6	4.6	2.9	25.4	4.0	19.7	0.5	—
	Mixed nuts													
1159	With peanuts, dry roasted	¼	cup(s)	34	0.6	203	5.9	8.7	3.1	17.6	2.4	10.8	3.7	—
32933	With peanuts, dry roasted, with salt added	¼	cup(s)	34	0.6	203	5.9	8.7	3.1	17.6	2.4	10.8	3.7	—
32906	Without peanuts, oil roasted, no salt added	¼	cup(s)	36	1.1	221	5.6	8.0	2.0	20.2	3.3	11.9	4.1	—
	Peanuts													
2807	Dry roasted	¼	cup(s)	37	0.6	214	8.6	7.9	2.9	18.1	2.5	9.0	5.7	—
2806	Dry roasted, salted	¼	cup(s)	37	0.6	214	8.6	7.9	2.9	18.1	2.5	9.0	5.7	—
1763	Oil roasted, salted	¼	cup(s)	36	0.5	216	10.1	5.5	3.4	18.9	3.1	9.4	5.5	—
1884	Peanut butter, chunky	1	tablespoon(s)	16	0.2	94	3.8	3.5	1.3	8.0	1.3	3.9	2.4	—
30303	Peanut butter, low sodium	1	tablespoon(s)	16	0.2	95	4.0	3.1	0.9	8.2	1.8	3.9	2.2	—
30305	Peanut butter, reduced fat	1	tablespoon(s)	18	0.2	94	4.7	6.4	0.9	6.1	1.3	2.9	1.8	—

Chol (mg)	Calc (mg)	Iron (mg)	Magn (mg)	Pota (mg)	Sodi (mg)	Zinc (mg)	Vit A (μg)	Thia (mg)	Vit E (mg α)	Ribo (mg)	Niac (mg)	Vit B$_6$ (mg)	Fola (μg)	Vit C (mg)	Vit B$_{12}$ (μg)	Sele (μg)
0	125	1.59	21.3	183.7	12.3	0.34	441.2	0.04	2.18	0.06	0.38	0.06	32.0	17.9	0	1.0
0	26	0.14	7.0	138.1	12.5	0.09	0	0.02	0.02	0.02	0.23	0.05	7.0	9.0	0	0.2
0	22	0.86	13.0	237.2	121.4	0.33	475.1	0.04	0.24	0.04	0.47	0.06	19.6	4.1	0	0.2
0	23	0.74	20.0	153.8	31.9	0.44	194.7	0.06	0.34	0.10	0.77	0.06	17.3	2.9	0	0.3
0	20	0.36	12.9	260.0	310.0	0.24	100.0	0.05	—	0.03	0.87	0.17	—	30.0	0	—
0	20	0.36	—	450.0	70.0	—	100.0	0.02	—	0.02	0.75	—	—	30.0	0	—
0	20	0.36	12.9	240.0	360.0	0.24	50.0	0.05	—	0.03	0.88	0.17	—	15.0	0	—
0	7	0.00		5.0	—	0	—	—	—	—	—	—	—	2.0	—	—
0	7	0.00	—	—	5.0	—	0	—	—	—	—	—	—	2.0	—	—
0	41	0.06	7.1	112.2	13.9	0.03	54.4	0.03	0.34	0.04	0.06	0.04	3.1	14.6	0	0.3
0	43	0.59	48.5	121.3	72.0	0.49	0	0.02	4.16	0.10	0.46	0.01	10.4	0.1	0	0.8
0	43	0.59	48.5	121.3	1.8	0.48	0	0.02	—	0.09	0.46	0.01	10.4	0.1	0	—
0	78	1.34	99.7	249.0	10.2	1.13	0	0.07	8.95	0.20	1.32	0.04	10.9	0	0	1.0
0	92	1.55	98.7	257.4	0.3	1.22	0	0.02	8.97	0.29	1.32	0.04	11.4	0	0	1.0
0	92	1.55	98.7	257.4	117.0	1.22	0	0.02	8.97	0.29	1.32	0.04	11.4	0	0	1.0
0	114	1.44	107.5	274.4	133.1	1.20	0	0.03	10.19	0.30	1.43	0.04	10.6	0	0	1.1
0	71	1.00	72.4	190.4	0.3	0.83	0	0.05	7.07	0.27	0.91	0.03	13.5	0	0	0.7
0	1	1.39	0	579.7	21.7	0.20	0	0.16	—	0.20	0.48	0.38	64.4	8.8	0	4.0
0	56	0.85	131.6	230.7	1.1	1.42	0	0.21	2.00	0.01	0.10	0.03	7.7	0.2	0	671.0
0	49	0.50	35.3	616.7	15.9	0.58	8.5	0.22	—	0.12	4.20	0.22	33.6	4.3	0	8.0
0	16	1.21	71.1	126.3	0.3	0.94	1.8	0.12	—	0.04	0.31	0.17	19.8	1.0	0	5.2
0	7	0.81	41.3	87.4	98.2	0.83	0	0.05	0.15	0.03	0.26	0.04	10.9	0	0	1.8
0	7	0.81	41.3	87.4	2.4	0.83	0	0.05	—	0.03	0.26	0.04	10.9	0	0	1.8
0	15	2.06	89.1	193.5	5.5	1.92	0	0.07	0.32	0.07	0.48	0.09	23.6	0	0	4.0
0	14	1.95	88.0	203.8	4.2	1.73	0	0.12	0.30	0.07	0.56	0.10	8.1	0.1	0	6.5
0	6	0.76	20.7	125.2	8.5	0.46	0	0.01	0.10	0.02	0.13	0.07	2.1	0.3	0	4.3
0	3	0.45	11.6	78.4	60.9	0.42	0	0.01	0.09	0.00	0.11	0.06	1.9	0.2	0	3.9
0	3	0.48	6.4	71.2	4.0	0.21	0	0.01	0.04	0.00	0.11	0.01	5.2	0.7	0	2.0
0	7	0.54	32.6	173.0	1.4	0.33	0	0.05	—	0.03	0.54	0.15	26.1	13.9	0	2.6
0	21	0.80	24.8	328.9	12.4	0.11	0.5	0.06	—	0.03	0.32	0.10	17.5	12.3	0	—
0	10	0.32	11.8	211.6	0.7	0.20	0.4	0.08	0.18	0.05	0.48	0.18	25.0	9.3	0	0.4
0	4	0.19	6.5	42.8	1.8	0.14	0.4	0.04	—	0.01	0.19	0.03	6.1	3.4	0	—
0	13	0.75	23.2	154.8	6.9	0.51	1.4	0.15	—	—	0.24	0.14	21.4	10.1	0	—
0	142	2.13	156.1	354.0	11.9	1.83	0	0.06	0.14	0.06	0.59	0.39	118.4	0.5	0	2.3
0	8	0.62	20.7	390.2	5.1	0.26	21.5	0.17	—	0.07	4.58	0.25	41.4	11.4	0	—
0	45	0.98	48.0	197.4	0	0.66	0.6	0.14	5.25	0.03	0.46	0.17	23.4	0.6	0	1.2
0	37	1.31	51.9	226.5	0	0.74	0.9	0.10	4.58	0.03	0.61	0.18	26.4	1.1	0	1.2
0	18	0.64	51.9	130.8	0.3	1.29	2.1	0.26	—	0.04	0.27	0.06	12.0	0.6	0	2.4
0	23	0.88	39.5	121.6	1.3	0.43	0	0.23	0.19	0.02	0.76	0.12	3.4	0.2	0	3.9
0	23	0.88	39.5	121.6	88.8	0.43	0	0.23	0.19	0.02	0.76	0.12	3.4	0.2	0	3.9
0	28	1.24	43.6	123.3	1.7	0.44	0	0.40	0.18	0.05	0.83	0.08	3.7	0.4	0	1.2
0	24	1.27	77.1	204.5	4.1	1.30	0.3	0.07	—	0.07	1.61	0.10	17.1	0.1	0	1.0
0	24	1.26	77.1	204.5	229.1	1.30	0	0.06	3.74	0.06	1.61	0.10	17.1	0.1	0	2.6
0	38	0.92	90.4	195.8	4.0	1.67	0.4	0.18	—	0.17	0.70	0.06	20.2	0.2	0	—
0	20	0.82	64.2	240.2	2.2	1.20	0	0.16	2.52	0.03	4.93	0.09	52.9	0	0	2.7
0	20	0.82	64.2	240.2	296.7	1.20	0	0.16	2.84	0.03	4.93	0.09	52.9	0	0	2.7
0	22	0.54	63.4	261.4	115.2	1.18	0	0.03	2.49	0.03	4.97	0.16	43.2	0.3	0	1.2
0	7	0.30	25.6	119.2	77.8	0.45	0	0.02	1.01	0.02	2.19	0.07	14.7	0	0	1.3
0	6	0.29	25.4	107.0	2.7	0.47	0	0.01	1.23	0.02	2.14	0.07	11.8	0	0	1.2
0	6	0.34	30.6	120.4	97.2	0.50	0	0.05	1.20	0.01	2.63	0.06	10.8	0	0	1.4

TABLE A-1 Table of Food Composition (*continued*) <small>(Computer code is for Cengage Diet Analysis program) (For purposes of calculations, use "0" for t, <1, <.1, <.01, etc.)</small>

DA+ Code	Food Description	Quantity	Measure	Wt (g)	H₂O (g)	Ener (kcal)	Prot (g)	Carb (g)	Fiber (g)	Fat (g)	Fat Breakdown (g) Sat	Mono	Poly	*Trans*
Nuts, Seeds, and Products—*continued*														
524	Peanut butter, smooth	1	tablespoon(s)	16	0.3	94	4.0	3.1	1.0	8.1	1.7	3.9	2.3	—
2804	Raw	¼	cup(s)	37	2.4	207	9.4	5.9	3.1	18.0	2.5	8.9	5.7	—
	Pecans													
32907	Dry roasted, no salt added	¼	cup(s)	28	0.3	198	2.6	3.8	2.6	20.7	1.8	12.3	5.7	—
32936	Dry roasted, with salt added	¼	cup(s)	27	0.3	192	2.6	3.7	2.5	20.0	1.7	11.9	5.6	—
1162	Oil roasted	¼	cup(s)	28	0.3	197	2.5	3.6	2.6	20.7	2.0	11.3	6.5	—
526	Raw	¼	cup(s)	27	1.0	188	2.5	3.8	2.6	19.6	1.7	11.1	5.9	—
12973	**Pine nuts or pignolia, dried**	1	tablespoon(s)	9	0.2	58	1.2	1.1	0.3	5.9	0.4	1.6	2.9	—
	Pistachios													
1164	Dry roasted	¼	cup(s)	31	0.6	176	6.6	8.5	3.2	14.1	1.7	7.4	4.3	—
32938	Dry roasted, with salt added	¼	cup(s)	32	0.6	182	6.8	8.6	3.3	14.7	1.8	7.7	4.4	—
1167	**Pumpkin or squash seeds, roasted**	¼	cup(s)	57	4.0	296	18.7	7.6	2.2	23.9	4.5	7.4	10.9	—
	Sesame													
32912	Sesame butter paste	1	tablespoon(s)	16	0.3	94	2.9	3.8	0.9	8.1	1.1	3.1	3.6	—
32941	Tahini or sesame butter	1	tablespoon(s)	15	0.5	89	2.6	3.2	0.7	8.0	1.1	3.0	3.5	—
1169	Whole, roasted, toasted	3	tablespoon(s)	10	0.3	54	1.6	2.4	1.3	4.6	0.6	1.7	2.0	—
	Soy nuts													
34173	Deep sea salted	¼	cup(s)	28	—	119	11.9	8.9	4.9	4.0	1.0	—	—	—
34174	Unsalted	¼	cup(s)	28	—	119	11.9	8.9	4.9	4.0	0	—	—	—
	Sunflower seeds													
528	Kernels, dried	1	tablespoon(s)	9	0.4	53	1.9	1.8	0.8	4.6	0.4	1.7	2.1	—
29721	Kernels, dry roasted, salted	1	tablespoon(s)	8	0.1	47	1.5	1.9	0.7	4.0	0.4	0.8	2.6	—
29723	Kernels, toasted, salted	1	tablespoon(s)	8	0.1	52	1.4	1.7	1.0	4.8	0.5	0.9	3.1	—
32928	Sunflower seed butter with salt added	1	tablespoon(s)	16	0.2	93	3.1	4.4	—	7.6	0.8	1.5	5.0	—
	Trail mix													
4646	Trail mix	¼	cup(s)	38	3.5	173	5.2	16.8	2.0	11.0	2.1	4.7	3.6	—
4647	Trail mix with chocolate chips	¼	cup(s)	38	2.5	182	5.3	16.8	—	12.0	2.3	5.1	4.2	—
4648	Tropical trail mix	¼	cup(s)	35	3.2	142	2.2	23.0	—	6.0	3.0	0.9	1.8	—
	Walnuts													
529	Dried black, chopped	¼	cup(s)	31	1.4	193	7.5	3.1	2.1	18.4	1.1	4.7	11.0	—
531	English or Persian	¼	cup(s)	29	1.2	191	4.5	4.0	2.0	19.1	1.8	2.6	13.8	—
Vegetarian Foods														
	Prepared													
34222	Brown rice and tofu stir-fry (vegan)	8	ounce(s)	227	244.4	302	16.5	18.0	3.2	21.0	1.7	4.7	13.4	0
34368	Cheese enchilada casserole (lacto)	8	ounce(s)	227	80.3	385	16.6	38.4	4.1	17.8	9.5	6.1	1.1	—
34247	Five bean casserole (vegan)	8	ounce(s)	227	175.8	178	5.9	26.6	6.0	5.8	1.1	2.5	1.9	0
34261	Lentil stew (vegan)	8	ounce(s)	227	227.9	188	11.5	35.9	11.0	0.7	0.1	0.1	0.3	0
34397	Macaroni and cheese (lacto)	8	ounce(s)	227	352.1	391	18.1	37.1	1.0	18.7	9.8	6.0	1.8	0
34238	Steamed rice and vegetables (vegan)	8	ounce(s)	227	222.9	587	11.2	87.9	5.8	23.1	4.1	8.7	9.1	0
34308	Tofu rice burgers (ovo-lacto)	1	piece(s)	218	77.6	435	22.4	68.6	5.6	8.4	1.7	2.4	3.5	—
34276	Vegan spinach enchiladas (vegan)	1	piece(s)	82	59.2	93	4.9	14.5	1.8	2.4	0.3	0.6	1.3	—
34243	Vegetable chow mein (vegan)	8	ounce(s)	227	163.3	166	6.5	22.1	2.0	6.4	0.7	2.7	2.5	0
34454	Vegetable lasagna (lacto)	8	ounce(s)	227	178.9	208	13.7	29.9	2.6	4.1	2.3	1.1	0.3	—
34339	Vegetable marinara (vegan)	8	ounce(s)	252	200.7	104	3.0	16.7	1.4	3.1	0.4	1.4	1.0	0
34356	Vegetable rice casserole (lacto)	8	ounce(s)	227	178.9	238	9.7	24.4	4.0	12.5	4.9	3.5	3.1	—
34311	Vegetable strudel (ovo-lacto)	8	ounce(s)	227	63.1	478	12.0	32.4	2.5	33.8	11.5	16.7	3.9	0
34371	Vegetable taco (lacto)	1	item(s)	85	46.5	117	4.2	13.6	2.9	5.6	2.1	1.9	1.3	—
34282	Vegetarian chili (vegan)	8	ounce(s)	227	191.4	115	5.6	21.4	7.1	1.5	0.2	0.3	0.7	0
34367	Vegetarian vegetable soup (vegan)	8	ounce(s)	227	257.9	111	3.2	16.0	3.2	5.0	1.0	2.1	1.6	0
	Boca burger													
32067	All American flamed grilled patty	1	item(s)	71	—	90	14.0	4.0	3.0	3.0	1.0	—	—	0
32074	Boca chik'n nuggets	4	item(s)	87	—	180	14.0	17.0	3.0	7.0	1.0	—	—	0
32075	Boca meatless ground burger	½	cup(s)	57	—	60	13.0	6.0	3.0	0.5	0	—	—	0
32072	Breakfast links	2	item(s)	45	—	70	8.0	5.0	2.0	3.0	0.5	—	—	0
32071	Breakfast patties	1	item(s)	38	—	60	7.0	5.0	2.0	2.5	0	—	—	0
35780	Cheeseburger meatless burger patty	1	item(s)	71	—	100	12.0	5.0	3.0	5.0	1.5	—	—	0
33958	Original meatless chik'n patties	1	item(s)	71	—	160	11.0	15.0	2.0	6.0	1.0	—	—	0

Chol (mg)	Calc (mg)	Iron (mg)	Magn (mg)	Pota (mg)	Sodi (mg)	Zinc (mg)	Vit A (µg)	Thia (mg)	Vit E (mg α)	Ribo (mg)	Niac (mg)	Vit B$_6$ (mg)	Fola (µg)	Vit C (mg)	Vit B$_{12}$ (µg)	Sele (µg)
0	7	0.30	24.6	103.8	73.4	0.47	0	0.01	1.44	0.02	2.14	0.09	11.8	0	0	0.9
0	34	1.67	61.3	257.3	6.6	1.19	0	0.23	3.04	0.04	4.40	0.12	87.6	0	0	2.6
0	20	0.78	36.8	118.3	0.3	1.41	1.9	0.12	0.35	0.03	0.32	0.05	4.5	0.2	0	1.1
0	19	0.75	35.6	114.5	103.4	1.36	1.9	0.11	0.34	0.03	0.31	0.05	4.3	0.2	0	1.1
0	18	0.68	33.3	107.8	0.3	1.23	1.4	0.13	0.70	0.03	0.33	0.05	4.1	0.2	0	1.7
0	19	0.69	33.0	111.7	0	1.23	0.8	0.18	0.38	0.04	0.32	0.06	6.0	0.3	0	1.0
0	1	0.47	21.6	51.3	0.2	0.55	0.1	0.03	0.80	0.02	0.37	0.01	2.9	0.1	0	0.1
0	34	1.29	36.9	320.4	3.1	0.71	4.0	0.26	0.59	0.05	0.44	0.39	15.4	0.7	0	2.9
0	35	1.34	38.4	333.4	129.6	0.73	4.2	0.26	0.61	0.05	0.45	0.40	16.0	0.7	0	3.0
0	24	8.48	303.0	457.4	10.2	4.22	10.8	0.12	0.00	0.18	0.99	0.05	32.3	1.0	0	3.2
0	154	3.07	57.9	93.1	1.9	1.17	0.5	0.04	—	0.03	1.07	0.13	16.0	0	0	0.9
0	21	0.66	14.3	68.9	5.3	0.69	0.5	0.24	—	0.02	0.85	0.02	14.7	0.6	0	0.3
0	94	1.40	33.8	45.1	1.0	0.68	0	0.07	—	0.02	0.43	0.07	9.3	0	0	0.5
0	59	1.07	—	—	148.1	—	0	—	—	—	—	—	—	0	—	—
0	59	1.07	—	—	9.9	—	0	—	—	—	—	—	—	0	—	—
0	7	0.47	29.3	58.1	0.8	0.45	0.3	0.13	2.99	0.03	0.75	0.12	20.4	0.1	0	4.8
0	6	0.30	10.3	68.0	32.8	0.42	0	0.01	2.09	0.02	0.56	0.06	19.0	0.1	0	6.3
0	5	0.57	10.8	41.1	51.3	0.44	0	0.03	—	0.02	0.35	0.07	19.9	0.1	0	5.2
0	20	0.76	59.0	11.5	83.2	0.85	0.5	0.05	—	0.05	0.85	0.13	37.9	0.4	0	—
0	29	1.14	59.3	256.9	85.9	1.20	0.4	0.17	—	0.07	1.76	0.11	26.6	0.5	0	—
2	41	1.27	60.4	243.0	45.4	1.17	0.8	0.15	—	0.08	1.65	0.09	24.4	0.5	0	—
0	20	0.92	33.6	248.2	3.5	0.41	0.7	0.15	—	0.04	0.51	0.11	14.7	2.7	0	—
0	19	0.97	62.8	163.4	0.6	1.05	0.6	0.01	0.56	0.04	0.14	0.18	9.7	0.5	0	5.3
0	29	0.85	46.2	129.0	0.6	0.90	0.3	0.10	0.20	0.04	0.32	0.15	28.7	0.4	0	1.4
0	353	6.34	118.3	501.4	142.2	2.03	—	0.23	0.07	0.14	1.49	0.36	51.8	24.8	0	14.8
39	441	2.44	34.6	191.2	1139.7	1.84	—	0.31	0.05	0.35	2.23	0.11	87.1	20.4	0.4	20.0
0	48	1.78	40.8	364.1	613.6	0.61	—	0.10	0.52	0.07	0.93	0.11	39.4	8.3	0	3.3
0	34	3.23	50.0	548.8	436.5	1.42	—	0.24	0.14	0.16	2.31	0.29	91.4	26.4	0	12.1
43	415	1.71	45.4	267.8	1641.0	2.32	—	0.32	0.27	0.48	2.18	0.13	74.2	0.9	0.8	33.3
0	91	3.31	153.1	810.1	3117.8	2.04	—	0.37	3.03	0.21	6.16	0.64	61.7	35.2	0	18.8
52	467	9.01	89.7	455.6	2449.5	2.06	—	0.27	0.12	0.26	3.43	0.29	106.6	2.0	0.1	43.0
0	117	1.13	40.4	170.5	134.2	0.68	—	0.07	—	0.07	0.53	0.10	52.1	1.8	0	5.1
0	189	3.70	28.0	310.3	372.7	0.76	—	0.13	0.05	0.11	1.43	0.14	45.6	8.0	0	6.5
10	176	1.86	41.9	470.0	759.4	1.14	—	0.26	0.05	0.25	2.49	0.22	64.7	19.0	0.4	21.8
0	17	0.94	19.1	189.9	439.6	0.42	—	0.15	0.55	0.08	1.36	0.12	40.6	23.5	0	10.8
17	190	1.28	29.3	414.2	626.0	1.24	—	0.16	0.35	0.29	2.00	0.19	72.6	56.0	0.2	5.8
29	200	2.15	24.5	181.0	512.1	1.24	—	0.28	0.20	0.31	2.88	0.11	88.3	17.4	0.2	19.7
7	77	0.88	26.3	174.1	280.7	0.59	—	0.08	0.04	0.06	0.49	0.08	38.7	4.6	0	3.0
0	65	1.98	41.0	543.1	390.7	0.74	—	0.14	0.15	0.10	1.31	0.18	59.3	20.3	0	4.4
0	46	1.87	34.9	550.3	729.5	0.56	—	0.13	0.55	0.09	1.99	0.27	47.8	29.9	0	1.4
5	150	1.80	—	—	280.0	—	0	—	—	—	—	—	—	0	—	—
0	40	1.44	—	—	500.0	—	—	—	—	—	—	—	—	0	—	—
0	60	1.80	—	—	270.0	—	0	—	—	—	—	—	—	0	—	—
0	20	1.44	—	—	330.0	—	0	—	—	—	—	—	—	0	—	—
0	20	1.08	—	—	280.0	—	0	—	—	—	—	—	—	0	—	—
5	80	1.80	—	—	360.0	—	—	—	—	—	—	—	—	0	—	—
0	40	1.80	—	—	430.0	—	—	—	—	—	—	—	—	0	—	—

TABLE A-1 Table of Food Composition (continued) (Computer code is for Cengage Diet Analysis program) (For purposes of calculations, use "0" for t, <1, <.1, <.01, etc.)

DA+ Code	Food Description	Quantity	Measure	Wt (g)	H₂O (g)	Ener (kcal)	Prot (g)	Carb (g)	Fiber (g)	Fat (g)	Fat Breakdown (g) Sat	Mono	Poly	Trans
Vegetarian Foods—continued														
32066	Original patty	1	item(s)	71	—	70	13.0	6.0	4.0	0.5	0	—	—	0
32068	Roasted garlic patty	1	item(s)	71	—	70	12.0	6.0	4.0	1.5	0	—	—	0
37814	Roasted onion meatless burger patty	1	item(s)	71	—	70	11.0	7.0	4.0	1.0	0	—	—	0
	Gardenburger													
37810	BBQ chik'n with sauce	1	item(s)	142	—	250	14.0	30.0	5.0	8.0	1.0	—	—	0
39661	Black bean burger	1	item(s)	71	—	80	8.0	11.0	4.0	2.0	0	—	—	0
39666	Buffalo chik'n wing	3	item(s)	95	—	180	9.0	8.0	5.0	12.0	1.5	—	—	0
39665	Country fried chicken with creamy pepper gravy	1	item(s)	142	—	190	9.0	16.0	2.0	9.0	1.0	—	—	0
37808	Flamed grilled chik'n	1	item(s)	71	—	100	13.0	5.0	3.0	2.5	0	—	—	0
37803	Garden vegan	1	item(s)	71	—	100	10.0	12.0	2.0	1.0	—	—	—	0
39663	Homestyle classic burger	1	item(s)	71	—	110	12.0	6.0	4.0	5.0	0.5	—	—	0
37807	Meatless breakfast sausage	1	item(s)	43	—	50	5.0	2.0	2.0	3.5	0	—	—	0
37809	Meatless meatballs	6	item(s)	85	—	110	12.0	8.0	4.0	4.5	1.0	—	—	0
37806	Meatless riblets with sauce	1	item(s)	142	—	160	17.0	11.0	4.0	5.0	0	—	—	0
29913	Original	1	item(s)	71	—	90	10.0	8.0	3.0	2.0	0.5	—	—	0
39662	Sun-dried tomato basil burger	1	item(s)	71	—	80	10.0	11.0	3.0	1.5	0.5	—	—	0
29915	Veggie medley	1	item(s)	71	—	90	9.0	11.0	4.0	2.0	0	—	—	0
	Loma Linda													
9311	Big franks, canned	1	item(s)	51	—	110	11.0	3.0	2.0	6.0	1.0	1.5	3.5	0
9323	Fried chik'n with gravy	2	piece(s)	80	45.9	150	12.0	5.0	2.0	10	1.5	2.5	5.0	0
9326	Linketts, canned	1	item(s)	35	21.0	70	7.0	1.0	1.0	4.0	0.5	1.0	2.5	0
9336	Redi-Burger patties, canned	1	slice(s)	85	50.5	120	18.0	7.0	4.0	2.5	0.5	0.5	1.5	0
9350	Swiss Stake pattie with gravy, frozen	1	piece(s)	92	65.7	130	9.0	9.0	3.0	6.0	1.0	1.5	3.5	0
9354	Tender Rounds meatball substitute, canned in gravy	6	piece(s)	80	53.9	120	13.0	6.0	1.0	4.5	0.5	1.5	2.5	0
	Morningstar Farms													
33707	America's Original Veggie Dog links	1	item(s)	57	—	80	11.0	6.0	1.0	0.5	0	—	—	0
9362	Better'n Eggs egg substitute	¼	cup(s)	57	50.3	20	5.0	0	0	0	0	0	0	0
9371	Breakfast bacon strips	2	item(s)	16	6.8	60	2.0	2.0	0.5	4.5	0.5	1.0	3.0	0
9368	Breakfast sausage links	2	item(s)	45	26.8	80	9.0	3.0	2.0	3.0	0.5	1.5	1.0	0
33705	Chik'n nuggets	4	piece(s)	86	—	190	12.0	18.0	2.0	7.0	1.0	2.0	4.0	0
11587	Chik patties	1	item(s)	71	36.3	150	9.0	16.0	2.0	6.0	1.0	1.5	2.5	0
2531	Garden veggie patties	1	item(s)	67	40.1	100	10.0	9.0	4.0	2.5	0.5	0.5	1.5	0
33702	Spicy black bean veggie burger	1	item(s)	78	—	140	12.0	15.0	3.0	4.0	0.5	1.0	2.5	0
9412	Vegetarian chili, canned	1	cup(s)	230	172.6	180	16.0	25.0	10.0	1.5	0.5	0.5	0.5	0
	Worthington													
9424	Chili, canned	1	cup(s)	230	167.0	280	24.0	25.0	8.0	10.0	1.5	1.5	7.0	0
9436	Diced chik, canned	¼	cup(s)	55	42.7	50	9.0	2.0	1.0	0	0	0	0	0
9440	Dinner roast, frozen	1	slice(s)	85	53.2	180	14.0	6.0	3.0	11.0	1.5	4.5	5.0	0
9420	Meatless chicken slices, frozen	3	slice(s)	57	38.9	90	9.0	2.0	0.5	4.5	1.0	1.0	2.5	0
36702	Meatless chicken style roll, frozen	1	slice(s)	55	—	90	9.0	2.0	1.0	4.5	1.0	1.0	2.5	0
9428	Meatless corned beef, sliced, frozen	3	slice(s)	57	31.2	140	10.0	5.0	0	9.0	1.0	2.0	5.0	0
9470	Meatless salami, sliced, frozen	3	slice(s)	57	32.4	120	12.0	3.0	2.0	7.0	1.0	1.0	5.0	0
9480	Meatless smoked turkey, sliced	3	slice(s)	57	—	140	10.0	4.0	0	9.0	1.5	2.0	5.0	0
9462	Prosage links	2	item(s)	45	26.8	80	9.0	3.0	2.0	3.0	0.5	0.5	2.0	0
9484	Stakelets patty beef steak substitute, frozen	1	piece(s)	71	41.5	150	14.0	7.0	2.0	7.0	1.0	2.5	3.5	0
9486	Stripples bacon substitute	2	item(s)	16	6.8	60	2.0	2.0	0.5	4.5	0.5	1.0	3.0	0
9496	Vegetable Skallops meat substitute, canned	½	cup(s)	85	—	90	17.0	4.0	3.0	1.0	0	0	0.5	0
Dairy														
	Cheese													
1433	Blue, crumbled	1	ounce(s)	28	12.0	100	6.1	0.7	0	8.1	5.3	2.2	0.2	—
884	Brick	1	ounce(s)	28	11.7	105	6.6	0.8	0	8.4	5.3	2.4	0.2	—
885	Brie	1	ounce(s)	28	13.7	95	5.9	0.1	0	7.8	4.9	2.3	0.2	—
34821	Camembert	1	ounce(s)	28	14.7	85	5.6	0.1	0	6.9	4.3	2.0	0.2	—
5	Cheddar, shredded	¼	cup(s)	28	10.4	114	7.0	0.4	0	9.4	6.0	2.7	0.3	—
888	Cheddar or colby	1	ounce(s)	28	10.8	112	6.7	0.7	0	9.1	5.7	2.6	0.3	—
32096	Cheddar or colby, low fat	1	ounce(s)	28	17.9	49	6.9	0.5	0	2.0	1.2	0.6	0.1	—
889	Edam	1	ounce(s)	28	11.8	101	7.1	0.4	0	7.9	5.0	2.3	0.2	—

PAGE KEY: A-6 = Breads/Baked Goods A-12 = Cereal/Rice/Pasta A-16 = Fruit A-20 = Vegetables/Legumes A-30 = Nuts/Seeds A-32 = Vegetarian A-34 = Dairy A-42 = Eggs A-42 = Seafood A-44 = Meats A-48 = Poultry A-48 = Processed Meats A-50 = Beverages A-54 = Fats/Oils A-56 = Sweets A-58 = Spices/Condiments/Sauces A-62 = Mixed Foods/Soups/Sandwiches A-66 = Fast Food A-86 = Convenience A-88 = Baby Foods

Chol (mg)	Calc (mg)	Iron (mg)	Magn (mg)	Pota (mg)	Sodi (mg)	Zinc (mg)	Vit A (µg)	Thia (mg)	Vit E (mg α)	Ribo (mg)	Niac (mg)	Vit B$_6$ (mg)	Fola (µg)	Vit C (mg)	Vit B$_{12}$ (µg)	Sele (µg)
0	60	1.80	—	—	280.0	—	0	—	—	—	—	—	—	0	—	—
0	60	1.80	—	—	370.0	—	0	—	—	—	—	—	—	0	—	—
0	100	2.70	—	—	300.0	—	—	—	—	—	—	—	—	0	—	—
0	150	1.08	—	—	890.0	—	—	—	—	—	—	—	—	0	—	—
0	40	1.44	—	—	330.0	—	—	—	—	—	—	—	—	0	—	—
0	40	0.72	—	—	1000.0	—	—	—	—	—	—	—	—	0	—	—
5	40	1.44	—	—	550.0	—	—	—	—	—	—	—	—	0	—	—
0	60	3.60	—	—	360.0	—	—	—	—	—	—	—	—	0	—	—
0	40	4.50	—	—	230.0	—	—	—	—	—	—	—	—	0	—	—
0	80	1.44	—	—	380.0	—	—	—	—	—	—	—	—	0	—	—
0	20	0.72	—	—	120.0	—	—	—	—	—	—	—	—	0	—	—
0	60	1.80	—	—	400.0	—	—	—	—	—	—	—	—	0	—	—
0	60	1.80	—	—	720.0	—	—	—	—	—	—	—	—	3.6	—	—
0	80	1.08	30.4	193.4	490.0	0.89	—	0.10	—	0.15	1.08	0.08	10.1	1.2	0.1	7.0
5	60	1.44	—	—	260.0	—	—	—	—	—	—	—	—	3.6	—	—
0	40	1.44	27.0	182.0	290.0	0.46	—	0.07	—	0.08	0.90	0.09	10.6	9.0	0	4.0
0	0	0.77	—	50.0	220.0	—	0	0.22	—	0.10	2.00	0.70	—	0	2.4	—
0	20	1.80	—	70.0	430.0	0.33	0	1.05	—	0.34	4.00	0.30	—	0	2.4	—
0	0	0.36	—	20.0	160.0	0.46	0	0.12	—	0.20	0.80	0.16	—	0	0.9	—
0	0	1.06	—	140.0	450.0	—	0	0.15	—	0.25	4.00	0.40	—	0	1.2	—
0	0	0.72	—	200.0	430.0	—	0	0.45	—	0.25	10.00	1.00	—	0	5.4	—
0	20	1.08	—	80.0	340.0	0.66	0	0.75	—	0.17	2.00	0.16	—	0	1.2	—
0	0	0.72	—	60.0	580.0	—	0	—	—	—	—	—	—	0	—	—
0	20	0.72	—	75.0	90.0	0.60	37.5	0.03	—	0.34	0.00	0.08	24.0	—	0.6	—
0	0	0.36	—	15.0	220.0	0.05	0	0.75	—	0.04	0.40	0.07	—	0	0.2	—
0	0	1.80	—	50.0	300.0	—	0	0.37	—	0.17	7.00	0.50	—	0	3.0	—
0	20	2.70	—	320.0	490.0	—	0	0.52	—	0.25	5.00	0.30	—	0	1.5	—
0	0	1.80	—	210.0	540.0	—	0	1.80	—	0.17	2.00	0.20	—	0	1.2	—
0	40	0.72	—	180.0	350.0	—	—	—	—	—	—	—	—	0	—	—
0	40	1.80	—	320.0	470.0	—	0	—	—	—	0.00	—	—	0	—	—
0	40	3.60	—	660.0	900.0	—	—	—	—	—	—	—	—	0	—	—
0	40	3.60	—	330.0	1130.0	—	0	0.30	—	0.13	2.00	0.70	—	0	1.5	—
0	0	1.08	—	100.0	220.0	0.24	0	0.06	—	0.10	4.00	0.08	—	0	0.2	—
0	20	1.80	—	120.0	580.0	0.64	0	1.80	—	0.25	6.00	0.60	—	0	1.5	—
0	250	1.80	—	250.0	250.0	0.26	0	0.37	—	0.13	4.00	0.30	—	0	1.8	—
0	100	1.08	—	240.0	240.0	—	0	0.37	—	0.13	4.00	0.30	—	0	1.8	—
0	0	1.80	—	130.0	460.0	0.26	0	0.45	—	0.17	5.00	0.30	—	0	1.8	—
0	0	1.08	—	95.0	800.0	0.30	0	0.75	—	0.17	4.00	0.20	—	0	0.6	—
0	60	2.70	—	60.0	450.0	0.23	0	1.80	—	0.17	6.00	0.40	—	0	3.0	—
0	0	1.44	—	50.0	320.0	0.36	0	1.80	—	0.17	2.00	0.30	—	0	3.0	—
0	40	1.08	—	130.0	480.0	0.50	0	1.20	—	0.13	3.00	0.30	—	0	1.5	—
0	0	0.36	—	15.0	220.0	0.05	0	0.75	—	0.03	0.40	0.08	—	0	0.2	—
0	0	0.36	—	10.0	390.0	0.67	0	0.03	—	0.03	0.00	0.01	—	0	0	—
21	150	0.08	6.5	72.6	395.5	0.75	56.1	0.01	0.07	0.10	0.28	0.04	10.2	0	0.3	4.1
27	191	0.12	6.8	38.6	158.8	0.73	82.8	0.00	0.07	0.10	0.03	0.01	5.7	0	0.4	4.1
28	52	0.14	5.7	43.1	178.3	0.67	49.3	0.02	0.06	0.14	0.10	0.06	18.4	0	0.5	4.1
20	110	0.09	5.7	53.0	238.7	0.67	68.3	0.01	0.06	0.14	0.18	0.06	17.6	0	0.4	4.1
30	204	0.19	7.9	27.7	175.4	0.87	74.9	0.01	0.08	0.10	0.02	0.02	5.1	0	0.2	3.9
27	194	0.21	7.4	36.0	171.2	0.87	74.8	0.00	0.07	0.10	0.02	0.02	5.1	0	0.2	4.1
6	118	0.11	4.5	18.7	173.5	0.51	17.0	0.00	0.01	0.06	0.01	0.01	3.1	0	0.1	4.1
25	207	0.12	8.5	53.3	273.6	1.06	68.9	0.01	0.06	0.11	0.02	0.02	4.5	0	0.4	4.1

TABLE A-1 Table of Food Composition (*continued*) (Computer code is for Cengage Diet Analysis program) (For purposes of calculations, use "0" for t, <1, <.1, <.01, etc.)

DA+ Code	Food Description	Quantity	Measure	Wt (g)	H₂O (g)	Ener (kcal)	Prot (g)	Carb (g)	Fiber (g)	Fat (g)	Sat	Mono	Poly	Trans
											Fat Breakdown (g)			

Dairy—*continued*

DA+ Code	Food Description	Quantity	Measure	Wt (g)	H₂O (g)	Ener (kcal)	Prot (g)	Carb (g)	Fiber (g)	Fat (g)	Sat	Mono	Poly	Trans
890	Feta	1	ounce(s)	28	15.7	75	4.0	1.2	0	6.0	4.2	1.3	0.2	—
891	Fontina	1	ounce(s)	28	10.8	110	7.3	0.4	0	8.8	5.4	2.5	0.5	—
8527	Goat cheese, soft	1	ounce(s)	28	17.2	76	5.3	0.3	0	6.0	4.1	1.4	0.1	—
893	Gouda	1	ounce(s)	28	11.8	101	7.1	0.6	0	7.8	5.0	2.2	0.2	—
894	Gruyere	1	ounce(s)	28	9.4	117	8.5	0.1	0	9.2	5.4	2.8	0.5	—
895	Limburger	1	ounce(s)	28	13.7	93	5.7	0.1	0	7.7	4.7	2.4	0.1	—
896	Monterey jack	1	ounce(s)	28	11.6	106	6.9	0.2	0	8.6	5.4	2.5	0.3	—
13	Mozzarella, part skim milk	1	ounce(s)	28	15.2	72	6.9	0.8	0	4.5	2.9	1.3	0.1	—
12	Mozzarella, whole milk	1	ounce(s)	28	14.2	85	6.3	0.6	0	6.3	3.7	1.9	0.2	—
897	Muenster	1	ounce(s)	28	11.8	104	6.6	0.3	0	8.5	5.4	2.5	0.2	—
898	Neufchatel	1	ounce(s)	28	17.6	74	2.8	0.8	0	6.6	4.2	1.9	0.2	—
14	Parmesan, grated	1	tablespoon(s)	5	1.0	22	1.9	0.2	0	1.4	0.9	0.4	0.1	—
17	Provolone	1	ounce(s)	28	11.6	100	7.3	0.6	0	7.5	4.8	2.1	0.2	—
19	Ricotta, part skim milk	¼	cup(s)	62	45.8	85	7.0	3.2	0	4.9	3.0	1.4	0.2	—
18	Ricotta, whole milk	¼	cup(s)	62	44.1	107	6.9	1.9	0	8.0	5.1	2.2	0.2	—
20	Romano	1	tablespoon(s)	5	1.5	19	1.6	0.2	0	1.3	0.9	0.4	0	—
900	Roquefort	1	ounce(s)	28	11.2	105	6.1	0.6	0	8.7	5.5	2.4	0.4	—
21	Swiss	1	ounce(s)	28	10.5	108	7.6	1.5	0	7.9	5.0	2.1	0.3	—
	Imitation cheese													
42245	Imitation American cheddar cheese	1	ounce(s)	28	15.1	68	4.7	3.3	0	4.0	2.5	1.2	0.1	—
53914	Imitation cheddar	1	ounce(s)	28	15.1	68	4.7	3.3	0	4.0	2.5	1.2	0.1	—
	Cottage cheese													
9	Low fat, 1% fat	½	cup(s)	113	93.2	81	14.0	3.1	0	1.2	0.7	0.3	0	—
8	Low fat, 2% fat	½	cup(s)	113	89.6	102	15.5	4.1	0	2.2	1.4	0.6	0.1	—
	Cream cheese													
11	Cream cheese	2	tablespoon(s)	29	15.6	101	2.2	0.8	0	10.1	6.4	2.9	0.4	—
17366	Fat-free cream cheese	2	tablespoon(s)	30	22.7	29	4.3	1.7	0	0.4	0.3	0.1	0	—
10438	Tofutti Better than Cream Cheese	2	tablespoon(s)	30	—	80	1.0	1.0	0	8.0	2.0	—	6.0	—
	Processed cheese													
24	American cheese food, processed	1	ounce(s)	28	12.3	94	5.2	2.2	0	7.1	4.2	2.0	0.3	—
25	American cheese spread, processed	1	ounce(s)	28	13.5	82	4.7	2.5	0	6.0	3.8	1.8	0.2	—
22	American cheese, processed	1	ounce(s)	28	11.1	106	6.3	0.5	0	8.9	5.6	2.5	0.3	—
9110	Kraft deluxe singles pasteurized process American cheese	1	ounce(s)	28	—	108	5.4	0	0	9.5	5.4	—	—	—
23	Swiss cheese, processed	1	ounce(s)	28	12.0	95	7.0	0.6	0	7.1	4.5	2.0	0.2	—
	Soy cheese													
10437	Galaxy Foods vegan grated parmesan cheese alternative	1	tablespoon(s)	8	—	23	3.0	1.5	0	0	0	0	0	0
10430	Nu Tofu cheddar flavored cheese alternative	1	ounce(s)	28	—	70	6.0	1.0	0	4.0	0.5	2.5	1.0	—
	Cream													
26	Half and half cream	1	tablespoon(s)	15	12.1	20	0.4	0.6	0	1.7	1.1	0.5	0.1	—
32	Heavy whipping cream, liquid	1	tablespoon(s)	15	8.7	52	0.3	0.4	0	5.6	3.5	1.6	0.2	—
28	Light coffee or table cream, liquid	1	tablespoon(s)	15	11.1	29	0.4	0.5	0	2.9	1.8	0.8	0.1	—
30	Light whipping cream, liquid	1	tablespoon(s)	15	9.5	44	0.3	0.4	0	4.6	2.9	1.4	0.1	—
34	Whipped cream topping, pressurized	1	tablespoon(s)	3	1.8	8	0.1	0.4	0	0.7	0.4	0.2	0	—
	Sour cream													
30556	Fat-free sour cream	2	tablespoon(s)	32	25.8	24	1.0	5.0	0	0	0	0	0	0
36	Sour cream	2	tablespoon(s)	24	17.0	51	0.8	1.0	0	5.0	3.1	1.5	0.2	—
	Imitation cream													
3659	Coffeemate nondairy creamer, liquid	1	tablespoon(s)	15	—	20	0	2.0	0	1.0	0	0.5	0	—
40	Cream substitute, powder	1	teaspoon(s)	2	0	11	0.1	1.1	0	0.7	0.7	0	0	—
904	Imitation sour cream	2	tablespoon(s)	29	20.5	60	0.7	1.9	0	5.6	5.1	0.2	0	—
35972	Nondairy coffee whitener, liquid, frozen	1	tablespoon(s)	15	11.7	21	0.2	1.7	0	1.5	0.3	1.1	0	—
35976	Nondairy dessert topping, frozen	1	tablespoon(s)	5	2.4	15	0.1	1.1	0	1.2	1.0	0.1	0	—
35975	Nondairy dessert topping, pressurized	1	tablespoon(s)	4	2.7	12	0	0.7	0	1.0	0.8	0.1	0	—

PAGE KEY: A-6 = Breads/Baked Goods A-12 = Cereal/Rice/Pasta A-16 = Fruit A-20 = Vegetables/Legumes A-30 = Nuts/Seeds A-32 = Vegetarian A-34 = Dairy A-42 = Eggs A-42 = Seafood A-44 = Meats A-48 = Poultry A-48 = Processed Meats A-50 = Beverages A-54 = Fats/Oils A-56 = Sweets A-58 = Spices/Condiments/Sauces A-62 = Mixed Foods/Soups/Sandwiches A-66 = Fast Food A-86 = Convenience A-88 = Baby Foods

Chol (mg)	Calc (mg)	Iron (mg)	Magn (mg)	Pota (mg)	Sodi (mg)	Zinc (mg)	Vit A (µg)	Thia (mg)	Vit E (mg α)	Ribo (mg)	Niac (mg)	Vit B$_6$ (mg)	Fola (µg)	Vit C (mg)	Vit B$_{12}$ (µg)	Sele (µg)
25	140	0.18	5.4	17.6	316.4	0.81	35.4	0.04	0.05	0.23	0.28	0.12	9.1	0	0.5	4.3
33	156	0.06	4.0	18.1	226.8	0.99	74.0	0.01	0.07	0.05	0.04	0.02	1.7	0	0.5	4.1
13	40	0.53	4.5	7.4	104.3	0.26	81.6	0.02	0.05	0.10	0.12	0.07	3.4	0	0.1	0.8
32	198	0.06	8.2	34.3	232.2	1.10	46.8	0.01	0.06	0.09	0.01	0.02	6.0	0	0.4	4.1
31	287	0.04	10.2	23.0	95.3	1.10	76.8	0.01	0.07	0.07	0.03	0.02	2.8	0	0.5	4.1
26	141	0.03	6.0	36.3	226.8	0.59	96.4	0.02	0.06	0.14	0.04	0.02	16.4	0	0.3	4.1
25	211	0.20	7.7	23.0	152.0	0.85	56.1	0.00	0.07	0.11	0.02	0.02	5.1	0	0.2	4.1
18	222	0.06	6.5	23.8	175.5	0.78	36.0	0.01	0.04	0.08	0.03	0.02	2.6	0	0.2	4.1
22	143	0.12	5.7	21.5	177.8	0.82	50.7	0.01	0.05	0.08	0.02	0.01	2.0	0	0.6	4.8
27	203	0.11	7.7	38.0	178.0	0.79	84.5	0.00	0.07	0.09	0.02	0.01	3.4	0	0.4	4.1
22	21	0.07	2.3	32.3	113.1	0.14	84.5	0.00	—	0.05	0.03	0.01	3.1	0	0.1	0.9
4	55	0.04	1.9	6.3	76.5	0.19	6.0	0.00	0.01	0.02	0.01	0.00	0.5	0	0.1	0.9
20	214	0.14	7.9	39.1	248.3	0.91	66.9	0.01	0.06	0.09	0.04	0.02	2.8	0	0.4	4.1
19	167	0.27	9.2	76.9	76.9	0.82	65.8	0.01	0.04	0.11	0.04	0.01	8.0	0	0.2	10.3
31	127	0.23	6.8	64.6	51.7	0.71	73.8	0.01	0.06	0.12	0.06	0.02	7.4	0	0.2	8.9
5	53	0.03	2.1	4.3	60	0.12	4.8	0.00	0.01	0.01	0.00	0.00	0.4	0	0.1	0.7
26	188	0.15	8.5	25.8	512.9	0.59	83.3	0.01	—	0.16	0.20	0.03	13.9	0	0.2	4.1
26	224	0.05	10.8	21.8	54.4	1.23	62.4	0.01	0.10	0.08	0.02	0.02	1.7	0	0.9	5.2
10	159	0.08	8.2	68.6	381.3	0.73	32.3	0.01	0.07	0.12	0.03	0.03	2.0	0	0.1	4.3
10	159	0.09	8.2	68.6	381.3	0.73	32.3	0.01	0.07	0.12	0.04	0.03	2.0	0	0.1	4.3
5	69	0.15	5.7	97.2	458.8	0.42	12.4	0.02	0.01	0.18	0.14	0.07	13.6	0	0.7	10.2
9	78	0.18	6.8	108.5	458.8	0.47	23.7	0.02	0.02	0.20	0.16	0.08	14.7	0	0.8	11.5
32	23	0.34	1.7	34.5	85.8	0.15	106.1	0.01	0.08	0.05	0.02	0.01	3.8	0	0.1	0.7
2	56	0.05	4.2	48.9	163.5	0.26	83.7	0.01	0.00	0.05	0.04	0.01	11.1	0	0.2	1.5
0	0	0.00	—	—	135.0	—	0	—	—	—	—	—	—	0	—	—
23	162	0.16	8.8	82.5	358.6	0.90	57.0	0.01	0.06	0.14	0.04	0.02	2.0	0	0.4	4.6
16	159	0.09	8.2	68.6	381.3	0.73	49.0	0.01	0.05	0.12	0.03	0.03	2.0	0	0.1	3.2
27	156	0.05	7.7	47.9	422.1	0.80	72.0	0.01	0.07	0.10	0.02	0.02	2.3	0	0.2	4.1
27	338	0.00	0	33.8	459.0	1.22	114.0	—	—	0.14	—	—	—	0	0.2	—
24	219	0.17	8.2	61.2	388.4	1.02	56.1	0.00	0.09	0.07	0.01	0.01	1.7	0	0.3	4.5
0	60	0.00	—	75.0	97.5	—	—	—	—	—	—	—	—	—	—	—
0	200	0.36	—	—	190.0	—	—	—	—	—	—	—	—	0	—	—
6	16	0.01	1.5	19.5	6.2	0.08	14.6	0.01	0.05	0.02	0.01	0.01	0.5	0.1	0	0.3
21	10	0.00	1.1	11.3	5.7	0.03	61.7	0.00	0.15	0.01	0.01	0.00	0.6	0.1	0	0.1
10	14	0.01	1.4	18.3	6.0	0.04	27.2	0.01	0.08	0.02	0.01	0.01	0.3	0.1	0	0.1
17	10	0.00	1.1	14.6	5.1	0.03	41.9	0.00	0.13	0.01	0.01	0.00	0.6	0.1	0	0.1
2	3	0.00	0.3	4.4	3.9	0.01	5.6	0.00	0.01	0.00	0.00	0.00	0.1	0	0	0
3	40	0.00	3.2	41.3	45.1	0.16	23.4	0.01	0.00	0.04	0.02	0.01	3.5	0	0.1	1.7
11	28	0.01	2.6	34.6	12.7	0.06	42.5	0.01	0.14	0.03	0.01	0.00	2.6	0.2	0.1	0.5
0	0	0.00	—	30.0	0	—	0	0.01	—	0.01	0.20	—	—	0	—	—
0	0	0.02	0.1	16.2	3.6	0.01	0	0.00	0.01	0.00	0.00	0.00	0	0	0	0
0	1	0.11	1.7	46.3	29.3	0.34	0	0.00	0.21	0.00	0.00	0.00	0	0	0	0.7
0	1	0.00	0	28.9	12.0	0.00	0.2	0.00	0.12	0.00	0.00	0.00	0	0	0	0.2
0	0	0.00	0.1	0.9	1.2	0.00	0.3	0.00	0.05	0.00	0.00	0.00	0	0	0	0.1
0	0	0.00	0	0.8	2.8	0.00	0.2	0.00	0.04	0.00	0.00	0.00	0	0	0	0.1

TABLE A-1 Table of Food Composition (*continued*) (Computer code is for Cengage Diet Analysis program) (For purposes of calculations, use "0" for t, <1, <.1, <.01, etc.

DA+ Code	Food Description	Quantity	Measure	Wt (g)	H₂O (g)	Ener (kcal)	Prot (g)	Carb (g)	Fiber (g)	Fat (g)	Fat Breakdown (g) Sat	Mono	Poly	*Trans*
Dairy—*continued*														
	Fluid milk													
60	Buttermilk, low fat	1	cup(s)	245	220.8	98	8.1	11.7	0	2.2	1.3	0.6	0.1	—
54	Low fat, 1%	1	cup(s)	244	219.4	102	8.2	12.2	0	2.4	1.5	0.7	0.1	—
55	Low fat, 1%, with nonfat milk solids	1	cup(s)	245	220.0	105	8.5	12.2	0	2.4	1.5	0.7	0.1	—
57	Nonfat, skim or fat free	1	cup(s)	245	222.6	83	8.3	12.2	0	0.2	0.1	0.1	0	—
58	Nonfat, skim or fat free with nonfat milk solids	1	cup(s)	245	221.4	91	8.7	12.3	0	0.6	0.4	0.2	0	—
51	Reduced fat, 2%	1	cup(s)	244	218.0	122	8.1	11.4	0	4.8	3.1	1.4	0.2	—
52	Reduced fat, 2%, with nonfat milk solids	1	cup(s)	245	217.7	125	8.5	12.2	0	4.7	2.9	1.4	0.2	—
50	Whole, 3.3%	1	cup(s)	244	215.5	146	7.9	11.0	0	7.9	4.6	2.0	0.5	—
	Canned milk													
62	Nonfat or skim evaporated	2	tablespoon(s)	32	25.3	25	2.4	3.6	0	0.1	0	0	0	—
63	Sweetened condensed	2	tablespoon(s)	38	10.4	123	3.0	20.8	0	3.3	2.1	0.9	0.1	—
61	Whole evaporated	2	tablespoon(s)	32	23.3	42	2.1	3.2	0	2.4	1.4	0.7	0.1	—
	Dried milk													
64	Buttermilk	¼	cup(s)	30	0.9	117	10.4	14.9	0	1.8	1.1	0.5	0.1	—
65	Instant nonfat with added vitamin A	¼	cup(s)	17	0.7	61	6.0	8.9	0	0.1	0.1	0	0	—
5234	Skim milk powder	¼	cup(s)	17	0.7	62	6.1	9.1	0	0.1	0.1	0	0	—
907	Whole dry milk	¼	cup(s)	32	0.8	159	8.4	12.3	0	8.5	5.4	2.5	0.2	—
909	**Goat milk**	1	cup(s)	244	212.4	168	8.7	10.9	0	10.1	6.5	2.7	0.4	—
	Chocolate milk													
33155	Chocolate syrup, prepared with milk	1	cup(s)	282	227.0	254	8.7	36.0	0.8	8.3	4.7	2.1	0.5	—
33184	Cocoa mix with aspartame, added sodium and vitamin A, no added calcium or phosphorus, prepared with water	1	cup(s)	192	177.4	56	2.3	10.8	1.2	0.4	0.3	0.1	0	—
908	Hot cocoa, prepared with milk	1	cup(s)	250	206.4	193	8.8	26.6	2.5	5.8	3.6	1.7	0.1	0.2
69	Low fat	1	cup(s)	250	211.3	158	8.1	26.1	1.3	2.5	1.5	0.8	0.1	—
68	Reduced fat	1	cup(s)	250	205.4	190	7.5	30.3	1.8	4.8	2.9	1.1	0.2	—
67	Whole	1	cup(s)	250	205.8	208	7.9	25.9	2.0	8.5	5.3	2.5	0.3	—
70	**Eggnog**	1	cup(s)	254	188.9	343	9.7	34.4	0	19.0	11.3	5.7	0.9	—
	Breakfast drinks													
10093	Carnation Instant Breakfast classic chocolate malt, prepared with skim milk, no sugar added	1	cup(s)	243	—	142	11.1	21.3	0.7	1.3	0.7	—	—	—
10092	Carnation Instant Breakfast classic French vanilla, prepared with skim milk, no sugar added	1	cup(s)	273	—	150	12.9	24.0	0	0.4	0.4	—	—	—
10094	Carnation Instant Breakfast stawberry sensation, prepared with skim milk, no sugar added	1	cup(s)	243	—	142	11.1	21.3	0	0.4	0.4	—	—	—
10091	Carnation Instant Breakfast strawberry sensation, prepared with skim milk	1	cup(s)	273	—	220	12.5	38.8	0	0.4	0.4	—	—	—
1417	Ovaltine rich chocolate flavor, prepared with skim milk	1	cup(s)	258	—	170	8.5	31.0	0	0	0	0	0	0
8539	**Malted milk, chocolate mix, fortified, prepared with milk**	1	cup(s)	265	215.8	223	8.9	28.9	1.1	8.6	5.0	2.2	0.5	—
	Milkshakes													
73	Chocolate	1	cup(s)	227	164.0	270	6.9	48.1	0.7	6.1	3.8	1.8	0.2	—
3163	Strawberry	1	cup(s)	226	167.8	256	7.7	42.8	0.9	6.3	3.9	—	—	—
74	Vanilla	1	cup(s)	227	169.2	254	8.8	40.3	0	6.9	4.3	2.0	0.3	—
	Ice cream													
4776	Chocolate	½	cup(s)	66	36.8	143	2.5	18.6	0.8	7.3	4.5	2.1	0.3	—
12137	Chocolate fudge, no sugar added	½	cup(s)	71	—	100	3.0	16.0	2.0	3.0	1.5	—	—	0
16514	Chocolate, soft serve	½	cup(s)	87	49.9	177	3.2	24.1	0.7	8.4	5.2	2.4	0.3	—
16523	Sherbet, all flavors	½	cup(s)	97	63.8	139	1.1	29.3	3.2	1.9	1.1	0.5	0.1	—
4778	Strawberry	½	cup(s)	66	39.6	127	2.1	18.2	0.6	5.5	3.4	—	—	—
76	Vanilla	½	cup(s)	72	43.9	145	2.5	17.0	0.5	7.9	4.9	2.1	0.3	—
12146	Vanilla chocolate swirl, fat-free, no sugar added	½	cup(s)	71	—	100	3.0	14.0	2.0	3.0	2.0	—	—	0
82	Vanilla, light	½	cup(s)	76	48.3	125	3.6	19.6	0.2	3.7	2.2	1.0	0.2	—
78	Vanilla, light, soft serve	½	cup(s)	88	61.2	111	4.3	19.2	0	2.3	1.4	0.7	0.1	—

Chol (mg)	Calc (mg)	Iron (mg)	Magn (mg)	Pota (mg)	Sodi (mg)	Zinc (mg)	Vit A (µg)	Thia (mg)	Vit E (mg α)	Ribo (mg)	Niac (mg)	Vit B$_6$ (mg)	Fola (µg)	Vit C (mg)	Vit B$_{12}$ (µg)	Sele (µg)
10	284	0.12	27.0	370.0	257.3	1.02	17.2	0.08	0.12	0.37	0.14	0.08	12.3	2.5	0.5	4.9
12	290	0.07	26.8	366.0	107.4	1.02	141.5	0.04	0.02	0.45	0.22	0.09	12.2	0	1.1	8.1
10	314	0.12	34.3	396.9	127.4	0.98	144.6	0.09	—	0.42	0.22	0.11	12.3	2.5	0.9	5.6
5	306	0.07	27.0	382.2	102.9	1.02	149.5	0.11	0.02	0.44	0.23	0.09	12.3	0	1.3	7.6
5	316	0.12	36.8	419.0	129.9	1.00	149.5	0.10	0.00	0.42	0.22	0.11	12.3	2.5	1.0	5.4
20	285	0.07	26.8	366.0	100.0	1.04	134.2	0.09	0.07	0.45	0.22	0.09	12.2	0.5	1.1	6.1
20	314	0.12	34.3	396.9	127.4	0.98	137.2	0.09	—	0.42	0.22	0.11	12.3	2.5	0.9	5.6
24	276	0.07	24.4	348.9	97.6	0.97	68.3	0.10	0.14	0.44	0.26	0.08	12.2	0	1.1	9.0
1	93	0.09	8.6	105.9	36.7	0.28	37.6	0.01	0.00	0.09	0.05	0.01	2.9	0.4	0.1	0.8
13	109	0.07	9.9	141.9	48.6	0.36	28.3	0.03	0.06	0.16	0.08	0.02	4.2	1.0	0.2	5.7
9	82	0.06	7.6	95.4	33.4	0.24	20.5	0.01	0.04	0.10	0.06	0.01	2.5	0.6	0.1	0.7
21	359	0.09	33.3	482.5	156.7	1.21	14.9	0.11	0.03	0.48	0.27	0.10	14.2	1.7	1.2	6.2
3	209	0.05	19.9	289.9	93.3	0.75	120.5	0.07	0.00	0.30	0.15	0.06	8.5	1.0	0.7	4.6
3	214	0.05	20.3	296.0	95.3	0.76	123.1	0.07	0.00	0.30	0.15	0.06	8.7	1.0	0.7	4.7
31	292	0.15	27.2	425.6	118.7	1.06	82.2	0.09	0.15	0.38	0.20	0.09	11.8	2.8	1.0	5.2
27	327	0.12	34.2	497.8	122.0	0.73	139.1	0.11	0.17	0.33	0.67	0.11	2.4	3.2	0.2	3.4
25	251	0.90	50.8	408.9	132.5	1.21	70.5	0.11	0.14	0.46	0.38	0.09	14.1	0	1.1	9.6
0	92	0.74	32.6	405.1	138.2	0.51	0	0.04	0.00	0.20	0.16	0.04	1.9	0	0.2	2.5
20	263	1.20	57.5	492.5	110.0	1.57	127.5	0.09	0.07	0.45	0.33	0.10	12.5	0.5	1.1	6.8
8	288	0.60	32.5	425.0	152.5	1.02	145.0	0.09	0.05	0.41	0.31	0.10	12.5	2.3	0.9	4.8
20	273	0.60	35.0	422.5	165.0	0.97	160.0	0.11	0.10	0.45	0.41	0.06	5.0	0	0.8	8.5
30	280	0.60	32.5	417.5	150.0	1.02	65.0	0.09	0.15	0.40	0.31	0.10	12.5	2.3	0.8	4.8
150	330	0.50	48.3	419.1	137.2	1.16	116.8	0.08	0.50	0.48	0.26	0.12	2.5	3.8	1.1	10.7
9	444	4.00	88.9	631.1	195.6	3.38	—	0.33	—	0.45	4.44	0.44	4.0	26.7	1.3	8.0
9	500	4.50	100.0	665.0	192.0	3.75	—	0.37	—	0.51	5.00	0.49	100.0	30.0	1.5	9.0
9	444	4.00	88.9	568.9	186.7	3.38	—	0.33	—	0.45	4.44	0.44	88.9	26.7	1.3	8.0
9	500	4.47	100.0	665.0	288.0	3.75	—	0.37	—	0.51	5.07	0.50	100.0	30.0	1.5	8.8
5	350	3.60	100.0	—	270.0	3.75	—	0.37	—	—	4.00	0.40	—	12.0	1.2	—
27	339	3.76	45.1	577.7	230.6	1.16	903.7	0.75	0.15	1.31	11.08	1.01	18.6	31.8	1.1	12.5
25	300	0.70	36.4	508.9	252.2	1.09	40.9	0.10	0.11	0.50	0.28	0.05	11.4	0	0.7	4.3
25	256	0.24	29.4	412.0	187.9	0.81	58.9	0.10	—	0.44	0.39	0.10	6.8	1.8	0.7	4.8
27	332	0.22	27.3	415.8	215.8	0.88	56.8	0.06	0.11	0.44	0.33	0.09	15.9	0	1.2	5.2
22	72	0.61	19.1	164.3	50.2	0.38	77.9	0.02	0.19	0.12	0.14	0.03	10.6	0.5	0.2	1.7
10	100	0.36	—	—	65.0	—	—	—	—	—	—	—	—	0	—	—
22	103	0.32	19.0	192.0	43.3	0.45	66.6	0.03	0.22	0.13	0.11	0.03	4.3	0.5	0.3	2.5
0	52	0.13	7.7	92.6	44.4	0.46	9.7	0.02	0.02	0.08	0.07	0.02	6.8	5.6	0.1	1.3
19	79	0.13	9.2	124.1	39.6	0.22	63.4	0.03	—	0.16	0.11	0.03	7.9	5.1	0.2	1.3
32	92	0.06	10.1	143.3	57.6	0.49	85.0	0.03	0.21	0.17	0.08	0.03	3.6	0.4	0.3	1.3
10	100	0.00	—	—	65.0	—	—	—	—	—	—	—	—	0	—	—
21	122	0.14	10.6	158.1	56.2	0.55	97.3	0.04	0.09	0.19	0.10	0.03	4.6	0.9	0.4	1.5
11	138	0.05	12.3	194.5	61.6	0.46	25.5	0.04	0.05	0.17	0.10	0.04	4.4	0.8	0.4	3.2

TABLE A-1 Table of Food Composition (*continued*) (Computer code is for Cengage Diet Analysis program) (For purposes of calculations, use "0" for t, <1, <.1, <.01, etc.)

DA+ Code	Food Description	Quantity	Measure	Wt (g)	H₂O (g)	Ener (kcal)	Prot (g)	Carb (g)	Fiber (g)	Fat (g)	Fat Breakdown (g) Sat	Mono	Poly	*Trans*
Dairy—*continued*														
	Soy desserts													
10694	Tofutti low fat vanilla fudge nondairy frozen dessert	½	cup(s)	70	—	140	2.0	24.0	0	4.0	1.0	—	—	—
15721	Tofutti premium chocolate supreme nondairy frozen dessert	½	cup(s)	70	—	180	3.0	18.0	0	11.0	2.0	—	—	—
15720	Tofutti premium vanilla non-dairy frozen dessert	½	cup(s)	70	—	190	2.0	20.0	0	11.0	2.0	—	—	—
	Ice milk													
16517	Chocolate	½	cup(s)	66	42.9	94	2.8	16.9	0.3	2.1	1.3	0.6	0.1	—
16516	Flavored, not chocolate	½	cup(s)	66	41.4	108	3.5	17.5	0.2	2.6	1.7	0.6	0.1	—
	Pudding													
25032	Chocolate	½	cup(s)	144	109.7	155	5.1	22.7	0.7	5.4	3.1	1.7	0.2	0
1923	Chocolate, sugar free, prepared with 2% milk	½	cup(s)	133	—	100	5.0	14.0	0.3	3.0	1.5	—	—	—
1722	Rice	½	cup(s)	113	75.6	151	4.1	29.9	0.5	1.9	1.1	0.5	0.1	—
4747	Tapioca, ready to eat	1	item(s)	142	102.0	185	2.8	30.8	0	5.5	1.4	3.6	0.1	—
25031	Vanilla	½	cup(s)	136	109.7	116	4.7	17.6	0	2.8	1.6	0.9	0.2	0
1924	Vanilla, sugar free, prepared with 2% milk	½	cup(s)	133	—	90	4.0	12.0	0.2	2.0	1.5	—	—	—
	Frozen yogurt													
4785	Chocolate, soft serve	½	cup(s)	72	45.9	115	2.9	17.9	1.6	4.3	2.6	1.3	0.2	—
1747	Fruit varieties	½	cup(s)	113	80.5	144	3.4	24.4	0	4.1	2.6	1.1	0.1	—
4786	Vanilla, soft serve	½	cup(s)	72	47.0	117	2.9	17.4	0	4.0	2.5	1.1	0.2	—
	Milk substitutes													
	Lactose free													
16081	Fat-free, calcium fortified [milk]	1	cup(s)	240	—	80	8.0	13.0	0	0	0	0	0	0
36486	Low fat milk	1	cup(s)	240	—	110	8.0	13.0	0	2.5	1.5	—	—	—
36487	Reduced fat milk	1	cup(s)	240	—	130	8.0	12.0	0	5.0	3.0	—	—	—
36488	Whole milk	1	cup(s)	240	—	150	8.0	12.0	0	8.0	5.0	—	—	—
	Rice													
10083	Rice Dream carob rice beverage	1	cup(s)	240	—	150	1.0	32.0	0	2.5	0	—	—	—
17089	Rice Dream original rice beverage, enriched	1	cup(s)	240	—	120	1.0	25.0	0	2.0	0	—	—	—
10087	Rice Dream vanilla enriched rice beverage	1	cup(s)	240	—	130	1.0	28.0	0	2.0	0	—	—	—
	Soy													
34750	Soy Dream chocolate enriched soy beverage	1	cup(s)	240	—	210	7.0	37.0	1.0	3.5	0.5	—	—	—
34749	Soy Dream vanilla enriched soy beverage	1	cup(s)	240	—	150	7.0	22.0	0	4.0	0.5	—	—	—
13840	Vitasoy light chocolate soymilk	1	cup(s)	240	—	100	4.0	17.0	0	2.0	0.5	0.5	1.0	—
13839	Vitasoy light vanilla soymilk	1	cup(s)	240	—	70	4.0	10.0	0	2.0	0.5	0.5	1.0	—
13836	Vitasoy rich chocolate soymilk	1	cup(s)	240	—	160	7.0	24.0	1.0	4.0	0.5	1.0	2.5	—
13835	Vitasoy vanilla delite soymilk	1	cup(s)	240	—	120	7.0	13.0	1.0	4.0	0.5	1.0	2.5	—
	Yogurt													
3615	Custard style, fruit flavors	6	ounce(s)	170	127.1	190	7.0	32.0	0	3.5	2.0	—	—	—
3617	Custard style, vanilla	6	ounce(s)	170	134.1	190	7.0	32.0	0	3.5	2.0	0.9	0.1	—
32101	Fruit, low fat	1	cup(s)	245	184.5	243	9.8	45.7	0	2.8	1.8	0.8	0.1	—
29638	Fruit, nonfat, sweetened with low-calorie sweetener	1	cup(s)	241	208.3	123	10.6	19.4	1.2	0.4	0.2	0.1	0	—
93	Plain, low fat	1	cup(s)	245	208.4	154	12.9	17.2	0	3.8	2.5	1.0	0.1	—
94	Plain, nonfat	1	cup(s)	245	208.8	137	14.0	18.8	0	0.4	0.3	0.1	0	—
32100	Vanilla, low fat	1	cup(s)	245	193.6	208	12.1	33.8	0	3.1	2.0	0.8	0.1	—
5242	Yogurt beverage	1	cup(s)	245	199.8	172	6.2	32.8	0	2.2	1.4	0.6	0.1	—
38202	Yogurt smoothie, nonfat, all flavors	1	item(s)	325	—	290	10.0	60.0	6.0	0	0	0	0	0
	Soy yogurt													
34617	Stonyfield Farm O'Soy strawberry-peach pack organic cultured soy yogurt	1	item(s)	113	—	100	5.0	16.0	3.0	2.0	0	—	—	0
34616	Stonyfield Farm O'Soy vanilla organic cultured soy yogurt	1	item(s)	170	—	150	7.0	26.0	4.0	2.0	0	—	—	0
10453	White Wave plain silk cultured soy yogurt	8	ounce(s)	227	—	140	5.0	22.0	1.0	3.0	0.5	—	—	0

PAGE KEY: A-6 = Breads/Baked Goods A-12 = Cereal/Rice/Pasta A-16 = Fruit A-20 = Vegetables/Legumes A-30 = Nuts/Seeds A-32 = Vegetarian A-34 = Dairy A-42 = Eggs A-42 = Seafood A-44 = Meats A-48 = Poultry
A-48 = Processed Meats A-50 = Beverages A-54 = Fats/Oils A-56 = Sweets A-58 = Spices/Condiments/Sauces A-62 = Mixed Foods/Soups/Sandwiches A-66 = Fast Food A-86 = Convenience A-88 = Baby Foods

Chol (mg)	Calc (mg)	Iron (mg)	Magn (mg)	Pota (mg)	Sodi (mg)	Zinc (mg)	Vit A (µg)	Thia (mg)	Vit E (mg α)	Ribo (mg)	Niac (mg)	Vit B$_6$ (mg)	Fola (µg)	Vit C (mg)	Vit B$_{12}$ (µg)	Sele (µg)
0	0	0.00	—	8.0	90.0	—	0	—	—	—	—	—	—	0	—	—
0	0	0.00	—	7.0	180.0	—	0	—	—	—	—	—	—	0	—	—
0	0	0.00	—	2.0	210.0	—	0	—	—	—	—	—	—	0	—	—
6	94	0.15	13.1	155.2	40.6	0.36	15.7	0.03	0.05	0.11	0.08	0.02	3.9	0.5	0.3	2.2
16	76	0.05	9.2	136.2	48.5	0.47	90.4	0.02	0.05	0.11	0.06	0.01	3.3	0.1	0.2	1.3
35	149	0.46	31.3	226.7	137.0	0.71	—	0.05	0.00	0.22	0.15	0.06	8.3	1.2	0.5	4.9
10	150	0.72	—	330.0	310.0	—	—	0.06	—	0.26	—	—	—	0	—	—
7	113	0.28	15.8	201.4	66.4	0.52	41.6	0.03	0.05	0.17	0.34	0.06	4.5	0.2	0.2	4.8
1	101	0.15	8.5	130.6	205.9	0.31	0	0.03	0.21	0.13	0.09	0.03	4.3	0.4	0.3	0
35	146	0.17	17.2	188.9	136.4	0.52	—	0.04	0.00	0.22	0.10	0.05	8.0	1.2	0.5	4.6
10	150	0.00	—	190.0	380.0	—	—	0.03	—	0.17	—	—	—	0	—	—
4	106	0.90	19.4	187.9	70.6	0.35	31.7	0.02	—	0.15	0.22	0.05	7.9	0.2	0.2	1.7
15	113	0.52	11.3	176.3	71.2	0.31	55.4	0.04	0.10	0.20	0.07	0.04	4.5	0.8	0.1	2.1
1	103	0.21	10.1	151.9	62.6	0.30	42.5	0.02	0.07	0.16	0.20	0.05	4.3	0.6	0.2	2.4
3	500	0.00	—	—	125.0	—	100.0	—	—	—	—	—	—	0	0	—
10	300	0.00	—	—	125.0	—	100.0	—	—	—	—	—	—	0	—	—
20	300	0.00	—	—	125.0	—	98.2	—	—	—	—	—	—	0	—	—
35	300	0.00	—	—	125.0	—	58.1	—	—	—	—	—	—	0	—	—
0	20	0.72	—	82.5	100.0	—	—	—	—	—	—	—	—	1.2	—	—
0	300	0.00	13.3	60.0	90.0	0.24	—	0.06	—	0.00	0.84	0.07	—	0	1.5	—
0	300	0.00	—	53.0	90.0	—	—	—	—	—	—	—	—	0	1.5	—
0	300	1.80	60.0	350.0	160.0	0.60	33.3	0.15	—	0.06	0.80	0.12	60.0	0	3.0	—
0	300	1.80	40.0	260.0	140.0	0.60	33.3	0.15	—	0.06	0.80	0.12	60.0	0	3.0	—
0	300	0.72	24.0	200.0	140.0	0.90	—	0.09	—	0.34	—	—	24.0	0	0.9	—
0	300	0.72	24.0	200.0	120.0	0.90	—	0.09	—	0.34	—	—	24.0	0	0.9	—
0	300	1.08	40.0	320.0	150.0	0.90	—	0.15	—	0.34	—	—	60.0	0	0.9	—
0	40	0.72	—	320.0	115.0	—	0	—	—	—	—	—	—	0	—	—
15	300	0.00	16.0	310.0	100.0	—	—	—	—	0.25	—	—	—	0	—	—
15	300	0.00	16.0	310.0	100.0	—	—	—	—	0.25	—	—	—	0	—	—
12	338	0.14	31.9	433.7	129.9	1.64	27.0	0.08	0.04	0.39	0.21	0.09	22.1	1.5	1.1	6.9
5	369	0.62	41.0	549.5	139.8	1.83	4.8	0.10	0.16	0.44	0.49	0.10	31.3	26.5	1.1	7.0
15	448	0.19	41.7	573.3	171.5	2.18	34.3	0.10	0.07	0.52	0.27	0.12	27.0	2.0	1.4	8.1
5	488	0.22	46.6	624.8	188.7	2.37	4.9	0.11	0.00	0.57	0.30	0.13	29.4	2.2	1.5	8.8
12	419	0.17	39.2	536.6	161.7	2.03	29.4	0.10	0.04	0.49	0.26	0.11	27.0	2.0	1.3	12.0
13	260	0.22	39.2	399.4	98.0	1.10	14.7	0.11	0.00	0.51	0.30	0.14	29.4	2.1	1.5	—
5	300	2.70	100.0	580.0	290.0	2.25	—	0.37	—	0.42	5.00	0.50	100.0	15.0	1.5	—
0	100	1.08	24.0	5.0	20.0	—	0	0.22	—	0.10	—	0.04	—	0	0	—
0	150	1.44	40.0	15.0	40.0	—	—	0.30	—	0.13	—	0.08	—	0	0	—
0	400	1.44	—	0	30.0	—	0	—	—	—	—	—	—	0	—	—

TABLE A-1 Table of Food Composition (*continued*) (Computer code is for Cengage Diet Analysis program) (For purposes of calculations, use "0" for t, <1, <.1, <.01, etc.)

DA+ Code	Food Description	Quantity	Measure	Wt (g)	H₂O (g)	Ener (kcal)	Prot (g)	Carb (g)	Fiber (g)	Fat (g)	Fat Breakdown (g)			
											Sat	Mono	Poly	*Trans*
Eggs														
	Eggs													
99	Fried	1	item(s)	46	31.8	90	6.3	0.4	0	7.0	2.0	2.9	1.2	—
100	Hard boiled	1	item(s)	50	37.3	78	6.3	0.6	0	5.3	1.6	2.0	0.7	—
101	Poached	1	item(s)	50	37.8	71	6.3	0.4	0	5.0	1.5	1.9	0.7	—
97	Raw, white	1	item(s)	33	28.9	16	3.6	0.2	0	0.1	0	0	0	—
96	Raw, whole	1	item(s)	50	37.9	72	6.3	0.4	0	5.0	1.5	1.9	0.7	—
98	Raw, yolk	1	item(s)	17	8.9	54	2.7	0.6	0	4.5	1.6	2.0	0.7	—
102	Scrambled, prepared with milk and butter	2	item(s)	122	89.2	204	13.5	2.7	0	14.9	4.5	5.8	2.6	0.7
	Egg substitute													
4028	Egg Beaters	¼	cup(s)	61	—	30	6.0	1.0	0	0	0	0	0	0
920	Frozen	¼	cup(s)	60	43.9	96	6.8	1.9	0	6.7	1.2	1.5	3.7	—
918	Liquid	¼	cup(s)	63	51.9	53	7.5	0.4	0	2.1	0.4	0.6	1.0	—
Seafood														
	Cod													
6040	Atlantic cod or scrod, baked or broiled	3	ounce(s)	85	64.6	89	19.4	0	0	0.7	0.1	0.1	0.2	—
1573	Atlantic cod, cooked, dry heat	3	ounce(s)	85	64.6	89	19.4	0	0	0.7	0.1	0.1	0.2	—
2905	Eel, raw	3	ounce(s)	85	58.0	156	15.7	0	0	9.9	2.0	6.1	0.8	—
	Fish fillets													
25079	Baked	3	ounce(s)	84	79.9	99	21.7	0	0	0.7	0.1	0.1	0.3	—
8615	Batter coated or breaded, fried	3	ounce(s)	85	45.6	197	12.5	14.4	0.4	10.5	2.4	2.2	5.3	—
25082	Broiled fish steaks	3	ounce(s)	85	68.1	128	24.2	0	0	2.6	0.4	0.9	0.8	—
25083	Poached fish steaks	3	ounce(s)	85	67.1	111	21.1	0	0	2.3	0.3	0.8	0.7	—
25084	Steamed	3	ounce(s)	85	72.2	79	17.2	0	0	0.6	0.1	0.1	0.2	—
25089	**Flounder, baked**	3	ounce(s)	85	64.4	113	14.8	0.4	0.1	5.5	1.1	2.2	1.4	—
1825	**Grouper, cooked, dry heat**	3	ounce(s)	85	62.4	100	21.1	0	0	1.1	0.3	0.2	0.3	—
	Haddock													
6049	Baked or broiled	3	ounce(s)	85	63.2	95	20.6	0	0	0.8	0.1	0.1	0.3	—
1578	Cooked, dry heat	3	ounce(s)	85	63.1	95	20.6	0	0	0.8	0.1	0.1	0.3	—
1886	**Halibut, Atlantic and Pacific, cooked, dry heat**	3	ounce(s)	85	61.0	119	22.7	0	0	2.5	0.4	0.8	0.8	—
1582	**Herring, Atlantic, pickled**	4	piece(s)	60	33.1	157	8.5	5.8	0	10.8	1.4	7.2	1.0	—
1587	**Jack mackerel, solids, canned, drained**	2	ounce(s)	57	39.2	88	13.1	0	0	3.6	1.1	1.3	0.9	—
8580	**Octopus, common, cooked, moist heat**	3	ounce(s)	85	51.5	139	25.4	3.7	0	1.8	0.4	0.3	0.4	—
1831	**Perch, mixed species, cooked, dry heat**	3	ounce(s)	85	62.3	100	21.1	0	0	1.0	0.2	0.2	0.4	—
1592	**Pacific rockfish, cooked, dry heat**	3	ounce(s)	85	62.4	103	20.4	0	0	1.7	0.4	0.4	0.5	—
	Salmon													
2938	Coho, farmed, raw	3	ounce(s)	85	59.9	136	18.1	0	0	6.5	1.5	2.8	1.6	—
1594	Broiled or baked with butter	3	ounce(s)	85	53.9	155	23.0	0	0	6.3	1.2	2.3	2.3	—
29727	Smoked chinook (lox)	2	ounce(s)	57	40.8	66	10.4	0	0	2.4	0.5	1.1	0.6	—
154	**Sardine, Atlantic with bones, canned in oil**	3	ounce(s)	85	50.7	177	20.9	0	0	9.7	1.3	3.3	4.4	—
	Scallops													
155	Mixed species, breaded, fried	3	item(s)	47	27.2	100	8.4	4.7	—	5.1	1.2	2.1	1.3	—
1599	Steamed	3	ounce(s)	85	64.8	90	13.8	2.0	0	2.6	0.4	1.0	0.8	—
1839	**Snapper, mixed species, cooked, dry heat**	3	ounce(s)	85	59.8	109	22.4	0	0	1.5	0.3	0.3	0.5	—
	Squid													
1868	Mixed species, fried	3	ounce(s)	85	54.9	149	15.3	6.6	0	6.4	1.6	2.3	1.8	—
16617	Steamed or boiled	3	ounce(s)	85	63.3	89	15.2	3.0	0	1.3	0.4	0.1	0.5	—
1570	**Striped bass, cooked, dry heat**	3	ounce(s)	85	62.4	105	19.3	0	0	2.5	0.6	0.7	0.9	—
1601	**Sturgeon, steamed**	3	ounce(s)	85	59.4	111	17.0	0	0	4.3	1.0	2.0	0.7	—
1840	**Surimi, formed**	3	ounce(s)	85	64.9	84	12.9	5.8	0	0.8	0.2	0.1	0.4	—
1842	**Swordfish, cooked, dry heat**	3	ounce(s)	85	58.5	132	21.6	0	0	4.4	1.2	1.7	1.0	—
1846	**Tuna, yellowfin or ahi, raw**	3	ounce(s)	85	60.4	92	19.9	0	0	0.8	0.2	0.1	0.2	—
	Tuna, canned													
159	Light, canned in oil, drained	2	ounce(s)	57	33.9	112	16.5	0	0	4.6	0.9	1.7	1.6	—
355	Light, canned in water, drained	2	ounce(s)	57	42.2	66	14.5	0	0	0.5	0.1	0.1	0.2	—
33211	Light, no salt, canned in oil, drained	2	ounce(s)	57	33.9	112	16.5	0	0	4.7	0.9	1.7	1.6	—
33212	Light, no salt, canned in water, drained	2	ounce(s)	57	42.6	66	14.5	0	0	0.5	0.1	0.1	0.2	—

PAGE KEY: A-6 = Breads/Baked Goods A-12 = Cereal/Rice/Pasta A-16 = Fruit A-20 = Vegetables/Legumes A-30 = Nuts/Seeds A-32 = Vegetarian A-34 = Dairy A-42 = Eggs A-42 = Seafood A-44 = Meats A-48 = Poultry A-48 = Processed Meats A-50 = Beverages A-54 = Fats/Oils A-56 = Sweets A-58 = Spices/Condiments/Sauces A-62 = Mixed Foods/Soups/Sandwiches A-66 = Fast Food A-86 = Convenience A-88 = Baby Foods

Chol (mg)	Calc (mg)	Iron (mg)	Magn (mg)	Pota (mg)	Sodi (mg)	Zinc (mg)	Vit A (µg)	Thia (mg)	Vit E (mg α)	Ribo (mg)	Niac (mg)	Vit B$_6$ (mg)	Fola (µg)	Vit C (mg)	Vit B$_{12}$ (µg)	Sele (µg)
210	27	0.91	6.0	67.6	93.8	0.55	91.1	0.03	0.56	0.23	0.03	0.07	23.5	0	0.6	15.7
212	25	0.59	5.0	63.0	62.0	0.52	84.5	0.03	0.51	0.25	0.03	0.06	22.0	0	0.6	15.4
211	27	0.91	6.0	66.5	147.0	0.55	69.5	0.02	0.48	0.20	0.03	0.06	17.5	0	0.6	15.8
0	2	0.02	3.6	53.8	54.8	0.01	0	0.00	0.00	0.14	0.03	0.00	1.3	0	0	6.6
212	27	0.91	6.0	67.0	70.0	0.55	70.0	0.03	0.48	0.23	0.03	0.07	23.5	0	0.6	15.9
210	22	0.46	0.9	18.5	8.2	0.39	64.8	0.03	0.43	0.09	0.00	0.06	24.8	0	0.3	9.5
429	87	1.46	14.6	168.4	341.6	1.22	174.5	0.06	1.33	0.53	0.09	0.14	36.6	0.2	0.9	27.5
0	20	1.08	4.0	85.0	115.0	0.60	112.5	0.15	—	0.85	0.20	0.08	60.0	0	1.2	—
1	44	1.18	9.0	127.8	119.4	0.58	6.6	0.07	0.95	0.23	0.08	0.08	9.6	0.3	0.2	24.8
1	33	1.32	5.6	207.1	111.1	0.82	11.3	0.07	0.17	0.19	0.07	0.00	9.4	0	0.2	15.6
47	12	0.41	35.7	207.5	66.3	0.49	11.9	0.07	0.68	0.06	2.13	0.24	6.8	0.8	0.9	32.0
47	12	0.41	35.7	207.5	66.3	0.49	11.9	0.07	0.68	0.06	2.13	0.24	6.8	0.9	0.9	32.0
107	17	0.42	17.0	231.3	43.4	1.37	887.0	0.13	3.40	0.03	2.97	0.05	12.8	1.5	2.6	5.5
44	8	0.31	29.1	489.0	86.1	0.48	—	0.02	—	0.05	2.47	0.46	8.1	3.0	1.0	44.3
29	15	1.79	20.4	272.2	452.5	0.37	9.4	0.09	—	0.09	1.78	0.08	14.5	0	0.9	7.7
37	55	0.97	96.7	524.3	62.9	0.49	—	0.05	—	0.08	6.47	0.36	12.6	0	1.2	42.5
32	48	0.85	84.0	455.6	54.7	0.42	—	0.05	—	0.07	5.92	0.33	11.5	0	1.1	37.0
41	12	0.29	24.7	319.3	41.7	0.34	—	0.06	—	0.06	1.89	0.21	6.1	0.8	0.8	32.0
44	19	0.34	47.3	224.7	280.2	0.20	—	0.06	0.40	0.07	2.02	0.18	7.4	2.8	1.6	33.5
40	18	0.96	31.5	404.0	45.1	0.43	42.5	0.06	—	0.01	0.32	0.29	8.5	0	0.6	39.8
63	36	1.15	42.5	339.4	74.0	0.40	16.2	0.03	0.42	0.03	3.94	0.29	6.8	0	1.2	34.4
63	36	1.14	42.5	339.3	74.0	0.40	16.2	0.03	—	0.03	3.93	0.29	11.1	0	1.2	34.4
35	51	0.91	91.0	489.9	58.7	0.45	45.9	0.05	—	0.07	6.05	0.33	11.9	0	1.2	39.8
8	46	0.73	4.8	41.4	522.0	0.31	154.8	0.02	1.02	0.08	1.98	0.10	1.2	0	2.6	35.1
45	137	1.15	21.0	110.0	214.9	0.57	73.7	0.02	0.58	0.12	3.50	0.11	2.8	0.5	3.9	21.4
82	90	8.11	51.0	535.8	391.2	2.85	76.5	0.04	1.02	0.06	3.21	0.55	20.4	6.8	30.6	76.2
98	87	0.98	32.3	292.6	67.2	1.21	8.5	0.06	—	0.10	1.61	0.11	5.1	1.4	1.9	13.7
37	10	0.45	28.9	442.3	65.5	0.45	60.4	0.03	1.32	0.07	3.33	0.22	8.5	0	1.0	39.8
43	10	0.29	26.4	382.7	40.0	0.36	47.6	0.08	—	0.09	5.79	0.56	11.1	0.9	2.3	10.7
40	15	1.02	26.9	376.6	98.6	0.56	—	0.13	1.14	0.05	8.33	0.18	4.2	1.8	2.3	41.0
13	6	0.48	10.2	99.2	1134.0	0.17	14.7	0.01	—	0.05	2.67	0.15	1.1	0	1.8	21.6
121	325	2.48	33.2	337.6	429.5	1.10	27.2	0.04	1.70	0.18	4.43	0.14	10.2	0	7.6	44.8
28	20	0.38	27.4	154.8	215.8	0.49	10.7	0.02	—	0.05	0.70	0.06	17.2	1.1	0.6	12.5
27	20	0.22	45.9	238.0	358.7	0.78	32.3	0.01	0.16	0.05	0.84	0.11	10.2	2.0	1.1	18.2
40	34	0.20	31.5	444.0	48.5	0.37	29.8	0.04	—	0.00	0.29	0.39	5.1	1.4	3.0	41.7
221	33	0.85	32.3	237.3	260.3	1.48	9.4	0.04	—	0.39	2.21	0.04	11.9	3.6	1.0	44.1
227	31	0.62	28.9	192.1	356.2	1.49	8.5	0.01	1.17	0.32	1.69	0.04	3.4	3.2	1.0	43.7
88	16	0.91	43.4	279.0	74.8	0.43	26.4	0.09	—	0.03	2.17	0.29	8.5	0	3.8	39.8
63	11	0.59	29.8	239.7	388.5	0.35	198.9	0.06	0.52	0.07	8.30	0.19	14.5	0	2.2	13.3
26	8	0.22	36.6	95.3	121.6	0.28	17.0	0.01	0.53	0.01	0.18	0.02	1.7	0	1.4	23.9
43	5	0.88	28.9	313.8	97.8	1.25	34.9	0.03	—	0.09	10.02	0.32	1.7	0.9	1.7	52.5
38	14	0.62	42.5	377.6	31.5	0.44	15.3	0.37	0.42	0.04	8.33	0.77	1.7	0.8	0.4	31.0
10	7	0.79	17.6	117.3	200.6	0.51	13.0	0.02	0.49	0.07	7.03	0.06	2.8	0	1.2	43.1
17	6	0.87	15.3	134.3	191.5	0.43	9.6	0.01	0.19	0.04	7.52	0.19	2.3	0	1.7	45.6
10	7	0.78	17.6	117.4	28.3	0.51	0	0.02	—	0.06	7.03	0.06	2.8	0	1.2	43.1
17	6	0.86	15.3	134.4	28.3	0.43	0	0.01	—	0.04	7.52	0.19	2.3	0	1.7	45.6

TABLE A-1 Table of Food Composition (continued) (Computer code is for Cengage Diet Analysis program) (For purposes of calculations, use "0" for t, <1, <.1, <.01, etc.)

DA+ Code	Food Description	Quantity	Measure	Wt (g)	H₂O (g)	Ener (kcal)	Prot (g)	Carb (g)	Fiber (g)	Fat (g)	Fat Breakdown (g) Sat	Mono	Poly	Trans
Seafood—*continued*														
2961	White, canned in oil, drained	2	ounce(s)	57	36.3	105	15.0	0	0	4.6	0.7	1.8	1.7	—
351	White, canned in water, drained	2	ounce(s)	57	41.5	73	13.4	0	0	1.7	0.4	0.4	0.6	—
33213	White, no salt, canned in oil, drained	2	ounce(s)	57	36.3	105	15.0	0	0	4.6	0.9	1.4	1.9	—
33214	White, no salt, canned in water, drained	2	ounce(s)	57	42.0	73	13.4	0	0	1.7	0.4	0.4	0.6	—
	Yellowtail													
8548	Mixed species, cooked, dry heat	3	ounce(s)	85	57.3	159	25.2	0	0	5.7	1.4	2.2	1.5	
2970	Mixed species, raw	2	ounce(s)	57	42.2	83	13.1	0	0	3.0	0.7	1.1	0.8	
	Shellfish, meat only													
1857	Abalone, mixed species, fried	3	ounce(s)	85	51.1	161	16.7	9.4	0	5.8	1.4	2.3	1.4	—
16618	Abalone, steamed or poached	3	ounce(s)	85	40.7	177	28.8	10.1	0	1.3	0.3	0.2	0.2	—
	Crab													
1851	Blue crab, canned	2	ounce(s)	57	43.2	56	11.6	0	0	0.7	0.1	0.1	0.2	—
1852	Blue crab, cooked, moist heat	3	ounce(s)	85	65.9	87	17.2	0	0	1.5	0.2	0.2	0.6	—
8562	Dungeness crab, cooked, moist heat	3	ounce(s)	85	62.3	94	19.0	0.8	0	1.1	0.1	0.2	0.3	—
1860	**Clams, cooked, moist heat**	3	ounce(s)	85	54.1	126	21.7	4.4	0	1.7	0.2	0.1	0.5	
1853	**Crayfish, farmed, cooked, moist heat**	3	ounce(s)	85	68.7	74	14.9	0	0	1.1	0.2	0.2	0.4	
	Oysters													
8720	Baked or broiled	3	ounce(s)	85	68.6	89	5.6	3.2	0	5.8	1.3	2.1	1.9	—
152	Eastern, farmed, raw	3	ounce(s)	85	73.3	50	4.4	4.7	0	1.3	0.4	0.1	0.5	—
8715	Eastern, wild, cooked, moist heat	3	ounce(s)	85	59.8	117	12.0	6.7	0	4.2	1.3	0.5	1.6	—
8584	Pacific, cooked, moist heat	3	ounce(s)	85	54.5	139	16.1	8.4	0	3.9	0.9	0.7	1.5	—
1865	Pacific, raw	3	ounce(s)	85	69.8	69	8.0	4.2	0	2.0	0.4	0.3	0.8	—
1854	**Lobster, northern, cooked, moist heat**	3	ounce(s)	85	64.7	83	17.4	1.1	0	0.5	0.1	0.1	0.1	—
1862	**Mussel, blue, cooked, moist heat**	3	ounce(s)	85	52.0	146	20.2	6.3	0	3.8	0.7	0.9	1.0	—
	Shrimp													
158	Mixed species, breaded, fried	3	ounce(s)	85	44.9	206	18.2	9.8	0.3	10.4	1.8	3.2	4.3	—
1855	Mixed species, cooked, moist heat	3	ounce(s)	85	65.7	84	17.8	0	0	0.9	0.2	0.2	0.4	—
Beef, Lamb, Pork														
	Beef													
4450	Breakfast strips, cooked	2	slice(s)	23	5.9	101	7.1	0.3	0	7.8	3.2	3.8	0.4	—
174	Corned beef, canned	3	ounce(s)	85	49.1	213	23.0	0	0	12.7	5.3	5.1	0.5	—
33147	Cured, thin siced	2	ounce(s)	57	32.9	100	15.9	3.2	0	2.2	0.9	1.0	0.1	—
4581	Jerky	1	ounce(s)	28	6.6	116	9.4	3.1	0.5	7.3	3.1	3.2	0.3	—
	Ground beef													
5898	Lean, broiled, medium	3	ounce(s)	85	50.4	202	21.6	0	0	12.2	4.8	5.3	0.4	—
5899	Lean, broiled, well done	3	ounce(s)	85	48.4	214	23.8	0	0	12.5	5.0	5.7	0.3	0.4
5914	Regular, broiled, medium	3	ounce(s)	85	46.1	246	20.5	0	0	17.6	6.9	7.7	0.6	—
5915	Regular, broiled, well done	3	ounce(s)	85	43.8	259	21.6	0	0	18.4	7.5	8.5	0.5	0.6
	Beef rib													
4241	Rib, small end, separable lean, 0" fat, broiled	3	ounce(s)	85	53.2	164	25.0	0	0	6.4	2.4	2.6	0.2	—
4183	Rib, whole, lean and fat, ¼" fat, roasted	3	ounce(s)	85	39.0	320	18.9	0	0	26.6	10.7	11.4	0.9	—
	Beef roast													
16981	Bottom round, choice, separable lean and fat, ⅛" fat, braised	3	ounce(s)	85	46.2	216	27.9	0	0	10.7	4.1	4.6	0.4	—
16979	Bottom round, separable lean and fat, ⅛" fat, roasted	3	ounce(s)	85	52.4	185	22.5	0	0	9.9	3.8	4.2	0.4	—
16924	Chuck, arm pot roast, separable lean and fat, ⅛" fat, braised	3	ounce(s)	85	42.9	257	25.6	0	0	16.3	6.5	7.0	0.6	—
16930	Chuck, blade roast, separable lean and fat, ⅛" fat, braised	3	ounce(s)	85	40.5	290	22.8	0	0	21.4	8.5	9.2	0.8	—
5853	Chuck, blade roast, separable lean, 0" trim, pot roasted	3	ounce(s)	85	47.4	202	26.4	0	0	9.9	3.9	4.3	0.3	—
4296	Eye of round, choice, separable lean, 0" fat, roasted	3	ounce(s)	85	56.5	138	24.4	0	0	3.7	1.3	1.5	0.1	—
16989	Eye of round, separable lean and fat, ⅛" fat, roasted	3	ounce(s)	85	52.2	180	24.2	0	0	8.5	3.2	3.6	0.3	—

AGE KEY: A-6 = Breads/Baked Goods A-12 = Cereal/Rice/Pasta A-16 = Fruit A-20 = Vegetables/Legumes A-30 = Nuts/Seeds A-32 = Vegetarian A-34 = Dairy A-42 = Eggs A-42 = Seafood A-44 = Meats A-48 = Poultry A-48 = Processed Meats A-50 = Beverages A-54 = Fats/Oils A-56 = Sweets A-58 = Spices/Condiments/Sauces A-62 = Mixed Foods/Soups/Sandwiches A-66 = Fast Food A-86 = Convenience A-88 = Baby Foods

Chol (mg)	Calc (mg)	Iron (mg)	Magn (mg)	Pota (mg)	Sodi (mg)	Zinc (mg)	Vit A (µg)	Thia (mg)	Vit E (mg α)	Ribo (mg)	Niac (mg)	Vit B6 (mg)	Fola (µg)	Vit C (mg)	Vit B12 (µg)	Sele (µg)
18	2	0.36	19.3	188.8	224.5	0.26	2.8	0.01	1.30	0.04	6.63	0.24	2.8	0	1.2	34.1
24	8	0.55	18.7	134.3	213.6	0.27	3.4	0.00	0.48	0.02	3.28	0.12	1.1	0	0.7	37.2
18	2	0.36	19.3	188.8	28.3	0.26	0	0.01	—	0.04	6.63	0.24	2.8	0	1.2	34.1
24	8	0.54	18.7	134.4	28.3	0.27	3.4	0.00	—	0.02	3.28	0.12	1.1	0	0.7	37.3
60	25	0.53	32.3	457.6	42.5	0.56	26.4	0.14	—	0.04	7.41	0.15	3.4	2.5	1.1	39.8
31	13	0.28	17.0	238.1	22.1	0.29	16.4	0.08	—	0.02	3.86	0.09	2.3	1.6	0.7	20.7
80	31	3.23	47.6	241.5	502.6	0.80	1.7	0.18	—	0.11	1.61	0.12	11.9	1.5	0.6	44.1
144	50	4.84	68.9	295.0	980.1	1.38	3.4	0.28	6.74	0.12	1.89	0.21	6.0	2.6	0.7	75.6
50	57	0.47	22.1	212.1	188.8	2.27	1.1	0.04	1.04	0.04	0.77	0.08	24.4	1.5	0.3	18.0
85	88	0.77	28.1	275.6	237.3	3.58	1.7	0.08	1.56	0.04	2.80	0.15	43.4	2.8	6.2	34.2
65	50	0.36	49.3	347.0	321.5	4.65	26.4	0.04	—	0.17	3.08	0.14	35.7	3.1	8.8	40.5
57	78	23.78	15.3	534.1	95.3	2.32	145.4	0.12	—	0.36	2.85	0.09	24.7	18.8	84.1	54.4
117	43	0.94	28.1	202.4	82.5	1.25	12.8	0.03	—	0.06	1.41	0.11	9.4	0.4	2.6	29.1
43	36	5.30	37.4	125.0	403.8	72.22	60.4	0.07	0.98	0.06	1.04	0.04	7.7	2.8	14.7	50.7
21	37	4.91	28.1	105.4	151.3	32.23	6.8	0.08	—	0.05	1.07	0.05	15.3	4.0	13.8	54.1
89	77	10.19	80.8	239.0	358.9	154.45	45.9	0.16	—	0.15	2.11	0.10	11.9	5.1	29.8	60.9
85	14	7.82	37.4	256.8	180.3	28.27	124.2	0.10	0.72	0.37	3.07	0.07	12.8	10.9	24.5	131.0
43	7	4.34	18.7	142.9	90.1	14.13	68.9	0.05	—	0.20	1.70	0.04	8.5	6.8	13.6	65.5
61	52	0.33	29.8	299.4	323.2	2.48	22.1	0.01	0.85	0.05	0.91	0.06	9.4	0	2.6	36.3
48	28	5.71	31.5	227.9	313.8	2.27	77.4	0.25	—	0.35	2.55	0.08	64.6	11.6	20.4	76.2
150	57	1.07	34.0	191.3	292.4	1.17	0	0.11	—	0.11	2.60	0.08	15.3	1.3	1.6	35.4
166	33	2.62	28.9	154.8	190.5	1.32	57.8	0.02	1.17	0.02	2.20	0.10	3.4	1.9	1.3	33.7
27	2	0.71	6.1	93.1	509.2	1.44	0	0.02	0.06	0.05	1.46	0.07	1.8	0	0.8	6.1
73	10	1.76	11.9	115.7	855.6	3.03	0	0.01	0.12	0.12	2.06	0.11	7.7	0	1.4	36.5
23	6	1.53	10.8	243.2	815.9	2.25	0	0.04	0.00	0.10	2.98	0.19	6.2	0	1.5	16.0
14	6	1.53	14.5	169.2	627.4	2.29	0	0.04	0.13	0.04	0.49	0.05	38.0	0	0.3	3.0
58	6	2.00	17.9	266.2	59.5	4.63	0	0.05	—	0.23	4.21	0.23	7.6	0	1.8	16.0
69	12	2.21	18.4	250.0	62.4	5.86	0	0.08	—	0.23	5.10	0.16	9.4	0	1.7	19.0
62	9	2.07	17.0	248.3	70.6	4.40	0	0.02	—	0.16	4.90	0.23	7.6	0	2.5	16.2
71	12	2.30	18.5	242.4	72.4	5.18	0	0.08	—	0.23	4.93	0.17	8.5	0	1.6	18.0
65	16	1.59	21.3	319.8	51.9	4.64	0	0.06	0.34	0.12	7.15	0.53	8.5	0	1.4	29.2
72	9	1.96	16.2	251.7	53.6	4.45	0	0.06	—	0.14	2.85	0.19	6.0	0	2.1	18.7
68	6	2.29	17.9	223.7	35.7	4.59	0	0.05	0.41	0.15	5.05	0.36	8.5	0	1.7	29.3
64	5	1.83	14.5	182.0	29.8	3.76	0	0.05	0.34	0.12	3.92	0.29	6.8	0	1.3	23.0
67	14	2.15	17.0	205.8	42.5	5.93	0	0.05	0.45	0.15	3.63	0.25	7.7	0	1.9	24.1
88	11	2.66	16.2	198.2	55.3	7.15	0	0.06	0.17	0.20	2.06	0.22	4.3	0	1.9	20.9
73	11	3.12	19.6	223.7	60.4	8.73	0	0.06	—	0.23	2.27	0.24	5.1	0	2.1	22.7
49	5	2.16	16.2	200.7	32.3	4.28	0	0.05	0.30	0.15	4.69	0.34	8.5	0	1.4	28.0
54	5	1.98	15.3	193.1	31.5	3.95	0	0.05	0.34	0.13	4.37	0.31	7.7	0	1.5	25.2

TABLE A-1 Table of Food Composition (*continued*) (Computer code is for Cengage Diet Analysis program) (For purposes of calculations, use "0" for t, <1, <.1, <.01, etc.

DA+ Code	Food Description	Quantity	Measure	Wt (g)	H₂O (g)	Ener (kcal)	Prot (g)	Carb (g)	Fiber (g)	Fat (g)	Fat Breakdown (g) Sat	Mono	Poly	Trans
	Beef, Lamb, Pork—*continued*													
	Beef steak													
4348	Short loin, t-bone steak, lean and fat, ¼" fat, broiled	3	ounce(s)	85	43.2	274	19.4	0	0	21.2	8.3	9.6	0.8	—
4349	Short loin, t-bone steak, lean, ¼" fat, broiled	3	ounce(s)	85	52.3	174	22.8	0	0	8.5	3.1	4.2	0.3	—
4360	Top loin, prime, lean and fat, ¼" fat, broiled	3	ounce(s)	85	42.7	275	21.6	0	0	20.3	8.2	8.6	0.7	—
	Beef variety													
188	Liver, pan fried	3	ounce(s)	85	52.7	149	22.6	4.4	0	4.0	1.3	0.5	0.5	0.2
4447	Tongue, simmered	3	ounce(s)	85	49.2	242	16.4	0	0	19.0	6.9	8.6	0.6	0.7
	Lamb chop													
3275	Loin, domestic, lean and fat, ¼" fat, broiled	3	ounce(s)	85	43.9	269	21.4	0	0	19.6	8.4	8.3	1.4	—
	Lamb leg													
3264	Domestic, lean and fat, ¼" fat, cooked	3	ounce(s)	85	45.7	250	20.9	0	0	17.8	7.5	7.5	1.3	—
	Lamb rib													
182	Domestic, lean and fat, ¼" fat, broiled	3	ounce(s)	85	40.0	307	18.8	0	0	25.2	10.8	10.3	2.0	—
183	Domestic, lean, ¼" fat, broiled	3	ounce(s)	85	50.0	200	23.6	0	0	11.0	4.0	4.4	1.0	—
	Lamb shoulder													
186	Shoulder, arm and blade, domestic, choice, lean and fat, ¼" fat, roasted	3	ounce(s)	85	47.8	235	19.1	0	0	17.0	7.2	6.9	1.4	—
187	Shoulder, arm and blade, domestic, choice, lean, ¼" fat, roasted	3	ounce(s)	85	53.8	173	21.2	0	0	9.2	3.5	3.7	0.8	—
3287	Shoulder, arm, domestic, lean and fat, ¼" fat, braised	3	ounce(s)	85	37.6	294	25.8	0	0	20.4	8.4	8.7	1.5	—
3290	Shoulder, arm, domestic, lean, ¼" fat, braised	3	ounce(s)	85	41.9	237	30.2	0	0	12.0	4.3	5.2	0.8	—
	Lamb variety													
3375	Brain, pan fried	3	ounce(s)	85	51.6	232	14.4	0	0	18.9	4.8	3.4	1.9	—
3406	Tongue, braised	3	ounce(s)	85	49.2	234	18.3	0	0	17.2	6.7	8.5	1.1	—
	Pork, cured													
29229	Bacon, Canadian style, cured	2	ounce(s)	57	37.9	89	11.7	1.0	0	4.0	1.3	1.8	0.4	—
161	Bacon, cured, broiled, pan fried or roasted	2	slice(s)	16	2.0	87	5.9	0.2	0	6.7	2.2	3.0	0.7	0
35422	Breakfast strips, cured, cooked	3	slice(s)	34	9.2	156	9.8	0.4	0	12.5	4.3	5.6	1.9	—
189	Ham, cured, boneless, 11% fat, roasted	3	ounce(s)	85	54.9	151	19.2	0	0	7.7	2.7	3.8	1.2	—
29215	Ham, cured, extra lean, 4% fat, canned	2	2 ounce(s)	57	41.7	68	10.5	0	0	2.6	0.9	1.3	0.2	—
1316	Ham, cured, extra lean, 5% fat, roasted	3	ounce(s)	85	57.6	123	17.8	1.3	0	4.7	1.5	2.2	0.5	—
16561	Ham, smoked or cured, lean, cooked	1	slice(s)	42	27.6	66	10.5	0	0	2.3	0.8	1.1	0.3	—
	Pork chop													
32671	Loin, blade, chops, lean and fat, pan fried	3	ounce(s)	85	42.5	291	18.3	0	0	23.6	8.6	10	2.6	—
32672	Loin, center cut, chops, lean and fat, pan fried	3	ounce(s)	85	45.1	236	25.4	0	0	14.1	5.1	6.0	1.6	—
32682	Loin, center rib, chops, boneless, lean and fat, braised	3	ounce(s)	85	49.5	217	22.4	0	0	13.4	5.2	6.1	1.1	—
32603	Loin, center rib, chops, lean, broiled	3	ounce(s)	85	55.4	158	21.9	0	0	7.1	2.4	3.0	0.8	0.1
32478	Loin, whole, lean and fat, braised	3	ounce(s)	85	49.6	203	23.2	0	0	11.6	4.3	5.2	1.0	—
32481	Loin, whole, lean, braised	3	ounce(s)	85	52.2	174	24.3	0	0	7.8	2.9	3.5	0.6	—
	Pork leg or ham													
32471	Pork leg or ham, rump portion, lean and fat, roasted	3	ounce(s)	85	48.3	214	24.6	0	0	12.1	4.5	5.4	1.2	—
32468	Pork leg or ham, whole, lean and fat, roasted	3	ounce(s)	85	46.8	232	22.8	0	0	15.0	5.5	6.7	1.4	—
	Pork ribs													
32693	Loin, country style, lean and fat, roasted	3	ounce(s)	85	43.3	279	19.9	0	0	21.6	7.8	9.4	1.7	—
32696	Loin, country style, lean, roasted	3	ounce(s)	85	49.5	210	22.6	0	0	12.6	4.5	5.5	0.9	—

Chol (mg)	Calc (mg)	Iron (mg)	Magn (mg)	Pota (mg)	Sodi (mg)	Zinc (mg)	Vit A (µg)	Thia (mg)	Vit E (mg α)	Ribo (mg)	Niac (mg)	Vit B_6 (mg)	Fola (µg)	Vit C (mg)	Vit B_{12} (µg)	Sele (µg)
58	7	2.56	17.9	233.9	57.8	3.56	0	0.07	0.18	0.17	3.29	0.27	6.0	0	1.8	10.0
50	5	3.11	22.1	278.1	65.5	4.34	0	0.09	0.11	0.21	3.93	0.33	6.8	0	1.9	8.5
67	8	1.88	19.6	294.3	53.6	3.85	0	0.06	—	0.15	3.96	0.31	6.0	0	1.6	19.5
324	5	5.24	18.7	298.5	65.5	4.44	6586.3	0.15	0.39	2.91	14.86	0.87	221.1	0.6	70.7	27.9
112	4	2.22	12.8	156.5	55.3	3.47	0	0.01	0.25	0.25	2.96	0.13	6.0	1.1	2.7	11.2
85	17	1.53	20.4	278.1	65.5	2.96	0	0.08	0.11	0.21	6.03	0.11	15.3	0	2.1	23.3
82	14	1.59	19.6	263.7	61.2	3.79	0	0.08	0.11	0.21	5.66	0.11	15.3	0	2.2	22.5
84	16	1.59	19.6	229.5	64.6	3.40	0	0.07	0.10	0.18	5.95	0.09	11.9	0	2.2	20.3
77	14	1.87	24.7	266.1	72.3	4.47	0	0.08	0.15	0.21	5.56	0.12	17.9	0	2.2	26.4
78	17	1.67	19.6	213.4	56.1	4.44	0	0.07	0.11	0.20	5.22	0.11	17.9	0	2.2	22.3
74	16	1.81	21.3	225.3	57.8	5.13	0	0.07	0.15	0.22	4.89	0.12	21.3	0	2.3	24.2
102	21	2.03	22.1	260.3	61.2	5.17	0	0.06	0.12	0.21	5.66	0.09	15.3	0	2.2	31.6
103	22	2.29	24.7	287.5	64.6	6.20	0	0.06	0.15	0.23	5.38	0.11	18.7	0	2.3	32.1
2130	18	1.73	18.7	304.5	133.5	1.70	0	0.14	—	0.31	3.87	0.19	6.0	19.6	20.5	10.2
161	9	2.23	13.6	134.4	57.0	2.54	0	0.06	—	0.35	3.13	0.14	2.6	6.0	5.4	23.8
28	5	0.38	9.6	195.0	798.9	0.78	0	0.42	0.11	0.09	3.53	0.22	2.3	0	0.4	14.2
18	2	0.22	5.3	90.4	369.6	0.56	1.8	0.06	0.04	0.04	1.76	0.04	0.3	0	0.2	9.9
36	5	0.67	8.8	158.4	713.7	1.25	0	0.25	0.08	0.12	2.58	0.11	1.4	0	0.6	8.4
50	7	1.13	18.7	347.7	1275.0	2.09	0	0.62	0.26	0.28	5.22	0.26	2.6	0	0.6	16.8
22	3	0.53	9.6	206.4	711.6	1.09	0	0.47	0.09	0.13	3.00	0.25	3.4	0	0.5	8.2
45	7	1.25	11.9	244.1	1023.1	2.44	0	0.64	0.21		3.42	0.34	2.6	0	0.6	16.6
23	3	0.39	9.2	132.7	557.3	1.07	0	0.28	0.10	0.10	2.10	0.19	1.7	0	0.3	10.7
72	26	0.74	17.9	282.4	57.0	2.71	1.7	0.52	0.17	0.25	3.35	0.28	3.4	0.5	0.7	29.7
78	23	0.77	24.7	361.5	68.0	1.96	1.7	0.96	0.21	0.25	4.76	0.39	5.1	0.9	0.6	33.2
62	4	0.78	14.5	329.1	34.0	1.76	1.7	0.44	—	0.20	3.66	0.26	3.4	0.3	0.4	28.4
56	22	0.57	21.3	291.7	48.5	1.91	0	0.48	0.08	0.18	6.68	0.57	0	0	0.4	38.6
68	18	0.91	16.2	318.1	40.8	2.02	1.7	0.53	0.20	0.21	3.75	0.31	2.6	0.5	0.5	38.5
67	15	0.96	17.0	329.1	42.5	2.10	1.7	0.56	0.17	0.22	3.90	0.32	3.4	0.5	0.5	41.0
82	10	0.89	23.0	318.1	52.7	2.39	2.6	0.63	0.18	0.28	3.95	0.26	2.6	0.2	0.6	39.8
80	12	0.85	18.7	299.4	51.0	2.51	2.6	0.54	0.18	0.26	3.89	0.34	8.5	0.3	0.6	38.5
78	21	0.90	19.6	292.6	44.2	2.00	2.6	0.75	—	0.29	3.67	0.37	4.3	0.3	0.7	31.6
79	25	1.09	20.4	296.8	24.7	3.24	1.7	0.48	—	0.29	3.96	0.37	4.3	0.3	0.7	36.0

TABLE A-1 Table of Food Composition (*continued*) (Computer code is for Cengage Diet Analysis program) (For purposes of calculations, use "0" for t, <1, <.1, <.01, etc.)

DA+ Code	Food Description	Quantity	Measure	Wt (g)	H₂O (g)	Ener (kcal)	Prot (g)	Carb (g)	Fiber (g)	Fat (g)	Fat Breakdown (g) Sat	Mono	Poly	*Trans*
Beef, Lamb, Pork—*continued*														
	Pork shoulder													
32626	Shoulder, arm picnic, lean and fat, roasted	3	ounce(s)	85	44.3	270	20.0	0	0	20.4	7.5	9.1	2.0	—
32629	Shoulder, arm picnic, lean, roasted	3	ounce(s)	85	51.3	194	22.7	0	0	10.7	3.7	5.1	1.0	—
	Rabbit													
3366	Domesticated, roasted	3	ounce(s)	85	51.5	168	24.7	0	0	6.8	2.0	1.8	1.3	—
3367	Domesticated, stewed	3	ounce(s)	85	50.0	175	25.8	0	0	7.2	2.1	1.9	1.4	—
	Veal													
3391	Liver, braised	3	ounce(s)	85	50.9	163	24.2	3.2	0	5.3	1.7	1.0	0.9	0.3
3319	Rib, lean only, roasted	3	ounce(s)	85	55.0	151	21.9	0	0	6.3	1.8	2.3	0.6	—
1732	Deer or venison, roasted	3	ounce(s)	85	55.5	134	25.7	0	0	2.7	1.1	0.7	0.5	—
Poultry														
	Chicken													
29562	Flaked, canned	2	ounce(s)	57	39.3	97	10.3	0.1	0	5.8	1.6	2.3	1.3	
	Chicken, fried													
29632	Breast, meat only, breaded, baked or fried	3	ounce(s)	85	44.3	193	25.3	6.9	0.2	6.6	1.6	2.7	1.7	
35327	Broiler breast, meat only, fried	3	ounce(s)	85	51.2	159	28.4	0.4	0	4.0	1.1	1.5	0.9	—
36413	Broiler breast, meat and skin, flour coated, fried	3	ounce(s)	85	48.1	189	27.1	1.4	0.1	7.5	2.1	3.0	1.7	—
36414	Broiler drumstick, meat and skin, flour coated, fried	3	ounce(s)	85	48.2	208	22.9	1.4	0.1	11.7	3.1	4.6	2.7	—
35389	Broiler drumstick, meat only, fried	3	ounce(s)	85	52.9	166	24.3	0	0	6.9	1.8	2.5	1.7	—
35406	Broiler leg, meat only, fried	3	ounce(s)	85	51.5	177	24.1	0.6	0	7.9	2.1	2.9	1.9	—
35484	Broiler wing, meat only, fried	3	ounce(s)	85	50.9	179	25.6	0	0	7.8	2.1	2.6	1.8	—
29580	Patty, fillet or tenders, breaded, cooked	3	ounce(s)	85	40.2	256	14.5	12.2	0	16.5	3.7	8.4	3.7	—
	Chicken, roasted, meat only													
35409	Broiler leg, meat only, roasted	3	ounce(s)	85	55.0	162	23.0	0	0	7.2	1.9	2.6	1.7	—
35486	Broiler wing, meat only, roasted	3	ounce(s)	85	53.4	173	25.9	0	0	6.9	1.9	2.2	1.5	—
35138	Roasting chicken, dark meat, meat only, roasted	3	ounce(s)	85	57.0	151	19.8	0	0	7.4	2.1	2.8	1.7	—
35136	Roasting chicken, light meat, meat only, roasted	3	ounce(s)	85	57.7	130	23.1	0	0	3.5	0.9	1.3	0.8	—
35132	Roasting chicken, meat only, roasted	3	ounce(s)	85	57.3	142	21.3	0	0	5.6	1.5	2.1	1.3	—
	Chicken, stewed													
1268	Gizzard, simmered	3	ounce(s)	85	57.8	124	25.8	0	0	2.3	0.6	0.4	0.3	0.1
1270	Liver, simmered	3	ounce(s)	85	56.8	142	20.8	0.7	0	5.5	1.8	1.2	1.7	0.1
3174	Meat only, stewed	3	ounce(s)	85	56.8	151	23.2	0	0	5.7	1.6	2.0	1.3	—
	Duck													
1286	Domesticated, meat and skin, roasted	3	ounce(s)	85	44.1	287	16.2	0	0	24.1	8.2	11.0	3.1	—
1287	Domesticated, meat only, roasted	3	ounce(s)	85	54.6	171	20.0	0	0	9.5	3.5	3.1	1.2	—
	Goose													
35507	Domesticated, meat and skin, roasted	3	ounce(s)	85	44.2	259	21.4	0	0	18.6	5.8	8.7	2.1	—
35524	Domesticated, meat only, roasted	3	ounce(s)	85	48.7	202	24.6	0	0	10.8	3.9	3.7	1.3	—
1297	Liver pate, smoked, canned	4	tablespoon(s)	52	19.3	240	5.9	2.4	0	22.8	7.5	13.3	0.4	—
	Turkey													
3256	Ground turkey, cooked	3	ounce(s)	85	50.5	200	23.3	0	0	11.2	2.9	4.2	2.7	—
3263	Patty, batter coated, breaded, fried	1	item(s)	94	46.7	266	13.2	14.8	0.5	16.9	4.4	7.0	4.4	—
219	Roasted, dark meat, meat only	3	ounce(s)	85	53.7	159	24.3	0	0	6.1	2.1	1.4	1.8	—
222	Roasted, fryer roaster breast, meat only	3	ounce(s)	85	58.2	115	25.6	0	0	0.6	0.2	0.1	0.2	—
220	Roasted, light meat, meat only	3	ounce(s)	85	56.4	134	25.4	0	0	2.7	0.9	0.5	0.7	—
1303	Turkey roll, light and dark meat	2	slice(s)	57	39.8	84	10.3	1.2	0	4.0	1.2	1.3	1.0	—
1302	Turkey roll, light meat	2	slice(s)	57	42.5	56	8.4	2.9	0	0.9	0.2	0.2	0.1	0
Processed Meats														
	Beef													
1331	Corned beef loaf, jellied, sliced	2	slice(s)	57	39.2	87	13.0	0	0	3.5	1.5	1.5	0.2	

PAGE KEY: A-6 = Breads/Baked Goods A-12 = Cereal/Rice/Pasta A-16 = Fruit A-20 = Vegetables/Legumes A-30 = Nuts/Seeds A-32 = Vegetarian A-34 = Dairy A-42 = Eggs A-42 = Seafood A-44 = Meats A-48 = Poultry
A-48 = Processed Meats A-50 = Beverages A-54 = Fats/Oils A-56 = Sweets A-58 = Spices/Condiments/Sauces A-62 = Mixed Foods/Soups/Sandwiches A-66 = Fast Food A-86 = Convenience A-88 = Baby Foods

Chol (mg)	Calc (mg)	Iron (mg)	Magn (mg)	Pota (mg)	Sodi (mg)	Zinc (mg)	Vit A (µg)	Thia (mg)	Vit E (mg α)	Ribo (mg)	Niac (mg)	Vit B_6 (mg)	Fola (µg)	Vit C (mg)	Vit B_{12} (µg)	Sele (µg)
80	16	1.00	14.5	276.4	59.5	2.93	1.7	0.44	—	0.25	3.33	0.29	3.4	0.2	0.6	28.6
81	8	1.20	17.0	298.5	68.0	3.46	1.7	0.49	—	0.30	3.66	0.34	4.3	0.3	0.7	32.7
70	16	1.93	17.9	325.7	40.0	1.93	0	0.07	—	0.17	7.17	0.40	9.4	0	7.1	32.7
73	17	2.01	17.0	255.1	31.5	2.01	0	0.05	0.37	0.14	6.09	0.28	7.7	0	5.5	32.7
435	5	4.34	17.0	279.8	66.3	9.55	8026	0.15	0.57	2.43	11.18	0.78	281.5	0.9	72.0	16.4
98	10	0.81	20.4	264.5	82.5	3.81	0	0.05	0.30	0.24	6.37	0.23	11.9	0	1.3	9.4
95	6	3.80	20.4	284.9	45.9	2.33	0	0.15	—	0.51	5.70	—	—	0	—	11.0
35	8	0.89	6.8	147.4	408.2	0.79	19.3	0.01	—	0.07	3.58	0.19	2.3	0	0.2	—
67	19	1.05	24.7	222.6	450.2	0.84	—	0.08	—	0.09	10.97	0.46	4.3	0	0.3	—
77	14	0.96	26.4	234.7	67.2	0.91	6.0	0.06	0.35	0.10	12.57	0.54	3.4	0	0.3	22.3
76	14	1.01	25.5	220.3	64.6	0.93	12.8	0.06	0.39	0.11	11.68	0.49	5.1	0	0.3	20.3
77	10	1.13	19.6	194.8	75.7	2.45	21.3	0.06	0.65	0.19	5.13	0.29	8.5	0	0.3	15.6
80	10	1.12	20.4	211.8	81.6	2.73	15.3	0.06	—	0.20	5.22	0.33	7.7	0	0.3	16.7
84	11	1.19	21.3	216.0	81.6	2.53	17.0	0.07	0.38	0.21	5.68	0.33	7.7	0	0.3	16.0
71	13	0.96	17.9	176.9	77.4	1.80	15.3	0.03	0.40	0.10	6.15	0.50	3.4	0	0.3	21.6
49	11	0.75	19.6	244.8	411.4	0.79	4.3	0.09	1.04	0.12	5.99	0.24	24.7	0	0.2	13.9
80	10	1.11	20.4	205.8	77.4	2.43	16.2	0.06	0.22	0.19	5.37	0.31	6.8	0	0.3	18.8
72	14	0.98	17.9	178.6	78.2	1.82	15.3	0.03	0.22	0.10	6.21	0.50	3.4	0	0.3	21.0
64	9	1.13	17.0	190.5	80.8	1.81	13.6	0.05	—	0.16	4.87	0.26	6.0	0	0.2	16.7
64	11	0.91	19.6	200.7	43.4	0.66	6.8	0.05	0.22	0.07	8.90	0.45	2.6	0	0.3	21.9
64	10	1.02	17.9	194.8	63.8	1.29	10.2	0.05	—	0.12	6.70	0.34	4.3	0	0.2	20.9
315	14	2.71	2.6	152.2	47.6	3.75	0	0.02	0.17	0.17	2.65	0.06	4.3	0	0.9	35.0
479	9	9.89	21.3	223.7	64.6	3.38	3385.8	0.24	0.69	1.69	9.39	0.64	491.6	23.7	14.3	70.1
71	12	0.99	17.9	153.1	59.5	1.69	12.8	0.04	0.22	0.13	5.20	0.22	5.1	0	0.2	17.8
71	9	2.29	13.6	173.5	50.2	1.58	53.6	0.14	0.59	0.22	4.10	0.15	5.1	0	0.3	17.0
76	10	2.29	17.0	214.3	55.3	2.21	19.6	0.22	0.59	0.39	4.33	0.21	8.5	0	0.3	19.1
77	11	2.40	18.7	279.8	59.5	2.22	17.9	0.06	1.47	0.27	3.54	0.31	1.7	0	0.3	18.5
82	12	2.44	21.3	330.0	64.6	2.69	10.2	0.07	—	0.33	3.47	0.39	10.2	0	0.4	21.7
78	36	2.86	6.8	71.8	362.4	0.47	520.5	0.04	—	0.15	1.30	0.03	31.2	0	4.9	22.9
87	21	1.64	20.4	229.6	91.0	2.43	0	0.04	0.28	0.14	4.09	0.33	6.0	0	0.3	31.6
71	13	2.06	14.1	258.5	752.0	1.35	9.4	0.09	0.87	0.17	2.16	0.18	38.5	0	0.2	20.8
72	27	1.98	20.4	246.6	67.2	3.79	0	0.05	0.54	0.21	3.10	0.30	7.7	0	0.3	34.8
71	10	1.30	24.7	248.3	44.2	1.48	0	0.03	0.07	0.11	6.37	0.47	5.1	0	0.3	27.3
59	16	1.14	23.8	259.4	54.4	1.73	0	0.05	0.07	0.11	5.81	0.45	5.1	0	0.3	27.3
31	18	0.76	10.2	153.1	332.3	1.13	0	0.05	0.19	0.16	2.72	0.15	2.8	0	0.1	16.6
19	4	0.21	10.8	242.1	590.8	0.50	0	0.01	0.07	0.08	4.05	0.23	2.3	0	0.2	7.4
27	6	1.15	6.2	57.3	540.4	2.31	0	0.00	—	0.06	0.99	0.06	4.5	0	0.7	9.8

TABLE A-1 Table of Food Composition (*continued*) <small>(Computer code is for Cengage Diet Analysis program) (For purposes of calculations, use "0" for t, <1, <.1, <.01, etc.</small>

DA+ Code	Food Description	Quantity	Measure	Wt (g)	H₂O (g)	Ener (kcal)	Prot (g)	Carb (g)	Fiber (g)	Fat (g)	Fat Breakdown (g)			
											Sat	Mono	Poly	*Trans*
Processed Meats—*continued*														
	Bologna													
13459	Beef	1	slice(s)	28	15.1	90	3.0	1.0	0	8.0	3.5	4.3	0.3	—
13461	Light, made with pork and chicken	1	slice(s)	28	18.2	60	3.0	2.0	0	4.0	1.0	2.0	0.4	—
13458	Made with chicken and pork	1	slice(s)	28	15.0	90	3.0	1.0	0	8.0	3.0	4.1	1.1	—
13565	Turkey bologna	1	slice(s)	28	19.0	50	3.0	1.0	0	4.0	1.0	1.1	1.0	0
	Chicken													
7125	Breast, smoked	1	slice(s)	10	—	10	1.8	0.3	0	0.2	0	—	—	—
	Ham													
7127	Deli-sliced, honey	1	slice(s)	10	—	10	1.7	0.3	0	0.3	0.1	—	—	—
7126	Deli-sliced, smoked	1	slice(s)	10	—	10	1.7	0.2	0	0.3	0.1	—	—	—
8614	**Beef and pork mortadella, sliced**	2	slice(s)	46	24.1	143	7.5	1.4	0	11.7	4.4	5.2	1.4	—
1323	**Pork olive loaf**	2	slice(s)	57	33.1	133	6.7	5.2	0	9.4	3.3	4.5	1.1	—
1324	**Pork pickle and pimento loaf**	2	slice(s)	57	34.2	128	6.4	4.8	0.9	9.1	3.0	4.0	1.6	—
	Sausages and frankfurters													
37296	Beerwurst beef, beer salami (bierwurst)	1	slice(s)	29	16.6	74	4.1	1.2	0	5.7	2.5	2.7	0.2	—
37257	Beerwurst pork, beer salami	1	slice(s)	21	12.9	50	3.0	0.4	0	4.0	1.3	1.9	0.5	—
35338	Berliner, pork and beef	1	ounce(s)	28	17.3	65	4.3	0.7	0	4.9	1.7	2.3	0.4	—
37298	Bratwurst pork, cooked	1	piece(s)	74	42.3	181	10.4	1.9	0	14.3	5.1	6.7	1.5	—
37299	Braunschweiger pork liver sausage	1	slice(s)	15	8.2	51	2.0	0.3	0	4.5	1.5	2.1	0.5	—
1329	Cheesefurter or cheese smokie, beef and pork	1	item(s)	43	22.6	141	6.1	0.6	0	12.5	4.5	5.9	1.3	—
1330	Chorizo, beef and pork	2	ounce(s)	57	18.1	258	13.7	1.1	0	21.7	8.2	10.4	2.0	—
8600	Frankfurter, beef	1	item(s)	45	23.4	149	5.1	1.8	0	13.3	5.3	6.4	0.5	—
202	Frankfurter, beef and pork	1	item(s)	45	25.2	137	5.2	0.8	0	12.4	4.8	6.2	1.2	—
1293	Frankfurter, chicken	1	item(s)	45	28.1	100	7.0	1.2	0.2	7.3	1.7	2.7	1.7	0.1
3261	Frankfurter, turkey	1	item(s)	45	28.3	100	5.5	1.7	0	7.8	1.8	2.6	1.8	0.4
37275	Italian sausage, pork, cooked	1	item(s)	68	32.0	234	13.0	2.9	0.1	18.6	6.5	8.1	2.2	—
37307	Kielbasa or kolbassa, pork and beef	1	slice(s)	30	18.5	67	5.0	1.0	0	4.7	1.7	2.2	0.5	—
1333	Knockwurst or knackwurst, beef and pork	2	ounce(s)	57	31.4	174	6.3	1.8	0	15.7	5.8	7.3	1.7	—
37285	Pepperoni, beef and pork	1	slice(s)	11	3.4	51	2.2	0.4	0.2	4.4	1.8	2.1	0.3	—
37313	Polish sausage, pork	1	slice(s)	21	11.4	60	2.8	0.7	0	5.0	1.8	2.3	0.5	—
206	Salami, beef, cooked, sliced	2	slice(s)	52	31.2	136	6.5	1.0	0	11.5	5.1	5.5	0.5	—
37272	Salami, pork, dry or hard	1	slice(s)	13	4.6	52	2.9	0.2	0	4.3	1.5	2.0	0.5	—
40987	Sausage, turkey, cooked	2	ounce(s)	57	36.9	111	13.5	0	0	5.9	1.3	1.7	1.5	0.2
8620	Smoked sausage, beef and pork	2	ounce(s)	57	30.6	181	6.8	1.4	0	16.3	5.5	6.9	2.2	0
8619	Smoked sausage, pork	2	ounce(s)	57	32.0	178	6.8	1.2	0	16.0	5.3	6.4	2.1	0.1
37273	Smoked sausage, pork link	1	piece(s)	76	29.8	295	16.8	1.6	0	24.0	8.6	11.1	2.8	—
1336	Summer sausage, thuringer, or cervelat, beef and pork	2	ounce(s)	57	25.6	205	9.9	1.9	0	17.3	6.5	7.4	0.7	—
37294	Vienna sausage, cocktail, beef and pork, canned	1	piece(s)	16	10.4	37	1.7	0.4	0	3.1	1.1	1.5	0.2	—
	Spreads													
1318	Ham salad spread	¼	cup(s)	60	37.6	130	5.2	6.4	0	9.3	3.0	4.3	1.6	—
32419	Pork and beef sandwich spread	4	tablespoon(s)	60	36.2	141	4.6	7.2	0.1	10.4	3.6	4.6	1.5	—
	Turkey													
13604	Breast, fat free, oven roasted	1	slice(s)	28	—	25	4.0	1.0	0	0	0	0	0	0
13606	Breast, hickory smoked fat free	1	slice(s)	28	—	25	4.0	1.0	0	0	0	0	0	0
16049	Breast, hickory smoked slices	1	slice(s)	56	—	50	11.0	1.0	0	0	0	0	0	0
16047	Breast, honey roasted slices	1	slice(s)	56	—	60	11.0	3.0	0	0	0	0	0	0
16048	Breast, oven roasted slices	1	slice(s)	56	—	50	11.0	1.0	0	0	0	0	0	0
7124	Breast, oven roasted	1	slice(s)	10	—	10	1.8	0.3	0	0.1	0	0	0	—
13567	Turkey ham, 10% water added	2	slice(s)	56	40.9	70	10.0	2.0	0	3.0	0	0.4	0.6	0
37270	Turkey pastrami	1	slice(s)	28	20.3	35	4.6	1.0	0	1.2	0.3	0.4	0.3	—
3262	Turkey salami	2	slice(s)	57	39.1	98	10.9	0.9	0.1	5.2	1.6	1.8	1.4	0
37318	Turkey salami, cooked	1	slice(s)	28	20.4	43	4.3	0.1	0	2.7	0.8	0.9	0.7	—
Beverages														
	Beer													
866	Ale, mild	12	fluid ounce(s)	360	332.3	148	1.1	13.3	0.4	0	0	0	0	0
686	Beer	12	fluid ounce(s)	356	327.7	153	1.6	12.7	0	0	0	0	0	0
16886	Beer, non alcoholic	12	fluid ounce(s)	360	328.1	133	0.8	29.0	0	0.4	0.1	0	0.2	0

Chol (mg)	Calc (mg)	Iron (mg)	Magn (mg)	Pota (mg)	Sodi (mg)	Zinc (mg)	Vit A (μg)	Thia (mg)	Vit E (mg α)	Ribo (mg)	Niac (mg)	Vit B_6 (mg)	Fola (μg)	Vit C (mg)	Vit B_{12} (μg)	Sele (μg)
20	0	0.36	3.9	47.0	310.0	0.56	0	0.01	—	0.03	0.67	0.04	3.6	0	0.4	—
20	40	0.36	5.6	45.6	300.0	0.45	0	—	—	—	—	—	—	0	—	—
30	20	0.36	5.9	43.1	300.0	0.39	0	—	—	—	—	—	—	0	—	—
20	40	0.36	6.2	42.6	270.0	0.51	0	—	—	—	—	—	—	0	—	—
4	0	0.00	—	—	100.0	—	0	—	—	—	—	—	—	0	—	—
4	0	0.12	—	—	100.0	—	0	—	—	—	—	—	—	0.6	—	—
4	0	0.12	—	—	103.3	—	0	—	—	—	—	—	—	0.6	—	—
26	8	0.64	5.1	75.0	573.2	0.96	0	0.05	0.10	0.07	1.23	0.06	1.4	0	0.7	10.4
22	62	0.30	10.8	168.7	842.9	0.78	34.1	0.16	0.14	0.14	1.04	0.13	1.1	0	0.7	9.3
33	62	0.75	19.3	210.7	740.7	0.95	44.3	0.22	0.22	0.06	1.41	0.23	21.0	4.4	0.3	4.5
18	3	0.44	3.5	66.5	264.9	0.71	0	0.02	0.05	0.03	0.98	0.04	0.9	0	0.6	4.7
12	2	0.15	2.7	53.3	261.0	0.36	0	0.11	0.03	0.04	0.68	0.07	0.6	0	0.2	4.4
13	3	0.32	4.3	80.2	367.7	0.70	0	0.10	—	0.06	0.88	0.05	1.4	0	0.8	4.0
44	33	0.95	11.1	156.9	412.2	1.70	0	0.37	0.01	0.13	2.36	0.15	1.5	0.7	0.7	15.7
24	1	1.42	1.7	27.5	131.5	0.42	641.0	0.03	0.05	0.23	1.27	0.05	6.7	0	3.1	8.8
29	25	0.46	5.6	88.6	465.3	0.96	20.2	0.10	0.10	0.06	1.24	0.05	1.3	0	0.7	6.8
50	5	0.90	10.2	225.7	700.2	1.93	0	0.35	0.12	0.17	2.90	0.30	1.1	0	1.1	12.0
24	6	0.67	6.3	70.2	513.0	1.10	0	0.01	0.09	0.06	1.06	0.04	2.3	0	0.8	3.7
23	5	0.51	4.5	75.2	504.0	0.82	8.1	0.09	0.11	0.05	1.18	0.05	1.8	0	0.6	6.2
43	33	0.52	9.0	90.9	379.8	0.50	0	0.02	0.09	0.11	2.10	0.14	3.2	0	0.2	10.4
35	67	0.66	6.3	176.4	485.1	0.82	0	0.01	0.27	0.08	1.65	0.06	4.1	0	0.4	6.8
39	14	0.97	12.2	206.7	820.8	1.62	6.8	0.42	0.17	0.15	2.83	0.22	3.4	0.1	0.9	15.0
20	13	0.44	4.9	84.4	283.0	0.61	0	0.06	0.06	0.06	0.87	0.05	1.5	0	0.5	5.4
34	6	0.37	6.2	112.8	527.3	0.94	0	0.19	0.32	0.07	1.55	0.09	1.1	0	0.7	7.7
13	2	0.15	2.0	34.7	196.7	0.30	0	0.05	0.00	0.02	0.59	0.04	0.7	0.1	0.2	2.4
15	2	0.29	2.9	37.3	199.3	0.40	0	0.10	0.04	0.03	0.71	0.03	0.4	0.2	0.2	3.7
37	3	1.14	6.8	97.8	592.8	0.92	0	0.04	0.08	0.08	1.68	0.08	1.0	0	1.6	7.6
10	2	0.16	2.8	48.4	289.3	0.53	0	0.11	0.02	0.04	0.71	0.07	0.3	0	0.4	3.3
52	12	0.84	11.9	169.0	377.1	2.19	7.4	0.04	0.10	0.14	3.24	0.18	3.4	0.4	0.7	0
33	7	0.42	7.4	101.5	516.5	0.71	7.4	0.10	0.07	0.06	1.66	0.09	1.1	0	0.3	0
35	6	0.33	6.2	273.9	468.9	0.74	0	0.12	0.14	0.10	1.59	0.10	0.6	0	0.4	10.4
52	23	0.87	14.4	254.6	1136.6	2.13	0	0.53	0.18	0.19	3.43	0.26	3.8	1.5	1.2	16.4
42	5	1.15	7.9	147.4	737.1	1.45	0	0.08	0.12	0.18	2.44	0.14	1.1	9.4	3.1	11.5
14	2	0.14	1.1	16.2	155.0	0.25	0	0.01	0.03	0.01	0.25	0.01	0.6	0	0.2	2.7
22	5	0.35	6.0	90.0	547.2	0.66	0	0.26	1.04	0.07	1.25	0.09	0.6	0	0.5	10.7
23	7	0.47	4.8	66.0	607.8	0.61	15.6	0.10	1.04	0.08	1.03	0.07	1.2	0	0.7	5.8
10	0	0.00	—	—	340.0	—	0	—	—	—	—	—	—	0	—	—
10	0	0.00	—	—	300.0	—	0	—	—	—	—	—	—	0	—	—
25	0	0.72	—	—	720.0	—	0	—	—	—	—	—	—	0	—	—
20	0	0.72	—	—	660.0	—	0	—	—	—	—	—	—	0	—	—
20	0	0.72	—	—	660.0	—	0	—	—	—	—	—	—	0	—	—
4	0	0.06	—	—	103.3	—	0	—	—	—	—	—	—	0	—	—
40	0	0.72	12.3	162.4	700.0	1.44	0	—	—	—	—	—	—	0	—	—
19	3	1.19	4.0	97.8	278.1	0.61	1.1	0.01	0.06	0.07	1.00	0.07	1.4	4.6	0.1	4.6
43	23	0.70	12.5	122.5	569.3	1.31	1.1	0.24	0.13	0.17	2.25	0.24	5.7	0	0.6	15.0
22	11	0.35	6.2	61.2	284.6	0.65	0.6	0.12	0.06	0.08	1.12	0.12	2.8	0	0.3	7.5
0	18	0.07	21.6	90.0	14.4	0.03	0	0.03	0.00	0.10	1.62	0.18	21.6	0	0.1	2.5
0	14	0.07	21.4	96.2	14.3	0.03	0	0.01	0.00	0.08	1.82	0.16	21.4	0	0.1	2.1
0	25	0.21	25.2	28.8	46.8	0.07	—	0.07	0.00	0.18	3.99	0.10	50.4	1.8	0.1	4.3

TABLE A-1 Table of Food Composition (*continued*) (Computer code is for Cengage Diet Analysis program) (For purposes of calculations, use "0" for t, <1, <.1, <.01, etc

DA+ Code	Food Description	Quantity	Measure	Wt (g)	H₂O (g)	Ener (kcal)	Prot (g)	Carb (g)	Fiber (g)	Fat (g)	Fat Breakdown (g) Sat	Mono	Poly	Trans
Beverages—*continued*														
31609	Bud Light beer	12	fluid ounce(s)	355	335.5	110	0.9	6.6	0	0	0	0	0	0
31608	Budweiser beer	12	fluid ounce(s)	355	327.7	145	1.3	10.6	0	0	0	0	0	0
869	Light beer	12	fluid ounce(s)	354	335.9	103	0.9	5.8	0	0	0	0	0	0
31613	Michelob beer	12	fluid ounce(s)	355	323.4	155	1.3	13.3	0	0	0	0	0	0
31614	Michelob Light beer	12	fluid ounce(s)	355	329.8	134	1.1	11.7	0	0	0	0	0	0
	Gin, rum, vodka, whiskey													
857	Distilled alcohol, 100 proof	1	fluid ounce(s)	28	16.0	82	0	0	0	0	0	0	0	0
687	Distilled alcohol, 80 proof	1	fluid ounce(s)	28	18.5	64	0	0	0	0	0	0	0	0
688	Distilled alcohol, 86 proof	1	fluid ounce(s)	28	17.8	70	0	0	0	0	0	0	0	0
689	Distilled alcohol, 90 proof	1	fluid ounce(s)	28	17.3	73	0	0	0	0	0	0	0	0
856	Distilled alcohol, 94 proof	1	fluid ounce(s)	28	16.8	76	0	0	0	0	0	0	0	0
	Liqueurs													
33187	Coffee liqueur, 53 proof	1	fluid ounce(s)	35	10.8	113	0	16.3	0	0.1	0	0	0	—
3142	Coffee liqueur, 63 proof	1	fluid ounce(s)	35	14.4	107	0	11.2	0	0.1	0	0	0	—
736	Cordials, 54 proof	1	fluid ounce(s)	30	8.9	106	0	13.3	0	0.1	0	0	0	—
	Wine													
861	California red wine	5	fluid ounce(s)	150	133.4	125	0.3	3.7	0	0	0	0	0	0
858	Domestic champagne	5	fluid ounce(s)	150	—	105	0.3	3.8	0	0	0	0	0	0
690	Sweet dessert wine	5	fluid ounce(s)	147	103.7	235	0.3	20.1	0	0	0	0	0	0
1481	White wine	5	fluid ounce(s)	148	128.1	121	0.1	3.8	0	0	0	0	0	0
1811	Wine cooler	10	fluid ounce(s)	300	267.4	159	0.3	20.2	0	0.1	0	0	0	0
	Carbonated													
31898	7 Up	12	fluid ounce(s)	360	321.0	140	0	39.0	0	0	0	0	0	0
692	Club soda	12	fluid ounce(s)	355	354.8	0	0	0	0	0	0	0	0	0
12010	Coca-Cola Classic cola soda	12	fluid ounce(s)	360	319.4	146	0	40.5	0	0	0	0	0	0
693	Cola	12	fluid ounce(s)	368	332.7	136	0.3	35.2	0	0.1	0	0	0	—
2391	Cola or pepper-type soda, low calorie with saccharin	12	fluid ounce(s)	355	354.5	0	0	0.3	0	0	0	0	0	0
9522	Cola soda, decaffeinated	12	fluid ounce(s)	372	333.4	153	0	39.3	0	0	0	0	0	0
9524	Cola, decaffeinated, low calorie with aspartame	12	fluid ounce(s)	355	354.3	4	0.4	0.5	0	0	0	0	0	0
1415	Cola, low calorie with aspartame	12	fluid ounce(s)	355	353.6	7	0.4	1.0	0	0.1	0	0	0	0
1412	Cream soda	12	fluid ounce(s)	371	321.5	189	0	49.3	0	0	0	0	0	0
31899	Diet 7 Up	12	fluid ounce(s)	360	—	0	0	0	0	0	0	0	0	0
12031	Diet Coke cola soda	12	fluid ounce(s)	360	—	2	0	0.2	0	0	0	0	0	0
29392	Diet Mountain Dew soda	12	fluid ounce(s)	360	—	0	0	0	0	0	0	0	0	0
29389	Diet Pepsi cola soda	12	fluid ounce(s)	360	—	0	0	0	0	0	0	0	0	0
12034	Diet Sprite soda	12	fluid ounce(s)	360	—	4	0	0	0	0	0	0	0	0
695	Ginger ale	12	fluid ounce(s)	366	333.9	124	0	32.1	0	0	0	0	0	0
694	Grape soda	12	fluid ounce(s)	372	330.3	160	0	41.7	0	0	0	0	0	0
1876	Lemon lime soda	12	fluid ounce(s)	368	330.8	147	0.2	37.4	0	0.1	0	0	0	—
29391	Mountain Dew soda	12	fluid ounce(s)	360	314.0	170	0	46.0	0	0	0	0	0	0
3145	Orange soda	12	fluid ounce(s)	372	325.9	179	0	45.8	0	0	0	0	0	0
1414	Pepper-type soda	12	fluid ounce(s)	368	329.3	151	0	38.3	0	0.4	0.3	0	0	—
29388	Pepsi regular cola soda	12	fluid ounce(s)	360	318.9	150	0	41.0	0	0	0	0	0	0
696	Root beer	12	fluid ounce(s)	370	330.0	152	0	39.2	0	0	0	0	0	0
12044	Sprite soda	12	fluid ounce(s)	360	321.0	144	0	39.0	0	0	0	0	0	0
	Coffee													
731	Brewed	8	fluid ounce(s)	237	235.6	2	0.3	0	0	0	0	0	0	0
9520	Brewed, decaffeinated	8	fluid ounce(s)	237	234.3	5	0.3	1.0	0	0	0	0	0	0
16882	Cappuccino	8	fluid ounce(s)	240	224.8	79	4.1	5.8	0.2	4.9	2.3	1.0	0.2	—
16883	Cappuccino, decaffeinated	8	fluid ounce(s)	240	224.8	79	4.1	5.8	0.2	4.9	2.3	1.0	0.2	—
16880	Espresso	8	fluid ounce(s)	237	231.8	21	0	3.6	0	0.4	0.2	0	0.2	0
16881	Espresso, decaffeinated	8	fluid ounce(s)	237	231.8	21	0	3.6	0	0.4	0.2	0	0.2	0
732	Instant, prepared	8	fluid ounce(s)	239	236.5	5	0.2	0.8	0	0	0	0	0	0
	Fruit drinks													
29357	Crystal Light sugar-free lemonade drink	8	fluid ounce(s)	240	—	5	0	0	0	0	0	0	0	0
6012	Fruit punch drink with added vitamin C, canned	8	fluid ounce(s)	248	218.2	117	0	29.7	0.5	0	0	0	0	0
31143	Gatorade Thirst Quencher, all flavors	8	fluid ounce(s)	240	—	50	0	14.0	0	0	0	0	0	0
260	Grape drink, canned	8	fluid ounce(s)	250	210.5	153	0	39.4	0	0	0	0	0	0
17372	Kool-Aid (lemonade/punch/ fruit drink)	8	fluid ounce(s)	248	220.0	108	0.1	27.8	0.2	0	0	0	0	0

PAGE KEY: A-6 = Breads/Baked Goods A-12 = Cereal/Rice/Pasta A-16 = Fruit A-20 = Vegetables/Legumes A-30 = Nuts/Seeds A-32 = Vegetarian A-34 = Dairy A-42 = Eggs A-42 = Seafood A-44 = Meats A-48 = Poultry
A-48 = Processed Meats A-50 = Beverages A-54 = Fats/Oils A-56 = Sweets A-58 = Spices/Condiments/Sauces A-62 = Mixed Foods/Soups/Sandwiches A-66 = Fast Food A-86 = Convenience A-88 = Baby Foods

Chol (mg)	Calc (mg)	Iron (mg)	Magn (mg)	Pota (mg)	Sodi (mg)	Zinc (mg)	Vit A (µg)	Thia (mg)	Vit E (mg α)	Ribo (mg)	Niac (mg)	Vit B_6 (mg)	Fola (µg)	Vit C (mg)	Vit B_{12} (µg)	Sele (µg)
0	18	0.14	17.8	63.9	9.0	0.10	0	0.03	—	0.10	1.39	0.12	14.6	0	0	4.0
0	18	0.10	21.3	88.8	9.0	0.07	0	0.02	—	0.09	1.60	0.17	21.3	0	0.1	4.0
0	14	0.10	17.7	74.3	14.2	0.03	0	0.01	0.00	0.05	1.38	0.12	21.2	0	0.1	1.4
0	18	0.10	21.3	88.8	9.0	0.07	0	0.02	—	0.09	1.60	0.17	21.3	0	0.1	4.0
0	18	0.14	17.8	63.9	9.0	0.10	0	0.03	—	0.10	1.39	0.12	14.6	0	0	4.0
0	0	0.01	0	0.6	0.3	0.01	0	0.00	—	0.00	0.00	0.00	0	0	0	0
0	0	0.01	0	0.6	0.3	0.01	0	0.00	0.00	0.00	0.00	0.00	0	0	0	0
0	0	0.01	0	0.6	0.3	0.01	0	0.00	0.00	0.00	0.00	0.00	0	0	0	0
0	0	0.01	0	0.6	0.3	0.01	0	0.00	0.00	0.00	0.00	0.00	0	0	0	0
0	0	0.01	0	0.6	0.3	0.01	0	0.00	—	0.00	0.00	0.00	0	0	0	0
0	0	0.02	1.0	10.4	2.8	0.01	0	0.00	—	0.00	0.05	0.00	0	0	0	0.1
0	0	0.02	1.0	10.4	2.8	0.01	0	0.00	—	0.00	0.05	0.00	0	0	0	0.1
0	0	0.02	0.6	4.5	2.1	0.01	0	0.00	—	0.00	0.02	0.00	0	0	0	0.1
0	12	1.43	16.2	170.6	15.0	0.14	0	0.01	0.00	0.04	0.11	0.05	1.5	0	0	—
0	—	—	—	—	—	—	—	—	—	—	—	—	—	0	0	—
0	12	0.34	13.2	135.4	13.2	0.10	0	0.01	0.00	0.01	0.30	0.00	0	0	0	0.7
0	13	0.39	14.8	104.7	7.4	0.18	0	0.01	0.00	0.01	0.15	0.06	1.5	0	0	0.1
0	18	0.75	15.0	129.0	24.0	0.18	—	0.01	0.03	0.03	0.13	0.03	3.0	5.4	0	0.6
0	—	—	—	0.6	75.0	—	0	—	—	—	—	—	—	0	—	—
0	18	0.03	3.5	7.1	74.6	0.35	0	0.00	0.00	0.00	0.00	0.00	0	0	0	0
0	—	—	—	0	49.5	—	0	—	—	—	—	—	—	0	—	—
0	7	0.41	0	7.4	14.7	0.06	0	0.00	0.00	0.00	0.00	0.00	0	0	0	0.4
0	14	0.06	3.5	14.2	56.8	0.11	0	0.00	0.00	0.00	0.00	0.00	0	0	0	0.3
0	7	0.08	0	11.2	14.9	0.03	0	0.00	0.00	0.00	0.00	0.00	0	0	0	0.4
0	11	0.06	0	24.9	14.2	0.03	0	0.02	0.00	0.08	0.00	0.00	0	0	0	0.3
0	11	0.39	3.5	28.4	28.4	0.03	0	0.02	0.00	0.08	0.00	0.00	0	0	0	0
0	19	0.18	3.7	3.7	44.5	0.26	0	0.00	0.00	0.00	0.00	0.00	0	0	0	0
0	—	—	—	77.0	45.0	—	—	—	—	—	—	—	—	—	—	—
0	—	—	—	18.0	42.0	—	0	—	—	—	—	—	—	0	—	—
0	—	—	—	70.0	35.0	—	—	—	—	—	—	—	—	—	—	—
0	—	—	—	30.0	35.0	—	—	—	—	—	—	—	—	—	—	—
0	—	—	—	109.5	36.0	—	0	—	—	—	—	—	—	0	—	—
0	11	0.65	3.7	3.7	25.6	0.18	0	0.00	0.00	0.00	0.00	0.00	0	0	0	0.4
0	11	0.29	3.7	3.7	55.8	0.26	0	0.00	0.00	0.00	0.00	0.00	0	0	0	0
0	7	0.41	3.7	3.7	33.2	0.14	0	0.00	0.00	0.00	0.05	0.00	0	0	0	0
0	—	—	—	0	70.0	—	—	—	—	—	—	—	—	—	—	—
0	19	0.21	3.7	7.4	44.6	0.36	0	0.00	—	0.00	0.00	0.00	0	0	0	0
0	11	0.14	0	3.7	36.8	0.14	0	0.00	—	0.00	0.00	0.00	0	0	0	0.4
0	—	—	—	0	35.0	—	—	—	—	—	—	—	—	—	—	—
0	18	0.18	3.7	3.7	48.0	0.26	0	0.00	0.00	0.00	0.00	0.00	0	0	0	0.4
0	—	—	—	0	70.5	—	0	—	—	—	—	—	—	0	—	—
0	5	0.02	7.1	116.1	4.7	0.04	0	0.03	0.02	0.18	0.45	0.00	4.7	0	0	0
0	7	0.14	11.8	108.9	4.7	0.00	0	0.00	0.00	0.03	0.66	0.00	0	0	0	0.5
12	144	0.19	14.4	232.8	50.4	0.50	33.6	0.04	0.09	0.27	0.13	0.04	7.2	0	0.4	4.6
12	144	0.19	14.4	232.8	50.4	0.50	33.6	0.04	0.09	0.27	0.13	0.04	7.2	0	0.4	4.6
0	5	0.30	189.6	272.6	33.2	0.11	0	0.00	0.04	0.42	12.34	0.00	2.4	0.5	0	0
0	5	0.30	189.6	272.6	33.2	0.11	0	0.00	0.04	0.42	12.34	0.00	2.4	0.5	0	0
0	10	0.09	9.5	71.6	9.5	0.01	0	0.00	0.00	0.00	0.56	0.00	0	0	0	0.2
0	0	0.00	—	160.0	40.0	—	0	—	—	—	—	—	—	0	—	—
0	20	0.22	7.4	62.0	94.2	0.02	5.0	0.05	0.04	0.05	0.05	0.02	9.9	89.3	0	0.5
0	0	0.00	—	30.0	110.0	—	0	—	—	—	—	—	—	0	—	—
0	130	0.17	2.5	30.0	40.0	0.30	0	0.00	0.00	0.01	0.02	0.01	0	78.5	0	0.3
0	14	0.45	5.0	49.6	31.0	0.19	—	0.03	—	0.05	0.04	0.01	4.3	41.6	0	1.0

TABLE A-1 Table of Food Composition (continued) (Computer code is for Cengage Diet Analysis program) (For purposes of calculations, use "0" for t, <1, <.1, <.01, etc.)

DA+ Code	Food Description	Quantity	Measure	Wt (g)	H₂O (g)	Ener (kcal)	Prot (g)	Carb (g)	Fiber (g)	Fat (g)	Fat Breakdown (g) Sat	Mono	Poly	Trans
Beverages—*continued*														
17225	Kool-Aid sugar free, low calorie tropical punch drink mix, prepared	8	fluid ounce(s)	240	—	5	0	0	0	0	0	0	0	0
266	Lemonade, prepared from frozen concentrate	8	fluid ounce(s)	248	221.6	99	0.2	25.8	0	0.1	0	0	0	—
268	Limeade, prepared from frozen concentrate	8	fluid ounce(s)	247	212.6	128	0	34.1	0	0	0	0	0	—
14266	Odwalla strawberry C monster smoothie blend	8	fluid ounce(s)	240	—	160	2.0	38.0	0	0	0	0	0	0
10080	Odwalla strawberry lemonade quencher	8	fluid ounce(s)	240	—	110	0	28.0	0	0	0	0	0	0
10099	Snapple fruit punch fruit drink	8	fluid ounce(s)	240	—	110	0	29.0	0	0	0	0	0	0
10096	Snapple kiwi strawberry fruit drink	8	fluid ounce(s)	240	211.2	110	0	28.0	0	0	0	0	0	0
	Slim Fast ready-to-drink shake													
16054	French vanilla ready to drink shake	11	fluid ounce(s)	325	—	220	10.0	40.0	5.0	2.5	0.5	1.5	0.5	—
40447	Optima rich chocolate royal ready-to-drink shake	11	fluid ounce(s)	330	—	180	10.0	24.0	5.0	5.0	1.0	3.5	0.5	0
16055	Strawberries n cream ready to drink shake	11	fluid ounce(s)	325	—	220	10.0	40.0	5.0	2.5	0.5	1.5	0.5	—
	Tea													
33179	Decaffeinated, prepared	8	fluid ounce(s)	237	236.3	2	0	0.7	0	0	0	0	0	0
1877	Herbal, prepared	8	fluid ounce(s)	237	236.1	2	0	0.5	0	0	0	0	0	0
735	Instant tea mix, lemon flavored with sugar, prepared	8	fluid ounce(s)	259	236.2	91	0	22.3	0.3	0.2	0	0	0	—
734	Instant tea mix, unsweetened, prepared	8	fluid ounce(s)	237	236.1	2	0.1	0.4	0	0	0	0	0	0
733	Tea, prepared	8	fluid ounce(s)	237	236.3	2	0	0.7	0	0	0	0	0	0
	Water													
1413	Mineral water, carbonated	8	fluid ounce(s)	237	236.8	0	0	0	0	0	0	0	0	0
33183	Poland spring water, bottled	8	fluid ounce(s)	237	237.0	0	0	0	0	0	0	0	0	0
1821	Tap water	8	fluid ounce(s)	237	236.8	0	0	0	0	0	0	0	0	0
1879	Tonic water	8	fluid ounce(s)	244	222.3	83	0	21.5	0	0	0	0	0	0
Fats and Oils														
	Butter													
104	Butter	1	tablespoon(s)	14	2.3	102	0.1	0	0	11.5	7.3	3.0	0.4	—
2522	Butter Buds, dry butter substitute	1	teaspoon(s)	2	—	5	0	2.0	0	0	0	0	0	0
921	Unsalted	1	tablespoon(s)	14	2.5	102	0.1	0	0	11.5	7.3	3.0	0.4	—
107	Whipped	1	tablespoon(s)	9	1.5	67	0.1	0	0	7.6	4.7	2.2	0.3	—
944	Whipped, unsalted	1	tablespoon(s)	11	2.0	82	0.1	0	0	9.2	5.9	2.4	0.3	—
	Fats, cooking													
2671	Beef tallow, semisolid	1	tablespoon(s)	13	0	115	0	0	0	12.8	6.4	5.4	0.5	—
922	Chicken fat	1	tablespoon(s)	13	0	115	0	0	0	12.8	3.8	5.7	2.7	—
5454	Household shortening with vegetable oil	1	tablespoon(s)	13	0	115	0	0	0	13.0	3.4	5.5	2.7	2.2
111	Lard	1	tablespoon(s)	13	0	115	0	0	0	12.8	5.0	5.8	1.4	—
	Margarine													
114	Margarine	1	tablespoon(s)	14	2.3	101	0	0.1	0	11.4	2.1	5.5	3.4	2.1
5439	Soft	1	tablespoon(s)	14	2.3	103	0.1	0.1	0	11.6	1.7	4.4	2.1	3.0
32329	Soft, unsalted, with hydroge-nated soybean and cottonseed oils	1	tablespoon(s)	14	2.5	101	0.1	0.1	0	11.3	2.0	5.4	3.5	
928	Unsalted	1	tablespoon(s)	14	2.6	101	0.1	0.1	0	11.3	2.1	5.2	3.5	—
119	Whipped	1	tablespoon(s)	9	1.5	64	0.1	0.1	0	7.2	1.2	3.2	2.5	—
	Spreads													
54657	I Can't Believe It's Not Butter!, tub, soya oil (non-hydrogenated)	1	tablespoon(s)	14	2.3	103	0.1	0.1	0	11.6	2.8	2.0	5.1	0.1
2708	Mayonnaise with soybean and safflower oils	1	tablespoon(s)	14	2.1	99	0.2	0.4	0	11.0	1.2	1.8	7.6	—
16157	Promise vegetable oil spread, stick	1	tablespoon(s)	14	4.2	90	0	0	0	10.0	2.5	2.0	4.0	—
	Oils													
2681	Canola	1	tablespoon(s)	14	0	120	0	0	0	13.6	1.0	8.6	3.8	0.1
120	Corn	1	tablespoon(s)	14	0	120	0	0	0	13.6	1.8	3.8	7.4	0
122	Olive	1	tablespoon(s)	14	0	119	0	0	0	13.5	1.9	9.9	1.4	—

AGE KEY: A-6 = Breads/Baked Goods A-12 = Cereal/Rice/Pasta A-16 = Fruit A-20 = Vegetables/Legumes A-30 = Nuts/Seeds A-32 = Vegetarian A-34 = Dairy A-42 = Eggs A-42 = Seafood A-44 = Meats A-48 = Poultry A-48 = Processed Meats A-50 = Beverages A-54 = Fats/Oils A-56 = Sweets A-58 = Spices/Condiments/Sauces A-62 = Mixed Foods/Soups/Sandwiches A-66 = Fast Food A-86 = Convenience A-88 = Baby Foods

Chol (mg)	Calc (mg)	Iron (mg)	Magn (mg)	Pota (mg)	Sodi (mg)	Zinc (mg)	Vit A (µg)	Thia (mg)	Vit E (mg α)	Ribo (mg)	Niac (mg)	Vit B_6 (mg)	Fola (µg)	Vit C (mg)	Vit B_{12} (µg)	Sele (µg)
0	0	0.00	—	10.1	10.1	—	0	—	—	—	—	—	—	6.0	—	—
0	10	0.39	5.0	37.2	9.9	0.05	0	0.01	0.02	0.05	0.04	0.01	2.5	9.7	0	0.2
0	5	0.00	4.9	24.7	7.4	0.02	0	0.01	0.00	0.01	0.02	0.01	2.5	7.7	0	0.2
0	20	0.72	—	0	20.0	—	0	—	—	—	—	—	—	600.0	0	—
0	0	0.00	—	70.0	10.0	—	0	—	—	—	—	—	—	54.0	0	—
0	0	0.00	—	20.0	10.0	—	0	—	—	—	—	—	—	0	0	—
0	0	0.00	—	40.0	10.0	—	0	—	—	—	—	—	—	0	0	—
5	400	2.70	140.0	600.0	220.0	2.25	—	0.52	—	0.59	7.00	0.70	120.0	60.0	2.1	17.5
5	1000	2.70	140.0	600.0	220.0	2.25	—	0.52	—	0.59	7.00	0.70	120.0	30.0	2.1	17.5
5	400	2.70	140.0	600.0	220.0	2.25	—	0.52	—	0.59	7.00	0.70	120.0	60.0	2.1	17.5
0	0	0.04	7.1	87.7	7.1	0.04	0	0.00	0.00	0.03	0.00	0.00	11.9	0	0	0
0	5	0.18	2.4	21.3	2.4	0.09	0	0.02	0.00	0.01	0.00	0.00	2.4	0	0	0
0	5	0.05	2.6	38.9	5.2	0.02	0	0.00	0.00	0.00	0.02	0.00	0	0	0	0.3
0	7	0.02	4.7	42.7	9.5	0.02	0	0.00	0.00	0.01	0.07	0.00	0	0	0	0
0	0	0.04	7.1	87.7	7.1	0.04	0	0.00	0.00	0.03	0.00	0.00	11.9	0	0	0
0	33	0.00	0	0	2.4	0.00	0	0.00	—	0.00	0.00	0.00	0	0	0	0
0	2	0.02	2.4	0	2.4	0.00	0	0.00	—	0.00	0.00	0.00	0	0	0	0
0	7	0.00	2.4	2.4	7.1	0.00	0	0.00	0.00	0.00	0.00	0.00	0	0	0	0
0	2	0.02	0	0	29.3	0.24	0	0.00	0.00	0.00	0.00	0.00	0	0	0	0
31	3	0.00	0.3	3.4	81.8	0.01	97.1	0.00	0.32	0.01	0.01	0.00	0.4	0	0	0.1
0	0	0.00	0	1.6	120.0	0.00	0	0.00	0.00	0.00	0.00	0.00	0	0	0	—
31	3	0.00	0.3	3.4	1.6	0.01	97.1	0.00	0.32	0.01	0.01	0.00	0.4	0	0	0.1
21	2	0.01	0.2	2.4	77.7	0.01	64.3	0.00	0.21	0.00	0.00	0.00	0.3	0	0	0.1
25	3	0.00	0.2	2.7	1.3	0.01	78.0	0.00	0.26	0.00	0.00	0.00	0.3	0	0	0.1
14	0	0.00	0	0	0	0.00	0	0.00	0.34	0.00	0.00	0.00	0	0	0	0
11	0	0.00	0	0	0	0.00	0	0.00	0.34	0.00	0.00	0.00	0	0	0	0
0	0	0.00	0	0	0	0.00	0	0.00	—	0.00	0.00	0.00	0	0	0	0
12	0	0.00	0	0	0	0.01	0	0.00	0.07	0.00	0.00	0.00	0	0	0	0
0	4	0.01	0.4	5.9	133.0	0.00	115.5	0.00	1.26	0.01	0.00	0.00	0.1	0	0	0
0	4	0.00	0.3	5.5	155.4	0.00	142.7	0.00	1.00	0.00	0.00	0.00	0.1	0	0	0
0	4	0.00	0.3	5.4	3.9	0.00	103.1	0.00	0.98	0.00	0.00	0.00	0.1	0	0	0
0	2	0.00	0.3	3.5	0.3	0.00	115.5	0.00	1.80	0.00	0.00	0.00	0.1	0	0	0
0	2	0.00	0.2	3.4	97.1	0.00	73.7	0.00	0.45	0.00	0.00	0.00	0.1	0	0	0
0	4	0.00	0.3	5.5	155.3	0.00	142.6	0.00	0.72	0.00	0.00	0.00	0.1	0	0	0
8	2	0.06	0.1	4.7	78.4	0.01	11.6	0.00	3.03	0.00	0.00	0.08	1.1	0	0	0.2
0	10	0.18	—	8.7	90.0	—	—	0.00	—	0.00	0.00	—	—	0.6	—	
0	0	0.00	0	0	0	0.00	0	0.00	2.37	0.00	0.00	0.00	0	0	0	0
0	0	0.00	0	0	0	0.00	0	0.00	1.94	0.00	0.00	0.00	0	0	0	0
0	0	0.07	0	0.1	0.3	0.00	0	0.00	1.93	0.00	0.00	0.00	0	0	0	0

TABLE A-1 Table of Food Composition (*continued*) (Computer code is for Cengage Diet Analysis program) (For purposes of calculations, use "0" for t, <1, <.1, <.01, etc

DA+ Code	Food Description	Quantity	Measure	Wt (g)	H₂O (g)	Ener (kcal)	Prot (g)	Carb (g)	Fiber (g)	Fat (g)	Fat Breakdown (g) Sat	Mono	Poly	Trans
Fats and Oils—*continued*														
124	Peanut	1	tablespoon(s)	14	0	119	0	0	0	13.5	2.3	6.2	4.3	—
2693	Safflower	1	tablespoon(s)	14	0	120	0	0	0	13.6	0.8	10.2	2.0	—
923	Sesame	1	tablespoon(s)	14	0	120	0	0	0	13.6	1.9	5.4	5.7	—
128	Soybean, hydrogenated	1	tablespoon(s)	14	0	120	0	0	0	13.6	2.0	5.8	5.1	—
130	Soybean, with soybean and cottonseed oil	1	tablespoon(s)	14	0	120	0	0	0	13.6	2.4	4.0	6.5	—
2700	Sunflower	1	tablespoon(s)	14	0	120	0	0	0	13.6	1.8	6.3	5.0	—
357	**Pam original no stick cooking spray**	1	serving(s)	0	0.2	0	0	0	0	0	0	0	0	—
	Salad dressing													
132	Blue cheese	2	tablespoon(s)	30	9.7	151	1.4	2.2	0	15.7	3.0	3.7	8.3	—
133	Blue cheese, low calorie	2	tablespoon(s)	32	25.4	32	1.6	0.9	0	2.3	0.8	0.6	0.8	—
1764	Caesar	2	tablespoon(s)	30	10.3	158	0.4	0.9	0	17.3	2.6	4.1	9.9	—
29654	Creamy, reduced calorie, fat-free, cholesterol-free, sour cream and/or buttermilk and oil	2	tablespoon(s)	32	23.9	34	0.4	6.4	0	0.9	0.2	0.2	0.5	—
29617	Creamy, reduced calorie, sour cream and/or buttermilk and oil	2	tablespoon(s)	30	22.2	48	0.5	2.1	0	4.2	0.6	1.0	2.4	—
134	French	2	tablespoon(s)	32	11.7	146	0.2	5.0	0	14.3	1.8	2.7	6.7	—
135	French, low fat	2	tablespoon(s)	32	17.4	74	0.2	9.4	0.4	4.3	0.4	1.9	1.6	—
136	Italian	2	tablespoon(s)	29	16.6	86	0.1	3.1	0	8.3	1.3	1.9	3.8	—
137	Italian, diet	2	tablespoon(s)	30	25.4	23	0.1	1.4	0	1.9	0.1	0.7	0.5	—
139	Mayonnaise-type	2	tablespoon(s)	29	11.7	115	0.3	7.0	0	9.8	1.4	2.6	5.3	—
942	Oil and vinegar	2	tablespoon(s)	32	15.2	144	0	0.8	0	16.0	2.9	4.7	7.7	—
1765	Ranch	2	tablespoon(s)	30	11.6	146	0.1	1.6	0	15.8	2.3	5.2	7.6	—
3666	Ranch, reduced calorie	2	tablespoon(s)	30	20.5	62	0.1	2.2	0	6.1	1.1	1.8	2.9	—
940	Russian	2	tablespoon(s)	30	11.6	107	0.5	9.3	0.7	7.8	1.2	1.8	4.4	—
939	Russian, low calorie	2	tablespoon(s)	32	20.8	45	0.2	8.8	0.1	1.3	0.2	0.3	0.7	—
941	Sesame seed	2	tablespoon(s)	30	11.8	133	0.9	2.6	0.3	13.6	1.9	3.6	7.5	—
142	Thousand Island	2	tablespoon(s)	32	14.9	118	0.3	4.7	0.3	11.2	1.6	2.5	5.8	—
143	Thousand Island, low calorie	2	tablespoon(s)	30	18.2	61	0.3	6.7	0.4	3.9	0.2	1.9	0.8	—
	Sandwich spreads													
138	Mayonnaise with soybean oil	1	tablespoon(s)	14	2.1	99	0.1	0.4	0	11.0	1.6	2.7	5.8	0
140	Mayonnaise, low calorie	1	tablespoon(s)	16	10.0	37	0	2.6	0	3.1	0.5	0.7	1.7	—
141	Tartar sauce	2	tablespoon(s)	28	8.7	144	0.3	4.1	0.1	14.4	2.2	3.8	7.7	—
Sweets														
4799	**Butterscotch or caramel topping**	2	tablespoon(s)	41	13.1	103	0.6	27.0	0.4	0	0	0	0	—
	Candy													
1786	Almond Joy candy bar	1	item(s)	45	4.3	220	2.0	27.0	2.0	12.0	8.0	3.3	0.7	0
1785	Bit-O-Honey candy	6	item(s)	40	—	190	1.0	39.0	0	3.5	2.5	—	—	—
33375	Butterscotch candy	2	piece(s)	12	0.6	47	0	10.8	0	0.4	0.2	0.1	0	—
1701	Chewing gum, stick	1	item(s)	3	0.1	7	0	2.0	0.1	0	0	0	0	—
33378	Chocolate fudge with nuts, prepared	2	piece(s)	38	2.9	175	1.7	25.8	1.0	7.2	2.5	1.5	2.9	0.1
1787	Jelly beans	15	item(s)	43	2.7	159	0	39.8	0.1	0	0	0	0	—
1784	Kit Kat wafer bar	1	item(s)	42	0.8	210	3.0	27.0	0.5	11.0	7.0	3.5	0.3	0
4674	Krackel candy bar	1	item(s)	41	0.6	210	2.0	28.0	0.5	10.0	6.0	3.9	0.4	0
4934	Licorice	4	piece(s)	44	7.3	154	1.1	35.1	0	1.0	0	0.1	0	—
1780	Life Savers candy	1	item(s)	2	—	8	0	2.0	0	0	0	0	0	—
1790	Lollipop	1	item(s)	28	—	108	0	28.0	0	0	0	0	0	0
4679	M & Ms peanut chocolate candy, small bag	1	item(s)	49	0.9	250	5.0	30.0	2.0	13.0	5.0	5.4	2.1	—
1781	M & Ms plain chocolate candy, small bag	1	item(s)	48	0.8	240	2.0	34.0	1.0	10.0	6.0	3.3	0.3	—
4673	Milk chocolate bar, Symphony	1	item(s)	91	0.9	483	7.7	52.8	1.5	27.8	16.7	7.2	0.6	—
1783	Milky Way bar	1	item(s)	58	3.7	270	2.0	41.0	1.0	10.0	5.0	3.5	0.3	—
1788	Peanut brittle	1½	ounce(s)	43	0.3	207	3.2	30.3	1.1	8.1	1.8	3.4	1.9	—
1789	Reese's peanut butter cups	2	piece(s)	51	0.8	280	6.0	19.0	2.0	15.5	6.0	7.2	2.7	0
4689	Reese's pieces candy, small bag	1	item(s)	43	1.1	220	5.0	26.0	1.0	11.0	7.0	0.9	0.4	0
33399	Semisweet chocolate candy, made with butter	½	ounce(s)	14	0.1	68	0.6	9.0	0.8	4.2	2.5	1.4	0	—
1782	Snickers bar	1	item(s)	59	3.2	280	4.0	35.0	1.0	14.0	5.0	6.1	2.9	—
4694	Special Dark chocolate bar	1	item(s)	41	0.4	220	2.0	25.0	3.0	12.0	8.0	4.6	0.4	0
4695	Starburst fruit chews, original fruits	1	package(s)	59	3.9	240	0	48.0	0	5.0	1.0	2.1	1.8	—

PAGE KEY: A-6 = Breads/Baked Goods A-12 = Cereal/Rice/Pasta A-16 = Fruit A-20 = Vegetables/Legumes A-30 = Nuts/Seeds A-32 = Vegetarian A-34 = Dairy A-42 = Eggs A-42 = Seafood A-44 = Meats A-48 = Poultry A-48 = Processed Meats A-50 = Beverages A-54 = Fats/Oils A-56 = Sweets A-58 = Spices/Condiments/Sauces A-62 = Mixed Foods/Soups/Sandwiches A-66 = Fast Food A-86 = Convenience A-88 = Baby Foods

Chol (mg)	Calc (mg)	Iron (mg)	Magn (mg)	Pota (mg)	Sodi (mg)	Zinc (mg)	Vit A (µg)	Thia (mg)	Vit E (mg α)	Ribo (mg)	Niac (mg)	Vit B_6 (mg)	Fola (µg)	Vit C (mg)	Vit B_{12} (µg)	Sele (µg)
0	0	0.00	0	0	0	0.00	0	0.00	2.11	0.00	0.00	0.00	0	0	0	0
0	0	0.00	0	0	0	0.00	0	0.00	4.63	0.00	0.00	0.00	0	0	0	0
0	0	0.00	0	0	0	0.00	0	0.00	0.19	0.00	0.00	0.00	0	0	0	0
0	0	0.00	0	0	0	0.00	0	0.00	1.10	0.00	0.00	0.00	0	0	0	0
0	0	0.00	0	0	0	0.00	0	0.00	1.64	0.00	0.00	0.00	0	0	0	0
0	0	0.00	0	0	0	0.00	0	0.00	5.58	0.00	0.00	0.00	0	0	0	0
0	0	0.00	0	0.3	1.5	0.01	0.1	0.00	0.00	0.00	0.00	0.00	0	0	0	0
5	24	0.06	0	11.1	328.2	0.08	20.1	0.00	1.80	0.03	0.03	0.01	7.8	0.6	0.1	0.3
0	28	0.16	2.2	1.6	384.0	0.08	—	0.01	0.08	0.03	0.01	0.01	1.0	0.1	0.1	0.5
1	7	0.05	0.6	8.7	323.4	0.03	0.6	0.00	1.56	0.00	0.01	0.00	0.9	0	0	0.5
0	12	0.08	1.6	42.6	320.0	0.05	0.3	0.00	0.21	0.01	0.01	0.01	1.9	0	0	0.5
0	2	0.03	0.6	10.8	306.9	0.01	—	0.00	0.71	0.00	0.01	0.01	0	0.1	0	0.5
0	8	0.25	1.6	21.4	267.5	0.09	7.4	0.01	1.60	0.01	0.06	0.00	0	0	0	0
0	4	0.27	2.6	34.2	257.3	0.06	8.6	0.01	0.09	0.01	0.14	0.01	0.6	0	0	0.5
0	2	0.18	0.9	14.1	486.3	0.03	0.6	0.00	1.47	0.01	0.00	0.01	0	0	0	0.6
2	3	0.19	1.2	25.5	409.8	0.05	0.3	0.00	0.06	0.00	0.00	0.02	0	0	0	2.4
8	4	0.05	0.6	2.6	209.0	0.05	6.2	0.00	0.60	0.01	0.00	0.01	1.8	0	0.1	0.5
0	0	0.00	0	2.6	0.3	0.00	0	0.00	1.46	0.00	0.00	0.00	0	0	0	0.5
1	4	0.03	1.2	8.4	354.0	0.01	5.4	0.00	1.84	0.01	0.00	0.00	0.3	0.1	0	0.1
0	5	0.01	1.5	8.4	413.7	0.01	0.9	0.00	0.72	0.01	0.00	0.00	0.3	0.1	0	0.1
0	6	0.20	3.0	51.9	282.3	0.06	13.2	0.01	0.98	0.01	0.16	0.02	1.5	1.4	0	0.5
2	6	0.18	0	50.2	277.8	0.02	0.6	0.00	0.12	0.00	0.00	0.00	1.0	1.9	0	0.5
0	6	0.18	0	47.1	300.0	0.02	0.6	0.00	1.50	0.00	0.00	0.00	0	0	0	0.5
8	5	0.37	2.6	34.2	276.2	0.08	4.5	0.46	1.28	0.01	0.13	0.00	0	0	0	0.5
0	5	0.27	2.1	60.6	249.3	0.05	4.8	0.01	0.30	0.01	0.13	0.00	0	0	0	0
5	1	0.03	0.1	1.7	78.4	0.02	11.2	0.01	0.72	0.01	0.00	0.08	0.7	0	0	0.2
4	0	0.00	0	1.6	79.5	0.01	0	0.00	0.32	0.00	0.00	0.00	0	0	0	0.3
8	6	0.20	0.8	10.1	191.5	0.05	20.2	0.00	0.97	0.00	0.01	0.07	2.0	0.1	0.1	0.5
0	22	0.08	2.9	34.4	143.1	0.07	11.1	0.01	—	0.03	0.01	0.01	0.8	0.1	0	0
0	18	0.33	30.3	126.5	65.0	0.36	0	0.01	—	0.06	0.21	—	—	0	—	—
0	20	0.00	—	—	150.0	—	0	—	—	—	—	—	—	0	—	—
1	0	0.00	0	0.4	46.9	0.01	3.4	0.00	0.01	0.00	0.00	0.00	0	0	0	0.1
0	0	0.00	0	0.1	0	0.00	0	0.00	0.00	0.00	0.00	0.00	0	0	0	0
5	22	0.74	20.9	69.5	14.8	0.54	14.4	0.02	0.09	0.03	0.12	0.03	6.1	0.1	0	1.1
0	1	0.05	0.9	15.7	21.3	0.02	0	0.00	0.00	0.01	0.00	0.00	0	0	0	0.5
3	60	0.36	16.4	126.0	30.0	0.51	0	0.07	—	0.22	1.07	0.05	59.6	0	0.1	2.0
3	40	0.36	—	168.8	50.0	—	0	—	—	—	—	—	—	0	—	—
0	0	0.22	2.6	28.2	126.3	0.07	0	0.01	0.07	0.01	0.04	0.00	0	0	0	—
0	0	0.00	—	0	0	—	0	0.00	—	0.00	0.00	0.00	—	0	—	0
0	0	0.00	—	—	10.8	—	0	0.00	—	0.00	0.00	—	—	0	—	1.0
5	40	0.36	36.5	170.6	25.0	1.13	14.8	0.03	—	0.06	1.60	0.04	17.3	0.6	0.1	1.9
5	40	0.36	19.6	127.4	30.0	0.46	14.8	0.02	—	0.06	0.10	0.01	2.9	0.6	0.1	1.4
22	228	0.82	61.0	398.6	91.9	1.00	0	0.06	—	0.25	0.14	0.10	10.9	2.0	0.4	—
5	60	0.18	19.8	140.1	95.0	0.41	15.1	0.02	—	0.06	0.20	0.02	5.8	0.6	0.2	3.3
5	11	0.51	17.9	71.4	189.2	0.37	16.6	0.05	1.08	0.01	1.12	0.03	19.6	0	0	1.1
3	40	0.72	45.4	217.4	180.0	0.93	0	0.12	—	0.08	2.35	0.07	28.1	0	0.1	2.3
0	20	0.00	18.9	169.9	80.0	0.32	0	0.04	—	0.06	1.22	0.03	12.0	0	0.1	0.8
3	5	0.44	16.3	51.7	1.6	0.23	0.4	0.00	—	0.01	0.06	0.01	0.4	0	0	0.5
5	40	0.36	42.3	—	140.0	1.37	15.3	0.03	—	0.06	1.60	0.05	23.5	0.6	0.1	2.7
0	0	1.80	45.5	136.0	50.0	0.59	0	0.01	—	0.02	0.16	0.01	0.8	0	0	1.2
0	10	0.18	0.6	1.2	0	0.00	—	0.00	—	0.00	0.00	0.00	0	30	0	0.5

TABLE A-1 Table of Food Composition (*continued*) (Computer code is for Cengage Diet Analysis program) (For purposes of calculations, use "0" for t, <1, <.1, <.01, etc.)

DA+ Code	Food Description	Quantity	Measure	Wt (g)	H₂O (g)	Ener (kcal)	Prot (g)	Carb (g)	Fiber (g)	Fat (g)	Sat	Mono	Poly	Trans
											Fat Breakdown (g)			

Sweets—*continued*

DA+ Code	Food Description	Quantity	Measure	Wt (g)	H₂O (g)	Ener (kcal)	Prot (g)	Carb (g)	Fiber (g)	Fat (g)	Sat	Mono	Poly	Trans
4698	Taffy	3	piece(s)	45	2.2	179	0	41.2	0	1.5	0.9	0.4	0.1	0.1
4699	Three Musketeers bar	1	item(s)	60	3.5	260	2.0	46.0	1.0	8.0	4.5	2.6	0.3	—
4702	Twix caramel cookie bars	2	item(s)	58	2.4	280	3.0	37.0	1.0	14.0	5.0	7.7	0.5	—
4705	York peppermint pattie	1	item(s)	39	3.9	160	0.5	32.0	0.5	3.0	1.5	1.2	0.1	0
	Frosting, icing													
4760	Chocolate frosting, ready to eat	2	tablespoon(s)	31	5.2	122	0.3	19.4	0.3	5.4	1.7	2.8	0.6	—
4771	Creamy vanilla frosting, ready to eat	2	tablespoon(s)	28	4.2	117	0	19.0	0	4.5	0.8	1.4	2.2	0
17291	Dec-A-Cake variety pack candy decoration	1	teaspoon(s)	4	—	15	0	3.0	0	0.5	0	—	0	0
536	White icing	2	tablespoon(s)	40	3.6	162	0.1	31.8	0	4.2	0.8	2.0	1.2	—
	Gelatin													
13697	Gelatin snack, all flavors	1	item(s)	99	96.8	70	1.0	17.0	0	0	0	0	0	0
2616	Sugar free, low calorie mixed fruit gelatin mix, prepared	½	cup(s)	121	—	10	1.0	0	0	0	0	0	0	0
548	**Honey**	1	tablespoon(s)	21	3.6	64	0.1	17.3	0	0	0	0	0	—
	Jams, jellies													
550	Jam or preserves	1	tablespoon(s)	20	6.1	56	0.1	13.8	0.2	0	0	0	0	—
42199	Jams, preserves, dietetic, all flavors, w/sodium saccharin	1	tablespoon(s)	14	6.4	18	0	7.5	0.4	0	0	0	0	—
552	Jelly	1	tablespoon(s)	21	6.3	56	0	14.7	0.2	0	0	0	0	—
545	**Marshmallows**	4	item(s)	29	4.7	92	0.5	23.4	0	0.1	0	0	0	—
4800	**Marshmallow cream topping**	2	tablespoon(s)	40	7.9	129	0.3	31.6	0	0.1	0	0	0	—
555	**Molasses**	1	tablespoon(s)	20	4.4	58	0	14.9	0	0	0	0	0	—
4780	**Popsicle or ice pop**	1	item(s)	59	47.5	47	0	11.3	0	0.1	0	0	0	—
	Sugar													
559	Brown sugar, packed	1	teaspoon(s)	5	0.1	17	0	4.5	0	0	0	0	0	0
563	Powdered sugar, sifted	⅓	cup(s)	33	0.1	130	0	33.2	0	0	0	0	0	—
561	White granulated sugar	1	teaspoon(s)	4	0	16	0	4.2	0	0	0	0	0	0
	Sugar substitute													
1760	Equal sweetener, packet size	1	item(s)	1	—	0	0	0.9	0	0	0	0	0	0
13029	Splenda granular no calorie sweetener	1	teaspoon(s)	1	—	0	0	0.5	0	0	0	0	0	0
1759	Sweet N Low sugar substitute, packet	1	item(s)	1	0.1	4	0	0.5	0	0	0	0	0	0
	Syrup													
3148	Chocolate syrup	2	tablespoon(s)	38	11.6	105	0.8	24.4	1.0	0.4	0.2	0.1	0	—
29676	Maple syrup	¼	cup(s)	80	25.7	209	0	53.7	0	0.2	0	0.1	0.1	—
4795	Pancake syrup	¼	cup(s)	80	30.4	187	0	49.2	0	0	0	0	0	0

Spices, Condiments, Sauces

DA+ Code	Food Description	Quantity	Measure	Wt (g)	H₂O (g)	Ener (kcal)	Prot (g)	Carb (g)	Fiber (g)	Fat (g)	Sat	Mono	Poly	Trans
	Spices													
807	Allspice, ground	1	teaspoon(s)	2	0.2	5	0.1	1.4	0.4	0.2	0	0	0	—
1171	Anise seeds	1	teaspoon(s)	2	0.2	7	0.4	1.1	0.3	0.3	0	0.2	0.1	—
729	Bakers' yeast, active	1	teaspoon(s)	4	0.3	12	1.5	1.5	0.8	0.2	0	0.1	0	—
683	Baking powder, double acting with phosphate	1	teaspoon(s)	5	0.2	2	0	1.1	0	0	0	0	0	0
1611	Baking soda	1	teaspoon(s)	5	0	0	0	0	0	0	0	0	0	0
8552	Basil	1	teaspoon(s)	1	0.8	0	0	0	0	0	0	0	0	0
34959	Basil, fresh	1	piece(s)	1	0.5	0	0	0	0	0	0	0	0	—
808	Basil, ground	1	teaspoon(s)	1	0.1	4	0.2	0.9	0.6	0.1	0	0	0	—
809	Bay leaf	1	teaspoon(s)	1	0	2	0	0.5	0.2	0.1	0	0	0	—
11720	Betel leaves	1	ounce(s)	28	—	17	1.8	2.4	0	0	—	—	—	—
730	Brewers' yeast	1	teaspoon(s)	3	0.1	8	1.0	1.0	0.8	0	0	0	0	0
11710	Capers	1	teaspoon(s)	5	—	0	0	0	0	0	0	0	0	0
1172	Caraway seeds	1	teaspoon(s)	2	0.2	7	0.4	1.0	0.8	0.3	0	0.2	0.1	—
1173	Celery seeds	1	teaspoon(s)	2	0.1	8	0.4	0.8	0.2	0.5	0	0.3	0.1	—
1174	Chervil, dried	1	teaspoon(s)	1	0	1	0.1	0.3	0.1	0	0	0	0	—
810	Chili powder	1	teaspoon(s)	3	0.2	8	0.3	1.4	0.9	0.4	0.1	0.1	0.2	—
8553	Chives, chopped	1	teaspoon(s)	1	0.9	0	0	0	0	0	0	0	0	—
51420	Cilantro (coriander)	1	teaspoon(s)	0	0.3	0	0	0	0	0	0	0	0	—
811	Cinnamon, ground	1	teaspoon(s)	2	0.2	6	0.1	1.9	1.2	0	0	0	0	—
812	Cloves, ground	1	teaspoon(s)	2	0.1	7	0.1	1.3	0.7	0.4	0.1	0	0.1	—
1175	Coriander leaf, dried	1	teaspoon(s)	1	0	2	0.1	0.3	0.1	0	0	0	0	—
1176	Coriander seeds	1	teaspoon(s)	2	0.2	5	0.2	1.0	0.8	0.3	0	0.2	0	—
1706	Cornstarch	1	tablespoon(s)	8	0.7	30	0	7.3	0.1	0	0	0	0	—

PAGE KEY: A-6 = Breads/Baked Goods A-12 = Cereal/Rice/Pasta A-16 = Fruit A-20 = Vegetables/Legumes A-30 = Nuts/Seeds A-32 = Vegetarian A-34 = Dairy A-42 = Eggs A-42 = Seafood A-44 = Meats A-48 = Poultry A-48 = Processed Meats A-50 = Beverages A-54 = Fats/Oils A-56 = Sweets A-58 = Spices/Condiments/Sauces A-62 = Mixed Foods/Soups/Sandwiches A-66 = Fast Food A-86 = Convenience A-88 = Baby Foods

Chol (mg)	Calc (mg)	Iron (mg)	Magn (mg)	Pota (mg)	Sodi (mg)	Zinc (mg)	Vit A (µg)	Thia (mg)	Vit E (mg α)	Ribo (mg)	Niac (mg)	Vit B_6 (mg)	Fola (µg)	Vit C (mg)	Vit B_{12} (µg)	Sele (µg)
4	4	0.00	0	1.4	23.4	0.09	12.2	0.01	0.04	0.01	0.00	0.00	0	0	0	0.3
5	20	0.36	17.5	80.3	110.0	0.33	14.5	0.01	—	0.03	0.20	0.01	0	0.6	0.1	1.5
5	40	0.36	18.5	116.8	115.0	0.45	15.0	0.09	—	0.13	0.69	0.01	13.9	0.6	0.1	1.2
0	0	0.33	23.4	66.1	10.0	0.28	0	0.01	—	0.03	0.31	0.01	1.5	0	0	—
0	2	0.44	6.4	60.0	56.1	0.09	0	0.00	0.48	0.00	0.03	0.00	0.3	0	0	0.2
0	1	0.04	0.3	9.5	51.5	0.01	0	0.00	0.43	0.08	0.06	0.00	2.2	0	0	0
0	0	0.00	—	—	15.0	—	0	—	—	—	—	—	—	0	—	—
0	4	0.01	0.4	5.6	76.4	0.01	44.4	0.00	0.32	0.01	0.00	0.00	0	0	0	0.3
0	0	0.00	—	0	40.0	—	0	—	—	—	—	—	—	0	—	—
0	0	0.00	0	0	50.0	0.00	0	0.00	0.00	0.00	0.00	0.00	0	0	0	—
0	1	0.08	0.4	10.9	0.8	0.04	0	0.00	0.00	0.01	0.02	0.01	0.4	0.1	0	0.2
0	4	0.10	0.8	15.4	6.4	0.01	0	0.00	0.02	0.02	0.01	0.00	2.2	1.8	0	0.4
0	1	0.56	0.7	9.7	0	0.01	0	0.00	0.01	0.00	0.00	0.00	1.3	0	0	0.2
0	1	0.04	1.3	11.3	6.3	0.01	0	0.00	0.00	0.01	0.01	0.00	0.4	0.2	0	0.1
0	1	0.06	0.6	1.4	23.0	0.01	0	0.00	0.00	0.00	0.02	0.00	0.3	0	0	0.5
0	1	0.08	0.8	2.0	32.0	0.01	0	0.00	0.00	0.00	0.03	0.00	0.4	0	0	0.7
0	41	0.94	48.4	292.8	7.4	0.05	0	0.01	0.00	0.00	0.18	0.13	0	0	0	3.6
0	0	0.31	0.6	8.9	4.1	0.08	0	0.00	0.00	0.00	0.00	0.00	0	0.4	0	0.1
0	4	0.03	0.4	6.1	1.3	0.00	0	0.00	0.00	0.00	0.01	0.00	0	0	0	0.1
0	0	0.01	0	0.7	0.3	0.00	0	0.00	0.00	0.00	0.00	0.00	0	0	0	0.2
0	0	0.00	0	0.1	0	0.00	0	0.00	0.00	0.00	0.00	0.00	0	0	0	0
0	0	0.00	0	0	0	0.00	0	0.00	0.00	0.00	0.00	0.00	0	0	0	0
0	0	0.00	—	—	0	—	—	0.00	—	0.00	0.00	—	—	0	0	—
0	0	0.00	—	—	0	—	0	—	0.00	—	—	—	—	0	0	—
0	5	0.79	24.4	84.0	27.0	0.27	0	0.00	0.01	0.01	0.12	0.00	0.8	0.1	0	0.5
0	54	0.96	11.2	163.2	7.2	3.32	0	0.01	0.00	0.01	0.02	0.00	0	0	0	0.5
0	2	0.02	1.6	12.0	65.6	0.06	0	0.01	0.00	0.01	0.00	0.00	0	0	0	0
0	13	0.13	2.6	19.8	1.5	0.01	0.5	0.00	—	0.00	0.05	0.00	0.7	0.7	0	0.1
0	14	0.77	3.6	30.3	0.3	0.11	0.3	0.01	—	0.01	0.06	0.01	0.2	0.4	0	0.1
0	3	0.66	3.9	80.0	2.0	0.25	0	0.09	0.00	0.21	1.59	0.06	93.6	0	0	1.0
0	339	0.51	1.8	0.2	363.1	0.00	0	0.00	0.00	0.00	0.00	0.00	0	0	0	0
0	0	0.00	0	0	1258.6	0.00	0	0.00	0.00	0.00	0.00	0.00	0	0	0	0
0	2	0.02	0.6	2.6	0	0.01	2.3	0.00	0.01	0.00	0.01	0.00	0.6	0.2	0	0
0	1	0.01	0.4	2.3	0	0.00	1.3	0.00	—	0.00	0.00	0.00	0.3	0.1	0	0
0	30	0.58	5.9	48.1	0.5	0.08	6.6	0.00	0.10	0.00	0.09	0.03	3.8	0.9	0	0
0	5	0.25	0.7	3.2	0.1	0.02	1.9	0.00	—	0.00	0.01	0.01	1.1	0.6	0	0
0	110	2.29	—	155.9	2.0	—	—	0.04	—	0.07	0.19	—	—	0.9	0	—
0	6	0.46	6.1	50.7	3.3	0.21	0	0.41	—	0.11	1.00	0.06	104.3	0	0	0
0	—	—	—	—	105.0	—	—	—	—	—	—	—	—	—	0	—
0	14	0.34	5.4	28.4	0.4	0.11	0.4	0.01	0.05	0.01	0.07	0.01	0.2	0.4	0	0.3
0	35	0.89	8.8	28.0	3.2	0.13	0.1	0.01	0.02	0.01	0.06	0.01	0.2	0.3	0	0.2
0	8	0.19	0.8	28.4	0.5	0.05	1.8	0.00	—	0.00	0.03	0.01	1.6	0.3	0	0.2
0	7	0.37	4.4	49.8	26.3	0.07	38.6	0.01	0.75	0.02	0.20	0.09	2.6	1.7	0	0.2
0	1	0.01	0.4	3.0	0	0.01	2.2	0.00	0.00	0.00	0.01	0.00	1.1	0.6	0	0
0	0	0.01	0.1	1.7	0.2	0.00	1.1	0.00	0.01	0.00	0.00	0.00	0.2	0.1	0	0
0	23	0.19	1.4	9.9	0.2	0.04	0.3	0.00	0.05	0.00	0.03	0.00	0.1	0.1	0	0.1
0	14	0.18	5.5	23.1	5.1	0.02	0.6	0.00	0.17	0.01	0.03	0.01	2.0	1.7	0	0.1
0	7	0.25	4.2	26.8	1.3	0.02	1.8	0.01	0.01	0.01	0.06	0.00	1.6	3.4	0	0.2
0	13	0.29	5.9	22.8	0.6	0.08	0	0.00	—	0.01	0.03	—	0	0.4	0	0.5
0	0	0.03	0.2	0.2	0.7	0.01	0	0.00	0.00	0.00	0.00	0.00	0	0	0	0.2

TABLE A-1 **Table of Food Composition (*continued*)** (Computer code is for Cengage Diet Analysis program) (For purposes of calculations, use "0" for t, <1, <.1, <.01, etc

DA+ Code	Food Description	Quantity	Measure	Wt (g)	H₂O (g)	Ener (kcal)	Prot (g)	Carb (g)	Fiber (g)	Fat (g)	Fat Breakdown (g) Sat	Mono	Poly	*Trans*
Spices, Condiments, Sauces—*continued*														
1177	Cumin seeds	1	teaspoon(s)	2	0.2	8	0.4	0.9	0.2	0.5	0	0.3	0.1	—
11729	Cumin, ground	1	teaspoon(s)	5	—	11	0.4	0.8	0.8	0.4	—	—	—	—
1178	Curry powder	1	teaspoon(s)	2	0.2	7	0.3	1.2	0.7	0.3	0	0.1	0.1	—
1179	Dill seeds	1	teaspoon(s)	2	0.2	6	0.3	1.2	0.4	0.3	0	0.2	0	—
1180	Dill weed, dried	1	teaspoon(s)	1	0.1	3	0.2	0.6	0.1	0	0	0	0	—
34949	Dill weed, fresh	5	piece(s)	1	0.9	0	0	0.1	0	0	0	0	0	—
4949	Fennel leaves, fresh	1	teaspoon(s)	1	0.9	0	0	0.1	0	0	—	—	—	—
1181	Fennel seeds	1	teaspoon(s)	2	0.2	7	0.3	1.0	0.8	0.3	0	0.2	0	—
1182	Fenugreek seeds	1	teaspoon(s)	4	0.3	12	0.9	2.2	0.9	0.2	0.1	—	—	—
11733	Garam masala, powder	1	ounce(s)	28	—	107	4.4	12.8	0	4.3	—	—	—	—
1067	Garlic clove	1	item(s)	3	1.8	4	0.2	1.0	0.1	0	0	0	0	—
813	Garlic powder	1	teaspoon(s)	3	0.2	9	0.5	2.0	0.3	0	0	0	0	—
1068	Ginger root	2	teaspoon(s)	4	3.1	3	0.1	0.7	0.1	0	0	0	0	—
1183	Ginger, ground	1	teaspoon(s)	2	0.2	6	0.2	1.3	0.2	0.1	0	0	0	—
35497	Leeks, bulb and lower-leaf, freeze-dried	¼	cup(s)	1	0	3	0.1	0.6	0.1	0	0	0	0	—
1184	Mace, ground	1	teaspoon(s)	2	0.1	8	0.1	0.9	0.3	0.6	0.2	0.2	0.1	—
1185	Marjoram, dried	1	teaspoon(s)	1	0	2	0.1	0.4	0.2	0	0	0	0	—
1186	Mustard seeds, yellow	1	teaspoon(s)	3	0.2	15	0.8	1.2	0.5	0.9	0	0.7	0.2	—
814	Nutmeg, ground	1	teaspoon(s)	2	0.1	12	0.1	1.1	0.5	0.8	0.6	0.1	0	—
2747	Onion flakes, dehydrated	1	teaspoon(s)	2	0.1	6	0.1	1.4	0.2	0	0	0	0	—
1187	Onion powder	1	teaspoon(s)	2	0.1	7	0.2	1.7	0.1	0	0	0	0	—
815	Oregano, ground	1	teaspoon(s)	2	0.1	5	0.2	1.0	0.6	0.2	0	0	0.1	—
816	Paprika	1	teaspoon(s)	2	0.2	6	0.3	1.2	0.8	0.3	0	0	0.2	—
817	Parsley, dried	1	teaspoon(s)	0	0	1	0.1	0.2	0.1	0	0	0	0	—
818	Pepper, black	1	teaspoon(s)	2	0.2	5	0.2	1.4	0.6	0.1	0	0	0	—
819	Pepper, cayenne	1	teaspoon(s)	2	0.1	6	0.2	1.0	0.5	0.3	0.1	0	0.2	—
1188	Pepper, white	1	teaspoon(s)	2	0.3	7	0.3	1.6	0.6	0.1	0	0	0	—
1189	Poppy seeds	1	teaspoon(s)	3	0.2	15	0.5	0.7	0.3	1.3	0.1	0.2	0.9	—
1190	Poultry seasoning	1	teaspoon(s)	2	0.1	5	0.1	1.0	0.2	0.1	0	0	0	—
1191	Pumpkin pie spice, powder	1	teaspoon(s)	2	0.1	6	0.1	1.2	0.3	0.2	0.1	0	0	—
1192	Rosemary, dried	1	teaspoon(s)	1	0.1	4	0.1	0.8	0.5	0.2	0.1	0	0	—
11723	Rosemary, fresh	1	teaspoon(s)	1	0.5	1	0	0.1	0.1	0	0	0	0	—
2722	Saffron powder	1	teaspoon(s)	1	0.1	2	0.1	0.5	0	0	0	0	0	—
11724	Sage	1	teaspoon(s)	1	—	1	0	0.1	0	0	—	—	—	—
1193	Sage, ground	1	teaspoon(s)	1	0.1	2	0.1	0.4	0.3	0.1	0	0	0	—
30189	Salt substitute	¼	teaspoon(s)	1	—	0	0	0	0	0	0	0	0	0
30190	Salt substitute, seasoned	¼	teaspoon(s)	1	—	1	0	0.1	0	0	0	—	—	—
822	Salt, table	¼	teaspoon(s)	2	0	0	0	0	0	0	0	0	0	—
1194	Savory, ground	1	teaspoon(s)	1	0.1	4	0.1	1.0	0.6	0.1	0	—	—	—
820	Sesame seed kernels, toasted	1	teaspoon(s)	3	0.1	15	0.5	0.7	0.5	1.3	0.2	0.5	0.6	—
11725	Sorrel	1	teaspoon(s)	3	—	1	0.1	0.1	0	0	0	—	—	—
11721	Spearmint	1	teaspoon(s)	2	1.6	1	0.1	0.2	0.1	0	0	0	0	—
35498	Sweet green peppers, freeze-dried	¼	cup(s)	2	0	5	0.3	1.1	0.3	0	0	0	0	—
11726	Tamarind leaves	1	ounce(s)	28	—	33	1.6	5.2	0	0.6	—	—	—	—
11727	Tarragon	1	ounce(s)	28	—	14	1.0	1.8	0	0.3	—	—	—	—
1195	Tarragon, ground	1	teaspoon(s)	2	0.1	5	0.4	0.8	0.1	0.1	0	0	0.1	—
11728	Thyme, fresh	1	teaspoon(s)	1	0.5	1	0	0.2	0.1	0	0	0	0	—
821	Thyme, ground	1	teaspoon(s)	1	0.1	4	0.1	0.9	0.5	0.1	0	0	0	—
1196	Turmeric, ground	1	teaspoon(s)	2	0.3	8	0.2	1.4	0.5	0.2	0.1	0	0	—
11995	Wasabi	1	tablespoon(s)	14	10.7	10	0.7	2.3	0.2	0	—	—	—	—
	Condiments													
674	Catsup or ketchup	1	tablespoon(s)	15	10.4	15	0.3	3.8	0	0	0	0	0	—
703	Dill pickle	1	ounce(s)	28	26.7	3	0.2	0.7	0.3	0	0	0	0	—
138	Mayonnaise with soybean oil	1	tablespoon(s)	14	2.1	99	0.1	0.4	0	11.0	1.6	2.7	5.8	0
140	Mayonnaise, low calorie	1	tablespoon(s)	16	10.0	37	0	2.6	0	3.1	0.5	0.7	1.7	—
1682	Mustard, brown	1	teaspoon(s)	5	4.1	5	0.3	0.3	0	0.3	—	—	—	—
700	Mustard, yellow	1	teaspoon(s)	5	4.1	3	0.2	0.3	0.2	0.2	0	0.1	0	0
706	Sweet pickle relish	1	tablespoon(s)	15	9.3	20	0.1	5.3	0.2	0.1	0	0	0	—
141	Tartar sauce	2	tablespoon(s)	28	8.7	144	0.3	4.1	0.1	14.4	2.2	3.8	7.7	—
	Sauces													
685	Barbecue sauce	2	tablespoon(s)	31	18.9	47	0	11.3	0.2	0.1	0	0	0.1	—
834	Cheese sauce	¼	cup(s)	63	44.4	110	4.2	4.3	0.3	8.4	3.8	2.4	1.6	—
32123	Chili enchilada sauce, green	2	tablespoon(s)	57	53.0	15	0.6	3.1	0.7	0.3	0	0	0.1	—
32122	Chili enchilada sauce, red	2	tablespoon(s)	32	24.5	27	1.1	5.0	2.1	0.8	0.1	0	0.4	0

PAGE KEY: A-6 = Breads/Baked Goods A-12 = Cereal/Rice/Pasta A-16 = Fruit A-20 = Vegetables/Legumes A-30 = Nuts/Seeds A-32 = Vegetarian A-34 = Dairy A-42 = Eggs A-42 = Seafood A-44 = Meats A-48 = Poultry A-48 = Processed Meats A-50 = Beverages A-54 = Fats/Oils A-56 = Sweets A-58 = Spices/Condiments/Sauces A-62 = Mixed Foods/Soups/Sandwiches A-66 = Fast Food A-86 = Convenience A-88 = Baby Foods

Chol (mg)	Calc (mg)	Iron (mg)	Magn (mg)	Pota (mg)	Sodi (mg)	Zinc (mg)	Vit A (µg)	Thia (mg)	Vit E (mg α)	Ribo (mg)	Niac (mg)	Vit B_6 (mg)	Fola (µg)	Vit C (mg)	Vit B_{12} (µg)	Sele (µg)
0	20	1.39	7.7	37.5	3.5	0.10	1.3	0.01	0.07	0.01	0.09	0.01	0.2	0.2	0	0.1
0	20	—	—	43.6	4.8	—	—	—	—	—	—	—	—	—	—	—
0	10	0.59	5.1	30.9	1.0	0.08	1.0	0.01	0.44	0.01	0.06	0.02	3.1	0.2	0	0.3
0	32	0.34	5.4	24.9	0.4	0.10	0.1	0.01	—	0.01	0.05	0.01	0.2	0.4	0	0.3
0	18	0.48	4.5	33.1	2.1	0.03	2.9	0.00	—	0.00	0.02	0.01	1.5	0.5	0	—
0	2	0.06	0.6	7.4	0.6	0.01	3.9	0.00	0.01	0.00	0.01	0.00	1.5	0.9	0	—
0	1	0.02	—	4.0	0.1	—	—	0.00	—	0.00	0.01	0.00	—	0.3	0	—
0	24	0.37	7.7	33.9	1.8	0.07	0.1	0.01	—	0.01	0.12	0.01	—	0.4	0	—
0	7	1.24	7.1	28.5	2.5	0.09	0.1	0.01	—	0.01	0.06	0.02	2.1	0.1	0	0.2
0	215	9.24	93.6	411.1	27.5	1.07	—	0.09	—	0.09	0.70	—	0	0	0	—
0	5	0.05	0.8	12.0	0.5	0.03	0	0.01	0.00	0.00	0.02	0.03	0.1	0.9	0	0.4
0	2	0.07	1.6	30.8	0.7	0.07	0	0.01	0.01	0.00	0.01	0.08	0.1	0.5	0	1.1
0	1	0.02	1.7	16.6	0.5	0.01	0	0.00	0.01	0.00	0.02	0.01	0.4	0.2	0	0
0	2	0.20	3.3	24.2	0.6	0.08	0.1	0.00	0.32	0.00	0.09	0.01	0.7	0.1	0	0.7
0	3	0.06	1.3	19.2	0.3	0.01	0.1	0.01	—	0.00	0.02	0.01	2.9	0.9	0	0
0	4	0.23	2.8	7.9	1.4	0.03	0.7	0.01	—	0.01	0.02	0.00	1.3	0.4	0	0
0	12	0.49	2.1	9.1	0.5	0.02	2.4	0.00	0.01	0.00	0.02	0.01	1.6	0.3	0	0
0	17	0.32	9.8	22.5	0.2	0.18	0.1	0.01	0.09	0.01	0.26	0.01	2.5	0.1	0	4.4
0	4	0.06	4.0	7.7	0.4	0.04	0.1	0.01	0.00	0.00	0.02	0.00	1.7	0.1	0	0
0	4	0.02	1.5	27.1	0.4	0.03	0	0.01	0.01	0.00	0.01	0.02	2.8	1.3	0	0.1
0	8	0.05	2.6	19.8	1.1	0.04	0	0.01	0.01	0.00	0.01	0.02	3.5	0.3	0	0
0	24	0.66	4.1	25.0	0.2	0.06	5.2	0.01	0.28	0.01	0.09	0.01	4.1	0.8	0	0.1
0	4	0.49	3.9	49.2	0.7	0.08	55.4	0.01	0.62	0.03	0.32	0.08	2.2	1.5	0	0.1
0	4	0.29	0.7	11.4	1.4	0.01	1.5	0.00	0.02	0.00	0.02	0.00	0.5	0.4	0	0.1
0	9	0.60	4.1	26.4	0.9	0.03	0.3	0.00	0.01	0.01	0.02	0.01	0.2	0.4	0	0.1
0	3	0.14	2.7	36.3	0.5	0.04	37.5	0.01	0.53	0.01	0.15	0.04	1.9	1.4	0	0.2
0	6	0.34	2.2	1.8	0.1	0.02	0	0.00	—	0.00	0.01	0.00	0.2	0.5	0	0.1
0	41	0.26	9.3	19.6	0.6	0.28	0	0.02	0.03	0.01	0.02	0.01	1.6	0.1	0	0
0	15	0.53	3.4	10.3	0.4	0.04	2.0	0.00	0.02	0.00	0.04	0.02	2.1	0.2	0	0.1
0	12	0.33	2.3	11.3	0.9	0.04	0.2	0.00	0.01	0.00	0.03	0.01	0.9	0.4	0	0.2
0	15	0.35	2.6	11.5	0.6	0.03	1.9	0.01	—	0.01	0.01	0.02	3.7	0.7	0	0.1
0	2	0.04	0.6	4.7	0.2	0.01	1.0	0.00	—	0.00	0.00	0.00	0.8	0.2	0	—
0	1	0.07	1.8	12.1	1.0	0.01	0.2	0.00	—	0.00	0.01	0.01	0.7	0.6	0	0
0	4	—	1.1	2.7	0	0.01	—	0.00	—	—	—	—	—	—	0	—
0	12	0.19	3.0	7.5	0.1	0.03	2.1	0.01	0.05	0.00	0.04	0.01	1.9	0.2	0	0
0	7	0.00	0	603.6	0.1	—	0	—	—	—	—	—	—	0	—	—
0	0	0.00	—	476.3	0.1	—	0	—	—	—	—	—	—	0	—	—
0	0	0.01	0	0.1	581.4	0.00	0	0.00	0.00	0.00	0.00	0.00	0	0	0	0
0	30	0.53	5.3	14.7	0.3	0.06	3.6	0.01	—	—	0.05	0.02	—	0.7	0	0.1
0	3	0.21	9.2	10.8	1.0	0.27	0.1	0.03	0.01	0.01	0.15	0.01	2.6	0	0	0
0	—	—	—	—	0.1	—	—	—	—	—	—	—	—	—	—	—
0	4	0.22	1.2	8.7	0.6	0.02	3.9	0.00	—	0.00	0.01	0.00	2.0	0.3	0	0
0	2	0.16	3.0	50.7	3.1	0.03	4.5	0.01	0.06	0.01	0.11	0.03	3.7	30.4	0	0.1
0	85	1.48	20.2	—	—	—	—	0.06	—	0.02	1.16	—	—	0.9	0	—
0	48	—	14.5	128.1	2.6	0.17	—	0.04	—	—	—	—	—	0.6	0	—
0	18	0.51	5.6	48.3	1.0	0.06	3.4	0.00	—	0.02	0.14	0.03	4.4	0.8	0	0.1
0	3	0.14	1.3	4.9	0.1	0.01	1.9	0.00	—	0.00	0.01	0.00	0.4	1.3	0	0
0	26	1.73	3.1	11.4	0.8	0.08	2.7	0.01	0.10	0.01	0.06	0.01	3.8	0.7	0	0.1
0	4	0.91	4.2	55.6	0.8	0.09	0	0.00	0.06	0.01	0.11	0.04	0.9	0.6	0	0.1
0	13	0.11	—	—	0.1	—	—	0.02	—	0.00	0.07	—	—	11.2	0	—
0	3	0.07	2.9	57.3	167.1	0.03	7.1	0.00	0.21	0.02	0.21	0.02	1.5	2.3	0	0
0	12	0.10	2.0	26.1	248.1	0.03	2.6	0.01	0.02	0.01	0.03	0.01	0.3	0.2	0	0
5	1	0.03	0.1	1.7	78.4	0.02	11.2	0.01	0.72	0.01	0.00	0.08	0.7	0	0	0.2
4	0	0.00	0	1.6	79.5	0.01	0	0.00	0.32	0.00	0.00	0.00	0	0	0	0.3
0	6	0.09	1.0	6.8	68.1	0.01	0	0.00	0.09	0.00	0.01	0.00	0.2	0.1	0	—
0	3	0.07	2.5	6.9	56.8	0.03	0.2	0.01	0.01	0.00	0.02	0.00	0.4	0.1	0	1.6
0	0	0.13	0.8	3.8	121.7	0.02	9.2	0.00	0.08	0.00	0.03	0.00	0.2	0.2	0	0
8	6	0.20	0.8	10.1	191.5	0.05	20.2	0.00	0.97	0.00	0.01	0.07	2.0	0.1	0.1	0.5
0	4	0.06	3.8	65.0	349.7	0.04	3.8	0.00	0.20	0.01	0.15	0.01	0.6	0.2	0	0.4
18	116	0.13	5.7	18.9	521.6	0.61	50.4	0.00	—	0.07	0.01	0.01	2.5	0.3	0.1	2.0
0	5	0.36	9.5	125.7	61.9	0.11	—	0.02	0.00	0.02	0.63	0.06	5.7	43.9	0	0
0	7	1.05	11.1	231.3	113.8	0.14	—	0.01	0.00	0.21	0.61	0.34	6.6	0.3	0	0.3

TABLE A-1 Table of Food Composition (*continued*) <small>(Computer code is for Cengage Diet Analysis program) (For purposes of calculations, use "0" for t, <1, <.1, <.01, etc.)</small>

DA+ Code	Food Description	Quantity	Measure	Wt (g)	H₂O (g)	Ener (kcal)	Prot (g)	Carb (g)	Fiber (g)	Fat (g)	Fat Breakdown (g) Sat	Mono	Poly	Trans
Spices, Condiments, Sauces—*continued*														
29688	Hoisin sauce	1	tablespoon(s)	16	7.1	35	0.5	7.1	0.4	0.5	0.1	0.2	0.3	—
1641	Horseradish sauce, prepared	1	teaspoon(s)	5	3.3	10	0.1	0.2	0	1.0	0.6	0.3	0	—
16670	Mole poblano sauce	½	cup(s)	133	102.7	156	5.3	11.4	2.7	11.3	2.6	5.1	3.0	—
29689	Oyster sauce	1	tablespoon(s)	16	12.8	8	0.2	1.7	0	0	0	0	0	—
1655	Pepper sauce or Tabasco	1	teaspoon(s)	5	4.8	1	0.1	0	0	0	0	0	0	—
347	Salsa	2	tablespoon(s)	32	28.8	9	0.5	2.0	0.5	0.1	0	0	0	—
52206	Soy sauce, tamari	1	tablespoon(s)	18	12.0	11	1.9	1.0	0.1	0	0	0	0	—
839	Sweet and sour sauce	2	tablespoon(s)	39	29.8	37	0.1	9.1	0.1	0	0	0	0	—
1613	Teriyaki sauce	1	tablespoon(s)	18	12.2	16	1.1	2.8	0	0	0	0	0	0
25294	Tomato sauce	½	cup(s)	150	132.8	63	2.2	11.9	2.6	1.8	0.2	0.4	0.9	0
728	White sauce, medium	¼	cup(s)	63	46.8	92	2.4	5.7	0.1	6.7	1.8	2.8	1.8	—
1654	Worcestershire sauce	1	teaspoon(s)	6	4.5	4	0	1.1	0	0	0	0	0	—
	Vinegar													
30853	Balsamic	1	tablespoon(s)	15	—	10	0	2.0	0	0	0	0	0	0
727	Cider	1	tablespoon(s)	15	14.0	3	0	0.1	0	0	0	0	0	0
1673	Distilled	1	tablespoon(s)	15	14.3	2	0	0.8	0	0	0	0	0	0
12948	Tarragon	1	tablespoon(s)	15	13.8	2	0	0.1	0	0	0	0	0	0
Mixed Foods, Soups, Sandwiches														
	Mixed dishes													
16652	Almond chicken	1	cup(s)	242	186.8	281	21.8	15.8	3.4	14.7	1.8	6.3	5.6	—
25224	Barbecued chicken	1	serving(s)	177	99.3	327	27.1	15.7	0.5	17.1	4.8	6.8	3.8	0
25227	Bean burrito	1	item(s)	149	81.8	326	16.1	33.0	5.6	14.8	8.3	4.7	0.9	—
9516	Beef and vegetable fajita	1	item(s)	223	143.9	397	22.4	35.3	3.1	18.0	5.9	8.0	2.5	—
16796	Beef or pork egg roll	2	item(s)	128	85.2	225	9.9	18.4	1.4	12.4	2.9	6.0	2.6	—
177	Beef stew with vegetables, prepared	1	cup(s)	245	201.0	220	16.0	15.0	3.2	11.0	4.4	4.5	0.5	—
30233	Beef stroganoff with noodles	1	cup(s)	256	190.1	343	19.7	22.8	1.5	19.1	7.4	5.7	4.4	—
16651	Cashew chicken	1	cup(s)	242	186.8	281	21.8	15.8	3.4	14.7	1.8	6.3	5.6	—
30274	Cheese pizza with vegetables, thin crust	2	slice(s)	140	76.6	298	12.7	35.4	2.5	12.0	4.9	4.7	1.6	—
30330	Cheese quesadilla	1	item(s)	54	18.3	190	7.7	15.3	1.0	10.8	5.2	3.6	1.3	—
215	Chicken and noodles, prepared	1	cup(s)	240	170.0	365	22.0	26.0	1.3	18.0	5.1	7.1	3.9	—
30239	Chicken and vegetables with broccoli, onion, bamboo shoots in soy based sauce	1	cup(s)	162	125.5	180	15.8	9.3	1.8	8.6	1.7	3.0	3.1	—
25093	Chicken cacciatore	1	cup(s)	244	175.7	284	29.9	5.7	1.3	15.3	4.3	6.2	3.3	0
28020	Chicken fried turkey steak	3	ounce(s)	492	276.2	706	77.1	68.7	3.6	12.0	3.4	2.9	3.9	—
218	Chicken pot pie	1	cup(s)	252	154.6	542	22.6	41.4	3.5	31.3	9.8	12.5	7.1	—
30240	Chicken teriyaki	1	cup(s)	244	158.3	364	51.0	15.2	0.7	7.0	1.8	2.0	1.7	—
25119	Chicken waldorf salad	½	cup(s)	100	67.2	179	14.0	6.8	1.0	10.8	1.8	3.1	5.2	—
25099	Chili con carne	¾	cup(s)	215	174.4	198	13.7	21.4	7.5	6.9	2.5	2.8	0.5	0
1062	Coleslaw	¾	cup(s)	90	73.4	70	1.2	11.2	1.4	2.3	0.3	0.6	1.2	—
1574	Crab cakes, from blue crab	1	item(s)	60	42.6	93	12.1	0.3	0	4.5	0.9	1.7	1.4	—
32144	Enchiladas with green chili sauce (enchiladas verdes)	1	item(s)	144	103.8	207	9.3	17.6	2.6	11.7	6.4	3.6	1.0	0
2793	Falafel patty	3	item(s)	51	17.7	170	6.8	16.2	—	9.1	1.2	5.2	2.1	—
28546	Fettuccine alfredo	1	cup(s)	244	88.7	279	13.1	46.1	1.4	4.2	2.2	1.0	0.4	0
32146	Flautas	3	item(s)	162	78.0	438	24.9	36.3	4.1	21.6	8.2	8.8	2.3	—
29629	Fried rice with meat or poultry	1	cup(s)	198	128.5	333	12.3	41.8	1.4	12.3	2.2	3.5	5.7	—
16649	General Tso chicken	1	cup(s)	146	91.0	296	18.7	16.4	0.9	17.0	4.0	6.3	5.3	—
1826	Green salad	¾	cup(s)	104	98.9	17	1.3	3.3	2.2	0.1	0	0	0	—
1814	Hummus	½	cup(s)	123	79.8	218	6.0	24.7	4.9	10.6	1.4	6.0	2.6	—
16650	Kung pao chicken	1	cup(s)	162	87.2	434	28.8	11.7	2.3	30.6	5.2	13.9	9.7	—
16622	Lamb curry	1	cup(s)	236	187.9	257	28.2	3.7	0.9	13.8	3.9	4.9	3.3	—
25253	Lasagna with ground beef	1	cup(s)	237	158.4	284	16.9	22.3	2.4	14.5	7.5	4.9	0.8	—
442	Macaroni and cheese, prepared	1	cup(s)	200	122.3	390	14.9	40.6	1.6	18.6	7.9	6.4	2.9	—
29637	Meat filled ravioli with tomato or meat sauce, canned	1	cup(s)	251	198.7	208	7.8	36.5	1.3	3.7	1.5	1.4	0.3	—
25105	Meat loaf	1	slice(s)	115	84.5	245	17.0	6.6	0.4	16.0	6.1	6.9	0.9	0
16646	Moo shi pork	1	cup(s)	151	76.8	512	18.9	5.3	0.6	46.4	6.9	15.8	21.2	—
16788	Nachos with beef, beans, cheese, tomatoes and onions	1	serving(s)	551	253.5	1576	59.1	137.5	20.4	90.8	32.6	41.9	9.4	—
6116	Pepperoni pizza	2	slice(s)	142	66.1	362	20.2	39.7	2.9	13.9	4.5	6.3	2.3	—
29601	Pizza with meat and vegetables, thin crust	2	slice(s)	158	81.4	386	16.5	36.8	2.7	19.1	7.7	8.1	2.2	—
655	Potato salad	½	cup(s)	125	95.0	179	3.4	14.0	1.6	10.3	1.8	3.1	4.7	—

Chol (mg)	Calc (mg)	Iron (mg)	Magn (mg)	Pota (mg)	Sodi (mg)	Zinc (mg)	Vit A (µg)	Thia (mg)	Vit E (mg α)	Ribo (mg)	Niac (mg)	Vit B6 (mg)	Fola (µg)	Vit C (mg)	Vit B12 (µg)	Sele (µg)
0	5	0.16	3.8	19.0	258.4	0.05	0	0.00	0.04	0.03	0.18	0.01	3.7	0.1	0	0.3
2	5	0.00	0.5	6.7	14.6	0.01	8.0	0.00	0.02	0.01	0.00	0.00	0.5	0.1	0	0.1
1	38	1.81	58.3	280.9	304.8	1.15	13.3	0.06	1.72	0.08	1.84	0.09	15.9	3.4	0.1	1.1
0	5	0.02	0.6	8.6	437.3	0.01	0	0.00	0.00	0.02	0.23	0.00	2.4	0	0.1	0.7
0	1	0.05	0.6	6.4	31.7	0.01	4.1	0.00	0.00	0.00	0.01	0.01	0.1	0.2	0	0
0	9	0.14	4.8	95.0	192.0	0.11	4.8	0.01	0.37	0.01	0.02	0.05	1.3	0.6	0	0.3
0	4	0.43	7.3	38.7	1018.9	0.08	0	0.01	0.00	0.03	0.72	0.04	3.3	0	0	0.1
0	5	0.20	1.2	8.2	97.5	0.01	0	0.00	—	0.01	0.11	0.03	0.2	0	0	—
0	5	0.30	11.0	40.5	689.9	0.01	0	0.01	0.00	0.01	0.22	0.01	1.4	0	0	0.2
0	23	1.24	28.9	536.8	268.6	0.36	—	0.08	0.52	0.08	1.64	0.20	23.2	32.0	0	1.0
4	74	0.20	8.8	97.5	221.3	0.25	—	0.04	—	0.11	0.25	0.02	3.1	0.5	0.2	—
0	6	0.30	0.7	45.4	55.6	0.01	0.3	0.00	0.00	0.01	0.03	0.00	0.5	0.7	0	0
0	0	0.00	—	—	0	—	0	—	—	—	—	—	—	0	—	—
0	1	0.03	0.7	10.9	0.7	0.01	0	0.00	0.00	0.00	0.00	0.00	0	0	0	0
0	1	0.09	0	2.3	0.1	0.00	0	0.00	0.00	0.00	0.00	0.00	0	0	0	5.0
0	0	0.07	—	2.3	0.7	—	—	0.07	—	0.07	0.07	—	—	0.3	0	—
41	68	1.86	58.1	539.7	510.6	1.50	31.5	0.07	4.11	0.22	9.57	0.43	26.6	5.1	0.3	13.6
120	26	1.70	32.4	419.7	500.9	2.67	—	0.09	0.01	0.24	6.87	0.40	15.0	7.9	0.3	19.5
38	333	3.01	52.5	447.6	510.6	1.98	—	0.28	0.01	0.30	1.92	0.19	122.9	8.2	0.3	15.9
45	85	3.65	37.9	475.0	756.0	3.52	17.8	0.38	0.80	0.29	5.33	0.39	69.1	23.4	2.1	28.3
74	31	1.68	20.5	248.3	547.8	0.89	25.6	0.32	1.28	0.24	2.55	0.18	38.4	4.0	0.3	17.5
71	29	2.90	—	613.0	292.0	—	—	0.15	0.51	0.17	4.70	—	—	17.0	0	15.0
74	69	3.25	35.8	391.7	816.6	3.63	69.1	0.21	1.25	0.30	3.80	0.21	48.6	1.3	1.8	27.9
41	68	1.86	58.1	539.7	510.6	1.50	31.5	0.07	4.11	0.22	9.57	0.43	26.6	5.1	0.3	13.6
17	249	2.78	28.0	294.0	739.2	1.42	47.6	0.29	1.05	0.33	2.84	0.14	61.6	15.3	0.4	18.6
23	190	1.04	13.5	75.6	469.3	0.86	58.3	0.11	0.43	0.15	0.89	0.02	21.6	2.4	0.1	9.2
103	26	2.20	—	149.0	600.0	—	—	0.05	—	0.17	4.30	—	—	0	—	29.0
42	28	1.19	22.7	299.7	620.5	1.32	81.0	0.07	1.11	0.14	5.28	0.36	16.2	22.5	0.2	12.0
109	47	1.97	40.0	489.3	492.1	2.13	—	0.11	0.00	0.20	9.81	0.57	16.1	14.0	0.3	22.6
156	423	8.79	110.3	1182.9	880.4	6.18	—	0.72	0.00	1.05	20.16	1.20	113.9	2.7	1.3	97.6
68	66	3.32	37.8	390.6	652.7	1.94	259.6	0.39	1.05	0.39	7.25	0.23	80.6	10.3	0.2	27.0
156	51	3.26	68.3	588.0	3208.6	3.75	31.7	0.15	0.58	0.36	16.68	0.88	24.4	2.0	0.5	36.1
42	20	0.82	23.9	202.5	246.5	1.13	—	0.05	0.62	0.09	4.06	0.25	15.8	2.5	0.2	10.7
27	42	2.83	50.6	636.8	864.8	2.36	—	0.15	0.01	0.22	3.18	0.19	58.1	10.3	0.6	7.3
7	41	0.53	9.0	162.9	20.7	0.18	47.7	0.06	—	0.05	0.24	0.11	24.3	29.4	0	0.6
90	63	0.64	19.8	194.4	198.0	2.45	34.2	0.05	—	0.04	1.74	0.10	31.8	1.7	3.6	24.4
27	266	1.07	38.5	251.4	276.3	1.26	—	0.07	0.02	0.16	1.27	0.17	44.6	59.3	0.2	6.0
0	28	1.74	41.8	298.4	149.9	0.76	0.5	0.07	—	0.08	0.53	0.06	47.4	0.8	0	0.5
9	218	1.83	38.4	163.9	472.9	1.24	—	0.41	0.00	0.35	2.85	0.09	96.2	1.6	0.4	38.4
73	146	2.66	61.3	222.9	885.7	3.43	0	0.10	0.10	0.16	3.00	0.26	95.7	0	1.2	36.7
103	38	2.77	33.7	196.0	833.6	1.34	41.6	0.33	1.60	0.18	4.17	0.27	97.0	3.4	0.3	22.0
66	26	1.46	23.4	248.2	849.7	1.40	29.2	0.10	1.62	0.18	6.28	0.28	23.4	12.0	0.2	19.9
0	13	0.65	11.4	178.0	26.9	0.21	59.0	0.03	—	0.05	0.56	0.08	38.3	24.0	0	0.4
0	60	1.91	35.7	212.8	297.7	1.34	0	0.10	0.92	0.06	0.49	0.49	72.6	9.7	0	3.0
65	50	1.96	63.2	427.7	907.2	1.50	38.9	0.15	4.32	0.14	13.22	0.58	42.1	7.5	0.3	23.0
90	38	2.95	40.1	493.2	495.6	6.60	—	0.08	1.29	0.28	8.03	0.21	28.3	1.4	2.9	30.4
68	233	2.22	40.1	420.1	433.6	2.70	—	0.21	0.21	0.29	3.06	0.22	50.4	15.0	0.8	21.4
34	310	2.06	40.0	258.0	784.0	2.06	180.0	0.27	0.72	0.43	2.18	0.08	64.0	0	0.5	30.6
15	35	2.10	20.1	283.6	1352.9	1.28	27.6	0.19	0.70	0.16	2.77	0.14	42.7	21.6	0.4	13.3
85	59	1.87	21.8	300.8	411.7	3.40	—	0.08	0.00	0.27	3.72	0.13	18.7	0.9	1.6	17.9
172	32	1.57	25.7	333.7	1052.5	1.82	49.8	0.49	5.39	0.36	2.88	0.31	21.1	8.0	0.8	30.0
154	948	7.32	242.4	1201.2	1862.4	10.68	259.0	0.29	7.71	0.81	6.39	1.09	148.8	16.0	2.6	44.1
28	129	1.87	17.0	305.3	533.9	1.03	105.1	0.26	—	0.46	6.09	0.11	73.8	3.3	0.4	26.1
36	258	3.14	31.6	352.3	971.7	2.02	49.0	0.37	1.13	0.37	3.77	0.19	64.8	15.6	0.6	22.8
85	24	0.81	18.8	317.5	661.3	0.38	40.0	0.09	—	0.07	1.11	0.17	8.8	12.5	0	5.1

TABLE A-1 Table of Food Composition (*continued*) (Computer code is for Cengage Diet Analysis program) (For purposes of calculations, use "0" for t, <1, <.1, <.01, etc.

DA+ Code	Food Description	Quantity	Measure	Wt (g)	H₂O (g)	Ener (kcal)	Prot (g)	Carb (g)	Fiber (g)	Fat (g)	Sat	Mono	Poly	Trans
												Fat Breakdown (g)		

Mixed Foods, Soups, Sandwiches—*continued*

DA+ Code	Food Description	Quantity	Measure	Wt (g)	H₂O (g)	Ener (kcal)	Prot (g)	Carb (g)	Fiber (g)	Fat (g)	Sat	Mono	Poly	Trans
25109	Salisbury steaks with mushroom sauce	1	serving(s)	135	101.8	251	17.1	9.3	0.5	15.5	6.0	6.7	0.8	0
16637	Shrimp creole with rice	1	cup(s)	243	176.6	309	27.0	27.7	1.2	9.2	1.7	3.6	2.9	—
497	Spaghetti and meatballs with tomato sauce, prepared	1	cup(s)	248	174.0	330	19.0	39.0	2.7	12.0	3.9	4.4	2.2	—
28585	Spicy thai noodles (pad thai)	8	ounce(s)	227	73.3	221	8.9	35.7	3.0	6.4	0.8	3.3	1.8	—
33073	Stir fried pork and vegetables with rice	1	cup(s)	235	173.6	348	15.4	33.5	1.9	16.3	5.6	6.9	2.6	0
28588	Stuffed shells	2½	item(s)	249	157.5	243	15.0	28.0	2.5	8.1	3.1	3.0	1.3	—
16821	Sushi with egg in seaweed	6	piece(s)	156	116.5	190	8.9	20.5	0.3	7.9	2.2	3.2	1.5	—
16819	Sushi with vegetables and fish	6	piece(s)	156	101.6	218	8.4	43.7	1.7	0.6	0.2	0.1	0.2	—
16820	Sushi with vegetables in seaweed	6	piece(s)	156	110.3	183	3.4	40.6	0.8	0.4	0.1	0.1	0.1	—
25266	Sweet and sour pork	¾	cup(s)	249	205.9	265	29.2	17.1	1.0	8.1	2.6	3.5	1.5	0
16824	Tabouli, tabbouleh or tabuli	1	cup(s)	160	123.7	198	2.6	15.9	3.7	14.9	2.0	10.9	1.6	—
25276	Three bean salad	½	cup(s)	99	82.2	95	1.9	9.7	2.6	5.9	0.8	1.4	3.5	0
160	Tuna salad	½	cup(s)	103	64.7	192	16.4	9.6	0	9.5	1.6	3.0	4.2	—
25241	Turkey and noodles	1	cup(s)	319	228.5	270	24.0	21.2	1.0	9.2	2.4	3.5	2.3	—
16794	Vegetable egg roll	2	item(s)	128	89.8	201	5.1	19.5	1.7	11.6	2.5	5.7	2.6	—
16818	Vegetable sushi, no fish	6	piece(s)	156	99.0	226	4.8	49.9	2.0	0.4	0.1	0.1	0.1	—
	Sandwiches													
1744	Bacon, lettuce and tomato with mayonnaise	1	item(s)	164	97.2	341	11.6	34.2	2.3	17.6	3.8	5.5	6.7	—
30287	Bologna and cheese with margarine	1	item(s)	111	45.6	345	13.4	29.3	1.2	19.3	8.1	7.0	2.4	—
30286	Bologna with margarine	1	item(s)	83	33.6	251	8.1	27.3	1.2	12.1	3.7	5.0	2.1	—
16546	Cheese	1	item(s)	83	31.0	261	9.1	27.6	1.2	12.7	5.4	4.2	2.1	—
8789	Cheeseburger, large, plain	1	item(s)	185	78.9	564	32.0	38.5	2.6	31.5	12.5	10.2	1.0	1.8
8624	Cheeseburger, large, with bacon, vegetables, and condiments	1	item(s)	195	91.4	550	30.8	36.8	2.5	30.9	11.9	10.6	1.3	1.5
1745	Club with bacon, chicken, tomato, lettuce, and mayonnaise	1	item(s)	246	137.5	546	31.0	48.9	3.0	24.5	5.3	7.5	9.4	—
1908	Cold cut submarine with cheese and vegetables	1	item(s)	228	131.8	456	21.8	51.0	2.0	18.6	6.8	8.2	2.3	—
30247	Corned beef	1	item(s)	130	74.9	265	18.2	25.3	1.6	9.6	3.6	3.5	1.0	—
25283	Egg salad	1	item(s)	126	72.1	278	10.7	28.0	1.4	13.5	2.9	4.2	5.0	—
16686	Fried egg	1	item(s)	96	49.7	226	10.0	26.2	1.2	8.6	2.3	3.2	1.9	—
16547	Grilled cheese	1	item(s)	83	27.5	291	9.2	27.9	1.2	15.8	6.0	5.7	3.0	—
16659	Gyro with onion and tomato	1	item(s)	105	68.3	163	12.0	20.0	1.1	3.5	1.3	1.3	0.5	—
1906	Ham and cheese	1	item(s)	146	74.2	352	20.7	33.3	2.0	15.5	6.4	6.7	1.4	—
31890	Ham with mayonnaise	1	item(s)	112	56.3	271	13.0	27.9	1.9	11.6	2.8	4.0	4.0	—
756	Hamburger, double patty, large, with condiments and vegetables	1	item(s)	226	121.5	540	34.3	40.3	—	26.6	10.5	10.3	2.8	—
8793	Hamburger, large, plain	1	item(s)	137	57.7	426	22.6	31.7	1.5	22.9	8.4	9.9	2.1	—
8795	Hamburger, large, with vegetables and condiments	1	item(s)	218	121.4	512	25.8	40.0	3.1	27.4	10.4	11.4	2.2	—
25134	Hot chicken salad	1	item(s)	98	48.4	242	15.2	23.8	1.3	9.2	2.9	2.5	3.0	—
25133	Hot turkey salad	1	item(s)	98	50.1	224	15.6	23.8	1.3	6.9	2.3	1.6	2.5	—
1411	Hotdog with bun, plain	1	item(s)	98	52.9	242	10.4	18.0	1.6	14.5	5.1	6.9	1.7	—
30249	Pastrami	1	item(s)	134	71.2	328	13.4	27.8	1.6	17.7	6.1	8.3	1.2	—
16701	Peanut butter	1	item(s)	93	23.6	345	12.2	37.6	3.3	17.4	3.4	7.7	5.2	—
30306	Peanut butter and jelly	1	item(s)	93	24.2	330	10.3	41.9	2.9	14.7	2.9	6.5	4.4	—
1909	Roast beef submarine with mayonnaise and vegetables	1	item(s)	216	127.4	410	28.6	44.3	—	13.0	7.1	1.8	2.6	—
1910	Roast beef, plain	1	item(s)	139	67.6	346	21.5	33.4	1.2	13.8	3.6	6.8	1.7	—
1907	Steak with mayonnaise and vegetables	1	item(s)	204	104.2	459	30.3	52.0	2.3	14.1	3.8	5.3	3.3	—
25288	Tuna salad	1	item(s)	179	102.2	415	24.5	28.4	1.6	22.4	3.5	6.2	11.4	—
30283	Turkey submarine with cheese, lettuce, tomato, and mayonnaise	1	item(s)	277	168.0	529	30.4	49.4	3.0	22.8	6.8	6.0	8.6	—
31891	Turkey with mayonnaise	1	item(s)	143	74.5	329	28.7	26.4	1.3	11.2	2.6	2.6	4.8	—
	Soups													
25296	Bean	1	cup(s)	301	253.1	191	13.8	29.0	6.5	2.3	0.7	0.8	0.5	0
711	Bean with pork, condensed, prepared with water	1	cup(s)	253	215.9	159	7.3	21.0	7.3	5.5	1.4	2.0	1.7	—

PAGE KEY: A-6 = Breads/Baked Goods A-12 = Cereal/Rice/Pasta A-16 = Fruit A-20 = Vegetables/Legumes A-30 = Nuts/Seeds A-32 = Vegetarian A-34 = Dairy A-42 = Eggs A-42 = Seafood A-44 = Meats A-48 = Poultry A-48 = Processed Meats A-50 = Beverages A-54 = Fats/Oils A-56 = Sweets A-58 = Spices/Condiments/Sauces A-62 = Mixed Foods/Soups/Sandwiches A-66 = Fast Food A-86 = Convenience A-88 = Baby Foods

Chol (mg)	Calc (mg)	Iron (mg)	Magn (mg)	Pota (mg)	Sodi (mg)	Zinc (mg)	Vit A (µg)	Thia (mg)	Vit E (mg α)	Ribo (mg)	Niac (mg)	Vit B_6 (mg)	Fola (µg)	Vit C (mg)	Vit B_{12} (µg)	Sele (µg)
60	74	1.94	23.8	314.5	360.5	3.45	—	0.10	0.00	0.27	3.95	0.13	20.8	0.7	1.6	17.4
180	102	4.68	63.2	413.1	330.5	1.72	94.8	0.29	2.06	0.11	4.75	0.21	75.3	12.9	1.2	49.3
89	124	3.70	—	665.0	1009.0	—	81.5	0.25	—	0.30	4.00	—	—	22.0	—	22.0
37	31	1.56	49.4	181.3	591.6	1.05	—	0.18	0.35	0.13	1.82	0.17	44.6	22.6	0.1	3.2
46	38	2.71	33.0	396.9	569.5	2.08	—	0.51	0.38	0.20	5.07	0.30	103.0	18.8	0.4	22.8
30	188	2.26	49.4	403.0	471.5	1.41	—	0.26	0.00	0.26	3.83	0.24	80.0	17.9	0.2	28.9
214	45	1.84	18.7	135.7	463.3	0.98	106.1	0.13	0.67	0.28	1.35	0.13	62.4	1.9	0.7	20.3
11	23	2.15	25.0	202.8	340.1	0.78	45.2	0.26	0.24	0.07	2.76	0.14	76.4	3.6	0.3	13.9
0	20	1.54	18.7	96.7	152.9	0.68	25.0	0.19	0.12	0.03	1.86	0.13	73.3	2.3	0	9.8
74	40	1.76	35.6	619.9	621.8	2.53	—	0.81	0.20	0.37	6.69	0.66	14.7	11.9	0.7	49.6
0	30	1.21	35.2	249.6	796.8	0.48	54.4	0.07	2.43	0.04	1.11	0.11	30.4	26.1	0	0.5
0	26	0.96	15.5	144.8	224.2	0.30	—	0.02	0.88	0.04	0.26	0.04	32.2	10.0	0	2.7
13	17	1.02	19.5	182.5	412.1	0.57	24.6	0.03	—	0.07	6.86	0.08	8.2	2.3	1.2	42.2
77	69	2.56	33.2	400.8	577.1	2.51	—	0.23	0.28	0.30	6.41	0.29	61.4	1.4	1.1	33.4
60	29	1.65	17.9	193.3	549.1	0.48	25.6	0.15	1.28	0.20	1.59	0.09	46.1	5.5	0.2	11.3
0	23	2.38	21.8	157.6	369.7	0.82	48.4	0.28	0.15	0.05	2.44	0.12	85.8	3.7	0	8.1
21	79	2.36	27.9	351.0	944.6	1.08	44.3	0.32	1.16	0.24	4.36	0.21	73.8	9.7	0.2	27.1
40	258	2.38	24.4	215.3	941.3	1.88	102.1	0.31	0.55	0.35	2.97	0.14	59.9	0.2	0.8	20.4
17	100	2.24	16.6	138.6	579.3	1.02	44.8	0.29	0.49	0.21	2.92	0.12	58.1	0.2	0.5	16.0
22	233	2.04	19.9	127.0	733.7	1.24	97.1	0.25	0.47	0.30	2.25	0.05	58.1	0	0.3	13.1
104	309	4.47	44.4	401.5	986.1	5.75	0	0.35	—	0.77	8.26	0.49	109.2	0	2.8	38.9
98	267	4.03	44.9	464.1	1314.3	5.20	0	0.33	—	0.67	8.25	0.47	95.6	1.4	2.4	6.6
71	157	4.57	46.7	464.9	1087.3	1.82	41.8	0.54	1.52	0.40	12.82	0.61	118.1	6.4	0.4	42.3
36	189	2.50	68.4	394.4	1650.7	2.57	70.7	1.00	—	0.79	5.49	0.13	86.6	12.3	1.1	30.8
46	81	3.04	19.5	127.4	1206.4	2.26	2.6	0.23	0.20	0.24	3.42	0.11	59.8	0.3	0.9	31.2
219	85	2.25	18.8	159.0	423.1	0.87	—	0.27	0.12	0.43	2.06	0.15	73.6	0.9	0.6	29.9
206	104	2.79	17.3	117.1	438.7	0.92	89.3	0.26	0.66	0.40	2.26	0.10	79.7	0	0.6	24.2
22	235	2.05	19.9	128.7	763.6	1.26	129.5	0.19	0.72	0.28	2.05	0.05	38.2	0	0.2	13.2
28	47	1.77	22.1	218.4	235.2	2.33	9.5	0.23	0.26	0.20	3.12	0.13	44.1	3.2	0.9	18.3
58	130	3.24	16.1	290.5	770.9	1.37	96.4	0.30	0.29	0.48	2.68	0.20	75.9	2.8	0.5	23.1
34	91	2.47	23.5	210.6	1097.6	1.13	5.6	0.57	0.50	0.26	3.80	0.25	60.5	2.2	0.2	20.2
122	102	5.85	49.7	569.5	791.0	5.67	0	0.36	—	0.38	7.57	0.54	76.8	1.1	4.1	25.5
71	74	3.57	27.4	267.2	474.0	4.11	0	0.28	—	0.28	6.24	0.23	60.3	0	2.1	27.1
87	96	4.92	43.6	479.6	824.0	4.88	0	0.41	—	0.37	7.28	0.32	82.8	2.6	2.4	33.6
39	115	1.88	20.0	172.4	505.1	1.19	—	0.23	0.28	0.22	4.84	0.19	46.4	0.5	0.2	19.9
37	114	1.99	21.3	189.0	494.5	1.07	—	0.22	0.28	0.20	4.26	0.22	46.4	0.5	0.2	23.4
44	24	2.31	12.7	143.1	670.3	1.98	0	0.23	—	0.27	3.64	0.04	48.0	0.1	0.5	26.0
51	80	3.02	22.8	182.2	1364.1	2.70	2.7	0.28	0.26	0.26	4.97	0.14	60.3	0.3	1.0	14.3
0	110	2.92	66.0	226.0	580.3	1.32	0	0.31	2.39	0.23	6.72	0.18	92.1	0	0	13.2
0	94	2.50	56.7	198.1	492.9	1.12	—	0.26	2.01	0.20	5.66	0.15	78.1	0.1	0	11.2
73	41	2.80	67.0	330.5	844.6	4.38	30.2	0.41	—	0.41	5.96	0.32	71.3	5.6	1.8	25.7
51	54	4.22	30.6	315.5	792.3	3.39	11.1	0.37	—	0.30	5.86	0.26	57.0	2.1	1.2	29.2
73	92	5.16	49.0	524.3	797.6	4.52	0	0.40	—	0.36	7.30	0.36	89.8	5.5	1.6	42.0
59	78	2.97	35.9	316.3	724.7	1.02	—	0.27	0.34	0.26	12.07	0.46	60.8	1.8	2.4	76.9
64	307	4.59	49.9	534.6	1759.0	2.74	74.8	0.49	1.19	0.65	3.91	0.31	121.9	10.5	0.6	42.1
67	100	3.46	34.3	304.6	564.9	3.00	5.7	0.28	0.74	0.32	6.84	0.46	64.4	0	0.3	40
5	79	3.05	61.8	588.8	689.0	1.41	—	0.27	0.02	0.15	3.63	0.23	140.1	3.6	0.2	7.9
3	78	1.89	43.0	371.9	883.0	0.96	43.0	0.08	1.08	0.03	0.52	0.03	30.4	1.5	0	7.8

TABLE A-1 Table of Food Composition (*continued*) (Computer code is for Cengage Diet Analysis program)   (For purposes of calculations, use "0" for t, <1, <.1, <.01, etc.)

DA+ Code	Food Description	Quantity	Measure	Wt (g)	H₂O (g)	Ener (kcal)	Prot (g)	Carb (g)	Fiber (g)	Fat (g)	Fat Breakdown (g) Sat	Mono	Poly	*Trans*
	Mixed Foods, Soups, Sandwiches—*continued*													
713	Beef noodle, condensed, prepared with water	1	cup(s)	244	224.9	83	4.7	8.7	0.7	3.0	1.1	1.2	0.5	—
825	Cheese, condensed, prepared with milk	1	cup(s)	251	206.9	231	9.5	16.2	1.0	14.6	9.1	4.1	0.5	—
826	Chicken broth, condensed, prepared with water	1	cup(s)	244	234.1	39	4.9	0.9	0	1.4	0.4	0.6	0.3	—
25297	Chicken noodle soup	1	cup(s)	286	258.4	117	10.8	10.9	0.9	2.9	0.8	1.1	0.7	—
827	Chicken noodle, condensed, prepared with water	1	cup(s)	241	226.1	60	3.1	7.1	0.5	2.3	0.6	1.0	0.6	0
724	Chicken noodle, dehydrated, prepared with water	1	cup(s)	252	237.3	58	2.1	9.2	0.3	1.4	0.3	0.5	0.4	—
823	Cream of asparagus, condensed, prepared with milk	1	cup(s)	248	213.3	161	6.3	16.4	0.7	8.2	3.3	2.1	2.2	—
824	Cream of celery, condensed, prepared with milk	1	cup(s)	248	214.4	164	5.7	14.5	0.7	9.7	3.9	2.5	2.7	—
708	Cream of chicken, condensed, prepared with milk	1	cup(s)	248	210.4	191	7.5	15.0	0.2	11.5	4.6	4.5	1.6	—
715	Cream of chicken, condensed, prepared with water	1	cup(s)	244	221.1	117	3.4	9.3	0.2	7.4	2.1	3.3	1.5	—
709	Cream of mushroom, condensed, prepared with milk	1	cup(s)	248	215.0	166	6.2	14.0	0	9.6	3.3	2.0	1.8	0.1
716	Cream of mushroom, condensed, prepared with water	1	cup(s)	244	224.6	102	1.9	8.0	0	7.0	1.6	1.3	1.7	—
25298	Cream of vegetable	1	cup(s)	285	250.7	165	7.2	15.2	1.9	8.6	1.6	4.6	1.9	—
16689	Egg drop	1	cup(s)	244	228.9	73	7.5	1.1	0	3.8	1.1	1.5	0.6	—
25138	Golden squash	1	cup(s)	258	223.9	145	7.6	20.4	0.4	4.1	0.8	2.2	0.9	—
16663	Hot and sour	1	cup(s)	244	209.7	161	15.0	5.4	0.5	7.9	2.7	3.4	1.1	—
28054	Lentil chowder	1	cup(s)	244	202.8	153	11.4	27.7	12.6	0.5	0.1	0.1	0.2	0
28560	Macaroni and bean	1	cup(s)	246	138.8	146	5.8	22.9	5.1	3.7	0.5	2.2	0.6	0
714	Manhattan clam chowder, condensed, prepared with water	1	cup(s)	244	225.1	73	2.1	11.6	1.5	2.1	0.4	0.4	1.2	—
28561	Minestrone	1	cup(s)	241	185.4	103	4.5	16.8	4.8	2.3	0.3	1.4	0.4	0
717	Minestrone, condensed, prepared with water	1	cup(s)	241	220.1	82	4.3	11.2	1.0	2.5	0.6	0.7	1.1	—
28038	Mushroom and wild rice	1	cup(s)	244	199.7	86	4.7	13.2	1.7	0.3	0	0	0.2	0
828	New England clam chowder, condensed, prepared with milk	1	cup(s)	248	212.2	151	8.0	18.4	0.7	5.0	2.1	0.7	0.6	0
28036	New England style clam chowder	1	cup(s)	244	227.5	61	3.8	8.8	1.8	0.2	0.1	0	0	0
28566	Old country pasta	1	cup(s)	252	183.3	146	6.5	18.3	3.6	4.5	2.0	2.4	0.9	0
725	Onion, dehydrated, prepared with water	1	cup(s)	246	235.7	30	0.8	6.8	0.7	0	0	0	0	0
16667	Shrimp gumbo	1	cup(s)	244	207.2	166	9.5	18.2	2.4	6.7	1.3	2.9	2.0	—
28037	Southwestern corn chowder	1	cup(s)	244	217.8	98	4.9	17.0	2.4	0.5	0.1	0.1	0.2	0
30282	Soybean (miso)	1	cup(s)	240	218.6	84	6.0	8.0	1.9	3.4	0.6	1.1	1.4	—
25140	Split pea	1	cup(s)	165	119.7	72	4.5	16.0	1.6	0.3	0.1	0	0.2	—
718	Split pea with ham, condensed, prepared with water	1	cup(s)	253	206.9	190	10.3	28.0	2.3	4.4	1.8	1.8	0.6	—
726	Tomato vegetable, dehydrated, prepared with water	1	cup(s)	253	238.4	56	2.0	10.2	0.8	0.9	0.4	0.3	0.1	0
710	Tomato, condensed, prepared with milk	1	cup(s)	248	213.4	136	6.2	22.0	1.5	3.2	1.8	0.9	0.3	—
719	Tomato, condensed, prepared with water	1	cup(s)	244	223.0	73	1.9	16.0	1.5	0.7	0.2	0.2	0.2	—
28595	Turkey noodle	1	cup(s)	244	216.9	114	8.1	15.1	1.9	2.4	0.3	1.1	0.7	—
28051	Turkey vegetable	1	cup(s)	244	220.8	96	12.2	6.6	2.0	1.1	0.3	0.2	0.3	0
25141	Vegetable	1	cup(s)	252	228.1	82	5.2	16.5	4.5	0.3	0	0	0.1	0
720	Vegetable beef, condensed, prepared with water	1	cup(s)	244	224.0	76	5.4	9.9	2.0	1.9	0.8	0.8	0.1	—
28598	Vegetable gumbo	1	cup(s)	252	184.5	170	4.4	28.9	3.6	4.7	0.7	3.2	0.5	0
721	Vegetarian vegetable, condensed, prepared with water	1	cup(s)	241	222.7	67	2.1	11.8	0.7	1.9	0.3	0.8	0.7	—
	Fast Food													
	Arby's													
36094	Au jus sauce	1	serving(s)	85	—	43	1.0	7.0	0	1.3	0.4	—	—	0.4
751	Beef 'n cheddar sandwich	1	item(s)	195	—	445	22.0	44.0	2.0	21.0	6.0	—	—	1.0
9279	Cheddar curly fries	1	serving(s)	198	—	631	8.0	73.0	7.0	37.4	6.8	—	—	5.7

Chol (mg)	Calc (mg)	Iron (mg)	Magn (mg)	Pota (mg)	Sodi (mg)	Zinc (mg)	Vit A (µg)	Thia (mg)	Vit E (mg α)	Ribo (mg)	Niac (mg)	Vit B₆ (mg)	Fola (µg)	Vit C (mg)	Vit B₁₂ (µg)	Sele (µg)
5	20	1.07	7.3	97.6	929.6	1.51	12.2	0.06	1.22	0.05	1.03	0.03	19.5	0.5	0.2	7.3
48	289	0.80	20.1	341.4	1019.1	0.67	358.9	0.06	—	0.33	0.50	0.07	10.0	1.3	0.4	7.0
0	10	0.51	2.4	209.8	775.9	0.24	0	0.01	0.04	0.07	3.34	0.02	4.9	0	0.2	0
24	25	1.38	16.4	340.1	774.5	0.77	—	0.15	0.02	0.16	5.57	0.13	37.2	1.8	0.3	10.2
12	14	1.59	9.6	53.0	638.7	0.38	26.5	0.13	0.07	0.10	1.30	0.04	19.3	0	0	11.6
10	5	0.50	7.6	32.8	577.1	0.20	2.5	0.20	0.12	0.07	1.08	0.02	17.6	0	0.1	9.6
22	174	0.86	19.8	359.6	1041.6	0.91	62.0	0.10	—	0.27	0.88	0.06	29.8	4.0	0.5	8.0
32	186	0.69	22.3	310.0	1009.4	0.19	114.1	0.07	—	0.24	0.43	0.06	7.4	1.5	0.5	4.7
27	181	0.67	17.4	272.8	1046.6	0.67	178.6	0.07	—	0.25	0.92	0.06	7.4	1.2	0.5	8.0
10	34	0.61	2.4	87.8	985.8	0.63	163.5	0.02	—	0.06	0.82	0.01	2.4	0.2	0.1	7.0
10	164	1.36	19.8	267.8	823.4	0.79	81.8	0.10	1.01	0.29	0.62	0.05	7.4	0.2	0.6	6.0
0	17	1.31	4.9	73.2	775.9	0.24	9.8	0.05	0.97	0.05	0.50	0.00	2.4	0	0	2.9
1	80	1.20	17.5	340.7	787.9	0.56	—	0.12	1.05	0.18	3.32	0.12	39.5	10.7	0.3	4.3
102	22	0.75	4.9	219.6	729.6	0.48	41.5	0.02	0.29	0.19	3.02	0.05	14.6	0	0.5	7.6
4	262	0.78	42.4	542.2	515.6	0.88	—	0.16	0.52	0.30	1.14	0.16	32.7	12.5	0.7	6.0
34	29	1.24	19.5	373.3	1561.6	1.43	—	0.26	0.12	0.24	4.96	0.20	14.6	0.5	0.4	19.3
0	48	4.38	59.3	626.2	26.7	1.57	—	0.24	0.06	0.12	1.87	0.32	176.3	16.1	0	3.5
0	59	1.90	32.4	275.9	531.0	0.51	—	0.16	0.37	0.12	1.44	0.10	58.2	9.1	0	8.8
2	27	1.56	9.8	180.6	551.4	0.87	48.8	0.02	1.22	0.03	0.77	0.09	9.8	3.9	3.9	9.0
0	62	1.70	29.9	287.5	442.7	0.42	—	0.09	0.23	0.09	0.70	0.07	47.3	13.3	0	3.5
2	34	0.91	7.2	313.3	911.0	0.74	118.1	0.05	—	0.04	0.94	0.09	36.2	1.2	0	8.0
0	30	1.38	27.3	376.9	283.8	1.00	—	0.06	0.07	0.23	3.21	0.14	18.1	3.7	0.1	4.7
17	169	3.00	29.8	456.3	887.8	0.99	91.8	0.20	0.54	0.43	1.96	0.17	22.3	5.2	11.9	10.9
3	89	1.30	29.2	503.7	256.8	0.52	—	0.06	0.02	0.10	1.30	0.15	24.2	11.8	3.0	3.8
5	57	2.43	51.9	500.4	355.7	0.78	—	0.21	0.01	0.14	2.64	0.20	80.0	22.0	0.1	10.3
0	22	0.12	9.8	76.3	851.2	0.12	0	0.03	0.02	0.03	0.15	0.06	0	0.2	0	0.5
51	105	2.85	48.8	461.2	441.6	0.90	80.5	0.18	1.90	0.12	2.52	0.19	85.4	17.6	0.3	14.9
1	83	1.03	26.3	434.4	217.4	0.57	—	0.08	0.09	0.13	1.81	0.21	32.1	39.6	0.2	1.7
0	65	1.87	36.0	362.4	988.8	0.86	232.8	0.06	0.96	0.16	2.61	0.15	57.6	4.6	0.2	1.0
0	28	1.26	29.8	328.1	602.4	0.52	—	0.10	0.00	0.07	1.50	0.16	49.5	8.1	0	0.7
8	23	2.27	48.1	399.7	1006.9	1.31	22.8	0.14	—	0.07	1.47	0.06	2.5	1.5	0.3	8.0
0	20	0.60	10.1	169.5	334.0	0.20	10.1	0.06	0.43	0.09	1.26	0.06	12.7	3.0	0.1	2.0
10	166	1.36	29.8	466.2	711.8	0.84	94.2	0.09	0.44	0.31	1.35	0.15	5.0	15.6	0.6	9.2
0	20	1.31	17.1	273.3	663.7	0.29	24.4	0.04	0.41	0.07	1.23	0.10	0	15.4	0	6.1
26	28	1.40	24.1	223.8	395.9	0.75	—	0.21	0.01	0.12	2.85	0.15	45.0	7.1	0.1	13.7
21	38	1.48	25.0	423.4	348.7	0.99	—	0.09	0.01	0.09	3.64	0.27	23.9	10.6	0.2	10.3
0	40	2.08	39.1	681.5	670.3	0.67	—	0.16	0.00	0.09	2.70	0.26	36.3	22.4	0	2.2
5	20	1.09	7.3	168.4	773.5	1.51	190.3	0.03	0.58	0.04	1.00	0.07	9.8	2.4	0.3	2.7
0	56	1.85	38.9	360.2	518.4	0.64	—	0.18	0.64	0.08	1.77	0.17	57.6	21.9	0	4.1
0	24	1.06	7.2	207.3	814.6	0.45	171.1	0.05	1.39	0.04	0.90	0.05	9.6	1.4	0	4.3
0	0	—	—	—	1510.0	—	—	—	—	—	—	—	—	—	—	—
51	80	3.96	—	—	1274.0	—	—	—	—	—	—	—	—	1.8	—	—
0	80	3.24	—	—	1476.0	—	—	—	—	—	—	—	—	9.6	—	—

TABLE A-1 Table of Food Composition (*continued*) (Computer code is for Cengage Diet Analysis program) (For purposes of calculations, use "0" for t, <1, <.1, <.01, etc.)

DA+ Code	Food Description	Quantity	Measure	Wt (g)	H₂O (g)	Ener (kcal)	Prot (g)	Carb (g)	Fiber (g)	Fat (g)	Sat	Mono	Poly	*Trans*
											\

Fat Breakdown (g) is the header spanning Sat, Mono, Poly, Trans columns.

DA+ Code	Food Description	Quantity	Measure	Wt (g)	H₂O (g)	Ener (kcal)	Prot (g)	Carb (g)	Fiber (g)	Fat (g)	Sat	Mono	Poly	*Trans*
Fast Food—*continued*														
34770	Chicken breast fillet sandwich, grilled	1	item(s)	233	—	414	32.0	36.0	3.0	17.0	3.0	—	—	0
36131	Chocolate shake, regular	1	serving(s)	397	—	507	13.0	83.0	0	13.0	8.0	—	—	0
36045	Curly fries, large size	1	serving(s)	198	—	631	8.0	73.0	7.0	37.0	7.0	—	—	6.0
36044	Curly fries, medium size	1	serving(s)	128	—	406	5.0	47.0	5.0	24.0	4.0	—	—	4.0
752	Ham 'n cheese sandwich	1	item(s)	167	—	304	23.0	35.0	1.0	7.0	2.0	—	—	0
36048	Homestyle fries, large size	1	serving(s)	213	—	566	6.0	82.0	6.0	37.0	7.0	—	—	5.0
36047	Homestyle fries, medium size	1	serving(s)	142	—	377	4.0	55.0	4.0	25.0	4.0	—	—	4.0
33465	Homestyle fries, small size	1	serving(s)	113	—	302	3.0	44.0	3.0	20.0	4.0	—	—	3.0
9249	Junior roast beef sandwich	1	item(s)	125	—	272	16.0	34.0	2.0	10.0	4.0	—	—	0
9251	Large roast beef sandwich	1	item(s)	281	—	547	42.0	41.0	3.0	28.0	12.0	—	—	2.0
39640	Market Fresh chicken salad with pecans sandwich	1	item(s)	322	—	769	30.0	79.0	9.0	39.0	10.0	—	—	0
39641	Market Fresh Martha's Vineyard salad, without dressing	1	serving(s)	330	—	277	26.0	24.0	5.0	8.0	4.0	—	—	0
34769	Market Fresh roast turkey and Swiss sandwich	1	serving(s)	359	—	725	45.0	75.0	5.0	30.0	8.0	—	—	1.0
9267	Market Fresh roast turkey ranch and bacon sandwich	1	serving(s)	382	—	834	49.0	75.0	5.0	38.0	11.0	—	—	1.0
39642	Market Fresh Santa Fe salad, without dressing	1	serving(s)	372	—	499	30.0	42.0	7.0	23.0	8.0	—	—	2.0
39650	Market Fresh Southwest chicken wrap	1	serving(s)	251	—	567	36.0	42.0	4.0	29.0	9.0	—	—	1.0
37021	Market Fresh Ultimate BLT sandwich	1	item(s)	294	—	779	23.0	75.0	6.0	45.0	11.0	—	—	1.0
750	Roast beef sandwich, regular	1	item(s)	154	—	320	21.0	34.0	2.0	14.0	5.0	—	—	1.0
36132	Strawberry shake, regular	1	serving(s)	397	—	498	13.0	81.0	0	13.0	8.0	—	—	0
2009	Super roast beef sandwich	1	item(s)	198	—	398	21.0	40.0	2.0	19.0	6.0	—	—	1.0
36130	Vanilla shake, regular	1	serving(s)	369	—	437	13.0	66.0	0	13.0	8.0	—	—	0
	Auntie Anne's													
35371	Cheese dipping sauce	1	serving(s)	35	—	100	3.0	4.0	0	8.0	4.0	—	—	0
35353	Cinnamon sugar soft pretzel	1	item(s)	120	—	350	9.0	74.0	2.0	2.0	0	—	—	0
35354	Cinnamon sugar soft pretzel with butter	1	item(s)	120	—	450	8.0	83.0	3.0	9.0	5.0	—	—	0
35372	Marinara dipping sauce	1	serving(s)	35	—	10	0	4.0	0	0	0	0	0	0
35357	Original soft pretzel	1	serving(s)	120	—	340	10.0	72.0	3.0	1.0	0	—	—	0
35358	Original soft pretzel with butter	1	item(s)	120	—	370	10.0	72.0	3.0	4.0	2.0	—	—	0
35359	Parmesan herb soft pretzel	1	item(s)	120	—	390	11.0	74.0	4.0	5.0	2.5	—	—	—
35360	Parmesan herb soft pretzel with butter	1	item(s)	120	—	440	10.0	72.0	9.0	13.0	7.0	—	—	0
35361	Sesame soft pretzel	1	item(s)	120	—	350	11.0	63.0	3.0	6.0	1.0	—	—	0
35362	Sesame soft pretzel with butter	1	item(s)	120	—	410	12.0	64.0	7.0	12.0	4.0	—	—	0
35364	Sour cream and onion soft pretzel	1	item(s)	120	—	310	9.0	66.0	2.0	1.0	0	—	—	0
35366	Sour cream and onion soft pretzel with butter	1	item(s)	120	—	340	9.0	66.0	2.0	5.0	3.0	—	—	0
35373	Sweet mustard dipping sauce	1	serving(s)	35	—	60	0.5	8.0	0	1.5	1.0	—	—	0
35367	Whole wheat soft pretzel	1	item(s)	120	—	350	11.0	72.0	7.0	1.5	0	—	—	0
35368	Whole wheat soft pretzel with butter	1	item(s)	120	—	370	11.0	72.0	7.0	4.5	1.5	—	—	0
	Boston Market													
34978	Butternut squash	¾	cup(s)	143	—	140	2.0	25.0	2.0	4.5	3.0	—	—	0
35006	Caesar side salad	1	serving(s)	71	—	40	3.0	3.0	1.0	20.0	2.0	—	—	1.5
35013	Chicken Carver sandwich with cheese and sauce	1	item(s)	321	—	700	44.0	68.0	3.0	29.0	7.0	—	—	0
34979	Chicken gravy	4	ounce(s)	113	—	15	1.0	4.0	0	0.5	0	—	—	0
35053	Chicken noodle soup	¾	cup(s)	283	—	180	13.0	16.0	1.0	7.0	2.0	—	—	0
34973	Chicken pot pie	1	item(s)	425	—	800	29.0	59.0	4.0	49.0	18.0	—	—	7.0
35054	Chicken tortilla soup with toppings	¾	cup(s)	227	—	340	12.0	24.0	1.0	22.0	7.0	—	—	0
35007	Cole slaw	¾	cup(s)	125	—	170	2.0	21.0	2.0	9.0	2.0	—	—	0
35057	Cornbread	1	item(s)	45	—	130	1.0	21.0	0	3.5	1.0	—	—	1.0
34980	Creamed spinach	¾	cup(s)	191	—	280	9.0	12.0	4.0	23.0	15.0	—	—	0
34998	Fresh vegetable stuffing	1	cup(s)	136	—	190	3.0	25.0	2.0	8.0	1.0	—	—	0
34991	Garlic dill new potatoes	¾	cup(s)	156	—	140	3.0	24.0	3.0	3.0	1.0	—	—	0
34983	Green bean casserole	¾	cup(s)	170	—	60	2.0	9.0	2.0	2.0	1.0	—	—	0
34982	Green beans	¾	cup(s)	91	—	60	2.0	7.0	3.0	3.5	1.5	—	—	0

AGE KEY: A-6 = Breads/Baked Goods A-12 = Cereal/Rice/Pasta A-16 = Fruit A-20 = Vegetables/Legumes A-30 = Nuts/Seeds A-32 = Vegetarian A-34 = Dairy A-42 = Eggs A-42 = Seafood A-44 = Meats A-48 = Poultry A-48 = Processed Meats A-50 = Beverages A-54 = Fats/Oils A-56 = Sweets A-58 = Spices/Condiments/Sauces A-62 = Mixed Foods/Soups/Sandwiches A-66 = Fast Food A-86 = Convenience A-88 = Baby Foods

Chol (mg)	Calc (mg)	Iron (mg)	Magn (mg)	Pota (mg)	Sodi (mg)	Zinc (mg)	Vit A (µg)	Thia (mg)	Vit E (mg α)	Ribo (mg)	Niac (mg)	Vit B$_6$ (mg)	Fola (µg)	Vit C (mg)	Vit B$_{12}$ (µg)	Sele (µg)
9	90	3.06	—	—	913.0	—	—	—	—	—	—	—	—	10.8	—	—
34	510	0.54	—	—	357.0	—	—	—	—	—	—	—	—	5.4	—	—
0	80	3.24	—	—	1476.0	—	—	—	—	—	—	—	—	9.6	—	—
0	50	1.98	—	—	949.0	—	—	—	—	—	—	—	—	6.0	—	—
35	160	2.70	—	—	1420.0	—	—	—	—	—	—	—	—	1.2	—	—
0	50	1.62	—	—	1029.0	—	—	—	—	—	—	—	—	12.6	—	—
0	30	1.08	—	—	686.0	—	—	—	—	—	—	—	—	8.4	—	—
0	30	0.90	—	—	549.0	—	—	—	—	—	—	—	—	6.6	—	—
29	60	3.06	—	—	740.0	0	—	—	—	—	—	—	—	0	—	—
102	70	6.30	—	—	1869.0	0	—	—	—	—	—	—	—	0.6	—	—
74	180	4.32	—	—	1240.0	—	—	—	—	—	—	—	—	30.0	—	—
72	200	1.62	—	—	454.0	—	—	—	—	—	—	—	—	33.6	—	—
91	360	5.22	—	—	1788.0	—	—	—	—	—	—	—	—	10.2	—	—
109	330	5.40	—	—	2258.0	—	—	—	—	—	—	—	—	11.4	—	—
59	420	3.60	—	—	1231.0	—	—	—	—	—	—	—	—	36.6	—	—
88	240	4.50	—	—	1451.0	—	—	—	—	—	—	—	—	7.8	—	—
51	170	4.68	—	—	1571.0	—	—	—	—	—	—	—	—	16.8	—	—
44	60	3.60	—	—	953.0	0	—	—	—	—	—	—	—	0	—	—
34	510	0.72	—	—	363.0	—	—	—	—	—	—	—	—	6.6	—	—
44	70	3.78	—	—	1060.0	—	—	—	—	—	—	—	—	6.0	—	—
34	510	0.36	—	—	350.0	—	—	—	—	—	—	—	—	5.4	—	—
10	100	0.00	—	—	510.0	—	—	—	—	—	—	—	—	0	—	—
0	20	1.98	—	—	410.0	0	—	—	—	—	—	—	—	0	—	—
25	30	2.34	—	—	430.0	—	—	—	—	—	—	—	—	0	—	—
0	0	0.00	—	—	180.0	0	—	—	—	—	—	—	—	0	—	—
0	30	2.34	—	—	900.0	0	—	—	—	—	—	—	—	0	—	—
10	30	2.16	—	—	930.0	—	—	—	—	—	—	—	—	0	—	—
10	80	1.80	—	—	780.0	—	—	—	—	—	—	—	—	1.2	—	—
30	60	1.80	—	—	660.0	—	—	—	—	—	—	—	—	1.2	—	—
0	20	2.88	—	—	840.0	0	—	—	—	—	—	—	—	0	—	—
15	20	2.70	—	—	860.0	—	—	—	—	—	—	—	—	0	—	—
0	30	1.98	—	—	920.0	—	—	—	—	—	—	—	—	0	—	—
10	40	2.16	—	—	930.0	—	—	—	—	—	—	—	—	0	—	—
40	0	0.00	—	—	120.0	0	—	—	—	—	—	—	—	0	—	—
0	30	1.98	—	—	1100.0	0	—	—	—	—	—	—	—	0	—	—
10	30	2.34	—	—	1120.0	—	—	—	—	—	—	—	—	0	—	—
10	59	0.80	—	—	35.0	—	—	—	—	—	—	—	—	22.2	—	—
0	60	0.43	—	—	75.0	—	—	—	—	—	—	—	—	5.4	—	—
90	211	2.85	—	—	1560.0	—	—	—	—	—	—	—	—	15.8	—	—
0	0	0.00	—	—	570.0	0	—	—	—	—	—	—	—	0	—	—
55	0	1.07	—	—	220.0	—	—	—	—	—	—	—	—	1.8	—	—
115	40	4.50	—	—	800.0	—	—	—	—	—	—	—	—	1.2	—	—
45	123	1.32	—	—	1310.0	—	—	—	—	—	—	—	—	18.4	—	—
10	41	0.48	—	—	270.0	—	—	—	—	—	—	—	—	24.5	—	—
5	0	0.71	—	—	220.0	0	—	—	—	—	—	—	—	0	—	—
70	264	2.84	—	—	580.0	—	—	—	—	—	—	—	—	9.5	—	—
0	41	1.48	—	—	580.0	—	—	—	—	—	—	—	—	2.5	—	—
0	0	0.85	—	—	120.0	0	—	—	—	—	—	—	—	14.3	—	—
5	20	0.72	—	—	620.0	—	—	—	—	—	—	—	—	2.4	—	—
0	43	0.38	—	—	180.0	—	—	—	—	—	—	—	—	5.1	—	—

TABLE A-1 Table of Food Composition (*continued*) (Computer code is for Cengage Diet Analysis program) (For purposes of calculations, use "0" for t, <1, <.1, <.01, etc.)

DA+ Code	Food Description	Quantity	Measure	Wt (g)	H₂O (g)	Ener (kcal)	Prot (g)	Carb (g)	Fiber (g)	Fat (g)	Sat	Mono	Poly	Trans
Fast Food—*continued*														
34984	Homestyle mashed potatoes	¾	cup(s)	221	—	210	4.0	29.0	3.0	9.0	6.0	—	—	0
34985	Homestyle mashed potatoes and gravy	1	cup(s)	334	—	225	5.0	33.0	3.0	9.5	6.0	—	—	0
34988	Hot cinnamon apples	¾	cup(s)	145	—	210	0	47.0	3.0	3.0	0	—	—	0
34989	Macaroni and cheese	¾	cup(s)	221	—	330	14.0	39.0	1.0	12.0	7.0	—	—	0.5
51193	Market chopped salad with dressing	1	item(s)	563	—	580	11.0	31.0	9.0	48.0	9.0	—	—	1.0
34970	Meatloaf	1	serving(s)	218	—	480	29.0	23.0	2.0	33.0	13.0	—	—	0
39383	Nestle Toll House chocolate chip cookie	1	item(s)	78	—	370	4.0	49.0	2.0	19.0	9.0	—	—	0
34965	Quarter chicken, dark meat, no skin	1	item(s)	134	—	260	30.0	2.0	0	13.0	4.0	—	—	0
34966	Quarter chicken, dark meat, with skin	1	item(s)	149	—	280	31.0	3.0	0	15.0	4.5	—	—	0
34963	Quarter chicken, white meat, no skin or wing	1	item(s)	173	—	250	41.0	4.0	0	8.0	2.5	—	—	0
34964	Quarter chicken, white meat, with skin and wing	1	item(s)	110	—	330	50.0	3.0	0	12.0	4.0	—	—	0
34968	Roasted turkey breast	5	ounce(s)	142	—	180	38.0	0	0	3.0	1.0	—	—	0
35011	Seasonal fresh fruit salad	1	serving(s)	142	—	60	1.0	15.0	1.0	0	0	0	0	0
51192	Spinach with garlic butter sauce	1	serving(s)	170	—	130	5.0	9.0	5.0	9.0	6.0	—	—	0
34969	Spiral sliced holiday ham	8	ounce(s)	227	—	450	40.0	13.0	0	26.0	10.0	—	—	0
35003	Steamed vegetables	1	cup(s)	136	—	50	2.0	8.0	3.0	2.0	0	—	—	0
35005	Sweet corn	¾	cup(s)	176	—	170	6.0	37.0	2.0	4.0	1.0	—	—	0
35004	Sweet potato casserole	¾	cup(s)	198	—	460	4.0	77.0	3.0	17.0	6.0	—	—	0
	Burger King													
29731	Biscuit with sausage, egg, and cheese	1	item(s)	191	—	610	20.0	33.0	1.0	45.0	15.0	—	—	1.0
14249	Cheeseburger	1	item(s)	133	—	330	17.0	31.0	1.0	16.0	7.0	—	—	0.5
14251	Chicken sandwich	1	item(s)	219	—	660	24.0	52.0	4.0	40.0	8.0	—	—	2.5
3808	Chicken Tenders, 8 pieces	1	serving(s)	123	—	340	19.0	21.0	0.5	20.0	5.0	—	—	3.0
14259	Chocolate shake, small	1	item(s)	315	—	470	8.0	75.0	1.0	14.0	9.0	—	—	0
29732	Croissanwich with sausage and cheese	1	item(s)	106	37.2	370	14.0	23.0	0.5	25.0	9.0	12.7	3.3	2.0
14261	Croissanwich with sausage, egg, and cheese	1	item(s)	159	71.4	470	19.0	26.0	0.5	32.0	11.0	15.8	6.1	2.5
3809	Double cheeseburger	1	item(s)	189	—	500	30.0	31.0	1.0	29.0	14.0	—	—	1.5
14244	Double Whopper sandwich	1	item(s)	373	—	900	47.0	51.0	3.0	57.0	19.0	—	—	2.0
14245	Double Whopper with cheese sandwich	1	item(s)	398	—	990	52.0	52.0	3.0	64.0	24.0	—	—	2.5
14250	Fish Filet sandwich	1	item(s)	250	—	630	24.0	67.0	4.0	30.0	6.0	—	—	2.5
14255	French fries, medium, salted	1	serving(s)	116	—	360	4.0	41.0	4.0	20.0	4.5	—	—	4.5
14262	French toast sticks, 5 pieces	1	serving(s)	112	37.6	390	6.0	46.0	2.0	20.0	4.5	10.6	2.9	4.5
14248	Hamburger	1	item(s)	121	—	290	15.0	30.0	1.0	12.0	4.5	—	—	0
14263	Hash brown rounds, small	1	serving(s)	75	27.1	230	2.0	23.0	2.0	15.0	4.0	—	—	5.0
14256	Onion rings, medium	1	serving(s)	91	—	320	4.0	40.0	3.0	16.0	4.0	—	—	3.5
39000	Tendercrisp chicken sandwich	1	item(s)	286	—	780	25.0	73.0	4.0	43.0	8.0	—	—	4.0
37514	TenderGrill chicken sandwich	1	item(s)	258	—	450	37.0	53.0	4.0	10.0	2.0	—	—	0
14258	Vanilla shake, small	1	item(s)	296	—	400	8.0	57.0	0	15.0	9.0	—	—	0
1736	Whopper sandwich	1	item(s)	290	—	670	28.0	51.0	3.0	39.0	11.0	—	—	1.5
14243	Whopper with cheese sandwich	1	item(s)	315	—	760	33.0	52.0	3.0	47.0	16.0	—	—	1.5
	Carl's Jr													
33962	Carl's bacon Swiss crispy chicken sandwich	1	item(s)	268	—	750	31.0	91.0	—	28.0	28.0	—	—	—
10801	Carl's Catch fish sandwich	1	item(s)	215	—	560	19.0	58.0	2.0	27.0	7.0	—	1.9	—
10862	Carl's Famous Star hamburger	1	item(s)	254	—	590	24.0	50.0	3.0	32.0	9.0	—	—	—
10785	Charbroiled chicken club sandwich	1	item(s)	270	—	550	42.0	43.0	4.0	23.0	7.0	—	2.9	—
10866	Charbroiled chicken salad	1	item(s)	437	—	330	34.0	17.0	5.0	7.0	4.0	—	1.0	—
10855	Charbroiled Santa Fe chicken sandwich	1	item(s)	266	—	610	38.0	43.0	4.0	32.0	8.0	—	—	—
10790	Chicken stars, 6 pieces	1	serving(s)	85	—	260	13.0	14.0	1.0	16.0	4.0	—	1.6	—
34864	Chocolate shake, small	1	serving(s)	595	—	540	15.0	98.0	0	11.0	7.0	—	—	—
10797	Crisscut fries	1	serving(s)	139	—	410	5.0	43.0	4.0	24.0	5.0	—	—	—
10799	Double Western Bacon cheeseburger	1	item(s)	308	—	920	51.0	65.0	2.0	50	21.0	—	6.6	—

PAGE KEY: A-6 = Breads/Baked Goods A-12 = Cereal/Rice/Pasta A-16 = Fruit A-20 = Vegetables/Legumes A-30 = Nuts/Seeds A-32 = Vegetarian A-34 = Dairy A-42 = Eggs A-42 = Seafood A-44 = Meats A-48 = Poultry A-48 = Processed Meats A-50 = Beverages A-54 = Fats/Oils A-56 = Sweets A-58 = Spices/Condiments/Sauces A-62 = Mixed Foods/Soups/Sandwiches A-66 = Fast Food A-86 = Convenience A-88 = Baby Foods

Chol (mg)	Calc (mg)	Iron (mg)	Magn (mg)	Pota (mg)	Sodi (mg)	Zinc (mg)	Vit A (µg)	Thia (mg)	Vit E (mg α)	Ribo (mg)	Niac (mg)	Vit B_6 (mg)	Fola (µg)	Vit C (mg)	Vit B_{12} (µg)	Sele (µg)
25	51	0.46	—	—	660.0	—	—	—	—	—	—	—	—	19.2	—	—
25	100	0.59	—	—	1230.0	—	—	—	—	—	—	—	—	24.9	—	—
0	16	0.28	—	—	15.0	—	—	—	—	—	—	—	—	0	—	—
30	345	1.65	—	—	1290.0	—	—	—	—	—	—	—	—	0	—	—
10	—	—	—	—	2010.0	—	—	—	—	—	—	—	—	—	—	—
125	140	3.77	—	—	970.0	—	—	—	—	—	—	—	—	1.8	—	—
20	0	1.32	—	—	340.0	—	—	—	—	—	—	—	—	0	—	—
155	0	1.52	—	—	260.0	0	—	—	—	—	—	—	—	0	—	—
155	0	2.14	—	—	660.0	0	—	—	—	—	—	—	—	0	—	—
125	0	0.89	—	—	480.0	0	—	—	—	—	—	—	—	0	—	—
165	0	0.78	—	—	960.0	0	—	—	—	—	—	—	—	0	—	—
70	20	1.80	—	—	620.0	0	—	—	—	—	—	—	—	0	—	—
0	16	0.29	—	—	20.0	—	—	—	—	—	—	—	—	29.5	—	—
20	—	—	—	—	200.0	—	—	—	—	—	—	—	—	—	—	—
140	0	1.73	—	—	2230.0	0	—	—	—	—	—	—	—	0	—	—
0	53	0.46	—	—	45.0	—	—	—	—	—	—	—	—	24.0	—	—
0	0	0.43	—	—	95.0	—	—	—	—	—	—	—	—	5.8	—	—
20	44	1.18	—	—	210.0	—	—	—	—	—	—	—	—	9.8	—	—
210	250	2.70	—	—	1620.0	—	89.9	—	—	—	—	—	—	0	—	—
55	150	2.70	—	—	780.0	—	—	0.24	—	0.31	4.17	—	—	1.2	—	—
70	64	2.89	—	—	1440.0	—	—	0.50	—	0.32	10.29	—	—	0	—	—
55	20	0.72	—	—	960.0	—	—	0.14	—	0.11	10.93	—	—	0	—	—
55	333	0.79	—	—	350.0	—	—	0.11	—	0.61	0.26	—	—	2.7	0	—
50	99	1.78	20.1	217.3	810.0	1.51	—	0.34	1.03	0.33	4.33	—	—	0	0.6	22.2
180	146	2.63	28.6	313.2	1060.0	2.08	—	0.38	1.66	0.51	4.72	0.28	—	0	1.1	38.0
105	250	4.50	—	—	1030.0	—	—	0.26	—	0.44	6.37	—	—	1.2	—	—
175	150	8.07	—	—	1090.0	—	—	0.39	—	0.59	11.05	—	—	9.0	—	—
195	299	8.08	—	—	1520.0	—	—	0.39	—	0.66	11.03	—	—	9.0	—	—
60	101	3.62	—	—	1380.0	—	—	—	—	—	—	—	—	3.6	—	—
0	20	0.71	—	—	590.0	—	0	0.15	—	0.48	2.30	—	—	8.9	—	—
0	60	1.80	21.3	124.3	440.0	0.57	—	0.31	0.98	0.19	2.88	0.05	—	0	0	13.7
40	80	2.70	—	—	560.0	—	—	0.25	—	0.28	4.25	—	—	1.2	—	—
0	0	0.36	—	—	450.0	—	0	0.11	0.83	0.06	1.35	0.17	—	1.2	—	—
0	100	0.00	—	—	460.0	—	0	0.14	—	0.09	2.32	—	—	0	—	—
75	79	4.43	—	—	1730.0	—	—	—	—	—	—	—	—	8.9	—	—
75	57	6.82	—	—	1210.0	—	—	—	—	—	—	—	—	5.7	—	—
60	348	0.00	—	—	240.0	—	—	0.11	—	0.63	0.21	—	—	2.4	0	—
51	100	5.38	—	—	1020.0	—	—	0.38	—	0.43	7.30	—	—	9.0	—	—
115	249	5.38	—	—	1450.0	—	—	0.38	—	0.51	7.28	—	—	9.0	—	—
80	200	5.40	—	—	1900.0	—	—	—	—	—	—	—	—	2.4	—	—
80	150	2.70	—	—	990.0	—	60.0	—	—	—	—	—	—	2.4	—	—
70	100	4.50	—	—	910.0	—	—	—	—	—	—	—	—	6.0	—	—
95	200	3.60	—	—	1330.0	—	—	—	—	—	—	—	—	9.0	—	—
75	200	1.80	—	—	880.0	—	—	—	—	—	—	—	—	30.0	—	—
100	200	3.60	—	—	1440.0	—	—	—	—	—	—	—	—	9.0	—	—
35	19	1.02	—	—	470.0	—	0	—	—	—	—	—	—	0	—	—
45	600	1.08	—	—	360.0	—	0	—	—	—	—	—	—	0	—	—
0	20	1.80	—	—	950.0	—	0	—	—	—	—	—	—	12.0	—	—
155	300	7.20	—	—	1730.0	—	—	—	—	—	—	—	—	1.2	—	—

TABLE A-1 **Table of Food Composition (*continued*)** (Computer code is for Cengage Diet Analysis program) (For purposes of calculations, use "0" for t, <1, <.1, <.01, etc.)

DA+ Code	Food Description	Quantity	Measure	Wt (g)	H₂O (g)	Ener (kcal)	Prot (g)	Carb (g)	Fiber (g)	Fat (g)	Fat Breakdown (g) Sat	Mono	Poly	*Trans*
Fast Food—*continued*														
14238	French fries, small	1	serving(s)	92	—	290	5.0	37.0	3.0	14.0	3.0	—	—	—
10798	French toast dips without syrup, 5 pieces	1	serving(s)	155	—	370	8.0	49.0	0	17.0	5.0	—	1.4	—
10802	Onion rings	1	serving(s)	128	—	440	7.0	53.0	3.0	22.0	5.0	—	0.8	—
34858	Spicy chicken sandwich	1	item(s)	198	—	480	14.0	48.0	2.0	26.0	5.0	—	—	—
34867	Strawberry shake, small	1	serving(s)	595	—	520	14.0	93.0	0	11.0	7.0	—	—	—
10865	Super Star hamburger	1	item(s)	348	—	790	41.0	52.0	3.0	47.0	14.0	—	—	—
38925	The Six Dollar burger	1	item(s)	429	—	1010	40.0	60.0	3.0	66.0	26.0	—	—	—
10818	Vanilla shake, small	1	item(s)	398	—	314	10.0	51.5	0	7.4	4.7	—	—	—
10770	Western Bacon cheeseburger	1	item(s)	225	—	660	32.0	64.0	2.0	30.0	12.0	—	4.8	—
	Chick Fil-A													
38746	Biscuit with bacon, egg, and cheese	1	item(s)	163	—	470	18.0	39.0	1.0	26.0	9.0	—	—	3.0
38747	Biscuit with egg	1	item(s)	135	—	350	11.0	38.0	1.0	16.0	4.5	—	—	3.0
38748	Biscuit with egg and cheese	1	item(s)	149	—	400	14.0	38.0	1.0	21.0	7.0	—	—	3.0
38753	Biscuit with gravy	1	item(s)	192	—	330	5.0	43.0	1.0	15.0	4.0	—	—	4.0
38752	Biscuit with sausage, egg, and cheese	1	item(s)	212	—	620	22.0	39.0	2.0	42.0	14.0	—	—	3.0
38771	Carrot and raisin salad	1	item(s)	113	—	170	1.0	28.0	2.0	6.0	1.0	—	—	0
38761	Chargrilled chicken Cool Wrap	1	item(s)	245	—	390	29.0	54.0	3.0	7.0	3.0	—	—	0
38766	Chargrilled chicken garden salad	1	item(s)	275	—	180	22.0	9.0	3.0	6.0	3.0	—	—	0
38758	Chargrilled chicken sandwich	1	item(s)	193	—	270	28.0	33.0	3.0	3.5	1.0	—	—	0
38742	Chicken biscuit	1	item(s)	145	—	420	18.0	44.0	2.0	19.0	4.5	—	—	3.0
38743	Chicken biscuit with cheese	1	item(s)	159	—	470	21.0	45.0	2.0	23.0	8.0	—	—	3.0
38762	Chicken Caesar Cool Wrap	1	item(s)	227	—	460	36.0	52.0	3.0	10.0	6.0	—	—	0
38757	Chicken deluxe sandwich	1	item(s)	208	—	420	28.0	39.0	2.0	16.0	3.5	—	—	0
38764	Chicken salad sandwich on wheat bun	1	item(s)	153	—	350	20.0	32.0	5.0	15.0	3.0	—	—	0
38756	Chicken sandwich	1	item(s)	170	—	410	28.0	38.0	1.0	16.0	3.5	—	—	0
38768	Chick-n-Strip salad	1	item(s)	327	—	400	34.0	21.0	4.0	20.0	6.0	—	—	0
38763	Chick-n-Strips	4	item(s)	127	—	300	28.0	14.0	1.0	15.0	2.5	—	—	0
38770	Cole slaw	1	item(s)	128	—	260	2.0	17.0	2.0	21.0	3.5	—	—	0
38776	Diet lemonade, small	1	cup(s)	255	—	25	0	5.0	0	0	0	0	0	0
38755	Hashbrowns	1	serving(s)	84	—	260	2.0	25.0	3.0	17.0	3.5	—	—	1.0
38765	Hearty breast of chicken soup	1	cup(s)	241	—	140	8.0	18.0	1.0	3.5	1.0	—	—	0
38741	Hot buttered biscuit	1	item(s)	79	—	270	4.0	38.0	1.0	12.0	3.0	—	—	3.0
38778	IceDream, small cone	1	item(s)	135	—	160	4.0	28.0	0	4.0	2.0	—	—	0
38774	IceDream, small cup	1	serving(s)	227	—	240	6.0	41.0	0	6.0	3.5	—	—	0
38775	Lemonade, small	1	cup(s)	255	—	170	0	41.0	0	0.5	0	—	—	0
38777	Nuggets	8	item(s)	113	—	260	26.0	12.0	0.5	12.0	2.5	—	—	0
38769	Side salad	1	item(s)	108	—	60	3.0	4.0	2.0	3.0	1.5	—	—	0
38767	Southwest chargrilled salad	1	item(s)	303	—	240	25.0	17.0	5.0	8.0	3.5	—	—	0
40481	Spicy chicken cool wrap	1	serving(s)	230	—	380	30.0	52.0	3.0	6.0	3.0	—	—	0
38772	Waffle potato fries, small, salted	1	serving(s)	85	—	270	3.0	34.0	4.0	13.0	3.0	—	—	1.5
	Cinnabon													
39572	Caramellata Chill w/whipped cream	16	fluid ounce(s)	480	—	406	10.0	61.0	0	14.0	8.0	—	—	0
39571	Cinnabon Bites	1	serving(s)	149	—	510	8.0	77.0	2.0	19.0	5.0	—	—	5.0
39570	Cinnabon Stix	5	item(s)	85	—	379	6.0	41.0	1.0	21.0	6.0	—	—	4.0
39567	Classic roll	1	item(s)	221	—	813	15.0	117.0	4.0	32.0	8.0	—	—	5.0
39568	Minibon	1	item(s)	92	—	339	6.0	49.0	2.0	13.0	3.0	—	—	2.0
39573	Mochalatta Chill w/whipped cream	16	fluid ounce(s)	480	—	362	9.0	55.0	0	13.0	8.0	—	—	0
39569	Pecanbon	1	item(s)	272	—	1100	16.0	141.0	8.0	56.0	10.0	—	—	5.0
	Dairy Queen													
1466	Banana split	1	item(s)	369	—	510	8.0	96.0	3.0	12.0	8.0	—	—	0
38552	Brownie Earthquake®	1	serving(s)	304	—	740	10.0	112.0	0	27.0	16.0	—	—	0.5
38561	Chocolate chip cookie dough blizzard,® small	1	item(s)	319	—	720	12.0	105.0	0	28.0	14.0	—	—	2.5
1464	Chocolate malt, small	1	item(s)	418	—	640	15.0	111.0	1.0	16.0	11.0	—	—	0.5
38541	Chocolate shake, small	1	item(s)	397	—	560	13.0	93.0	1.0	15.0	10.0	—	—	0.5
17257	Chocolate soft serve	½	cup(s)	94	—	150	4.0	22.0	0	5.0	3.5	—	—	0
1463	Chocolate sundae, small	1	item(s)	163	—	280	5.0	49.0	0	7.0	4.5	—	—	0

PAGE KEY: A-6 = Breads/Baked Goods A-12 = Cereal/Rice/Pasta A-16 = Fruit A-20 = Vegetables/Legumes A-30 = Nuts/Seeds A-32 = Vegetarian A-34 = Dairy A-42 = Eggs A-42 = Seafood A-44 = Meats A-48 = Poultry A-48 = Processed Meats A-50 = Beverages A-54 = Fats/Oils A-56 = Sweets A-58 = Spices/Condiments/Sauces A-62 = Mixed Foods/Soups/Sandwiches A-66 = Fast Food A-86 = Convenience A-88 = Baby Foods

Chol (mg)	Calc (mg)	Iron (mg)	Magn (mg)	Pota (mg)	Sodi (mg)	Zinc (mg)	Vit A (µg)	Thia (mg)	Vit E (mg α)	Ribo (mg)	Niac (mg)	Vit B_6 (mg)	Fola (µg)	Vit C (mg)	Vit B_{12} (µg)	Sele (µg)
0	0	1.08	—	—	170.0	—	0	—	—	—	—	—	—	21.0	—	—
3	0	0.00	—	—	470.0	—	0	0.25	—	0.23	2.00	—	—	0	—	—
0	20	0.72	—	—	700.0	—	0	—	—	—	—	—	—	3.6	—	—
40	100	3.60	—	—	1220.0	—	—	—	—	—	—	—	—	6.0	—	—
45	600	0.00	—	—	340.0	—	0	—	—	—	—	—	—	0	—	—
130	100	7.20	—	—	980.0	—	—	—	—	—	—	—	—	9.0	—	—
145	279	4.29	—	—	1960.0	—	—	—	—	—	—	—	—	16.7	—	—
30	401	0.00	—	—	234.0	—	0	—	—	—	—	—	—	0	—	—
85	200	5.40	—	—	1410.0	—	60.0	—	—	—	—	—	—	1.2	—	—
270	150	2.70	—	—	1190.0	—	—	—	—	—	—	—	—	0	—	—
240	80	2.70	—	—	740.0	—	—	—	—	—	—	—	—	0	—	—
255	150	2.70	—	—	970.0	—	—	—	—	—	—	—	—	0	—	—
5	60	1.80	—	—	930.0	—	0	—	—	—	—	—	—	0	—	—
300	200	3.60	—	—	1360.0	—	—	—	—	—	—	—	—	0	—	—
10	40	0.36	—	—	110.0	—	—	—	—	—	—	—	—	4.8	—	—
65	200	3.60	—	—	1020.0	—	—	—	—	—	—	—	—	6.0	—	—
65	150	0.72	—	—	620.0	—	—	—	—	—	—	—	—	30	—	—
65	80	2.70	—	—	940.0	—	—	—	—	—	—	—	—	6.0	—	—
35	60	2.70	—	—	1270.0	—	0	—	—	—	—	—	—	0	—	—
50	150	2.70	—	—	1500.0	—	—	—	—	—	—	—	—	0	—	—
80	500	3.60	—	—	1350.0	—	—	—	—	—	—	—	—	1.2	—	—
60	100	2.70	—	—	1300.0	—	—	—	—	—	—	—	—	2.4	—	—
65	150	1.80	—	—	880.0	—	—	—	—	—	—	—	—	0	—	—
60	100	2.70	—	—	1300.0	—	—	—	—	—	—	—	—	0	—	—
80	150	1.44	—	—	1070.0	—	—	—	—	—	—	—	—	6.0	—	—
65	40	1.44	—	—	940.0	—	—	—	—	—	—	—	—	0	—	—
25	60	0.36	—	—	220.0	—	—	—	—	—	—	—	—	36.0	—	—
0	0	0.36	—	—	5.0	—	0	—	—	—	—	—	—	15.0	—	—
5	20	0.72	—	—	380.0	—	—	—	—	—	—	—	—	0	—	—
25	40	1.08	—	—	900.0	—	—	—	—	—	—	—	—	0	—	—
0	60	1.80	—	—	660.0	—	0	—	—	—	—	—	—	0	—	—
15	100	0.36	—	—	80.0	—	—	—	—	—	—	—	—	0	—	—
25	200	0.36	—	—	105.0	—	—	—	—	—	—	—	—	0	—	—
0	0	0.36	—	—	10.0	—	0	—	—	—	—	—	—	15.0	—	—
70	40	1.08	—	—	1090.0	—	0	—	—	—	—	—	—	0	—	—
10	100	0.00	—	—	75.0	—	—	—	—	—	—	—	—	15.0	—	—
60	200	1.08	—	—	770.0	—	—	—	—	—	—	—	—	24.0	—	—
60	200	3.60	—	—	1090.0	—	—	—	—	—	—	—	—	3.6	—	—
0	20	1.08	—	—	115.0	—	0	—	—	—	—	—	—	1.2	—	—
46	—	—	—	—	187.0	—	—	—	—	—	—	—	—	—	—	—
35	—	—	—	—	530.0	—	—	—	—	—	—	—	—	—	—	—
16	—	—	—	—	413.0	—	—	—	—	—	—	—	—	—	—	—
67	—	—	—	—	801.0	—	—	—	—	—	—	—	—	—	—	—
27	—	—	—	—	337.0	—	—	—	—	—	—	—	—	—	—	—
46	—	—	—	—	252.0	—	—	—	—	—	—	—	—	—	—	—
63	—	—	—	—	600.0	—	—	—	—	—	—	—	—	—	—	—
30	250	1.80	—	—	180.0	—	—	—	—	—	—	—	—	15.0	—	—
50	250	1.80	—	—	350.0	—	—	—	—	—	—	—	—	0	—	—
50	350	2.70	—	—	370.0	—	—	—	—	—	—	—	—	1.2	—	—
55	450	1.80	—	—	340.0	—	—	—	—	—	—	—	—	2.4	—	—
50	450	1.44	—	—	280.0	—	—	—	—	—	—	—	—	2.4	—	—
15	100	0.72	—	—	75.0	—	—	—	—	—	—	—	—	0	—	—
20	200	1.08	—	—	140.0	—	—	—	—	—	—	—	—	0	—	—

TABLE A-1 Table of Food Composition (*continued*) (Computer code is for Cengage Diet Analysis program) (For purposes of calculations, use "0" for t, <1, <.1, <.01, etc.

DA+ Code	Food Description	Quantity	Measure	Wt (g)	H₂O (g)	Ener (kcal)	Prot (g)	Carb (g)	Fiber (g)	Fat (g)	Fat Breakdown (g) Sat	Mono	Poly	Trans
Fast Food—*continued*														
1462	Dipped cone, small	1	item(s)	156	—	340	6.0	42.0	1.0	17.0	9.0	4.0	3.0	1.0
38555	Oreo cookies blizzard, small	1	item(s)	283	—	570	11.0	83.0	0.5	21.0	10.0	—	—	2.5
38547	Royal Treats Peanut Buster® Parfait	1	item(s)	305	—	730	16.0	99.0	2.0	31.0	17.0	—	—	0
17256	Vanilla soft serve	½	cup(s)	94	—	140	3.0	22.0	0	4.5	3.0	—	—	0
Domino's														
31606	Barbeque buffalo wings	1	item(s)	25	—	50	6.0	2.0	0	2.5	0.5	—	—	—
31604	Breadsticks	1	item(s)	30	—	115	2.0	12.0	0	6.3	1.1	—	—	—
37551	Buffalo Chicken Kickers	1	item(s)	24	—	47	4.0	3.0	0	2.0	0.5	—	—	—
37548	CinnaStix	1	item(s)	30	—	123	2.0	15.0	1.0	6.1	1.1	—	—	—
37549	Dot, cinnamon	1	item(s)	28	7.6	99	1.9	14.9	0.7	3.7	0.7	—	—	—
31605	Double cheesy bread	1	item(s)	35	—	123	4.0	13.0	0	6.5	1.9	—	—	—
31607	Hot buffalo wings	1	item(s)	25	—	45	5.0	1.0	0	2.5	0.5	—	—	—
Domino's Classic hand tossed pizza														
31573	America's favorite feast, 12"	1	slice(s)	102	—	257	10.0	29.0	2.0	11.5	4.5	—	—	—
31574	America's favorite feast, 14"	1	slice(s)	141	—	353	14.0	39.0	2.0	16.0	6.0	—	—	—
37543	Bacon cheeseburger feast, 12"	1	slice(s)	99	—	273	12.0	28.0	2.0	13.0	5.5	—	—	—
37545	Bacon cheeseburger feast, 14"	1	slice(s)	137	—	379	17.0	38.0	2.0	18.0	8.0	—	—	—
37546	Barbeque feast, 12"	1	slice(s)	96	—	252	11.0	31.0	1.0	10.0	4.5	—	—	—
37547	Barbeque feast, 14"	1	slice(s)	131	—	344	14.0	43.0	2.0	13.5	6.0	—	—	—
31569	Cheese, 12"	1	slice(s)	55	—	160	6.0	28.0	1.0	3.0	1.0	—	—	0
31570	Cheese, 14"	1	slice(s)	75	—	220	8.0	38.0	2.0	4.0	1.0	—	—	0
37538	Deluxe feast, 12"	1	slice(s)	201	101.8	465	19.5	57.4	3.5	18.2	7.7	—	—	—
37540	Deluxe feast, 14"	1	slice(s)	273	138.4	627	26.4	78.3	4.7	24.1	10.2	—	—	—
31685	Deluxe, 12"	1	slice(s)	100	—	234	9.0	29.0	2.0	9.5	3.5	—	—	—
31694	Deluxe, 14"	1	slice(s)	136	—	316	13.0	39.0	2.0	12.5	5.0	—	—	—
31686	Extravaganzza, 12"	1	slice(s)	122	—	289	13.0	30.0	2.0	14.0	5.5	—	—	—
31695	Extravaganzza, 14"	1	slice(s)	165	—	388	17.0	40.0	3.0	18.5	7.5	—	—	—
31575	Hawaiian feast, 12"	1	slice(s)	102	—	223	10.0	30.0	2.0	8.0	3.5	—	—	—
31576	Hawaiian feast, 14"	1	slice(s)	141	—	309	14.0	41.0	2.0	11.0	4.5	—	—	—
31687	Meatzza, 12"	1	slice(s)	108	—	281	13.0	29.0	2.0	13.5	5.5	—	—	—
31696	Meatzza, 14"	1	slice(s)	146	—	378	17.0	39.0	2.0	18.0	7.5	—	—	—
31571	Pepperoni feast, extra pepperoni and cheese, 12"	1	slice(s)	98	—	265	11.0	28.0	2.0	12.5	5.0	—	—	—
31572	Pepperoni feast, extra pepperoni and cheese, 14"	1	slice(s)	135	—	363	16.0	39.0	2.0	17.0	7.0	—	—	—
31577	Vegi feast, 12"	1	slice(s)	102	—	218	9.0	29.0	2.0	8.0	3.5	—	—	—
31578	Vegi feast, 14"	1	slice(s)	139	—	300	13.0	40.0	3.0	11.0	4.5	—	—	—
Domino's thin crust pizza														
31583	America's favorite, 12"	1	slice(s)	72	—	208	8.0	15.0	1.0	13.5	5.0	—	—	—
31584	America's favorite, 14"	1	slice(s)	100	—	285	11.0	20.0	2.0	18.5	7.0	—	—	—
31579	Cheese, 12"	1	slice(s)	49	—	137	5.0	14.0	1.0	7.0	2.5	—	—	—
31580	Cheese, 14"	1	slice(s)	68	27.0	214	8.8	19.0	1.4	11.4	4.6	2.9	2.5	—
31688	Deluxe, 12"	1	slice(s)	70	—	185	7.0	15.0	1.0	11.5	4.0	—	—	—
31697	Deluxe, 14"	1	slice(s)	94	—	248	10.0	20.0	2.0	15.0	5.5	—	—	—
31689	Extravaganzza, 12"	1	slice(s)	92	—	240	11.0	16.0	1.0	15.5	6.0	—	—	—
31698	Extravaganzza, 14"	1	slice(s)	123	—	320	14.0	21.0	2.0	20.5	8.0	—	—	—
31585	Hawaiian, 12"	1	slice(s)	71	—	174	8.0	16.0	1.0	9.5	3.5	—	—	—
31586	Hawaiian, 14"	1	slice(s)	100	—	240	11.0	21.0	2.0	13.0	5.0	—	—	—
31690	Meatzza, 12"	1	slice(s)	78	—	232	11.0	15.0	1.0	15.0	6.0	—	—	—
31699	Meatzza, 14"	1	slice(s)	104	—	310	14.0	20.0	2.0	20	8.0	—	—	—
31581	Pepperoni, extra pepperoni and cheese, 12"	1	slice(s)	68	—	216	9.0	14.0	1.0	14.0	5.5	—	—	—
31582	Pepperoni, extra pepperoni and cheese, 14"	1	slice(s)	93	—	295	13.0	20.0	1.0	19.0	7.5	—	—	—
31587	Vegi, 12"	1	slice(s)	71	—	168	7.0	15.0	1.0	9.5	3.5	—	—	—
31588	Vegi, 14"	1	slice(s)	97	—	231	10.0	21.0	2.0	13.5	5.0	—	—	—
Domino's Ultimate deep dish pizza														
31596	America's favorite, 12"	1	slice(s)	115	—	309	12.0	29.0	2.0	17.0	6.0	—	—	—
31702	America's favorite, 14"	1	slice(s)	162	—	433	17.0	42.0	3.0	23.5	8.0	—	—	—
31590	Cheese, 12"	1	slice(s)	90	—	238	9.0	28.0	2.0	11.0	3.5	—	—	—
31591	Cheese, 14"	1	slice(s)	128	53.9	351	14.5	41.0	2.9	13.2	5.2	3.8	2.5	—
31589	Cheese, 6"	1	item(s)	215	—	598	22.9	68.4	3.9	27.6	9.9	—	—	—
31691	Deluxe, 12"	1	slice(s)	122	—	287	11.0	29.0	2.0	15.0	5.0	—	—	—

PAGE KEY: A-6 = Breads/Baked Goods A-12 = Cereal/Rice/Pasta A-16 = Fruit A-20 = Vegetables/Legumes A-30 = Nuts/Seeds A-32 = Vegetarian A-34 = Dairy A-42 = Eggs A-42 = Seafood A-44 = Meats A-48 = Poultry A-48 = Processed Meats A-50 = Beverages A-54 = Fats/Oils A-56 = Sweets A-58 = Spices/Condiments/Sauces A-62 = Mixed Foods/Soups/Sandwiches A-66 = Fast Food A-86 = Convenience A-88 = Baby Foods

Chol (mg)	Calc (mg)	Iron (mg)	Magn (mg)	Pota (mg)	Sodi (mg)	Zinc (mg)	Vit A (μg)	Thia (mg)	Vit E (mg α)	Ribo (mg)	Niac (mg)	Vit B$_6$ (mg)	Fola (μg)	Vit C (mg)	Vit B$_{12}$ (μg)	Sele (μg)
20	200	1.08	—	—	130.0	—	—	—	—	—	—	—	—	1.2	—	—
40	350	2.70	—	—	430.0	—	—	—	—	—	—	—	—	1.2	—	—
35	300	1.80	—	—	400.0	—	—	—	—	—	—	—	—	1.2	—	—
15	150	0.72	—	—	70.0	—	—	—	—	—	—	—	—	0	—	—
26	10	0.36	—	—	175.5	—	—	—	—	—	—	—	—	0	—	—
0	0	0.72	—	—	122.1	—	—	—	—	—	—	—	—	0	—	—
9	0	0.00	—	—	162.5	—	—	—	—	—	—	—	—	0	—	—
0	0	0.72	—	—	111.4	—	—	—	—	—	—	—	—	0	—	—
0	6	0.59	—	—	85.7	—	—	—	—	—	—	—	—	0	—	—
6	40	0.72	—	—	162.3	—	—	—	—	—	—	—	—	0	—	—
26	10	0.36	—	—	254.5	—	—	—	—	—	—	—	—	1.2	—	—
22	100	1.80	—	—	625.5	—	—	—	—	—	—	—	—	0.6	—	—
31	140	2.52	—	—	865.5	—	—	—	—	—	—	—	—	0.6	—	—
27	140	1.80	—	—	634.0	—	—	—	—	—	—	—	—	0	—	—
38	190	2.52	—	—	900.0	—	—	—	—	—	—	—	—	0	—	—
20	140	1.62	—	—	600.0	—	—	—	—	—	—	—	—	0.6	—	—
27	190	2.16	—	—	831.5	—	—	—	—	—	—	—	—	0.6	—	—
0	0	1.80	—	—	110.0	—	0	—	—	—	—	—	—	0	—	—
0	0	2.70	—	—	150.0	—	0	—	—	—	—	—	—	0	—	—
40	199	3.56	—	—	1063.1	—	—	—	—	—	—	—	—	1.4	—	—
53	276	4.84	—	—	1432.2	—	—	—	—	—	—	—	—	1.8	—	—
17	100	1.80	—	—	541.5	—	—	—	—	—	—	—	—	0.6	—	—
23	130	2.34	—	—	728.5	—	—	—	—	—	—	—	—	1.2	—	—
28	140	1.98	—	—	764.0	—	—	—	—	—	—	—	—	0.6	—	—
37	190	2.70	—	—	1014.0	—	—	—	—	—	—	—	—	1.2	—	—
16	130	1.62	—	—	546.5	—	—	—	—	—	—	—	—	1.2	—	—
23	180	2.34	—	—	765.0	—	—	—	—	—	—	—	—	1.2	—	—
28	130	1.80	—	—	739.5	—	—	—	—	—	—	—	—	0	—	—
37	190	2.52	—	—	983.5	—	—	—	—	—	—	—	—	0	—	—
24	130	1.62	—	—	670.0	—	70.9	—	—	—	—	—	—	0	—	—
33	180	2.34	—	—	920.0	—	104.7	—	—	—	—	—	—	0	—	—
13	130	1.62	—	—	489.0	—	—	—	—	—	—	—	—	0.6	—	—
18	180	2.34	—	—	678.0	—	—	—	—	—	—	—	—	0.6	—	—
23	100	0.90	—	—	533.0	—	—	—	—	—	—	—	—	2.4	—	—
32	140	1.26	—	—	736.5	—	—	—	—	—	—	—	—	3.0	—	—
10	90	0.54	—	—	292.5	—	60.0	—	—	—	—	—	—	1.8	—	—
14	151	0.48	17.7	125.1	338.0	0.02	64.6	0.05	1.01	0.07	0.69	—	—	2.4	0.5	24.1
19	100	0.90	—	—	449.0	—	—	—	—	—	—	—	—	2.4	—	—
24	130	1.08	—	—	601.0	—	—	—	—	—	—	—	—	3.6	—	—
29	140	1.08	—	—	671.5	—	—	—	—	—	—	—	—	2.4	—	—
38	190	1.44	—	—	886.5	—	—	—	—	—	—	—	—	3.6	—	—
17	130	0.72	—	—	454.0	—	—	—	—	—	—	—	—	3.0	—	—
24	180	0.90	—	—	637.5	—	—	—	—	—	—	—	—	3.6	—	—
29	140	0.90	—	—	647.0	—	—	—	—	—	—	—	—	1.8	—	—
38	190	1.26	—	—	865.5	—	—	—	—	—	—	—	—	2.4	—	—
26	130	0.72	—	—	577.0	—	80.0	—	—	—	—	—	—	1.8	—	—
35	80	1.08	—	—	792.5	—	105.8	—	—	—	—	—	—	2.4	—	—
14	130	0.72	—	—	396.5	—	—	—	—	—	—	—	—	2.4	—	—
19	180	1.08	—	—	550.5	—	—	—	—	—	—	—	—	3.0	—	—
25	120	2.34	—	—	796.5	—	—	—	—	—	—	—	—	0.6	—	—
34	170	3.24	—	—	1110.0	—	—	—	—	—	—	—	—	0.6	—	—
11	110	1.98	—	—	555.5	—	70.0	—	—	—	—	—	—	0	—	—
18	189	3.78	32.0	209.9	718.1	1.75	99.8	0.29	1.13	0.31	5.44	—	—	0	0.6	45.6
36	295	4.67	—	—	1341.4	—	174.0	—	—	—	—	—	—	0.5	—	—
20	120	2.16	—	—	712.0	—	—	—	—	—	—	—	—	1.2	—	—

TABLE A-1 Table of Food Composition (*continued*) (Computer code is for Cengage Diet Analysis program) (For purposes of calculations, use "0" for t, <1, <.1, <.01, etc.)

DA+ Code	Food Description	Quantity	Measure	Wt (g)	H₂O (g)	Ener (kcal)	Prot (g)	Carb (g)	Fiber (g)	Fat (g)	Sat	Mono	Poly	Trans
Fast Food—*continued*														
31700	Deluxe, 14"	1	slice(s)	156	—	396	15.0	42.0	3.0	20.0	7.0	—	—	—
31692	Extravaganzza, 12"	1	slice(s)	136	—	341	14.0	30.0	2.0	19.0	7.0	—	—	—
31701	Extravaganzza, 14"	1	slice(s)	186	—	468	20.0	43.0	3.0	25.5	9.5	—	—	—
31599	Hawaiian, 12"	1	slice(s)	114	—	275	12.0	30.0	2.0	13.0	5.0	—	—	—
31600	Hawaiian, 14"	1	slice(s)	162	—	389	17.0	43.0	3.0	18.0	6.5	—	—	—
31693	Meatzza, 12"	1	slice(s)	121	—	333	14.0	29.0	2.0	19.0	7.0	—	—	—
31703	Meatzza, 14"	1	slice(s)	167	—	458	19.0	42.0	3.0	25.0	9.5	—	—	—
31593	Pepperoni, extra pepperoni and cheese, 12"	1	slice(s)	110	—	317	13.0	29.0	2.0	17.5	6.5	—	—	—
31594	Pepperoni, extra pepperoni and cheese, 14"	1	slice(s)	155	—	443	18.0	42.0	3.0	24.0	9.0	—	—	—
31602	Vegi, 12"	1	slice(s)	114	—	270	11.0	30.0	2.0	13.5	5.0	—	—	—
31603	Vegi, 14"	1	slice(s)	159	—	380	15.0	43.0	3.0	18.0	6.5	—	—	—
31598	With ham and pineapple tidbits, 6"	1	item(s)	430	—	619	25.2	69.9	4.0	28.3	10.2	—	—	—
31595	With Italian sausage, 6"	1	item(s)	430	—	642	24.8	69.6	4.2	31.1	11.3	—	—	—
31592	With pepperoni, 6"	1	item(s)	430	—	647	25.1	68.5	3.9	32.0	11.7	—	—	—
31601	With vegetables, 6"	1	item(s)	430	—	619	23.4	70.8	4.6	28.7	10.1	—	—	—
In-n-Out Burger														
34391	Cheeseburger with mustard and ketchup	1	serving(s)	268	—	400	22.0	41.0	3.0	18.0	9.0	—	—	0.5
34374	Cheeseburger	1	serving(s)	268	—	480	22.0	39.0	3.0	27.0	10.0	—	—	0.5
34390	Cheeseburger, lettuce leaves instead of buns	1	serving(s)	300	—	330	18.0	11.0	3.0	25.0	9.0	—	—	0
34377	Chocolate shake	1	serving(s)	425	—	690	9.0	83.0	0	36.0	24.0	—	—	1.0
34375	Double-Double cheeseburger	1	serving(s)	330	—	670	37.0	39.0	3.0	41.0	18.0	—	—	1.0
34393	Double-Double cheeseburger with mustard and ketchup	1	serving(s)	330	—	590	37.0	41.0	3.0	32.0	17.0	—	—	1.0
34392	Double-Double cheeseburger, lettuce leaves instead of buns	1	serving(s)	362	—	520	33.0	11.0	3.0	39.0	17.0	—	—	1.0
34376	French fries	1	serving(s)	125	—	400	7.0	54.0	2.0	18.0	5.0	—	—	0
34373	Hamburger	1	item(s)	243	—	390	16.0	39.0	3.0	19.0	5.0	—	—	0
34389	Hamburger with mustard and ketchup	1	serving(s)	243	—	310	16.0	41.0	3.0	10.0	4.0	—	—	0
34388	Hamburger, lettuce leaves instead of buns	1	serving(s)	275	—	240	13.0	11.0	3.0	17.0	4.0	—	—	0
34379	Strawberry shake	1	serving(s)	425	—	690	9.0	91.0	0	33.0	22.0	—	—	0.5
34378	Vanilla shake	1	serving(s)	425	—	680	9.0	78.0	0	37.0	25.0	—	—	1.0
Jack in the Box														
30392	Bacon ultimate cheeseburger	1	item(s)	338	—	1090	46.0	53.0	2.0	77.0	30.0	—	—	3.0
1740	Breakfast Jack	1	item(s)	125	—	290	17.0	29.0	1.0	12.0	4.5	—	—	0
14074	Cheeseburger	1	item(s)	131	—	350	18.0	31.0	1.0	17.0	8.0	—	—	1.0
14106	Chicken breast strips, 4 pieces	1	serving(s)	201	—	500	35.0	36.0	3.0	25.0	6.0	—	—	6.0
37241	Chicken club salad, plain, without salad dressing	1	serving(s)	431	—	300	27.0	13.0	4.0	15.0	6.0	—	—	0
14064	Chicken sandwich	1	item(s)	145	—	400	15.0	38.0	2.0	21.0	4.5	—	—	2.5
14111	Chocolate ice cream shake, small	1	serving(s)	414	—	880	14.0	107.0	1.0	45.0	31.0	—	—	2.0
14073	Hamburger	1	item(s)	118	—	310	16.0	30.0	1.0	14.0	6.0	—	—	1.0
14090	Hash browns	1	serving(s)	57	—	150	1.0	13.0	2.0	10.0	2.5	—	—	3.0
14072	Jack's Spicy Chicken sandwich	1	item(s)	270	—	620	25.0	61.0	4.0	31.0	6.0	—	—	3.0
1468	Jumbo Jack hamburger	1	item(s)	261	—	600	21.0	51.0	3.0	35.0	12.0	—	—	1.5
1469	Jumbo Jack hamburger with cheese	1	item(s)	286	—	690	25.0	54.0	3.0	42.0	16.0	—	—	1.5
14099	Natural cut french fries, large	1	serving(s)	196	—	530	8.0	69.0	5.0	25.0	6.0	—	—	7.0
14098	Natural cut french fries, medium	1	serving(s)	133	—	360	5.0	47.0	4.0	17.0	4.0	—	—	5.0
1470	Onion rings	1	serving(s)	119	—	500	6.0	51.0	3.0	30.0	6.0	—	—	10
33141	Sausage, egg, and cheese biscuit	1	item(s)	234	—	740	27.0	35.0	2.0	55.0	17.0	—	—	6.0
14095	Seasoned curly fries, medium	1	serving(s)	125	—	400	6.0	45.0	5.0	23.0	5.0	—	—	7.0
14077	Sourdough Jack	1	item(s)	245	—	710	27.0	36.0	3.0	51.0	18.0	—	—	3.0
37249	Southwest chicken salad, plain, without salad dressing	1	serving(s)	488	—	300	24.0	29.0	7.0	11.0	5.0	—	—	0
14112	Strawberry ice cream shake, small	1	serving(s)	417	—	880	13.0	105.0	0	44.0	31.0	—	—	2.0

PAGE KEY: A-6 = Breads/Baked Goods A-12 = Cereal/Rice/Pasta A-16 = Fruit A-20 = Vegetables/Legumes A-30 = Nuts/Seeds A-32 = Vegetarian A-34 = Dairy A-42 = Eggs A-42 = Seafood A-44 = Meats A-48 = Poultry
A-48 = Processed Meats A-50 = Beverages A-54 = Fats/Oils A-56 = Sweets A-58 = Spices/Condiments/Sauces A-62 = Mixed Foods/Soups/Sandwiches A-66 = Fast Food A-86 = Convenience A-88 = Baby Foods

Chol (mg)	Calc (mg)	Iron (mg)	Magn (mg)	Pota (mg)	Sodi (mg)	Zinc (mg)	Vit A (µg)	Thia (mg)	Vit E (mg α)	Ribo (mg)	Niac (mg)	Vit B6 (mg)	Fola (µg)	Vit C (mg)	Vit B12 (µg)	Sele (µg)
26	170	3.06	—	—	974.5	—	—	—	—	—	—	—	—	1.2	—	—
31	160	2.52	—	—	934.5	—	—	—	—	—	—	—	—	1.2	—	—
40	220	3.42	—	—	1260.0	—	—	—	—	—	—	—	—	1.2	—	—
19	150	1.98	—	—	717.0	—	—	—	—	—	—	—	—	1.2	—	—
26	210	2.88	—	—	1011.0	—	—	—	—	—	—	—	—	1.8	—	—
31	160	2.34	—	—	910.5	—	—	—	—	—	—	—	—	0	—	—
40	220	3.24	—	—	1230.0	—	—	—	—	—	—	—	—	0.6	—	—
27	150	2.16	—	—	840.5	—	86.5	—	—	—	—	—	—	0	—	—
37	220	3.06	—	—	1166.0	—	115.4	—	—	—	—	—	—	0.6	—	—
15	150	2.16	—	—	659.5	—	—	—	—	—	—	—	—	0.6	—	—
21	220	3.06	—	—	924.0	—	—	—	—	—	—	—	—	1.2	—	—
43	298	4.84	—	—	1497.8	—	—	—	—	—	—	—	—	1.5	—	—
45	302	4.89	—	—	1478.1	—	—	—	—	—	—	—	—	0.6	—	—
47	299	4.81	—	—	1523.7	—	167.9	—	—	—	—	—	—	0.6	—	—
36	307	5.10	—	—	1472.5	—	—	—	—	—	—	—	—	4.7	—	—
60	200	3.60	—	—	1080.0	—	—	—	—	—	—	—	—	12.0	—	—
60	200	3.60	—	—	1000.0	—	—	—	—	—	—	—	—	9.0	—	—
60	200	2.70	—	—	720.0	—	—	—	—	—	—	—	—	12.0	—	—
95	300	0.72	—	—	350.0	—	—	—	—	—	—	—	—	0	—	—
120	350	5.40	—	—	1440.0	—	—	—	—	—	—	—	—	9.0	—	—
115	350	5.40	—	—	1520.0	—	—	—	—	—	—	—	—	12.0	—	—
120	350	4.50	—	—	1160.0	—	—	—	—	—	—	—	—	12.0	—	—
0	20	1.80	—	—	245.0	—	0	—	—	—	—	—	—	0	—	—
40	40	3.60	—	—	650.0	—	—	—	—	—	—	—	—	9.0	—	—
35	40	3.60	—	—	730.0	—	—	—	—	—	—	—	—	12.0	—	—
40	40	2.70	—	—	370.0	—	—	—	—	—	—	—	—	12.0	—	—
85	300	0.00	—	—	280.0	—	—	—	—	—	—	—	—	0	—	—
90	300	0.00	—	—	390.0	—	—	—	—	—	—	—	—	0	—	—
140	308	7.38	—	540.0	2040.0	—	—	—	—	—	—	—	—	0.6	—	—
220	145	3.48	—	210.0	760.0	—	—	—	—	—	—	—	—	3.5	—	—
50	151	3.61	—	270.0	790.0	—	40.2	—	—	—	—	—	—	0	—	—
80	18	1.60	—	530.0	1260.0	—	—	—	—	—	—	—	—	1.1	—	—
65	280	3.35	—	560.0	880.0	—	—	—	—	—	—	—	—	50.4	—	—
35	100	2.70	—	240.0	730.0	—	—	—	—	—	—	—	—	4.8	—	—
135	460	0.47	—	840.0	330.0	—	—	—	—	—	—	—	—	0	—	—
40	100	3.60	—	250.0	600.0	—	0	—	—	—	—	—	—	0	—	—
0	10	0.18	—	190.0	230.0	—	0	—	—	—	—	—	—	0	—	—
50	150	1.80	—	450.0	1100.0	—	—	—	—	—	—	—	—	9.0	—	—
45	164	4.92	—	380.0	940.0	—	—	—	—	—	—	—	—	9.8	—	—
70	234	4.20	—	410.0	1310.0	—	—	—	—	—	—	—	—	8.4	—	—
0	20	1.42	—	1240.0	870.0	—	0	—	—	—	—	—	—	8.9	—	—
0	19	1.01	—	840.0	590.0	—	0	—	—	—	—	—	—	5.6	—	—
0	40	2.70	—	140.0	420.0	—	40.0	—	—	—	—	—	—	18.0	—	—
280	88	2.36	—	310.0	1430.0	—	—	—	—	—	—	—	—	0	—	—
0	40	1.80	—	580.0	890.0	—	—	—	—	—	—	—	—	0	—	—
75	200	4.50	—	430.0	1230.0	—	—	—	—	—	—	—	—	9.0	—	—
55	274	4.10	—	670.0	860.0	—	—	—	—	—	—	—	—	43.8	—	—
135	466	0.00	—	750.0	290.0	—	—	—	—	—	—	—	—	0	—	—

TABLE A-1 Table of Food Composition (*continued*) (Computer code is for Cengage Diet Analysis program) (For purposes of calculations, use "0" for t, <1, <.1, <.01, etc.

DA+ Code	Food Description	Quantity	Measure	Wt (g)	H₂O (g)	Ener (kcal)	Prot (g)	Carb (g)	Fiber (g)	Fat (g)	Sat	Mono	Poly	*Trans*
Fast Food—*continued*														
14078	Ultimate cheeseburger	1	item(s)	323	—	1010	40.0	53.0	2.0	71.0	28.0	—	—	3.0
14110	Vanilla ice cream shake, small	1	serving(s)	379	—	790	13.0	83.0	0	44.0	31.0	—	—	2.0
	Jamba Juice													
31645	Aloha Pineapple smoothie	24	fluid ounce(s)	730	—	500	8.0	117.0	4.0	1.5	1.0	—	—	—
31646	Banana Berry smoothie	24	fluid ounce(s)	719	—	480	5.0	112.0	4.0	1.0	0	—	—	—
31656	Berry Lime Sublime smoothie	24	fluid ounce(s)	728	—	460	3.0	106.0	5.0	2.0	1.0	—	—	—
31647	Carribean Passion smoothie	24	fluid ounce(s)	730	—	440	4.0	102.0	4.0	2.0	1.0	—	—	—
38422	Carrot juice	16	fluid ounce(s)	472	—	100	3.0	23.0	0	0.5	0	—	—	—
31648	Chocolate Moo'd smoothie	24	fluid ounce(s)	634	—	720	17.0	148.0	3.0	8.0	5.0	—	—	—
31649	Citrus Squeeze smoothie	24	fluid ounce(s)	727	—	470	5.0	110.0	4.0	2.0	1.0	—	—	—
31651	Coldbuster smoothie	24	fluid ounce(s)	724	—	430	5.0	100.0	5.0	2.5	1.0	—	—	—
31652	Cranberry Craze smoothie	24	fluid ounce(s)	793	—	460	6.0	104.0	4.0	0.5	0	—	—	—
31654	Jamba Powerboost smoothie	24	fluid ounce(s)	738	—	440	6.0	105.0	6.0	1.0	0	—	—	—
38423	Lemonade	16	fluid ounce(s)	483	—	300	1.0	75.0	0	0	0	0	0	0
31657	Mango-a-go-go smoothie	24	fluid ounce(s)	690	—	440	3.0	104.0	4.0	1.5	0.5	—	—	—
38424	Orange juice, freshly squeezed	16	fluid ounce(s)	496	—	220	3.0	52.0	0.5	1.0	0	—	—	—
38426	Orange/carrot juice	16	fluid ounce(s)	484	—	160	3.0	37.0	0	1.0	0	—	—	—
31660	Orange-a-peel smoothie	24	fluid ounce(s)	726	—	440	8.0	102.0	5.0	1.5	0	—	—	—
31662	Peach Pleasure smoothie	24	fluid ounce(s)	720	—	460	4.0	108.0	4.0	2.0	1.0	—	—	—
31665	Protein Berry Pizzaz smoothie	24	fluid ounce(s)	710	—	440	20.0	92.0	5.0	1.5	0	—	—	—
31668	Razzmatazz smoothie	24	fluid ounce(s)	730	—	480	3.0	112.0	4.0	2.0	1.0	—	—	—
31669	Strawberries Wild smoothie	24	fluid ounce(s)	725	—	450	6.0	105.0	4.0	0.5	0	—	—	—
38421	Strawberry Tsunami smoothie	24	fluid ounce(s)	740	—	530	4.0	128.0	4.0	2.0	1.0	—	—	—
38427	Vibrant C juice	16	fluid ounce(s)	448	—	210	2.0	50.0	1.0	0	0	0	0	0
38428	Wheatgrass juice, freshly squeezed	1	ounce(s)	28	—	5	0.5	1.0	0	0	0	0	0	0
	Kentucky Fried Chicken (KFC)													
31850	BBQ baked beans	1	serving(s)	136	—	220	8.0	45.0	7.0	1.0	0	—	—	0
31853	Biscuit	1	item(s)	57	—	220	4.0	24.0	1.0	11.0	2.5	—	—	3.5
51223	Boneless Fiery Buffalo Wings	6	item(s)	211	—	530	30.0	44.0	3.0	26.0	5.0	—	—	2.5
39386	Boneless Honey BBQ Wings	6	item(s)	213	—	570	30.0	54.0	5.0	26.0	5.0	—	—	2.5
51224	Boneless Sweet & Spicy Wings	6	item(s)	203	—	550	30.0	50.0	3.0	26.0	5.0	—	—	2.5
31851	Cole slaw	1	serving(s)	130	—	180	1.0	22.0	3.0	10.0	1.5	—	—	0
31842	Colonel's Crispy Strips	3	item(s)	151	—	370	28.0	17.0	1.0	20.0	4.0	—	—	2.5
31849	Corn on the cob	1	item(s)	162	—	150	5.0	26.0	7.0	3.0	1.0	—	—	0
51221	Double Crunch sandwich	1	item(s)	213	—	520	27.0	39.0	3.0	29.0	5.0	—	—	1.5
3761	Extra Crispy chicken, breast	1	item(s)	162	—	370	33.0	10.0	2.0	22.0	5.0	—	—	1.5
3762	Extra Crispy chicken, drumstick	1	item(s)	60	—	150	12.0	4.0	0	10.0	2.5	—	—	1.0
3763	Extra Crispy chicken, thigh	1	item(s)	114	—	290	17.0	16.0	1.0	18.0	4.0	—	—	1.5
3764	Extra Crispy chicken, whole wing	1	item(s)	52	—	150	11.0	11.0	1.0	7.0	1.5	—	—	0
51218	Famous Bowls mashed potatoes with gravy	1	serving(s)	531	—	720	26.0	79.0	6.0	34.0	9.0	—	—	3.5
51219	Famous Bowls rice with gravy	1	serving(s)	384	—	610	25.0	67.0	5.0	27.0	8.0	—	—	2.5
31841	Honey BBQ chicken sandwich	1	item(s)	147	—	290	23.0	40.0	2.0	4.0	1.0	—	—	0
31833	Honey BBQ wing pieces	6	item(s)	157	—	460	27.0	26.0	3.0	27.0	6.0	—	—	2.0
10859	Hot wings pieces	6	piece(s)	134	—	450	26.0	19.0	2.0	30.0	7.0	—	—	2.0
42382	KFC Snacker sandwich	1	serving(s)	119	—	320	14.0	29.0	2.0	17.0	3.0	—	—	1.0
31848	Macaroni and cheese	1	serving(s)	136	—	180	8.0	18.0	0	8.0	3.5	—	—	1.0
31847	Mashed potatoes with gravy	1	serving(s)	151	—	140	2.0	20.0	1.0	5.0	1.0	—	—	0.5
10825	Original Recipe chicken, breast	1	item(s)	161	—	340	38.0	9.0	2.0	17.0	4.0	—	—	1.0
10826	Original Recipe chicken, drumstick	1	item(s)	59	—	140	13.0	3.0	0	8.0	2.0	—	—	0.5
10827	Original Recipe chicken, thigh	1	item(s)	126	—	350	19.0	7.0	1.0	27.0	7.0	—	—	1.0
10828	Original Recipe chicken, whole wing	1	item(s)	47	—	140	10.0	4.0	0	9.0	2.0	—	—	0.5
51222	Oven roasted Twister chicken wrap	1	item(s)	269	—	520	30.0	46.0	4.0	23.0	3.5	—	—	0
31844	Popcorn chicken, small or individual	1	item(s)	114	—	370	19.0	21.0	2.0	24.0	4.5	—	—	2.5
31852	Potato salad	1	serving(s)	128	—	180	2.0	22.0	2.0	9.0	1.5	—	—	0
10845	Potato wedges, small	1	serving(s)	102	—	250	4.0	32.0	3.0	12.0	2.0	—	—	1.5
31839	Tender Roast chicken sandwich with sauce	1	item(s)	236	—	430	37.0	29.0	2.0	18.0	3.5	—	—	0

PAGE KEY: A-6 = Breads/Baked Goods A-12 = Cereal/Rice/Pasta A-16 = Fruit A-20 = Vegetables/Legumes A-30 = Nuts/Seeds A-32 = Vegetarian A-34 = Dairy A-42 = Eggs A-42 = Seafood A-44 = Meats A-48 = Poultry A-48 = Processed Meats A-50 = Beverages A-54 = Fats/Oils A-56 = Sweets A-58 = Spices/Condiments/Sauces A-62 = Mixed Foods/Soups/Sandwiches A-66 = Fast Food A-86 = Convenience A-88 = Baby Foods

Chol (mg)	Calc (mg)	Iron (mg)	Magn (mg)	Pota (mg)	Sodi (mg)	Zinc (mg)	Vit A (µg)	Thia (mg)	Vit E (mg α)	Ribo (mg)	Niac (mg)	Vit B$_6$ (mg)	Fola (µg)	Vit C (mg)	Vit B$_{12}$ (µg)	Sele (µg)
125	308	7.39	—	480.0	1580.0	—	—	—	—	—	—	—	—	0.6	—	—
135	532	0.00	—	750.0	280.0	—	—	—	—	—	—	—	—	0	—	—
5	200	1.80	60.0	1000.0	30.0	0.30	—	0.37	—	0.34	2.00	0.60	60.0	102.0	0	1.4
0	200	1.44	40.0	1010.0	115.0	0.60	—	0.09	—	0.25	0.80	0.70	24.0	15.0	0.2	1.4
5	200	1.80	16.0	510.0	35.0	0.30	—	0.06	—	0.25	6.00	0.70	140.0	54.0	0	1.4
5	100	1.80	24.0	810.0	60.0	0.30	—	0.09	—	0.25	5.00	0.50	100.0	78.0	0	1.4
0	150	2.70	80.0	1030.0	250.0	0.90	—	0.52	—	0.25	5.00	0.70	80.0	18.0	0	5.6
30	500	1.08	60.0	810.0	380.0	1.50	—	0.22	—	0.76	0.40	0.16	16.0	6.0	1.5	4.2
5	100	1.80	80.0	1170.0	35.0	0.30	—	0.37	—	0.34	1.90	0.60	100.0	180.0	0	1.4
5	100	1.08	60.0	1260.0	35.0	16.50	—	0.37	—	0.34	3.00	0.40	121.5	1302.0	0	1.4
0	250	1.44	16.0	500.0	50.0	0.30	—	0.03	—	0.25	5.00	0.60	120.0	54.0	0	1.4
0	1200		480.0	1070.0	45.0	16.50	—	5.55	—	6.12	68.00	7.40	640.0	288.0	10.8	77.0
0	20	0.00	8.0	200.0	10.0	0.00	—	0.03	—	0.17	14.00	1.80	320.0	36.0	0	0
5	100	1.08	24.0	780.0	50.0	0.30	—	0.15	—	0.25	5.00	0.70	120.0	72.0	0	1.4
0	60	1.08	60.0	990.0	0	0.30	—	0.45	—	0.13	2.00	0.20	160.0	246.0	0	0
0	100	1.80	60.0	1010.0	125.0	0.60	—	0.45	—	0.25	3.00	0.50	120.0	132.0	0	2.8
0	250	1.80	80.0	1380.0	160.0	0.90	—	0.45	—	0.42	2.00	0.50	140.0	240.0	0.6	1.4
5	100	0.72	32.0	740.0	60.0	0.30	—	0.06	—	0.25	4.00	0.60	80.0	18.0	0	1.4
0	1100	2.62	60.0	650.0	240.0	0.58	—	0.08	—	0.17	1.20	0.70	58.3	60.0	0	5.6
5	150	1.80	32.0	810.0	70.0	0.30	—	0.09	—	0.34	6.00	1.00	160.0	60.0	0	1.4
5	250	1.80	40.0	1050.0	180.0	0.90	—	0.12	—	0.34	0.80	0.40	40.0	60.0	0.6	1.4
5	100	1.08	24.0	480.0	10.0	0.30	—	0.06	—	0.34	14.00	1.80	320.0	90.0	0	1.4
0	20	1.08	40.0	720.0	0	0.30	—	0.30	—	0.10	1.60	0.40	80.0	678.0	0	0
0	0	1.80	8.0	80.0	0	0.00	0	0.03	—	0.03	0.40	0.04	16.0	3.6	0	2.8
0	100	2.70	—	—	730.0	—	—	—	—	—	—	—	—	1.2	—	—
0	40	1.80	—	—	640.0	—	—	—	—	—	—	—	—	0	—	—
65	40	1.80	—	—	2670.0	—	—	—	—	—	—	—	—	1.2	—	—
65	40	1.80	—	—	2210.0	—	—	—	—	—	—	—	—	1.2	—	—
65	60	1.80	—	—	2000.0	—	—	—	—	—	—	—	—	1.2	—	—
5	40	0.72	—	—	270.0	—	—	—	—	—	—	—	—	12.0	—	—
65	40	1.44	—	—	1220.0	—	0	—	—	—	—	—	—	1.2	—	—
0	60	1.08	—	—	10.0	—	—	—	—	—	—	—	—	6.0	—	—
55	100	2.70	—	—	1220.0	—	—	—	—	—	—	—	—	6.0	—	—
85	20	2.70	—	—	1020.0	—	—	—	—	—	—	—	—	1.2	—	—
55	0	1.44	—	—	300.0	—	0	—	—	—	—	—	—	0	—	—
95	20	2.70	—	—	700.0	—	—	—	—	—	—	—	—	—	—	—
45	20	1.08	—	—	340.0	—	—	—	—	—	—	—	—	0	—	—
35	200	5.40	—	—	2330.0	—	—	—	—	—	—	—	—	6.0	—	—
35	200	4.50	—	—	2130.0	—	—	—	—	—	—	—	—	6.0	—	—
60	80	2.70	—	—	710.0	—	—	—	—	—	—	—	—	2.4	—	—
140	40	1.80	—	—	970.0	—	—	—	—	—	—	—	—	21.0	—	—
115	40	1.44	—	—	990.0	—	—	—	—	—	—	—	—	1.2	—	—
25	60	2.70	—	—	690.0	—	—	—	—	—	—	—	—	2.4	—	—
15	150	0.72	—	—	800.0	—	—	—	—	—	—	—	—	1.2	—	—
0	40	1.44	—	—	560.0	—	—	—	—	—	—	—	—	1.2	—	—
135	20	2.70	—	—	960.0	—	—	—	—	—	—	—	—	6.0	—	—
70	20	1.08	—	—	340.0	—	—	—	—	—	—	—	—	0	—	—
110	20	2.70	—	—	870.0	—	—	—	—	—	—	—	—	1.2	—	—
50	20	1.44	—	—	350.0	—	0	—	—	—	—	—	—	1.2	—	—
60	40	6.30	—	—	1380.0	—	—	—	—	—	—	—	—	15.0	—	—
25	40	1.80	—	—	1110.0	—	0	—	—	—	—	—	—	0	—	—
5	0	0.36	—	—	470.0	—	—	—	—	—	—	—	—	6.0	—	—
0	20	1.08	—	—	700.0	—	0	—	—	—	—	—	—	0	—	—
80	80	2.70	—	—	1180.0	—	—	—	—	—	—	—	—	9.0	—	—

TABLE A-1 **Table of Food Composition (*continued*)** <small>(Computer code is for Cengage Diet Analysis program)</small>   <small>(For purposes of calculations, use "0" for t, <1, <.1, <.01, etc.,)</small>

DA+ Code	Food Description	Quantity	Measure	Wt (g)	H₂0 (g)	Ener (kcal)	Prot (g)	Carb (g)	Fiber (g)	Fat (g)	Fat Breakdown (g) Sat	Mono	Poly	Trans
Fast Food—*continued*														
	Long John Silver													
39392	Baked cod	1	serving(s)	101	—	120	22.0	1.0	0	4.5	1.0	—	—	0
3777	Batter dipped fish sandwich	1	item(s)	177	—	470	18.0	48.0	3.0	23.0	5.0	—	—	4.5
37568	Battered fish	1	item(s)	92	—	260	12.0	17.0	0.5	16.0	4.0	—	—	4.5
37569	Breaded clams	1	serving(s)	85	—	240	8.0	22.0	1.0	13.0	2.0	—	—	2.5
37566	Chicken plank	1	item(s)	52	—	140	8.0	9.0	0.5	8.0	2.0	—	—	2.5
39404	Clam chowder	1	item(s)	227	—	220	9.0	23.0	0	10.0	4.0	—	—	1.0
39398	Cocktail sauce	1	ounce(s)	28	—	25	0	6.0	0	0	0	0	0	0
3770	Coleslaw	1	serving(s)	113	—	200	1.0	15.0	3.0	15.0	2.5	1.8	4.1	0
39400	French fries, large	1	item(s)	142	—	390	4.0	56.0	5.0	17.0	4.0	—	—	5.0
3774	Fries, regular	1	serving(s)	85	—	230	3.0	34.0	3.0	10.0	2.5	—	—	3.0
3779	Hushpuppy	1	piece(s)	23	—	60	1.0	9.0	1.0	2.5	0.5	—	—	1.0
3781	Shrimp, batter-dipped, 1 piece	1	piece(s)	14	—	45	2.0	3.0	0	3.0	1.0	—	—	1.0
39399	Tartar sauce	1	ounce(s)	28	—	100	0	4.0	0	9.0	1.5	—	—	—
39395	Ultimate Fish sandwich	1	item(s)	199	—	530	21.0	49.0	3.0	28.0	8.0	—	—	5.0
	McDonald's													
50828	Asian salad with grilled chicken	1	item(s)	362	—	290	31.0	23.0	6.0	10.0	1.0	—	—	0
2247	Barbecue sauce	1	item(s)	28	—	45	0	11.0	0	0	0	0	0	0
737	Big Mac hamburger	1	item(s)	219	—	560	25.0	47.0	3.0	30.0	10.0	—	—	1.5
29777	Caesar salad dressing	1	package(s)	44	—	150	1.0	5.0	0	13.0	2.5	—	—	—
38391	Caesar salad with grilled chicken, no dressing	1	serving(s)	278	230.6	181	26.4	10.5	3.1	6.0	2.9	1.7	0.8	0.2
38393	Caesar salad without chicken, no dressing	1	serving(s)	190	170.4	84	6.0	8.1	3.0	3.9	2.2	0.9	0.3	0.1
738	Cheeseburger	1	item(s)	119	—	310	15.0	35.0	1.0	12.0	6.0	—	—	1.0
29775	Chicken McGrill sandwich	1	item(s)	213	—	400	27.0	38.0	3.0	16.0	3.0	—	—	0
1873	Chicken McNuggets, 6 piece	1	serving(s)	96	—	250	15.0	15.0	0	15.0	3.0	—	—	1.5
3792	Chicken McNuggets, 4 piece	1	serving(s)	64	—	170	10.0	10.0	0	10.0	2.0	—	—	1.0
29774	Crispy chicken sandwich	1	item(s)	232	121.8	500	27.0	63.0	3.0	16.0	3.0	5.7	7.4	1.5
743	Egg McMuffin	1	item(s)	139	76.8	300	17.0	30.0	2.0	12.0	4.5	3.8	2.5	0
742	Filet-O-Fish sandwich	1	item(s)	141	—	400	14.0	42.0	1.0	18.0	4.0	—	—	1.0
2257	French fries, large	1	serving(s)	170	—	570	6.0	70.0	7.0	30.0	6.0	—	—	8.0
1872	French fries, small	1	serving(s)	74	—	250	2.0	30.0	3.0	13.0	2.5	—	—	3.5
33822	Fruit 'n Yogurt Parfait	1	item(s)	149	111.2	160	4.0	31.0	1.0	2.0	1.0	0.2	0.1	0
739	Hamburger	1	item(s)	105	—	260	13.0	33.0	1.0	9.0	3.5	—	—	0.5
2003	Hash browns	1	item(s)	53	—	140	1.0	15.0	2.0	8.0	1.5	—	—	2.0
2249	Honey sauce	1	item(s)	14	—	50	0	12.0	0	0	0	0	0	0
38397	Newman's Own creamy caesar salad dressing	1	item(s)	59	32.5	190	2.0	4.0	0	18.0	3.5	4.6	9.6	0
38398	Newman's Own low fat balsamic vinaigrette salad dressing	1	item(s)	44	29.1	40	0	4.0	0	3.0	0	1.0	1.2	0
38399	Newman's Own ranch salad dressing	1	item(s)	59	30.1	170	1.0	9.0	0	15.0	2.5	9.0	3.7	0
1874	Plain Hotcakes with syrup and margarine	3	item(s)	221	—	600	9.0	102.0	2.0	17.0	4.0	—	—	4.0
740	Quarter Pounder hamburger	1	item(s)	171	—	420	24.0	40.0	3.0	18.0	7.0	—	—	1.0
741	Quarter Pounder hamburger with cheese	1	item(s)	199	—	510	29.0	43.0	3.0	25.0	12.0	—	—	1.5
2005	Sausage McMuffin with egg	1	item(s)	165	82.4	450	20.0	31.0	2.0	27.0	10.0	10.9	4.6	0.5
50831	Side salad	1	item(s)	87	—	20	1.0	4.0	1.0	0	0	0	0	0
	Pizza Hut													
39009	Hot chicken wings	2	item(s)	57	—	110	11.0	1.0	0	6.0	2.0	—	—	0.3
14025	Meat Lovers hand tossed pizza	1	slice(s)	118	—	300	15.0	29.0	2.0	13.0	6.0	—	—	0.5
14026	Meat Lovers pan pizza	1	slice(s)	123	—	340	15.0	29.0	2.0	19.0	7.0	—	—	0.5
31009	Meat Lovers stuffed crust pizza	1	slice(s)	169	—	450	21.0	43.0	3.0	21.0	10.0	—	—	1.0
14024	Meat Lovers thin 'n crispy pizza	1	slice(s)	98	—	270	13.0	21.0	2.0	14.0	6.0	—	—	0.5
14031	Pepperoni Lovers hand tossed pizza	1	slice(s)	113	—	300	15.0	30.0	2.0	13.0	7.0	—	—	0.5
14032	Pepperoni Lovers pan pizza	1	slice(s)	118	—	340	15.0	29.0	2.0	19.0	7.0	—	—	0.5
31011	Pepperoni Lovers stuffed crust pizza	1	slice(s)	163	—	420	21.0	43.0	3.0	19.0	10.0	—	—	1.0
14030	Pepperoni Lovers thin 'n crispy pizza	1	slice(s)	92	—	260	13.0	21.0	2.0	14.0	7.0	—	—	0.5
10834	Personal Pan pepperoni pizza	1	slice(s)	61	—	170	7.0	18.0	0.5	8.0	3.0	—	—	1.0
10842	Personal Pan supreme pizza	1	slice(s)	77	—	190	8.0	19.0	1.0	9.0	3.5	—	—	1.0

Chol (mg)	Calc (mg)	Iron (mg)	Magn (mg)	Pota (mg)	Sodi (mg)	Zinc (mg)	Vit A (µg)	Thia (mg)	Vit E (mg α)	Ribo (mg)	Niac (mg)	Vit B$_6$ (mg)	Fola (µg)	Vit C (mg)	Vit B$_{12}$ (µg)	Sele (µg)
90	20	0.72	—	—	240.0	—	—	—	—	—	—	—	—	0	—	—
45	60	2.70	—	—	1210.0	—	—	—	—	—	—	—	—	2.4	—	—
35	20	0.72	—	—	790.0	—	—	—	—	—	—	—	—	4.8	—	—
10	20	1.08	—	—	1110.0	—	0	—	—	—	—	—	—	0	—	—
20	0	0.72	—	—	480.0	—	0	—	—	—	—	—	—	2.4	—	—
25	150	0.72	—	—	810.0	—	—	—	—	—	—	—	—	0	—	—
0	0	0.00	—	—	250.0	—	—	—	—	—	—	—	—	0	—	—
20	40	0.36	—	222.7	340.0	0.70	—	0.07	—	0.08	2.34	—	—	18.0	—	—
0	0	0.00	—	—	580.0	—	0	—	—	—	—	—	—	24.0	—	—
0	0	0.00	—	370.0	350.0	0.30	0	0.09	—	0.01	1.60	—	—	15.0	—	—
0	20	0.36	—	—	200.0	—	0	—	—	—	—	—	—	0	—	—
15	0	0.00	—	—	160.0	—	0	—	—	—	—	—	—	1.2	—	—
15	0	0.00	—	—	250.0	—	0	—	—	—	—	—	—	0	—	—
60	150	2.70	—	—	1400.0	—	—	—	—	—	—	—	—	4.8	—	—
65	150	3.60	—	—	890.0	—	—	—	—	—	—	—	—	54.0	—	—
0	0	0.00	—	55.0	260.0	—	—	—	—	—	—	—	—	0	—	—
80	250	4.50	—	400.0	1010.0	—	—	—	—	—	—	—	—	1.2	—	—
10	40	0.18	—	30.0	400.0	—	—	—	—	—	—	—	—	0.6	—	—
67	178	1.77	—	708.9	767.3	—	—	0.15	—	0.19	10.62	—	127.9	29.2	0.2	—
10	163	1.15	17.1	410.4	157.7	—	—	0.08	—	0.07	0.40	—	102.6	26.8	0	0.4
40	200	2.70	—	240.0	740.0	—	60.0	—	—	—	—	—	—	1.2	—	—
70	150	2.70	—	510.0	1010.0	—	—	—	—	—	—	—	—	6.0	—	—
35	20	0.72	—	240.0	670.0	—	—	—	—	—	—	—	—	1.2	—	—
25	0	0.36	—	160.0	450.0	—	—	—	—	—	—	—	—	1.2	—	—
60	80	3.60	62.6	526.6	1380.0	1.53	41.8	0.46	2.27	0.39	12.85	—	104.4	6.0	0.4	—
230	300	2.70	26.4	218.2	860.0	1.59	—	0.36	0.82	0.51	4.31	0.20	109.8	1.2	0.9	—
40	150	1.80	—	250.0	640.0	—	36.2	—	—	—	—	—	—	0	—	—
0	20	1.80	—	—	330.0	—	0	—	—	—	—	—	—	9.0	—	—
0	20	0.72	—	—	140.0	—	0	—	—	—	—	—	—	3.6	—	—
5	150	0.67	20.9	248.8	85.0	0.53	0	0.06	—	0.17	0.35	—	19.4	9.0	0.3	—
30	150	2.70	—	210.0	530.0	—	5.0	—	—	—	—	—	—	1.2	—	—
0	0	0.36	—	210.0	290.0	—	0	—	—	—	—	—	—	1.2	—	—
0	0	0.00	—	0	0	—	0	—	—	—	—	—	—	0	—	—
20	61	0.00	3.0	16.0	500.0	0.20	—	0.01	15.43	0.02	0.01	0.64	2.4	0	0.1	0.1
0	4	0.00	1.3	8.8	730.0	0.01	—	0.00	0.00	0.00	0.00	0.00	0	2.4	0	0
0	40	0.00	1.8	70.4	530.0	0.03	0	0.01	—	0.08	0.01	0.02	0.6	0	0	0.2
20	150	2.70	—	280.0	620.0	—	—	—	—	—	—	—	—	0	—	—
70	150	4.50	—	390.0	730.0	—	10.0	—	—	—	—	—	—	1.2	—	—
95	300	4.50	—	440.0	1150.0	—	100.0	—	—	—	—	—	—	1.2	—	—
255	300	3.60	29.7	282.2	950.0	2.01	—	0.43	0.82	0.56	4.83	0.24	—	0	1.2	—
0	20	0.72	—	—	10.0	—	—	—	—	—	—	—	—	15.0	—	—
70	0	0.36	—	—	450.0	—	—	—	—	—	—	—	—	0	—	—
35	150	1.80	—	—	760.0	—	—	—	—	—	—	—	—	6.0	—	—
35	150	2.70	—	—	750.0	—	—	—	—	—	—	—	—	6.0	—	—
55	250	2.70	—	—	1250.0	—	—	—	—	—	—	—	—	9.0	—	—
35	150	1.44	—	—	740.0	—	—	—	—	—	—	—	—	6.0	—	—
40	200	1.80	—	—	710.0	—	57.7	—	—	—	—	—	—	2.4	—	—
40	200	2.70	—	—	700.0	—	57.7	—	—	—	—	—	—	2.4	—	—
55	300	2.70	—	—	1120.0	—	—	—	—	—	—	—	—	3.6	—	—
40	200	1.44	—	—	690.0	—	58.0	—	—	—	—	—	—	2.4	—	—
15	80	1.44	—	—	340.0	—	38.5	—	—	—	—	—	—	1.4	—	—
20	80	1.86	—	—	420.0	—	—	—	—	—	—	—	—	3.6	—	—

TABLE A-1 Table of Food Composition (*continued*) (Computer code is for Cengage Diet Analysis program) (For purposes of calculations, use "0" for t, <1, <.1, <.01, etc.)

DA+ Code	Food Description	Quantity	Measure	Wt (g)	H₂O (g)	Ener (kcal)	Prot (g)	Carb (g)	Fiber (g)	Fat (g)	Sat	Mono	Poly	Trans
												Fat Breakdown (g)		

Fast Food—*continued*

39013	Personal Pan Veggie Lovers pizza	1	slice(s)	69	—	150	6.0	19.0	1.0	6.0	2.0	—	—	0.5
14028	Veggie Lovers hand tossed pizza	1	slice(s)	118	—	220	10.0	31.0	2.0	6.0	3.0	—	—	0.3
14029	Veggie Lovers pan pizza	1	slice(s)	119	—	260	10.0	30.0	2.0	12.0	4.0	—	—	0.3
31010	Veggie Lovers stuffed crust pizza	1	slice(s)	172	—	360	16.0	45.0	3.0	14.0	7.0	—	—	0.5
14027	Veggie Lovers thin 'n crispy pizza	1	slice(s)	101	—	180	8.0	23.0	2.0	7.0	3.0	—	—	0.5
39012	Wing blue cheese dipping sauce	1	item(s)	43	—	230	2.0	2.0	0	24.0	5.0	—	—	1.0
39011	Wing ranch dipping sauce	1	item(s)	43	—	210	0.5	4.0	0	22.0	3.5	—	—	0.5

Starbucks

38052	Cappuccino, tall	12	fluid ounce(s)	360	—	120	7.0	10.0	0	6.0	4.0	—	—	—
38053	Cappuccino, tall nonfat	12	fluid ounce(s)	360	—	80	7.0	11.0	0	0	0	0	0	0
38054	Cappuccino, tall soymilk	12	fluid ounce(s)	360	—	100	5.0	13.0	0.5	2.5	0	—	—	—
38059	Cinnamon spice mocha, tall nonfat w/o whipped cream	12	fluid ounce(s)	360	—	170	11.0	32.0	0	0.5	—	—	—	—
38057	Cinnamon spice mocha, tall w/whipped cream	12	fluid ounce(s)	360	—	320	10.0	31.0	0	17.0	11.0	—	—	—
38051	Espresso, single shot	1	fluid ounce(s)	30	—	5	0	1.0	0	0	0	0	0	0
38088	Flavored syrup, 1 pump	1	serving(s)	10	—	20	0	5.0	0	0	0	0	0	0
32562	Frappuccino bottled coffee drink, mocha	9½	fluid ounce(s)	298	—	190	6.0	39.0	3.0	3.0	2.0	—	—	—
32561	Frappuccino coffee drink, all bottled flavors	9½	fluid ounce(s)	281	—	190	7.0	35.0	0	3.5	2.5	—	—	—
38073	Frappuccino, mocha	12	fluid ounce(s)	360	—	220	5.0	44.0	0	3.0	1.5	—	—	—
38067	Frappuccino, tall caramel w/o whipped cream	12	fluid ounce(s)	360	—	210	4.0	43.0	0	2.5	1.5	—	—	—
38070	Frappuccino, tall coffee	12	fluid ounce(s)	360	—	190	4.0	38.0	0	2.5	1.5	—	—	—
39894	Frappuccino, tall coffee, light blend	12	fluid ounce(s)	360	—	110	5.0	22.0	2.0	1.0	0	—	—	—
38071	Frappuccino, tall espresso	12	fluid ounce(s)	360	—	160	4.0	33.0	0	2.0	1.5	—	—	—
39897	Frappuccino, tall mocha, light blend	12	fluid ounce(s)	360	—	140	5.0	28.0	3.0	1.5	0	—	—	—
39887	Frappuccino, tall Strawberries and Creme, w/o whipped cream	12	fluid ounce(s)	360	—	330	10.0	65.0	0	3.5	1.0	—	—	—
38063	Frappuccino, tall Tazo chai creme w/o whipped cream	12	fluid ounce(s)	360	—	280	10.0	52.0	0	3.5	1.0	—	—	—
38066	Frappuccino, tall Tazoberry	12	fluid ounce(s)	360	—	140	0.5	36.0	0.5	0	0	0	0	0
38065	Frappuccino, tall Tazoberry Crème	12	fluid ounce(s)	360	—	240	4.0	54.0	0.5	1.0	0	—	—	—
38080	Frappuccino, tall vanilla w/o whipped cream	12	fluid ounce(s)	360	—	270	10.0	51.0	0	3.5	1.0	—	—	—
39898	Frappuccino, tall white chocolate mocha, light blend	12	fluid ounce(s)	360	—	160	6.0	32.0	2.0	2.0	1.0	—	—	—
38074	Frappuccino, tall white chocolate w/o whipped cream	12	fluid ounce(s)	360	—	240	5.0	48.0	0	3.5	2.5	—	—	—
39883	Java Chip Frappuccino, tall w/o whipped cream	12	fluid ounce(s)	360	—	270	5.0	51.0	1.0	7.0	4.5	—	—	—
33111	Latte, tall w/nonfat milk	12	fluid ounce(s)	360	335.3	120	12.0	18.0	0	0	0	0	0	0
33112	Latte, tall w/whole milk	12	fluid ounce(s)	360	—	200	11.0	16.0	0	11.0	7.0	—	—	—
33109	Macchiato, tall caramel w/nonfat milk	12	fluid ounce(s)	360	—	170	11.0	30.0	0	1.0	0	—	—	—
33110	Macchiato, tall caramel w/whole milk	12	fluid ounce(s)	360	—	240	10.0	28.0	0	10.0	6.0	—	—	—
33107	Mocha coffee drink, tall nonfat, w/o whipped cream	12	fluid ounce(s)	360	—	170	11.0	33.0	1.0	1.5	0	—	—	—
38089	Mocha syrup	1	serving(s)	17	—	25	1.0	6.0	0	0.5	0	—	—	—
33108	Mocha, tall mocha w/whole milk	12	fluid ounce(s)	360	—	310	10.0	32.0	1.0	17.0	10.0	—	—	—
38042	Steamed apple cider, tall	12	fluid ounce(s)	360	—	180	0	45.0	0	0	0	0	0	0
38087	Tazo chai black tea, soymilk, tall	12	fluid ounce(s)	360	—	190	4.0	39.0	0.5	2.0	0	—	—	—
38084	Tazo chai black tea, tall	12	fluid ounce(s)	360	—	210	6.0	36.0	0	5.0	3.5	—	—	—
38083	Tazo chai black tea, tall nonfat	12	fluid ounce(s)	360	—	170	6.0	37.0	0	0	0	—	—	—
38076	Tazo iced tea, tall	12	fluid ounce(s)	360	—	60	0	16.0	0	0	0	0	0	0
38077	Tazo tea, grande lemonade	16	fluid ounce(s)	480	—	120	0	31.0	0	0	0	0	0	0

Chol (mg)	Calc (mg)	Iron (mg)	Magn (mg)	Pota (mg)	Sodi (mg)	Zinc (mg)	Vit A (µg)	Thia (mg)	Vit E (mg α)	Ribo (mg)	Niac (mg)	Vit B₆ (mg)	Fola (µg)	Vit C (mg)	Vit B₁₂ (µg)	Sele (µg)
10	80	1.80	—	—	280.0	—	—	—	—	—	—	—	—	3.6	—	—
15	150	1.80	—	—	490.0	—	—	—	—	—	—	—	—	9.0	—	—
15	150	2.70	—	—	470.0	—	—	—	—	—	—	—	—	9.0	—	—
35	250	2.70	—	—	980.0	—	—	—	—	—	—	—	—	9.0	—	—
15	150	1.44	—	—	480.0	—	—	—	—	—	—	—	—	9.0	—	—
25	20	0.00	—	—	550.0	—	0	—	—	—	—	—	—	0	—	—
10	0	0.00	—	—	340.0	—	0	—	—	—	—	—	—	0	—	—
25	250	0.00	—	—	95.0	—	—	—	—	—	—	—	—	1.2	0	—
3	200	0.00	—	—	100.0	—	—	—	—	—	—	—	—	0	0	—
0	250	0.72	—	—	75.0	—	—	—	—	—	—	—	—	0	0	—
5	300	0.72	—	—	150.0	—	—	—	—	—	—	—	—	0	0	—
70	350	1.08	—	—	140.0	—	—	—	—	—	—	—	—	2.4	0	—
0	0	0.00	—	—	0	—	0	—	—	—	—	—	—	0	0	—
0	0	0.00	—	—	0	—	0	—	—	—	—	—	—	0	0	—
12	219	1.08	—	530.0	110.0	—	—	—	—	—	—	—	—	0	—	—
15	250	0.36	—	510.0	105.0	—	—	—	—	—	—	—	—	0	—	—
10	150	0.72	—	—	180.0	—	—	—	—	—	—	—	—	0	0	—
10	150	0.00	—	—	180.0	—	—	—	—	—	—	—	—	0	0	—
10	150	0.00	—	—	180.0	—	—	—	—	—	—	—	—	0	0	—
0	150	0.00	—	—	220.0	—	—	—	—	—	—	—	—	0	—	—
10	100	0.00	—	—	160.0	—	—	—	—	—	—	—	—	0	0	—
0	150	0.72	—	—	220.0	—	—	—	—	—	—	—	—	0	—	—
3	350	0.00	—	—	270.0	—	—	—	—	—	—	—	—	21.0	—	—
3	350	0.00	—	—	270.0	—	—	—	—	—	—	—	—	3.6	0	—
0	0	0.00	—	—	30.0	—	0	—	—	—	—	—	—	0	0	—
0	150	0.00	—	—	125.0	—	0	—	—	—	—	—	—	1.2	0	—
3	350	0.00	—	—	370.0	—	—	—	—	—	—	—	—	3.6	0	—
3	150	0.00	—	—	250.0	—	—	—	—	—	—	—	—	0	—	—
10	150	0.00	—	—	210.0	—	—	—	—	—	—	—	—	0	0	—
10	150	1.44	—	—	220.0	—	—	—	—	—	—	—	—	0	—	—
5	350	0.00	39.8	—	170.0	1.35	—	0.12	—	0.47	0.36	0.13	17.5	0	1.3	—
45	400	0.00	46.6	—	160.0	1.28	—	0.12	—	0.54	0.34	0.14	16.8	2.4	1.2	—
5	300	0.00	—	—	160.0	—	—	—	—	—	—	—	—	1.2	—	—
30	300	0.00	—	—	135.0	—	—	—	—	—	—	—	—	2.4	—	—
5	300	2.70	—	—	135.0	—	—	—	—	—	—	—	—	0	—	—
0	0	0.72	—	—	0	—	0	—	—	—	—	—	—	0	0	—
55	300	2.70	—	—	115.0	—	—	—	—	—	—	—	—	0	—	—
0	0	1.08	—	—	15.0	—	0	—	—	—	—	—	—	0	0	—
0	200	0.72	—	—	70.0	—	—	—	—	—	—	—	—	0	0	—
20	200	0.36	—	—	85.0	—	—	—	—	—	—	—	—	1.2	0	—
5	200	0.36	—	—	95.0	—	—	—	—	—	—	—	—	0	0	—
0	0	0.00	—	—	0	—	0	—	—	—	—	—	—	0	0	—
0	0	0.00	—	—	15.0	—	0	—	—	—	—	—	—	4.8	0	—

TABLE A-1 Table of Food Composition (*continued*) <small>(Computer code is for Cengage Diet Analysis program)</small> <small>(For purposes of calculations, use "0" for t, <1, <.1, <.01, etc.</small>

DA+ Code	Food Description	Quantity	Measure	Wt (g)	H₂O (g)	Ener (kcal)	Prot (g)	Carb (g)	Fiber (g)	Fat (g)	Sat	Mono	Poly	Trans
Fast Food—*continued*														
38045	Vanilla crème steamed nonfat milk, tall w/whipped cream	12	fluid ounce(s)	360	—	260	11.0	33.0	0	8.0	5.0	—	—	—
38046	Vanilla crème steamed soymilk, tall w/whipped cream	12	fluid ounce(s)	360	—	300	8.0	37.0	1.0	12.0	6.0	—	—	—
38044	Vanilla crème steamed whole milk, tall w/whipped cream	12	fluid ounce(s)	360	—	330	10.0	31.0	0	18.0	11.0	—	—	—
38090	Whipped cream	1	serving(s)	27	—	100	0	2.0	0	9.0	6.0	—	—	—
38062	White chocolate mocha, tall nonfat w/o whipped cream	12	fluid ounce(s)	360	—	260	12.0	45.0	0	4.0	3.0	—	—	—
38061	White chocolate mocha, tall w/whipped cream	12	fluid ounce(s)	360	—	410	11.0	44.0	0	20.0	13.0	—	—	—
38048	White hot chocolate, tall non-fat w/o whipped cream	12	fluid ounce(s)	360	—	300	15.0	51.0	0	4.5	3.5	—	—	—
38050	White hot chocolate, tall soy-milk w/whipped cream	12	fluid ounce(s)	360	—	420	11.0	56.0	1.0	16.0	9.0	—	—	—
38047	White hot chocolate, tall w/whipped cream	12	fluid ounce(s)	360	—	460	13.0	50.0	0	22.0	15.0	—	—	—
	Subway													
15842	Cheese steak sandwich, 6", wheat bread	1	item(s)	250	—	360	24.0	47.0	5.0	10.0	4.5	—	—	0
40478	Chicken and bacon ranch sandwich, 6", white or wheat bread	1	serving(s)	297	—	540	36.0	47.0	5.0	25.0	10.0	—	—	0.5
38622	Chicken and bacon ranch wrap with cheese	1	item(s)	257	—	440	41.0	18.0	9.0	27.0	10.0	—	—	0.5
32045	Chocolate chip cookie	1	item(s)	45	—	210	2.0	30.0	1.0	10.0	6.0	—	—	0
32048	Chocolate chip M&M cookie	1	item(s)	45	—	210	2.0	32.0	0.5	10.0	5.0	—	—	0
32049	Chocolate chunk cookie	1	item(s)	45	—	220	2.0	30.0	0.5	10.0	5.0	—	—	0
4024	Classic Italian B.M.T. sandwich, 6", white bread	1	item(s)	236	—	440	22.0	45.0	2.0	21.0	8.5	—	—	0
15838	Classic tuna sandwich, 6", wheat bread	1	item(s)	250	—	530	22.0	45.0	4.0	31.0	7.0	—	—	0.5
15837	Classic tuna sandwich, 6", white bread	1	item(s)	243	—	520	21.0	43.0	2.0	31.0	7.5	—	—	0.5
16397	Club salad, no dressing and croutons	1	item(s)	412	—	160	18.0	15.0	4.0	4.0	1.5	—	—	—
3422	Club sandwich, 6", white bread	1	item(s)	250	—	310	23.0	45.0	2.0	6.0	2.5	—	—	0
4030	Cold cut combo sandwich, 6", white bread	1	item(s)	242	—	400	20.0	45.0	2.0	17.0	7.5	—	—	0.5
34030	Ham and egg breakfast sandwich	1	item(s)	142	—	310	16.0	35.0	3.0	13.0	3.5	—	—	0
3885	Ham sandwich, 6", white bread	1	item(s)	238	—	310	17.0	52.0	2.0	5.0	2.0	—	—	0
3888	Meatball marinara sandwich, 6", wheat bread	1	item(s)	377	—	560	24.0	63.0	7.0	24.0	11.0	—	—	1.0
4651	Meatball sandwich, 6", white bread	1	item(s)	370	—	550	23.0	61.0	5.0	24.0	11.5	—	—	1.0
15839	Melt sandwich, 6", white bread	1	item(s)	260	—	410	25.0	47.0	4.0	15.0	5.0	—	—	—
32046	Oatmeal raisin cookie	1	item(s)	45	—	200	3.0	30.0	1.0	8.0	4.0	—	—	0
16379	Oven-roasted chicken breast sandwich, 6", wheat bread	1	item(s)	238	—	330	24.0	48.0	5.0	5.0	1.5	—	—	0
32047	Peanut butter cookie	1	item(s)	45	—	220	4.0	26.0	1.0	12.0	5.0	—	—	0
4655	Roast beef sandwich, 6", wheat bread	1	item(s)	224	—	290	19.0	45.0	4.0	5.0	2.0	—	—	0
3957	Roast beef sandwich, 6", white bread	1	item(s)	217	—	280	18.0	43.0	2.0	5.0	2.5	—	—	0
16378	Roasted chicken breast, 6", white bread	1	item(s)	231	—	320	23.0	46.0	3.0	5.0	2.0	—	—	0
34028	Southwest steak and cheese sandwich, 6", Italian bread	1	item(s)	271	—	450	24.0	48.0	6.0	20.0	6.0	—	—	0
4032	Spicy Italian sandwich, 6", white bread	1	item(s)	220	—	470	20.0	43.0	2.0	25.0	9.5	—	—	0
4031	Steak and cheese sandwich, 6", white bread	1	item(s)	243	—	350	23.0	45.0	3.0	10.0	5.0	—	—	0
32050	Sugar cookie	1	item(s)	45	—	220	2.0	28.0	0.5	12.0	6.0	—	—	0
40477	Sweet onion chicken teriyaki sandwich, 6", white or wheat bread	1	serving(s)	281	—	370	26.0	59.0	4.0	5.0	1.5	—	—	0
38623	Turkey breast and bacon melt wrap with chipotle sauce	1	item(s)	228	—	380	31.0	20.0	9.0	24.0	7.0	—	—	0

PAGE KEY: A-6 = Breads/Baked Goods A-12 = Cereal/Rice/Pasta A-16 = Fruit A-20 = Vegetables/Legumes A-30 = Nuts/Seeds A-32 = Vegetarian A-34 = Dairy A-42 = Eggs A-42 = Seafood A-44 = Meats A-48 = Poultry A-48 = Processed Meats A-50 = Beverages A-54 = Fats/Oils A-56 = Sweets A-58 = Spices/Condiments/Sauces A-62 = Mixed Foods/Soups/Sandwiches A-66 = Fast Food A-86 = Convenience A-88 = Baby Foods

Chol (mg)	Calc (mg)	Iron (mg)	Magn (mg)	Pota (mg)	Sodi (mg)	Zinc (mg)	Vit A (µg)	Thia (mg)	Vit E (mg α)	Ribo (mg)	Niac (mg)	Vit B$_6$ (mg)	Fola (µg)	Vit C (mg)	Vit B$_{12}$ (µg)	Sele (µg)
35	350	0.00	—	—	170.0	—	—	—	—	—	—	—	—	0	0	—
30	400	1.44	—	—	130.0	—	—	—	—	—	—	—	—	0	0	—
65	350	0.00	—	—	140.0	—	—	—	—	—	—	—	—	0	0	—
40	0	0.00	—	—	10.0	—	—	—	—	—	—	—	—	0	0	—
5	400	0.00	—	—	210.0	—	—	—	—	—	—	—	—	0	0	—
70	400	0.00	—	—	210.0	—	—	—	—	—	—	—	—	2.4	0	—
10	450	0.00	—	—	250.0	—	—	—	—	—	—	—	—	0	0	—
35	500	1.44	—	—	210.0	—	—	—	—	—	—	—	—	0	0	—
75	500	0.00	—	—	250.0	—	—	—	—	—	—	—	—	3.6	0	—
35	150	8.10	—	—	1090.0	—	—	—	—	—	—	—	—	18.0	—	—
90	250	4.50	—	—	1400.0	—	—	—	—	—	—	—	—	21.0	—	—
90	300	2.70	—	—	1680.0	—	—	—	—	—	—	—	—	9.0	—	—
15	0	1.08	—	—	150.0	—	—	—	—	—	—	—	—	0	—	—
10	20	1.00	—	—	100.0	—	—	—	—	—	—	—	—	0	—	—
10	0	1.00	—	—	100.0	—	—	—	—	—	—	—	—	0	—	—
55	150	2.70	—	—	1770.0	—	—	—	—	—	—	—	—	16.8	—	—
45	100	5.40	—	—	1030.0	—	—	—	—	—	—	—	—	21.0	—	—
45	100	3.60	—	—	1010.0	—	—	—	—	—	—	—	—	16.8	—	—
35	60	3.60	—	—	880.0	—	—	—	—	—	—	—	—	30.0	—	—
35	60	3.60	—	—	1290.0	—	—	—	—	—	—	—	—	13.8	—	—
60	150	3.60	—	—	1530.0	—	—	—	—	—	—	—	—	16.8	—	—
190	80	4.50	—	—	720.0	—	66.7	—	—	—	—	—	—	3.6	—	—
25	60	2.70	—	—	1375.0	—	—	—	—	—	—	—	—	13.8	—	—
45	200	7.20	—	—	1610.0	—	—	—	—	—	—	—	—	36.0	—	—
45	200	5.40	—	—	1590.0	—	—	—	—	—	—	—	—	31.8	—	—
45	150	5.40	—	—	1720.0	—	—	—	—	—	—	—	—	24.0	—	—
15	20	1.08	—	—	170.0	—	—	—	—	—	—	—	—	0	—	—
45	60	4.50	—	—	1020.0	—	—	—	—	—	—	—	—	18.0	—	—
15	20	0.72	—	—	200.0	—	—	—	—	—	—	—	—	0	—	—
20	60	6.30	—	—	920.0	—	—	—	—	—	—	—	—	18.0	—	—
20	60	4.50	—	—	900.0	—	—	—	—	—	—	—	—	13.8	—	—
45	60	2.70	—	—	1000.0	—	—	—	—	—	—	—	—	13.8	—	—
45	150	8.10	—	—	1310.0	—	—	—	—	—	—	—	—	21.0	—	—
55	60	2.70	—	—	1650.0	—	—	—	—	—	—	—	—	16.8	—	—
35	150	6.30	—	—	1070.0	—	—	—	—	—	—	—	—	13.8	—	—
15	0	0.72	—	—	140.0	—	—	—	—	—	—	—	—	0	—	—
50	80	4.50	—	—	1220.0	—	—	—	—	—	—	—	—	24.0	—	—
50	200	2.70	—	—	1780.0	—	—	—	—	—	—	—	—	6.0	—	—

TABLE A-1 Table of Food Composition (*continued*) (Computer code is for Cengage Diet Analysis program) (For purposes of calculations, use "0" for t, <1, <.1, <.01, etc.)

DA+ Code	Food Description	Quantity	Measure	Wt (g)	H₂O (g)	Ener (kcal)	Prot (g)	Carb (g)	Fiber (g)	Fat (g)	Fat Breakdown (g) Sat	Mono	Poly	*Trans*
Fast Food—*continued*														
15834	Turkey breast and ham sandwich, 6", white bread	1	item(s)	227	—	280	19.0	45.0	2.0	5.0	2.0	—	—	0
16376	Turkey breast sandwich, 6", white bread	1	item(s)	217	—	270	17.0	44.0	2.0	4.5	2.0	—	—	0
15841	Veggie Delite sandwich, 6", wheat bread	1	item(s)	167	—	230	9.0	44.0	4.0	3.0	1.0	—	—	0
16375	Veggie Delite, 6", white bread	1	item(s)	160	—	220	8.0	42.0	2.0	3.0	1.5	—	—	0
32051	White chip macadamia nut cookie	1	item(s)	45	—	220	2.0	29.0	0.5	11.0	5.0	—	—	0
	Taco Bell													
29906	7-Layer burrito	1	item(s)	283	—	490	17.0	65.0	9.0	18.0	7.0	—	—	1.0
744	Bean burrito	1	item(s)	198	—	340	13.0	54.0	8.0	9.0	3.5	—	—	0.5
749	Beef burrito supreme	1	item(s)	248	—	410	17.0	51.0	7.0	17.0	8.0	—	—	1.0
33417	Beef Chalupa Supreme	1	item(s)	153	—	380	14.0	30.0	3.0	23.0	7.0	—	—	0.5
34474	Beef Gordita Baja	1	item(s)	153	—	340	13.0	29.0	4.0	19.0	5.0	—	—	0
29910	Beef Gordita Supreme	1	item(s)	153	—	310	14.0	29.0	3.0	16.0	6.0	—	—	0.5
2014	Beef soft taco	1	item(s)	99	—	200	10.0	21.0	3.0	9.0	4.0	—	—	0
10860	Beef soft taco supreme	1	item(s)	135	—	250	11.0	23.0	3.0	13.0	6.0	—	—	0.5
34472	Chicken burrito supreme	1	item(s)	248	—	390	20.0	49.0	6.0	13.0	6.0	—	—	0.5
33418	Chicken Chalupa Supreme	1	item(s)	153	—	360	17.0	29.0	2.0	20.0	5.0	—	—	0
34475	Chicken Gordita Baja	1	item(s)	153	—	320	17.0	28.0	3.0	16.0	3.5	—	—	0
29909	Chicken quesadilla	1	item(s)	184	—	520	28.0	40.0	3.0	28.0	12.0	—	—	0.5
29907	Chili cheese burrito	1	item(s)	156	—	390	16.0	40.0	3.0	18.0	9.0	—	—	1.5
10794	Cinnamon twists	1	serving(s)	35	—	170	1.0	26.0	1.0	7.0	0	—	—	0
29911	Grilled chicken Gordita Supreme	1	item(s)	153	—	290	17.0	28.0	2.0	12.0	5.0	—	—	0
14463	Grilled chicken soft taco	1	item(s)	99	—	190	14.0	19.0	1.0	6.0	2.5	—	—	—
29912	Grilled Steak Gordita Supreme	1	item(s)	153	—	290	15.0	28.0	2.0	13.0	5.0	—	—	0
29904	Grilled steak soft taco	1	item(s)	128	—	270	12.0	20.0	2.0	16.0	4.5	—	—	0
29905	Grilled steak soft taco supreme	1	item(s)	135	—	235	13.0	21.0	1.0	11.0	6.0	—	—	—
2021	Mexican pizza	1	serving(s)	216	—	530	20.0	42.0	7.0	30.0	8.0	—	—	1.0
29894	Mexican rice	1	serving(s)	131	—	170	6.0	23.0	1.0	11.0	3.0	—	—	0
10772	Meximelt	1	serving(s)	128	—	280	15.0	22.0	3.0	14.0	7.0	—	—	0.5
2011	Nachos	1	serving(s)	99	—	330	4.0	32.0	2.0	21.0	3.5	—	—	2.0
2012	Nachos Bellgrande	1	serving(s)	308	—	770	19.0	77.0	12.0	44.0	9.0	—	—	3.0
2023	Pintos 'n cheese	1	serving(s)	128	—	150	9.0	19.0	7.0	6.0	3.0	—	—	0.5
34473	Steak burrito supreme	1	item(s)	248	—	380	18.0	49.0	6.0	14.0	7.0	—	—	0.5
33419	Steak Chalupa Supreme	1	item(s)	153	—	360	15.0	28.0	2.0	21.0	6.0	—	—	0
747	Taco	1	item(s)	78	—	170	8.0	13.0	3.0	10.0	3.5	—	—	0
2015	Taco salad with salsa, with shell	1	serving(s)	548	—	840	30.0	80.0	15.0	45.0	11.0	—	—	1.5
14459	Taco supreme	1	item(s)	113	—	210	9.0	15.0	3.0	13.0	6.0	—	—	0
748	Tostada	1	item(s)	170	—	230	11.0	27.0	7.0	10.0	3.5	—	—	0.5
Convenience Meals														
	Banquet													
29961	Barbeque chicken meal	1	item(s)	281	—	330	16.0	37.0	2.0	13.0	3.0	—	—	—
14788	Boneless white fried chicken meal	1	item(s)	286	—	310	10.0	21.0	4.0	20.0	5.0	—	—	—
29960	Fish sticks meal	1	item(s)	207	—	470	13.0	58.0	1.0	20.0	3.5	—	—	—
29957	Lasagna with meat sauce meal	1	item(s)	312	—	320	15.0	46.0	7.0	9.0	4.0	—	—	—
14777	Macaroni and cheese meal	1	item(s)	340	—	420	15.0	57.0	5.0	14.0	8.0	—	—	—
1741	Meatloaf meal	1	item(s)	269	—	240	14.0	20.0	4.0	11.0	4.0	—	—	—
39418	Pepperoni pizza meal	1	item(s)	191	—	480	11.0	56.0	5.0	23.0	8.0	—	—	—
33759	Roasted white turkey meal	1	item(s)	255	—	230	14.0	30.0	5.0	6.0	2.0	—	—	—
1743	Salisbury steak meal	1	item(s)	269	196.9	380	12.0	28.0	3.0	24.0	12.0	—	—	—
	Budget Gourmet													
1914	Cheese manicotti with meat sauce entrée	1	item(s)	284	194.0	420	18.0	38.0	4.0	22.0	11.0	6.0	1.3	—
1915	Chicken with fettucini entrée	1	item(s)	284	—	380	20.0	33.0	3.0	19.0	10.0	—	—	—
3986	Light beef stroganoff entrée	1	item(s)	248	177.0	290	20.0	32.0	3.0	7.0	4.0	—	—	—
3996	Light sirloin of beef in herb sauce entrée	1	item(s)	269	214.0	260	19.0	30.0	5.0	7.0	4.0	2.3	0.3	—
3987	Light vegetable lasagna entrée	1	item(s)	298	227.0	290	15.0	36.0	4.8	9.0	1.8	0.9	0.6	—

Chol (mg)	Calc (mg)	Iron (mg)	Magn (mg)	Pota (mg)	Sodi (mg)	Zinc (mg)	Vit A (µg)	Thia (mg)	Vit E (mg α)	Ribo (mg)	Niac (mg)	Vit B_6 (mg)	Fola (µg)	Vit C (mg)	Vit B_{12} (µg)	Sele (µg)
25	60	2.70	—	—	1210.0	—	—	—	—	—	—	—	—	13.8	—	—
20	60	2.70	—	—	1000.0	—	—	—	—	—	—	—	—	13.8	—	—
0	60	4.50	—	—	520.0	—	—	—	—	—	—	—	—	18.0	—	—
0	60	2.70	—	—	500.0	—	—	—	—	—	—	—	—	13.8	—	—
15	20	0.72	—	—	160.0	—	—	—	—	—	—	—	—	0	—	—
25	250	5.40	—	—	1350.0	—	—	—	—	—	—	—	—	15.0	—	—
5	200	4.50	—	—	1190.0	—	5.9	—	—	—	—	—	—	4.8	—	—
40	200	4.50	—	—	1340.0	—	9.9	—	—	—	—	—	—	6.0	—	—
40	150	2.70	—	—	620.0	—	—	—	—	—	—	—	—	3.6	—	—
35	100	2.70	—	—	780.0	—	—	—	—	—	—	—	—	2.4	—	—
40	150	2.70	—	—	620.0	—	—	—	—	—	—	—	—	3.6	—	—
25	100	1.80	—	—	630.0	—	—	—	—	—	—	—	—	1.2	—	—
40	150	2.70	—	—	650.0	—	—	—	—	—	—	—	—	3.6	—	—
45	200	4.50	—	—	1360.0	—	—	—	—	—	—	—	—	9.0	—	—
45	100	2.70	—	—	650.0	—	—	—	—	—	—	—	—	4.8	—	—
40	100	1.80	—	—	800.0	—	—	—	—	—	—	—	—	3.6	—	—
75	450	3.60	—	—	1420.0	—	—	—	—	—	—	—	—	1.2	—	—
40	300	1.80	—	—	1080.0	—	—	—	—	—	—	—	—	0	—	—
0	0	0.37	—	—	200.0	—	0	—	—	—	—	—	—	0	—	—
45	150	1.80	—	—	650.0	—	—	—	—	—	—	—	—	4.8	—	—
30	100	1.08	—	—	550.0	—	14.6	—	—	—	—	—	—	1.2	—	—
40	100	2.70	—	—	530.0	—	—	—	—	—	—	—	—	3.6	—	—
35	100	2.70	—	—	660.0	—	—	—	—	—	—	—	—	3.6	—	—
35	120	1.44	—	—	565.0	—	29.2	—	—	—	—	—	—	3.6	—	—
40	350	3.60	—	—	1000.0	—	—	—	—	—	—	—	—	4.8	—	—
15	100	1.44	—	—	790.0	—	—	—	—	—	—	—	—	3.6	—	—
40	250	2.70	—	—	880.0	—	—	—	—	—	—	—	—	2.4	—	—
3	80	0.71	—	—	530.0	—	0	—	—	—	—	—	—	0	—	—
35	200	3.60	—	—	1280.0	—	—	—	—	—	—	—	—	4.8	—	—
15	150	1.44	—	—	670.0	—	—	—	—	—	—	—	—	3.6	—	—
35	200	4.50	—	—	1250.0	—	9.9	—	—	—	—	—	—	9.0	—	—
40	100	2.70	—	—	530.0	—	—	—	—	—	—	—	—	3.6	—	—
25	80	1.08	—	—	350.0	—	—	—	—	—	—	—	—	1.2	—	—
65	450	7.20	—	—	1780.0	—	—	—	—	—	—	—	—	12.0	—	—
40	100	1.08	—	—	370.0	—	—	—	—	—	—	—	—	3.6	—	—
15	200	1.80	—	—	730.0	—	—	—	—	—	—	—	—	4.8	—	—
																—
50	40	1.08	—	—	1210.0	—	0	—	—	—	—	—	—	4.8	—	—
45	80	1.44	—	—	1200.0	—	—	—	—	—	—	—	—	18.0	—	—
55	20	1.44	—	—	710.0	—	—	—	—	—	—	—	—	0	—	—
20	100	2.70	—	—	1170.0	—	—	—	—	—	—	—	—	0	—	—
20	150	1.44	—	—	1330.0	—	0	—	—	—	—	—	—	0	—	—
30	0	1.80	—	—	1040.0	—	0	—	—	—	—	—	—	0	—	—
35	150	1.80	—	—	870.0	—	0	—	—	—	—	—	—	0	—	—
25	60	1.80	—	—	1070.0	—	—	—	—	—	—	—	—	3.6	—	—
60	40	1.44	—	—	1140.0	—	0	—	—	—	—	—	—	0	—	—
85	300	2.70	45.4	484.0	810.0	2.29	—	0.45	—	0.51	4.00	0.22	30.7	0	0.7	—
85	100	2.70	—	—	810.0	—	—	0.15	—	0.42	6.00	—	—	0	—	—
35	40	1.80	38.9	280.0	580.0	4.71	—	0.17	—	0.36	4.28	0.27	18.9	2.4	2.5	—
30	40	1.80	57.7	540.0	850.0	4.81	—	0.15	—	0.29	5.53	0.37	38.4	6.0	1.6	—
15	283	3.03	78.5	420.0	780.0	1.39	—	0.22	—	0.45	3.13	0.32	74.8	59.1	0.2	—

TABLE A-1 Table of Food Composition (*continued*) <small>(Computer code is for Cengage Diet Analysis program)</small> <small>(For purposes of calculations, use "0" for t, <1, <.1, <.01, etc.</small>

DA+ Code	Food Description	Quantity	Measure	Wt (g)	H₂O (g)	Ener (kcal)	Prot (g)	Carb (g)	Fiber (g)	Fat (g)	Fat Breakdown (g)			
											Sat	Mono	Poly	*Trans*
Convenience Meals—*continued*														
	Healthy Choice													
9425	Cheese French bread pizza	1	item(s)	170	—	340	22.0	51.0	5.0	5.0	1.5	—	—	—
9306	Chicken enchilada suprema meal	1	item(s)	320	251.5	360	13.0	59.0	8.0	7.0	3.0	2.0	2.0	—
3821	Familiar Favorites lasagna bake with meat sauce entrée	1	item(s)	255	—	270	13.0	38.0	4.0	7.0	2.5	—	—	—
13744	Familiar Favorites sesame chicken with vegetables and rice entrée	1	item(s)	255	—	260	17.0	34.0	4.0	6.0	2.0	2.0	2.0	—
9316	Lemon pepper fish meal	1	item(s)	303	—	280	11.0	49.0	5.0	5.0	2.0	1.0	2.0	—
9322	Traditional salisbury steak meal	1	item(s)	354	250.3	360	23.0	45.0	5.0	9.0	3.5	4.0	1.0	—
9359	Traditional turkey breasts meal	1	item(s)	298	—	330	21.0	50.0	4.0	5.0	2.0	1.5	1.5	—
	Stouffers													
2313	Cheese French bread pizza	1	serving(s)	294	—	380	15.0	43.0	3.0	16.0	6.0	—	—	—
11138	Cheese manicotti with tomato sauce entrée	1	item(s)	255	—	360	18.0	41.0	2.0	14.0	6.0	—	—	—
2366	Chicken pot pie entrée	1	item(s)	284	—	740	23.0	56.0	4.0	47.0	18.0	12.4	10.5	—
11116	Homestyle baked chicken breast with mashed potatoes and gravy entrée	1	item(s)	252	—	270	21.0	21.0	2.0	11.0	3.5			
11146	Homestyle beef pot roast and potatoes entrée	1	item(s)	252	—	260	16.0	24.0	3.0	11.0	4.0	—	—	—
11152	Homestyle roast turkey breast with stuffing and mashed potatoes entrée	1	item(s)	273	—	290	16.0	30.0	2.0	12.0	3.5	—	—	—
11043	Lean Cuisine Comfort Classics baked chicken and whipped potatoes and stuffing entrée	1	item(s)	245	—	240	15.0	34.0	3.0	4.5	1.0	2.0	1.0	0
11046	Lean Cuisine Comfort Classics honey mustard chicken with rice pilaf entrée	1	item(s)	227	—	250	17.0	37.0	1.0	4.0	1.0	1.0	1.0	0
9479	Lean Cuisine Deluxe French bread pizza	1	item(s)	174	—	310	16.0	44.0	3.0	9.0	3.5	0.5	0.5	0
360	Lean Cuisine One Dish Favorites chicken chow mein with rice	1	item(s)	255	—	190	13.0	29.0	2.0	2.5	0.5	1.0	0.5	0
11054	Lean Cuisine One Dish Favorites chicken enchilada Suiza with Mexican-style rice	1	serving(s)	255	—	270	10.0	47.0	3.0	4.5	2.0	1.5	1.0	0
9467	Lean Cuisine One Dish Favorites fettucini alfredo entrée	1	item(s)	262	—	270	13.0	39.0	2.0	7.0	3.5	2.0	1.0	0
11055	Lean Cuisine One Dish Favorites lasagna with meat sauce entrée	1	item(s)	298	—	320	19.0	44.0	4.0	7.0	3.0	2.0	0.5	0
	Weight Watchers													
11164	Smart Ones chicken enchiladas suiza entrée	1	item(s)	255	—	340	12.0	38.0	3.0	10.0	4.5	—	—	—
39763	Smart Ones chicken oriental entrée	1	item(s)	255	—	230	15.0	34.0	3.0	4.5	1.0	—	—	—
11187	Smart Ones pepperoni pizza	1	item(s)	198	—	400	22.0	58.0	4.0	9.0	3.0	—	—	—
39765	Smart Ones spaghetti bolognese entrée	1	item(s)	326	—	280	17.0	43.0	5.0	5.0	2.0	—	—	—
31512	Smart Ones spicy szechuan style vegetables and chicken	1	item(s)	255	—	220	11.0	34.0	4.0	5.0	1.0	—	—	—
Baby Foods														
787	Apple juice	4	fluid ounce(s)	127	111.6	60	0	14.8	0.1	0.1	0	0	0	—
778	Applesauce, strained	4	tablespoon(s)	64	56.7	26	0.1	6.9	1.1	0.1	0	0	0	—
779	Bananas with tapioca, strained	4	tablespoon(s)	60	50.4	34	0.2	9.2	1.0	0	0	0	0	—
604	Carrots, strained	4	tablespoon(s)	56	51.7	15	0.4	3.4	1.0	0.1	0	0	0	—
770	Chicken noodle dinner, strained	4	tablespoon(s)	64	54.8	42	1.7	5.8	1.3	1.3	0.4	0.5	0.3	—
801	Green beans, strained	4	tablespoon(s)	60	55.1	16	0.7	3.8	1.3	0.1	0	0	0	—
910	Human milk, mature	2	fluid ounce(s)	62	53.9	43	0.6	4.2	0	2.7	1.2	1.0	0.3	—
760	Mixed cereal, prepared with whole milk	4	ounce(s)	113	84.6	128	5.4	18.0	1.5	4.0	2.2	1.2	0.4	—
772	Mixed vegetable dinner, strained	2	ounce(s)	57	50.3	23	0.7	5.4	0.8	0	—	—	0	—
762	Rice cereal, prepared with whole milk	4	ounce(s)	113	84.6	130	4.4	18.9	0.1	4.1	2.6	1.0	0.2	—
758	Teething biscuits	1	item(s)	11	0.7	44	1.0	8.6	0.2	0.6	0.2	0.2	0.1	—

PAGE KEY: A-6 = Breads/Baked Goods A-12 = Cereal/Rice/Pasta A-16 = Fruit A-20 = Vegetables/Legumes A-30 = Nuts/Seeds A-32 = Vegetarian A-34 = Dairy A-42 = Eggs A-42 = Seafood A-44 = Meats A-48 = Poultry A-48 = Processed Meats A-50 = Beverages A-54 = Fats/Oils A-56 = Sweets A-58 = Spices/Condiments/Sauces A-62 = Mixed Foods/Soups/Sandwiches A-66 = Fast Food A-86 = Convenience A-88 = Baby Foods

Chol (mg)	Calc (mg)	Iron (mg)	Magn (mg)	Pota (mg)	Sodi (mg)	Zinc (mg)	Vit A (µg)	Thia (mg)	Vit E (mg α)	Ribo (mg)	Niac (mg)	Vit B$_6$ (mg)	Fola (µg)	Vit C (mg)	Vit B$_{12}$ (µg)	Sele (µg)
10	350	3.60	—	—	600.0	—	—	—	—	—	—	—	—	0	—	—
30	40	1.44	—	—	580.0	—	—	—	—	—	—	—	—	3.6	—	—
20	100	1.80	—	—	600.0	—	—	—	—	—	—	—	—	0	—	—
35	18	0.72	—	—	580.0	—	—	—	—	—	—	—	—	12.0	—	—
35	20	0.36	—	—	580.0	—	—	—	—	—	—	—	—	30.0	—	—
45	80	2.70	—	—	580.0	—	—	—	—	—	—	—	—	21.0	—	—
35	40	1.80	—	—	600.0	—	—	—	—	—	—	—	—	0	—	—
30	200	1.80	—	230.0	660.0	—	—	—	—	—	—	—	—	2.4	—	—
70	250	1.44	—	550.0	920.0	—	—	—	—	—	—	—	—	6.0	—	—
65	150	2.70	—	—	1170.0	—	—	—	—	—	—	—	—	2.4	—	—
55	20	0.72	—	490.0	770.0	—	0	—	—	—	—	—	—	0	—	—
35	20	1.80	—	800.0	960.0	—	—	—	—	—	—	—	—	6.0	—	—
45	40	1.08	—	490.0	970.0	—	—	—	—	—	—	—	—	3.6	—	—
25	40	1.16	—	500.0	650.0	—	—	—	—	—	—	—	—	3.6	—	—
30	64	0.38	—	370.0	650.0	—	—	—	—	—	—	—	—	0	—	—
20	150	2.70	—	300.0	700.0	—	—	—	—	—	—	—	—	15.0	—	—
25	40	0.72	—	380.0	650.0	—	—	—	—	—	—	—	—	2.4	—	—
20	150	0.72	—	350.0	510.0	—	—	—	—	—	—	—	—	2.4	—	—
15	200	0.72	—	290.0	690.0	—	0	—	—	—	—	—	—	0	—	—
30	250	1.47	—	610.0	690.0	—	—	—	—	—	—	—	—	2.4	—	—
40	200	0.72	—	—	800.0	—	—	—	—	—	—	—	—	2.4	—	—
35	40	0.72	—	—	790.0	—	—	—	—	—	—	—	—	6.0	—	—
15	200	1.08	—	401.0	700.0	—	69.1	—	—	—	—	—	—	4.8	—	—
15	150	3.60	—	—	670.0	—	—	—	—	—	—	—	—	9.0	—	—
10	40	1.44	—	—	890.0	—	—	—	—	—	—	—	—	0	—	—
0	5	0.72	3.8	115.4	3.8	0.03	1.3	0.01	0.76	0.02	0.10	0.03	0	73.4	0	0.1
0	3	0.12	1.9	45.4	1.3	0.01	0.6	0.01	0.36	0.02	0.04	0.02	1.3	24.5	0	0.2
0	3	0.12	6.0	52.8	5.4	0.04	1.2	0.01	0.36	0.02	0.08	0.04	3.6	10.0	0	0.4
0	12	0.20	5.0	109.8	20.7	0.08	320.9	0.01	0.29	0.02	0.25	0.04	8.4	3.2	0	0.1
10	17	0.40	9.0	89.0	14.7	0.32	70.4	0.03	0.12	0.04	0.44	0.04	7.0	0	0	2.4
0	23	0.40	12.0	87.6	3.0	0.12	10.8	0.02	0.04	0.04	0.20	0.02	14.4	0.2	0	0
9	20	0.02	1.8	31.4	10.5	0.10	37.6	0.01	0.04	0.02	0.10	0.01	3.1	3.1	0	1.1
12	249	11.82	30.6	225.7	53.3	0.80	28.4	0.49	—	0.65	6.54	0.07	12.5	1.4	0.3	
—	12	0.18	6.2	68.6	4.5	0.08	77.1	0.01	—	0.02	0.28	0.04	4.5	1.6	0	0.4
12	271	13.82	51.0	215.5	52.2	0.72	24.9	0.52	—	0.56	5.90	0.12	9.1	1.4	0.3	4.0
0	11	0.39	3.9	35.5	28.4	0.10	3.1	0.02	0.02	0.05	0.47	0.01	5.4	1.0	0	2.6

WHO: Nutrition Recommendations Canada: Guidelines and Meal Planning

This appendix presents nutrition recommendations from the World Health Organization (WHO) and details for Canadians on the *Eating Well with Canada's Food Guide* and the *Beyond the Basics* meal-planning system.

Nutrition Recommendations from WHO

The World Health Organization (WHO) has assessed the relationships between diet and the development of chronic diseases. Its recommendations include:

- Energy: sufficient to support growth, physical activity, and a healthy body weight (BMI between 18.5 and 24.9) and to avoid weight gain greater than 11 pounds (5 kilograms) during adult life
- Total fat: 15 to 30 percent of total energy
- Saturated fatty acids: <10 percent of total energy
- Polyunsaturated fatty acids: 6 to 10 percent of total energy
- Omega-6 polyunsaturated fatty acids: 5 to 8 percent of total energy
- Omega-3 polyunsaturated fatty acids: 1 to 2 percent of total energy
- *Trans*-fatty acids: <1 percent of total energy
- Total carbohydrate: 55 to 75 percent of total energy
- Sugars: <10 percent of total energy
- Protein: 10 to 15 percent of total energy
- Cholesterol: <300 mg per day
- Salt (sodium): <5 g salt per day (<2 g sodium per day), appropriately iodized
- Fruits and vegetables: ≥400 g per day (about 1 pound)
- Total dietary fiber: >25 g per day from foods
- Physical activity: one hour of moderate-intensity activity, such as walking, on most days of the week

Eating Well with Canada's Food Guide

Figure B-1 presents the 2007 *Eating Well with Canada's Food Guide*. Additional publications, which are available from Health Canada (✚) through its website, provide many more details.

✚ Search for "Canada's food guide" at Health Canada: www.hc-sc.gc.ca

FIGURE B-1 | Eating Well with Canada's Food Guide

 Health Canada   Santé Canada   *Your health and safety... our priority.*   *Votre santé et votre sécurité... notre priorité.*

Eating Well with
Canada's Food Guide

Canada

Eating Well with Canada's Food Guide *(Continued)*

Recommended Number of **Food Guide Servings** *per Day*

	Children			Teens		Adults			
Age in Years	2-3	4-8	9-13	14-18		19-50		51+	
Sex	Girls and Boys			Females	Males	Females	Males	Females	Males
Vegetables and Fruit	4	5	6	7	8	7-8	8-10	7	7
Grain Products	3	4	6	6	7	6-7	8	6	7
Milk and Alternatives	2	2	3-4	3-4	3-4	2	2	3	3
Meat and Alternatives	1	1	1-2	2	3	2	3	2	3

The chart above shows how many Food Guide Servings you need from each of the four food groups every day.

Having the amount and type of food recommended and following the tips in *Canada's Food Guide* will help:

- Meet your needs for vitamins, minerals and other nutrients.
- Reduce your risk of obesity, type 2 diabetes, heart disease, certain types of cancer and osteoporosis.
- Contribute to your overall health and vitality.

What is One Food Guide Serving?
Look at the examples below.

Fresh, frozen or canned vegetables
125 mL (½ cup)

Leafy vegetables
Cooked: 125 mL (½ cup)
Raw: 250 mL (1 cup)

Fresh, frozen or canned fruits
1 fruit or 125 mL (½ cup)

100% Juice
125 mL (½ cup)

Bread
1 slice (35 g)

Bagel
½ bagel (45 g)

Flat breads
½ pita or ½ tortilla (35 g)

Cooked rice, bulgur or quinoa
125 mL (½ cup)

Cereal
Cold: 30 g
Hot: 175 mL (¾ cup)

Cooked pasta or couscous
125 mL (½ cup)

Milk or powdered milk (reconstituted)
250 mL (1 cup)

Canned milk (evaporated)
125 mL (½ cup)

Fortified soy beverage
250 mL (1 cup)

Yogurt
175 g
(¾ cup)

Kefir
175 g
(¾ cup)

Cheese
50 g (1 ½ oz.)

Cooked fish, shellfish, poultry, lean meat
75 g (2 ½ oz.)/125 mL (½ cup)

Cooked legumes
175 mL (¾ cup)

Tofu
150 g or
175 mL (¾ cup)

Eggs
2 eggs

Peanut or nut butters
30 mL (2 Tbsp)

Shelled nuts and seeds
60 mL (¼ cup)

Oils and Fats
- Include a small amount – 30 to 45 mL (2 to 3 Tbsp) – of unsaturated fat each day. This includes oil used for cooking, salad dressings, margarine and mayonnaise.
- Use vegetable oils such as canola, olive and soybean.
- Choose soft margarines that are low in saturated and trans fats.
- Limit butter, hard margarine, lard and shortening.

Make each Food Guide Serving count...
wherever you are – at home, at school, at work or when eating out!

▸ **Eat at least one dark green and one orange vegetable each day.**
- Go for dark green vegetables such as broccoli, romaine lettuce and spinach.
- Go for orange vegetables such as carrots, sweet potatoes and winter squash.

▸ **Choose vegetables and fruit prepared with little or no added fat, sugar or salt.**
- Enjoy vegetables steamed, baked or stir-fried instead of deep-fried.

▸ **Have vegetables and fruit more often than juice.**

▸ **Make at least half of your grain products whole grain each day.**
- Eat a variety of whole grains such as barley, brown rice, oats, quinoa and wild rice.
- Enjoy whole grain breads, oatmeal or whole wheat pasta.

▸ **Choose grain products that are lower in fat, sugar or salt.**
- Compare the Nutrition Facts table on labels to make wise choices.
- Enjoy the true taste of grain products. When adding sauces or spreads, use small amounts.

▸ **Drink skim, 1%, or 2% milk each day.**
- Have 500 mL (2 cups) of milk every day for adequate vitamin D.
- Drink fortified soy beverages if you do not drink milk.

▸ **Select lower fat milk alternatives.**
- Compare the Nutrition Facts table on yogurts or cheeses to make wise choices.

▸ **Have meat alternatives such as beans, lentils and tofu often.**

▸ **Eat at least two Food Guide Servings of fish each week.***
- Choose fish such as char, herring, mackerel, salmon, sardines and trout.

▸ **Select lean meat and alternatives prepared with little or no added fat or salt.**
- Trim the visible fat from meats. Remove the skin on poultry.
- Use cooking methods such as roasting, baking or poaching that require little or no added fat.
- If you eat luncheon meats, sausages or prepackaged meats, choose those lower in salt (sodium) and fat.

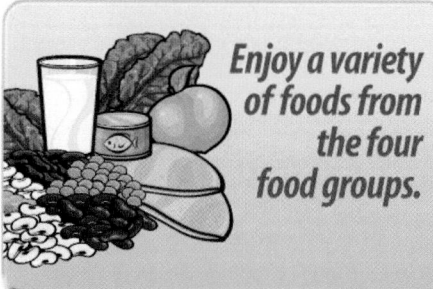

Enjoy a variety of foods from the four food groups.

Satisfy your thirst with water!

Drink water regularly. It's a calorie-free way to quench your thirst. Drink more water in hot weather or when you are very active.

* Health Canada provides advice for limiting exposure to mercury from certain types of fish. Refer to www.hc-sc.gc.ca for the latest information.

FIGURE B-1 | Eating Well with Canada's Food Guide *(Continued)*

Advice for different ages and stages...

Children

Following *Canada's Food Guide* helps children grow and thrive.

Young children have small appetites and need calories for growth and development.

- Serve small nutritious meals and snacks each day.

- Do not restrict nutritious foods because of their fat content. Offer a variety of foods from the four food groups.

- Most of all... be a good role model.

Women of childbearing age

All women who could become pregnant and those who are pregnant or breastfeeding need a multivitamin containing **folic acid** every day. Pregnant women need to ensure that their multivitamin also contains **iron**. A health care professional can help you find the multivitamin that's right for you.

Pregnant and breastfeeding women need more calories. Include an extra 2 to 3 Food Guide Servings each day.

Here are two examples:
- Have fruit and yogurt for a snack, or

- Have an extra slice of toast at breakfast and an extra glass of milk at supper.

Men and women over 50

The need for **vitamin D** increases after the age of 50.

In addition to following *Canada's Food Guide*, everyone over the age of 50 should take a daily vitamin D supplement of 10 μg (400 IU).

How do I count Food Guide Servings in a meal?

Here is an example:

Vegetable and beef stir-fry with rice, a glass of milk and an apple for dessert		
250 mL (1 cup) mixed broccoli, carrot and sweet red pepper	=	2 **Vegetables and Fruit** Food Guide Servings
75 g (2 ½ oz.) lean beef	=	1 **Meat and Alternatives** Food Guide Serving
250 mL (1 cup) brown rice	=	2 **Grain Products** Food Guide Servings
5 mL (1 tsp) canola oil	=	part of your **Oils and Fats** intake for the day
250 mL (1 cup) 1% milk	=	1 **Milk and Alternatives** Food Guide Serving
1 apple	=	1 **Vegetables and Fruit** Food Guide Serving

Eat well and be active today and every day!

The benefits of eating well and being active include:

- Better overall health.
- Lower risk of disease.
- A healthy body weight.
- Feeling and looking better.
- More energy.
- Stronger muscles and bones.

Be active

To be active every day is a step towards better health and a healthy body weight.

Canada's Physical Activity Guide recommends building 30 to 60 minutes of moderate physical activity into daily life for adults and at least 90 minutes a day for children and youth. You don't have to do it all at once. Add it up in periods of at least 10 minutes at a time for adults and five minutes at a time for children and youth.

Start slowly and build up.

Eat well

Another important step towards better health and a healthy body weight is to follow *Canada's Food Guide* by:

- Eating the recommended amount and type of food each day.
- Limiting foods and beverages high in calories, fat, sugar or salt (sodium) such as cakes and pastries, chocolate and candies, cookies and granola bars, doughnuts and muffins, ice cream and frozen desserts, french fries, potato chips, nachos and other salty snacks, alcohol, fruit flavoured drinks, soft drinks, sports and energy drinks, and sweetened hot or cold drinks.

Read the label

- Compare the Nutrition Facts table on food labels to choose products that contain less fat, saturated fat, trans fat, sugar and sodium.
- Keep in mind that the calories and nutrients listed are for the amount of food found at the top of the Nutrition Facts table.

Nutrition Facts
Per 0 mL (0 g)

Amount	% Daily Value
Calories 0	
Fat 0 g	0 %
Saturates 0 g	0 %
+ Trans 0 g	
Cholesterol 0 mg	
Sodium 0 mg	0 %
Carbohydrate 0 g	0 %
Fibre 0 g	0 %
Sugars 0 g	
Protein 0 g	

Vitamin A	0 %	Vitamin C	0 %
Calcium	0 %	Iron	0 %

Limit trans fat

When a Nutrition Facts table is not available, ask for nutrition information to choose foods lower in trans and saturated fats.

Take a step today...

✓ Have breakfast every day. It may help control your hunger later in the day.

✓ Walk wherever you can – get off the bus early, use the stairs.

✓ Benefit from eating vegetables and fruit at all meals and as snacks.

✓ Spend less time being inactive such as watching TV or playing computer games.

✓ Request nutrition information about menu items when eating out to help you make healthier choices.

✓ Enjoy eating with family and friends!

✓ Take time to eat and savour every bite!

For more information, interactive tools, or additional copies visit Canada's Food Guide on-line at: www.hc-sc.gc.ca

or contact:

Publications
Health Canada
Ottawa, Ontario K1A 0K9
E-Mail: publications@hc-sc.gc.ca
Tel.: 1-866-225-0709
Fax: (613) 941-5366
TTY: 1-800-267-1245

Également disponible en français sous le titre :
Bien manger avec le Guide alimentaire canadien

This publication can be made available on request on diskette, large print, audio-cassette and braille.

Beyond the Basics: Meal Planning for Healthy Eating, Diabetes Prevention and Management

Beyond the Basics: Meal Planning for Healthy Eating, Diabetes Prevention and Management is Canada's system of meal planning.[1] Similar to the U.S. exchange system, *Beyond the Basics* sorts foods into groups and defines portion sizes to help people manage their blood glucose and maintain a healthy weight. Because foods that contain carbohydrate raise blood glucose, the food groups are organized into two sections—those that contain carbohydrate (presented in Table B-1) and those that contain little or no carbohydrate (shown in Table B-2). One portion from any of the food groups listed in Table B-1 provides about 15 grams of available carbohydrate (total carbohydrate minus fiber) and counts as one carbohydrate choice. Within each group, foods are identified as those to "choose more often" (generally higher in vitamins, minerals, and fiber) and those to "choose less often" (generally higher in sugar, saturated fat, or *trans* fat).

[1]The tables for the Canadian meal planning system are adapted from *Beyond the Basics: Meal Planning for Healthy Eating, Diabetes Prevention and Management,* copyright 2005, with permission of the Canadian Diabetes Association. Additional information is available from www.diabetes.ca.

TABLE B-1 Food Groups that Contain Carbohydrate

1 serving = 15 g carbohydrate or 1 carbohydrate choice

KEY
● Choose more often
▲ Choose less often

Food	Measure
Grains and starches: 15 g carbohydrate, 3 g protein, 0 g fat, 286 kJ (68 kcal)	
▲ Bagel, large (11 cm, 4.5″)	¼
▲ Bagel, small (8 cm, 3″)	½
▲ Bannock, fried	1.5″ × 2.5″
● Bannock, whole grain baked	1.5″ × 2.5″
● Barley, pearled, cooked	125 mL (½ c)
▲ Bread, white	1 slice (30 g)
● Bread, whole grain	1 slice (30 g)
● Bulghur, cooked	125 mL (½ c)
▲ Bun, hamburger or hotdog	½
▲ Cereal, flaked unsweetened	125 mL (½ c)
● Cream of Wheat, cooked	175 mL (¾ c)
● Red River, cooked	125 mL (½ c)
● Chapati (15 cm, 6″)	1 (44 g)
● Corn	125 mL (½ c)
● Couscous, cooked	125 mL (½ c)
▲ Crackers, soda type	7
▲ Croutons	175 mL (¾ c)
● English muffin, whole grain	½ (28 g)
▲ French fries	10 (50 g)
● Millet, cooked	⅓ c (75 mL)
▲ Naan bread (15 cm, 6″)	¼
▲ Pancake (10 cm, 4″)	1
● Pasta, cooked	125 mL (½ c)
▲ Pita bread, white (15 cm, 6″)	½
● Pita bread, whole wheat (15 cm, 6″)	½
▲ Pizza crust (30 cm, 12″)	¹⁄₁₂ (90 g)

(continued)

● Choose more often
▲ Choose less often

TABLE B-1 Food Groups that Contain Carbohydrate (*continued*)

Food	Measure
Grains and starches: 15 g carbohydrate, 3 g protein, 0 g fat, 286 kJ (68 kcal)—continued	
● Plantain, cooked, mashed	⅓ c (75 mL)
● Potatoes, boiled or baked	½ medium (84 g)
● Rice, white or brown, cooked	⅓ c (75 mL)
● Roti (15 cm, 6″)	1 (44 g)
● Soup, thick, chunky type	250 mL (1 c)
● Sweet potato, mashed	⅓ c (75 mL)
▲ Taco shells (13 cm, 5″)	2 (17 g)
● Tortilla, wheat flour (25 cm, 10″)	½
▲ Waffle (medium)	1 (39 g)
Fruits: 15 g carbohydrate, 1–2 g protein, 0 g fat, 269 kJ (64 kcal)	
● Apple	1 medium (138 g)
● Applesauce, unsweetened	125 mL (½ c)
● Banana	1 small or ½ large
● Blackberries	500 mL (2 c)
● Cherries	15 (102 g)
● Fruit, canned in juice	125 mL (½ c)
▲ Fruit, dried	60 mL (¼ c)
● Grapefruit	1 small
● Grapes	15 or ½ c (80 g)
● Kiwi	2 medium (150 g)
▲ Juice	125 mL (½ c)
● Mango	½ medium
● Melon	250 mL (1 c)
● Orange	1 medium
● Other berries	250 mL (1 c)
● Pear	1 medium
● Pineapple	175 mL (¾ c)
● Plum	2 medium
● Raspberries	500 mL (2 c)
● Strawberries	500 mL (2 c)
Milk and alternatives: 15 g carbohydrate, 7 g protein, variable fat, 386–651 kJ (92–155 kcal)	
● Evaporated milk, canned	125 mL (½ c)
● Milk, fluid	250 mL (1 c)
● Milk powder, skim	60 mL (4 tbs)
● Soy beverage, flavoured	125 mL (½ c)
● Soy beverage, plain	250 mL (1 c)
● Soy yogourt, flavoured	75 mL (⅓ c)
● Yogourt, nonfat, plain	175 mL (¾ c)
● Yogourt, skim, artificially sweetened	250 mL (1 c)
Other choices (sweet foods and snacks): 15 g carbohydrate, variable protein and fat	
▲ Brownies, unfrosted	5 cm × 5 cm (2″ × 2″)
▲ Cake, unfrosted	5 cm × 5 cm (2″ × 2″)
▲ Cookies, arrowroot or gingersnap	3–4
▲ Jam, jelly, marmalade	15 mL (1 tbs)

(continued)

TABLE B-1 Food Groups that Contain Carbohydrate (*continued*)

Food	Measure
Other choices (sweet foods and snacks): 15 g carbohydrate, variable protein and fat—continued	
● Milk pudding, skim, no sugar added	125 mL (½ c)
▲ Muffin, plain	1 small (45 g)
▲ Oatmeal granola bar	1 (28 g)
● Popcorn, low fat, air popped	750 mL (3 c)
▲ Pretzels, low fat, large	7
▲ Pretzels, low fat, sticks	30
▲ Sugar, white	15 mL (1 tbs, 3 tsp, or 3 packets)
▲ Syrup, honey, molasses	1 tbs (15 mL)

KEY
● Choose more often
▲ Choose less often

TABLE B-2 Food Groups that Contain Little or No Carbohydrate

Food	Measure
Vegetables: To encourage consumption, most vegetables are considered "free"	
▲ Artichokes, Jerusalem[a]	
● Asparagus	
● Beans, yellow or green	
● Bean sprouts	
● Beets	
● Broccoli	
● Cabbage	
● Carrots	
● Cauliflower	
● Celery	
● Cucumber	
● Eggplant	
● Kale	
● Leeks	
● Mushrooms	
● Okra	
● Onions	
▲ Parsnips[a]	
▲ Peas[a]	
● Peppers	
● Rutabagas	
● Salad vegetables	
▲ Squash, Hubbard, pumpkin, spaghetti	
▲ Squash, acorn[a], butternut[a]	
● Tomatoes, fresh	
● Tomatoes, canned, regular	
▲ Tomatoes, canned, stewed[a]	
● Turnips	

(continued)

[a]These vegetables contain enough carbohydrate to be counted as one carbohydrate choice (15 g of available carbohydrate) when the portion size eaten is 1 cup (250 mL) or more.

TABLE B-2 **Food Groups that Contain Little or No Carbohydrate (*continued*)**

Food	Measure
Meat and alternatives: 0 g carbohydrate, 7 g protein, 3–5 g fat, 307 kJ (73 kcal)	
● Cheese, skim (<7% milk fat)	2.5 cm × 2.5 cm × 2.5 cm (1″ × 1″ × 1″)
● Cheese, light (<20% milk fat)	2.5 cm × 2.5 cm × 2.5 cm (1″ × 1″ × 1″)
▲ Cheese, regular (≥21% milk fat)	2.5 cm × 2.5 cm × 2.5 cm (1″ × 1″ × 1″)
● Cottage cheese (1–2% milk fat)	60 mL (¼ c)
● Egg	1 medium-large
● Fish, canned in oil or water	60 mL (¼ c)
● Fish, fresh or frozen, cooked	30 g (1 oz)
● Hummus	90 g (⅓ c)
● Legumes, cooked	125 mL (½ c)
● Meat, game, cooked	30 g (1 slice)
● Meat, ground, lean or extra lean, cooked	30 g (2 tbs)
● Meat, lean, cooked	30 g (1 slice)
● Meat, organ or tripe, cooked	30 g (1 slice)
● Meat, prepared, low fat	30 g (1–3 slices)
▲ Meat, prepared, regular fat	30 g (1–3 slices)
▲ Meat, regular, cooked	30 g (1–3 slices)
● Peameal/back bacon, cooked	30 g (1–2 slices)
● Poultry, ground, lean, cooked	30 g (2 tbs)
● Poultry, skinless, cooked	30 g (1 slice)
▲ Poultry/wings, skin on, cooked	45 g (2)
● Shellfish, cooked	30 g (3 medium)
● Tofu (soybean)	½ block (100 g)
● Vegetarian meat alternatives	30 g (1 oz)
Fats: 0 g carbohydrate, 0 g protein, 5 g fat, 189 kJ (45 kcal)	
▲ Avocado	34 g (⅙)
▲ Bacon	30 g (1 slice)
▲ Butter	5 mL (1 tsp)
▲ Cheese, spreadable	15 mL (1 tbs)
▲ Margarine, non-hydrogenated, regular	5 mL (1 tsp)
▲ Mayonnaise, light	15 mL (1 tbs)
▲ Nuts	15 mL (1 tbs)
▲ Oil, canola or olive	5 mL (1 tsp)
▲ Salad dressing, regular	5 mL (1 tsp)
▲ Seeds	15 g (1 tbs)
▲ Tahini	8 mL (½ tbs)
Extras: <5 g carbohydrate, 84 kJ (20 kcal)	
Broth	
Coffee	
Herbs and spices	
Ketchup	
Mustard	
Relish	
Sugar-free gelatin	
Sugar-free soft drinks	
Tea	

Exchange Lists for Diabetes

Chapter 20 introduces the exchange system, and this appendix provides details from the 2008 Choose Your Foods: Exchange Lists for Diabetes. Appendix B presents Canada's meal-planning system.

Exchange lists can help people with diabetes to manage their blood glucose levels by controlling the amount and kinds of carbohydrates they consume. These lists can also help in planning diets for weight management by controlling kcalorie and fat intake.

The Exchange System

The exchange system sorts foods into groups by their proportions of carbohydrate, fat, and protein (Table C-1 on p. C-2). These groups may be organized into several exchange lists of foods (Tables C-2 through C-12 on pp. C-3–C-16). For example, the carbohydrate group includes these exchange lists:

- Starch
- Fruits
- Milk (fat-free, reduced-fat, and whole)
- Sweets, Desserts, and Other Carbohydrates
- Nonstarchy Vegetables

Then any food on a list can be "exchanged" for any other on that same list. Another group for alcohol has been included as a reminder that these beverages often deliver substantial carbohydrate and kcalories, and therefore warrant their own list.

Serving Sizes

The serving sizes have been carefully adjusted and defined so that a serving of any food on a given list provides roughly the same amount of carbohydrate, fat, and protein, and, therefore, total energy. Any food on a list can thus be exchanged, or traded, for any other food on the same list without significantly affecting the diet's energy-nutrient balance or total kcalories. For example, a person may select 17 small grapes or ½ large grapefruit as one fruit exchange, and either choice would provide roughly 15 grams of carbohydrate and 60 kcalories. A whole grapefruit, however, would count as 2 fruit exchanges.

To apply the system successfully, users must become familiar with the specified serving sizes. A convenient way to remember the serving sizes and energy values is to keep in mind a typical item from each list (review TABLE C-1).

The Foods on the Lists

Foods do not always appear on the exchange list where you might first expect to find them. They are grouped according to their energy-nutrient contents rather than by their source (such as milks), their outward appearance, or their vitamin and mineral contents. For example, cheeses are grouped with meats (not milk) because, like meats, cheeses contribute energy from protein and fat but provide negligible carbohydrate.

For similar reasons, starchy vegetables such as corn, green peas, and potatoes are found on the Starch list with breads and cereals, not with the vegetables. Likewise, bacon is grouped with the fats and oils, not with the meats.

Diet planners learn to view mixtures of foods, such as casseroles and soups, as combinations of foods from different exchange lists. They also learn to interpret food labels with the exchange system in mind.

Controlling Energy, Fat, and Sodium

The exchange lists help people control their energy intakes by paying close attention to serving sizes. People wanting to lose weight can limit foods from the Sweets, Desserts, and Other Carbohydrates and Fats lists, and they might choose to avoid the Alcohol list altogether. The Free Foods list provide low-kcalorie choices.

By assigning items like bacon to the Fats list, the exchange lists alert consumers to foods that are unexpectedly high in fat. Even the Starch list specifies which grain products contain added fat (such as biscuits, cornbread, and waffles) by marking them with a symbol to indicate added fat (the symbols are explained in the table keys). In addition, the exchange lists encourage users to think of fat-free milk as milk and of whole milk as milk with added fat, and to think of lean meats as meats and of medium-fat and high-fat meats as meats with added fat. To that end, foods on the milk and meat lists are separated into categories based on their fat contents (review Table C-1). The Milk list is subdivided for fat-free, reduced fat, and whole; the meat list is subdivided for lean, medium fat, and high fat. The meat list also includes plant-based proteins, which tend to be rich in fiber. Notice that many of these foods (p. C-11) bear the symbol for "high fiber."

People wanting to control the sodium in their diets can begin by eliminating any foods bearing the "high sodium" symbol. In most cases, the symbol identifies foods that, in one serving, provide 480 milligrams or more of sodium. Foods on the Combination Foods or Fast Foods lists that bear the symbol provide more than 600 milligrams of

TABLE C-1 The Food Lists

Lists	Typical Item/Portion Size	Carbohydrate (g)	Protein (g)	Fat (g)	Energy[a] (kcal)
Carbohydrates					
Starch[b]	1 slice bread	15	0–3	0–1	80
Fruits	1 small apple	15	—	—	60
Milk					
Fat-free, low-fat, 1%	1 c fat-free milk	12	8	0–3	100
Reduced-fat, 2%	1 c reduced-fat milk	12	8	5	120
Whole	1 c whole milk	12	8	8	160
Sweets, desserts, and other carbohydrates[c]	2 small cookies	15	varies	varies	varies
Nonstarchy vegetables	½ c cooked carrots	5	2	—	25
Meat and Meat Substitutes					
Lean	1 oz chicken (no skin)	—	7	0–3	45
Medium-fat	1 oz ground beef	—	7	4–7	75
High-fat	1 oz pork sausage	—	7	8+	100
Plant-based proteins	½ c tofu	varies	7	varies	varies
Fats	1 tsp butter	—	—	5	45
Alcohol	12 oz beer	varies	—	—	100

[a]The energy value for each exchange list represents an approximate average for the group and does not reflect the precise number of grams of carbohydrate, protein, and fat. For example, a slice of bread contains 15 grams of carbohydrate (60 kcalories), 3 grams protein (12 kcalories), and a little fat—rounded to 80 kcalories for ease in calculating. A ½ cup of vegetables (not including starchy vegetables) contains 5 grams carbohydrate (20 kcalories) and 2 grams protein (8 more), which has been rounded down to 25 kcalories.
[b]The Starch list includes cereals, grains, breads, crackers, snacks, starchy vegetables (such as corn, peas, and potatoes), and legumes (dried beans, peas, and lentils).
[c]The Sweets, Desserts, and Other Carbohydrates list includes foods that contain added sugars and fats such as sodas, candy, cakes, cookies, doughnuts, ice cream, pudding, syrup, and frozen yogurt.

sodium. Other foods may also contribute substantially to sodium (consult Chapter 9 for details).

Planning a Healthy Diet

To obtain a daily variety of foods that provide healthful amounts of carbohydrate, protein, and fat, as well as vitamins, minerals, and fiber, the meal plan for adults and teenagers should include at least:

- Two to three servings of nonstarchy vegetables
- Two servings of fruits
- Six servings of grains (at least three of whole grains), beans, and starchy vegetables
- Two servings of low-fat or fat-free milk
- About 6 ounces of meat or meat substitutes
- *Small* amounts of fat and sugar

The actual amounts are determined by age, gender, activity levels, and other factors that influence energy needs.

TABLE C-2 Starch

The Starch list includes bread, cereals and grains, starchy vegetables, crackers and snacks, and legumes (dried beans, peas, and lentils). 1 starch choice = 15 grams carbohydrate, 0–3 grams protein, 0–1 grams fat, and 80 kcalories.

NOTE: In general, one starch exchange is ½ cup cooked cereal, grain, or starchy vegetable; ⅓ cup cooked rice or pasta; 1 ounce of bread product; ¾ ounce to 1 ounce of most snack foods.

Bread

Food	Serving Size
Bagel, large (about 4 oz)	¼ (1 oz)
▽ Biscuit, 2½ inches across	1
Bread	
☺ reduced-kcalorie	2 slices (1½ oz)
white, whole-grain, pumpernickel, rye, unfrosted raisin	1 slice (1 oz)
Chapatti, small, 6 inches across	1
▽ Cornbread, 1¾ inch cube	1 (1½ oz)
English muffin	½
Hot dog bun or hamburger bun	½ (1 oz)
Naan, 8 inches by 2 inches	¼
Pancake, 4 inches across, ¼ inch thick	1
Pita, 6 inches across	½
Roll, plain, small	1 (1 oz)
▽ Stuffing, bread	⅓ cup
▽ Taco shell, 5 inches across	2
Tortilla, corn, 6 inches across	1
Tortilla, flour, 6 inches across	1
Tortilla, flour, 10 inches across	⅓
▽ Waffle, 4-inch square or 4 inches across	1

Cereals and Grains

Food	Serving Size
Barley, cooked	⅓ cup
Bran, dry	
☺ oat	¼ cup
☺ wheat	½ cup
☺ Bulgur (cooked)	½ cup
Cereals	
☺ bran	½ cup
cooked (oats, oatmeal)	½ cup
puffed	1½ cups
shredded wheat, plain	½ cup
sugar-coated	½ cup
unsweetened, ready-to-eat	¾ cup
Couscous	⅓ cup
Granola	
low-fat	¼ cup
▽ regular	¼ cup
Grits, cooked	½ cup
Kasha	½ cup
Millet, cooked	⅓ cup

(continued)

KEY

☺ = More than 3 grams of dietary fiber per serving.

▽ = Extra fat, or prepared with added fat. (Count as 1 starch + 1 fat.)

▤ = 480 milligrams or more of sodium per serving.

TABLE C-2 Starch (*continued*)

Cereals and Grains—continued

Food	Serving Size
Muesli	¼ cup
Pasta, cooked	⅓ cup
Polenta, cooked	⅓ cup
Quinoa, cooked	⅓ cup
Rice, white or brown, cooked	⅓ cup
Tabbouleh (tabouli), prepared	½ cup
Wheat germ, dry	3 Tbsp
Wild rice, cooked	½ cup

Starchy Vegetables

Food	Serving Size
Cassava	⅓ cup
Corn	½ cup
on cob, large	½ cob (5 oz)
☺ Hominy, canned	¾ cup
☺ Mixed vegetables with corn, peas, or pasta	1 cup
☺ Parsnips	½ cup
☺ Peas, green	½ cup
Plantain, ripe	⅓ cup
Potato	
baked with skin	¼ large (3 oz)
boiled, all kinds	½ cup or ½ medium (3 oz)
▽ mashed, with milk and fat	½ cup
french fried (oven-baked)[a]	1 cup (2 oz)
☺ Pumpkin, canned, no sugar added	1 cup
Spaghetti/pasta sauce	½ cup
☺ Squash, winter (acorn, butternut)	1 cup
☺ Succotash	½ cup
Yam, sweet potato, plain	½ cup

Crackers and Snacks[b]

Food	Serving Size
Animal crackers	8
Crackers	
▽ round-butter type	6
saltine-type	6
▽ sandwich-style, cheese or peanut butter filling	3
▽ whole-wheat regular	2–5 (¾ oz)
☺ whole-wheat lower fat or crispbreads	2–5 (¾ oz)
Graham cracker, 2½-inch square	3
Matzoh	¾ oz
Melba toast, about 2-inch by 4-inch piece	4
Oyster crackers	20
Popcorn	3 cups
▽ ☺ with butter	3 cups
☺ no fat added	3 cups
☺ lower fat	3 cups
Pretzels	¾ oz
Rice cakes, 4 inches across	2
Snack chips	
fat-free or baked (tortilla, potato), baked pita chips	15–20 (¾ oz)
▽ regular (tortilla, potato)	9–13 (¾ oz)

Beans, Peas, and Lentils[c]

The choices on this list count as 1 starch + 1 lean meat.

Food	Serving Size
☺ Baked beans	⅓ cup
☺ Beans, cooked (black, garbanzo, kidney, lima, navy, pinto, white)	½ cup
☺ Lentils, cooked (brown, green, yellow)	½ cup
☺ Peas, cooked (black-eyed, split)	½ cup
🧂 ☺ Refried beans, canned	½ cup

KEY

☺ = More than 3 grams of dietary fiber per serving.

▽ = Extra fat, or prepared with added fat. (Count as 1 starch + 1 fat.)

🧂 = 480 milligrams or more of sodium per serving.

[a] Restaurant-style french fries are on the Fast Foods list.
[b] For other snacks, see the Sweets, Desserts, and Other Carbohydrates list. For a quick estimate of serving size, an open handful is equal to about 1 cup or 1 to 2 ounces of snack food.
[c] Beans, peas, and lentils are also found on the Meat and Meat Substitutes list.

TABLE C-3 Fruits

Fruit[a]

The Fruits list includes fresh, frozen, canned, and dried fruits and fruit juices. 1 fruit choice = 15 grams carbohydrate, 0 grams protein, 0 grams fat, and 60 kcalories.

NOTE: In general, one fruit exchange is ½ cup canned or fresh fruit or unsweetened fruit juice; 1 small fresh fruit (4 ounces); 2 tablespoons dried fruit.

Food	Serving Size	Food	Serving Size
Apple, unpeeled, small	1 (4 oz)	Nectarine, small	1 (5 oz)
Apples, dried	4 rings	☻ Orange, small	1 (6½ oz)
Applesauce, unsweetened	½ cup	Papaya	½ or 1 cup cubed (8 oz)
Apricots		Peaches	
canned	½ cup	canned	½ cup
dried	8 halves	fresh, medium	1 (6 oz)
☻ fresh	4 whole (5½ oz)	Pears	
Banana, extra small	1 (4 oz)	canned	½ cup
☻ Blackberries	¾ cup	fresh, large	½ (4 oz)
Blueberries	¾ cup	Pineapple	
Cantaloupe, small	⅓ melon or 1 cup cubed (11 oz)	canned	½ cup
		fresh	¾ cup
Cherries		Plums	
sweet, canned	½ cup	canned	½ cup
sweet fresh	12 (3 oz)	dried (prunes)	3
Dates	3	small	2 (5 oz)
Dried fruits (blueberries, cherries, cranberries, mixed fruit, raisins)	2 Tbsp	☻ Raspberries	1 cup
		☻ Strawberries	1¼ cup whole berries
Figs		☻ Tangerines, small	2 (8 oz)
dried	1½	Watermelon	1 slice or 1¼ cups cubes (13½ oz)
☻ fresh	1½ large or 2 medium (3½ oz)		
Fruit cocktail	½ cup		

Fruit Juice

Food	Serving Size
Grapefruit	
large	½ (11 oz)
sections, canned	¾ cup
Grapes, small	17 (3 oz)
Honeydew melon	1 slice or 1 cup cubed (10 oz)
☻ Kiwi	1 (3½ oz)
Mandarin oranges, canned	¾ cup
Mango, small	½ (5½ oz) or ½ cup

Food	Serving Size
Apple juice/cider	½ cup
Fruit juice blends, 100% juice	⅓ cup
Grape juice	⅓ cup
Grapefruit juice	½ cup
Orange juice	½ cup
Pineapple juice	½ cup
Prune juice	⅓ cup

KEY

☻ = More than 3 grams of dietary fiber per serving.

▽! = Extra fat, or prepared with added fat. (Count as 1 starch + 1 fat.)

🧂 = 480 milligrams or more of sodium per serving.

[a]The weight listed includes skin, core, seeds, and rind.

TABLE C-4 **Milk**

The Milk list groups milks and yogurts based on the amount of fat they have (fat-free/low fat, reduced fat, and whole). Cheeses are found on the Meat and Meat Substitutes list and cream and other dairy fats are found on the Fats list.

NOTE: In general, one milk choice is 1 cup (8 fluid ounces or ½ pint) milk or yogurt.

Milk and Yogurts

Food	Serving Size
Fat-free or low-fat (1%)	
1 fat-free/low-fat milk choice = 12 g carbohydrate, 8 g protein, 0–3 g fat, and 100 kcal.	
Milk, buttermilk, acidophilus milk, Lactaid	1 cup
Evaporated milk	½ cup
Yogurt, plain or flavored with an artificial sweetener	⅔ cup (6 oz)
Reduced-fat (2%)	
1 reduced-fat milk choice = 12 g carbohydrate, 8 g protein, 5 g fat, and 120 kcal.	
Milk, acidophilus milk, kefir, Lactaid	1 cup
Yogurt, plain	⅔ cup (6 oz)
Whole	
1 whole milk choice = 12 g carbohydrate, 8 g protein, 8 g fat, and 160 kcal.	
Milk, buttermilk, goat's milk	1 cup
Evaporated milk	½ cup
Yogurt, plain	8 oz

Dairy-Like Foods

Food	Serving Size	Count as
Chocolate milk		
fat-free	1 cup	1 fat-free milk + 1 carbohydrate
whole	1 cup	1 whole milk + 1 carbohydrate
Eggnog, whole milk	½ cup	1 carbohydrate + 2 fats
Rice drink		
flavored, low fat	1 cup	2 carbohydrates
plain, fat-free	1 cup	1 carbohydrate
Smoothies, flavored, regular	10 oz	1 fat-free milk + 2½ carbohydrates
Soy milk		
light	1 cup	1 carbohydrate + ½ fat
regular, plain	1 cup	1 carbohydrate + 1 fat
Yogurt		
and juice blends	1 cup	1 fat-free milk + 1 carbohydrate
low carbohydrate (less than 6 grams carbohydrate per choice)	⅔ cup (6 oz)	½ fat-free milk
with fruit, low-fat	⅔ cup (6 oz)	1 fat-free milk + 1 carbohydrate

TABLE C-5 **Sweets, Desserts, and Other Carbohydrates**

1 other carbohydrate choice = 15 grams carbohydrate, variable grams protein, variable grams fat, and variable kcalories.

NOTE: In general, one choice from this list can substitute for foods on the Starch, Fruits, or Milk lists.

Beverages, Soda, and Energy/Sports Drinks

Food	Serving Size	Count as
Cranberry juice cocktail	½ cup	1 carbohydrate
Energy drink	1 can (8.3 oz)	2 carbohydrates
Fruit drink or lemonade	1 cup (8 oz)	2 carbohydrates

(continued)

TABLE C-5 Sweets, Desserts, and Other Carbohydrates (*continued*)

Beverages, Soda, and Energy/Sports Drinks—continued

Food	Serving Size	Count as
Hot chocolate		
regular	1 envelope added to 8 oz water	1 carbohydrate + 1 fat
sugar-free or light	1 envelope added to 8 oz water	1 carbohydrate
Soft drink (soda), regular	1 can (12 oz)	2½ carbohydrates
Sports drink	1 cup (8 oz)	1 carbohydrate

Brownies, Cake, Cookies, Gelatin, Pie, and Pudding

Food	Serving Size	Count as
Brownie, small, unfrosted	1¼-inch square, ⅞ inch high (about 1 oz)	1 carbohydrate + 1 fat
Cake		
angel food, unfrosted	1/12 of cake (about 2 oz)	2 carbohydrates
frosted	2-inch square (about 2 oz)	2 carbohydrates + 1 fat
unfrosted	2-inch square (about 2 oz)	1 carbohydrate + 1 fat
Cookies		
chocolate chip	2 cookies (2¼ inches across)	1 carbohydrate + 2 fats
gingersnap	3 cookies	1 carbohydrate
sandwich, with crème filling	2 small (about ⅔ oz)	1 carbohydrate + 1 fat
sugar-free	3 small or 1 large (¾–1 oz)	1 carbohydrate + 1–2 fats
vanilla wafer	5 cookies	1 carbohydrate + 1 fat
Cupcake, frosted	1 small (about 1¾ oz)	2 carbohydrates + 1–1½ fats
Fruit cobbler	½ cup (3½ oz)	3 carbohydrates + 1 fat
Gelatin, regular	½ cup	1 carbohydrate
Pie		
commercially prepared fruit, 2 crusts	⅙ of 8-inch pie	3 carbohydrates + 2 fats
pumpkin or custard	⅛ of 8-inch pie	1½ carbohydrates + 1½ fats
Pudding		
regular (made with reduced-fat milk)	½ cup	2 carbohydrates
sugar-free or sugar- and fat-free (made with fat-free milk)	½ cup	1 carbohydrate

Candy, Spreads, Sweets, Sweeteners, Syrups, and Toppings

Food	Serving Size	Count as
Candy bar, chocolate/peanut	2 "fun size" bars (1 oz)	1½ carbohydrates + 1½ fats
Candy, hard	3 pieces	1 carbohydrate
Chocolate "kisses"	5 pieces	1 carbohydrate + 1 fat
Coffee creamer		
dry, flavored	4 tsp	½ carbohydrate + ½ fat
liquid, flavored	2 Tbsp	1 carbohydrate
Fruit snacks, chewy (pureed fruit concentrate)	1 roll (¾ oz)	1 carbohydrate
Fruit spreads, 100% fruit	1½ Tbsp	1 carbohydrate
Honey	1 Tbsp	1 carbohydrate
Jam or jelly, regular	1 Tbsp	1 carbohydrate
Sugar	1 Tbsp	1 carbohydrate
Syrup		
chocolate	2 Tbsp	2 carbohydrates
light (pancake type)	2 Tbsp	1 carbohydrate
regular (pancake type)	1 Tbsp	1 carbohydrate

(continued)

TABLE C-5 Sweets, Desserts, and Other Carbohydrates (*continued*)

Condiments and Sauces[a]

Food	Serving Size	Count as
Barbeque sauce	3 Tbsp	1 carbohydrate
Cranberry sauce, jellied	¼ cup	1½ carbohydrates
🧂 Gravy, canned or bottled	½ cup	½ carbohydrate + ½ fat
Salad dressing, fat-free, low-fat, cream-based	3 Tbsp	1 carbohydrate
Sweet and sour sauce	3 Tbsp	1 carbohydrate

Doughnuts, Muffins, Pastries, and Sweet Breads

Food	Serving Size	Count as
Banana nut bread	1-inch slice (1 oz)	2 carbohydrates + 1 fat
Doughnut		
cake, plain	1 medium (1½ oz)	1½ carbohydrates + 2 fats
yeast type, glazed	3¾ inches across (2 oz)	2 carbohydrates + 2 fats
Muffin (4 oz)	¼ muffin (1 oz)	1 carbohydrate + ½ fat
Sweet roll or Danish	1 (2½ oz)	2½ carbohydrates + 2 fats

Frozen Bars, Frozen Desserts, Frozen Yogurt, and Ice Cream

Food	Serving Size	Count as
Frozen pops	1	½ carbohydrate
Fruit juice bars, frozen, 100% juice	1 bar (3 oz)	1 carbohydrate
Ice cream		
fat-free	½ cup	1½ carbohydrates
light	½ cup	1 carbohydrate + 1 fat
no sugar added	½ cup	1 carbohydrate + 1 fat
regular	½ cup	1 carbohydrate + 2 fats
Sherbet, sorbet	½ cup	2 carbohydrates
Yogurt, frozen		
fat-free	⅓ cup	1 carbohydrate
regular	½ cup	1 carbohydrate + 0–1 fat

Granola Bars, Meal Replacement Bars/Shakes, and Trail Mix

Food	Serving Size	Count as
Granola or snack bar, regular or low-fat	1 bar (1 oz)	1½ carbohydrates
Meal replacement bar	1 bar (1⅓ oz)	1½ carbohydrates + 0–1 fat
Meal replacement bar	1 bar (2 oz)	2 carbohydrates + 1 fat
Meal replacement shake, reduced kcalorie	1 can (10–11 oz)	1½ carbohydrates + 0–1 fat
Trail mix		
candy/nut-based	1 oz	1 carbohydrate + 2 fats
dried fruit-based	1 oz	1 carbohydrate + 1 fat

KEY

🧂 = 480 milligrams or more of sodium per serving.

[a] You can also check the Fats list and Free Foods list for other condiments.

TABLE C-6 Nonstarchy Vegetables

The Nonstarchy Vegetables list includes vegetables that have few grams of carbohydrates or kcalories; starchy vegetables are found on the Starch list. 1 nonstarchy vegetable choice = 5 grams carbohydrate, 2 grams protein, 0 grams fat, and 25 kcalories.

NOTE: In general, one nonstarchy vegetable choice is ½ cup cooked vegetables or vegetable juice or 1 cup raw vegetables. Count 3 cups of raw vegetables or 1½ cups of cooked vegetables as one carbohydrate choice.

Nonstarchy Vegetables[a]

Amaranth or Chinese spinach	Kohlrabi
Artichoke	Leeks
Artichoke hearts	Mixed vegetables (without corn, peas, or pasta)
Asparagus	Mung bean sprouts
Baby corn	Mushrooms, all kinds, fresh
Bamboo shoots	Okra
Beans (green, wax, Italian)	Onions
Bean sprouts	Oriental radish or daikon
Beets	Pea pods
🧂 Borscht	😊 Peppers (all varieties)
Broccoli	Radishes
😊 Brussels sprouts	Rutabaga
Cabbage (green, bok choy, Chinese)	🧂 Sauerkraut
😊 Carrots	Soybean sprouts
Cauliflower	Spinach
Celery	Squash (summer, crookneck, zucchini)
😊 Chayote	Sugar pea snaps
Coleslaw, packaged, no dressing	😊 Swiss chard
Cucumber	Tomato
Eggplant	Tomatoes, canned
Gourds (bitter, bottle, luffa, bitter melon)	🧂 Tomato sauce
Green onions or scallions	🧂 Tomato/vegetable juice
Greens (collard, kale, mustard, turnip)	Turnips
Hearts of palm	Water chestnuts
Jicama	Yard-long beans

KEY

😊 = More than 3 grams of dietary fiber per serving.

🧂 = 480 milligrams or more of sodium per serving.

[a]Salad greens (like chicory, endive, escarole, lettuce, romaine, spinach, arugula, radicchio, watercress) are on the Free Foods list.

TABLE C-7 Meat and Meat Substitutes

The Meat and Meat Substitutes list groups foods based on the amount of fat they have (lean meat, medium-fat meat, high-fat meat, and plant-based proteins).

Lean Meats and Meat Substitutes

1 lean meat choice = 0 grams carbohydrate, 7 grams protein, 0–3 grams fat, and 100 kcalories.

Food	Amount
Beef: Select or Choice grades trimmed of fat: ground round, roast (chuck, rib, rump), round, sirloin, steak (cubed, flank, porterhouse, T-bone), tenderloin	1 oz
Beef jerky	1 oz
Cheeses with 3 grams of fat or less per oz	1 oz
Cottage cheese	¼ cup
Egg substitutes, plain	¼ cup
Egg whites	2
Fish, fresh or frozen, plain: catfish, cod, flounder, haddock, halibut, orange roughy, salmon, tilapia, trout, tuna	1 oz
Fish, smoked: herring or salmon (lox)	1 oz
Game: buffalo, ostrich, rabbit, venison	1 oz
Hot dog with 3 grams of fat or less per oz (8 dogs per 14 oz package) Note: May be high in carbohydrate.	1
Lamb: chop, leg, or roast	1 oz
Organ meats: heart, kidney, liver Note: May be high in cholesterol.	1 oz
Oysters, fresh or frozen	6 medium
Pork, lean	
Canadian bacon	1 oz
rib or loin chop/roast, ham, tenderloin	1 oz
Poultry, without skin: Cornish hen, chicken, domestic duck or goose (well-drained of fat), turkey	1 oz
Processed sandwich meats with 3 grams of fat or less per oz: chipped beef, deli thin-sliced meats, turkey ham, turkey kielbasa, turkey pastrami	1 oz
Salmon, canned	1 oz
Sardines, canned	2 medium
Sausage with 3 grams of fat or less per oz	1 oz
Shellfish: clams, crab, imitation shellfish, lobster, scallops, shrimp	1 oz
Tuna, canned in water or oil, drained	1 oz
Veal, lean chop, roast	1 oz

Medium-Fat Meat and Meat Substitutes

1 medium-fat meat choice = 0 grams carbohydrate, 7 grams protein, 4–7 grams fat, and 130 kcalories.

Food	Amount
Beef: corned beef, ground beef, meatloaf, Prime grades trimmed of fat (prime rib), short ribs, tongue	1 oz

Medium-Fat Meat and Meat Substitutes—continued

Food	Amount
Cheeses with 4–7 grams of fat per oz: feta, mozzarella, pasteurized processed cheese spread, reduced-fat cheeses, ' string	1 oz
Egg Note: High in cholesterol, so limit to 3 per week.	1
Fish, any fried product	1 oz
Lamb: ground, rib roast	1 oz
Pork: cutlet, shoulder roast	1 oz
Poultry: chicken with skin; dove, pheasant, wild duck, or goose; fried chicken; ground turkey	1 oz
Ricotta cheese	2 oz or ¼ cup
Sausage with 4–7 grams of fat per oz	1 oz
Veal, cutlet (no breading)	1 oz

High-Fat Meat and Meat Substitutes

1 high-fat meat choice = 0 grams carbohydrate, 7 grams protein, 8+ grams fat, and 150 kcalories. These foods are high in saturated fat, cholesterol, and kcalories and may raise blood cholesterol levels if eaten on a regular basis. Try to eat 3 or fewer servings from this group per week.

Food	Amount
Bacon	
pork	2 slices (16 slices per lb or 1 oz each, before cooking)
turkey	3 slices (½ oz each before cooking)
Cheese, regular: American, bleu, brie, cheddar, hard goat, Monterey jack, queso, and Swiss	1 oz
Hot dog: beef, pork, or combination (10 per lb-sized package)	1
Hot dog: turkey or chicken (10 per lb-sized package)	1
Pork: ground, sausage, spareribs	1 oz
Processed sandwich meats with 8 grams of fat or more per oz: bologna, pastrami, hard salami	1 oz
Sausage with 8 grams fat or more per oz: bratwurst, chorizo, Italian, knockwurst, Polish, smoked, summer	1 oz

(continued)

KEY

☺ = More than 3 grams of dietary fiber per serving.

▽ = Extra fat, or prepared with added fat. (Count as 1 starch + 1 fat.)

▯ = 480 milligrams or more of sodium per serving.

TABLE C-7 Meat and Meat Substitutes (*continued*)

Plant-Based Proteins

1 plant-based protein choice = variable grams carbohydrate, 7 grams protein, variable grams fat, and variable kcalories.

Because carbohydrate content varies among plant-based proteins, you should read the food label.

Food	Serving Size	Count as
"Bacon" strips, soy-based	3 strips	1 medium-fat meat
☺ Baked beans	⅓ cup	1 starch + 1 lean meat
☺ Beans, cooked: black, garbanzo, kidney, lima, navy, pinto, white[a]	½ cup	1 starch + 1 lean meat
☺ "Beef" or "sausage" crumbles, soy-based	2 oz	½ carbohydrate + 1 lean meat
"Chicken" nuggets, soy-based	2 nuggets (1½ oz)	½ carbohydrate + 1 medium-fat meat
☺ Edamame	½ cup	½ carbohydrate + 1 lean meat
Falafel (spiced chickpea and wheat patties)	3 patties (about 2 inches across)	1 carbohydrate + 1 high-fat meat
Hot dog, soy-based	1 (1½ oz)	½ carbohydrate + 1 lean meat
☺ Hummus	⅓ cup	1 carbohydrate + 1 high-fat meat
☺ Lentils, brown, green, or yellow	½ cup	1 carbohydrate + 1 lean meat
☺ Meatless burger, soy-based	3 oz	½ carbohydrate + 2 lean meats
☺ Meatless burger, vegetable- and starch-based	1 patty (about 2½ oz)	1 carbohydrate + 2 lean meats
Nut spreads: almond butter, cashew butter, peanut butter, soy nut butter	1 Tbsp	1 high-fat meat
☺ Peas, cooked: black-eyed and split peas	½ cup	1 starch + 1 lean meat
🥫 ☺ Refried beans, canned	½ cup	1 starch + 1 lean meat
"Sausage" patties, soy-based	1 (1½ oz)	1 medium-fat meat
Soy nuts, unsalted	¾ oz	½ carbohydrate + 1 medium-fat meat
Tempeh	¼ cup	1 medium-fat meat
Tofu	4 oz (½ cup)	1 medium-fat meat
Tofu, light	4 oz (½ cup)	1 lean meat

KEY

☺ = More than 3 grams of dietary fiber per serving.

▽ = Extra fat, or prepared with added fat. (Add an additional fat choice to this food.)

🥫 = 480 milligrams or more of sodium per serving (based on the sodium content of a typical 3-oz serving of meat, unless 1 or 2 oz is the normal serving size).

[a]Beans, peas, and lentils are also found on the Starch list; nut butters in smaller amounts are found in the Fats list.

TABLE C-8 Fats

Fats and oils have mixtures of unsaturated (polyunsaturated and monounsaturated) and saturated fats. Foods on the Fats list are grouped together based on the major type of fat they contain. 1 fat choice = 0 grams carbohydrate, 0 grams protein, 5 grams fat, and 45 kcalories.

NOTE: In general, one fat exchange is 1 teaspoon of regular margarine, vegetable oil, or butter; 1 tablespoon of regular salad dressing.

When used in large amounts, bacon and peanut butter are counted as high-fat meat choices (see Meat and Meat Substitutes list). Fat-free salad dressings are found on the Sweets, Desserts, and Other Carbohydrates list. Fat-free products such as margarines, salad dressings, mayonnaise, sour cream, and cream cheese are found on the Free Foods list.

Monounsaturated Fats

Food	Serving Size
Avocado, medium	2 Tbsp (1 oz)
Nut butters (trans fat-free): almond butter, cashew butter, peanut butter (smooth or crunchy)	1½ tsp
Nuts	
almonds	6 nuts
Brazil	2 nuts
cashews	6 nuts
filberts (hazelnuts)	5 nuts
macadamia	3 nuts
mixed (50% peanuts)	6 nuts
peanuts	10 nuts
pecans	4 halves
pistachios	16 nuts
Oil: canola, olive, peanut	1 tsp
Olives	
black (ripe)	8 large
green, stuffed	10 large

Polyunsaturated Fats

Food	Serving Size
Margarine: lower-fat spread (30%–50% vegetable oil, trans fat-free)	1 Tbsp
Margarine: stick, tub (trans fat-free) or squeeze (trans fat-free)	1 tsp
Mayonnaise	
reduced-fat	1 Tbsp
regular	1 tsp
Mayonnaise-style salad dressing	
reduced-fat	1 Tbsp
regular	2 tsp
Nuts	
Pignolia (pine nuts)	1 Tbsp
walnuts, English	4 halves
Oil: corn, cottonseed, flaxseed, grape seed, safflower, soybean, sunflower	1 tsp
Oil: made from soybean and canola oil—Enova	1 tsp
Plant stanol esters	
light	1 Tbsp
regular	2 tsp

Polyunsaturated Fats—continued

Food	Serving Size
Salad dressing	
🥫 reduced-fat Note: May be high in carbohydrate.	2 Tbsp
🥫 regular	1 Tbsp
Seeds	
flaxseed, whole	1 Tbsp
pumpkin, sunflower	1 Tbsp
sesame seeds	1 Tbsp
Tahini or sesame paste	2 tsp

Saturated Fats

Food	Serving Size
Bacon, cooked, regular or turkey	1 slice
Butter	
reduced-fat	1 Tbsp
stick	1 tsp
whipped	2 tsp
Butter blends made with oil	
reduced-fat or light	1 Tbsp
regular	1½ tsp
Chitterlings, boiled	2 Tbsp (½ oz)
Coconut, sweetened, shredded	2 Tbsp
Coconut milk	
light	⅓ cup
regular	1½ Tbsp
Cream	
half and half	2 Tbsp
heavy	1 Tbsp
light	1½ Tbsp
whipped	2 Tbsp
whipped, pressurized	¼ cup
Cream cheese	
reduced-fat	1½ Tbsp (¾ oz)
regular	1 Tbsp (½ oz)
Lard	1 tsp
Oil: coconut, palm, palm kernel	1 tsp
Salt pork	¼ oz
Shortening, solid	1 tsp
Sour cream	
reduced-fat or light	3 Tbsp
regular	2 Tbsp

KEY

🥫 = 480 milligrams or more of sodium per serving.

TABLE C-9 Free Foods

A "free" food is any food or drink choice that has less than 20 kcalories and 5 grams or less of carbohydrate per serving.

- Most foods on this list should be limited to 3 servings (as listed here) per day. Spread out the servings throughout the day. If you eat all 3 servings at once, it could raise your blood glucose level.
- Food and drink choices listed here without a serving size can be eaten whenever you like.

Low Carbohydrate Foods

Food	Serving Size
Cabbage, raw	½ cup
Candy, hard (regular or sugar-free)	1 piece
Carrots, cauliflower, or green beans, cooked	¼ cup
Cranberries, sweetened with sugar substitute	½ cup
Cucumber, sliced	½ cup
Gelatin	
dessert, sugar-free	
unflavored	
Gum	
Jam or jelly, light or no sugar added	2 tsp
Rhubarb, sweetened with sugar substitute	½ cup
Salad greens	
Sugar substitutes (artificial sweeteners)	
Syrup, sugar-free	2 Tbsp

Modified Fat Foods with Carbohydrate

Food	Serving Size
Cream cheese, fat-free	1 Tbsp (½ oz)
Creamers	
nondairy, liquid	1 Tbsp
nondairy, powdered	2 tsp
Margarine spread	
fat-free	1 Tbsp
reduced-fat	1 tsp
Mayonnaise	
fat-free	1 Tbsp
reduced-fat	1 tsp
Mayonnaise-style salad dressing	
fat-free	1 Tbsp
reduced-fat	1 tsp
Salad dressing	
fat-free or low-fat	1 Tbsp
fat-free, Italian	2 Tbsp
Sour cream, fat-free or reduced-fat	1 Tbsp
Whipped topping	
light or fat-free	2 Tbsp
regular	1 Tbsp

Condiments

Food	Serving Size
Barbecue sauce	2 tsp
Catsup (ketchup)	1 Tbsp
Honey mustard	1 Tbsp

Condiments—continued

Food	Serving Size
Horseradish	
Lemon juice	
Miso	1½ tsp
Mustard	
Parmesan cheese, freshly grated	1 Tbsp
Pickle relish	1 Tbsp
Pickles	
🖥 dill	1½ medium
sweet, bread and butter	2 slices
sweet, gherkin	¾ oz
Salsa	¼ cup
🖥 Soy sauce, light or regular	1 Tbsp
Sweet and sour sauce	2 tsp
Sweet chili sauce	2 tsp
Taco sauce	1 Tbsp
Vinegar	
Yogurt, any type	2 Tbsp

Drinks/Mixes

Any food on the list—without a serving size listed—can be consumed in any moderate amount.

- 🖥 Bouillon, broth, consommé
- Bouillon or broth, low-sodium
- Carbonated or mineral water
- Club soda
- Cocoa powder, unsweetened (1 Tbsp)
- Coffee, unsweetened or with sugar substitute
- Diet soft drinks, sugar-free
- Drink mixes, sugar-free
- Tea, unsweetened or with sugar substitute
- Tonic water, diet
- Water
- Water, flavored, carbohydrate free

Seasonings

Any food on this list can be consumed in any moderate amount.

- Flavoring extracts (for example, vanilla, almond, peppermint)
- Garlic
- Herbs, fresh or dried
- Nonstick cooking spray
- Pimento
- Spices
- Hot pepper sauce
- Wine, used in cooking
- Worcestershire sauce

KEY

🖥 = 480 milligrams or more of sodium per serving.

TABLE C-10 Combination Foods

Many foods are eaten in various combinations, such as casseroles. Because "combination" foods do not fit into any one choice list, this list of choices provides some typical combination foods.

Entrees

Food	Serving Size	Count as
🧂 Casserole type (tuna noodle, lasagna, spaghetti with meatballs, chili with beans, macaroni and cheese)	1 cup (8 oz)	2 carbohydrates + 2 medium-fat meats
🧂 Stews (beef/other meats and vegetables)	1 cup (8 oz)	1 carbohydrate + 1 medium-fat meat + 0–3 fats
Tuna salad or chicken salad	½ cup (3½ oz)	½ carbohydrate + 2 lean meats + 1 fat

Frozen Meals/Entrees

Food	Serving Size	Count as
🧂 ☺ Burrito (beef and bean)	1 (5 oz)	3 carbohydrates + 1 lean meat + 2 fats
🧂 Dinner-type meal	generally 14–17 oz	3 carbohydrates + 3 medium-fat meats + 3 fats
🧂 Entrée or meal with less than 340 kcalories	about 8–11 oz	2–3 carbohydrates + 1–2 lean meats
Pizza		
🧂 cheese/vegetarian, thin crust	¼ of a 12 inch (4½–5 oz)	2 carbohydrates + 2 medium-fat meats
🧂 meat topping, thin crust	¼ of a 12 inch (5 oz)	2 carbohydrates + 2 medium-fat meats + 1½ fats
🧂 Pocket sandwich	1 (4½ oz)	3 carbohydrates + 1 lean meat + 1–2 fats
🧂 Pot pie	1 (7 oz)	2½ carbohydrates + 1 medium-fat meat + 3 fats

Salads (Deli-Style)

Food	Serving Size	Count as
Coleslaw	½ cup	1 carbohydrate + 1½ fats
Macaroni/pasta salad	½ cup	2 carbohydrates + 3 fats
🧂 Potato salad	½ cup	1½–2 carbohydrates + 1–2 fats

Soups

Food	Serving Size	Count as
🧂 Bean, lentil, or split pea	1 cup	1 carbohydrate + 1 lean meat
🧂 Chowder (made with milk)	1 cup (8 oz)	1 carbohydrate + 1 lean meat + 1½ fats
🧂 Cream (made with water)	1 cup (8 oz)	1 carbohydrate + 1 fat
🧂 Instant	6 oz prepared	1 carbohydrate
🧂 with beans or lentils	8 oz prepared	2½ carbohydrates + 1 lean meat
🧂 Miso soup	1 cup	½ carbohydrate + 1 fat
🧂 Oriental noodle	1 cup	2 carbohydrates + 2 fats
Rice (congee)	1 cup	1 carbohydrate
🧂 Tomato (made with water)	1 cup (8 oz)	1 carbohydrate
🧂 Vegetable beef, chicken noodle, or other broth-type	1 cup (8 oz)	1 carbohydrate

KEY

☺ = More than 3 grams of dietary fiber per serving.

▽ = Extra fat, or prepared with added fat.

🧂 = 600 milligrams or more of sodium per serving (for combination food main dishes/meals).

TABLE C-11 Fast Foods

The choices in the Fast Foods list are not specific fast-food meals or items, but are estimates based on popular foods. Ask the restaurant or check its website for nutrition information about your favorite fast foods.

Breakfast Sandwiches

Food	Serving Size	Count as
🧂 Egg, cheese, meat, English muffin	1 sandwich	2 carbohydrates + 2 medium-fat meats
🧂 Sausage biscuit sandwich	1 sandwich	2 carbohydrates + 2 high-fat meats + 3½ fats

Main Dishes/Entrees

Food	Serving Size	Count as
🧂 ☺ Burrito (beef and beans)	1 (about 8 oz)	3 carbohydrates + 3 medium-fat meats + 3 fats
🧂 Chicken breast, breaded and fried	1 (about 5 oz)	1 carbohydrate + 4 medium-fat meats
Chicken drumstick, breaded and fried	1 (about 2 oz)	2 medium-fat meats
🧂 Chicken nuggets	6 (about 3½ oz)	1 carbohydrate + 2 medium-fat meats + 1 fat
🧂 Chicken thigh, breaded and fried	1 (about 4 oz)	½ carbohydrate + 3 medium-fat meats + 1½ fats
🧂 Chicken wings, hot	6 (5 oz)	5 medium-fat meats + 1½ fats

Oriental

Food	Serving Size	Count as
🧂 Beef/chicken/shrimp with vegetables in sauce	1 cup (about 5 oz)	1 carbohydrate + 1 lean meat + 1 fat
🧂 Egg roll, meat	1 (about 3 oz)	1 carbohydrate + 1 lean meat + 1 fat
Fried rice, meatless	½ cup	1½ carbohydrates + 1½ fats
🧂 Meat and sweet sauce (orange chicken)	1 cup	3 carbohydrates + 3 medium-fat meats + 2 fats
🧂 ☺ Noodles and vegetables in sauce (chow mein, lo mein)	1 cup	2 carbohydrates + 1 fat

Pizza

Food	Serving Size	Count as
Pizza		
🧂 cheese, pepperoni, regular crust	⅛ of a 14 inch (about 4 oz)	2½ carbohydrates + 1 medium-fat meat + 1½ fats
🧂 cheese/vegetarian, thin crust	¼ of a 12 inch (about 6 oz)	2½ carbohydrates + 2 medium-fat meats + 1½ fats

Sandwiches

Food	Serving Size	Count as
🧂 Chicken sandwich, grilled	1	3 carbohydrates + 4 lean meats
🧂 Chicken sandwich, crispy	1	3½ carbohydrates + 3 medium-fat meats + 1 fat
Fish sandwich with tartar sauce	1	2½ carbohydrates + 2 medium-fat meats + 2 fats
Hamburger		
🧂 large with cheese	1	2½ carbohydrates + 4 medium-fat meats + 1 fat
regular	1	2 carbohydrates + 1 medium-fat meat + 1 fat
🧂 Hot dog with bun	1	1 carbohydrate + 1 high-fat meat + 1 fat
Submarine sandwich		
🧂 less than 6 grams fat	6-inch sub	3 carbohydrates + 2 lean meats
🧂 regular	6-inch sub	3½ carbohydrates + 2 medium-fat meats + 1 fat
Taco, hard or soft shell (meat and cheese)	1 small	1 carbohydrate + 1 medium-fat meat + 1½ fats

(continued)

KEY

☺ = More than 3 grams of dietary fiber per serving.

▽ = Extra fat, or prepared with added fat.

🧂 = 600 milligrams or more of sodium per serving (for fast-food main dishes/meals).

TABLE C-11 Fast Foods (*continued*)

Salads

Food	Serving Size	Count as
🧂 🙂 Salad, main dish (grilled chicken type, no dressing or croutons)		1 carbohydrate + 4 lean meats
Salad, side, no dressing or cheese	Small (about 5 oz)	1 vegetable

Sides/Appetizers

Food	Serving Size	Count as
▽ French fries, restaurant style	small	3 carbohydrates + 3 fats
	medium	4 carbohydrates + 4 fats
	large	5 carbohydrates + 6 fats
🧂 Nachos with cheese	small (about 4½ oz)	2½ carbohydrates + 4 fats
🧂 Onion rings	1 serving (about 3 oz)	2½ carbohydrates + 3 fats

Desserts

Food	Serving Size	Count as
Milkshake, any flavor	12 oz	6 carbohydrates + 2 fats
Soft-serve ice cream cone	1 small	2½ carbohydrates + 1 fat

KEY

🙂 = More than 3 grams of dietary fiber per serving.

▽ = Extra fat, or prepared with added fat.

🧂 = 600 milligrams or more of sodium per serving (for fast-food main dishes/meals).

TABLE C-12 Alcohol

1 alcohol equivalent = variable grams carbohydrate, 0 grams protein, 0 grams fat, and 100 kcalories.

NOTE: In general, one alcohol choice (½ ounce absolute alcohol) has about 100 kcalories. For those who choose to drink alcohol, guidelines suggest limiting alcohol intake to 1 drink or less per day for women, and 2 drinks or less per day for men. To reduce your risk of low blood glucose (hypoglycemia), especially if you take insulin or a diabetes pill that increases insulin, always drink alcohol with food. While alcohol, by itself, does not directly affect blood glucose, be aware of the carbohydrate (for example, in mixed drinks, beer, and wine) that may raise your blood glucose.

Alcoholic Beverage	Serving Size	Count as
Beer		
light (4.2%)	12 fl oz	1 alcohol equivalent + ½ carbohydrate
regular (4.9%)	12 fl oz	1 alcohol equivalent + 1 carbohydrate
Distilled spirits: vodka, rum, gin, whiskey, 80 or 86 proof	1½ fl oz	1 alcohol equivalent
Liqueur, coffee (53 proof)	1 fl oz	1 alcohol equivalent + 1 carbohydrate
Sake	1 fl oz	½ alcohol equivalent
Wine		
dessert (sherry)	3½ fl oz	1 alcohol equivalent + 1 carbohydrate
dry, red or white (10%)	5 fl oz	1 alcohol equivalent

Physical Activity and Energy Requirements

Chapter 6 described how to calculate your estimated energy requirements by using an equation that accounts for your gender, age, weight, height, and physical activity level. This appendix first helps you determine the correct physical activity factor to use in the equation, either by calculating your physical activity level or by guesstimating it. Then the appendix presents tables that provide a shortcut to estimating total energy expenditure.*

Calculating Your Physical Activity Level

To calculate your physical activity level, record all of your activities for a typical 24-hour day, noting the type of activity, the level of intensity, and the duration. Then, using a copy of Table D-1, find your activity in the first column (or an activity that is reasonably similar) and multiply the number of minutes spent on that activity by the factor in the third column. Put your answer in the last column and total the accumulated values for the day. Now add the subtotal of the last column to 1.1 (to account for basal energy and the thermic effect of food) as shown. This score indicates your level of physical activity. Using Table D-2, find the PA (physical activity) factor for your gender that correlates with your physical activity level score and use it in the energy equation presented on p. 139 of Chapter 6.

Guesstimating Your Physical Activity Level

As an alternative to recording your activities for a day, you can use the first two columns of Table D-3 to decide if your daily activity is sedentary, low active, active, or very active. Find the PA factor for your gender that correlates with your typical physical activity level and use it in the energy equation presented on p. 139.

Using a Shortcut to Estimate Total Energy Expenditure

The DRI committee has developed estimates of total energy expenditure based on the equations presented in Chapter 6. These estimates are presented in Table D-4 for women and Table D-5 for men. You can use these tables to estimate your energy requirementis, the number of kcalories needed to maintain your current body weight. On the table appropriate for your gender, find your height in meters (or inches) in the left-hand column. Then follow the row across to find your weight in kilograms (or pounds). (If you can't find your exact

---

*This appendix, including the tables, is adapted from Committee on Dietary Reference Intakes, Food and Nutrition Board, Institute of Medicine, *Dietary Reference Intakes for Energy, Carbohydrate, Fiber, Fat, Fatty Acids, Cholesterol, Protein, and Amino Acids* (Washington, D.C.: National Academies Press, 2002).

TABLE D-1	Physical Activities and Their Scores		
If your activity was equivalent to this…	**Then list the number of minutes here and…**	**Multiply by this factor…**	**Add this column to get your physical activity level score:**
Activities of Daily Living			
Gardening (no lifting)		0.0032	
Household tasks (moderate effort)		0.0024	
Lifting items continuously		0.0029	
Loading/unloading car		0.0019	
Lying quietly		0.0000	
Mopping		0.0024	
Mowing lawn (power mower)		0.0033	
Raking lawn		0.0029	
Riding in a vehicle		0.0000	
Sitting (idle)		0.0000	
Sitting (doing light activity)		0.0005	
Taking out trash		0.0019	
Vacuuming		0.0024	
Walking the dog		0.0019	
Walking from house to car or bus		0.0014	
Watering plants		0.0014	
Additional Activities			
Billiards		0.0013	
Calisthenics (no weight)		0.0029	
Canoeing (leisurely)		0.0014	
Chopping wood		0.0037	

TABLE
D-1

TABLE D-1	Physical Activities and Their Scores (Continued)		
If your activity was equivalent to this…	**Then list the number of minutes here and…**	**Multiply by this factor…**	**Add this column to get your physical activity level score:**
Climbing hills (carrying 11 lb load)		0.0061	
Climbing hills (no load)		0.0056	
Cycling (leisurely)		0.0024	
Cycling (moderately)		0.0045	
Dancing (aerobic or ballet)		0.0048	
Dancing (ballroom, leisurely)		0.0018	
Dancing (fast ballroom or square)		0.0043	
Golf (with cart)		0.0014	
Golf (without cart)		0.0032	
Horseback riding (walking)		0.0012	
Horseback riding (trotting)		0.0053	
Jogging (6 mph)		0.0088	
Music (playing accordion)		0.0008	
Music (playing cello)		0.0012	
Music (playing flute)		0.0010	
Music (playing piano)		0.0012	
Music (playing violin)		0.0014	
Rope skipping		0.0105	
Skating (ice)		0.0043	
Skating (roller)		0.0052	
Skiing (water or downhill)		0.0055	
Squash		0.0106	

(Continued)

TABLE D-1	Physical Activities and Their Scores (Continued)		
If your activity was equivalent to this...	Then list the number of minutes here and...	Multiply by this factor...	Add this column to get your physical activity level score:
Surfing		0.0048	
Swimming (slow)		0.0033	
Swimming (fast)		0.0057	
Tennis (doubles)		0.0038	
Tennis (singles)		0.0057	
Volleyball (noncompetitive)		0.0018	
Walking (2 mph)		0.0014	
Walking (3 mph)		0.0022	
Walking (4 mph)		0.0033	
Walking (5 mph)		0.0067	
Subtotal			
Factor for basal energy and the thermic effect of food			1.1
Your physical activity level score			

TABLE D-2 | Physical Activity Level Scores and Their PA Factors

Physical Activity Level Score	Description	Men: PA Factor	Women: PA Factor
1.0 to 1.39	Sedentary	1.0	1.0
1.4 to 1.59	Low active	1.11	1.12
1.6 to 1.89	Active	1.25	1.27
1.9 and above	Very active	1.48	1.45

TABLE D-3 | Physical Activity Equivalents and Their PA Factors

Description	Physical Activity Equivalents	Men: PA Factor	Women: PA Factor
Sedentary	Only those physical activities required for normal independent living	1.0	1.0
	Activities equivalent to walking at a pace of 2–4 mph for the following distances:		
Low active	1.5 to 3.0 miles/day	1.11	1.12
Active	3 to 10 miles/day	1.25	1.27
Very active	10 or more miles/day	1.48	1.45

| TABLE D-4 | Total Energy Expenditure (TEE in kCalories per Day) for Women 30 Years of Age[a] at Various Levels of Activity and Various Heights and Weights |

Height m (in)	Physical Activity Level	Weight[b] kg (lb)					
1.45 (57)		38.9 (86)	45.2 (100)	52.6 (116)	63.1 (139)	73.6 (162)	84.1 (185)
		kCalories					
	Sedentary	1564	1623	1698	1813	1927	2042
	Low active	1734	1800	1912	2043	2174	2304
	Active	1946	2021	2112	2257	2403	2548
	Very active	2201	2287	2387	2553	2719	2886
1.50 (59)		41.6 (92)	48.4 (107)	56.3 (124)	67.5 (149)	78.8 (174)	90.0 (198)
		kCalories					
	Sedentary	1625	1689	1771	1894	2017	2139
	Low active	1803	1874	1996	2136	2276	2415
	Active	2025	2105	2205	2360	2516	2672
	Very active	2291	2382	2493	2671	2849	3027
1.55 (61)		44.4 (98)	51.7 (114)	60.1 (132)	72.1 (159)	84.1 (185)	96.1 (212)
		kCalories					
	Sedentary	1688	1756	1846	1977	2108	2239
	Low active	1873	1949	2081	2230	2380	2529
	Active	2104	2190	2299	2466	2632	2798
	Very active	2382	2480	2601	2791	2981	3171
1.60 (63)		47.4 (104)	55.0 (121)	64.0 (141)	76.8 (169)	89.6 (197)	102.4 (226)
		kCalories					
	Sedentary	1752	1824	1922	2061	2201	2340
	Low active	1944	2025	2168	2327	2486	2645
	Active	2185	2276	2396	2573	2750	2927
	Very active	2474	2578	2712	2914	3116	3318
1.65 (65)		50.4 (111)	58.5 (129)	68.1 (150)	81.7 (180)	95.3 (210)	108.9 (240)
		kCalories					
	Sedentary	1816	1893	1999	2148	2296	2444
	Low active	2016	2102	2556	2425	2594	2763
	Active	2267	2364	2494	2682	2871	3059
	Very active	2567	2678	2824	3039	3254	3469
1.70 (67)		53.5 (118)	62.1 (137)	72.3 (159)	86.7 (191)	101.2 (223)	115.6 (255)
		kCalories					
	Sedentary	1881	1963	2078	2235	2393	2550
	Low active	2090	2180	2345	2525	2705	2884
	Active	2350	2453	2594	2794	2994	3194
	Very active	2662	2780	2938	3166	3395	3623

TABLE D-4	Total Energy Expenditure (TEE in kCalories per Day) for Women 30 Years of Age[a] at Various Levels of Activity and Various Heights and Weights *(Continued)*					

Height m (in)	Physical Activity Level	Weight[b] kg (lb)					
1.75 (69)		56.7 (125)	65.8 (145)	76.6 (169)	91.9 (202)	107.2 (236)	122.5 (270)
		kCalories					
	Sedentary	1948	2034	2158	2325	2492	2659
	Low active	2164	2260	2437	2627	2817	3007
	Active	2434	2543	2695	2907	3119	3331
	Very active	2758	2883	3054	3296	3538	3780
1.80 (71)		59.9 (132)	69.7 (154)	81.0 (178)	97.2 (214)	113.4 (250)	129.6 (285)
		kCalories					
	Sedentary	2015	2106	2239	2416	2593	2769
	Low active	2239	2341	2529	2731	2932	3133
	Active	2519	2634	2799	3023	3247	3472
	Very active	2855	2987	3172	3428	3684	3940
1.85 (73)		63.3 (139)	73.6 (162)	85.6 (189)	102.7 (226)	119.8 (264)	136.9 (302)
		kCalories					
	Sedentary	2083	2179	2322	2509	2695	2882
	Low active	2315	2422	2624	2836	3049	3262
	Active	2605	2727	2904	3141	3378	3615
	Very active	2954	3093	3292	3562	3833	4103
1.90 (75)		66.8 (147)	77.6 (171)	90.3 (199)	108.3 (239)	126.4 (278)	144.4 (318)
		kCalories					
	Sedentary	2151	2253	2406	2603	2800	2996
	Low active	2392	2505	2720	2944	3168	3393
	Active	2693	2821	3011	3261	3511	3760
	Very active	3053	3200	3414	3699	3984	4270
1.95 (77)		70.3 (155)	81.8 (180)	95.1 (209)	114.1 (251)	133.1 (293)	152.1 (335)
		kCalories					
	Sedentary	2221	2328	2492	2699	2906	3113
	Low active	2470	2589	2817	3053	3290	3526
	Active	2781	2917	3119	3383	3646	3909
	Very active	3154	3309	3538	3838	4139	4439

[a]For each year below 30, add 7 kcalories/day to TEE. For each year above 30, subtract 7 kcalories/day from TEE.

[b]These columns represent a BMI of 18.5, 22.5, 25, 30, 35, and 40, respectively.

TABLE D-5 | Total Energy Expenditure (TEE in kCalories per Day) for Men 30 Years of Age[a] at Various Levels of Activity and Various Heights and Weights

Height m (in)	Physical Activity Level	Weight[b] kg (lb)					
1.45 (57)		38.9 (86)	47.3 (100)	52.6 (116)	63.1 (139)	73.6 (163)	84.1 (185)
				kCalories			
	Sedentary	1777	1911	2048	2198	2347	2496
	Low active	1931	2080	2225	2393	2560	2727
	Active	2127	2295	2447	2636	2826	3015
	Very active	2450	2648	2845	3075	3305	3535
1.50 (59)		41.6 (92)	50.6 (107)	56.3 (124)	67.5 (149)	78.8 (174)	90.0 (198)
				kCalories			
	Sedentary	1848	1991	2126	2286	2445	2605
	Low active	2009	2168	2312	2491	2670	2849
	Active	2215	2394	2545	2748	2951	3154
	Very active	2554	2766	2965	3211	3457	3703
1.55 (61)		44.4 (98)	54.1 (114)	60.1 (132)	72.1 (159)	84.1 (185)	96.1 (212)
				kCalories			
	Sedentary	1919	2072	2205	2376	2546	2717
	Low active	2089	2259	2401	2592	2783	2974
	Active	2305	2496	2646	2862	3079	3296
	Very active	2660	2887	3087	3349	3612	3875
1.60 (63)		47.4 (104)	57.6 (121)	64.0 (141)	76.8 (169)	89.6 (197)	102.4 (226)
				kCalories			
	Sedentary	1993	2156	2286	2468	2650	2831
	Low active	2171	2351	2492	2695	2899	3102
	Active	2397	2601	2749	2980	3210	3441
	Very active	2769	3010	3211	3491	3771	4051
1.65 (65)		50.4 (111)	61.3 (129)	68.1 (150)	81.7 (180)	95.3 (210)	108.9 (240)
				kCalories			
	Sedentary	2068	2241	2369	2562	2756	2949
	Low active	2254	2446	2585	2801	3017	3234
	Active	2490	2707	2854	3099	3345	3590
	Very active	2880	3136	3339	3637	3934	4232
1.70 (67)		53.5 (118)	65.0 (137)	72.3 (159)	86.7 (191)	101.2 (223)	115.6 (255)
				kCalories			
	Sedentary	2144	2328	2454	2659	2864	3069
	Low active	2338	2542	2679	2909	3139	3369
	Active	2586	2816	2961	3222	3483	3743
	Very active	2992	3265	3469	3785	4101	4417

| TABLE D-5 | Total Energy Expenditure (TEE in kCalories per Day) for Men 30 Years of Age[a] at Various Levels of Activity and Various Heights and Weights (Continued) |

Height m (in)	Physical Activity Level	Weight[b] kg (lb)					
1.75 (69)		56.7 (125)	68.9 (145)	76.6 (169)	91.9 (202)	107.2 (236)	122.5 (270)
		kCalories					
	Sedentary	2222	2416	2540	2757	2975	3192
	Low active	2425	2641	2776	3020	3263	3507
	Active	2683	2927	3071	3347	3623	3900
	Very active	3108	3396	3602	3937	4272	4607
1.80 (71)		59.9 (132)	72.9 (154)	81.0 (178)	97.2 (214)	113.4 (250)	129.6 (285)
		kCalories					
	Sedentary	2301	2507	2628	2858	3088	3318
	Low active	2513	2741	2875	3132	3390	3648
	Active	2782	3040	3183	3475	3767	4060
	Very active	3225	3530	3738	4092	4447	4801
1.85 (73)		63.3 (139)	77.0 (162)	85.6 (189)	102.7 (226)	119.8 (264)	136.9 (302)
		kCalories					
	Sedentary	2382	2599	2718	2961	3204	3447
	Low active	2602	2844	2976	3248	3520	3792
	Active	2883	3155	3297	3606	3915	4223
	Very active	3344	3667	3877	4251	4625	4999
1.90 (75)		66.8 (147)	81.2 (171)	90.3 (199)	108.3 (239)	126.4 (278)	144.4 (318)
		kCalories					
	Sedentary	2464	2693	2810	3066	3322	3579
	Low active	2693	2948	3078	3365	3652	3939
	Active	2986	3273	3414	3739	4065	4390
	Very active	3466	3806	4018	4413	4807	5202
1.95 (77)		70.3 (155)	85.6 (180)	95.1 (209)	114.1 (251)	133.1 (293)	152.1 (335)
		kCalories					
	Sedentary	2547	2789	2903	3173	3443	3713
	Low active	2786	3055	3183	3485	3788	4090
	Active	3090	3393	3533	3875	4218	4561
	Very active	3590	3948	4162	4578	4993	5409

[a]For each year below 30, add 10 kcalories/day to TEE. For each year above 30, subtract 10 kcalories/day from TEE.

[b]These columns represent a BMI of 18.5, 22.5, 25, 30, 35, and 40, respectively.

height and weight, choose a value between the two closest ones.) Look down the column to find the number of kcalories that corresponds to your activity level.

Importantly, the values given in the tables are for 30-year-old people. Women 19 to 29 should add 7 kcalories per day for each year below age 30; older women should subtract 7 kcalories per day for each year above age 30. Similarly, men 19 to 29 should add 10 kcalories per day for each year below age 30; older men should subtract 10 kcalories per day for each year above age 30.

Nutrition Assessment: Supplemental Information

Chapter 13 described data from nutrition assessments that help health professionals evaluate patients' nutrition status and nutrient needs. This appendix provides additional information that may be useful for complete assessments.

Weight Gain during Pregnancy

Chapter 10 described desirable weight-gain patterns during pregnancy. Figure E-1 shows prenatal weight-gain grids, which are used to plot the rate of weight gain during pregnancy.

Growth Charts

Health professionals evaluate physical development by monitoring growth rates of children and comparing these rates with those on standard growth charts. Standard charts compare length or height to age, weight to age, weight to length, head circumference to

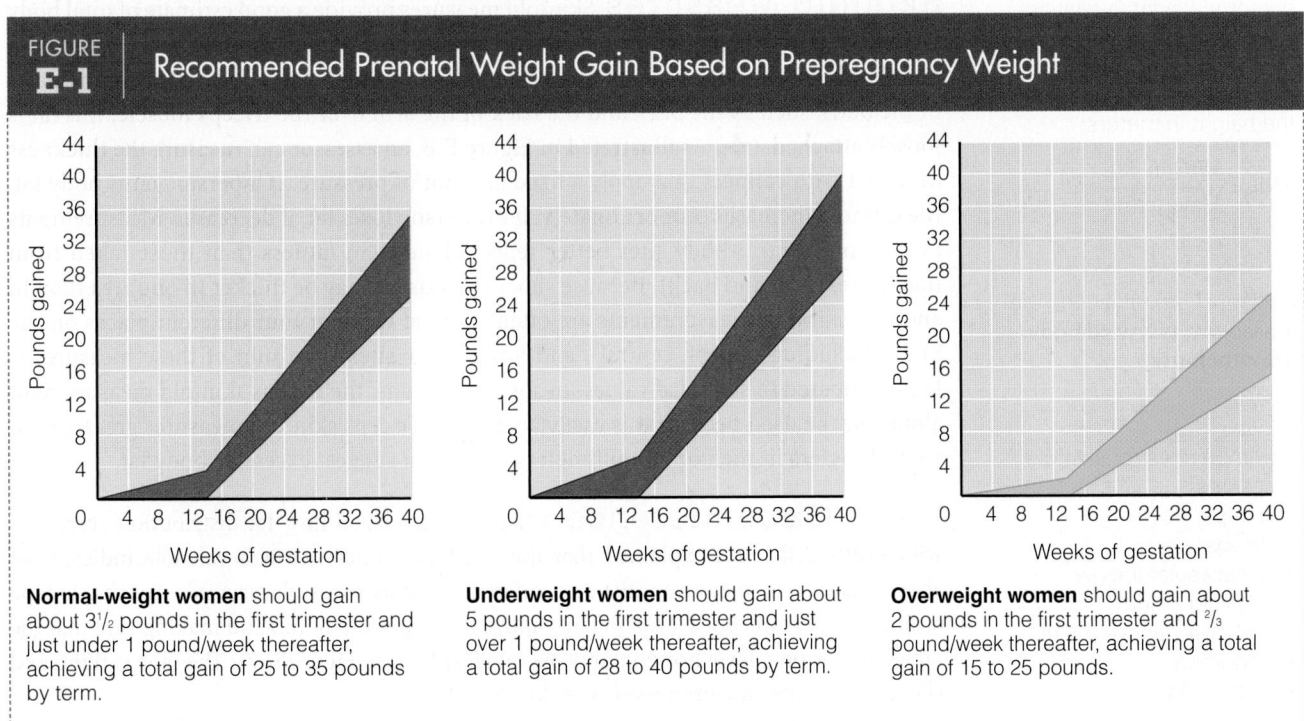

FIGURE E-1 Recommended Prenatal Weight Gain Based on Prepregnancy Weight

Normal-weight women should gain about 3½ pounds in the first trimester and just under 1 pound/week thereafter, achieving a total gain of 25 to 35 pounds by term.

Underweight women should gain about 5 pounds in the first trimester and just over 1 pound/week thereafter, achieving a total gain of 28 to 40 pounds by term.

Overweight women should gain about 2 pounds in the first trimester and ⅔ pound/week thereafter, achieving a total gain of 15 to 25 pounds.

age, and body mass index (BMI) (✚) to age. Although individual growth patterns vary, a child's growth curve will generally stay at about the same percentile throughout childhood. In children whose growth has been retarded, nutrition rehabilitation will ideally cause height and weight to increase to higher percentiles. In overweight children, the goal is for weight to remain stable as height increases, until weight becomes appropriate for height.

To evaluate growth in infants, an assessor uses a chart such as those in Figures E-2 (A and B) through E-5 (A and B). (✚) For example, the assessor follows these steps to determine the weight percentile:

- Select the appropriate chart based on age and gender.
- Locate the child's age along the horizontal axis on the bottom of the chart.
- Locate the child's weight in pounds or kilograms along the vertical axis.
- Mark the chart where the age and weight lines intersect, and read off the percentile.

For other measures, the assessor follows a similar procedure, using the appropriate chart. (When length is measured, use the chart for birth to 36 months; when height is measured, use the chart for 2 to 20 years.) Once all of the measures are plotted on growth charts, a skilled clinician can begin to interpret the data. Ideally, the height, weight, and head circumference should be in roughly the same percentile.

Head circumference is generally measured in children under two years of age. Since the brain grows rapidly before birth and during early infancy, extreme and chronic malnutrition during these times can impair brain development, curtailing the number of brain cells and the size of head circumference. Nonnutritional factors, such as certain disorders and genetic variation, can also influence head circumference.

Measures of Body Fat and Lean Tissue

Significant weight changes in both children and adults can reflect overnutrition or undernutrition with respect to energy and protein. To estimate the degree to which fat stores or lean tissues are affected by malnutrition, several anthropometric measurements are useful.

Skinfold Measures Skinfold measures provide a good estimate of total body fat and a fair assessment of the fat's location. Most body fat lies directly beneath the skin, and the thickness of this subcutaneous fat correlates with total body fat. In some parts of the body, such as the back and the back of the arm over the triceps muscle, this fat is loosely attached. (✚) As illustrated in Figure E-6, an assessor can measure the thickness of the fat with calipers that apply a fixed amount of pressure. If a person gains body fat, the skinfold increases proportionately; if the person loses fat, it decreases. Measurements taken from central-body sites better reflect changes in fatness than those taken from upper sites (arm and back). Because subcutaneous fat may be thicker in one area than in another, skinfold measurements are often taken at three or four different places on the body (including upper-, central-, and lower-body sites); the sum of these measures is then compared to standard values. In some situations, the triceps skinfold measurement alone may be used because it is easily accessible. Triceps skinfold measures greater than 15 millimeters in men or 25 millimeters in women suggest excessive body fat.

Waist Circumference Chapter 6 described how fat distribution correlates with health risks and explained that the waist circumference is a valuable indicator of abdominal fat. To measure waist circumference, the assessor places a nonstretchable tape around the person's body, crossing just above the upper hip bones and making sure that the tape remains on a level horizontal plane on all sides (see Figure E-7). The tape is tightened slightly, but without compressing the skin.

✚ Reminder: The *body mass index (BMI)* is an index of a person's weight in relation to height, determined by dividing the weight in kilograms by the square of the height in meters:

$$BMI = \frac{Weight\ (kg)}{Height\ (m)^2}$$

✚ Additional growth charts are available at **www.cdc.gov/growthcharts**

✚ Common sites for skinfold measures:
- Triceps
- Biceps
- Subscapular (below shoulder blade)
- Suprailiac (above hip bone)
- Abdomen
- Upper thigh

FIGURE E-2 (A and B) Length-for-Age and Weight-for-Age Percentiles

FIGURE E-3 | (A and B) Head Circumference-for-Age and Weight-for-Length Percentiles

Head Circumference-for-Age and Weight-for-Length Percentiles: Girls, Birth to 36 Months

Published May 30, 2000 (modified 10/16/00).
SOURCE: Developed by the National Center for Health Statistics in collaboration with the National Center for Chronic Disease Prevention and Health Promotion (2000).
www.cdc.gov/growthcharts.

Head Circumference-for-Age and Weight-for-Length Percentiles: Boys, Birth to 36 Months

Published May 30, 2000 (modified 10/16/00).
SOURCE: Developed by the National Center for Health Statistics in collaboration with the National Center for Chronic Disease Prevention and Health Promotion (2000).
www.cdc.gov/growthcharts.

FIGURE E-4 | (A and B) Stature-for-Age and Weight-for-Age Percentiles

Stature-for-Age and Weight-for-Age Percentiles: Boys, 2 to 20 Years

Stature-for-Age and Weight-for-Age Percentiles: Girls, 2 to 20 Years

FIGURE E-5 (A and B) Body Mass Index-for-Age Percentiles

FIGURE E-6 | How to Measure the Triceps Skinfold

Clavicle
Acromion process
Midpoint
Olecranon process

A. Find the midpoint of the arm:
1. Ask the subject to bend his or her arm at the elbow and lay the hand across the stomach. (If he or she is right-handed, measure the left arm, and vice versa.)
2. Feel the shoulder to locate the acromion process. It helps to slide your fingers along the clavicle to find the acromion process. The olecranon process is the tip of the elbow.
3. Place a measuring tape from the acromion process to the tip of the elbow.

Divide this measurement by 2 and mark the midpoint of the arm with a pen.
B. Measure the skinfold:
1. Ask the subject to let his or her arm hang loosely to the side.
2. Grasp a fold of skin and subcutaneous fat between the thumb and forefinger slightly above the midpoint mark. Gently pull the skin away from the underlying muscle. (This step takes a lot of practice. If you want to be sure you don't have muscle as well as fat, ask the subject to

contract and relax the muscle. You should be able to feel if you are pinching muscle.)
3. Place the calipers over the skinfold at the midpoint mark, and read the measurement to the nearest 1.0 millimeter in two to three seconds. (If using plastic calipers, align pressure lines, and read the measurement to the nearest 1.0 millimeter in two to three seconds.)
4. Repeat steps 2 and 3 twice more. Add the three readings, and then divide by 3 to find the average.

FIGURE E-7 | How to Measure Waist Circumference

Place the measuring tape around the waist just above the bony crest of the hip. The tape runs parallel to the floor and is snug (but does not compress the skin). The measurement is taken at the end of normal expiration.

Source: National Institutes of Health Obesity Education Initiative, *Clinical Guidelines on the Identification, Evaluation, and Treatment of Overweight and Obesity in Adults* (Washington, D.C.: U.S. Department of Health and Human Services, 1998), p. 59.

✚ The calculation of waist-to-hip ratio in a woman with a 28-inch waist and 38-inch hips is 28 ÷ 38 = 0.74.

Waist-to-Hip Ratio

The waist-to-hip ratio assesses abdominal obesity, but it offers no advantage over the waist circumference alone. To calculate the waist-to-hip ratio, divide the waistline measurement by the hip measurement. (✚) In general, women with a waist-to-hip ratio of 0.8 or greater and men with a waist-to-hip ratio of 0.9 or greater have an increased risk of developing diabetes and cardiovascular diseases.

Hydrodensitometry

To estimate body density using hydrodensitometry, the person is weighed twice—first on land and then again when submerged in water. Underwater weighing usually generates a good estimate of body fat and is useful in research, although the technique has drawbacks: it requires bulky, expensive, and nonportable equipment. Furthermore, submerging some people in water (especially those who are very young, very old, ill, or fearful) is difficult and not well tolerated.

Bioelectrical Impedance

To measure body fat using the bioelectrical impedance method, a very-low-intensity electrical current is briefly sent through the body by way of electrodes placed on the wrist and ankle. Fat impedes the flow of electricity; thus, the magnitude of the current is influenced by the body fat content. Recent food intake and hydration status can influence results. As with other anthropometric methods, bioelectrical impedance requires standardized procedures and calibrated instruments.

A number of other methods are sometimes used to estimate the body's content of body fat. Table E-1 describes common techniques often used in the clinical or research setting.

TABLE E-1	Selected Methods for Estimating Body Fat Content
Method	**Description**
Air-displacement plethysmography (Bod Pod®)	Estimates body density by measuring the body's volume (density = mass/volume); the density value allows derivation of the body's fat and lean tissue contents
Bioelectrical impedance assay	Measures the magnitude of an electrical current passed through the body; electrical conductivity is higher in lean tissues than in fat tissue
Dual energy X-ray absorptiometry	Analyzes the change in X-rays after they contact body tissues; fat and lean tissues have different effects on X-rays, allowing quantification of the various tissues
Hydrodensitometry (underwater weighing)	Estimates body density by comparing the body's weight on land and in water or by measuring the body's volume (density = mass/volume); the density value allows derivation of the body's fat and lean tissue contents
Isotope dilution—deuterated water	Measures total body water content by analyzing the dilution of heavy water (water with a heavy form of hydrogen) in body tissues; allows an estimate of lean tissue and body fat content
Skinfolds	Estimates subcutaneous fat in several regions of the body by using calipers to measure skinfold thicknesses
Ultrasound	Estimates subcutaneous fat in several regions of the body by using ultrasound to measure skinfold thicknesses

Nutritional Anemias

Anemia, a symptom of a wide variety of nutrition- and nonnutrition-related disorders, is characterized by the reduced oxygen-carrying capacity of blood. Iron, folate, and vitamin B_{12} deficiencies—caused by inadequate intake, poor absorption, or abnormal metabolism of these nutrients—are the most common causes of nutritional anemias. Table E-2 lists laboratory tests that distinguish among the various nutrition-related anemias. Some non-nutrition-related causes of anemia include massive blood loss, infections, hereditary blood disorders such as sickle-cell anemia, and chronic liver or kidney disease.

TABLE E-2	Laboratory Tests Useful in Evaluating Nutrition-Related Anemias
Test or Test Result	**What It Reflects**
For Anemia (general)	
Hemoglobin (Hg)	Total amount of hemoglobin in the red blood cells (RBC)
Hematocrit (Hct)	Percentage of RBC in the total blood volume
Red blood cell (RBC) count	Number of RBC
Mean corpuscular volume (MCV)	RBC size; helps to determine is anemia is microcytic (iron deficiency) or macrocytic (folate or vitamin B_{12} deficiency)
Mean corpuscular hemoglobin concentration (MCHC)	Hemoglobin concentration within the average RBC; helps to determine if anemia is hypochromic (iron deficiency) or normochromic (folate or vitamin B_{12} deficiency)
Bone marrow aspiration	The manufacture of blood cells in different developmental states
For Iron-Deficiency Anemia	
↓ Serum ferritin	Early deficiency state with depleted iron stores
↓ Transferrin saturation	Progressing deficiency state with diminished transport iron
↓ Erythrocyte protoporphyrin	Later deficiency state with limited hemoglobin production
For Folate-Deficiency Anemia	
↓ Serum folate	Progressing deficiency state
↓ RBC folate	Later deficiency state
For Vitamin B_{12}-Deficiency Anemia	
↓ Serum vitamin B_{12}	Progressing deficiency state
Schilling test	Absorption of vitamin B_{12}

Assessment of Iron Status

Chapter 9 described the progression of iron deficiency in detail, (✚) as well as the roles of some of the proteins involved in iron metabolism. This section describes the various tests that assess iron status, and Table E-3 provides acceptable values. Although other tests are more specific for detecting the early stages of iron deficiency, hemoglobin and hematocrit are most often used to detect iron-deficiency anemia because they are inexpensive and easily measured.

Serum Ferritin In the initial stage of iron deficiency, iron stores diminish. Iron is stored in the protein ferritin, which is located in the liver, spleen, and bone marrow. Serum ferritin values provide a noninvasive estimate of iron stores, because the ferritin levels in blood reflect the amounts stored in the tissues. Serum ferritin is not a reliable indicator of iron deficiency, however, because its concentrations are increased by infection, inflammation, alcohol consumption, and liver disease.

Serum Iron and Total Iron-Binding Capacity (TIBC) Early stages of iron deficiency are characterized by reduced levels of serum iron, which represent the amount of iron bound to transferrin, the iron transport protein. Total iron-binding capacity (TIBC) is a measure of the total amount of iron that the transferrin in blood can carry; thus, it is an indirect measure of the transferrin content of blood. During iron deficiency, the liver produces more transferrin in an effort to increase iron transport capacity, and therefore iron depletion is characterized by an increase in TIBC. TIBC reflects liver function as well as changes in iron metabolism.

TABLE E-3 | Criteria for Assessing Iron Status

Laboratory Test	Acceptable Values	Effect of Iron Deficiency
Serum ferritin	Male: 20-250 ng/mL Female: 10-120 ng/mL	Lower than normal
Serum iron	Male: 60-175 μg/dL Female: 50-170 μg/dL	Lower than normal
Total iron-binding capacity	250-450 μg/dL	Higher than normal
Transferrin saturation	Male: 20-50% Female: 15-50%	Lower than normal
Erythrocyte protoporphyrin	<70 μg/dL red blood cells	Higher than normal
Hemoglobin (Hb)	Male: 13.5-17.5 g/dL Female: 12.0-16.0 g/dL	Lower than normal
Hematocrit (Hct)	Male: 39-49% Female: 35-45%	Lower than normal
Mean corpuscular volume (MCV)	80-100 fL	Lower than normal

Note: ng = nanogram, μg = microgram, dL = deciliter, nmol = nanomole, fL=femtoliter

Sources: L. Goldman and D. Ausiello, coeditors, *Cecil Medicine* (Philadelphia: Saunders, 2008), pp. 2983–2991; R. J. Wood and A. G. Ronnenberg, Iron, in M. E. Shils and coeditors, *Modern Nutrition in Health and Disease* (Baltimore: Lippincott Williams & Wilkins, 2006), pp. 248–270.

Transferrin Saturation The percentage of transferrin that is saturated with iron is an indirect measure derived from the serum iron and total iron-binding capacity measures, as follows:

$$\%\text{Transferrin} = \frac{\text{serum iron}}{\text{total iron-binding capacity}} \times 100$$

During iron deficiency, transferrin saturation decreases. The transferrin saturation value is a useful indicator of iron status because it includes information about both the iron and transferrin content of blood.

Erythrocyte Protoporphyrin The iron-containing molecule in hemoglobin is heme, which is formed from iron and protoporphyrin. Protoporphyrin accumulates in the blood when iron supplies are inadequate for the formation of heme. However, levels of protoporphyrin may increase when hemoglobin synthesis is impaired for other reasons, such as lead poisoning or inflammation.

Hemoglobin When iron stores become depleted, hemoglobin production is impaired, and symptoms of anemia may eventually develop. Hemoglobin's usefulness in evaluating iron status is limited, however, because hemoglobin concentrations drop fairly late in the development of iron deficiency, and other nutrient deficiencies and medical conditions can also alter hemoglobin concentrations.

Hematocrit The hematocrit is the percentage of the total blood volume occupied by red blood cells. To measure the hematocrit, a clinician spins the blood samples in a centrifuge to separate the red blood cells from the plasma. Low values indicate a reduced number or size of red blood cells. Although this test is not specific for iron status, it can help to detect the presence of iron-deficiency anemia.

Mean Corpuscular Volume (MCV) The hematocrit value divided by the red blood cell count provides a measure of the average size of a red blood cell, referred to as the mean corpuscular volume (MCV). Such a measure helps to classify the type of anemia that is present. In iron deficiency, the red blood cells are smaller than average (microcytic cells).

Assessment of Folate and Vitamin B$_{12}$ Status

Folate deficiency and vitamin B$_{12}$ deficiency present a similar clinical picture—an anemia characterized by abnormally large, misshapen, and immature red blood cells (megaloblastic cells). Distinguishing between folate and vitamin B$_{12}$ deficiency is essential, however, because their treatments differ. Giving folate to a person with vitamin B$_{12}$ deficiency improves many of the test results indicative of vitamin B$_{12}$ deficiency, but this would be a dangerous treatment because vitamin B$_{12}$ deficiency causes nerve damage that folate cannot correct. Thus, inappropriate folate administration masks vitamin B$_{12}$-deficiency anemia, and nerve damage worsens. For this reason, it is critical to determine whether the anemia results from a folate deficiency or from a vitamin B$_{12}$ deficiency. Several of the following assessment measures help to make this distinction.

Mean Corpuscular Volume (MCV) As previously mentioned, MCV is a measure of red blood cell size. In folate and vitamin B$_{12}$ deficiencies, the red blood cells are larger than average, or macrocytic. Macrocytic cells are not necessarily indicative of nutrient deficiency, however, as they may also result from a high alcohol intake, liver disease, and various medications.

Serum Folate and Vitamin B$_{12}$ Levels Analyses of serum folate and vitamin B$_{12}$ levels are usually among the first tests conducted to determine the cause of macrocytic red blood cells. The presence of low serum levels of either nutrient is consistent with a deficiency of that

TABLE E-4	Criteria for Assessing Folate and Vitamin B_{12} Status	
Laboratory Test	**Acceptable Range**	**Effect of Folate or Vitamin B_{12} Deficiency**
Serum folate	3-16 ng/mL	Reduced in folate deficiency
Erythrocyte folate	140-628 ng/mL packed cells	Reduced in folate deficiency
Serum vitamin B_{12}	200-835 pg/mL	Reduced in vitamin B_{12} deficiency
Serum methylmalonic acid	70-270 nmol/L	Increased in vitamin B_{12} deficiency
Serum homocysteine	5-14 µmol/L	Increased in folate or vitamin B_{12} deficiency

Note: ng = nanogram, pg = picogram, nmol = nanomole, µmol = micromole

Sources: L. Goldman and D. Ausiello, coeditors, *Cecil Medicine* (Philadelphia: Saunders, 2008), p. 1238 and pp. 2983–2991.

nutrient, whereas adequate levels can help to rule out deficiency. Folate levels are not a specific measure of folate status, however; they may increase after folate consumption, and decrease due to alcohol consumption, pregnancy, or use of anticonvulsants. The folate levels in red blood cells (called erythrocyte folate) correlate well with folate stores and can help to diagnose folate deficiency, but the more reliable testing methods are not widely available. Table E-4 shows the acceptable ranges for these tests.

Methylmalonic Acid and Homocysteine Levels To determine whether a nutrient deficiency is present, clinicians can measure the levels of substances that accumulate when the functions of that nutrient are impaired. For example, blood levels of the amino acid homocysteine are usually increased by both folate and vitamin B_{12} deficiency, because both nutrients are needed for its metabolism. Methylmalonic acid, a breakdown product of several amino acids, requires vitamin B_{12} for its metabolism; hence, its levels accumulate in serum as a result of vitamin B_{12} deficiency. Because methylmalonic acid levels are not influenced by folate status, this measure is useful in distinguishing between folate and vitamin B_{12} deficiency.

Schilling test As Chapter 8 explained, vitamin B_{12} deficiency most often results from malabsorption, not poor intake. The Schilling test helps to diagnose malabsorption of vitamin B_{12}. After the patient takes an oral dose of radioactive vitamin B_{12}, a urine test determines whether the vitamin B_{12} was absorbed. More extensive testing can determine the cause of malabsorption.

Cautions about Nutrition Assessment

The tests outlined in this appendix yield information that becomes meaningful only when they are conducted and interpreted by a skilled clinician. Potential sources of error may be introduced at any step, from the collection of samples to the analysis and reporting of data. Equipment must be regularly calibrated to ensure accuracy of measurements. In addition, the assessor must keep in mind that few tests may be specific to the nutrient of interest alone, and lab results may reflect physiological processes other than the ones being tested. Furthermore, because many tests are not sensitive enough to detect the early stages of deficiency, follow-up testing is often necessary to identify a nutrition problem.

Aids to Calculations

Many mathematical problems have been worked out in the "How to" sections of the text. These pages provide additional help and examples.

Conversion Factors

A *conversion factor* is a fraction that converts a measurement expressed in one unit to another unit; for example, the fraction may be used to convert pounds to kilograms or feet to inches. To create a conversion factor, an equality (such as *1 kilogram = 2.2 pounds*) is expressed as a fraction:

$$\frac{1 \text{ kg}}{2.2 \text{ lb}} \text{ and } \frac{2.2 \text{ lb}}{1 \text{ kg}}.$$

Because a conversion factor has a value of *1* (the value in the numerator is equal to the value in the denominator), it can be used as a multiplier to change the *unit* of measure without changing the *value* of the measurement. To convert the units of a measurement, the fraction must have the desired unit in the numerator, as the unit in the denominator will cancel out the original unit.

Example 1 Convert the weight of 130 pounds to kilograms.
- Multiply 130 pounds by a conversion factor (fraction) that includes both pounds and kilograms and is arranged so that the desired unit (kilograms) is in the numerator:

$$130 \text{ lb} \times \frac{1 \text{ kg}}{2.2 \text{ lb}} = \frac{130 \text{ kg}}{2.2} = 59 \text{ kg}.$$

As this example shows, the unit for *pounds* cancels out and the unit for *kilograms* remains in the solution.

Example 2 The food label on a bottle of apple juice shows the contents in both fluid ounces and liters. How many liters are contained in a bottle that holds 64 fluid ounces?
- Multiply 64 ounces by a conversion factor that includes both fluid ounces and liters, with the desired unit (liters) in the numerator:

$$64 \text{ fl oz} \times \frac{1 \text{ L}}{33.8 \text{ fl oz}} = \frac{64 \text{ L}}{33.8} = 1.89 \text{ L}.$$

Percentages

A percentage expresses a fraction that has 100 in the denominator; for example, the term *50 percent* is equivalent to the fraction 50/100. Similar to other fractions, percentages are used to express a *proportion* of the *whole*; therefore, the units in the numerator and denominator must be similar. Any fraction can be expressed in hundredths and converted to a percentage by dividing the numerator by the denominator and multiplying by 100:

$$¼ = 0.25.$$
$$0.25 \times 100 = 25\%.$$

Example 3 Suppose your energy intake for the day is 2000 kcalories (kcal) and your recommended energy intake is 2400 kcalories. What percent of the recommended energy intake did you consume?

- Divide your intake by the recommended intake:

$$200 \text{ kcal (your intake)} \div$$
$$2400 \text{ kcal (recommended intake)} = 0.83.$$

- Multiply by 100 to express the decimal as a percentage:

$$0.83 \times 100 = 83\%$$

Example 4 A percentage can also be more than 100. Suppose your intake of vitamin C is 120 milligrams and your RDA (male) is 90 milligrams. What percent of the RDA for vitamin C did you consume?

$$120 \text{ mg (your intake)} \div 90 \text{ mg (RDA)} = 1.33.$$
$$1.33 \times 100 = 133\%.$$

Weights and Measures

LENGTH

1 meter (m) = 39 in.
1 centimeter (cm) = 0.4 in.
1 inch (in) = 2.5 cm.
1 foot (ft) = 30 cm.

TEMPERATURE

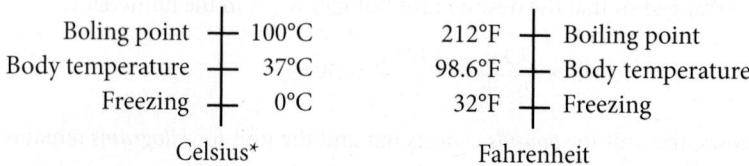

Boling point	100°C		212°F	Boiling point
Body temperature	37°C		98.6°F	Body temperature
Freezing	0°C		32°F	Freezing
	Celsius*			Fahrenheit

- To find degrees Fahrenheit (°F) when you know degrees Celsius (°C), multiply by 9/5 and then add 32.
- To find degrees Celsius (°C) when you know degrees Fahrenheit (°F), subtract 32 and then multiply by 5/9.

VOLUME

1 liter (L) = 1000 mL, 0.26 gal, 1.06 qt, 2.1 pt, or 33.8 fl. oz.
1 milliliter (mL) = 1/1000 L or 0.03 fluid oz.
1 gallon (gal) = 128 oz, 8 c, or 3.8 L.
1 quart (qt) = 32 oz, 4 c, or 0.95 L.
1 pint (pt) = 16 oz, 2 c, or 0.47 L.
1 cup (c) = 8 oz, 16 tbs, about 250 mL, or 0.25 L.
1 ounce (oz) = 30 mL.
1 tablespoon (tbs) = 3 tsp or 15 mL.
1 teaspoon (tsp) = 5 mL.

---

*Also known as *centigrade*.

WEIGHT

1 kilogram (kg) = 1000 g or 2.2 lb.
1 gram (g) = 1/1000 kg, 1000 mg, or 0.035 oz.
1 milligram (mg) = 1/1000 g or 1000 µg.
1 microgram (µg) = 1/1000 mg.
1 pound (lb) = 16 oz, 454 g, or 0.45 kg.
1 ounce (oz) = about 28 g.

ENERGY

1 kilojoule (kJ) = 0.24 kcal.
1 millijoule (mJ) = 240 kcal.
1 kcalorie (kcal) = 4.2 kJ.
1 g carbohydrate = 4 kcal = 17 kJ.
1 g fat = 9 kcal = 37 kJ.
1 g protein = 4 kcal = 17 kJ.
1 g alcohol = 7 kcal = 29 kJ.

Enteral Formulas

The large number of enteral formulas available allows patients to meet a wide variety of medical needs. The first step in narrowing the choice of formulas is to determine the patient's ability to digest and absorb nutrients. Table G–1 on pp. G-2 through G-3 lists examples of standard formulas for patients who can adequately digest and absorb nutrients, and Table G–2 on p. G-4 provides examples of elemental formulas for patients with a limited ability to digest or absorb nutrients. Each formula is listed only once, although a formula may have more than one use. A high-protein formula, for example, may also be a fiber-containing formula. Tables G–3 and G–4 on p. G-5 list modules that can be used to prepare modular formulas or enhance enteral formulas.

The information shown in this appendix reflects the literature provided by manufacturers and does not suggest endorsement by the authors. Manufacturers frequently add new formulas, discontinue old ones, and change formula composition. Consult the manufacturers' literature and websites for updates and additional examples of enteral formulas.[a] The following products are listed in this appendix:

- *Abbott Nutrition:* Glucerna 1.0 Cal, Jevity 1 Cal, Jevity 1.5 Cal, Nepro with Carb Steady, Optimental, Osmolite 1 Cal, Oxepa, Pivot 1.5 Cal, Polycose Powder, Promote, Promote with Fiber, Pulmocare, Suplena with Carb Steady
- *Nestlé Nutrition:* Compleat, Compleat Pediatric, Crucial, Diabetisource AC, Fibersource HN, Impact, Impact 1.5, Impact Glutamine, Isosource HN, MCT Oil, Microlipid, Novasource Renal, Nutren 1.0, Nutren 1.0 Fiber, Nutren 1.5, Nutren 2.0, Nutren Glytrol, Nutren Junior, Nutren Pulmonary, Nutren Replete, Nutren Replete Fiber, NutriHep, Peptamen, Peptamen Junior, Resource Beneprotein Instant Protein Powder, Vivonex Pediatric, Vivonex T.E.N.

[a]Sources for the information in this appendix: Abbott Nutrition, **www.abbottnutrition.com**, Nestlé Nutrition, **www.nestle-nutrition.com**.

TABLE G-1 | Standard Formulas

Product	Volume to Meet 100% RDI[a] (mL)	Energy (kcal/mL)	Protein or Amino Acids (g/L)	Carbohydrate (g/L)	Fat (g/L)	Notes
Lactose-Free, Standard Formulas						
Compleat	1313	1.07	48	128	40	Blenderized formula, 6 g fiber/L
Nutren 1.0	1500	1.00	40	127	38	25% fat from MCT
Osmolite 1 Cal	1321	1.06	44	144	35	20% fat from MCT
Lactose-Free, Fiber-Enhanced Formulas						
Jevity 1 Cal	1321	1.06	44	155	35	14 g fiber/L
Nutren 1.0 Fiber	1500	1.00	40	127	38	14 g fiber/L
Promote with Fiber	1000	1.00	63	138	28	14 g fiber/L
Lactose-Free, High-kCalorie Formulas						
Jevity 1.5 Cal	1500	1.50	64	216	50	22 g fiber/L
Nutren 1.5	1000	1.50	60	169	68	50% fat from MCT
Nutren 2.0	750	2.00	80	196	104	75% fat from MCT
Lactose-Free, High-Protein Formulas						
Fibersource HN	1165	1.20	53	160	39	20% fat from MCT, 10 g fiber/L
Isosource HN	1165	1.20	53	160	39	20% fat from MCT, low residue
Promote	1000	1.00	63	130	26	20% fat from MCT, low residue
Specialized Formulas: Pediatric (1 to 10 years)						
Compleat Pediatric	Varies[b]	1.00	38	130	39	Blenderized formula, 7 g fiber/L
Nutren Junior	Varies[b]	1.00	30	110	50	21% fat from MCT

(Continued)

TABLE G-1	Standard Formulas (Continued)					
Product	Volume to Meet 100% RDI[a] (mL)	Energy (kcal/mL)	Protein or Amino Acids (g/L)	Carbohydrate (g/L)	Fat (g/L)	Notes
Specialized Formulas: Glucose Intolerance						
Diabetisource AC	1250	1.20	60	100	59	36% kcal from carbohydrate, 15 g fiber/L
Glucerna 1.0 Cal	1420	1.00	42	96	54	34% kcal from carbohydrate, 14 g fiber/L
Nutren Glytrol	1400	1.00	45	100	48	40% kcal from carbohydrate, 15 g fiber/L
Specialized Formulas: Immune System Support						
Impact	1500	1.00	56	130	28	Enriched with arginine, nucleic acids, and omega-3 fatty acids
Impact 1.5	1250	1.50	84	140	69	Same as above
Impact Glutamine	1000	1.30	78	150	43	Same as above, and enriched with glutamine
Specialized Formulas: Chronic Kidney Disease (CKD)						
Nepro with Carb Steady	948	1.80	81	167	96	Low potassium, low phosphorus; to be used after dialysis has been instituted
Novasource Renal	1000	2.00	74	200	100	Low in electrolytes; to be used after dialysis has been instituted
Suplena with Carb Steady	948	1.80	45	205	96	Low in protein and electrolytes; for patients with CKD (stage 3 or 4)

(Continued)

| TABLE G-1 | Standard Formulas (Continued) |

Product	Volume to Meet 100% RDI[a] (mL)	Energy (kcal/mL)	Protein or Amino Acids (g/L)	Carbohydrate (g/L)	Fat (g/L)	Notes
Specialized Formulas: Respiratory Insufficiency						
Nutren Pulmonary	1000	1.50	68	100	95	55% kcal from fat, 40% fat from MCT
Oxepa	946	1.50	63	105	94	Enriched with omega-3 fatty acids and antioxidants; for mechanically ventilated patients
Pulmocare	947	1.50	63	106	93	55% kcal from fat, 20% fat from MCT, enriched with antioxidant nutrients
Specialized Formulas: Wound Healing						
Nutren Replete	1000	1.00	62	113	34	Enhanced with vitamins and minerals; for patients recovering from surgery, burns, and pressure ulcers
Nutren Replete Fiber	1000	1.00	62	113	34	Same as above; 14 g fiber/L

Note: MCT = Medium-chain triglycerides

[a] RDI = Reference Daily Intakes, which are labeling standards for vitamins, minerals, and protein. Consuming 100 percent of the RDI will meet the nutrient needs of most people using the product.

[b] Depends on age of child

TABLE G-2 | Elemental Formulas

Product	Volume to Meet 100% RDI[a] (mL)	Energy (kcal/mL)	Protein or Amino Acids (g/L)	Carbohydrate (g/L)	Fat (g/L)	Notes
Specialized Elemental Formula: Hepatic Insufficiency						
NutriHep	1000	1.50	40	290	21	Free amino acids, high in branched-chain amino acids and low in aromatic amino acids
Specialized Elemental Formulas: Immune System Support						
Crucial	1000	1.50	94	134	68	Enriched with arginine, omega-3 fatty acids, antioxidant nutrients, and zinc
Pivot 1.5 Cal	1500	1.50	94	172	51	Enriched with arginine, glutamine, omega-3 fatty acids, and antioxidant nutrients
Specialized Elemental Formulas: Malabsorption						
Optimental	1422	1.00	51	139	28	Contains MCT and arginine, enriched with antioxidants and omega-3 fatty acids
Peptamen	1500	1.00	40	127	39	70% fat from MCT
Vivonex T.E.N.	2000	1.00	38	210	3	Powder form, 100% free amino acids, enriched with glutamine
Specialized Elemental Formulas: Pediatric (1 to 10 years)						
Peptamen Junior	Varies[b]	1.00	30	138	38	60% fat from MCT
Vivonex Pediatric	Varies[b]	0.80	24	130	24	Powder form, 100% free amino acids

Note: MCT = Medium-chain triglycerides

[a] RDI = Reference Daily Intakes, which are labeling standards for vitamins, minerals, and protein. Consuming 100 percent of the RDI will meet the nutrient needs of most people using the product.

[b] Depends on age of child

TABLE G-3	Protein and Carbohydrate Modules			
Product	Major Ingredient	Energy (kcal/g)	Nutrient Content (g/100 g)
Resource Beneprotein Instant Protein Powder	Whey protein	3.6	86 g protein
Polycose Powder	Hydrolyzed cornstarch	3.8	94 g carbohydrate

TABLE G-4	Fat Modules			
Product	Major Ingredient	Energy (kcal/mL)	Fat Content (g/100 mL)
MCT Oil	Coconut oil	7.7	93
Microlipid	Safflower oil	4.5	50

Answers to Self Check Questions

Chapter 1
1. d, 2. d, 3. c, 4. d, 5. c, 6. b, 7. c, 8. b, 9. c, 10. c

Chapter 2
1. b, 2. a, 3. d, 4. a, 5. c, 6. a, 7. d, 8. c, 9. d, 10. d

Chapter 3
1. b, 2. b, 3. c, 4. a, 5. a, 6. a, 7. b, 8. a, 9. d, 10. c

Chapter 4
1. b, 2. c, 3. a, 4. d, 5. a, 6. a, 7. d, 8. d, 9. b, 10. a

Chapter 5
1. c, 2. b, 3. d, 4. d, 5. a, 6. d, 7. c, 8. b, 9. c, 10. d

Chapter 6
1. b, 2. c, 3. d, 4. d, 5. b, 6. a, 7. a, 8. b, 9. c, 10. c

Chapter 7
1. b, 2. a, 3. a, 4. c, 5. b, 6. c, 7. d, 8. b, 9. c, 10. b

Chapter 8
1. d, 2. d, 3. c, 4. a, 5. d, 6. d, 7. b, 8. c, 9. c, 10. a

Chapter 9
1. d, 2. b, 3. a, 4. d, 5. c, 6. d, 7. a, 8. d, 9. d, 10. b

Chapter 10
1. a, 2. d, 3. c, 4. c, 5. b, 6. d, 7. c, 8. d, 9. d, 10. c

Chapter 11
1. b, 2. a, 3. b, 4. d, 5. c, 6. d, 7. c, 8. b, 9. c, 10. d

Chapter 12
1. d, 2. c, 3. d, 4. d, 5. d, 6. d, 7. b, 8. b, 9. a, 10. b

Chapter 13
1. b, 2. d, 3. c, 4. d, 5. a, 6. d, 7. b, 8. d, 9. a, 10. a

Chapter 14
1. c, 2. b, 3. c, 4. b, 5. d, 6. a, 7. d, 8. c, 9. d, 10. a

Chapter 15
1. c, 2. a, 3. b, 4. c, 5. d, 6. b, 7. a, 8. c, 9. a, 10. d

Chapter 16
1. d, 2. a, 3. b, 4. c, 5. d, 6. b, 7. c, 8. c, 9. d, 10. a

Chapter 17
1. c, 2. b, 3. a, 4. d, 5. a, 6. c, 7. d, 8. b, 9. b, 10. c

Chapter 18
1. d, 2. c, 3. b, 4. b, 5. c, 6. c, 7. a, 8. d, 9. a, 10. d

Chapter 19
1. d, 2. a, 3. d, 4. b, 5. a, 6. b, 7. c, 8. d, 9. c, 10. a

Chapter 20
1. b, 2. d, 3. d, 4. c, 5. a, 6. c, 7. d, 8. c, 9. a, 10. b

Chapter 21
1. a, 2. d, 3. c., 4. a, 5. d, 6. c, 7. d, 8. b, 9. c, 10. d

Chapter 22
1. a, 2. c, 3. b, 4. d, 5. c, 6. a, 7. b, 8. b, 9. c, 10. d

Chapter 23
1. d, 2. c, 3. c, 4. b, 5. d, 6. b, 7. b, 8. a, 9. a, 10. d

Glossary

24-hour recall a record of foods consumed in the previous 24 hours; sometimes modified to include foods consumed in a typical day.

2-in-1 solution a parenteral solution that contains dextrose and amino acids, but excludes lipids.

abscesses (AB-sess-es) accumulations of pus

Acceptable Daily Intake (ADI) the amount of an artificial sweetener that individuals can safely consume each day over the course of a lifetime without adverse effect. It includes a 100-fold safety factor.

Acceptable Macronutrient Distribution Ranges (AMDR) ranges of intakes for the energy-yielding nutrients that provide adequate energy and nutrients and reduce the risk of chronic disease.

acetone breath a distinctive fruity odor on the breath of a person with ketosis.

achalasia (ack-ah-LAY-zhah) an esophageal disorder characterized by weakened peristalsis and impaired relaxation of the lower esophageal sphincter.

achlorhydria (AY-clor-HIGH-dree-ah) an absence of gastric acid secretions.

acid-base balance the balance maintained between acid and base concentrations in the blood and body fluids.

acidosis acid accumulation in the blood and body fluids; depresses the central nervous system and can lead to disorientation and, eventually, coma.

acids compounds that release hydrogen ions in a solution.

acquired immune deficiency syndrome (AIDS) the late stage of illness caused by infection with the human immunodeficiency virus (HIV); characterized by severe damage to immune function.

acute kidney injury abrupt decline in kidney function over a period of hours or days; also known as *acute renal failure.*

acute respiratory distress syndrome (ARDS) respiratory failure triggered by severe lung injury; a medical emergency that causes dyspnea and pulmonary edema and usually requires mechanical ventilation.

added sugars sugars and syrups added to a food for any purpose, such as to add sweetness or bulk or to aid in browning (baked foods). Also called *carbohydrate sweeteners,* they include glucose, fructose, corn syrup, concentrated fruit juice, and other sweet carbohydrates.

adequacy the characteristic of a diet that provides all the essential nutrients, fiber, and energy necessary to maintain health and body weight.

Adequate Intakes (AI) a set of values that are used as guides for nutrient intakes when scientific evidence is insufficient to determine an RDA.

adipokines (AD-ih-poh-kynz) protein hormones made and released by adipose tissue (fat) cells.

adiponectin a protein produced by the fat cells that inhibits inflammation and protects against insulin resistance, type 2 diabetes, and cardiovascular disease.

adipose tissue the body's fat, which consists of masses of fat-storing cells called adipose cells.

adolescence the period of growth from the beginning of puberty until full maturity. Timing of adolescence varies from person to person.

advanced glycation end products (AGEs) reactive compounds formed after glucose combines with protein; AGEs can damage tissues and lead to diabetic complications.

adverse reactions unusual responses to food (including intolerances and allergies).

aerobic physical activity activity in which the body's large muscles move in a rhythmic manner for a sustained period of time. Aerobic activity, also called *endurance activity*, improves cardiorespiratory fitness. Brisk walking, running, swimming, and bicycling are examples.

AIDS-defining illnesses diseases and complications associated with the later stages of an HIV infection, including wasting, recurrent bacterial pneumonia, opportunistic infections, and certain cancers.

alcohol-related birth defects (ARBD) a condition caused by prenatal alcohol exposure. ARBD is diagnosed when there is a history of substantial, regular maternal alcohol intake or heavy episodic drinking and birth defects known to be associated with alcohol exposure.

alcohol-related neurodevelopmental disorder (ARND) a condition caused by prenatal alcohol exposure. ARND is diagnosed when there is a confirmed history of substantial, regular maternal alcohol intake or heavy episodic drinking and behavioral, cognitive, or central nervous system abnormalities known to be associated with alcohol exposure.

aldosterone (al-DOS-ter-own) a hormone secreted by the adrenal glands that stimulates the reabsorption of sodium by the kidneys; also regulates chloride and potassium concentrations.

alkalosis excessive base in the blood and body fluids.

alpha-lactalbumin (lackt-AL-byoo-min) the chief protein in human breast milk, as **casein (CAY-seen)** is the chief protein in cow's milk.

alveoli (al-VEE-oh-lie) air sacs in the lungs. One air sac is an *alveolus.*

Alzheimer's disease a progressive, degenerative disease that attacks the brain and impairs thinking, behavior, and memory.

amino (a-MEEN-oh) acids building blocks of protein. Each contains an amino group, an acid group, a hydrogen atom, and a distinctive side group, all attached to a central carbon atom.

amniotic (am-nee-OTT-ic) sac the "bag of waters" in the uterus in which the fetus floats.

anaphylactic (AN-ah-feh-LAC-tic) shock a life-threatening whole-body allergic reaction to an offending substance.

anencephaly (AN-en-SEF-a-lee) an uncommon and always fatal type of neural tube defect; characterized by the absence of a brain.

aneurysm (AN-you-rih-zum) an abnormal enlargement or bulging of a blood vessel (usually an artery) caused by weakness in the blood vessel wall.

angina (an-JYE-nah or AN-ji-nah) pectoris a condition caused by ischemia in the heart muscle that results in discomfort or dull pain in the chest region. The pain often radiates to the left shoulder and arm or to the back, neck, and lower jaw.

anthropometric (AN-throw-poe-MEH-trik) related to physical measurements of the human body, such as height, weight, body circumferences, and percentage of body fat.

antibodies large proteins of the blood and body fluids, produced in response to invasion of the body by unfamiliar molecules (mostly proteins) called *antigens*. Antibodies inactivate the invaders and so protect the body.

antidiuretic hormone (ADH) a hormone released by the pituitary gland in response to high salt concentrations in the blood. The kidneys respond by reabsorbing water.

antioxidant (anti-OX-ih-dant) a compound that protects other compounds from oxygen by itself reacting with oxygen. *Oxidation* is a potentially damaging effect of normal cell chemistry involving oxygen. As a food additive, a preservative that delays or prevents rancidity of foods and other damage to food caused by oxygen.

appetite the psychological desire to eat; a learned motivation that is experienced as a pleasant sensation that accompanies the sight, smell, or thought of appealing foods.

artery a vessel that carries blood away from the heart.

arthritis inflammation of a joint, usually accompanied by pain, swelling, and structural changes.

artificial fats zero-energy fat replacers that are chemically synthesized to mimic the sensory and cooking qualities of naturally occurring fats but are totally or partially resistant to digestion.

artificial sweeteners noncarbohydrate, nonkcaloric synthetic sweetening agents; sometimes called *nonnutritive sweeteners*.

ascites (ah-SIGH-teez) an abnormal accumulation of fluid in the abdominal cavity.

ascorbic acid one of the two active forms of vitamin C. Many people refer to vitamin C by this name.

aspiration pneumonia a lung disease resulting from the abnormal entry of foreign material; caused by either bacterial infection or irritation of the lower airways.

aspiration drawing in by suction or breathing; a common complication of enteral feedings in which foreign material enters the lungs, often from GI secretions or the reflux of stomach contents.

atherogenic able to initiate or promote atherosclerosis.

atherosclerosis (ATH-er-oh-scler-OH-sis) a type of artery disease characterized by accumulations of lipid-containing (fatty) material on the inner walls of arteries.

atrophic gastritis (a-TRO-fik gas-TRI-tis) a condition characterized by chronic inflammation of the stomach accompanied by a diminished size and functioning of the mucosa and glands.

autoimmune an immune response directed against the body's own tissues.

bacterial overgrowth excessive bacterial colonization of the stomach and small intestine; may be due to low gastric acidity, altered GI motility, mucosal damage, or contamination.

balance the dietary characteristic of providing foods of a number of types in proportion to each other, such that foods rich in some nutrients do not crowd out foods that are rich in other nutrients.

bariatric (BAH-ree-AH-trik) surgery surgery that treats severe obesity.

Barrett's esophagus a condition in which esophageal cells damaged by chronic exposure to stomach acid are replaced by cells that resemble those in the stomach or small intestine, sometimes becoming cancerous.

basal metabolic rate (BMR) the rate of energy use for metabolism under specified conditions after a 12-hour fast and restful sleep, without any physical activity or emotional excitement, and in a comfortable setting. It is usually expressed as kcalories per kilogram of body weight per hour.

basal metabolism the energy needed to maintain life when a person is at complete digestive, physical, and emotional rest. Basal metabolism is normally the largest part of a person's daily energy expenditure.

bases compounds that accept hydrogen ions in a solution.

behavior modification the changing of behavior by the manipulation of *antecedents* (cues or environmental factors that trigger behavior), the behavior itself, and *consequences* (the penalties or rewards attached to behavior).

beriberi the thiamin-deficiency disease; characterized by loss of sensation in the hands and feet, muscular weakness, advancing paralysis, and abnormal heart action.

beta-carotene a vitamin A precursor made by plants and stored in human fat tissue; an orange pigment.

BHA, BHT preservatives commonly used to slow the development of "off" flavors, odors, and color changes caused by oxidation.

bifidus (BIFF-id-us, by-FEED-us) factors factors in colostrum and breast milk that favor the growth of the "friendly" bacterium *Lactobacillus* (lack-toe-ba-SILL-us) *bifidus* in the infant's intestinal tract. These bacteria prevent other, less desirable intestinal inhabitants from flourishing.

binders chemical compounds in foods that combine with nutrients (especially minerals) to form complexes the body cannot absorb. Examples include phytates and oxalates.

bioavailability the rate and extent to which a nutrient is absorbed and used.

blastocyst (BLASS-toe-sist) the developmental stage of the zygote when it is about five days old and ready for implantation.

blenderized formulas enteral formulas that are prepared by using a food blender to mix and puree whole foods.

body mass index (BMI) an index of a person's weight in relation to height; determined by dividing the weight (in kilograms) by the square of the height (in meters).

bolus (BOH-lus) feeding delivery of about 250 to 500 milliliters of formula in less than 20 minutes.

bolus (BOH-lus) the portion of food swallowed at one time.

bone marrow transplant a procedure that replaces bone marrow that has been destroyed by cancer treatment; it is also used to treat certain types of cancers and blood disorders. Also called *hematopoietic stem cell transplantation*.

Bowman's (BOE-minz) capsule a cuplike component of the nephron that surrounds the glomerulus and collects the filtrate that is passed to the tubules.

bronchi (BRON-key), bronchioles (BRON-key-oles) the main airways of the lungs. The singular form of bronchi is *bronchus*.

buffalo hump the accumulation of fatty tissue at the base of the neck.

buffers compounds that can reversibly combine with hydrogen ions to help keep a solution's acidity or alkalinity constant.

built environment the buildings, roads, utilities, homes, fixtures, parks, and all other man-made entities that form the physical characteristics of a community.

calcium rigor hardness or stiffness of the muscles caused by high blood calcium.

calcium tetany intermittent spasms of the extremities due to nervous and muscular excitability caused by low blood calcium.

calories units by which energy is measured. Food energy is measured in **kilocalories** (1000 calories equal 1 kilocalorie), abbreviated **kcalories** or kcal. One kcalorie is the amount of heat necessary to raise the temperature of 1 kilogram (kg) of water 1°C. The scientific use of the term *kcalorie* is the same as the popular use of the term *calorie*.

cancer cachexia (ka-KEK-see-ah) a wasting syndrome associated with cancer that is characterized by anorexia, muscle wasting, weight loss, and fatigue.

cancers diseases characterized by the uncontrolled growth of a group of cells, which can destroy adjacent tissues and spread to other areas of the body via lymph or blood.

capillaries small vessels that branch from an artery. Capillaries connect arteries to veins. Oxygen, nutrients, and waste materials are exchanged across capillary walls.

carbohydrates energy nutrients composed of monosaccharides.

carbohydrate-to-insulin ratio the amount of carbohydrate that can be handled per unit of insulin. On average, every 15 grams of carbohydrate requires about 1 unit of rapid- or short-acting insulin.

carcinogenesis (CAR-sin-oh-JEN-eh-sis) the process of cancer development.

carcinogens (CAR-sin-oh-jenz or car-SIN-oh-jenz) substances that can cause cancer (the adjective is *carcinogenic*).

cardiac cachexia a condition of severe malnutrition that develops in heart failure patients; characterized by weight loss and tissue wasting.

cardiac output the volume of blood pumped by the heart within a specified period of time.

cardiovascular disease (CVD) a general term for all diseases of the heart and blood vessels.

cataracts thickenings of the eye lenses that impair vision and can lead to blindness.

cathartics (ca-THART-ics) strong laxatives.

catheter a thin tube placed within a narrow lumen (such as a blood vessel) or body cavity; can be used to infuse or withdraw fluids or keep a passage open.

celiac (SEE-lee-ack) disease an immune disorder characterized by an abnormal immune response to the dietary protein gluten; also called *gluten-sensitive enteropathy* or *celiac sprue*.

cellulite (SELL-you-light or SELL-you-leet) supposedly, a lumpy form of fat; actually, a fraud. Fatty areas of the body may appear lumpy when the strands of connective tissue that attach the skin to underlying muscles pull tight where the fat is thick. The fat itself is the same as fat anywhere else in the body. If the fat in these areas is lost, the lumpy appearance disappears.

central obesity excess fat around the trunk of the body; also called *abdominal fat* or *upper-body fat*.

central veins the large-diameter veins located close to the heart.

cerebral cortex the outer surface of the cerebrum, which is the largest part of the brain.

Certified Diabetes Educator (CDE) a health care professional who specializes in diabetes management education. Certification is obtained from the National Certification Board for Diabetes Educators.

chemotherapy the use of drugs to arrest or destroy cancer cells; these drugs are called *antineoplastic agents*.

choline a nonessential nutrient that can be made in the body from an amino acid.

chronic bronchitis (bron-KYE-tis) a lung disorder characterized by persistent inflammation and excessive secretions of mucus in the main airways of the lungs; diagnosis is based on the presence of a chronic, productive cough for at least three months of the year for two successive years.

chronic diseases degenerative diseases characterized by deterioration of the body organs. Examples include heart disease, cancer, and diabetes.

chronic hypertension in pregnant women, hypertension that is present and documented before pregnancy; in women whose prepregnancy blood pressure is unknown, the presence of sustained hypertension before 20 weeks of gestation.

chronic kidney disease a kidney disease characterized by gradual, irreversible deterioration of the kidneys; also known as *chronic renal failure*.

chronic obstructive pulmonary disease (COPD) a group of lung diseases characterized by persistent obstructed airflow through the lungs and airways; includes chronic bronchitis and emphysema.

chronological age a person's age in years from his or her date of birth.

chylomicrons (kye-lo-MY-crons) the lipoproteins that transport lipids from the intestinal cells into the body. The cells of the body remove the lipids they need from the chylomicrons, leaving chylomicron remnants to be picked up by the liver cells.

chyme (KIME) the semiliquid mass of partly digested food expelled by the stomach into the duodenum (the top portion of the small intestine).

cirrhosis (sih-ROE-sis) an advanced stage of liver disease in which extensive scarring replaces healthy liver tissue, causing impaired liver function and eventual liver failure.

claudication (CLAW-dih-KAY-shun) pain in the legs while walking; usually due to an inadequate supply of blood to muscles.

clear liquid diet a diet that consists of foods that are liquid at room temperature, require minimal digestion, and leave little residue (undigested material) in the colon.

clinically severe obesity a BMI of 40 or greater or a BMI of 35 or greater and one or more serious conditions such as hypertension. Another term used to describe the same condition is *morbid obesity*.

closed feeding system a delivery system in which the formula comes prepackaged in a container that can be attached directly to the feeding tube for administration.

coenzyme (co-EN-zime) a small molecule that works with an enzyme to promote the enzyme's activity. Many coenzymes have B vitamins as part of their structure.

cofactor a mineral element that, like a coenzyme, works with an enzyme to facilitate a chemical reaction.

cognitive skills as taught in behavior therapy, changes to conscious thoughts with the goal of improving adherence to lifestyle modifications; examples are problem-solving skills or the correction of false negative thoughts, termed *cognitive restructuring*.

colectomy removal of a portion or all of the colon.

collagen the characteristic protein of connective tissue.

collaterals blood vessels that enlarge to allow an alternative pathway for diverted blood.

colostomy (co-LAH-stoe-me) a surgical passage through the abdominal wall into the colon.

colostrum (co-LAHS-trum) a milklike secretion from the breasts that is rich in protective factors. Colostrum is present during the first day or so after delivery, before milk appears.

complementary proteins two or more proteins whose amino acid assortments complement each other in such a way that the essential amino acids missing from one are supplied by the other.

conditionally essential amino acid an amino acid that is normally nonessential but must be supplied by the diet in special circumstances when the need for it becomes greater than the body's ability to produce it.

continuous feedings slow delivery of formula at a constant rate over an 8- to 24-hour period.

continuous parenteral nutrition continuous administration of parenteral solutions over a 24-hour period.

cornea (KOR-nee-uh) the hard, transparent membrane covering the outside of the eye.

coronary heart disease (CHD) a chronic, progressive disease characterized by obstructed blood flow in the coronary arteries; also called *coronary artery disease*.

cretinism (CREE-tin-ism) an iodine-deficiency disease characterized by mental and physical retardation.

critical pathways coordinated programs of treatment that merge the care plans of different health practitioners; also called *clinical pathways*.

critical period a finite period during development in which certain events occur that will have irreversible effects on later developmental stages; usually a period of rapid cell division.

Crohn's disease an inflammatory bowel disease that usually occurs in the lower portion of the small intestine and the colon. Inflammation may pervade the entire intestinal wall.

cryptosporidiosis (KRIP-toe-spor-ih-dee-OH-sis) a foodborne illness caused by the parasite *Cryptosporidium parvum*.

cyanosis (sigh-ah-NOH-sis) a bluish cast in the skin due to the color of deoxygenated hemoglobin. Cyanosis is most evident in individuals with lighter, thinner skin; it is mostly seen on lips, cheeks, and ears and under the nails.

cyclic parenteral nutrition administration of parenteral solutions over a 10- to 16-hour period each day.

cystic fibrosis an inherited disease characterized by the presence of abnormally viscous exocrine secretions; often leads to respiratory illness and pancreatic insufficiency.

cystinuria (SIS-tin-NOO-ree-ah) an inherited disorder characterized by elevated urinary excretion of several amino acids, including cystine.

Daily Values reference values developed by the FDA specifically for use on food labels.

dawn phenomenon morning hyperglycemia that is caused by the early-morning release of growth hormone, which counteracts insulin's glucose-lowering effects.

debridement the surgical removal of dead, damaged, or contaminated tissue resulting from burns or wounds; helps to prevent infection and hasten healing.

deficient in regard to nutrient intake, describes the amount below which almost all healthy people can be expected, over time, to experience deficiency symptoms.

dehydration the loss of water from the body that occurs when water output exceeds water input. The symptoms progress rapidly from thirst, to weakness, to exhaustion and delirium and end in death if not corrected.

denaturation (dee-nay-cher-AY-shun) the change in a protein's shape brought about by heat, acid, or other agents. Past a certain point, denaturation is irreversible.

dental caries the gradual decay and disintegration of a tooth.

dermatitis herpetiformis (DERM-ah-TYE-tis HER-peh-tih-FOR-mis) a gluten-sensitive disorder characterized by a severe skin rash.

diabetes (DYE-ah-BEE-teez) mellitus a group of metabolic disorders characterized by hyperglycemia and disordered insulin metabolism.

diabetic coma a coma that occurs in uncontrolled diabetes; may be due to diabetic ketoacidosis, the hyperosmolar hyperglycemic syndrome, or severe hypoglycemia.

diabetic nephropathy (neh-FRAH-pah-thee) damage to the kidneys that results from long-term diabetes.

diabetic neuropathy (nur-RAH-pah-thee) complications of diabetes that cause damage to nerves.

diabetic retinopathy (REH-tih-NAH-pah-thee) retinal damage that results from long-term diabetes.

dialysate (dye-AL-ih-sate) the solution used in dialysis to draw wastes and fluids from the blood.

dialysis (dye-AH-lih-sis) a treatment that removes wastes and excess fluid from the blood after the kidneys have stopped functioning. The most common types of dialysis are *hemodialysis* and *peritoneal dialysis* (see Nutrition in Practice 22).

dialyzer (DYE-ah-LYE-zer) a machine used in hemodialysis to filter the blood; also called an *artificial kidney*.

diet manual a resource that specifies the exact foods or preparation methods to include or exclude in modified diets and provides sample menus.

diet orders specific instructions concerning dietary management including the type, amount, and frequency of feedings; also called *diet prescriptions* or *nutrition prescriptions*.

diet progression a change in diet as a patient's tolerances permit.

dietary antioxidants compounds typically found in plant foods that significantly decrease the adverse effects of oxidation on living tissues. The major antioxidant vitamins are vitamin E, vitamin C, and beta-carotene.

dietary fibers a general term denoting in plant foods the polysaccharides cellulose, hemicellulose, pectins, gums and mucilages, as well as the nonpolysaccharide lignins, that are not digested by human digestive enzymes, although some are digested by GI tract bacteria.

dietary folate equivalents (DFE) the amount of folate available to the body from naturally occurring sources, fortified foods, and supplements, accounting for differences in bioavailability from each source.

Dietary Reference Intakes (DRI) a set of values for the dietary nutrient intakes of healthy people in the United States and Canada. These values are used for planning and assessing diets.

differentiation the development of specific functions different from those of the original.

digestion the process by which complex food particles are broken down to smaller absorbable particles.

digestive system all the organs and glands associated with the ingestion and digestion of food.

dipeptide two amino acids bonded together.

disaccharides (dye-SACK-uh-rides) a pair of sugar units bonded together.

discretionary kcalorie allowance the kcalories remaining in a person's energy allowance after consuming enough nutrient-dense foods to meet all nutrient needs for a day.

diuresis (DYE-uh-REE-sis) increased urine production.

diuretics (dye-yoo-RET-ics) medications that promote the excretion of water through the kidneys. Not all diuretics increase the urinary loss of potassium. Some, called potassium-sparing diuretics, are less likely to result in a potassium deficiency (see Chapter 21).

diverticulitis (DYE-ver-tic-you-LYE-tis) an inflammation or infection involving diverticula.

diverticulosis (DYE-ver-tic-you-LOH-sis) an intestinal condition characterized by the presence of small herniations (called diverticula) in the intestinal wall.

dumping syndrome symptoms that result from the rapid emptying of an osmotic load from the stomach into the small intestine. Early symptoms include nausea, abdominal cramping, and diarrhea; later symptoms are those of hypoglycemia and include confusion, headache, and hunger.

dysentery (DIS-en-terry) an infection of the gastrointestinal tract caused by an amoeba or bacterium that gives rise to severe diarrhea.

dyspepsia a feeling of pain, bloating, or discomfort in the upper abdominal area, often called *indigestion;* a symptom of illness rather than a disease itself.

dysphagia difficulty swallowing.

dyspnea (DISP-nee-ah) shortness of breath.

eclampsia (eh-KLAMP-see-ah) a severe complication during pregnancy in which seizures occur.

edema (eh-DEEM-uh) the swelling of body tissue caused by leakage of fluid from the blood vessels and accumulation of the fluid in the interstitial spaces.

electrolyte solutions solutions that can conduct electricity.

electrolyte a salt that dissolves in water and dissociates into charged particles called ions.

elemental formulas enteral formulas that contain carbohydrates and proteins that are partially or fully hydrolyzed; also called *hydrolyzed, chemically defined,* or *monomeric formulas.*

embolism (EM-boh-lizm) the obstruction of a blood vessel by an embolus, causing sudden tissue death.

embolus (EM-boh-lus) an abnormal particle, such as a blood clot or air bubble, that travels in the blood.

embryo (EM-bree-oh) the developing infant from two to eight weeks after conception.

emphysema (EM-fih-ZEE-mah) a progressive lung condition characterized by the breakdown of the lungs' elastic structure and destruction of the walls of the bronchioles and alveoli, reducing the surface area involved in respiration.

empty-kcalorie foods a popular term used to denote foods that contribute energy but lack protein, vitamins, and minerals.

emulsifier a substance that mixes with both fat and water and that disperses the fat in the water, forming an emulsion.

end-stage renal disease (ESRD) an advanced stage of chronic kidney disease in which dialysis or a kidney transplant is necessary to sustain life.

energy density a measure of the energy a food provides relative to the amount of food (kcalories per gram).

energy-yielding nutrients the nutrients that break down to yield energy the body can use. The three energy-yielding nutrients are carbohydrate, protein, and fat.

enrichment the addition to a food of nutrients to meet a specified standard. In the case of refined bread or cereal, five nutrients have been added thiamin, riboflavin, niacin, and folate in amounts approximately equivalent to, or higher than, those originally present and iron in amounts to alleviate the prevalence of iron-deficiency anemia.

enteral (EN-ter-al) nutrition the provision of nutrients using the GI tract, including the use of tube feedings and oral diets.

enteric coated refers to medications or enzyme preparations that are coated to withstand stomach acidity and dissolve only at the higher pH of the small intestine.

environmental tobacco smoke (ETS) the combination of exhaled smoke (mainstream smoke) and smoke from lighted cigarettes, pipes, or cigars (sidestream smoke) that enters the air and may be inhaled by other people.

enzymes protein catalysts. A catalyst is a compound that facilitates chemical reactions without itself being changed in the process.

EPA, DHA omega-3 fatty acids made from linolenic acid. The full name for EPA is *eicosapentaenoic* (EYE-cosa-PENTA-ee-NO-ick) *acid.* The full name for DHA is *docosahexaenoic* (DOE-cosa-HEXA-ee-NO-ick) *acid.*

epinephrine one of the stress hormones secreted whenever emergency action is needed; prescribed therapeutically to relax the bronchioles during allergy or asthma attacks.

epithelial (ep-i-THEE-lee-ul) cells cells on the surface of the skin and mucous membranes.

epithelial tissue tissue composing the layers of the body that serve as selective barriers between the body's interior and the environment (examples are the cornea, the skin, the respiratory lining, and the lining of the digestive tract).

erythrocyte (er-REETH-ro-cite) hemolysis (he-MOLL-uh-sis) rupture of the red blood cells, caused by vitamin E deficiency.

erythrocyte protoporphyrin (PRO-toh-PORE-fe-rin) a precursor to hemoglobin

erythropoietin (eh-RITH-ro-POY-eh-tin) a hormone made by the kidneys that stimulates red blood cell production.

esophageal (eh-SOF-ah-JEE-al) involving the esophagus.

esophageal dysphagia an inability to move food through the esophagus; usually caused by an obstruction or a motility disorder.

essential amino acids amino acids that the body cannot synthesize in amounts sufficient to meet physiological need; also called *indispensable amino acids*. Nine amino acids are known to be essential for human adults.

essential fatty acids fatty acids that the body requires but cannot make in amounts sufficient to meet its physiological needs.

essential nutrients nutrients a person must obtain from food because the body cannot make them for itself in sufficient quantities to meet physiological needs.

Estimated Average Requirements (EAR) the average daily nutrient intake levels estimated to meet the requirements of half of the healthy individuals in a given age and gender group; used in nutrition research and policymaking and as the basis on which RDA values are set.

Estimated Energy Requirement (EER) the dietary energy intake level that is predicted to maintain energy balance in a healthy adult of a defined age, gender, weight, and physical activity level consistent with good health.

ethnic diets foodways and cuisines typical of national origins, races, cultural heritages, or geographic locations.

exclusive breastfeeding an infant's consumption of human milk with no supplementation of any type (no water, no juice, no nonhuman milk, and no foods) except for vitamins, minerals, and medications.

exocrine pertains to external secretions, such as those of the mucous membranes or the skin. Opposite of *endocrine*, which pertains to hormonal secretions into the blood.

expected outcomes patient-oriented goals that are derived from nursing diagnoses.

extracellular fluid fluid residing outside the cells; includes the fluid between the cells (interstitial fluid), plasma, and the water of structures such as the skin and bones. Extracellular fluid accounts for about one-third of the body's water.

fasting hyperglycemia hyperglycemia that develops after an overnight fast of at least eight hours.

fat replacers ingredients that replace some or all of the functions of fat in foods and may or may not provide energy.

fats lipids that are solid at room temperature (70°F or 21°C).

fatty acids organic compounds composed of a chain of carbon atoms with hydrogens attached and an acid group at one end.

fatty liver an accumulation of fat in liver tissue; also called *hepatic steatosis*.

fertility the capacity of a woman to produce a normal ovum periodically and of a man to produce normal sperm; the ability to reproduce.

fetal alcohol spectrum disorders (FASD) a spectrum of physical, behavioral, and cognitive disabilities caused by prenatal alcohol exposure.

fetal alcohol syndrome (FAS) the cluster of symptoms seen in an infant or child whose mother consumed excessive alcohol during her pregnancy. FAS includes, but is not limited to, brain damage, growth retardation, mental retardation, and facial abnormalities.

fetus (FEET-us) the developing infant from eight weeks after conception until its birth.

filtrate the substances that pass through the glomerulus and travel through the nephron's tubules, eventually forming urine.

fistulas (FIST-you-luz) abnormal passages between organs or tissues (or between an internal organ and the body's surface) that permit the passage of fluids or secretions.

flatulence the condition of having excessive intestinal gas, which causes abdominal discomfort.

fluid and electrolyte balance maintenance of the necessary amounts and types of fluid and minerals in each compartment of the body fluids.

fluorapatite (floor-APP-uh-tite) the stabilized form of bone and tooth crystal, in which fluoride has replaced the hydroxy portion of hydroxyapatite.

fluorosis (floor-OH-sis) mottling of the tooth enamel from ingestion of too much fluoride during tooth development.

follicle (FOLL-i-cul) a group of cells in the skin from which a hair grows.

food allergy an adverse reaction to food that involves an immune response; also called *food-hypersensitivity reactions*.

food aversions strong desires to avoid particular foods.

food cravings deep longings for particular foods.

food frequency questionnaire a survey of foods routinely consumed. Some questionnaires ask about the types of food eaten and yield only qualitative information, whereas others include questions about portions consumed and yield semiquantitative data as well.

food group plan a diet-planning tool that sorts foods into groups based on nutrient content and then specifies that people should eat certain amounts of food from each group.

food intolerances adverse reactions to foods or food additives that do not involve the immune system.

food record a detailed log of food eaten during a specified time period, usually several days; also called a *food diary*. A food record may also include information regarding medications, disease symptoms, and physical activity.

foodways the eating habits and culinary practices of a people, region, or historical period.

fortification the addition to a food of nutrients that were either not originally present or present in insignificant amounts. Fortification can be used to correct or prevent a widespread nutrient deficiency, to balance the total nutrient profile of a food, or to restore nutrients lost in processing.

free radicals highly reactive chemical forms that can cause destructive changes in nearby compounds, sometimes setting up a chain reaction.

French units units of measure used to indicate a feeding tube's outer diameter; 1 French unit equals ⅓ millimeter.

fructosamine test a measurement of glycated serum proteins; used to analyze glycemic control over the preceding two weeks. Also known as the *glycated albumin test* or the *glycated serum protein test*.

fructose a monosaccharide; sometimes known as *fruit sugar*. It is abundant in fruits, honey, and saps.

functional foods foods that may provide health benefits beyond their nutrient contributions. Functional foods may include whole foods, fortified foods, and modified foods.

galactose a monosaccharide; part of the disaccharide lactose.

gangrene death of tissue due to a deficient blood supply and/or infection.

gastrectomy (gah-STREK-ta-mee) the surgical removal of part of the stomach (partial gastrectomy) or the entire stomach (total gastrectomy).

gastric banding a surgical means of producing weight loss by restricting stomach size with a constricting band; used in people whose severe obesity brings extreme health risks.

gastric bypass surgery that restricts stomach size and reroutes food from the stomach to the lower part of the small intestine; creates a chronic, lifelong state of malabsorption by preventing normal digestion and absorption of nutrients.

gastric decompression the removal of the stomach contents (including swallowed saliva, stomach secretions, and gas) of patients with motility disorders or obstructions that prevent stomach emptying.

gastric outlet obstruction an obstruction that prevents the normal emptying of stomach contents into the duodenum.

gastric residual volume the volume of formula remaining in the stomach from a previous feeding.

gastritis inflammation of stomach tissue.

gastrointestinal (GI) tract the digestive tract. The principal organs are the stomach and intestines.

gastrointestinal motility spontaneous motion in the digestive tract accomplished by involuntary muscular contractions.

gastroparesis (GAS-troe-pah-REE-sis) delayed stomach emptying.

gatekeeper with respect to nutrition, a key person who controls other people's access to foods and thereby exerts a profound impact on their nutrition. Examples are the spouse who buys and cooks the food, the parent who feeds the children, and the caregiver in a day-care center.

gestation the period of about 40 weeks (three trimesters) from conception to birth; the term of a pregnancy.

gestational diabetes glucose intolerance with first onset or first recognition during pregnancy.

gestational hypertension high blood pressure that develops in the second half of pregnancy and usually resolves after childbirth.

ghrelin (GRELL-in) a hormone produced primarily by the stomach cells. It signals the hypothalamus of the brain to stimulate appetite and food intake.

glands single cells or groups of cells that secrete materials for special uses in the body. Glands may be *exocrine glands*, secreting their materials "out" (into the digestive tract or onto the surface of the skin), or *endocrine glands*, secreting their materials "in" (into the blood).

glomerular filtration rate (GFR) the rate at which filtrate is formed within the kidneys, normally approximately 125 mL/min.

glomerulus (gloh-MEHR-yoo-lus) a tuft of capillaries within the nephron that filters water and solutes from blood as urine production begins (plural *glomeruli*).

glucagon (GLOO-ka-gon) a hormone that is secreted by special cells in the pancreas in response to low blood glucose concentration and elicits release of glucose from storage.

glucose a monosaccharide, the sugar common to all disaccharides and polysaccharides; also called *blood sugar* or *dextrose*.

gluten (GLU-ten) a group of water-insoluble proteins in wheat, rye, and barley.

glycated hemoglobin (HbA1c) hemoglobin molecules that have been nonenzymatically attached to glucose; the level of HbA1c in blood helps to evaluate long-term glycemic control. Also called *glycosylated hemoglobin*.

glycemic (gly-SEE-mic) pertaining to blood glucose.

glycemic index a method of classifying foods according to their potential for raising blood glucose.

glycemic response the extent to which a food raises the blood glucose concentration and elicits an insulin response.

glycerol (GLISS-er-ol) an organic compound, three carbons long, that can form the backbone of triglycerides and phospholipids.

glycogen (GLY-co-gen) a polysaccharide composed of glucose, made and stored by liver and muscle tissues of human beings and animals as a storage form of glucose. Glycogen is not a significant food source of carbohydrate and is not counted as one of the polysaccharides in foods.

glycosuria (GLY-co-SOOR-ee-ah) an abnormal amount of glucose in urine.

goiter (GOY-ter) an enlargement of the thyroid gland due to an iodine deficiency, malfunction of the gland, or overconsumption of a thyroid antagonist. Goiter caused by iodine deficiency is sometimes called simple goiter.

goitrogen (GOY-troh-jen) a substance that enlarges the thyroid gland and causes toxic goiter. Goitrogens occur naturally in such foods as cabbage, kale, brussels sprouts, cauliflower, broccoli, and kohlrabi.

gout (GOWT) a metabolic disorder characterized by elevated uric acid levels in the blood and urine and the deposition of uric acid in and around the joints, causing acute joint inflammation.

HACCP (Hazard Analysis and Critical Control Points) systems of food or formula preparation that identify food safety hazards and critical control points during foodservice procedures; pronounced *hassip*.

health claims statements that characterize the relationship between a nutrient or other substance in food and a disease or health-related condition.

health a range of states with physical, mental, emotional, spiritual, and social components. At a minimum, health means freedom from physical disease, mental disturbances, emotional distress, spiritual discontent, social maladjustment, and other negative states. At a maximum, health means "wellness."

Healthy People a national public health initiative under the jurisdiction of the U.S. Department of Health and Human Services (DHHS) that identifies the most significant preventable threats to health and focuses efforts toward eliminating them.

heart failure a condition with various causes that is characterized by the heart's inability to pump adequate blood to the body's cells, resulting in fluid accumulation in the tissues; also called *congestive heart failure*.

Helicobacter pylori a species of bacterium that colonizes gastric mucosa; a primary cause of gastritis and peptic ulcer disease.

helper T cells lymphocytes that have a specific protein called CD4 on their surfaces and therefore are also known as *CD4+ T cells*; the cells most affected in HIV infection.

hematocrit (hee-MAT-oh-crit) measurement of the volume of the red blood cells packed by centrifuge in a given volume of blood.

hematuria (HE-mah-TOO-ree-ah) blood in the urine.

hemochromatosis (heem-oh-crome-a-TOH-sis) iron overload characterized by deposits of iron-containing pigment in many tissues, with tissue damage. Hemochromatosis is usually caused by a hereditary defect in iron absorption.

hemodialysis (HE-moe-dye-AL-ih-sis) a treatment that removes fluids and wastes from the blood by passing the blood through a dialyzer.

hemoglobin the oxygen-carrying protein of the red blood cells.

hemolytic (HE-moh-LIT-ick) anemia the condition of having too few red blood cells as a result of erythrocyte hemolysis.

hemorrhagic (hem-oh-RAJ-ik) disease the vitamin K–deficiency disease in which blood fails to clot.

hemorrhagic strokes strokes caused by bleeding within the brain, which destroys or compresses brain tissue.

hepatic coma loss of consciousness resulting from severe liver disease.

hepatic encephalopathy (en-sef-ah-LOP-ah-thie) a condition that develops in advanced liver disease that is characterized by altered neurological functioning, including changes in personality and behavior, reduced mental abilities, and disturbances in motor function.

hepatic portal vein the vein that collects blood from the GI tract and conducts it to capillaries in the liver.

hepatic vein the vein that collects blood from the liver capillaries and returns it to the heart.

hepatitis (hep-ah-TYE-tis) inflammation of the liver.

hepatomegaly (HEP-ah-toe-MEG-ah-lee) enlargement of the liver.

herpes simplex virus a common virus that can cause blisterlike lesions on the lips and in the mouth.

hiatal hernia a condition in which the upper portion of the stomach protrudes above the diaphragm; most cases are asymptomatic.

high-density lipoproteins (HDL) the type of lipoproteins that transport cholesterol back to the liver from peripheral cells; composed primarily of protein.

high-quality proteins dietary proteins containing all the essential amino acids in relatively the same amounts that human beings require. They may also contain nonessential amino acids.

high-risk pregnancy a pregnancy characterized by risk factors that make it likely the birth will be surrounded by problems such as premature delivery, difficult birth, retarded growth, birth defects, and early infant death.

histamine-2 receptor blockers a class of drugs that suppress acid secretion by inhibiting receptors on acid-producing cells; commonly called *H2 blockers.* Examples include cimetidine (Tagamet), ranitidine (Zantac), and famotidine (Pepcid).

HIV (human immunodeficiency virus) the virus that causes acquired immune deficiency syndrome (AIDS). HIV destroys immune cells and progressively impedes the body's ability to fight infections and certain cancers.

HIV-lipodystrophy (LIP-oh-DIS-tro-fee) syndrome a group of abnormalities in fat and glucose metabolism that may result from drug treatments for HIV infection; changes include body fat redistribution, abnormal blood lipid levels, and insulin resistance. The accumulation of abdominal fat is sometimes called *protease paunch.*

homeostasis (HOME-ee-oh-STAY-sis) the maintenance of constant internal conditions (such as chemistry, temperature, and blood pressure) by the body's control system.

hormones chemical messengers. Hormones are secreted by a variety of glands in the body in response to altered conditions. Each travels to one or more target tissues or organs and elicits specific responses to restore normal conditions.

hunger the physiological need to eat, experienced as a drive to obtain food; an unpleasant sensation that demands relief.

hydrogenation (high-dro-gen-AY-shun) a chemical process by which hydrogens are added to monounsaturated or polyunsaturated fats to reduce the number of double bonds, making the fats more saturated (solid) and more resistant to oxidation (protecting against rancidity). Hydrogenation produces *trans*-fatty acids.

hyperactivity inattentive and impulsive behavior that is more frequent and severe than is typical of others of a similar age; professionally called **attention deficit/hyperactivity disorder (ADHD)**.

hypercalcemia (HIGH-per-kal-SEE-me-ah) elevated serum calcium levels.

hypercalciuria (HIGH-per-kal-see-YOO-ree-ah) elevated urinary calcium levels.

hypercapnia (high-per-CAP-nee-ah) excessive carbon dioxide in the blood.

hyperglycemia elevated blood glucose concentrations. Normal fasting plasma glucose levels are less than 100 mg/dL. Fasting plasma glucose levels between 100 and 125 mg/dL suggest prediabetes; values of 126 mg/dL and above suggest diabetes.

hyperinsulinemia abnormally high levels of insulin in the blood.

hyperkalemia (HIGH-per-ka-LEE-me-ah) elevated serum potassium levels.

hyperosmolar hyperglycemic syndrome extreme hyperglycemia associated with dehydration, hyperosmolar blood, and altered mental status; sometimes called the *hyperosmolar hyperglycemic nonketotic state.*

hyperoxaluria (HIGH-per-ox-ah-LOO-ree-ah) elevated urinary oxalate levels.

hyperphosphatemia (HIGH-per-fos-fa-TEE-me-ah) elevated serum phosphate levels.

hypertension high blood pressure.

hypertonic formula a formula with an osmolality greater than that of blood serum.

hypochlorhydria (HIGH-poe-clor-HIGH-dree-ah) abnormally low gastric acid secretions.

hypoglycemia abnormally low concentrations of blood glucose. In diabetes, hypoglycemia is treated when plasma glucose levels fall below 70 mg/dL.

hypokalemia (HIGH-po-ka-LEE-me-ah) low serum potassium levels.

hyponatremia (HIGH-po-na-TREE-me-ah) a decreased concentration of sodium in the blood.

hypothalamus (high-poh-THALL-uh-mus) a part of the brain that helps regulate many body balances, including fluid balance.

hypoxemia (high-pock-SEE-me-ah) a low level of oxygen in the blood.

hypoxia (high-POCK-see-ah) a low amount of oxygen in body tissues.

ileostomy (ill-ee-AH-stoe-me) a surgical passage through the abdominal wall into the ileum.

implantation the stage of development in which the blastocyst embeds itself in the wall of the uterus and begins to develop; occurs during the first two weeks after conception.

inflammation an immunological response to cellular injury characterized by an increase in white blood cells.

inorganic not containing carbon or pertaining to living things.

insoluble fibers the tough, fibrous structures of fruits, vegetables, and grains; indigestible food components that do not dissolve in water.

insulin resistance the condition in which a normal of amount of insulin produces a subnormal effect in muscle, adipose, and liver cells, resulting in an elevated fasting glucose; a metabolic consequence of obesity that precedes type 2 diabetes.

insulin a hormone secreted by the pancreas in response to high blood glucose. It promotes cellular glucose uptake for use or storage.

intermittent claudication (claw-dih-KAY-shun) severe pain and weakness in the legs (especially the calves) caused by inadequate blood supply to the muscles; it usually occurs with walking and subsides during rest.

intermittent feedings delivery of about 250 to 400 milliliters of formula over 20 to 40 minutes.

intestinal adaptation the process of intestinal recovery following resection that leads to improved absorptive capacity.

intestinal flora the bacterial inhabitants of the GI tract.

intractable vomiting vomiting that is not easily managed or controlled.

intractable not easily managed or controlled.

intradialytic parenteral nutrition the infusion of nutrients during hemodialysis, often providing amino acids, dextrose, lipids, and some trace minerals.

intravenous feedings the provision of nutrients through a vein, bypassing the intestine; also called *parenteral nutrition*.

intrinsic factor a factor inside the system. Anemia that reflects a vitamin B12 deficiency caused by lack of intrinsic factor is known as *pernicious anemia*.

iron deficiency the condition of having depleted iron stores.

iron overload toxicity from excess iron.

iron-deficiency anemia a blood iron deficiency characterized by small, pale red blood cells; also called microcytic hypochromic anemia.

irritable bowel syndrome an intestinal disorder of unknown cause that disturbs the functioning of the lower bowel; symptoms include abdominal pain, flatulence, diarrhea, and constipation.

ischemia (iss-KEE-mee-a) inadequate blood supply within tissues due to obstructed blood flow in the arteries.

ischemic strokes strokes caused by the obstruction of blood flow to brain tissue.

isotonic formula a formula with an osmolality similar to that of blood serum (about 300 milliosmoles per kilogram).

jaundice (JAWN-dis) yellow discoloration of the skin and eyes due to an accumulation of bilirubin, a breakdown product of hemoglobin that normally exits the body via bile secretions.

Joint Commission a nonprofit organization that sets standards for health care performance and safety and confers accreditation to health care organizations and programs that meet those standards.

Kaposi's (kah-POH-seez) sarcoma a common cancer in HIV-infected persons that is characterized by lesions in the skin, lungs, and GI tract.

kcalorie (energy) control management of food energy intake.

kcalorie counts estimates of food energy (and often, protein) consumed by patients for one or more days.

keratin (KERR-uh-tin) a water-insoluble protein; the normal protein of hair and nails. Keratin-producing cells may replace mucus-producing cells in vitamin A deficiency.

ketoacidosis (KEY-toe-ass-ih-DOE-sis) an acidosis (lowering of blood pH) that results from the excessive production of ketone bodies.

ketones (KEY-tones) acidic, fat-related compounds formed from the incomplete breakdown of fat when carbohydrate is not available; technically known as *ketone* bodies.

ketonuria (KEY-toe-NOOR-ee-ah) the presence of ketone bodies in the urine.

kidney stones crystalline masses that form in the urinary tract; also called *renal calculi* or *nephrolithiasis*.

kwashiorkor (kwash-ee-OR-core or kwash-ee-or-CORE) a severe form of PEM that occurs more frequently after 18 months of age. Kwashiorkor is characterized by failure to grow and develop, changes in the pigmentation of the hair and skin, edema, and fatty liver. Kwashiorkor is associated with inadequate protein intake and infections.

lactadherin (lack-tad-HAIR-in) a protein in breast milk that attacks diarrhea-causing viruses.

lactation production and secretion of breast milk for the purpose of nourishing an infant.

lactoferrin (lack-toe-FERR-in) protein in breast milk that binds iron and keeps it from supporting the growth of the infant's intestinal bacteria.

lactose a disaccharide composed of glucose and galactose; commonly known as *milk sugar*.

laparoscopic weight-loss surgery a procedure in which surgeons gain access to the abdomen via several small incisions.A tiny video camera is inserted through one of the incisions and surgical instruments through the others. The surgeons watch their work on a large-screen monitor.

lapses periods of returning to old habits.

latent the period in the course of a disease when the condition is present but the symptoms have not begun to appear.

lecithins one type of phospholipid.

legumes (lay-GYOOMS, LEG-yooms) plants of the bean and pea family, with seeds that are rich in protein compared with other plant-derived foods.

leptin a hormone produced by fat cells under the direction of the (*ob*) gene. It decreases appetite and increases energy expenditure.

life expectancy the average number of years lived by people in a given society.

life span the maximum number of years of life attainable by a member of a species.

limiting amino acid an essential amino acid that is present in dietary protein in the shortest supply relative to the amount needed for protein synthesis in the body.

linoleic acid, linolenic acid polyunsaturated fatty acids that are essential for human beings.

lipids a family of compounds that includes triglycerides (fats and oils), phospholipids, and sterols. Lipids are characterized by their insolubility in water.

lipomas (lih-POE-muz) benign tumors composed of fatty tissue.

lipoprotein lipase (LPL) an enzyme mounted on the surface of fat cells (and other cells). It hydrolyzes triglycerides in the blood into fatty acids and glycerol for absorption into the cells. There they are metabolized or reassembled for storage.

lipoproteins clusters of lipids associated with proteins that serve as transport vehicles for lipids in the lymph and blood.

listeriosis a serious foodborne infection that can cause severe brain infection or death in a fetus or newborn; caused by the bacterium *Listeria monocytogenes*, which is found in soil and water.

longevity long duration of life.

low birthweight (LBW) a birthweight less than 5½ lb (2500 g); indicates probable poor health in the newborn and poor nutrition status of the mother during pregnancy. Optimal birthweight for a full-term infant is 6.8 to 7.9 lb (about 3100 to 3600 g).

Low-birthweight infants are of two different types. Some are **premature**; they are born early and are of a weight **appropriate for gestational age (AGA)**. Others have suffered growth failure in the uterus; they may or may not be born early, but they are **small for gestational age (SGA)**.

low-density lipoproteins (LDL) the type of lipoproteins derived from VLDL as cells remove triglycerides from them. LDL carry cholesterol and triglycerides from the liver to the cells of the body and are composed primarily of cholesterol.

low-risk pregnancy a pregnancy characterized by factors that make it likely the birth will be normal and the infant healthy.

lymph (LIMF) the body fluid found in lymphatic vessels. Lymph consists of all the constituents of blood except red blood cells.

lymphatic system a loosely organized system of vessels and ducts that conveys the products of digestion toward the heart.

macrosomia (MAK-roh-SOH-mee-ah) the condition of having an abnormally large body; in infants, refers to birth weights of 4000 grams (8 pounds 13 ounces) and above.

macrovascular complications disorders that affect the large blood vessels, including the coronary arteries and arteries of the limbs.

macular (MACK-you-lar) degeneration deterioration of the macular area of the eye that can lead to loss of central vision and eventual blindness. The **macula** is a small, oval, yellowish region in the center of the retina that provides the sharp, straight-ahead vision so critical to reading and driving.

major minerals essential mineral nutrients required in the adult diet in amounts greater than 100 milligrams per day.

malignant (ma-LIG-nent) describes a cancerous cell or tumor, which can injure healthy tissue and spread cancer to other regions of the body.

malnutrition any condition caused by deficient or excess energy or nutrient intake or by an imbalance of nutrients.

maltose a disaccharide composed of two glucose units; sometimes known as malt sugar.

marasmus (ma-RAZZ-mus) the most common form of severe PEM before one year of age. Marasmus is characterized by generalized muscle wasting associated with extreme deprivation, or impaired absorption, of energy, protein, vitamins, and minerals.

medical nutrition therapy nutrition care provided by a registered dietitian; includes assessment of nutrition status, diagnosis of nutrition problems, development of nutrition care plans, and provision of dietary counseling and nutrition education.

medium-chain triglycerides (MCT) triglycerides that contain fatty acids that are 8 to 10 carbons in length. MCT do not require digestion and can be absorbed in the absence of lipase or bile.

metastasize (meh-TAS-tah-size) to spread from one part of the body to another; refers to cancer cells.

microalbuminuria the presence of albumin (a blood protein) in the urine, a sign of diabetic nephropathy.

microvascular complications disorders that affect the small blood vessels and capillaries, including those in the retina and kidneys.

microvilli (MY-cro-VILL-ee or MY-cro-VILL-eye) tiny, hairlike projections on each cell of every villus that can trap nutrient particles and transport them into the cells. The singular form is **microvillus**.

moderate-intensity physical activity physical activity that requires some increase in breathing and/or heart rate and expends 3.5 to 7 kcalories per minute. Walking at a speed of 3 to 4.5 miles per hour (about 15 to 20 minutes to walk one mile) is an example.

moderation providing enough, but not too much, of a substance.

modified diet a diet that contains foods altered in texture, consistency, or nutrient content or that includes or omits specific foods; also called a *therapeutic diet*.

modular formulas enteral formulas prepared in the hospital from *modules* that contain single macronutrients; used for people with unique nutrient needs.

molybdenum (mo-LIB-duh-num) a trace element.

monosaccharides (mon-oh-SACK-uh-rides) a single sugar units.

monounsaturated fatty acid (MUFA) a fatty acid that has one point of unsaturation; for example, the oleic acid found in olive oil.

mucous membrane membrane composed of mucus-secreting cells that lines the surfaces of body tissues. (Reminder *Mucus* is the smooth, slippery substance secreted by these cells.)

myocardial (MY-oh-CAR-dee-al) infarction (in-FARK-shun), or MI death of heart muscle caused by a sudden reduction in coronary blood flow; also called a **heart attack** or *cardiac arrest*.

myoglobin the oxygen-carrying protein of the muscle cells.

naturally occurring sugars sugars that are not added to a food but are present as its original constituents, such as the sugars of fruit or milk.

nephron (NEF-ron) the functional unit of the kidneys, consisting of a glomerulus and tubules.

nephrotic (neh-FROT-ik) syndrome a syndrome associated with kidney disorders that cause urinary protein losses exceeding 3 g/day; symptoms include low serum albumin, elevated blood lipids, and edema.

nephrotoxic toxic to the kidneys.

neural tube defects (NTD) malformations of the brain, spinal cord, or both that occur during embryonic development; a serious central nervous system birth defect that often results in lifelong disability or death.

neural tube the embryonic tissue that later forms the brain and spinal cord.

neurofibrillary tangles snarls of the threadlike strands that extend from the nerve cells, commonly found in the brains of people with Alzheimer's dementia.

neurons nerve cells; the structural and functional units of the nervous system. Neurons initiate and conduct nerve transmissions.

niacin equivalents (NE) the amount of niacin present in food, including the niacin that can theoretically be made from tryptophan, its precursor, present in the food.

night blindness the slow recovery of vision after exposure to flashes of bright light at night; an early symptom of vitamin A deficiency.

nitrogen balance the amount of nitrogen consumed (N in) as compared with the amount of nitrogen excreted (N out) in a given period of time. The laboratory scientist can estimate the protein in a sample of food, body tissue, or excreta by measuring the nitrogen in it.

nonessential amino acids amino acids that the body can synthesize.

nonselective menus menus that do not allow choices and list only preselected food items.

nursing bottle tooth decay extensive tooth decay due to prolonged tooth contact with formula, milk, fruit juice, or other carbohydrate-rich liquid offered to an infant in a bottle.

nursing diagnoses clinical judgments about actual or potential health problems that provide the basis for selecting appropriate nursing interventions.

nutrient claims statements that characterize the quantity of a nutrient in a food.

nutrient density a measure of the nutrients a food provides relative to the energy it provides. The more nutrients and the fewer kcalories, the higher the nutrient density.

nutrients substances obtained from food and used in the body to provide energy and structural materials and to serve as regulating agents to promote growth, maintenance, and repair. Nutrients may also reduce the risks of some diseases.

nutrition care plans strategies for meeting an individual's nutritional needs.

nutrition care process a problem-solving method that dietetics professionals use to evaluate and treat nutrition-related problems.

nutrition screening a brief assessment of health-related variables to identify patients who are malnourished or at risk for malnutrition.

nutrition support teams health care professionals responsible for the provision of nutrients by tube feeding or intravenous infusion.

nutrition support the delivery of nutrients using a feeding tube or intravenous infusions.

nutrition the science of foods and the nutrients and other substances they contain, and of their ingestion, digestion, absorption, transport, metabolism, interaction, storage, and excretion. A broader definition includes the study of the environment and of human behavior as it relates to these processes.

nutritive sweeteners sweeteners that yield energy, including both the sugars and the sugar alcohols.

obesity overweight with adverse health effects; BMI 30 or higher.

oils lipids that are liquid at room temperature (70°F or 21°C).

olestra a synthetic fat made from sucrose and fatty acids that provides zero kcalories per gram; also known as *sucrose polyester*.

oliguria (OL-lih-GOO-ree-ah) an abnormally low amount of urine, often less than 400 mL/day.

omega-3 fatty acids polyunsaturated fatty acids in which the endmost double bond is three carbons back from the end of the carbon chain; relatively newly recognized as important in nutrition. Linolenic acid is an example.

omega-6 fatty acid a polyunsaturated fatty acid with its endmost double bond six carbons back from the end of its carbon chain; long recognized as important in nutrition. Linoleic acid is an example.

open feeding system a delivery system that requires the formula to be transferred from its original packaging to a feeding container before being administered through the feeding tube.

opportunistic infections infections from microorganisms that normally do not cause disease in healthy people, but are damaging to persons with compromised immune function.

opsin (OP-sin) the protein portion of the visual pigment molecule.

oral glucose tolerance test a test that evaluates a person's ability to tolerate an oral glucose load.

organic carbon containing. The four organic nutrients are carbohydrate, fat, protein, and vitamins.

oropharyngeal (OR-oh-fah-ren-JEE-al) involving the mouth and pharynx.

oropharyngeal dysphagia an inability to transfer food from the mouth and pharynx to the esophagus; usually caused by a neurological or muscular disorder.

osmolality (OZ-moe-LAL-ih-tee) the concentration of osmotically active solutes in a solution, expressed as milliosmoles (mOsm) per kilogram of solvent.

osmolarity the concentration of osmotically active solutes in a solution, expressed as milliosmoles per liter of solution (mOsm/L). *Osmolality* (mOsm/kg)is an alternative term used to describe a solution's osmotic properties.

osteoarthritis a painful, chronic disease of the joints that occurs when the cushioning cartilage in a joint breaks down; joint structure is usually altered, with loss of function; also called *degenerative arthritis*.

osteomalacia (os-tee-oh-mal-AY-shuh) a bone disease characterized by softening of the bones. Symptoms include bending of the spine and bowing of the legs. The disease occurs most often in adults with renal failure or malabsorption disorders.

osteoporosis (os-tee-oh-pore-OH-sis) literally, porous bones; reduced density of the bones, also known as *adult bone loss*.

overnutrition overconsumption of food energy or nutrients sufficient to cause disease or increased susceptibility to disease; a form of malnutrition.

overt out in the open, full-blown.

overweight body weight above some standard of acceptable weight that is usually defined in relation to height (such as BMI); BMI 25 to 29.9.

ovum (OH-vum) the female reproductive cell, capable of developing into a new organism upon fertilization; commonly referred to as an egg.

oxidation (OKS-ee-day-shun) the process of a substance combining with oxygen.

paracentesis (pah-rah-sen-TEE-sis) a surgical puncture of a body cavity with an aspirator to draw out excess fluid.

parenteral (par-EN-ter-al) nutrition the intravenous provision of nutrients that bypasses the GI tract.

pellagra (pell-AY-gra) the niacin-deficiency disease. Symptoms include the "4 Ds" diarrhea, dermatitis, dementia, and, ultimately, death.

peptic ulcer an open sore in the gastrointestinal mucosa resulting from the destructive effects of gastric acid and pepsin; may develop in the esophagus, stomach, or duodenum.

peripheral parenteral nutrition (PPN) the infusion of nutrient solutions into peripheral veins, usually a vein in the arm or back of the hand.

peripheral veins the small-diameter veins that carry blood from the arms and legs.

peristalsis (peri-STALL-sis) successive waves of involuntary muscular contractions passing along the walls of the GI tract that push the contents along.

peritoneal (PEH-rih-toe-NEE-al) dialysis a treatment that removes fluids and wastes from the blood by using the body's peritoneal membrane as a filter.

peritoneovenous (PEH-rih-toe-NEE-oh-VEE-nus) shunt a surgical passage created between the peritoneum and the jugular vein to divert fluid and relieve ascites. The peritoneum is the membrane that surrounds the abdominal cavity.

pernicious (per-NISH-us) anemia a vitamin B12-deficiency disease caused by lack of intrinsic factor and characterized by large, immature red blood cells and damage to the nervous system (*pernicious* means "highly injurious or destructive").

pH the concentration of hydrogen ions. The lower the pH, the stronger the acid. Thus pH 2 is a strong acid; pH 6 is a weak acid; pH 7 is neutral; and a pH above 7 is alkaline.

phlebitis (fleh-BYE-tiss) inflammation of a vein.

phospholipids one of the three main classes of lipids; compounds that are similar to triglycerides but have choline (or another compound) and a phosphorus-containing acid in place of one of the fatty acids.

physiological age a person's age as estimated from her or his body's health and probable life expectancy.

phytates nonnutrient components of grains, legumes, and seeds. Phytates can bind minerals such as iron, zinc, calcium, and magnesium in insoluble complexes in the intestine, and the body excretes them unused.

phytochemicals nonnutrient compounds in plant-derived foods that have biological activity in the body.

pica (PIE-ka) a craving for nonfood substances; also known as geophagia (jee-oh-FAY-jee-uh) when referring to clay-eating behavior.

piggyback the administration of a second solution using a separate port in an intravenous catheter.

pigment a molecule capable of absorbing certain wavelengths of light so that it reflects only those that we perceive as a certain color.

pituitary (pit-TOO-ih-tary) gland in the brain, the "king gland" that regulates the operation of many other glands.

placenta (pla-SEN-tuh) an organ that develops inside the uterus early in pregnancy, in which maternal and fetal blood circulate in close proximity and exchange materials. The fetus receives nutrients and oxygen across the placenta; the mother's blood picks up carbon dioxide and other waste materials to be excreted via her lungs and kidneys.

plaque (PLACK) an accumulation of fatty deposits, smooth muscle cells, and fibrous connective tissue in blood vessels.

polycystic kidney disease a hereditary disorder characterized by the formation of multiple cysts in the kidneys.

polydipsia (POL-ee-DIP-see-ah) excessive thirst.

polypeptide ten or more amino acids bonded together. An intermediate strand of between four and ten amino acids is an *oligopeptide*.

polyphagia (POL-ee-FAY-jee-ah) excessive appetite or food intake.

polysaccharides long chains of monosaccharide units arranged as starch, glycogen, or fiber.

polyunsaturated fatty acids (PUFA) fatty acids with two or more points of unsaturation. For example, linoleic acid has two such points, and linolenic acid has three. Thus polyunsaturated *fat* is composed of triglycerides containing a high percentage of PUFA.

polyuria (POL-ee-YOOR-ree-ah) excessive urine production.

portal hypertension elevated blood pressure in the portal vein due to obstructed blood flow through the liver.

precursors compounds that can be converted into other compounds; with regard to vitamins, compounds that can be converted into active vitamins; also known as provitamins.

prediabetes the condition in which blood glucose levels are higher than normal but not high enough to be diagnosed as diabetes.

preeclampsia (PRE-ee-KLAMP-see-ah) a condition characterized by hypertension and protein in the urine.

preformed vitamin A vitamin A in its active form.

prehypertension blood pressure values that predict hypertension.

pressure sores regions of damaged skin and tissue due to prolonged pressure on the affected area by an external object, such as a bed, wheelchair, or cast; vulnerable areas of the body include buttocks, hips, and heels. Also called *decubitus* (deh-KYU-bih-tus)*ulcers*.

primary hypertension hypertension with an unknown cause; also known as **essential hypertension.**

protein digestibility a measure of the amount of amino acids absorbed from a given protein intake.

protein isolates proteins that have been isolated from foods.

protein turnover the continuous breakdown and synthesis of body proteins involving the recycling of amino acids.

protein-energy malnutrition (PEM) a deficiency of protein and food energy; the world's most widespread malnutrition problem, including both marasmus and kwashiorkor.

proteins compounds made from strands of amino acids composed of carbon, hydrogen, oxygen, and nitrogen atoms. Some amino acids also contain sulfur atoms.

proteinuria (PRO-teen-NOO-ree-ah) loss of protein, mostly albumin, in the urine; also known as *albuminuria.*

proton-pump inhibitors a class of drugs that inhibit the enzyme that pumps hydrogen ions (protons) into the stomach. Examples include omeprazole (Prilosec) and lansoprazole (Prevacid).

puberty the period in life in which a person becomes physically capable of reproduction.

purines (PYOO-reens) products of nucleotide metabolism that degrade to uric acid.

quality of life a person's perceived physical and mental well-being.

radiation enteritis inflammation of intestinal tissue caused by radiation therapy.

radiation therapy the use of X-rays, gamma rays, or atomic particles to destroy cancer cells.

rancid the term used to describe fats when they have deteriorated, usually by oxidation. Rancid fats often have an "off" odor.

rebound hyperglycemia hyperglycemia that results from the release of counterregulatory hormones following nighttime hypoglycemia; also called the **Somogyi effect.**

Recommended Dietary Allowances (RDA) a set of values reflecting the average daily amounts of nutrients considered adequate to meet the known nutrient needs of practically all healthy people in a particular life stage and gender group; a goal for dietary intake by individuals.

refeeding syndrome a condition that sometimes develops when a severely malnourished person is aggressively fed; characterized by electrolyte and fluid imbalances and hyperglycemia.

refined grain a product from which the bran, germ, and husk have been removed, leaving only the endosperm.

reflux esophagitis inflammation in the esophagus that is related to the reflux of acidic stomach contents.

renal (REE-nal) pertaining to the kidneys.

renal colic the intense pain that occurs when a kidney stone passes through the ureter.

renal osteodystrophy a bone disorder that develops in patients with chronic kidney disease as a consequence of increased secretion of parathyroid hormone, reduced serum calcium, acidosis, and impaired vitamin D activation by the kidneys.

renal threshold the blood concentration of a substance that exceeds the kidneys' capacity for reabsorption, causing the substance to be passed into the urine.

requirement the lowest continuing intake of a nutrient that will maintain a specified criterion of adequacy.

resection the surgical removal of part of an organ or body structure.

residue material left in the intestine after digestion; includes mostly dietary fiber and undigested starches and proteins.

resistance training the use of free weights or weight machines to provide resistance for developing muscle strength, power, and endurance; also called *weight training*. A person's own body weight may also be used to provide resistance as when a person does push-ups, pull-ups, or abdominal crunches.

resistant starches starches that escape digestion and absorption in the small intestine of healthy people.

resting metabolic rate (RMR) a measure of the energy use of a person at rest in a comfortable setting; similar to the BMR but with less stringent criteria for recent food intake and physical activity. Consequently, the RMR is slightly higher than the BMR.

retina (RET-in-uh) the layer of light-sensitive nerve cells lining the back of the inside of the eye; consists of rods and cones.

retinol activity equivalents (RAE) a measure of vitamin A activity; the amount of retinol that the body will derive from a food containing preformed retinol or its precursor beta-carotene.

retinol-binding protein (RBP) the specific protein responsible for transporting retinol.

rheumatoid arthritis a disease of the immune system involving painful inflammation of the joints and related structures.

rhodopsin (ro-DOP-sin) a light-sensitive pigment of the retina; contains the retinal from of vitamin A and the protein opsin.

rickets the vitamin D–deficiency disease in children.

salts compounds composed of charged particles (ions). An example of a salt is potassium chloride (K+Cl-).

sarcopenia (SAR-koh-PEE-nee-ah) loss of skeletal muscle mass, strength, and quality.

saturated fatty acid a fatty acid carrying the maximum possible number of hydrogen atoms (having no points of unsaturation).

scurvy the vitamin C–deficiency disease.

secondary hypertension hypertension that results from a known physiological abnormality.

segmentation a periodic squeezing or partitioning of the intestine by its circular muscles that both mixes and slowly pushes the contents along.

selective menus menus that provide choices in some or all menu categories.

self-efficacy a person's belief in his or her ability to succeed in an undertaking.

self-monitoring of blood glucose home monitoring of blood glucose levels using a glucose meter.

semiselective menus menus that combine aspects of both selective and nonselective menus.

senile dementia the loss of brain function beyond the normal loss of physical adeptness and memory that occurs with aging.

senile plaques clumps of the protein fragment beta-amyloid on the nerve cells, commonly found in the brains of people with Alzheimer's dementia.

set-point theory the theory that proposes that the body tends to maintain a certain weight by means of its own internal controls.

short bowel syndrome the malabsorption syndrome that follows resection of the small intestine, which results in inadequate absorptive capacity in the remaining intestine.

sinusoids the small, capillary-like passages that carry blood through liver tissue.

Sjögren's (SHOW-grenz) syndrome an autoimmune disease characterized by the destruction of secretory glands, resulting in dry mouth and dry eyes.

skinfold measure a clinical estimate of total body fatness in which the thickness of a fold of skin on the back of the arm (over the triceps muscle), below the shoulder blade (subscapular), or in other places is measured with a caliper.

soaps chemical compounds formed from fatty acids and positively charged minerals.

soluble fibers indigestible food components that readily dissolve in water and often impart gummy or gel-like characteristics to foods. An example is pectin from fruit, which is used to thicken jellies.

spasm a sudden, forceful, and involuntary muscle contraction.

Special Supplemental Nutrition Program for Women, Infants, and Children (WIC) a high-quality, cost-effective health care and nutrition services program administered by the U.S. Department of Agriculture for low-income women, infants, and children who are nutritionally at risk. WIC provides supplemental foods, nutrition education, and referrals to health care and other social services.

specialized formulas enteral formulas designed to meet the nutrient needs of patients with specific illnesses; also called *disease-specific formulas*.

sphincter (SFINK-ter) a circular muscle surrounding, and able to close, a body opening.

sphincter = band (binder)

spina (SPY-nah) bifida (BIFF-ih-dah) one of the most common types of neural tube defects; characterized by the incomplete closure of the spinal cord and its bony encasement.

standard diet a diet that includes all foods and meets the nutrient needs of healthy people; also called a *regular diet*.

standard formulas enteral formulas that contain mostly intact proteins and polysaccharides; also called *polymeric formulas*.

starch a plant polysaccharide composed of glucose and digestible by human beings.

steatohepatitis (STEE-ah-to-HEP-ah-TYE-tis) liver inflammation that is associated with fatty liver.

steatorrhea (stee-AT-or-REE-ah) excessive fat in the stools resulting from fat malabsorption; characterized by stools that are loose, frothy, and foul smelling due to a high fat content.

sterile free of microorganisms, such as bacteria.

steroids (STARE-oids) medications used to reduce tissue inflammation, to suppress the immune response, or to replace certain steroid hormones in people who cannot synthesize them.

sterols one of the main classes of lipids; include cholesterol, vitamin D, and the sex hormones (such as testosterone).

stoma (STOE-ma) a surgically created opening in a body tissue or organ.

stricture abnormal narrowing of a passageway; often due to inflammation, scarring, or a congenital abnormality.

stroke a sudden injury to brain tissue resulting from impaired blood flow through an artery that supplies blood to the brain; also called a *cerebrovascular accident*.

struvite (STROO-vite) crystals of magnesium ammonium phosphate.

subcutaneous (sub-cue-TAY-nee-us) beneath the skin.

subcutaneous fat fat stored directly under the skin.

sucrose a disaccharide composed of glucose and fructose; commonly known as *table sugar*, *beet sugar*, or *cane sugar*.

sugar alcohols sugarlike compounds. Like sugars, they are sweet to taste but yield 2 to 3 kcal per gram, slightly less than sucrose. Examples are maltitol, mannitol, sorbitol, isomalt, lactitol, and xylitol.

syringes devices used for injecting medications. A syringe consists of a hypodermic needle attached to a hollow tube with a plunger inside.

tannins compounds in tea (especially black tea) and coffee that bind iron.

teratogenic (ter-AT-oh-jen-ik) causing abnormal fetal development and birth defects.
The tubules are surrounded by capillaries that reabsorb substances retained by tubule cells.

thermic effect of food an estimation of the energy required to process food (digest, absorb, transport, metabolize, and store ingested nutrients).

thrombosis (throm-BOH-sis) the formation or presence of a blood clot in blood vessels. A *coronary thrombosis* occurs in a coronary artery, and a *cerebral thrombosis* occurs in an artery that supplies blood to the brain.

thrombus a blood clot formed within a blood vessel that remains attached to its place of origin.

thrush a fungal infection of the mouth and throat, most often caused by *Candida albicans*.

tissue rejection destruction of donor tissue by the recipient's immune system, which recognizes the donor cells as foreign.

tocopherol (tuh-KOFF-er-ol) a general term for several chemically related compounds, one of which has vitamin E activity.

Tolerable Upper Intake Levels (UL) a set of values reflecting the highest average daily nutrient intake levels that are likely to pose no risk of toxicity to almost all healthy individuals in a particular life stage and gender group. As intake increases above the UL, the potential risk of adverse health effects increases.

tolerance level the maximum amount of residue permitted in a food when a pesticide is used according to the label directions.

total nutrient admixture (TNA) a parenteral solution that contains dextrose, amino acids, and lipids; also called a **3-in-1 solution** or an **all-in-one solution.**

total parenteral nutrition (TPN) the infusion of nutrient solutions into a central vein.

trace minerals essential mineral nutrients required in the adult diet in amounts less than 100 milligrams per day.

trans-fatty acids fatty acids in which the hydrogens next to the double bond are on opposite sides of the carbon chain.

transferrin (trans-FERR-in) the body's iron-carrying protein.

transient ischemic attacks (TIAs) brief ischemic strokes that cause short-term neurological symptoms.

triglycerides (try-GLISS-er-rides) one of the main classes of lipids the chief form of fat in foods and the major storage form of fat in the body; composed of glycerol with three fatty acids attached.

trimester a period representing one-third of the term of gestation. A trimester is about 13 to 14 weeks.

tripeptide three amino acids bonded together.

tube feedings liquid formulas delivered through a tube placed in the stomach or intestine.

tubules tubelike structures of the nephron that process filtrate during urine production.

tumor an abnormal tissue mass that has no physiological function; also called a *neoplasm* (NEE-oh-plazm).

type 1 diabetes the type of diabetes that accounts for 5 to 10 percent of diabetes cases and usually results from autoimmune destruction of pancreatic beta cells.

type 2 diabetes the type of diabetes that accounts for 90 to 95 percent of diabetes cases and usually results from insulin resistance coupled with insufficient insulin secretion.

ulcerative colitis (ko-LY-tis) an inflammatory bowel disease that involves the colon. Inflammation affects the mucosa and submucosa of the intestinal wall.

umbilical (um-BIL-ih-cul) cord the ropelike structure through which the fetus's veins and arteries reach the placenta; the route of nourishment and oxygen into the fetus and the route of waste disposal from the fetus.

undernutrition underconsumption of food energy or nutrients severe enough to cause disease or increased susceptibility to disease; a form of malnutrition.

underweight body weight below some standard of acceptable weight that is usually defined in relation to height (such as BMI); BMI below 18.5.

unsaturated fatty acid a fatty acid with one or more points of unsaturation where hydrogens are missing (includes monounsaturated and polyunsaturated fatty acids).

uremia (you-REE-me-ah) the abnormal accumulation of nitrogen-containing substances, especially urea, in the blood; also called *azotemia*(AZE-oh-TEE-me-ah).

uremic syndrome the cluster of symptoms associated with a GFR below 15 mL/min, including uremia, anemia, bone disease, hormonal imbalances, bleeding impairment, increased cardiovascular disease risk, and reduced immunity.

USDA Food Guide the USDA's food group plan for ensuring dietary adequacy that assigns foods to five major food groups.

uterus (YOO-ter-us) the womb, the muscular organ within which the infant develops before birth.

varices (VAH-rih-seez) abnormally dilated blood vessels (singular *varix*).

variety (dietary) eating a wide selection of foods within and among the major food groups (the opposite of monotony).

vein a vessel that carries blood back to the heart.

very-low-density lipoproteins (VLDL) the type of lipoproteins made primarily by liver cells to transport lipids to various tissues in the body; composed primarily of triglycerides.

vigorous-intensity physical activity physical activity that requires a large increase in breathing and/or heart rate and expends more than 7 kcalories per minute. Walking at a very brisk pace (>4.5 miles per hour) or running at a pace of at least 5 miles per hour are examples.

villi (VILL-ee or VILL-eye) fingerlike projections from the folds of the small intestine. The singular form is *villus*.

visceral fat fat stored within the abdominal cavity in association with the internal abdominal organs, as opposed to fat stored directly under the skin (subcutaneous fat); also called *intra-abdominal fat*.

viscous a gel-like consistency.

vitamin A a fat-soluble vitamin. Its three chemical forms are *retinol* (the alcohol form), *retinal* (the aldehyde form), and *retinoic acid* (the acid form).

vitamins essential, nonkaloric, organic nutrients needed in tiny amounts in the diet.

voluntary activities the component of a person's daily energy expenditure that involves conscious and deliberate muscular work¾walking, lifting, climbing, and other physical activities. Voluntary activities normally require less energy in a day than basal metabolism does.

waist circumference a measurement used to assess a person's abdominal fat.

wasting the gradual atrophy (loss) of body tissues; associated with protein-energy malnutrition or chronic illness.

water balance the balance between water intake and water excretion that keeps the body's water content constant.

water intoxication the rare condition in which body water contents are too high. The symptoms may include confusion, convulsion, coma, and even death in extreme cases.

wean to gradually replace breast milk with infant formula or other foods appropriate to an infant's diet.

wellness maximum well-being; the top range of health states; the goal of the person who strives toward realizing his or her full potential physically, mentally, emotionally, spiritually, and socially.

xerostomia (ZEE-roh-STOE-me-ah) dry mouth caused by reduced salivary flow.

zygote (ZY-goat) the product of the union of ovum and sperm; a fertilized ovum.

Index

This index lists primarily topics that received significant mention in the text. Inclusive pages (for example, 53–56) indicate major discussions; pages in **bold-face** refer to defined terms; pages in *italics* refer to figures, diagrams, or chemical structures; pages followed by a "t" refer to tables; pages followed by an "n" refer to notes.

nutrition risk factors for, 650–652, 651t
nutrition therapy for, 656–659, 657t
phytochemicals and, 3
reducing risk of, 653t
selenium and, 259
surgery and, 654, 654t
treatments for, 654–659
vitamin C and, 222
wasting associated with, 652

Cancer cachexia, **652**

Cancers, **649**

CAPD. *See* Continuous ambulatory peritoneal dialysis

Capillaries, **49**

Capsaicin, 231t

Carbohydrates, **64**
acute stress and, 475
alternative sweeteners and, 72–76
AMDR and, 9–10
chemist's view of, 64–67
childhood and, 318
cirrhosis and, 552t, 553
counting of, 573–575
diabetes mellitus and, 77–78, 572, 573–575, 574t, *575*
Dietary Guidelines for Americans and, 14t
disaccharides, 64, 65, 65t
food labels and, 82
food sources for, 80–82
gastrointestinal tract and, *39*
kCalorie measurement of, 6–7
late adulthood and, 363
monosaccharides, 64–65, 65t
parenteral solutions and, 452
polysaccharides, 64, 65–67
pregnancy and, 277–278
recommendations/disease prevention and, 77–80
role of, 6, 64
storing excess, 142, *143*
sugars, 67–72
terms used on labels regarding, 28t
weight management and, 178t, 179

Carbohydrate-to-insulin ratio, **578**

Carcinogenesis, **649**

Carcinogens, **649**

Carcinomas, 649

Cardiac cachexia, **611**

Cardiac output, **600**

Cardiopulmonary resuscitation (CPR), **670**, 671

Cardiovascular disease (CVD), **98**, **347**, **592**
alcohol and, 560–561
Alzheimer's disease and, 360
atherosclerosis, 592–594
beginnings of, 348
breakdown of deaths from, *592*

CHD and, 595–604
checklist for, 613
childhood obesity and, 347–351
cholesterol and, 99–100
diet-drug interactions and, 603
fat guidelines regarding, 101–102
fats and, 98–102, 112–115
genetics and, 347–348
harmful fats and, 114–115
heart failure, 610–611
heart-healthy diet for, 601
heart-healthy fats and, 112–113
hypertension, 604–609
hypertriglyceridemia and, 600, 602
LDL and, 114, *115*
metabolic syndrome and, 588
nephrotic syndrome and, 623
omegas and, 100–101
overview of, 592, *592*
prevention of, 106, 349
risk assessment for, 595–596, 596t, 597
stroke, 612
websites regarding, 614

Care planning, 407, 407t, 408t, 409

Cariogenic foods, **509**

Carnitine, 221

Carotenoids, 229, **230**, 231t, 232

Cataracts, **358**
website resources for, 372

Catecholamines, 470, 470t

Cathartic, **192**, **197**, **245**

Catheter, **451**, 454, 455t

Catholic Relief Services, 379t

CDC. *See* Centers for Disease Control

CDE. *See* Certified Diabetes Educator

Celiac disease, **525**
consequences of, 525
nutrition therapy for, 526–527, 526t, *527*

Cell differentiation, 203–204

Cells, water balance in, 238

Cellulite, **175**

Cellulose, 66, *76*

Centers for Disease Control (CDC), **54**

Central obesity, **152–153**, *153*

Central veins, **450**

Cerebral cortex, **359**

Certified Diabetes Educator (CDE), **570**

Channel blockers, 603

Chaparral, 429, 430t

CHD. *See* Coronary heart disease

Cheater's Diet, 163t

Cheese
fats in, 103
protein and, 132t

USDA Food Guide and, 17, *19*, 20t, *23*

Chemotherapy, 654, 655t

Childhood
anthropometric data and, 393
appetite, 317–318
blood cholesterol and, 348–349, 349t, 350
body shape and, 317, *317*
chronic disease development in, 347–351
cigarette smoking and, 350–351
CVD and, 347–351
dietary guidelines for, 349–350, 350t
energy and, 318, 321t
food allergies and, 325–326
food choices and, 5, 321
food/eating skills, 334t
food patterns in, 319, *320*, 321, 321t
hunger and, 321–322
hypertension and, 349
iron needs in, 318–319, 319t, 322
lead poisoning and, 322–324
malnutrition in, 321, 322, 323t
mealtimes at home, 332–336
MyPyramid for, 319, *320*
nutrient needs in, 317–321
nutrition checklist for, 342
obesity, 327–332, 347–351
parental role modeling during, 335–336
physical activity and, 328–329, 330–331, 330t, *331*, 349
power struggle avoidance during, 333
school nutrition and, 336–338
snacks and, 334, 335t
stages of growth regarding, 317
type 2 diabetes and, 566
vitamins/minerals and, 318–319
website resources regarding, 343–344

Chinese medicine. *See* Traditional Chinese medicine

Chiropractic, **431–432**

Chitosan, 174t

Chloride, *243*, 244–245, 253t

Cholesterol
CHD and, 595–596, 598–599
childhood/adolescence and, 348–349, 349t, 350
CVD and, 99–100
functional foods and, 234–235
mono/polyunsaturated fatty acids and, 100
obesity/childhood, and, 348–350
saturated fats and, 99
sterols and, 97
synthesis of, 97
terms used on labels regarding, 27t
trans-fatty acids and, 99
transport of, 97
website resources regarding, 109

Fats, **92**. *See also* Lipids (*Continued*)
  figuring out, 111–117
  in foods, 102–107
  gastrointestinal tract and, *40*
  glycemic index and, 88
  health effects/recommended intakes
    of, 98–102
  heart health and, 106
  heart-healthy diet and, 601
  kCalorie measurement of, 6–7
  late adulthood and, 363
  malabsorption of, 518–519, 518t, *519*,
    520t, *521*
  nephrotic syndrome and, 624
  pregnancy and, 278
  replacement of, 105–107
  revised recommendations for, 111–112
  role of, 6
  storing excess, 142, *143*
  subcutaneous, 153
  terms used on labels regarding, 27t
  visceral, 152–153, *153*
  website resources regarding, 109
  weight management and, 178t, 179

Fat-soluble vitamins, 202–213
  overview of, 202
  summary of, 213t
  vitamin A, *203*, 203–207, *206*, 213t
  vitamin D, 207–210, *208*, 213t
  vitamin E, 210–211, 213t
  vitamin K, 211–212, *212*, 213t

Fatty acids, **93**. *See also* Omega-3 fatty acid;
    Omega-6 fatty acid; *Trans*-fatty acids
  childhood and, 318
  cholesterol and, 99–100
  factors influencing, 95
  foods sources of, 116t
  monounsaturated, *94*, 95, 100, 116t, 598
  polyunsaturated, *94*, 95, 100, 210, 598
  saturated, *94*, *94*
  trans- vs. *cis-*, 95, *96*
  triglyceride formation and, 93, *94*
  types of, *94*, 94–96
  unsaturated, *94*, 94–95, 117t
  vegetarian diets and, 140

Fatty liver, **127**, **545**

Fatty streaks, *347*, 348

FDA. *See* Food and Drug
    Administration (FDA)

Feasting, 142–143, *143*

Feeding America, 379t

Feeding disabilities
  conditions leading to, 617t
  family life and, 620
  health professionals and, 618
  interventions for, 618t
  overview of, 617
  special equipment for, 618–620, *619*

Feeding route selection, 436, *436*

Feeding tubes, 442–443. *See also*
    Tube feeding

Female athlete triad, **192**, *193*, **193**

Fertility, **272**

Fetal alcohol spectrum disorder (FASD),
    290–291

Fetal alcohol syndrome (FAS), **291**

Fetal origins of disease, 348

Fetus, **274**, *275*

Feverfew, 430t, 431t

Fiber
  CHD and, 599
  childhood and, 318
  diabetes mellitus and, 572
  dietary, 66–67
  disease prevention and, 77–80
  effects of excessive, 79
  enteral formulas and, 437
  food labels and, 82
  glycemic index and, 88
  health effects of, 77–82
  late adulthood and, 363
  pregnancy and, 278
  recommended intakes of, 79–80
  restricted diet, 414
  in selected foods, *81*
  terms used on labels regarding, 28t
  website resources regarding, 84
  weight management and, 78–79, 178t, 179

Fibrinogen, **587**

Filtrate, **622**

Fish oils
  benefits of, 113
  CHD and, 599
  commonly eaten fish and, 114t
  contaminants in, 100
  hypertriglyceridemia and, 602
  supplementation of, 100–101

Fistulas, **440**, **527**

Fitness. *See also* Physical activity
  benefits of, 15–17
  Dietary Guidelines for Americans
    and, 14t
  Physical Activity Guidelines for
    Americans and, 15, 15t, 16t

Flatulence, **515**–516, 516t

Flavonoids, **229**, **230**, 231t

Flaxseed, **230**, **233**

Flexibility, 16t

Flora, **541**

Fluid balance, **124**

Fluorapatite, **261**

Fluoride
  deficiency, 261
  dental tissues and, 510

  pregnancy and, 281
  public water systems and, *262*
  sources, 261–262
  summary regarding, 263t

Fluorosis, **262**

Folate
  alcohol and, 560
  CHD and, 602
  estimating dietary equivalents of, 219
  in foods, 218–219
  late adulthood and, 364
  methotrexate and, 421, *422*, 654
  neural tube defects and, 218
  overview of, 225t
  pregnancy and, *279*, 279–280, 280t
  vitamin B12 and, 219–220, 279–280

Follicle, **205**

Food activity diary, *183*

Food allergy, **325**

Food and Agriculture Organization
    (FAO), 379t

Food and Drug Administration (FDA)
  foodborne illness and, 57
  food labels and, *24*, 24–29, 26t, 27t–28t,
    28t–29t

Food assistance programs
  for older adults, 367–368, 368t
  for pregnancy, 282–283
  school, 336

Food aversions, **286**

Food bank, **377**, **380**

Foodborne illness, **54**
  food safety and, 54–62
  late adulthood and, 368
  overview of, 54, 57
  pregnancy and, 290
  preventing, 58–62
  programs preventing, 57
  refrigerator storage and, 62t
  symptoms of, 54t
  transmission of, 57
  travel and, 62

Food choices
  adolescence, 5, 340–341
  factors in, 3–5
  for older seniors, 369–370

Food combining, myth of, 48

Food cravings, **286**

Food frequency questionnaire, **388**–390,
    389t, *390*

Food group plan, **17**

Food groups, 14t

Food history, 387t

Food history recall, 388

Food insecurity, *375*, **375**, 376t

Retinol-binding protein (RBP), **203**, 397

Rheumatoid arthritis, **359**

Rhodopsin, **203**

Riboflavin, 216, 224t

Rickets, *208*, **208**

Risk factors for malnutrition in older adults.
See Determine

Rooting reflex, **313**

Saccharin, 73, 74t, 75, **75**

Safety. *See* Food safety

Saliva, dental caries and, 510

Salivary glands, **44**

Salmonellosis, 56t

Salts
  cutting intake of, 245
  electrolyte balance and, **241**
  hypertension and, 243–244, 606

Saponins (glucosides), 232t

Sarcomas, 649

Sarcopenia, **361**–362, *362*

Saturated fats
  blood cholesterol and, 99
  CHD and, 596, 598, 598t
  foods high in, 114–115, 116t, 117t
  recommendations regarding, 101–102,
    111–112

Saturated fatty acid, *94*, **94**

Saw palmetto, 430t

Schiavo, Terri, 671–672

School
  lunch patterns, 337t
  nutrition at, 336–338
  nutrition standards and, 337, 338t
  recess followed by lunch in, 333

Science
  junk, 33t
  research and, 33

Scurvy, **221**

Secondary amenorrhea, **192**

Secretory diarrhea, 516

Segmentation, *42*, **42**–43

Selective menus, **417**

Selenium
  deficiency/toxicity, 259
  in human body, *243*
  recommendation, 260
  summary regarding, 263t

Self-efficacy, **184**

Self-monitoring of blood glucose, **570**

Semipermeable membrane, **644**

Semiselective menus, **418**

Senile dementia, **359**–361, 360t

Senile plaques, **360**

Senior Farmers Market Nutrition Program, 368t

Sepsis, **469**, 472
  as MODS risk factor, 486, 486t
  MODS/SIRS and, *485*, 485–486

Serum electrolytes, 396t

Serum enzymes, 396t

Serum proteins, 395, 395t–396t

Serving sizes
  measuring, 25, 25t
  nutrition facts panel and, *24*, 25

Set-point theory, **170**

Shear stress, 593

Shigellosis, 56t

Shock, **469**, 472

Short bowel syndrome, *531*, **531**–532

Sibutramine, 175

Silicon, 262

Single-nucleotide polymorphism, **404**

Sinusoids, **549**

SIRS. *See* Systemic inflammatory response
  syndrome

Sjögren's syndrome, **489**

Skin
  malnutrition and, 398t
  tube feeding and, 448t

Skinfold measure, **154**

Small intestine, **38**, **41**
  absorption in, 46, *47*, 48
  celiac disease and, 525–527
  conditions affecting, 525–532
  digestion in, *39–40*, 41–43, *42*, 45–46
  inflammatory bowel diseases and, 527–531
  peristalsis/segmentation in, 41–43, *42*
  specialization and, 48

Snacks
  adolescents and, 341
  childhood and, 334, 335t

SNAP. *See* Supplemental Nutrition
  Assistance Program

Soaps, **518**–519

Social history, 387, 387t

Society of St. Andrew, 379t

Sodium
  blood pressure and, 243–244, 609
  CHD and, 599
  chronic kidney disease and, 633
  cirrhosis and, 552t, 553–554
  controlled diet, 414, 625t
  cutting intake of, 245
  Dietary Guidelines for Americans and, 14t
  food processing and, *244*
  in human body, *243*

lithium and, 422–423
  nephrotic syndrome and, 624
  recommendations, 243
  reduction, 609
  summary regarding, 253t
  terms used on labels regarding, 28t

Sodium-controlled diet, 414, 625t

Soft diets, 413t

Soluble fibers, **67**

Sonoma Diet, 163t

Soup kitchens, **377**, **378**

South Beach Diet, 164t

Spasm, **595**

Specialized formulas, **437**

Special Supplemental Nutrition Program
  for Women, Infants, and Children
  (WIC), **282**–283

Sphincter, **38**, **41**

Spina bifida, **278**, *279*, **279**–280, 308

Spot reducing, 182

St. John's wort, 429, 430t, 431t

Standard diet, **410**

Standard formulas, **437**

Stanols, 599

Staphylococcal food poisoning, 56t

Starch, **66**
  food labels and, 82
  glycemic index and, 88
  health effects of, 77–82
  intake recommendations for, 79–80
  resistant, 67
  structure of, *66*, 66

Statins, 603

Steatohepatitis, **545**

Steatorrhea, **518**, 523

Sterile, **212**

Steroids, 245

Sterols, **97**
  phyto, 229, 230
  plant, 599

Stevia, 74t, 76

Stoma, **535**

Stomach, **38**, **41**
  actions of, *39–40*, 43
  bariatric surgery and, 499,
    503–505
  conditions affecting, 496–498
  digestion in, 44–45
  dyspepsia and, 496
  gastrectomy and, 499–502
  gastritis and, 497, 497t
  muscles of, 43, *43*
  nausea/vomiting and, 496–497
  peptic ulcer and, 497–498

Strength training, 15t, 16t

Stress. *See also* Acute stress; Metabolic stress; Respiratory stress
  body's response to, 469–472
  checklist, 481–482
  hormonal responses to, 470, 470t
  inflammatory response and, *471,* 471–472
  nutrition for respiratory, 476–481
  overview of, 469
  respiratory failure and, 480–481
  shear, 593
  treatment of acute, 472–476

Stress fractures, **192,** 193

Stress response, **469**

Stricture, **490**

Stroke, **592,** 612
  feeding disabilities and, 617–620
  percentage of deaths from, *592*
  websites regarding, 614

Structure-function claims, **29**

Struvite, **639**

Struvite stones, 639, 640

Subcutaneous, **576,** 577

Subcutaneous fat, **153**

Subjective global assessment, 385t

Sucralose, 74t, **75, 76**

Sucrose, **65**

Sugar alcohols, **72,** 73t

Sugars
  added, 67–69, *68*
  alternative sweeteners, 72–76
  dental caries and, 69
  diabetes mellitus and, 572
  glycemic index of, 87t
  health effects of, 67–72
  intake recommendations, 70
  naturally occurring, 68
  nutrients in, 69, 71t
  obesity and, 69
  recognizing, 70–72
  terms used on labels regarding, 28t

Sulfate, *243,* 252, 253t

Sulfonylureas, 579t, 580

Supplemental Nutrition Assistance Program (SNAP), 283, 368t, 377–378

Supplement history, 387, 387t

Supplement labels, 269, 269–270

Surgery
  bariatric, 499, *503,* 503–505
  cancer, 654, 654t
  obesity, 176, 332, 503–505

Surrogate, **670**

Sushi, **54, 58**

Symptomatic allergy, 325

Syringes, **576,** 577

Systemic, **469,** 472

Systemic inflammatory response syndrome (SIRS), **469,** 472
  as MODS risk factor, 486, 486t
  MODS/sepsis and, *485,* 485–486

Tagatose, 74t, **75, 76**

Tannins, 232t, **256**

TCM. *See* Traditional Chinese medicine

Teratogenic, **205**

Tetracycline, 419

Therapeutic Lifestyle Changes (TLC), 596, 598–600, 598t, 601

Therapeutic touch, **432**

Thermic effect of food, **146**

Thiamin
  alcohol and, 560
  in foods, 215–216
  need for, 215, 222
  overview of, 224t

Thiazolidinediones, 579t, 580

3-in-1 solution, **453**

Thrifty meals, planning, 378

Thrombosis, **592,** 593

Thrombus, **592,** 593

Thrush, **661,** *662*

TIAs. *See* Transient ischemic attacks

Tissue rejection, **655**

TLC. *See* Therapeutic Lifestyle Changes

TNA. *See* Total nutrient admixture

Tocopherol, **210**

Tofu, **230, 232**

Tolerable Upper Intake Levels (UL), **8, 9**

Tolerance level, **326**

Total nutrient admixture (TNA), **453**–454

Total parenteral nutrition (TPN), *451,* **451,** 659

TPN. *See* Total parenteral nutrition

Trace minerals, **242,** 242t
  acute stress and, 475
  chromium, 262, 263t
  copper, *243,* 260–261, 263t
  fluoride, 261–262, *262,* 263t
  in human body, *243*
  iodine, *243,* 260, 263t
  iron, *243,* 252, 254–257, 258, 263t
  manganese, *243,* 261, 263t
  other, 262
  overview of, 252
  parenteral solutions and, 453
  selenium, *243,* 259–260, 263t
  summary of, 263t
  websites regarding, 265

zinc, *243,* 257–259, 263t

Traditional Chinese medicine (TCM), **428,** 428t

Transcription factors, **404**

Trans-fatty acids, **95,** *96*
  blood cholesterol and, 99
  CHD and, 599
  foods high in, 115, 116t

Transferrin, **252,** 254, 395t, 397

Transient ischemic attacks (TIAs), **612**

Transnasal route, *440,* **441,** 442t

Transplantation
  bone marrow, 654–655, 659
  kidney, 635–637, 637t
  liver, 555

Traveler's diarrhea, **54, 62**

Triglycerides, **48, 93**
  formation of, 93, *94*
  hypertriglyceridemia and, 600, 602

Trimester, **275**

Trimethoprim, 421

Tripeptide, **120**

Tube feeding, **416**
  administration of, 443–446
  candidates of, 440
  complications, 447, 448t–449t
  formula delivery methods in, 445
  helping patients cope with, 444
  medication delivery via, 446–447
  preparing for, 444–445
  route comparisons, 442t
  routes, *440,* 440–442
  route selection, 442
  safe handling in, 443
  safety guidelines, 443–444
  schedule planning, 445
  transition to oral diet from, 447
  tubes, 442–443
  water needs and, 446

Tubules, *622,* **622**

Tumor, **649**

Turbinado sugar, **70**

24-hour recall, **388,** 389t

2-in-1 solution, **453**

Type 1 diabetes, **564**
  body weight concerns and, 571
  chronic complications of, 568–569
  conventional *vs.* intensive therapies for, 569–570, 570t
  diabetic ketoacidosis in, 566–567
  features of, 564–565, 565t
  hypoglycemia and, 567
  insulin therapy, 576–578, 576t, *577*
  meal planning strategies, 573–576
  nutrient recommendations, 571–573
  physical activity and, 579–580

Daily Values for Food Labels

The Daily Values are standard values developed by the Food and Drug Administration (FDA) for use on food labels. The values are based on 2000 kcalories a day for adults and children over 4 years old.

Proteins, Vitamins, and Minerals

Nutrient	Amount
Protein[a]	50 g
Thiamin	1.5 mg
Riboflavin	1.7 mg
Niacin	20 mg NE
Biotin	300 µg
Pantothenic acid	10 mg
Vitamin B$_6$	2 mg
Folate	400 µg
Vitamin B$_{12}$	6 µg
Vitamin C	60 mg
Vitamin A	5000 IU[b]
Vitamin D	400 IU[b]
Vitamin E	30 IU[b]
Vitamin K	80 µg
Calcium	1000 mg
Iron	18 mg
Zinc	15 mg
Iodine	150 µg
Copper	2 mg
Chromium	120 µg
Selenium	70 µg
Molybdenum	75 µg
Manganese	2 mg
Chloride	3400 mg
Magnesium	400 mg
Phosphorus	1000 mg

[a]The Daily Values for protein vary for different groups of people: pregnant women, 60 g; nursing mothers, 65 g; infants under 1 year, 14 g; children 1 to 4 years, 16 g.

[b]Equivalent values for nutrients expressed as IU are: vitamin A, 1500 RAE (assumes a mixture of 40% retinol and 60% beta-carotene); vitamin D, 10 µg; vitamin E, 20 mg.

Nutrients and Food Components

Food Component	Amount	Calculation Factors
Fat	65 g	30% of kcalories
Saturated fat	20 g	10% of kcalories
Cholesterol	300 mg	Same regardless of kcalories
Carbohydrate (total)	300 g	60% of kcalories
Fiber	25 g	11.5 g per 1000 kcalories
Protein	50 g	10% of kcalories
Sodium	2400 mg	Same regardless of kcalories
Potassium	3500 mg	Same regardless of kcalories

GLOSSARY OF NUTRIENT MEASURES

kcal: kcalories; a unit by which energy is measured (Chapter 1 provides more details).

g: grams; a unit of weight equivalent to about 0.03 ounces.

mg: milligrams; one-thousandth of a gram.

µg: micrograms; one-millionth of a gram.

IU: international units; an old measure of vitamin activity determined by biological methods (as opposed to new measures that are determined by direct chemical analyses). Many fortified foods and supplements use IU on their labels.
- For vitamin A, 1 IU = 0.3 µg retinol, 3.6 µg β-carotene, or 7.2 µg other vitamin A carotenoids.
- For vitamin D, 1 IU = 0.025 µg cholecalciferol.
- For vitamin E, 1 IU = 0.67 natural α-tocopherol (other conversion factors are used for different forms of vitamin E).

mg NE: milligrams niacin equivalents; a measure of niacin activity (Chapter 10 provides more details).
- 1 NE = 1 mg niacin.
  = 60 mg tryptophan (an amino acid).

µg DFE: micrograms dietary folate equivalents; a measure of folate activity (Chapter 10 provides more details).
- 1 µg DFE = 1 µg food folate.
  = 0.6 µg fortified food or supplement folate.
  = 0.5 µg supplement folate taken on an empty stomach.

µg RAE: micrograms retinol activity equivalents; a measure of vitamin A activity (Chapter 11 provides more details).
- 1 µg RAE = 1 µg retinol.
  = 12 µg β-carotene.
  = 24 µg other vitamin A carotenoids.

mmol: millimoles; one-thousanth of a mole, the molecular weight of a substance. To convert mmol to mg, multiply by the atomic weight of the substance.
- For sodium, mmol × 23 = mg Na.
- For chloride, mmol × 35.5 = mg Cl.
- For sodium chloride, mmol × 58.5 = mg NaCl.